TUBERCULOSIS

AND THE

TUBERCLE BACILLUS

2ND EDITION

TUBERCULOSIS

── AND THE ──

TUBERCLE BACILLUS

── 2ND EDITION ──

EDITED BY

William R. Jacobs, Jr.
Department of Immunology and Microbiology, Albert Einstein School of Medicine, Bronx, New York

Helen McShane
Cellular Immunology and Vaccine Development Group, Nuffield Department of Medicine, Jenner Institute, University of Oxford, Oxford, United Kingdom

Valerie Mizrahi
Institute of Infectious Disease and Molecular Medicine, University of Cape Town, Faculty of Health Sciences, Rondebosch, South Africa

Ian M. Orme
Department of Microbiology, Immunology, and Pathology, Colorado State University, Fort Collins, Colorado

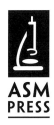

ASM
PRESS

AMERICAN SOCIETY FOR MICROBIOLOGY
WASHINGTON, DC

Library of Congress Cataloging-in-Publication Data

Names: Jacobs, William R., Jr., editor.
Title: Tuberculosis and the tubercle bacillus / edited by William R. Jacobs, Jr., Department of Immunology and Microbiology, Albert Einstein School of Medicine, Bronx, New York, Helen McShane, Cellular Immunology and Vaccine Development Group, Nuffield Department of Medicine, Jenner Institute, University of Oxford, Oxford, United Kingdom, Valerie Mizrahi, Institute of Infectious Disease and Molecular Medicine, University of Cape Town, Faculty of Health Sciences, Rondebosch, South Africa, Ian M. Orme, Department of Microbiology, Immunology, and Pathology, Colorado State University, Fort Collins, Colorado.
Description: 2nd edition. | Washington, DC : ASM Press, [2018] | Includes bibliographical references and index.
Identifiers: LCCN 2017038089 (print) | LCCN 2017040375 (ebook) | ISBN 9781555819569 (ebook) | ISBN 9781555819552 (print)
Subjects: LCSH: Tuberculosis.
Classification: LCC QR201.T6 (ebook) | LCC QR201.T6 T83 2018 (print) | DDC 614.5/42--dc23
LC record available at https://lccn.loc.gov/2017038089

doi:10.1128/9781555819569

Printed in Canada

10 9 8 7 6 5 4 3 2 1

Address editorial correspondence to: ASM Press, 1752 N St., N.W., Washington, DC 20036-2904, USA.
Send orders to: ASM Press, P.O. Box 605, Herndon, VA 20172, USA.
Phone: 800-546-2416; 703-661-1593. Fax: 703-661-1501.
E-mail: books@asmusa.org
Online: http://www.asmscience.org

Contents

Contributors   ix
Preface   xiii

SECTION I

TOWARDS EDWARD JENNER'S
REVENGE: DEVELOPING AN EFFECTIVE
TUBERCULOSIS VACCINE / 1

A. BASIC IMMUNOLOGY

1   Innate Immune Responses to
Tuberculosis / 3
JEFFREY S. SCHOREY AND LARRY S. SCHLESINGER

2   Cytokines and Chemokines in
Mycobacterium tuberculosis Infection / 33
RACQUEL DOMINGO-GONZALEZ, OLIVER PRINCE,
ANDREA COOPER, AND SHABAANA KHADER

3   Regulation of Immunity to Tuberculosis / 73
SUSANNA BRIGHENTI AND DIANE J. ORDWAY

4   The Memory Immune Response to
Tuberculosis / 95
JOANNA R. KIRMAN, MARCELA I. HENAO-TAMAYO,
AND ELSE MARIE AGGER

5   Pathology of Tuberculosis: How the
Pathology of Human Tuberculosis Informs
and Directs Animal Models / 117
RANDALL J. BASARABA AND ROBERT L. HUNTER

B. ANIMAL MODELS

6   Animal Models of Tuberculosis:
An Overview / 131
ANN WILLIAMS AND IAN M. ORME

7   Mouse and Guinea Pig Models of
Tuberculosis / 143
IAN M. ORME AND DIANE J. ORDWAY

8   Non-Human Primate Models of
Tuberculosis / 163
JULIET C. PEÑA AND WEN-ZHE HO

9   Experimental Infection Models of
Tuberculosis in Domestic Livestock / 177
BRYCE M. BUDDLE, H. MARTIN VORDERMEIER,
AND R. GLYN HEWINSON

C. VACCINES

10   Clinical Testing of Tuberculosis Vaccine
Candidates / 193
MARK HATHERILL, DERECK TAIT,
AND HELEN MCSHANE

D. HUMAN IMMUNOLOGY

11   Human Immunology of Tuberculosis / 213
THOMAS J. SCRIBA, ANNA K. COUSSENS,
AND HELEN A. FLETCHER

v

12 The Immune Interaction between HIV-1 Infection and *Mycobacterium tuberculosis* / 239
ELSA DU BRUYN AND ROBERT JOHN WILKINSON

SECTION II

DRUG DISCOVERY AND DEVELOPMENT: STATE OF THE ART AND FUTURE DIRECTIONS / 269

13 Preclinical Efficacy Testing of New Drug Candidates / 271
ERIC L. NUERMBERGER

14 Oxidative Phosphorylation as a Target Space for Tuberculosis: Success, Caution, and Future Directions / 295
GREGORY M. COOK, KIEL HARDS, ELYSE DUNN, ADAM HEIKAL, YOSHIO NAKATANI, CHRIS GREENING, DEAN C. CRICK, FABIO L. FONTES, KEVIN PETHE, ERIK HASENOEHRL, AND MICHAEL BERNEY

15 Targeting Phenotypically Tolerant *Mycobacterium tuberculosis* / 317
BEN GOLD AND CARL NATHAN

SECTION III

BIOMARKERS AND DIAGNOSTICS / 361

16 Tuberculosis Diagnostics: State of the Art and Future Directions / 363
MADHUKAR PAI, MARK P. NICOL, AND CATHARINA C. BOEHME

17 Latent *Mycobacterium tuberculosis* Infection and Interferon-Gamma Release Assays / 379
MADHUKAR PAI AND MARCEL BEHR

18 Impact of the GeneXpert MTB/RIF Technology on Tuberculosis Control / 389
WENDY SUSAN STEVENS, LESLEY SCOTT, LARA NOBLE, NATASHA GOUS, AND KEERTAN DHEDA

SECTION IV

HOST AND STRAIN DIVERSITY / 411

19 The Role of Host Genetics (and Genomics) in Tuberculosis / 413
VIVEK NARANBHAI

20 The Evolutionary History, Demography, and Spread of the *Mycobacterium tuberculosis* Complex / 453
MAXIME BARBIER AND THIERRY WIRTH

21 Impact of Genetic Diversity on the Biology of *Mycobacterium tuberculosis* Complex Strains / 475
STEFAN NIEMANN, MATTHIAS MERKER, THOMAS KOHL, AND PHILIP SUPPLY

22 Evolution of *Mycobacterium tuberculosis:* New Insights into Pathogenicity and Drug Resistance / 495
EVA C. BORITSCH AND ROLAND BROSCH

SECTION V

THE SIGNATURE PROBLEM OF TUBERCULOSIS PERSISTENCE / 517

23 Acid-Fast Positive and Acid-Fast Negative *Mycobacterium tuberculosis:* The Koch Paradox / 519
CATHERINE VILCHÈZE AND LAURENT KREMER

24 Mycobacterial Biofilms: Revisiting Tuberculosis Bacilli in Extracellular Necrotizing Lesions / 533
RANDALL J. BASARABA AND ANIL K. OJHA

25 Killing *Mycobacterium tuberculosis In Vitro:* What Model Systems Can Teach Us / 541
TRACY L. KEISER AND GEORGIANA E. PURDY

26 Epigenetic Phosphorylation Control of *Mycobacterium tuberculosis* Infection and Persistence / 557
MELISSA RICHARD-GREENBLATT AND YOSSEF AV-GAY

27 DNA Replication in *Mycobacterium tuberculosis* / 581
ZANELE DITSE, MEINDERT H. LAMERS, AND DIGBY F. WARNER

28 The Sec Pathways and Exportomes of *Mycobacterium tuberculosis* / 607
BRITTANY K. MILLER, KATELYN E. ZULAUF, AND MIRIAM BRAUNSTEIN

29 The Role of ESX-1 in *Mycobacterium tuberculosis* Pathogenesis / 627
KA-WING WONG

30 The Minimal Unit of Infection:
    Mycobacterium tuberculosis in the
    Macrophage / 635
    BRIAN C. VANDERVEN, LU HUANG,
    KYLE H. ROHDE, AND DAVID G. RUSSELL

31 Metabolic Perspectives on Persistence / 653
    TRAVIS E. HARTMAN, ZHE WANG,
    ROBERT S. JANSEN, SUSANA GARDETE,
    AND KYU Y. RHEE

32 Phenotypic Heterogeneity in *Mycobacterium
    tuberculosis* / 671
    NEERAJ DHAR, JOHN MCKINNEY, AND
    GIULIA MANINA

33 *Mycobacterium tuberculosis* in the Face of
    Host-Imposed Nutrient Limitation / 699
    MICHAEL BERNEY AND LINDA BERNEY-MEYER

Index / 717

Contributors

Else Marie Agger
Department of Infectious Disease Immunology, Statens Serum Institut, Artillerivej 5, Copenhagen, Denmark

Yossef Av-Gay
Division of Infectious Diseases, Department of Medicine, University of British Columbia, Vancouver, Canada

Maxime Barbier
Laboratoire Biologie Intégrative des Populations, Evolution Moléculaire; Institut de Systématique, Evolution, Biodiversité, UMR-CNRS 7205, Muséum National d'Histoire Naturelle, Univ. Pierre et Marie Curie, EPHE, Sorbonne Universités, Paris, France

Randall J. Basaraba
Department of Microbiology, Immunology, and Pathology, College of Veterinary Medicine and Biomedical Sciences, Colorado State University, Fort Collins, Colorado

Marcel Behr
McGill International TB Centre & Department of Epidemiology & Biostatistics, McGill University, Montreal, Canada

Michael Berney
Albert Einstein College of Medicine, Department of Microbiology and Immunology, New York, New York

Linda Berney-Meyer
Albert Einstein College of Medicine, Department of Microbiology and Immunology, New York, New York

Catharina C. Boehme
FIND, Geneva, Switzerland

Eva C. Boritsch
Institut Pasteur, Unit for Integrated Mycobacterial Pathogenomics, Paris, France

Miriam Braunstein
Department of Microbiology and Immunology, University of North Carolina – Chapel Hill, Chapel Hill, North Carolina

Susanna Brighenti
Center for Infectious Medicine (CIM), F59, Department of Medicine, Karolinska Institutet, Karolinska University Hospital Huddinge, Stockholm, Sweden

Roland Brosch
Institut Pasteur, Unit for Integrated Mycobacterial Pathogenomics, Paris, France

Bryce M. Buddle
AgResearch, Hopkirk Research Institute, Palmerston North, New Zealand

Gregory M. Cook
University of Otago, Department of Microbiology and Immunology, Otago School of Medical Sciences, Dunedin, New Zealand, and Maurice Wilkins Center for Molecular Biodiscovery, The University of Auckland, Auckland, New Zealand

Andrea Cooper
University of Leicester, Infection Immunity and Inflammation, Leicester, Leicestershire, United Kingdom

Anna K. Coussens
Clinical Infectious Diseases Research Initiative, Division of Medical Microbiology, Department of Pathology, and Institute of Infectious Disease and Molecular Medicine, University of Cape Town, Cape Town, South Africa

Dean C. Crick
Colorado State University, Department of Microbiology, Immunology, and Pathology, Fort Collins, Colorado

Neeraj Dhar
Global Health Institute, École Polytechnique Fédérale de Lausanne, Lausanne, Switzerland

Keertan Dheda
Lung Infection and Immunity Unit, Division of Pulmonology and UCT Lung Institute, Department of Medicine, University of Cape Town, Cape Town, South Africa

Zanele Ditse
MRC/NHLS/UCT Molecular Mycobacteriology Research Unit, DST/NRF Centre of Excellence for Biomedical TB Research, Department of Pathology, Faculty of Health Sciences, University of Cape Town, Cape Town, South Africa

Racquel Domingo-Gonzalez
Department of Molecular Microbiology, Washington University in St. Louis, St. Louis, Missouri

Elsa du Bruyn
Clinical Infectious Diseases Research Initiative, Institute of Infectious Diseases and Molecular Medicine, University of Cape Town, Observatory, Republic of South Africa

Elyse Dunn
University of Otago, Department of Microbiology and Immunology, Otago School of Medical Sciences, Dunedin, New Zealand

Helen A. Fletcher
Immunology and Infection Department, London School of Hygiene & Tropical Medicine, London, United Kingdom

Fabio L. Fontes
Colorado State University, Department of Microbiology, Immunology, and Pathology, Fort Collins, Colorado

Susana Gardete
Department of Medicine, Division of Infectious Diseases, Weill Cornell Medical College, New York, New York

Ben Gold
Department of Microbiology and Immunology, Weill Cornell Medical College, New York, New York

Natasha Gous
Department of Molecular Medicine and Haematology, Faculty of Health Sciences, University of the Witwatersrand, National Health Laboratory Service and National Priority Program of the National Health Laboratory Service, Johannesburg, South Africa

Chris Greening
The Commonwealth Scientific and Industrial Research Organization, Land and Water Flagship, Acton, Australia, and Monash University, School of Biological Sciences, Clayton, Victoria, Australia

Kiel Hards
University of Otago, Department of Microbiology and Immunology, Otago School of Medical Sciences, Dunedin, New Zealand

Travis E. Hartman
Department of Medicine, Division of Infectious Diseases, Weill Cornell Medical College, New York, New York

Erik Hasenoehrle
Albert Einstein College of Medicine, Department of Microbiology and Immunology, Bronx, New York

Mark Hatherill
South African Tuberculosis Vaccine Initiative (SATVI) and Institute of Infectious Disease & Molecular Medicine

(IDM), University of Cape Town, Wernher & Beit South Building, Anzio Road, Observatory, Cape Town, South Africa

Adam Heikal
University of Otago, Department of Microbiology and Immunology, Otago School of Medical Sciences, Dunedin, New Zealand, and Maurice Wilkins Center for Molecular Biodiscovery, The University of Auckland, Auckland, New Zealand

Marcela I. Henao-Tamayo
Department of Microbiology, Immunology and Pathology, Mycobacteria Research Laboratory, Colorado State University, Fort Collins, Colorado

R. Glyn Hewinson
Animal and Plant Health Agency – Weybridge, Addlestone, Surrey, United Kingdom

Wen-Zhe Ho
Animal Biosafety Level III Laboratory, Center for Animal Experiment, State Key Laboratory of Virology, Wuhan University, Wuhan, China; Department of Pathology and Laboratory Medicine, Temple University Lewis Katz School of Medicine, Philadelphia, Pennsylvania

Lu Huang
Microbiology and Immunology, College of Veterinary Medicine, Cornell University, Ithaca, New York

Robert L. Hunter
Department of Pathology and Laboratory Medicine, McGovern Medical School, University of Texas Health Science Center at Houston, Houston, Texas

Robert S. Jansen
Department of Medicine, Division of Infectious Diseases, Weill Cornell Medical College, New York, New York

Tracy L. Keiser
Department of Microbiology and Immunology, Albert Einstein College of Medicine, Bronx, New York

Shabaana Khader
Department of Molecular Microbiology, Washington University in St. Louis, St. Louis, Missouri

Joanna R. Kirman
Department of Microbiology and Immunology, University of Otago, Dunedin, New Zealand

Thomas Kohl
Molecular Mycobacteriology, Forschungszentrum Borstel, Leibniz-Zentrum für Medizin und Biowissenschaften, Borstel, Germany

Laurent Kremer
IRIM (ex-CPBS) UMR 9004, Infectious Disease Research Institute of Montpellier (IDRIM), Université de Montpellier, CNRS, Montpellier, France

Giulia Manina
Microbial Individuality and Infection Group, Institut Pasteur, 25 rue du Docteur Roux, Paris, France

John McKinney
Global Health Institute, École Polytechnique Fédérale de Lausanne, Lausanne, Switzerland

Helen McShane
The Jenner Institute, University of Oxford, Old Road Campus Research Building, Roosevelt Drive, Oxford, United Kingdom

Matthias Merker
Molecular Mycobacteriology, Forschungszentrum Borstel, Leibniz-Zentrum für Medizin und Biowissenschaften, Borstel, Germany

Brittany K. Miller
Department of Microbiology and Immunology, University of North Carolina – Chapel Hill, Chapel Hill, North Carolina

Yoshio Nakatani
University of Otago, Department of Microbiology and Immunology, Otago School of Medical Sciences, Dunedin, New Zealand, and Maurice Wilkins Center for Molecular Biodiscovery, The University of Auckland, Auckland, New Zealand

Vivek Naranbhai
Wellcome Trust Centre for Human Genetics, Nuffield Department of Medicine, University of Oxford, Oxford, United Kingdom, and Centre for the AIDS Programme of Research in South Africa, University of KwaZulu Natal, Durban, South Africa

Carl Nathan
Department of Microbiology and Immunology, Weill Cornell Medical College, New York, New York

Mark P. Nicol
University of Cape Town, Cape Town, South Africa

Stefan Niemann
Molecular Mycobacteriology, Forschungszentrum Borstel, Leibniz-Zentrum für Medizin und Biowissenschaften, and German Center for Infection Research (DZIF), partner site Borstel, Borstel, Germany

Lara Noble
Department of Molecular Medicine and Haematology, Faculty of Health Sciences, University of the Witwatersrand, Johannesburg, Gauteng, South Africa

Eric L. Nuermberger
Center for Tuberculosis Research, Department of Medicine, Johns Hopkins University School of Medicine, and Department of International Health, Johns Hopkins Bloomberg School of Public Health, Baltimore, Maryland

Anil K. Ojha
Wadsworth Center, NY State Department of Health and University at Albany, Albany, New York

Diane J. Ordway
Mycobacteria Research Laboratories, Department of Microbiology, Immunology and Pathology, Colorado State University, Fort Collins, Colorado

Ian M. Orme
Colorado State University, Fort Collins, Colorado

Madhukar Pai
McGill International TB Centre & Department of Epidemiology & Biostatistics, McGill University, Montreal, Canada

Juliet C. Peña
Department of Pathology and Laboratory Medicine, Temple University Lewis Katz School of Medicine, 3500 N. Broad St., MERB 843, Philadelphia, Pennsylvania

Kevin Pethe
Lee Kong Chian School of Medicine, Nanyang Technological University, Singapore

Oliver Prince
Department of Molecular Microbiology, Washington University in St. Louis, St. Louis, Missouri

Georgiana E. Purdy
Department of Microbiology and Immunology, Oregon Health Sciences University, Portland, Oregon

Kyu Y. Rhee
Department of Medicine and Department of Microbiology & Immunology, Division of Infectious Diseases, Weill Cornell Medical College, New York, New York

Melissa Richard-Greenblatt
Division of Infectious Diseases, Department of Medicine, University of British Columbia, Vancouver, Canada

Kyle H. Rohde
Burnett School of Biomedical Sciences, College of Medicine, University of Central Florida, Orlando, Florida

David G. Russell
Microbiology and Immunology, College of Veterinary Medicine, Cornell University, Ithaca, New York

Larry S. Schlesinger
Department of Microbial Infection and Immunity, Center for Microbial Interface Biology, The Ohio State University, Columbus, Ohio

Jeffrey S. Schorey
Department of Biological Sciences, Eck Institute for Global Health, Center for Rare and Neglected Diseases, University of Notre Dame, Notre Dame, Indiana

Lesley Scott
Department of Molecular Medicine and Haematology, Faculty of Health Sciences, University of the Witwatersrand, Johannesburg, Gauteng, South Africa

Thomas J. Scriba
South African Tuberculosis Vaccine Initiative, Division of
Immunology, Department of Pathology, and Institute of
Infectious Disease and Molecular Medicine, University of
Cape Town, Cape Town, South Africa

Wendy Susan Stevens
Department of Molecular Medicine and Haematology,
Faculty of Health Sciences, University of the Witwatersrand,
National Health Laboratory Service, and National Priority
Program of the National Health Laboratory Service,
Johannesburg, South Africa

Philip Supply
INSERM U1019; CNRS UMR 8204; Institut Pasteur
de Lille, Center for Infection and Immunity of Lille; and
Université Lille Nord de France, Lille, France

Dereck Tait
Aeras, Blackriver Park, First Floor, Observatory, Cape Town,
South Africa

Brian C. VanderVen
Microbiology and Immunology, College of Veterinary
Medicine, Cornell University, Ithaca, New York

Catherine Vilchèze
Howard Hughes Medical Institute, Department of
Microbiology and Immunology, Albert Einstein College of
Medicine, Bronx, New York

H. Martin Vordermeier
Animal and Plant Health Agency – Weybridge, Addlestone,
Surrey, United Kingdom

Zhe Wang
Department of Medicine, Division of Infectious Diseases,
Weill Cornell Medical College, New York, New York

Digby F. Warner
MRC/NHLS/UCT Molecular Mycobacteriology Research
Unit, Department of Pathology, and Institute of Infectious
Disease and Molecular Medicine, Faculty of Health Sciences,
University of Cape Town, Rondebosch, South Africa

Robert John Wilkinson
Department of Medicine, Imperial College London, and The
Francis Crick Institute Mill Hill Laboratory, London, United
Kingdom

Ann Williams
Health UK, Porton Down, Salisbury, United Kingdom

Thierry Wirth
Laboratoire Biologie Intégrative des Populations,
Evolution Moléculaire; Institut de Systématique, Evolution,
Biodiversité, UMR-CNRS 7205, Muséum National
d'Histoire Naturelle, Univ. Pierre et Marie Curie, EPHE,
Sorbonne Universités, Paris, France

Ka-Wing Wong
Shanghai Public Health Clinical Center, Key Laboratory
of Medical Molecular Virology, School of Basic Medical
Sciences, Shanghai Medical College of Fudan University,
Shanghai, People's Republic of China

Katelyn E. Zulauf
Department of Microbiology and Immunology, University of
North Carolina – Chapel Hill, Chapel Hill, North Carolina

Preface: Combating Tuberculosis: Edward Jenner's Revenge

It is the height of irony that the man who discovered the smallpox vaccine, Edward Jenner, lost both his wife and son to tuberculosis (TB). By the time smallpox was essentially eradicated, it is estimated that over 300 million people had died from this disease over the preceding century. Its eventual prevention—by a simple vaccine—clearly illustrates the power of scientific discovery and how its application can affect human health. Hundreds of millions of people have been spared death and suffering from infectious diseases because of the development of vaccines and chemotherapeutic agents in the last 100 years. Millions of lives have been saved with the use of the TB vaccine, BCG, and the development of chemotherapeutic regimens for TB. Depressingly, despite these effective interventions, TB remains one of the most challenging problems of global health, with over 9 million new cases and 1.6 million deaths each year. This crisis has been further compounded by the emergence of the HIV epidemic, as this explosive and deadly combination has dramatically increased the global spread of TB, including increasing numbers of cases of multidrug-resistant (MDR) and extensively drug-resistant (XDR) TB.

Historically, mycobacterial disease has long been at the forefront of scientific discovery for infectious diseases. The leprosy bacillus, *Mycobacterium leprae*, the first bacterium to be associated with human disease, was initially visualized by Gerhard Armauer Hansen in 1873. Earlier, Jean Antoine Villemin was the first person to realize that lung tubercles were infectious and not cancerous. By the 1880s, Robert Koch, aware of both of these discoveries, not only observed the tubercle bacilli in tubercles, but developed a growth medium of heated serum to cultivate the tubercle bacillus out-

side of humans. He went on to repeat the transfer experiment of Villemin and transferred the disease of TB to numerous animal species, establishing the experimental paradigm ("the postulates") of how to prove that an infectious agent is a cause of a disease. Koch's findings led Albert Calmette and Camille Guérin to follow Jenner's approach of developing an attenuated pathogen for use as a vaccine, using the bovine tubercle bacillus to develop the bacille Calmette-Guérin (BCG) vaccine that bears their names and is still used to this day.

It is noteworthy that Paul Ehrlich was sitting in the lecture hall when Robert Koch presented his work in 1882; he later went on to help Koch improve his staining techniques. By observing the selective staining of various cell types, including human cells and different bacteria, Ehrlich also developed the idea of chemotherapy—"magic bullets" that could kill microbial pathogens. He tried for years to develop a chemical that could kill the tubercle bacillus, with little success, though at the same time was far more successful in developing a treatment for syphilis. In the 1930s, his protégé Gerhard Domagk discovered the first sulfonamide to treat bacterial infections such as streptococcus, and as this fledgling field expanded, para-amino salicylic acid and isoniazid were discovered to be active against the TB bacillus. Parallel studies by Salman Waksman and Albert Schatz in the 1950s led to the discovery of streptomycin, the first bactericidal drug for the tubercle bacilli.

Despite these many historical advances, the TB bacillus—*Mycobacterium tuberculosis*—has proven to be a formidable adversary against numerous interventions. Nevertheless, despite the arduous challenges of working with this dangerous pathogen, the field continues to persevere, and our continued success in the pursuit of knowledge would, we suspect, be applauded by Koch, Ehrlich, Calmette, and many others, as we strive to find and apply more effective cures for this dreadful disease. In this spirit, this textbook is a collection of state-of-the-art research aimed at understanding the TB bacillus, the way it infects its host, the mechanisms by which it persists in the face of host immunity, and current intervention and therapeutic methods. The contributors of this book believe that such continued and dedicated research efforts will eventually lead to better vaccines, better chemotherapies, and ultimately the eradication of TB—Edward Jenner's revenge.

WILLIAM R. JACOBS, JR.
HELEN MCSHANE
VALERIE MIZRAHI
IAN M. ORME

Towards Edward Jenner's Revenge: Developing an Effective Tuberculosis Vaccine

I

A. BASIC IMMUNOLOGY

B. ANIMAL MODELS

C. VACCINES

D. HUMAN IMMUNOLOGY

Tuberculosis and the Tubercle Bacillus, 2nd ed.
Edited by William R. Jacobs, Jr., Helen McShane, Valerie Mizrahi, and Ian M. Orme
© 2018 American Society for Microbiology, Washington, DC
doi:10.1128/microbiolspec.TBTB2-0010-2016

A. BASIC IMMUNOLOGY

Innate Immune Responses to Tuberculosis

1

Jeffrey S. Schorey[1] and Larry S. Schlesinger[2]

INTRODUCTION

Tuberculosis (TB) remains one of the leading causes of death by an infectious agent, accounting for approximately 1.3 million deaths per year (1). Despite its clinical significance, there are still significant gaps in our understanding of *Mycobacterium tuberculosis* pathogenesis and the host mechanisms that limit active disease to approximately 10% of those infected. Nevertheless, we continue to gain insight into the dynamic interplay between pathogen and host, with much of the focus centered on the lung microenvironment because this is the initial and primary site of infection. The lung as the initial "battlefield" provides unique challenges to both the host and pathogen because the host must balance the inflammatory response to limit the damage to lung tissue while inducing a sufficient immune response to control the infection. In contrast, the *M. tuberculosis* organism must avoid or circumvent the initial defensive barriers present within the respiratory tract to gain access to its host cell, the alveolar macrophage (AM). The AM response to infection as well as the reaction of other lung immune and nonimmune cells and noncellular components is critical to determining whether the host will directly eliminate the pathogen or will in concert with the acquired immune system develop a protective granulomatous response. In addition, since bacteria disseminate during the early events in infection, engagement of innate immune components outside of the lung is also critical in shaping the host response. These early host processes which constitute the innate immune system will be the focus of this article.

LUNG

The lung is responsible for mediating gas exchange across a respiratory surface of 130 m^2, which is more than 60 times the surface of the body (2–4) (Fig. 1). On average, this involves inhalation of 14,000 liters of air each day (5) and processing not only of CO_2 and O_2, but also of pollutants, allergens, and microbes from the inhaled air. Efficient gas exchange requires a thin barrier between the air and blood; in some instances this barrier is composed of only one endothelial cell and one epithelial cell and is less than 2 m thick. The lung must maintain this thin barrier while clearing inhaled insults (2–4).

The lung uses multiple defenses to clear contaminants from the air (discussed in more detail below). Briefly, basic instincts such as the coughing and sneezing reflex remove particulates from the lung. Mucus, together with cilia, forms the mucociliary escalator which transfers particles up the trachea for removal. Also, epithelial cells in the airway secrete antimicrobials including lysozyme and antimicrobial peptides such as defensins and cathelicidins (6, 7). These defenses clear particulates ≥5 μm. Anything smaller passes through the conducting system with velocity, eventually settling in the alveoli, where alveolar cells become responsible for their clearance.

The main three cell types in the alveolus are type I and type II alveolar epithelial cells (AECs) and AMs. These cells are coated by alveolar fluid and surfactant. External to the alveolus is the alveolar septum, which contains blood vessels, fibroblasts, protein fibers, and

[1]Department of Biological Sciences, Eck Institute for Global Health, Center for Rare and Neglected Diseases, University of Notre Dame, Notre Dame, IN 46556; [2]Department of Microbial Infection and Immunity, Center for Microbial Interface Biology, The Ohio State University, Columbus, OH 43210.

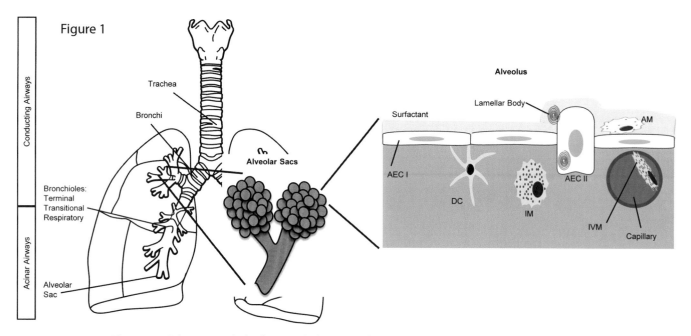

Figure 1 Schematic of the lung and the role of pulmonary innate immune cells during *M. tuberculosis* infection. From left to right: branching of the airways, culminating in the alveolar sacs and the alveolus. Also depicted are the cells in the alveolus. Abbreviations: AEC I and II, type I and II alveolar epithelial cell; AM, alveolar macrophage; DC, dendritic cell; IM, interstitial macrophage; IVM, intravascular macrophage.

pores of Kohn. The fibers are responsible for the structural integrity of the alveolus. The pores of Kohn are holes in the septum that connect alveoli to each other, are filled with surfactant, and provide a passage for cells to migrate between alveoli (2, 8).

Lung Cellular Components
AECs
Although type I AECs constitute only 8% of peripheral lung cells (a third of the cells in the alveolus), they cover ~95% of the alveolar surface. Their thin flat shape, as well as their contact with endothelial cells of the pulmonary capillaries, provides the necessary thin surface for gas exchange to occur (2, 3). The cuboidal type II AECs constitute about 15% of peripheral lung cells, cover 5% of the alveolar surface, and have a smaller surface area than type I AECs—250 μm^2 compared to 5,000 μm^2 (9, 10). Type II AECs contain distinctive lamellar bodies and have apical microvilli. These cells secrete surfactant phospholipids and proteins, as well as lysozyme and antimicrobial peptides in lamellar bodies (7, 9). Following lung damage, type II AECs can serve as precursors to type I cells and self-renew (2, 3, 7). These cells also express HLA class I and II molecules (9), and murine cells can present mycobacterial antigens (11).

Lung macrophages
AMs constitute the majority of cells collected from bronchoalveolar lavage (≥90%). They maintain the alveolar microenvironment, removing debris, dead cells, and microbes. They are long lived, with a half-life of 1 to 8 months (12, 13); about 40% of total AMs turn over each year (14). AMs are thought to originate from peripheral blood monocytes following migration into the lung (15) but may also originate from lung macrophages in response to inflammation (12, 16–20).

AMs must exert tightly regulated pro- and anti-inflammatory actions to control infection without damaging the fragile alveolar environment (14, 21). Thus, they exhibit characteristics of M1 (classically activated) and M2 (alternatively activated) macrophages (22). They express high levels of mannose receptor (MR), scavenger receptor-A, Toll-like receptor 9 (TLR9), and the nuclear receptor peroxisome proliferator-associated receptor gamma (PPARγ), and low levels of TLR2 and the costimulatory molecules CD80 and CD86 (14, 21, 23). PPARγ expression may be important for differentiation of AMs (24), which are highly phagocytic (25) but have a limited oxidative burst relative to neutrophils or peripheral blood mononuclear cells (PBMCs) (25, 26) and are weakly bactericidal (12). AMs are poor antigen presenters (27) and downregulate the ability of dendritic cells (DCs) to present antigen (28) and suppress lymphocyte activation (29).

The lung contains three types of macrophages, named based on their location: AMs, intravascular macrophages (IVMs), and interstitial macrophages (IMs). IVMs are located in the capillaries on endothelial cells, and IMs are in the interstitial space between alveoli (30, 31). The IVMs and IMs are less well understood than AMs, likely due to the difficulty isolating them. AMs are readily isolated from bronchoalveolar lavage following only a few washes, while IMs are obtained from the bronchoalveolar lavage following many washes (31), and many animals such as mice and humans (in contrast to pigs and horses, for example) may not constitutively produce IVMs (30). In rhesus macaques IMs were shown to have a higher turnover rate and be shorter lived than AMs (32). IMs are thought to regulate tissue fibrosis, inflammation, and antigen presentation (33) and be more proinflammatory than AMs (32). IVMs are phagocytic and may clear erythrocytes and fibrin from the blood (30).

DCs

A few DCs are located in the alveoli interstitial space, but most are in the conducting airways (2, 34). In the alveoli, they sit below the AECs and extend membrane protrusions to sample the inner surface of the airway lumen (35). Following antigen processing and presentation, DCs migrate to local lymph nodes (36) and inducible bronchus-associated lymphoid tissue that forms in response to infection or inflammation (37, 38). There are few lymphatic vessels around the alveoli, so alveolar DCs must migrate through the interstitium to access sites of lymphatic drainage (2). Other immune cells, including T and B cells, are found in low amounts in the interstitium.

Mucosal associated invariant T (MAIT) cells

Major histocompatibility complex (MHC)-related protein 1-restricted MAIT cells are unconventional CD8 T cells (39) and are present in the lung airways. MAIT cells detect antigen-presenting cells infected with fungi and bacteria, including *M. tuberculosis*. Following stimulation, MAIT cells produce gamma interferon (IFN-γ) and tumor necrosis factor (TNF) and lyse infected cells (40–42). They are important *in vivo* during mycobacterial infection. MHC-related protein 1 knockout mice show elevated bacillus Calmette-Guérin (BCG) growth compared to wild-type mice (43). Individuals with active TB have reduced levels of MAIT cells in the peripheral blood and enhanced levels in the lung compared with healthy individuals (40).

Neutrophils

Although under conditions of health lung alveoli contain predominantly macrophages, rapid recruitment of neutrophils is well known to be a key determinant of the innate immune response to bacterial pathogens (44). Neutrophils possess potent extracellular and intracellular killing mechanisms. However, severe bacterial lung infections are caused by excessive neutrophil-mediated inflammation. Neutrophils sense bacteria and/or their components and migrate across epithelia along a chemotactic gradient. Neutrophil sequestration is an essential antibacterial defense mechanism in the lung, which involves multiple steps, including activation of transcription factors, production of chemokines, upregulation of cell adhesion molecules, and enhancement of cell-cell interactions.

Mucus and Surfactant

Mucins are the main glycoproteins in mucus and are either tethered to epithelial cells or secreted. They are produced by submucosal glands and goblet cells, club cells, and alveolar cells in the conducting and peripheral airways. They bind particles and microbes to prevent their adherence to host cells and thus mediate clearance via the mucociliary escalator (7).

Pulmonary surfactant is produced by type II AECs in the alveoli and is a complex mixture of lipids and proteins that bathe cells in the alveolus and reduce surface tension to prevent alveolar collapse during expiration. Dipalmitoyl phosphatidylcholine is the most abundant phospholipid in surfactant (45), but surfactant also contains surfactant proteins (SPs) SP-A, SP-B, SP-C, and SP-D (46, 47). In general, SP-B and SP-C maintain stability of the surfactant lipids, while SP-A and SP-D are immunomodulators (7, 48). SP-A enhances apoptotic cell clearance by macrophages and regulates MR activity, the oxidative burst, and negative regulators of inflammation (49–54); SP-A also enhances macrophage phagocytosis of *M. tuberculosis* (55–58). In contrast, SP-D agglutinates *M. tuberculosis*, which decreases macrophage phagocytosis. However, the bacteria that are still phagocytosed show enhanced phagosome lysosome (PL) fusion and killing (59–61).

Soluble Components in the Surfactant Hypophase

Below the surfactant lipid monolayer is an aqueous hyphase of alveolar lining fluid (ALF) that contains substances with intrinsic antimicrobial properties which contribute to the innate immune response to pathogens within this environment (62). These include complement, antibody, defensins, lysozyme, phospholipases, protease inhibitors, and homeostatic hydrolases that can affect the *M. tuberculosis* cell wall and host responses (63). ALF is generated, secreted, and recycled by AECs and is essential for maintaining lung function (64). Components of the complement system are produced by AECs (65) and macrophages in the lung (66). The complement system is active in the alveolar space and plays an important role in the microbe-macrophage encounter (67–71). TB is increased in the elderly, and recent studies show how the pulmonary environment, particularly ALF, in old age can potentially modify mucosal immune responses, including those in response to *M. tuberculosis* (72).

M. TUBERCULOSIS INTERACTION WITH THE LUNG

Initial Interactions Following Inhalation

Human ALF contains hydrolases that alter the *M. tuberculosis* cell wall, reducing exposure of mannose-capped lipoarabinomannan (ManLAM) and trehalose 6,6′-dimycolate (TDM; cord factor). ALF treatment of *M. tuberculosis* reduced its association with and intracellular replication in human macrophages and led to increased TNF-α release by macrophages (73). Thus, initial exposure to surfactant may alter the *M. tuberculosis* cell wall before interaction with AMs or AECs and affect subsequent interactions with the host, perhaps by altering the receptor primarily engaged by the bacteria.

Interactions with the Macrophage

Phagocytic receptors

The MR (CD206; MRC1) is highly expressed by AMs and subsets of DCs but not by monocytes (74–78) (Fig. 2). It is the dominant C-type lectin on human AMs and monocyte-derived macrophages, and it recognizes endogenous N-linked glycoproteins (79, 80) and mannose-containing pathogen-associated molecular patterns (PAMPs) (81) via its carbohydrate recognition domains. The MR discriminates between mannose-containing PAMPs based on the degree and nature of mannan motifs. It binds to the mannose caps of ManLAM (82, 83) and the higher-order phosphatidylinositol mannosides (PIMs) that are more mannosylated and found in greater amounts on pathogenic mycobacteria (84), thus differentiating among *M. tuberculosis* strains (85, 86). *M. tuberculosis* is thought to use molecular mimicry to bind the MR and mediate favorable entry into macrophages, and usage of the MR may be a marker of host adaptation (83). Binding

to the MR mediates phagocytosis of *M. tuberculosis* and leads to decreased PL fusion (84, 87, 88), acidification (89, 90), and oxidative burst (91), as well as release of anti-inflammatory cytokines (92). MR engagement also leads to increased PPARγ activity, which allows for enhanced survival of *M. tuberculosis* in the macrophage, which is discussed in more detail below (23). The MR can facilitate presentation of lipids and ManLAM and serves as a prototypic pattern recognition receptor (PRR) linking innate and adaptive immunity, which has been exploited to deliver DNA vaccines to antigen-presenting cells (22) and is being used to modulate the immune system for therapeutic and vaccine purposes (93). The MR may also contribute to chronic stages of *M. tuberculosis* infection by mediating homotypic cellular adhesion and giant cell formation (94), which are characteristic of TB granulomas (95, 96).

DC-specific intercellular adhesion molecule 3 grabbing nonintegrin (DC-SIGN) is expressed by DCs and subsets of macrophages (77, 97) (Fig. 2). Its expression by human macrophages is generally low but can be induced following *M. tuberculosis* infection (98) or other stimulation (99). DC-SIGN recognizes mannosylated glycoconjugates such as *M. tuberculosis* ManLAM and PIMs (84, 100, 101). DC-SIGN activation during *M. tuberculosis* infection leads to PL fusion (contrary to the MR) and impedes DC maturation (100, 102).

Macrophage-inducible C-type lectin (Mincle; Clec4e, Clecsf9) is expressed on leukocytes at low levels before activation but is highly expressed on mouse macrophages following stimulation (103) (Fig. 2). Mincle recognizes damaged cells and fungi (104, 105). It also recognizes *M. tuberculosis* TDM, resulting in enhanced inflammatory cytokine production and granuloma formation (106, 107), but is not required for control of *M. tuberculosis* infection in mice (108).

Dectin-1 is a nonclassical C-type lectin that recognizes β-glucans (109) (Fig. 2). It is highly expressed on DCs, macrophages, monocytes, neutrophils, and a subset of T cells (110). Dectin-1 activation in conjunction with TLR4 during *M. tuberculosis* infection induces an interleukin (IL)-17A response (111). Similar to the MR, Dectin-1 differentiates between mycobacterium strains; activation by nonpathogenic (*Mycobacterium smegmatis*, *Mycobacterium phlei*) and attenuated (*Mycobacterium bovis* BCG, *M. tuberculosis* H37Ra) mycobacteria, but not virulent *M. tuberculosis* H37Rv, enhances TNF-α, IL-6, and RANTES production by macrophages (112, 113). Dectin-1 activation inhibits replication of BCG, but not virulent *M. tuberculosis*, in human macrophages (114). Dectin-2 recognizes mannose-

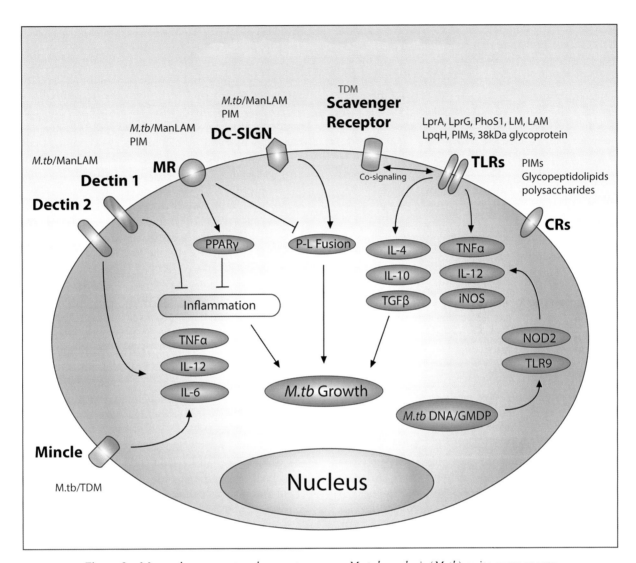

Figure 2 Macrophage receptors known to engage *M. tuberculosis* (*M.tb*) or its components and the downstream effects of receptor engagement on cytokine production, phagosome-lysosome fusion, and inflammation. Engagement of different receptors results in a macrophage response that can either promote or limit host immunity to *M. tuberculosis* infection.

containing lipids and is expressed by DC subsets and macrophages (115). Its stimulation by ManLAM induces pro- and anti-inflammatory responses and promotes T cell-mediated adaptive immunity in mice (116). Dectin-3 (also called MCL and Clec4d) recognizes TDM and is required for TDM-induced Mincle expression and production (117, 118).

Complement receptors CR1 (CD35), CR3 (CD11b/CD18), and CR4 (CD11c/CD18) are major phagocytic receptors expressed by monocytes, macrophages, neutrophils, and some lymphocytes, and their expression and activities change in a tissue- and differentiation-specific manner (Fig. 2). For example, CR4 expression increases during differentiation of monocytes into mac-

rophages and is the prominent CR on AMs (119, 120). CRs mediate phagocytosis of opsonized and nonopsonized *M. tuberculosis* by human macrophages (67, 68, 121, 122) and recognize surface polysaccharides, PIMs, and glycopeptidolipids of nonopsonized *M. tuberculosis* (123, 124).

FcγRs play a role in the phagocytosis of *M. tuberculosis* following opsonization of bacteria with immune-specific antibody (67); this can lead to increased PL fusion (125).

TLRs
TLRs are a highly conserved family of transmembrane PRRs that are expressed by many cells, including AMs

and DCs (126–130) (Fig. 2). They are surface exposed (e.g., TLR2 and TLR4) and intracellular (e.g., TLR9) (127) and are classically thought of as proinflammatory through NFκB activation (131–133) but can also act through the negative regulators TRIF, IRF, and IRAK-M (134, 135). Recognition of *M. tuberculosis* occurs via TLRs 2, 4, and 9. Mycobacterial lipids (phosphor-*myo*-inositol-capped LAM, PIM$_2$, and PIM$_6$) and 19-kDa lipoprotein are TLR2 agonists (136, 137). TLR4 recognizes heat shock protein 65 (136), and TLR9 recognizes *M. tuberculosis* CpG motifs (138). Studies in TLR knockout mice with *M. tuberculosis* have yielded contradictory results. Single and double knockout mice exhibit a range of phenotypes in response to *M. tuberculosis* infection including enhanced mortality and defective IL-12p40 and IFN-γ responses (139–142). Conversely, triple knockout TLR2/4/9 mice exhibited no loss of protective T cell responses, and growth of *M. tuberculosis* was similar in wild-type and knockout mice (143). Myeloid differentiation factor 88 (MyD88), an adaptor used by most TLRs, was reported to be indispensable for control of mycobacterial growth (143, 144), although MyD88's role may be tied to its importance in IL-1β signaling (145).

SRs

There are at least eight classes of SRs, which cooperate with other receptors to mediate their function (146) (Fig. 2). AMs express at least four different SRs: the class A scavenger receptor-A isoforms I and II (SRA-I/II), macrophage receptor with collagenous structure (MARCO), and the class B receptor CD36. SRA-I/II bind to most polyanionic molecules (147, 148), MARCO removes unopsonized particles in the lung (149), and CD36 removes apoptotic cells and oxidized LDL (150). SRs mediate *M. tuberculosis* binding to macrophages (151). MARCO cooperates with TLR2 and CD14 to initiate cytokine release following recognition of *M. tuberculosis* TDM (152). CD36 contributes to foam cell generation during *M. tuberculosis* infection (153) and PPARγ production during BCG infection (154). PPARγ induces CD36 expression in human AMs (155). The specific role of different SRs during *M. tuberculosis* infection is unclear, likely due to a redundancy in scavenger receptor expression (156). Infection of SRA-I/II (157, 158) and MARCO (159) single knockout mice indicates that these SRs may play a role in limiting inflammation and resistance to pulmonary pathogens. CD36 knockout mice are more resistant to *M. tuberculosis* infection (160). Further work is needed to understand the role of SRs during *M. tuberculosis* infection.

Phagosome maturation

Typical phagosome maturation involves sequential fusion of the phagosome with early endosomes, late endosomes, and lysosomes, during which process the pH decreases to 4.5 to 5.0 through the actions of a vacuolar ATPase. The phagosome also acquires antimicrobial peptides and proteases, including cathepsins that are activated by the low pH in the phagosome. These factors all contribute to the bactericidal nature of the mature phagosome and mediate clearance of the ingested particle (161). However, some pathogens, including *M. tuberculosis*, modify the phagosome such that it becomes a niche for intracellular replication (Fig. 3). *M. tuberculosis* phagosomes do not fully acidify, reaching a pH of 6.2, and do not fuse with lysosomes (Rab5, but not Rab7, is acquired). Many *M. tuberculosis* components interfere with this maturation, including ESAT-6/CFP-10 (early secretory antigenic target 6/culture filtrate protein 10), SecA1/2, ManLAM, and TDM (102, 162–165). ManLAM inhibits PL fusion through the macrophage MR (87). Recent work showed that a mycobacterial lipoprotein, LprG, binds ManLAM and controls its distribution in the mycobacterial envelope. Mutants of *M. tuberculosis* lacking LprG have less ManLAM on their surface and are less able to inhibit PL fusion (166, 167).

It has been proposed that *M. tuberculosis* can escape the phagosome and reside in the cytosol. This is controversial, with debate as to whether *M. tuberculosis* replicates in the cytosol or is released in conjunction with macrophage cell death (168). Cytosolic localization has been proposed because experiments in the 1980s to 1990s provide electron microscopy images showing intracellular *M. tuberculosis* independent of phagosome membranes (169–171), and components of *M. tuberculosis* are detected in the cytosol following infection in a region of difference-1 (RD-1) and ESAT-6-dependent manner (172–174). An explanation for the latter observation, besides complete phagosome membrane dissolution, is that the RD-1-dependent ESX-1 secretion system perforates, but does not destroy, the phagosome membrane, resulting in a "leaky," or porous, phagosome (175, 176). This leaky phagosome would allow *M. tuberculosis* components access to the cytosol and explain how *M. tuberculosis* infection leads to activation of cytosolic immune sensors.

Autophagy

Macroautophagy is a major form of autophagy, hereafter referred to simply as autophagy, which involves the entrapment of cytosolic compounds into double-membrane vesicles that fuse with lysosomes to mediate

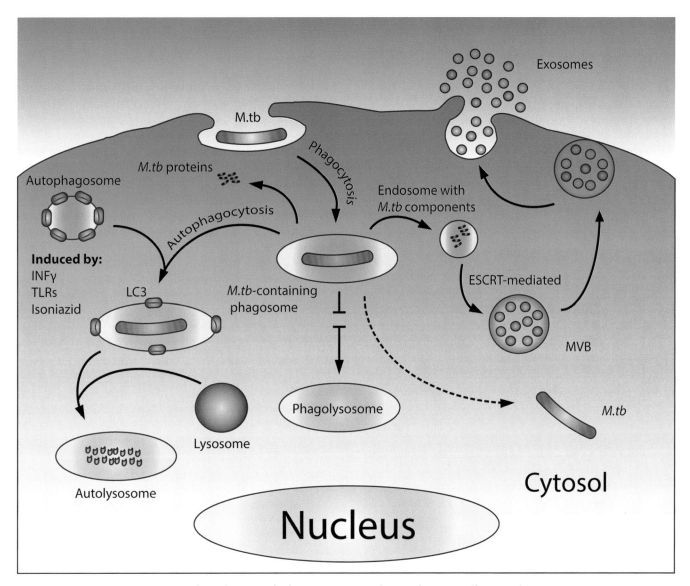

Figure 3 *M. tuberculosis* (*M.tb*) fate upon macrophage infection. Following phagocytosis, *M. tuberculosis* resides within a modified phagosome which may allow mycobacterial components to enter the cytosol in an ESX-1-dependent manner. The *M. tuberculosis* phagosome is also connected to the early endosomal network because membrane compartments can both fuse and bud from the phagosome, allowing exposure to important nutrients such as iron as well as removal of mycobacterial components. Endosomes containing mycobacterial components can fuse with multivesicular bodies (MVBs), leading to their incorporation into intraluminal vesicles, and upon MVB fusion with the plasma membrane, they can be released within exosomes (indicated as red circles in the figure). The *M. tuberculosis* phagosome has limited fusion with lysosomes, but with activation by IFN-γ or antibiotic treatment the *M. tuberculosis*-containing phagosome may undergo autophagosome formation and following lysosome fusion can limit *M. tuberculosis* growth, a process known as autophagy. There are also data suggesting that *M. tuberculosis* can escape into the cytosol, although this has been observed in only a limited number of studies.

degradation. This process is involved in cell maintenance and can also be used to limit infection (177–179).
Starvation, rapamycin, TLRs, 2′-5′ cyclic GMP-AMP,
IL-1, and IFN-γ can all induce autophagy (180). Recent
publications have indicated that the host AMP-activated
protein kinase-PPARγ, coactivator 1α pathway (AMPK-
PPARGC1A; PGC-1), and membrane occupation and
recognition nexus repeat containing 2 (MORN2) are involved in autophagy induction and regulate *M. tuberculosis* infection (181, 182) (Fig. 3). *M. tuberculosis*
has various components that regulate autophagy, including ESAT-6 (176, 183) and the enhanced intracellular survival (*eis*) gene (184). If autophagy is induced,
M. tuberculosis colocalizes with the autophagy marker
LC3, PL fusion occurs, and *M. tuberculosis* growth
is limited (185, 186). Autophagy is important *in vivo*;
autophagy-deficient mice show increased *M. tuberculosis* growth, lung pathology, and reduced survival compared to wild-type mice (176, 187). Two frontline TB
drugs, isoniazid and pyrazinamide, induce autophagy
in *M. tuberculosis*-infected macrophages and are more
inhibitory toward *M. tuberculosis* growth if the autophagy machinery is intact (188). Manipulation of autophagy is being pursued as a treatment option for TB
(189–192).

Intracellular receptors

Intracellular receptors include the transmembrane
TLRs and cytosolic nucleotide-binding oligomerization
domain-containing protein (NOD)-like receptors (NLRs),
RIG-I-like receptors, AIM2-like receptors (ALRs), and
other cytosolic DNA sensors (193–197). Some of these
receptors have been shown to recognize *M. tuberculosis*
ligands and play a role during *M. tuberculosis* infection.

NOD1 recognizes D-glutamyl-meso-diaminopimelic
acid, while NOD2 recognizes muramyl dipeptide
(MDP) and a glycolated form of MDP (GMDP) produced by *M. tuberculosis* (198–200). NOD2 regulates
M. tuberculosis growth in human and murine macrophages (201–203), perhaps via release of antimicrobial
peptides and autophagy, since MDP increases LL-37,
IRGM, and LC3 expression and *M. tuberculosis* killing
in AMs (204). *M. tuberculosis* infection also activates
NLRP3, but NLRP3 function during infection is unclear since NLRP3-deficient mice show a similar susceptibility to *M. tuberculosis* infection as wild-type
mice. On the other hand, mice lacking the adaptor protein PYCARD/ASC, which (like NLRP3) is involved
in caspase-1 activation, are more susceptible to *M. tuberculosis* infection (205). AIM2 and the ALR IFI204
recognize DNA and may play a role during *M. tuberculosis* infection (175, 206); AIM2-deficient mice have a

higher bacterial burden and succumb to infection more
quickly than wild-type mice (207).

PPARγ

The PPARs are a family of nuclear receptor-associated
transcription factors. They include PPARα, PPARβ/δ, and
PPARγ (208, 209). PPARγ is highly expressed by AMs,
and its deletion leads to increased expression of IFN-γ,
IL-12, macrophage inflammatory protein 1 alpha, and
inducible nitric oxide synthase (210). PPARγ expression
is induced in macrophages through the MR and TLR2
by *M. tuberculosis* and BCG, but not by the avirulent
M. smegmatis (23, 211). PPARγ inhibition or knockdown leads to reduced *M. tuberculosis* intracellular replication and lipid body formation and enhanced TNF-α
production (23, 153, 211). PPARγ is actively being pursued as a drug target, and efforts are ongoing to increase our understanding regarding its activities (209).

microRNAs (miRNAs)

miRNAs are endogenous, noncoding small RNAs that
are typically transcribed from intergenic or intragenic
regions of the genome in the pri-miRNA form. Following processing into miRNAs, they bind target mRNAs
and typically mediate translational repression or mRNA
degradation (212–214). Recent attention has focused on
the specific regulation and function of miRNAs in the
lung, particularly regarding cancer and inflammatory
responses (215, 216). miRNAs serve several potential
functions during *M. tuberculosis* infection: regulating
TLR signaling, NFκB activation, cytokine release, autophagy, and apoptosis to alter *M. tuberculosis* infection
and host survival (22, 217, 218). For example, miR-
124 downregulates expression of MyD88, TRAF6, and
TLR6 (219), and miR-let-7f targets a negative regulator
of NFκB, A20, to increase cytokine and nitrite production and reduce *M. tuberculosis* infection (217). miR-
132 and miR-26a negatively regulate the transcriptional
coactivator p300 and IFN-γ signaling (220). Expression of miRNAs can be altered in *M. tuberculosis*-
infected patients or cells (220–226), sometimes in a
virulence-dependent manner; e.g., *M. tuberculosis*, but
not *M. smegmatis*, infection induces expression of miR-
125b (227). miRNA activity can also be cell-type specific, because miR-19a-3p may regulate expression
of 5-lipoxygenase in primary human T cells, but not B
cells (228). Targeting of miRNAs is a promising host-
directed therapy (229).

Macrophage release of exosomes

miRNAs are also transported between cells via exosomes. Exosomes are membrane-bound vesicles of endo-

cytic origin that are released from most nucleated cells and function in intercellular communication and immune cell activation and serve as a source of disease biomarkers (230). In the context of an *M. tuberculosis* infection, exosomes released from infected macrophages can carry mycobacterial components including LAM, 19-KDa lipoprotein, and over 40 bacterial proteins, many of which are known immuno-dominant antigens (231, 232) (Fig. 3). The exosomes released from infected compared to uninfected macrophages also differ in their RNA content, and this has functional consequences on the exosome-recipient cell (233). Moreover, exosomes released from infected macrophages elicit both innate and acquired immune responses *in vitro* and *in vivo* and when used as a vaccine can protect mice against an aerosolized infection (231, 234, 235). However, whether exosomes released from infected macrophages function in regulating the immune response in humans during an *M. tuberculosis* infection remains an open question.

Macrophage cell death

Cell death can be an important step in controlling infection, and as such, many pathogens manipulate host cell death pathways to enhance their survival (236). The two cell death pathways that have been most studied are apoptosis, which is commonly thought of as anti-inflammatory and is characterized by retention of cell membrane integrity, and necrosis, which is typically proinflammatory and characterized by loss of membrane integrity (237, 238). Pyroptosis has characteristics of necrosis and apoptosis; pyroptotic cells lose membrane integrity similar to necrotic cells, but cell death is caspase-dependent, similar to apoptosis (239). Virulent *M. tuberculosis* inhibits apoptosis and instead induces necrosis to exacerbate infection. Apoptosis prevents *M. tuberculosis* dissemination and enhances antigen presentation to DCs and T cell priming. Necrosis and necroptosis mediate *M. tuberculosis* exit and dissemination from the infected cell, propagating infection; *M. tuberculosis* may downregulate pyroptosis, but this is not clear (240–242). *M. tuberculosis* components involved in regulating cell death include SodA, NuoG, ESX-1, and ESX-5 (243).

Interaction with DCs

DCs are a unique subset of immune cells which under steady-state conditions function as sentinels of the immune system. Immature DCs phagocytose *M. tuberculosis* at the site of infection, mature, migrate to secondary lymphoid organs, and prime T cells. DCs are equipped with a repertoire of PRRs for PAMPs

and damage-associated molecular pattern molecules (DAMPs) (Fig. 4). Engagement of individual receptors can ultimately dictate downstream DC responses. TLRs 2, 4, and 9 and DC-SIGN recognize *M. tuberculosis* surface molecules, as discussed above. The interaction between DC-SIGN and ManLAM expressed on virulent mycobacteria is exploited by *M. tuberculosis* to its benefit, with *M. tuberculosis* using DC-SIGN as a portal into DCs; once engulfed, bacteria are targeted to late endosomes/lysosomes expressing lysosomal-associated membrane protein 1 (LAMP1) (100). DC-SIGN-mediated entry leads to IL-10 production and inhibition of DC maturation (100), which in turn causes inefficient T cell priming and a state of antigenic tolerance (244). Mycobacteria are able to persist in DCs (245, 246). Other mycobacterial products such as Hip1, a serine hydrolase, modulate DC responses and intracellular survival of the pathogen. Hip1 mutants of *M. tuberculosis* induce high levels of IL-12 and increased expression of MHC-II in a MyD88- and TLR2/9-dependent manner (247). *M. tuberculosis* is also able to retain coronin-1 on the vesicular membrane, which interferes with phagosome maturation and promotes survival of the pathogen (245). Lung DCs encompass three major subsets of cells: conventional DCs, plasmacytoid DCs, and monocyte-derived DCs, with each subset having specific and interrelating functions in the host (248). Data from mouse studies show that monocyte-derived DCs are rapid responders and are detected in the lung as early as 48 hours postinfection (249, 250). DCs undergo phenotypic changes following engulfment of mycobacteria which include upregulation of MHC-I/II, CD40, CD80, and CD86 (251); increased production of IL-12, TNF-α, IL-1, and IL-6 (252–254); and increased migration to lymph nodes for T cell antigen presentation (255).

In specialized microenvironments, migratory DCs are able to efficiently prime CD4 T cells (256) and activate CD8 T cells by the endosome-cytosol (257) or "detour" (258) antigen presentation pathway. DCs possess a pathway capable of transferring exogenous antigens from the endosome to the cytosol, leading to the presentation of antigens via the classical MHC-I pathway (173, 257). As part of the "detour pathway" uninfected DCs engulf apoptotic vesicles released from *M. tuberculosis*-infected macrophages and present antigens from these extracellular vesicles to CD8 T cells (258).

DCs (in addition to macrophages) are key initiators of the immune response and are thought of as Trojan horses providing a reservoir for *M. tuberculosis* to survive and escape immune surveillance (259, 260). Char-

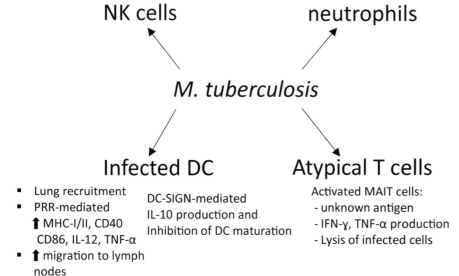

- BCG vaccination: ↑ IFN-γ
- *M.tb* antigens: ↑ IFN-γ, IL-22
- Lysis and killing of *M.tb* within MΦ
- Activation of DCs, CD8+ and gamma-delta T cells
- Inhibit proliferation of regulatory T cells

NK cells

- IL-8, LTB4-mediated recruitment of neutrophils
- Phagocytosis of *M.tb* (opsonin dependent and independent)
- Killing of ingested *M.tb*? Genetic variation?
- IL-8, TNF-α, IL-10 production: recruitment of MΦ, M1 vs M2 phenotype?
- Promotes/inhibits DC activation and presentation of antigen to T cells?
- Correlation between neutrophilia and disease severity

neutrophils

M. tuberculosis

Infected DC

- Lung recruitment
- PRR-mediated
  ↑ MHC-I/II, CD40
  CD86, IL-12, TNF-α
- ↑ migration to lymph nodes

DC-SIGN-mediated
IL-10 production and
Inhibition of DC maturation

Atypical T cells

Activated MAIT cells:
- unknown antigen
- IFN-γ, TNF-α production
- Lysis of infected cells

Figure 4 Responses of innate immune cells to *M. tuberculosis* (*M.tb*), *M. bovis* BCG, or their products, demonstrating both the beneficial and detrimental roles these cells have on controlling an *M. tuberculosis* infection.

acterizing the role of different DC subsets will enhance our understanding of the immune response to *M. tuberculosis*, aiding in the design of a better vaccine.

Interaction with NK Cells

Because resident immune cells present within the lung alveolar space, NK cells have received significant attention in the context of an *M. tuberculosis* infection (Fig. 4). This interest stems from their ability to produce cytokines which can regulate both the innate and acquired immune response, their ability to lyse infected cells, and their production of antibacterial mediators (e.g., nitric oxide and α-defensins) (261). NK cells are not homogeneous in their protein profile and function. In humans, NK cells are usually subdivided into two major groups: CD56^{bright} and CD56^{dim}, with CD56^{bright} NK cells being the most abundant NK cell present in lymph nodes and tissue. Upon stimulation, even at low concentrations of IL-2, CD56^{bright} NK cells can produce cytokines such as IFN-γ, TNF-α, and GM-CSF among others. However, they appear to have intrinsically low cytotoxic activity. In contrast, CD56^{dim} NK cells comprise approximately 90% of the NK cells in the peripheral blood and are found to be less stimu-

latory in the context of cytokine production but have a higher potential for cytotoxic activity compared to CD56^{bright} NK cells (262, 263).

Activation of NK cells is complex and involves both activating and inhibiting signals. The best-characterized inhibitory receptors are the immunoglobin-like receptors (KIRs), which upon binding MHC class I molecules inhibit NK cytotoxic functions. Examples of activating NK receptors include NKp30, NKp44, and NKp46. These receptors bind ligands on target cells, some of which are downregulated in tumor or infected cells (e.g., MHC class I) or to ligands which are upregulated in tumor or infected cells (264, 265). Recent studies indicate that some NK cells can also express PRRs such as TLR2 and TLR5, which upon binding PAMPs such as *Escherichia coli* flagellin are stimulated to produce IFN-γ and have upregulated α-defensin production (266, 267). This discovery suggests that NK cells may play a previously unappreciated role in directly recognizing and responding to microbial pathogens (266).

In the context of mycobacterial infections, initial studies in mice suggested that NK cells may not play a significant role in controlling an *M. tuberculosis* infection because NK cell-depleted mice did not show increased susceptibility to infection (268). However, in T cell-depleted mice such as RAG$^{-/-}$, NK cells were found to be a major source of IFN-γ upon *M. tuberculosis* infection (269). Although these studies suggested that NK cells are not required during a murine *M. tuberculosis* infection, caution must be maintained in extrapolating the conclusion to human infections since mice lack expression of both NKp30 and NKp44, which are key proteins in NK cell activation in humans (270). Studies in TB patients have shown NK cells to be present in high numbers in the pleural fluid (271). This increased NK cell number was not observed in other lung pathologies. A number of studies have assessed the cytolytic activity of NK cells isolated from the blood of TB patients and found that upon stimulation *ex vivo* these NK cells had impaired cytotoxic activity against well-characterized tumor target cell lines (272–274). However, the cytolytic activity was restored following successful drug treatment, suggesting that *M. tuberculosis* infection may suppress NK cell activity systemically (272, 273). Recent studies also suggest that increased expression of the coinhibitory receptor TIM-3 on NK cells might be tied to diminished NK cell function in TB patients (275). Whether suppression of NK cells occurs within a granuloma and how its activity differs between the different "types" of granulomas are presently unknown.

Nevertheless, studies in BCG-vaccinated infants suggest that NK cells are an important source of IFN-γ upon vaccination, and production of this cytokine is essential for driving the memory response associated with BCG vaccination (276). NK cells may also be involved in the "trained immunity" observed in BCG-vaccinated individuals (277). *In vitro* studies have shown that human NK cells produce cytokines such as IFN-γ upon exposure to *M. tuberculosis* antigens (278). IL-22 is also produced by activated NK cells and may play a role in killing of *M. tuberculosis* by promoting PL fusion within infected macrophages (279). A number of studies have shown that NK cells can lyse macrophages infected with *M. tuberculosis* (280), *Mycobacterium avium* complex (281), and *M. bovis* BCG (282) and that killing is enhanced by the presence of IL-2 and IL-12 (280). This NK cell-mediated killing is dependent on direct contact between the NK cell and infected macrophage but not on Fas-FasL interaction or release of cytotoxic granules (283). In addition to this direct NK cell-mediated killing, there appears to be a contact-independent/cytokine-dependent mechanism (284).

The effect of NK cells is not limited to mycobacteria-infected macrophages since studies have shown that human NK cells can also interact directly with *M. tuberculosis* and *M. bovis* BCG (285). The addition of purified human NK cells to BCG or mycobacterial cell wall preparations stimulated NK cell expression of CD69 as well as increased their cytotoxic activity and production of IFN-γ (286, 287). However, other studies have not confirmed these results (288). An explanation for these different experimental outcomes may stem from the source of human NK cells because studies have shown significant variation between individual donors in their NK cell response to intact mycobacteria (289). Variation in an individual's prior exposure to BCG or environmental mycobacteria and the potential for NK cells to maintain some form of immunological memory (290) may also be responsible for some of the observed variation between donors. Further support for a direct interaction between mycobacteria and NK cells stems from studies that have defined the NK cell receptors and *M. tuberculosis* ligands (291). This binding appeared specific to mycobacteria (and *Pseudomonas aeruginosa* and *Nocardia farcinica*) because the chimera did not bind other Gram-positive or Gram-negative bacteria. This chimera could bind the mycobacteria cell wall components mycolyl-arabinogalactan-peptidoglycan (mAGP) as well as mycolic acid and arabinogalactan from *M. tuberculosis* (292). Together, the data suggest that engagement of TLR2 by PG or components containing PG may be important in driving the initial NK cell response to the mycobacteria including IFN-γ production and upregulation of NKp44, which can then bind to other mycobacterial components, further promoting NK cell activation. The consequences of prolonged NK cell activation at the site of an infection are unclear because they could promote a protective response or could be a driver of immunopathology or a combination of both.

In the context of a mycobacterial infection, NK cells may also modulate other cells of the immune system in addition to macrophages. *In vitro* studies have shown that NK cells exposed to *M. tuberculosis* can activate immature DCs (iDCs), and this was dependent on both NK-DC interaction and cytokines produced by the NK cells (293). Reciprocally, DCs exposed to killed *M. tuberculosis* were activated and capable of inducing increased CD69 expression on human NK cells and increased cytotoxic activity against the Daudi cell line (293). Whether NK cells and DCs interact *in vivo* during a mycobacterial infection, promoting their reciprocal activation, is presently unclear, although they would be expected to have overlapping locations during a mycobacterial infection (i.e., inflammatory sites of the lung and draining lymph nodes). T cell activity has also been shown to be regulated by NK cells. Previous studies showed that depletion of NK cells from PBMCs isolated from healthy sensitized donors resulted in a diminished ability of gamma delta T cells to proliferate in the presence of *M. tuberculosis* antigens (294, 295). The NK cell activity was dependent on both direct NK cell-T cell contact and NK cell-derived cytokines but not IFN-γ. Similarly, CD8+ T cells from tuberculin-positive individuals were diminished in lysis of *M. tuberculosis*-infected macrophages when NK cells were removed from the PBMCs prior to incubation of the T cells with the infected macrophages (296). However, in this case, the CD8+ T cell activity was dependent on NK cell-derived IFN-γ. In contrast to T cell activation by NK cells, Roy et al. found that NK cells could inhibit proliferation of T regulatory cells in the context of an *M. tuberculosis* infection (297). Whether NK cells play a role in suppressing Tregs during the course of an *M. tuberculosis* infection is unclear but warrants further investigation.

In summary, the *in vitro* data and limited *in vivo* data suggest that NK cells may play an important role in promoting an effective immune response to an *M. tuberculosis* infection. This includes promoting macrophage activation and subsequent killing of phagocytosed bacilli, stimulating DC maturation and antigen presentation, activation of gamma delta T cells and antigen-specific CD8+ T cells, and inhibition of Tregs, all supporting a likely positive effect of NK cells on an immune response to *M. tuberculosis*. However, a potential negative consequence associated with excessive NK cell activation should not be ignored.

Interaction with Granulocytes

Neutrophils are the most studied granulocyte in the context of an *M. tuberculosis* infection (Fig. 4). However, despite the numerous studies both in mice and in humans, the role of neutrophils is still a subject of debate. Part of the issue lies with the difficulty of studying neutrophil function because they are easily activated, leading to skewed results and interpretations. More confounding is the likely bifunctional role played by neutrophils during the course of an *M. tuberculosis* infection: having a potential protective role during the early stages but promoting pathology at later stages. A number of studies support this bifunctionality. Studies by Barrios-Payán showed that depletion of neutrophils prior to an infection with *M. tuberculosis* resulted in higher bacterial load in the lung and spleen compared to mice with normal neutrophil levels (298). Similar results have been observed in other neutrophil depletion studies (299, 300), although this has not been uni-

versally true (301). In contrast, depletion of neutrophils during the chronic stage of a mouse *M. tuberculosis* infection led to a decrease in bacterial numbers over time (302). Moreover, in humans higher neutrophil counts are associated with poorer prognosis (303), again suggesting that neutrophils may contribute to TB disease pathology.

Neutrophils are actively recruited to the site of an *M. tuberculosis* infection (304, 305), and this response is dependent on production of cytokines/inflammatory mediators such as IL-8 and LTB4, among others (306). Mice or humans presensitized by either prior infection or BCG immunization show a significant recruitment of neutrophils at the site of new *M. tuberculosis* infection (307). Although this enhanced recruitment of neutrophils in sensitized individuals has been known since the early 20th century, only recently has a potential mechanism been identified. The cytokines IL-17 and IL-23 may be key mediators of this response and are likely produced by memory T helper (Th17) cells created during the initial infection/immunization (308). The recruitment of neutrophils from either a primary infection or reinfection can affect bacterial numbers, because previous studies have shown that neutrophils are capable of phagocytosing *M. tuberculosis* through opsonin-dependent and -independent mechanisms (309). Moreover, the recruited neutrophils produce antimicrobial compounds such as reactive oxygen species and cytokines and chemokines that further promote neutrophil recruitment and drive the inflammatory response (310–312). This early influx of neutrophils could function to limit the bacterial growth at the initial stages of an infection.

However, whether activated neutrophils can kill ingested virulent *M. tuberculosis* is still a matter of debate, and there is evidence to both support (313, 314) and refute (315, 316) killing by neutrophils. Factors that may influence which path is taken may reside in differences in experimental design, but evidence also suggests a genetic component. In studies using isolated human neutrophils Kisich et al. found that killing of ingested *M. tuberculosis* varied among donors (313) and that the ability to be activated by the 19-kDa lipoprotein also varied between donors (317). Therefore, some of the controversy surrounding the role of neutrophils during an *M. tuberculosis* infection may reside in whether the initial influx of neutrophils can limit bacterial growth. In the zebra fish infection model, neutrophil-mediated killing of *Mycobacterium marinum* was observed (318), suggesting that a slowing of the infection process may occur, allowing other components of the immune response to take hold and eventually leading to a controlled infection. However, in *M. tuberculosis*-infected cynomolgus macaques, Mattila et al. observed that, at the level of a single granuloma, increased levels of grzB+ neutrophils correlated with higher bacterial loads (319).

Neutrophils may also influence both recruitment and activation of macrophages during an *M. tuberculosis* infection. The initial production of cytokines and chemokines by neutrophils will promote macrophage recruitment and help define the macrophage M1 and M2 phenotype (320). Guinea pig neutrophils were found to produce IL-8 and TNF-α upon infection with *M. tuberculosis* and could drive macrophage activation in a TNF-α dependent manner (321). Alternatively, neutrophil production of IL-10 could dampen the inflammatory response and thus limit macrophage recruitment (322, 323). In addition, neutrophils which die *in situ* are ingested by recruited macrophages. Although uptake of apoptotic neutrophils by macrophages usually induces an anti-inflammatory response, ingestion of infected neutrophils which have died by apoptosis or necrosis may lead to a different macrophage response. Macrophage ingestion of apoptotic neutrophils previously infected with *M. bovis* BCG induced an anti-inflammatory response (324), while similar experiments with *M. tuberculosis* induced macrophage production of TNF-α and a proinflammatory response (325, 326). This differential response by the phagocytosing macrophage may be dependent on whether the neutrophil has killed the ingested mycobacteria prior to its own death, with macrophage ingestion of dead neutrophil/mycobacteria leading to a more anti-inflammatory response while the opposite is observed with live *M. tuberculosis*. Therefore, the variability of human neutrophils to kill *M. tuberculosis* as mentioned above may have consequences beyond the direct effect on neutrophils and likely influences the macrophage response and potentially the subsequent acquired immune response.

Independent of its effect on macrophages, neutrophils may function in regulating an acquired immune response to an *M. tuberculosis* infection. Following an *M. tuberculosis* or *M. bovis* BCG infection, neutrophils can produce cytokines and chemokines such as IL-12, macrophage inflammatory protein 1 alpha, and monocyte chemotactic protein, which can promote T cell recruitment and activation (327, 328), or IL-10, which can dampen the T cell response (323). The direction of the neutrophil response is likely dependent on many host and microbial components and is still not well understood. Neutrophils may also be a source of TB antigen. Studies with BCG have shown that DCs are more potent activators of both CD4+ and CD8+ T cells if they were exposed to infected neutrophils prior to their incubation with the T cells (329). Cross-presentation of antigen from neutrophils to DCs and enhanced T cell proliferation have also been observed in the context of an *in vitro M. tuberculosis* infection (330). Further, DC migration may be enhanced following exposure to infected neutrophils, and depletion of neutrophils in mice resulted in reduced migration of DCs to lymph nodes and delayed T cell activation following an *M. tuberculosis* infection (331). However, excess neutrophil influx has also been associated with impaired T cell activation and protection against an *M. tuberculosis* infection (332). Despite these studies, the role of neutrophils in promoting or limiting a T cell response remains an open question and is complicated by its potential direct effect on T cells and its effects on macrophages and DCs with subsequent effects on T cell responses. Moreover, the number of neutrophils recruited to the infection site, their activation state, their ability to kill ingested mycobacteria, etc. are all important factors in defining how neutrophils may regulate the initial T cell response.

Neutrophil activity has also been linked to TB pathology, since in both human and mouse models neutrophils are present within the granulomas and the extent of local neutrophilia appears to correlate with the severity of disease (333, 334). Moreover, a higher number of neutrophils in peripheral blood at the time of disease diagnosis is associated with poor prognosis and longer drug treatment times required to reach negative sputum cultures (303, 335). With the use of genetically susceptible mouse strains, knockout mice that have altered immune responses or comparing virulent to less virulent strains, there is again a strong reverse correlation between disease outcome and local neutrophilia (269, 336, 337). This suggests that, in general, a lack of protective immune response results in neutrophilia. The cause of this neutrophilia stems from an inadequate mononuclear phagocyte or acquired immune response with a "compensatory" neutrophil influx. It may also be due to a dysfunction of the neutrophil itself, with limited killing of ingested mycobacteria and/or prolonged production of inflammatory mediators again leading to an elevated neutrophil influx. In either case, the neutrophilia leads to increased tissue destruction and pathology, supporting the perception that neutrophils have a negative effect on the adaptive immune response.

In summary, although there are still significant gaps in our understanding of neutrophil function in the setting of an *M. tuberculosis* infection, we have begun to define their potential beneficial role, particularly at the early stages of infection, but also their association with disease pathology. In the context of an active disease neutrophils may be one of the drivers of disease pathology, or their increased numbers may be a consequence of some other underlying immune dysfunction.

M. TUBERCULOSIS GRANULOMA

Granulomas are the histopathologic hallmark of TB, and the terms "granulomas" and "tubercles" were described before the causative agent of TB was identified. The link to tubercles was acknowledged in the naming of *M. tuberculosis* (338). The TB granuloma has been classically thought of as the host response to contain and limit *M. tuberculosis* infection. However, granulomas also provide a niche that is recalcitrant to anti-TB treatment and allows for bacterial persistence.

The center of the classic granuloma consists of different types of macrophages. These include differentiated foamy macrophages and epithelioid cells and large multinucleated giant cells (fused macrophages). There are occasional NK cells, DCs, and neutrophils mixed with the macrophages. These cells are surrounded by B and T cells, which make up 1 to 10% and 15 to 50%, respectively, of leukocytes in the murine lung (339). TB-infected individuals typically have cavitating, necrotic granulomas. Large cavitating granulomas contain loose cellular accumulation and numerous neutrophils and macrophages, along with the characteristic acellular caseous (milky, thick substance) necrotic material, while noncavitating closed granulomas contain a central necrotic area that is fully acellular (340, 341). Granulomas are heterogeneous, dynamic structures that contain motile cells and change in size during infection (342–345).

Animal models to study TB granulomas are diverse, and each has its benefits and drawbacks (reviewed in reference 340). The most common animal model employed is the mouse, which does not generate necrotic granulomas or granuloma structures similar to those found in humans. However, genetically altered mouse models exist that have granuloma structures that more closely resemble the granulomas in humans, for example, mice that overexpress IL-13 (346) or lack IL-10 (347) or the *sst1* locus, i.e., C3HeB/FeJ mice (348). Guinea pigs, rabbits, and non-human primates also generate necrotic, caseating granulomas (349–351).

In vitro PBMC models are also being developed; these lack the ultrastructure provided by the lung but represent more tractable human systems for study (352, 353). Recent work with a PBMC granuloma model shows that granuloma formation and response are fundamentally different in PBMCs collected from people with latent TB infection compared to naive individuals

and that *M. tuberculosis* has a unique transcriptional profile in these latent TB infection-generated granulomas (352). Finally, *in silico* models of granuloma formation provide additional insight into the mechanisms at play (354, 355).

INNATE IMMUNITY AND EARLY BACTERIAL CLEARANCE

Previous studies have found that exposure to *M. tuberculosis* does not necessarily lead to a positive IFN-γ response assay (IGRA) test in immune-competent individuals. This observation has been known for many years, as illustrated in a 1941 study which found that despite long-term and significant exposure to *M. tuberculosis* by a group of nursing students, a significant number remained tuberculin skin test negative (356). Case contact studies indicate that approximately half of those significantly exposed (e.g., household contacts of an active TB patient) remained tuberculin skin test negative (357). What is responsible for the elimination of the pathogen in the absence of an acquired immune response? Although we do not have an answer to this important question, and indeed the mechanism may vary from case to case, we do have some insight into what components of the innate immune response may be involved.

Studies have found variation between individuals in the innate immune response to mycobacteria as observed in whole-blood stimulation assays (358), indicating that there are intrinsic differences in a person's ability to control an initial *M. tuberculosis* infection. AMs, which are the initial cells infected with *M. tuberculosis*, may play a critical role in early clearance. Differences in macrophage activation through early exposure to cytokines such as IFN-γ and TNF-α produced by MAIT cells, gamma-delta T cells, NK cells, or neutrophils could lead to varied responses by infected AMs. Variation in vitamin D3 or its receptor expression could also result in differences in the macrophage activation state. Polymorphisms in the vitamin D3 receptor have been associated with susceptibility to infection (359), and a number of polymorphisms in innate immune genes have been found (360). In addition to AMs, neutrophils may function in early clearance, because they are rapidly recruited to the lung upon infection and can both phagocytose and kill ingested *M. tuberculosis* (314, 361, 362), although the ability to kill ingested bacilli seems to vary significantly among individuals (313). Studies by Martineau et al. indicate that among household contacts of TB patients in London there was a statistically significant association between a positive IFN-γ response assay and low peripheral blood neutrophil counts (363). The authors hypothesize that neutrophils may play a role in the clearance of *M. tuberculosis* infection in household contacts that did not convert to a positive IGRA; however, there is no direct support of this hypothesis presently.

Accumulating evidence suggests that immunological memory is not specific to the acquired immune response; some aspects of memory can be associated with the innate immune response. This has been shown most clearly in arthropod studies such as those in *Anopheles* mosquitoes and *Drosophila melanogaster* (364–366). However, it is unclear whether in higher vertebrates such innate memory responses function in long-term protection and whether these memory cells can be induced by vaccination. Nevertheless, BCG infection has been shown to induce NOD2-dependent epigenetic changes in monocytes that lasted up to 3 months postinfection and resulted in sustained upregulation of key proinflammatory genes, so-called trained immunity (367, 368). As indicated above, BCG vaccination also leads to an increased number of IFN-γ-expressing NK cells, and depletion of the NK cells postvaccination resulted in reduced vaccine efficacy following an *M. tuberculosis* challenge (276). Gamma delta T cells also expand during BCG vaccination and have been shown to restrict *M. tuberculosis* growth (369, 370). Together, the data suggest that when evaluating a TB vaccine it is important to consider its effect on the innate immunity and its potential to induce longer-term changes in the innate immune response.

CONCLUSION

As an airborne pathogen, it is essential that we fully understand the nature of transmissible *M. tuberculosis* and its encounter with innate immune constituents of the lung as well as the impact of these events on subsequent granuloma formation and persistence. Our failure to completely understand these events creates a critical barrier in our attempts to develop new effective treatment and vaccine strategies that target the lung (e.g., drug delivery, optimal vaccine responses). The host response to *M. tuberculosis* occurs within host tissues of the lung and elsewhere. In this regard, the granuloma is a specialized tissue microenvironment, akin to the cancer microenvironment, with specialized cells and soluble factors that greatly influence both host and *M. tuberculosis* biology. Although parts of this chapter summarize findings directly applicable to the lung, much of our knowledge is still extrapolated from experiments using cells, and in some cases surro-

gate bacteria, in systems not representative of the lung environment. As models of the lung become more refined, we will gain valuable new insight into the mechanisms at play, aiding our attempts to improve treatment delivery and activity at the site of infection in the lung.

Our current understanding of the role of macrophages in TB, although incomplete, clearly demonstrates the central role these cells play both in the host protective immune response and control of infection and in the maintenance of chronic infection and its associated tissue damage and pathology. As we gain more knowledge about macrophage responses in the context of organ-specific microenvironments, our understanding of the molecular details underlying the pivotal *M. tuberculosis*-macrophage interactions that occur during TB infection will become more defined. In future studies, it is critical that we better understand these interactions during the entire spectrum of TB from primary infection, dissemination, microbial growth within granulomas, control of infection, and latency and reactivation of disease. It is clear that the nature of the macrophage receptor recognition, signaling, inflammation, and antigen presentation pathways differ during different stages of infection and disease and that the nature of the infecting *M. tuberculosis* strain also contributes to this diversity of responses.

In addition to macrophages, our knowledge is increasing with respect to a number of other soluble and cellular components of the innate immune system in response to *M. tuberculosis* which can be both protective and detrimental to the host, depending upon the tissue context. Recent studies on "trained immunity" indicate that that effects of *M. tuberculosis* on the innate immune system may be longer-lived than once imagined.

Since recent publications have highlighted the major differences in immune response among humans and different animal models, future studies must focus on comparative biology among mammalian hosts, with an eye toward the use of animal models that better recapitulate what is seen in human disease. In addition, an important future focus will be studies of human clinical samples and the use of platform technologies to maximize our understanding of human TB to develop rational approaches to find critically needed new biomarkers, therapies, and vaccines.

Acknowledgments. The authors thank Yong Cheng at the University of Notre Dame and Eusondia Arnett at the Ohio State University for their help with manuscript preparation and figures.

Citation. Schorey JS, Schlesinger LS. 2016. Innate immune responses to tuberculosis. Microbiol Spectrum 4(6):TBTB2-0010-2016.

References

1. **WHO.** 2015. *Global tuberculosis report 2015*, 20th ed. http://www.who.int/tb/publications/global_report/en/.

2. **Hasenberg M, Stegemann-Koniszewski S, Gunzer M.** 2013. Cellular immune reactions in the lung. *Immunol Rev* **251:**189–214.

3. **Weibel ER.** 2009. What makes a good lung? *Swiss Med Wkly* **139:**375–386.

4. **Burri PH.** 2011. Development and growth of the human lung, p 1–46. *In* Reich M (ed), *Comprehensive Physiology, Supplement 10. Handbook of Physiology: The Respiratory System, Circulation, and Nonrespiratory Functions*, 10th ed. John Wiley and Sons Hoboken, NJ.

5. **Hartung GH, Myhre LG, Nunneley SA.** 1980. Physiological effects of cold air inhalation during exercise. *Aviat Space Environ Med* **51:**591–594.

6. **Ryu J-H, Kim C-H, Yoon J-H.** 2010. Innate immune responses of the airway epithelium. *Mol Cells* **30:**173–183.

7. **Whitsett JA, Alenghat T.** 2015. Respiratory epithelial cells orchestrate pulmonary innate immunity. *Nat Immunol* **16:**27–35.

8. **Bastacky J, Goerke J.** 1992. Pores of Kohn are filled in normal lungs: low-temperature scanning electron microscopy. *J Appl Physiol (1985)* **73:**88–95.

9. **Mason RJ.** 2006. Biology of alveolar type II cells. *Respirology* **11**(Suppl):S12–S15.

10. **Guillot L, Nathan N, Tabary O, Thouvenin G, Le Rouzic P, Corvol H, Amselem S, Clement A.** 2013. Alveolar epithelial cells: master regulators of lung homeostasis. *Int J Biochem Cell Biol* **45:**2568–2573.

11. **Debbabi H, Ghosh S, Kamath AB, Alt J, Demello DE, Dunsmore S, Behar SM.** 2005. Primary type II alveolar epithelial cells present microbial antigens to antigen-specific CD4+ T cells. *Am J Physiol Lung Cell Mol Physiol* **289:**L274–L279.

12. **Fels AO, Cohn ZA.** 1986. The alveolar macrophage. *J Appl Physiol (1985)* **60:**353–369.

13. **Murphy J, Summer R, Wilson AA, Kotton DN, Fine A.** 2008. The prolonged life-span of alveolar macrophages. *Am J Respir Cell Mol Biol* **38:**380–385.

14. **Hussell T, Bell TJ.** 2014. Alveolar macrophages: plasticity in a tissue-specific context. *Nat Rev Immunol* **14:**81–93.

15. **van oud Alblas AB, van Furth R.** 1979. Origin, kinetics, and characteristics of pulmonary macrophages in the normal steady state. *J Exp Med* **149:**1504–1518.

16. **Bitterman PB, Saltzman LE, Adelberg S, Ferrans VJ, Crystal RG.** 1984. Alveolar macrophage replication. One mechanism for the expansion of the mononuclear phagocyte population in the chronically inflamed lung. *J Clin Invest* **74:**460–469.

17. **Landsman L, Jung S.** 2007. Lung macrophages serve as obligatory intermediate between blood monocytes and alveolar macrophages. *J Immunol* **179:**3488–3494.

18. **Kopf M, Schneider C, Nobs SP.** 2015. The development and function of lung-resident macrophages and dendritic cells. *Nat Immunol* **16:**36–44.

19. **Epelman S, Lavine KJ, Randolph GJ.** 2014. Origin and functionsof tissue macrophages. *Immunity* **41:**21–35.

20. **Ginhoux F.** 2014. Fate PPAR-titioning: PPAR-γ 'instructs' alveolar macrophage development. *Nat Immunol* **15:**1005–1007.

21. **Lambrecht BN.** 2006. Alveolar macrophage in the driver's seat. *Immunity* **24:**366–368.

22. **Rajaram MVS, Ni B, Dodd CE, Schlesinger LS.** 2014. Macrophage immunoregulatory pathways in tuberculosis. *Semin Immunol* **26:**471–485.

23. **Rajaram MVS, Brooks MN, Morris JD, Torrelles JB, Azad AK, Schlesinger LS.** 2010. *Mycobacterium tuberculosis* activates human macrophage peroxisome proliferator-activated receptor gamma linking mannose receptor recognition to regulation of immune responses. *J Immunol* **185:**929–942.

24. **Schneider C, Nobs SP, Kurrer M, Rehrauer H, Thiele C, Kopf M.** 2014. Induction of the nuclear receptor PPAR-γ by the cytokine GM-CSF is critical for the differentiation of fetal monocytes into alveolar macrophages. *Nat Immunol* **15:**1026–1037.

25. **Hoidal JR, Schmeling D, Peterson PK.** 1981. Phagocytosis, bacterial killing, and metabolism by purified human lung phagocytes. *J Infect Dis* **144:**61–71.

26. **Greening AP, Lowrie DB.** 1983. Extracellular release of hydrogen peroxide by human alveolar macrophages: the relationship to cigarette smoking and lower respiratory tract infections. *Clin Sci (Lond)* **65:**661–664.

27. **Lyons CR, Ball EJ, Toews GB, Weissler JC, Stastny P, Lipscomb MF.** 1986. Inability of human alveolar macrophages to stimulate resting T cells correlates with decreased antigen-specific T cell-macrophage binding. *J Immunol* **137:**1173–1180.

28. **Holt PG, Oliver J, Bilyk N, McMenamin C, McMenamin PG, Kraal G, Thepen T.** 1993. Downregulation of the antigen presenting cell function(s) of pulmonary dendritic cells *in vivo* by resident alveolar macrophages. *J Exp Med* **177:**397–407.

29. **Roth MD, Golub SH.** 1993. Human pulmonary macrophages utilize prostaglandins and transforming growth factor beta 1 to suppress lymphocyte activation. *J Leukoc Biol* **53:**366–371.

30. **Schneberger D, Aharonson-Raz K, Singh B.** 2012. Pulmonary intravascular macrophages and lung health: what are we missing? *Am J Physiol Lung Cell Mol Physiol* **302:**L498–L503.

31. **Lohmann-Matthes M-L, Steinmüller C, Franke-Ullmann G.** 1994. Pulmonary macrophages. *Eur Respir J* **7:**1678–1689.

32. **Cai Y, Sugimoto C, Arainga M, Alvarez X, Didier ES, Kuroda MJ.** 2014. *In vivo* characterization of alveolar and interstitial lung macrophages in rhesus macaques: implications for understanding lung disease in humans. *J Immunol* **192:**2821–2829.

33. **Schneberger D, Aharonson-Raz K, Singh B.** 2011. Monocyte and macrophage heterogeneity and Toll-like receptors in the lung. *Cell Tissue Res* **343:**97–106.

34. **Guilliams M, Lambrecht BN, Hammad H.** 2013. Division of labor between lung dendritic cells and macro-

phages in the defense against pulmonary infections. *Mucosal Immunol* 6:464–473.

35. Thornton EE, Looney MR, Bose O, Sen D, Sheppard D, Locksley R, Huang X, Krummel MF. 2012. Spatiotemporally separated antigen uptake by alveolar dendritic cells and airway presentation to T cells in the lung. *J Exp Med* 209:1183–1199.

36. Vermaelen KY, Carro-Muino I, Lambrecht BN, Pauwels RA. 2001. Specific migratory dendritic cells rapidly transport antigen from the airways to the thoracic lymph nodes. *J Exp Med* 193:51–60.

37. Halle S, Dujardin HC, Bakocevic N, Fleige H, Danzer H, Willenzon S, Suezer Y, Hämmerling G, Garbi N, Sutter G, Worbs T, Förster R. 2009. Induced bronchus-associated lymphoid tissue serves as a general priming site for T cells and is maintained by dendritic cells. *J Exp Med* 206:2593–2601.

38. Randall TD. 2010. Pulmonary dendritic cells: thinking globally, acting locally. *J Exp Med* 207:451–454.

39. Gold MC, Napier RJ, Lewinsohn DM. 2015. MR1-restricted mucosal associated invariant T (MAIT) cells in the immune response to *Mycobacterium tuberculosis*. *Immunol Rev* 264:154–166.

40. Gold MC, Cerri S, Smyk-Pearson S, Cansler ME, Vogt TM, Delepine J, Winata E, Swarbrick GM, Chua W-J, Yu YYL, Lantz O, Cook MS, Null MD, Jacoby DB, Harriff MJ, Lewinsohn DA, Hansen TH, Lewinsohn DM. 2010. Human mucosal associated invariant T cells detect bacterially infected cells. *PLoS Biol* 8:e1000407.

41. Le Bourhis L, Martin E, Péguillet I, Guihot A, Froux N, Coré M, Lévy E, Dusseaux M, Meyssonnier V, Premel V, Ngo C, Riteau B, Duban L, Robert D, Huang S, Rottman M, Soudais C, Lantz O. 2010. Antimicrobial activity of mucosal-associated invariant T cells. *Nat Immunol* 11:701–708. (Erratum 11:969.)

42. Le Bourhis L, Dusseaux M, Bohineust A, Bessoles S, Martin E, Premel V, Coré M, Sleurs D, Serriari N-E, Treiner E, Hivroz C, Sansonetti P, Gougeon M-L, Soudais C, Lantz O. 2013. MAIT cells detect and efficiently lyse bacterially-infected epithelial cells. *PLoS Pathog* 9:e1003681.

43. Chua W-J, Truscott SM, Eickhoff CS, Blazevic A, Hoft DF, Hansen TH. 2012. Polyclonal mucosa-associated invariant T cells have unique innate functions in bacterial infection. *Infect Immun* 80:3256–3267.

44. Craig A, Mai J, Cai S, Jeyaseelan S. 2009. Neutrophil recruitment to the lungs during bacterial pneumonia. *Infect Immun* 77:568–575.

45. Wright JR. 1997. Immunomodulatory functions of surfactant. *Physiol Rev* 77:931–962.

46. Wright JR. 2005. Immunoregulatory functions of surfactant proteins. *Nat Rev Immunol* 5:58–68.

47. Mason RJ, Voelker DR. 1998. Regulatory mechanisms of surfactant secretion. *Biochim Biophys Acta* 1408:226–240

48. Crouch E, Wright JR. 2001. Surfactant proteins a and d and pulmonary host defense. *Annu Rev Physiol* 63:521–554

49. Beharka AA, Gaynor CD, Kang BK, Voelker DR, McCormack FX, Schlesinger LS. 2002. Pulmonary surfactant protein A up-regulates activity of the mannose receptor, a pattern recognition receptor expressed on human macrophages. *J Immunol* 169:3565–3573.

50. Crowther JE, Kutala VK, Kuppusamy P, Ferguson JS, Beharka AA, Zweier JL, McCormack FX, Schlesinger LS. 2004. Pulmonary surfactant protein a inhibits macrophage reactive oxygen intermediate production in response to stimuli by reducing NADPH oxidase activity. *J Immunol* 172:6866–6874.

51. Nguyen HA, Rajaram MVS, Meyer DA, Schlesinger LS. 2012. Pulmonary surfactant protein A and surfactant lipids upregulate IRAK-M, a negative regulator of TLR-mediated inflammation in human macrophages. *Am J Physiol Lung Cell Mol Physiol* 303:L608–L616.

52. van Iwaarden F, Welmers B, Verhoef J, Haagsman HP, van Golde LM. 1990. Pulmonary surfactant protein A enhances the host-defense mechanism of rat alveolar macrophages. *Am J Respir Cell Mol Biol* 2:91–98.

53. Haagsman HP. 1998. Interactions of surfactant protein A with pathogens. *Biochim Biophys Acta* 1408:264–277.

54. Carlson TK, Brooks MN, Rajaram MVS, Henning LN, Meyer DA, Schlesinger LS. 2010. Pulmonary innate immunity: soluble and cellular host defenses of the lung, p 167–211. *In* Marsh CB, Hunter, Tridandapani S, Piper MG (ed), *Regulation of Innate Immune Function*. Transworld Research Signpost, STM Books.

55. Gaynor CD, McCormack FX, Voelker DR, McGowan SE, Schlesinger LS. 1995. Pulmonary surfactant protein A mediates enhanced phagocytosis of *Mycobacterium tuberculosis* by a direct interaction with human macrophages. *J Immunol* 155:5343–5351.

56. Downing JF, Pasula R, Wright JR, Twigg HL III, Martin WJ II. 1995. Surfactant protein a promotes attachment of *Mycobacterium tuberculosis* to alveolar macrophages during infection with human immunodeficiency virus. *Proc Natl Acad Sci USA* 92:4848–4852.

57. Pasula R, Downing JF, Wright JR, Kachel DL, Davis TE Jr, Martin WJ II. 1997. Surfactant protein A (SP-A) mediates attachment of *Mycobacterium tuberculosis* to murine alveolar macrophages. *Am J Respir Cell Mol Biol* 17:209–217.

58. Sidobre S, Nigou J, Puzo G, Rivière M. 2000. Lipoglycans are putative ligands for the human pulmonary surfactant protein A attachment to mycobacteria. Critical role of the lipids for lectin-carbohydrate recognition. *J Biol Chem* 275:2415–2422.

59. Ferguson JS, Voelker DR, McCormack FX, Schlesinger LS. 1999. Surfactant protein D binds to *Mycobacterium tuberculosis* bacilli and lipoarabinomannan via carbohydrate-lectin interactions resulting in reduced phagocytosis of the bacteria by macrophages. *J Immunol* 163:312–321.

60. Ferguson JS, Martin JL, Azad AK, McCarthy TR, Kang PB, Voelker DR, Crouch EC, Schlesinger LS. 2006. Surfactant protein D increases fusion of *Mycobacterium tuberculosis*-containing phagosomes with lysosomes in human macrophages. *Infect Immun* 74:7005–7009.

61. Ferguson JS, Voelker DR, Ufnar JA, Dawson AJ, Schlesinger LS. 2002. Surfactant protein D inhibition of human macrophage uptake of *Mycobacterium tuberculosis* is independent of bacterial agglutination. *J Immunol* **168**:1309–1314.

62. Ferguson JS, Schlesinger LS. 2000. Pulmonary surfactant in innate immunity and the pathogenesis of tuberculosis. *Tuber Lung Dis* **80**:173–184.

63. Arcos J, Diangelo LE, Scordo JM, Sasindran SJ, Moliva JI, Turner J, Torrelles JB. 2015. Lung mucosa lining fluid modification of *Mycobacterium tuberculosis* to reprogram human neutrophil killing mechanisms. *J Infect Dis* **212**:948–958.

64. Herzog EL, Brody AR, Colby TV, Mason R, Williams MC. 2008. Knowns and unknowns of the alveolus. *Proc Am Thorac Soc* **5**:778–782.

65. Strunk RC, Eidlen DM, Mason RJ. 1988. Pulmonary alveolar type II epithelial cells synthesize and secrete proteins of the classical and alternative complement pathways. *J Clin Invest* **81**:1419–1426.

66. Cole FS, Matthews WJ Jr, Rossing TH, Gash DJ, Lichtenberg NA, Pennington JE. 1983. Complement biosynthesis by human bronchoalveolar macrophages. *Clin Immunol Immunopathol* **27**:153–159.

67. Schlesinger LS, Bellinger-Kawahara CG, Payne NR, Horwitz MA. 1990. Phagocytosis of *Mycobacterium tuberculosis* is mediated by human monocyte complement receptors and complement component C3. *J Immunol* **144**:2771–2780.

68. Ferguson JS, Weis JJ, Martin JL, Schlesinger LS. 2004. Complement protein C3 binding to *Mycobacterium tuberculosis* is initiated by the classical pathway in human bronchoalveolar lavage fluid. *Infect Immun* **72**: 2564–2573.

69. Figueroa JE, Densen P. 1991. Infectious diseases associated with complement deficiencies. *Clin Microbiol Rev* **4**:359–395.

70. Mold C. 1999. Role of complement in host defense against bacterial infection. *Microbes Infect* **1**:633–638.

71. Tedesco F. 2008. Inherited complement deficiencies and bacterial infections. *Vaccine* **26**(Suppl 8):I3–I8.

72. Moliva JI, Rajaram MVS, Sidiki S, Sasindran SJ, Guirado E, Pan XJ, Wang S-H, Ross P Jr, Lafuse WP, Schlesinger LS, Turner J, Torrelles JB. 2014. Molecular composition of the alveolar lining fluid inthe aging lung. *Age (Dordr)* **36**:9633.

73. Arcos J, Sasindran SJ, Fujiwara N, Turner J, Schlesinger LS, Torrelles JB. 2011. Human lung hydrolases delineate *Mycobacterium tuberculosis*-macrophage interactions and the capacity to control infection. *J Immunol* **187**: 372–381.

74. Stahl PD. 1990. The macrophage mannose receptor: current status. *Am J Respir Cell Mol Biol* **2**:317–318.

75. Speert DP, Silverstein SC. 1985. Phagocytosis of unopsonized zymosan by human monocyte-derived macrophages: maturation and inhibition by mannan. *J Leukoc Biol* **38**:655–658.

76. Wileman TE, Lennartz MR, Stahl PD. 1986. Identification of the macrophage mannose receptor as a 175-kDa membrane protein. *Proc Natl Acad Sci USA* **83**:2501–2505.

77. McGreal EP, Miller JL, Gordon S. 2005. Ligand recognition by antigen-presenting cell C-type lectin receptors. *Curr Opin Immunol* **17**:18–24.

78. Stahl PD, Ezekowitz RA. 1998. The mannose receptor is a pattern recognition receptor involved in host defense. *Curr Opin Immunol* **10**:50–55.

79. Martinez-Pomares L, Linehan SA, Taylor PR, Gordon S. 2001. Binding properties of the mannose receptor. *Immunobiology* **204**:527–535.

80. Lee SJ, Evers S, Roeder D, Parlow AF, Risteli J, Risteli L, Lee YC, Feizi T, Langen H, Nussenzweig MC. 2002. Mannose receptor-mediated regulation of serum glycoprotein homeostasis. *Science* **295**:1898–1901.

81. Medzhitov R, Janeway C Jr. 2000. Innate immunity. *N Engl J Med* **343**:338–344.

82. Schlesinger LS, Hull SR, Kaufman TM. 1994. Binding of the terminal mannosyl units of lipoarabinomannan from a virulent strain of *Mycobacterium tuberculosis* to human macrophages. *J Immunol* **152**:4070–4079.

83. Torrelles JB, Schlesinger LS. 2010. Diversity in *Mycobacterium tuberculosis* mannosylated cell wall determinants impacts adaptation to the host. *Tuberculosis (Edinb)* **90**:84–93.

84. Torrelles JB, Azad AK, Schlesinger LS. 2006. Fine discrimination in the recognition of individual species of phosphatidyl-myo-inositol mannosides from *Mycobacterium tuberculosis* by C-type lectin pattern recognition receptors. *J Immunol* **177**:1805–1816.

85. Schlesinger LS, Kaufman TM, Iyer S, Hull SR, Marchiando LK. 1996. Differences in mannose receptor-mediated uptake of lipoarabinomannan from virulent and attenuated strains of *Mycobacterium tuberculosis* by human macrophages. *J Immunol* **157**:4568–4575.

86. Torrelles JB, Knaup R, Kolareth A, Slepushkina T, Kaufman TM, Kang P, Hill PJ, Brennan PJ, Chatterjee D, Belisle JT, Musser JM, Schlesinger LS. 2008. Identification of *Mycobacterium tuberculosis* clinical isolates with altered phagocytosis by human macrophages due to a truncated lipoarabinomannan. *J Biol Chem* **283**: 31417–31428.

87. Kang PB, Azad AK, Torrelles JB, Kaufman TM, Beharka A, Tibesar E, DesJardin LE, Schlesinger LS. 2005. The human macrophage mannose receptor directs *Mycobacterium tuberculosis* lipoarabinomannan-mediated phagosome biogenesis. *J Exp Med* **202**:987–999.

88. Aderem A, Underhill DM. 1999. Mechanisms of phagocytosis in macrophages. *Annu Rev Immunol* **17**: 593–623.

89. Singh CR, Moulton RA, Armitige LY, Bidani A, Snuggs M, Dhandayuthapani S, Hunter RL, Jagannath C. 2006. Processing and presentation of a mycobacterial antigen 85B epitope by murine macrophages is dependent on the phagosomal acquisition of vacuolar proton ATPase and *in situ* activation of cathepsin D. *J Immunol* **177**:3250–3259.

90. Sturgill-Koszycki S, Schlesinger PH, Chakraborty P, Haddix PL, Collins HL, Fok AK, Allen RD, Gluck SL,

Heuser J, Russell DG. 1994. Lack of acidification in *Mycobacterium* phagosomes produced by exclusion of the vesicular proton-ATPase. *Science* **263**:678–681.

91. Astarie-Dequeker C, N'Diaye EN, Le Cabec V, Rittig MG, Prandi J, Maridonneau-Parini I. 1999. The mannose receptor mediates uptake of pathogenic and nonpathogenic mycobacteria and bypasses bactericidal responses in human macrophages. *Infect Immun* **67**:469–477.

92. Chieppa M, Bianchi G, Doni A, Del Prete A, Sironi M, Laskarin G, Monti P, Piemonti L, Biondi A, Mantovani A, Introna M, Allavena P. 2003. Cross-linking of the mannose receptor on monocyte-derived dendritic cells activates an anti-inflammatory immunosuppressive program. *J Immunol* **171**:4552–4560.

93. Azad AK, Rajaram MVS, Schlesinger LS. 2014. Exploitation of the macrophage mannose receptor (CD206) in infectious disease diagnostics and therapeutics. *J Cytol Mol Biol* **1**:1000003.

94. McNally AK, DeFife KM, Anderson JM. 1996. Interleukin-4-induced macrophage fusion is prevented by inhibitors of mannose receptor activity. *Am J Pathol* **149**:975–985.

95. Gordon S, Martinez FO. 2010. Alternative activation of macrophages: mechanism and functions. *Immunity* **32**:593–604.

96. Gordon S, Keshav S, Stein M. 1994. BCG-induced granuloma formation in murine tissues. *Immunobiology* **191**:369–377.

97. Bleijs DA, Geijtenbeek TB, Figdor CG, van Kooyk Y. 2001. DC-SIGN and LFA-1: a battle for ligand. *Trends Immunol* **22**:457–463.

98. Tailleux L, Pham-Thi N, Bergeron-Lafaurie A, Herrmann J-L, Charles P, Schwartz O, Scheinmann P, Lagrange PH, de Blic J, Tazi A, Gicquel B, Neyrolles O. 2005. DC-SIGN induction in alveolar macrophages defines privileged target host cells for mycobacteria in patients with tuberculosis. *PLoS Med* **2**:e381.

99. Puig-Kröger A, Serrano-Gómez D, Caparrós E, Domínguez-Soto A, Relloso M, Colmenares M, Martínez-Muñoz L, Longo N, Sánchez-Sánchez N, Rincon M, Rivas L, Sánchez-Mateos P, Fernández-Ruiz E, Corbí AL. 2004. Regulated expression of the pathogen receptor dendritic cell-specific intercellular adhesion molecule 3 (ICAM-3)-grabbing nonintegrin in THP-1 human leukemic cells, monocytes, and macrophages. *J Biol Chem* **279**:25680–25688.

100. Geijtenbeek TBH, Van Vliet SJ, Koppel EA, Sanchez-Hernandez M, Vandenbroucke-Grauls CMJE, Appelmelk B, Van Kooyk Y. 2003. Mycobacteria target DC-SIGN to suppress dendritic cell function. *J Exp Med* **197**:7–17.

101. Tailleux L, Schwartz O, Herrmann JL, Pivert E, Jackson M, Amara A, Legres L, Dreher D, Nicod LP, Gluckman JC, Lagrange PH, Gicquel B, Neyrolles O. 2003. DC-SIGN is the major *Mycobacterium tuberculosis* receptor on human dendritic cells. *J Exp Med* **197**:121–127.

102. Guirado E, Schlesinger LS, Kaplan G. 2013. Macrophages in tuberculosis: friend or foe. *Semin Immunopathol* **35**:563–583.

103. Matsumoto M, Tanaka T, Kaisho T, Sanjo H, Copeland NG, Gilbert DJ, Jenkins NA, Akira S. 1999. A novel LPS-inducible C-type lectin is a transcriptional target of NF-IL6 in macrophages. *J Immunol* **163**:5039–5048.

104. Yamasaki S, Matsumoto M, Takeuchi O, Matsuzawa T, Ishikawa E, Sakuma M, Tateno H, Uno J, Hirabayashi J, Mikami Y, Takeda K, Akira S, Saito T. 2009. C-type lectin Mincle is an activating receptor for pathogenic fungus, *Malassezia*. *Proc Natl Acad Sci USA* **106**:1897–1902.

105. Yamasaki S, Ishikawa E, Sakuma M, Hara H, Ogata K, Saito T. 2008. Mincle is an ITAM-coupled activating receptor that senses damaged cells. *Nat Immunol* **9**:1179–1188.

106. Ishikawa E, Ishikawa T, Morita YS, Toyonaga K, Yamada H, Takeuchi O, Kinoshita T, Akira S, Yoshikai Y, Yamasaki S. 2009. Direct recognition of the mycobacterial glycolipid, trehalose dimycolate, by C-type lectin Mincle. *J Exp Med* **206**:2879–2888.

107. Schoenen H, Bodendorfer B, Hitchens K, Manzanero S, Werninghaus K, Nimmerjahn F, Agger EM, Stenger S, Andersen P, Ruland J, Brown GD, Wells C, Lang R. 2010. Cutting edge: mincle is essential for recognition and adjuvanticity of the mycobacterial cord factor and its synthetic analog trehalose-dibehenate. *J Immunol* **184**:2756–2760.

108. Heitmann L, Schoenen H, Ehlers S, Lang R, Hölscher C. 2013. Mincle is not essential for controlling *Mycobacterium tuberculosis* infection. *Immunobiology* **218**:506–516.

109. Tsoni SV, Brown GD. 2008. beta-Glucans and dectin-1. *Ann N Y Acad Sci* **1143**:45–60

110. Taylor PR, Brown GD, Reid DM, Willment JA, Martinez-Pomares L, Gordon S, Wong SY. 2002. The β-glucan receptor, dectin-1, is predominantly expressed on the surface of cells of the monocyte/macrophage and neutrophil lineages. *J Immunol* **169**:3876–3882.

111. van de Veerdonk FL, Teirlinck AC, Kleinnijenhuis J, Kullberg BJ, van Crevel R, van der Meer JWM, Joosten LAB, Netea MG. 2010. *Mycobacterium tuberculosis* induces IL-17A responses through TLR4 and dectin-1 and is critically dependent on endogenous IL-1. *J Leukoc Biol* **88**:227–232.

112. Rothfuchs AG, Báfica A, Feng CG, Egen JG, Williams DL, Brown GD, Sher A. 2007. Dectin-1 interaction with *Mycobacterium tuberculosis* leads to enhanced IL-12p40 production by splenic dendritic cells. *J Immunol* **179**:3463–3471.

113. Yadav M, Schorey JS. 2006. The beta-glucan receptor dectin-1 functions together with TLR2 to mediate macrophage activation by mycobacteria. *Blood* **108**:3168–3175.

114. Betz BE, Azad AK, Morris JD, Rajaram MVS, Schlesinger LS. 2011. β-Glucans inhibit intracellular growth of *Mycobacterium bovis* BCG but not virulent *Mycobacterium tuberculosis* in human macrophages. *Microb Pathog* **51**:233–242.

115. Taylor PR, Reid DM, Heinsbroek SEM, Brown GD, Gordon S, Wong SYC. 2005. Dectin-2 is predominantly myeloid restricted and exhibits unique activation-dependent expression on maturing inflammatory monocytes elicited *in vivo*. *Eur J Immunol* **35**:2163–2174.

116. Yonekawa A, Saijo S, Hoshino Y, Miyake Y, Ishikawa E, Suzukawa M, Inoue H, Tanaka M, Yoneyama M, Oh-Hora M, Akashi K, Yamasaki S. 2014. Dectin-2 is a direct receptor for mannose-capped lipoarabinomannan of mycobacteria. *Immunity* **41**:402–413.

117. Zhao X-Q, Zhu L-L, Chang Q, Jiang C, You Y, Luo T, Jia X-M, Lin X. 2014. C-type lectin receptor dectin-3 mediates trehalose 6,6′-dimycolate (TDM)-induced Mincle expression through CARD9/Bcl10/MALT1-dependent nuclear factor (NF)-κB activation. *J Biol Chem* **289**:30052–30062.

118. Miyake Y, Toyonaga K, Mori D, Kakuta S, Hoshino Y, Oyamada A, Yamada H, Ono K, Suyama M, Iwakura Y, Yoshikai Y, Yamasaki S. 2013. C-type lectin MCL is an FcRγ-coupled receptor that mediates the adjuvanticity of mycobacterial cord factor. *Immunity* **38**:1050–1062.

119. Myones BL, Dalzell JG, Hogg N, Ross GD. 1988. Neutrophil and monocyte cell surface p150,95 has iC3b-receptor (CR4) activity resembling CR3. *J Clin Invest* **82**:640–651.

120. Arnaout MA. 1990. Structure and function of the leukocyte adhesion molecules CD11/CD18. *Blood* **75**:1037–1050.

121. Schlesinger LS, Azad AK. 2008. Determinants of phagocytosis, phagosome biogenesis and autophagy for *Mycobacterium tuberculosis*, p 1–22. *In* Kaufmann SHE, Britton WJ (ed), *Handbook of Tuberculosis: Immunology and Cell Biology*. Wiley VCH Publishers, Weinheim, Germany.

122. Schlesinger LS. 1993. Macrophage phagocytosis of virulent but not attenuated strains of *Mycobacterium tuberculosis* is mediated by mannose receptors in addition to complement receptors. *J Immunol* **150**:2920–2930.

123. Cywes C, Hoppe HC, Daffé M, Ehlers MR. 1997. Nonopsonic binding of *Mycobacterium tuberculosis* to complement receptor type 3 is mediated by capsular polysaccharides and is strain dependent. *Infect Immun* **65**:4258–4266.

124. Villeneuve C, Gilleron M, Maridonneau-Parini I, Daffé M, Astarie-Dequeker C, Etienne G. 2005. Mycobacteria use their surface-exposed glycolipids to infect human macrophages through a receptor-dependent process. *J Lipid Res* **46**:475–483.

125. Armstrong JA, Hart PD. 1975. Phagosome-lysosome interactions in cultured macrophages infected with virulent tubercle bacilli. Reversal of the usual nonfusion pattern and observations on bacterial survival. *J Exp Med* **142**:1–16.

126. Basu S, Fenton MJ. 2004. Toll-like receptors: function and roles in lung disease. *Am J Physiol Lung Cell Mol Physiol* **286**:L887–L892.

127. Pandey S, Kawai T, Akira S. 2015. Microbial sensing by Toll-like receptors and intracellular nucleic acid sensors. *Cold Spring Harb Perspect Biol* **7**:a016246.

128. Kawasaki T, Kawai T. 2014. Toll-like receptor signaling pathways. *Front Immunol* **5**:461.

129. Kawai T, Akira S. 2011. Toll-like receptors and their crosstalk with other innate receptors in infection and immunity. *Immunity* **34**:637–650.

130. Cambi A, Koopman M, Figdor CG. 2005. How C-type lectins detect pathogens. *Cell Microbiol* **7**:481–488.

131. Poltorak A, He X, Smirnova I, Liu MY, Van Huffel C, Du X, Birdwell D, Alejos E, Silva M, Galanos C, Freudenberg M, Ricciardi-Castagnoli P, Layton B, Beutler B. 1998. Defective LPS signaling in C3H/HeJ and C57BL/10ScCr mice: mutations in Tlr4 gene. *Science* **282**:2085–2088.

132. Malhotra R, Thiel S, Reid KB, Sim RB. 1990. Human leukocyte C1q receptor binds other soluble proteins with collagen domains. *J Exp Med* **172**:955–959.

133. Akira S, Uematsu S, Takeuchi O. 2006. Pathogen recognition and innate immunity. *Cell* **124**:783–801.

134. Yamamoto M, Takeda K, Akira S. 2004. TIR domain-containing adaptors define the specificity of TLR signaling. *Mol Immunol* **40**:861–868.

135. Kobayashi K, Hernandez LD, Galán JE, Janeway CA Jr, Medzhitov R, Flavell RA. 2002. IRAK-M is a negative regulator of Toll-like receptor signaling. *Cell* **110**:191–202.

136. Means TK, Lien E, Yoshimura A, Wang S, Golenbock DT, Fenton MJ. 1999. The CD14 ligands lipoarabinomannan and lipopolysaccharide differ in their requirement for Toll-like receptors. *J Immunol* **163**:6748–6755.

137. Jones BW, Means TK, Heldwein KA, Keen MA, Hill PJ, Belisle JT, Fenton MJ. 2001. Different Toll-like receptor agonists induce distinct macrophage responses. *J Leukoc Biol* **69**:1036–1044.

138. Kindrachuk J, Potter J, Wilson HL, Griebel P, Babiuk LA, Napper S. 2008. Activation and regulation of toll-like receptor 9: CpGs and beyond. *Mini Rev Med Chem* **8**:590–600.

139. Báfica A, Scanga CA, Feng CG, Leifer C, Cheever A, Sher A. 2005. TLR9 regulates Th1 responses and cooperates with TLR2 in mediating optimal resistance to *Mycobacterium tuberculosis*. *J Exp Med* **202**:1715–1724.

140. Drennan MB, Nicolle D, Quesniaux VJF, Jacobs M, Allie N, Mpagi J, Frémond C, Wagner H, Kirschning C, Ryffel B. 2004. Toll-like receptor 2-deficient mice succumb to *Mycobacterium tuberculosis* infection. *Am J Pathol* **164**:49–57.

141. Abel B, Thieblemont N, Quesniaux VJF, Brown N, Mpagi J, Miyake K, Bihl F, Ryffel B. 2002. Toll-like receptor 4 expression is required to control chronic *Mycobacterium tuberculosis* infection in mice. *J Immunol* **169**:3155–3162.

142. Reiling N, Hölscher C, Fehrenbach A, Kröger S, Kirschning CJ, Goyert S, Ehlers S. 2002. Cutting edge: toll-like receptor (TLR)2- and TLR4-mediated pathogen recognition in resistance to airborne infection with *Mycobacterium tuberculosis*. *J Immunol* **169**:3480–3484.

143. Hölscher C, Reiling N, Schaible UE, Hölscher A, Bathmann C, Korbel D, Lenz I, Sonntag T, Kröger S, Akira S, Mossmann H, Kirschning CJ, Wagner H, Freudenberg M, Ehlers S. 2008. Containment of aerogenic *Mycobacterium tuberculosis* infection in mice does not require MyD88 adaptor function for TLR2, -4 and -9. *Eur J Immunol* **38**:680–694.

144. Fremond CM, Yeremeev V, Nicolle DM, Jacobs M, Quesniaux VF, Ryffel B. 2004. Fatal *Mycobacterium tuberculosis* infection despite adaptive immune response in the absence of MyD88. *J Clin Invest* **114:**1790–1799.

145. Mayer-Barber KD, Barber DL, Shenderov K, White SD, Wilson MS, Cheever A, Kugler D, Hieny S, Caspar P, Núñez G, Schlueter D, Flavell RA, Sutterwala FS, Sher A. 2010. Caspase-1 independent IL-1beta production is critical for host resistance to *Mycobacterium tuberculosis* and does not require TLR signaling *in vivo*. *J Immunol* **184:**3326–3330.

146. Canton J, Neculai D, Grinstein S. 2013. Scavenger receptors in homeostasis and immunity. *Nat Rev Immunol* **13:**621–634.

147. Doi T, Higashino K, Kurihara Y, Wada Y, Miyazaki T, Nakamura H, Uesugi S, Imanishi T, Kawabe Y, Itakura H, Yazaki Y, Matsumoto A, Kodama T. 1993. Charged collagen structure mediates the recognition of negatively charged macromolecules by macrophage scavenger receptors. *J Biol Chem* **268:**2126–2133.

148. Yamamoto K, Nishimura N, Doi T, Imanishi T, Kodama T, Suzuki K, Tanaka T. 1997. The lysine cluster in the collagen-like domain of the scavenger receptor provides for its ligand binding and ligand specificity. *FEBS Lett* **414:**182–186.

149. Arredouani MS, Palecanda A, Koziel H, Huang Y-C, Imrich A, Sulahian TH, Ning YY, Yang Z, Pikkarainen T, Sankala M, Vargas SO, Takeya M, Tryggvason K, Kobzik L. 2005. MARCO is the major binding receptor for unopsonized particles and bacteria on human alveolar macrophages. *J Immunol* **175:**6058–6064.

150. Reddy RC. 2008. Immunomodulatory role of PPAR-gamma in alveolar macrophages. *J Investig Med* **56:**522–527.

151. Zimmerli S, Edwards S, Ernst JD. 1996. Selective receptor blockade during phagocytosis does not alter the survival and growth of *Mycobacterium tuberculosis* in human macrophages. *Am J Respir Cell Mol Biol* **15:**760–770.

152. Bowdish DME, Sakamoto K, Kim M-J, Kroos M, Mukhopadhyay S, Leifer CA, Tryggvason K, Gordon S, Russell DG. 2009. MARCO, TLR2, and CD14 are required for macrophage cytokine responses to mycobacterial trehalose dimycolate and *Mycobacterium tuberculosis*. *PLoS Pathog* **5:**e1000474.

153. Mahajan S, Dkhar HK, Chandra V, Dave S, Nanduri R, Janmeja AK, Agrewala JN, Gupta P. 2012. *Mycobacterium tuberculosis* modulates macrophage lipid-sensing nuclear receptors PPARγ and TR4 for survival. *J Immunol* **188:**5593–5603.

154. Almeida PE, Roque NR, Magalhães KG, Mattos KA, Teixeira L, Maya-Monteiro C, Almeida CJ, Castro-Faria-Neto HC, Ryffel B, Quesniaux VFJ, Bozza PT. 2014. Differential TLR2 downstream signaling regulates lipid metabolism and cytokine production triggered by *Mycobacterium bovis* BCG infection. *Biochim Biophys Acta* **1841:**97–107.

155. Asada K, Sasaki S, Suda T, Chida K, Nakamura H. 2004. Antiinflammatory roles of peroxisome proliferator-activated receptor γ in human alveolar macrophages. *Am J Respir Crit Care Med* **169:**195–200.

156. Court N, Vasseur V, Vacher R, Frémond C, Shebzukhov Y, Yeremeev VV, Maillet I, Nedospasov SA, Gordon S, Fallon PG, Suzuki H, Ryffel B, Quesniaux VFJ. 2010. Partial redundancy of the pattern recognition receptors, scavenger receptors, and C-type lectins for the long-term control of *Mycobacterium tuberculosis* infection. *J Immunol* **184:**7057–7070.

157. Arredouani MS, Yang Z, Imrich A, Ning Y, Qin G, Kobzik L. 2006. The macrophage scavenger receptor SR-AI/II and lung defense against pneumococci and particles. *Am J Respir Cell Mol Biol* **35:**474–478.

158. Hollifield M, Bou Ghanem E, de Villiers WJS, Garvy BA. 2007. Scavenger receptor A dampens induction of inflammation in response to the fungal pathogen *Pneumocystis carinii*. *Infect Immun* **75:**3999–4005.

159. Arredouani M, Yang Z, Ning Y, Qin G, Soininen R, Tryggvason K, Kobzik L. 2004. The scavenger receptor MARCO is required for lung defense against pneumococcal pneumonia and inhaled particles. *J Exp Med* **200:**267–272.

160. Hawkes M, Li X, Crockett M, Diassiti A, Finney C, Min-Oo G, Liles WC, Liu J, Kain KC. 2010. CD36 deficiency attenuates experimental mycobacterial infection. *BMC Infect Dis* **10:**299

161. Flannagan RS, Jaumouillé V, Grinstein S. 2012. The cell biology of phagocytosis. *Annu Rev Pathol* **7:**61–98.

162. Russell DG. 2001. *Mycobacterium tuberculosis*: here today, and here tomorrow. *Nat Rev Mol Cell Biol* **2:**569–577.

163. Reiner NE. 1994. Altered cell signaling and mononuclear phagocyte deactivation during intracellular infection. *Immunol Today* **15:**374–381.

164. Deretic V, Singh S, Master S, Harris J, Roberts E, Kyei G, Davis A, de Haro S, Naylor J, Lee H-H, Vergne I. 2006. *Mycobacterium tuberculosis* inhibition of phagolysosome biogenesis and autophagy as a host defence mechanism. *Cell Microbiol* **8:**719–727.

165. Lugo-Villarino G, Neyrolles O. 2014. Manipulation of the mononuclear phagocyte system by *Mycobacterium tuberculosis*. *Cold Spring Harb Perspect Med* **4:**a018549.

166. Shukla S, Richardson ET, Athman JJ, Shi L, Wearsch PA, McDonald D, Banaei N, Boom WH, Jackson M, Harding CV. 2014. *Mycobacterium tuberculosis* lipoprotein LprG binds lipoarabinomannan and determines its cell envelope localization to control phagolysosomal fusion. *PLoS Pathog* **10:**e1004471. (Correction **10:**e1004596.)

167. Gaur RL, Ren K, Blumenthal A, Bhamidi S, González-Nilo FD, Jackson M, Zare RN, Ehrt S, Ernst JD, Banaei N. 2014. LprG-mediated surface expression of lipoarabinomannan is essential for virulence of *Mycobacterium tuberculosis*. *PLoS Pathog* **10:**e1004376. (Errata **10:**e1004489, **10:**e1004494.)

168. Welin A, Lerm M. 2012. Inside or outside the phagosome? The controversy of the intracellular localization of *Mycobacterium tuberculosis*. *Tuberculosis (Edinb)* **92:**113–120.

169. Leake ES, Myrvik QN, Wright MJ. 1984. Phagosomal membranes of *Mycobacterium bovis* BCG-immune

alveolar macrophages are resistant to disruption by *Mycobacterium tuberculosis* H37Rv. *Infect Immun* 45: 443–446.

170. **McDonough KA, Kress Y, Bloom BR.** 1993. Pathogenesis of tuberculosis: interaction of *Mycobacterium tuberculosis* with macrophages. *Infect Immun* 61:2763–2773.

171. **Myrvik QN, Leake ES, Wright MJ.** 1984. Disruption of phagosomal membranes of normal alveolar macrophages by the H37Rv strain of *Mycobacterium tuberculosis*. A correlate of virulence. *Am Rev Respir Dis* 129: 322–328.

172. **Simeone R, Bobard A, Lippmann J, Bitter W, Majlessi L, Brosch R, Enninga J.** 2012. Phagosomal rupture by *Mycobacterium tuberculosis* results in toxicity and host cell death. *PLoS Pathog* 8:e1002507.

173. **van der Wel N, Hava D, Houben D, Fluitsma D, van Zon M, Pierson J, Brenner M, Peters PJ.** 2007. *M. tuberculosis* and *M. leprae* translocate from the phagolysosome to the cytosol in myeloid cells. *Cell* 129:1287–1298.

174. **Houben D, Demangel C, van Ingen J, Perez J, Baldeón L, Abdallah AM, Caleechurn L, Bottai D, van Zon M, de Punder K, van der Laan T, Kant A, Bossers-de Vries R, Willemsen P, Bitter W, van Soolingen D, Brosch R, van der Wel N, Peters PJ.** 2012. ESX-1-mediated translocation to the cytosol controls virulence of mycobacteria. *Cell Microbiol* 14:1287–1298.

175. **Manzanillo PS, Shiloh MU, Portnoy DA, Cox JS.** 2012. *Mycobacterium tuberculosis* activates the DNA-dependent cytosolic surveillance pathway within macrophages. *Cell Host Microbe* 11:469–480.

176. **Watson RO, Manzanillo PS, Cox JS.** 2012. Extracellular *M. tuberculosis* DNA targets bacteria for autophagy by activating the host DNA-sensing pathway. *Cell* 150: 803–815.

177. **Shen H-M, Mizushima N.** 2014. At the end of the autophagic road: an emerging understanding of lysosomal functions in autophagy. *Trends Biochem Sci* 39:61–71.

178. **Mizushima N, Komatsu M.** 2011. Autophagy: renovation of cells and tissues. *Cell* 147:728–741.

179. **Levine B, Mizushima N, Virgin HW.** 2011. Autophagy in immunity and inflammation. *Nature* 469:323–335.

180. **Deretic V.** 2014. Autophagy in tuberculosis. *Cold Spring Harb Perspect Med* 4:a018481.

181. **Yang C-S, Kim J-J, Lee H-M, Jin HS, Lee S-H, Park J-H, Kim SJ, Kim J-M, Han Y-M, Lee M-S, Kweon GR, Shong M, Jo E-K.** 2014. The AMPK-PPARGC1A pathway is required for antimicrobial host defense through activation of autophagy. *Autophagy* 10:785–802.

182. **Abnave P, Mottola G, Gimenez G, Boucherit N, Trouplin V, Torre C, Conti F, Ben Amara A, Lepolard C, Djian B, Hamaoui D, Mettouchi A, Kumar A, Pagnotta S, Bonatti S, Lepidi H, Salvetti A, Abi-Rached L, Lemichez E, Mege J-L, Ghigo E.** 2014. Screening in planarians identifies MORN2 as a key component in LC3-associated phagocytosis and resistance to bacterial infection. *Cell Host Microbe* 16:338–350.

183. **Romagnoli A, Etna MP, Giacomini E, Pardini M, Remoli ME, Corazzari M, Falasca L, Goletti D, Gafa V,** Simeone R, Delogu G, Piacentini M, Brosch R, Fimia GM, Coccia EM. 2012. ESX-1 dependent impairment of autophagic flux by *Mycobacterium tuberculosis* in human dendritic cells. *Autophagy* 8:1357–1370.

184. **Shin D-M, Jeon B-Y, Lee H-M, Jin HS, Yuk J-M, Song C-H, Lee S-H, Lee Z-W, Cho S-N, Kim J-M, Friedman RL, Jo E-K.** 2010. *Mycobacterium tuberculosiseis* regulates autophagy, inflammation, and cell death through redox-dependent signaling. *PLoS Pathog* 6:e1001230.

185. **Gutierrez MG, Master SS, Singh SB, Taylor GA, Colombo MI, Deretic V.** 2004. Autophagy is a defense mechanism inhibiting BCG and *Mycobacterium tuberculosis* survival in infected macrophages. *Cell* 119:753–766.

186. **Fabri M, Stenger S, Shin D-M, Yuk J-M, Liu PT, Realegeno S, Lee H-M, Krutzik SR, Schenk M, Sieling PA, Teles R, Montoya D, Iyer SS, Bruns H, Lewinsohn DM, Hollis BW, Hewison M, Adams JS, Steinmeyer A, Zügel U, Cheng G, Jo E-K, Bloom BR, Modlin RL.** 2011. Vitamin D is required for IFN-gamma-mediated antimicrobial activity of human macrophages. *Sci Transl Med* 3:104ra102.

187. **Castillo EF, Dekonenko A, Arko-Mensah J, Mandell MA, Dupont N, Jiang S, Delgado-Vargas M, Timmins GS, Bhattacharya D, Yang H, Hutt J, Lyons CR, Dobos KM, Deretic V.** 2012. Autophagy protects against active tuberculosis by suppressing bacterial burden and inflammation. *Proc Natl Acad Sci USA* 109:E3168–E3176.

188. **Kim J-J, Lee H-M, Shin D-M, Kim W, Yuk J-M, Jin HS, Lee S-H, Cha G-H, Kim J-M, Lee Z-W, Shin SJ, Yoo H, Park YK, Park JB, Chung J, Yoshimori T, Jo E-K.** 2012. Host cell autophagy activated by antibiotics is required for their effective antimycobacterial drug action. *Cell Host Microbe* 11:457–468.

189. **Bento CF, Empadinhas N, Mendes V.** 2015. Autophagy in the fight against tuberculosis. *DNA Cell Biol* 34: 228–242.

190. **Stanley SA, Barczak AK, Silvis MR, Luo SS, Sogi K, Vokes M, Bray M-A, Carpenter AE, Moore CB, Siddiqi N, Rubin EJ, Hung DT.** 2014. Identification of host-targeted small molecules that restrict intracellular *Mycobacterium tuberculosis* growth. *PLoS Pathog* 10: e1003946.

191. **Hu D, Wu J, Zhang R, Chen L, Chen Z, Wang X, Xu L, Xiao J, Hu F, Wu C.** 2014. Autophagy-targeted vaccine of LC3-LpqH DNA and its protective immunity in a murine model of tuberculosis. *Vaccine* 32:2308–2314.

192. **Olive AJ, Sassetti CM.** 2014. New TB treatments hiding in plain sight. *EMBO Mol Med* 7:125–126.

193. **Ting JP-Y, Duncan JA, Lei Y.** 2010. How the non-inflammasome NLRs function in the innate immune system. *Science* 327:286–290.

194. **Franchi L, Eigenbrod T, Muñoz-Planillo R, Nuñez G.** 2009. The inflammasome: a caspase-1-activation platform that regulates immune responses and disease pathogenesis. *Nat Immunol* 10:241–247.

195. **Werner JL, Steele C.** 2014. Innate receptors and cellular defense against pulmonary infections. *J Immunol* 193:3842–3850.

196. Killick KE, Ní Cheallaigh C, O'Farrelly C, Hokamp K, MacHugh DE, Harris J. 2013. Receptor-mediated recognition of mycobacterial pathogens. *Cell Microbiol* 15: 1484–1495.

197. dos Santos G, Kutuzov MA, Ridge KM. 2012. The inflammasome in lung diseases. *Am J Physiol Lung Cell Mol Physiol* 303:L627–L633.

198. Hansen JM, Golchin SA, Veyrier FJ, Domenech P, Boneca IG, Azad AK, Rajaram MVS, Schlesinger LS, Divangahi M, Reed MB, Behr MA. 2014. N-glycolylated peptidoglycan contributes to the immunogenicity but not pathogenicity of *Mycobacterium tuberculosis*. *J Infect Dis* 209:1045–1054.

199. Coulombe F, Divangahi M, Veyrier F, de Léséleuc L, Gleason JL, Yang Y, Kelliher MA, Pandey AK, Sassetti CM, Reed MB, Behr MA. 2009. Increased NOD2-mediated recognition of N-glycolyl muramyl dipeptide. *J Exp Med* 206:1709–1716.

200. Inohara N, Ogura Y, Fontalba A, Gutierrez O, Pons F, Crespo J, Fukase K, Inamura S, Kusumoto S, Hashimoto M, Foster SJ, Moran AP, Fernandez-Luna JL, Nuñez G. 2003. Host recognition of bacterial muramyl dipeptide mediated through NOD2. Implications for Crohn's disease. *J Biol Chem* 278:5509–5512.

201. Brooks MN, Rajaram MVS, Azad AK, Amer AO, Valdivia-Arenas MA, Park J-H, Núñez G, Schlesinger LS. 2011. NOD2 controls the nature of the inflammatory response and subsequent fate of *Mycobacterium tuberculosis* and *M. bovis* BCG in human macrophages. *Cell Microbiol* 13:402–418.

202. Divangahi M, Mostowy S, Coulombe F, Kozak R, Guillot L, Veyrier F, Kobayashi KS, Flavell RA, Gros P, Behr MA. 2008. NOD2-deficient mice have impaired resistance to *Mycobacterium tuberculosis* infection through defective innate and adaptive immunity. *J Immunol* 181:7157–7165.

203. Gandotra S, Jang S, Murray PJ, Salgame P, Ehrt S. 2007. Nucleotide-binding oligomerization domain protein 2-deficient mice control infection with *Mycobacterium tuberculosis*. *Infect Immun* 75:5127–5134.

204. Juárez E, Carranza C, Hernández-Sánchez F, León-Contreras JC, Hernández-Pando R, Escobedo D, Torres M, Sada E. 2012. NOD2 enhances the innate response of alveolar macrophages to *Mycobacterium tuberculosis* in humans. *Eur J Immunol* 42:880–889.

205. McElvania Tekippe E, Allen IC, Hulseberg PD, Sullivan JT, McCann JR, Sandor M, Braunstein M, Ting JP-Y. 2010. Granuloma formation and host defense in chronic *Mycobacterium tuberculosis* infection requires PYCARD/ASC but not NLRP3 or caspase-1. *PLoS One* 5:e12320.

206. Shah S, Bohsali A, Ahlbrand SE, Srinivasan L, Rathinam VAK, Vogel SN, Fitzgerald KA, Sutterwala FS, Briken V. 2013. Cutting edge: *Mycobacterium tuberculosis* but not nonvirulent mycobacteria inhibits IFN-β and AIM2 inflammasome-dependent IL-1β production via its ESX-1 secretion system. *J Immunol* 191:3514–3518.

207. Saiga H, Kitada S, Shimada Y, Kamiyama N, Okuyama M, Makino M, Yamamoto M, Takeda K. 2012. Critical role of AIM2 in *Mycobacterium tuberculosis* infection. *Int Immunol* 24:637–644.

208. Glass CK, Ogawa S. 2006. Combinatorial roles of nuclear receptors in inflammation and immunity. *Nat Rev Immunol* 6:44–55.

209. Ahmadian M, Suh JM, Hah N, Liddle C, Atkins AR, Downes M, Evans RM. 2013. PPARγ signaling and metabolism: the good, the bad and the future. *Nat Med* 19:557–566.

210. Malur A, Mccoy AJ, Arce S, Barna BP, Kavuru MS, Malur AG, Thomassen MJ. 2009. Deletion of PPAR gamma in alveolar macrophages is associated with a Th-1 pulmonary inflammatory response. *J Immunol* 182:5816–5822.

211. Almeida PE, Silva AR, Maya-Monteiro CM, Töröcsik D, D'Avila H, Dezsö B, Magalhães KG, Castro-Faria-Neto HC, Nagy L, Bozza PT. 2009. *Mycobacterium bovis* bacillus Calmette-Guérin infection induces TLR2-dependent peroxisome proliferator-activated receptor gamma expression and activation: functions in inflammation, lipid metabolism, and pathogenesis. *J Immunol* 183:1337–1345.

212. Guo H, Ingolia NT, Weissman JS, Bartel DP. 2010. Mammalian microRNAs predominantly act to decrease target mRNA levels. *Nature* 466:835–840.

213. Bartel DP. 2004. MicroRNAs: genomics, biogenesis, mechanism, and function. *Cell* 116:281–297.

214. He L, Hannon GJ. 2004. MicroRNAs: small RNAs with a big role in gene regulation. *Nat Rev Genet* 5:522–531.

215. Foster PS, Plank M, Collison A, Tay HL, Kaiko GE, Li J, Johnston SL, Hansbro PM, Kumar RK, Yang M, Mattes J. 2013. The emerging role of microRNAs in regulating immune and inflammatory responses in the lung. *Immunol Rev* 253:198–215.

216. Sittka A, Schmeck B. 2013. MicroRNAs in the lung. *Adv Exp Med Biol* 774:121–134.

217. Kumar M, Sahu SK, Kumar R, Subuddhi A, Maji RK, Jana K, Gupta P, Raffetseder J, Lerm M, Ghosh Z, van Loo G, Beyaert R, Gupta UD, Kundu M, Basu J. 2015. MicroRNA let-7 modulates the immune response to *Mycobacterium tuberculosis* infection via control of A20, an inhibitor of the NF-κB pathway. *Cell Host Microbe* 17:345–356.

218. Kumar R, Sahu SK, Kumar M, Jana K, Gupta P, Gupta UD, Kundu M, Basu J. 2015. MicroRNA 17-5p regulates autophagy in *Mycobacterium tuberculosis*-infected macrophages by targeting Mcl-1 and STAT3. *Cell Microbiol* 18:679–691.

219. Ma C, Li Y, Li M, Deng G, Wu X, Zeng J, Hao X, Wang X, Liu J, Cho WCS, Liu X, Wang Y. 2014. MicroRNA-124 negatively regulates TLR signaling in alveolar macrophages in response to mycobacterial infection. *Mol Immunol* 62:150–158.

220. Ni B, Rajaram MVS, Lafuse WP, Landes MB, Schlesinger LS. 2014. *Mycobacterium tuberculosis* decreases human macrophage IFN-γ responsiveness through miR-132 and miR-26a. *J Immunol* 193:4537–4547.

221. Dorhoi A, Iannaccone M, Farinacci M, Faé KC, Schreiber J, Moura-Alves P, Nouailles G, Mollenkopf H-J, Oberbeck-Müller D, Jörg S, Heinemann E, Hahnke K, Löwe D, Del Nonno F, Goletti D, Capparelli R, Kaufmann SH. 2013. MicroRNA-223 controls suscepti-

bility to tuberculosis by regulating lung neutrophil recruitment. *J Clin Invest* **123**:4836–4848.

222. Liu Y, Wang X, Jiang J, Cao Z, Yang B, Cheng X. 2011. Modulation of T cell cytokine production by miR-144* with elevated expression in patients with pulmonary tuberculosis. *Mol Immunol* **48**:1084–1090.

223. Ma F, Xu S, Liu X, Zhang Q, Xu X, Liu M, Hua M, Li N, Yao H, Cao X. 2011. The microRNA miR-29 controls innate and adaptive immune responses to intracellular bacterial infection by targeting interferon-γ. *Nat Immunol* **12**:861–869.

224. Yi Z, Fu Y, Ji R, Li R, Guan Z. 2012. Altered microRNA signatures in sputum of patients with active pulmonary tuberculosis. *PLoS One* **7**:e43184.

225. Singh Y, Kaul V, Mehra A, Chatterjee S, Tousif S, Dwivedi VP, Suar M, Van Kaer L, Bishai WR, Das G. 2013. *Mycobacterium tuberculosis* controls microRNA-99b (miR-99b) expression in infected murine dendritic cells to modulate host immunity. *J Biol Chem* **288**:5056–5061.

226. Wang J, Yang K, Zhou L, Minhaowu, Wu Y, Zhu M, Lai X, Chen T, Feng L, Li M, Huang C, Zhong Q, Huang X. 2013. MicroRNA-155 promotes autophagy to eliminate intracellular mycobacteria by targeting Rheb. *PLoS Pathog* **9**:e1003697.

227. Rajaram MVS, Ni B, Morris JD, Brooks MN, Carlson TK, Bakthavachalu B, Schoenberg DR, Torrelles JB, Schlesinger LS. 2011. *Mycobacterium tuberculosis* lipomannan blocks TNF biosynthesis by regulating macrophage MAPK-activated protein kinase 2 (MK2) and microRNA miR-125b. *Proc Natl Acad Sci USA* **108**:17408–17413.

228. Busch S, Auth E, Scholl F, Huenecke S, Koehl U, Suess B, Steinhilber D. 2015. 5-lipoxygenase is a direct target of miR-19a-3p and miR-125b-5p. *J Immunol* **194**:1646–1653

229. Iannaccone M, Dorhoi A, Kaufmann SHE. 2014. Host-directed therapy of tuberculosis: what is in it for microRNA? *Expert Opin Ther Targets* **18**:491–494.

230. Schorey JS, Cheng Y, Singh PP, Smith VL. 2015. Exosomes and other extracellular vesicles in host-pathogen interactions. *EMBO Rep* **16**:24–43.

231. Bhatnagar S, Schorey JS. 2007. Exosomes released from infected macrophages contain *Mycobacterium avium* glycopeptidolipids and are proinflammatory. *J Biol Chem* **282**:25779–25789.

232. Giri PK, Kruh NA, Dobos KM, Schorey JS. 2010. Proteomic analysis identifies highly antigenic proteins in exosomes from *M. tuberculosis*-infected and culture filtrate protein-treated macrophages. *Proteomics* **10**:3190–3202.

233. Singh PP, Li L, Schorey JS. 2015. Exosomal RNA from *Mycobacterium tuberculosis*-infected cells is functional in recipient macrophages. *Traffic* **16**:555–571.

234. Cheng Y, Schorey JS. 2013. Exosomes carrying mycobacterial antigens can protect mice against *Mycobacterium tuberculosis* infection. *Eur J Immunol* **43**:3279–3290.

235. Ramachandra L, Qu Y, Wang Y, Lewis CJ, Cobb BA, Takatsu K, Boom WH, Dubyak GR, Harding CV. 2010. *Mycobacterium tuberculosis* synergizes with ATP to induce release of microvesicles and exosomes containing major histocompatibility complex class II molecules capable of antigen presentation. *Infect Immun* **78**:5116–5125.

236. Lamkanfi M, Dixit VM. 2010. Manipulation of host cell death pathways during microbial infections. *Cell Host Microbe* **8**:44–54.

237. Duprez L, Wirawan E, Vanden Berghe T, Vandenabeele P. 2009. Major cell death pathways at a glance. *Microbes Infect* **11**:1050–1062.

238. Golstein P, Kroemer G. 2007. Cell death by necrosis: towards a molecular definition. *Trends Biochem Sci* **32**:37–43.

239. Bergsbaken T, Fink SL, Cookson BT. 2009. Pyroptosis: host cell death and inflammation. *Nat Rev Microbiol* **7**:99–109.

240. Divangahi M, Behar SM, Remold H. 2013. Dying to live: how the death modality of the infected macrophage affects immunity to tuberculosis. *Adv Exp Med Biol* **783**:103–120.

241. Srinivasan L, Ahlbrand S, Briken V. 2014. Interaction of *Mycobacterium tuberculosis* with host cell death pathways. *Cold Spring Harb Perspect Med* **4**:a022459.

242. Behar SM, Martin CJ, Booty MG, Nishimura T, Zhao X, Gan H-X, Divangahi M, Remold HG. 2011. Apoptosis is an innate defense function of macrophages against *Mycobacterium tuberculosis*. *Mucosal Immunol* **4**:279–287.

243. Briken V. 2013. *Mycobacterium tuberculosis* genes involved in regulation of host cell death. *Adv Exp Med Biol* **783**:93–102.

244. Jonuleit H, Schmitt E, Schuler G, Knop J, Enk AH. 2000. Induction of interleukin 10-producing, nonproliferating CD4(+) T cells with regulatory properties by repetitive stimulation with allogeneic immature human dendritic cells. *J Exp Med* **192**:1213–1222.

245. Tailleux L, Neyrolles O, Honoré-Bouakline S, Perret E, Sanchez F, Abastado J-P, Lagrange PH, Gluckman JC, Rosenzwajg M, Herrmann J-L. 2003. Constrained intracellular survival of *Mycobacterium tuberculosis* in human dendritic cells. *J Immunol* **170**:1939–1948.

246. Buettner M, Meinken C, Bastian M, Bhat R, Stössel E, Faller G, Cianciolo G, Ficker J, Wagner M, Röllinghoff M, Stenger S. 2005. Inverse correlation of maturity and antibacterial activity in human dendritic cells. *J Immunol* **174**:4203–4209.

247. Madan-Lala R, Sia JK, King R, Adekambi T, Monin L, Khader SA, Pulendran B, Rengarajan J. 2014. *Mycobacterium tuberculosis* impairs dendritic cell functions through the serine hydrolase Hip1. *J Immunol* **192**:4263–4272.

248. Kopf M, Schneider C, Nobs SP. 2015. The development and function of lung-resident macrophages and dendritic cells. *Nat Immunol* **16**:36–44.

249. Reljic R, Di Sano C, Crawford C, Dieli F, Challacombe S, Ivanyi J. 2005. Time course of mycobacterial infection of dendritic cells in the lungs of intranasally infected mice. *Tuberculosis (Edinb)* **85**:81–88.

250. Lagranderie M, Nahori M-A, Balazuc A-M, Kiefer-Biasizzo H, Lapa e Silva JR, Milon G, Marchal G, Vargaftig BB. 2003. Dendritic cells recruited to the lung shortly after intranasal delivery of *Mycobacterium bovis* BCG drive the primary immune response towards a type 1 cytokine production. *Immunology* 108:352–364.

251. Henderson RA, Watkins SC, Flynn JL. 1997. Activation of human dendritic cells following infection with *Mycobacterium tuberculosis*. *J Immunol* 159:635–643.

252. Giacomini E, Iona E, Ferroni L, Miettinen M, Fattorini L, Orefici G, Julkunen I, Coccia EM. 2001. Infection of human macrophages and dendritic cells with *Mycobacterium tuberculosis* induces a differential cytokine gene expression that modulates T cell response. *J Immunol* 166:7033–7041.

253. Cooper AM, Solache A, Khader SA. 2007. Interleukin-12 and tuberculosis: an old story revisited. *Curr Opin Immunol* 19:441–447.

254. Hickman SP, Chan J, Salgame P. 2002. *Mycobacterium tuberculosis* induces differential cytokine production from dendritic cells and macrophages with divergent effects on naive T cell polarization. *J Immunol* 168:4636–4642.

255. Humphreys IR, Stewart GR, Turner DJ, Patel J, Karamanou D, Snelgrove RJ, Young DB. 2006. A role for dendritic cells in the dissemination of mycobacterial infection. *Microbes Infect* 8:1339–1346.

256. Khader SA, Partida-Sánchez S, Bell G, Jelley-Gibbs DM, Swain S, Pearl JE, Ghilardi N, Desauvage FJ, Lund FE, Cooper AM. 2006. Interleukin 12p40 is required for dendritic cell migration and T cell priming after *Mycobacterium tuberculosis* infection. *J Exp Med* 203:1805–1815.

257. Rodriguez A, Regnault A, Kleijmeer M, Ricciardi-Castagnoli P, Amigorena S. 1999. Selective transport of internalized antigens to the cytosol for MHC class I presentation in dendritic cells. *Nat Cell Biol* 1:362–368.

258. Schaible UE, Winau F, Sieling PA, Fischer K, Collins HL, Hagens K, Modlin RL, Brinkmann V, Kaufmann SHE. 2003. Apoptosis facilitates antigen presentation to T lymphocytes through MHC-I and CD1 in tuberculosis. *Nat Med* 9:1039–1046.

259. Kaufmann SHE, Schaible UE. 2003. A dangerous liaison between two major killers: *Mycobacterium tuberculosis* and HIV target dendritic cells through DC-SIGN. *J Exp Med* 197:1–5.

260. van Kooyk Y, Appelmelk B, Geijtenbeek TBH. 2003. A fatal attraction: *Mycobacterium tuberculosis* and HIV-1 target DC-SIGN to escape immune surveillance. *Trends Mol Med* 9:153–159.

261. Campbell KS, Hasegawa J. 2013. Natural killer cell biology: an update and future directions. *J Allergy Clin Immunol* 132:536–544.

262. Cooper MA, Fehniger TA, Caligiuri MA. 2001. The biology of human natural killer-cell subsets. *Trends Immunol* 22:633–640.

263. Moretta L. 2010. Dissecting CD56dim human NK cells. *Blood* 116:3689–3691.

264. Kruse PH, Matta J, Ugolini S, Vivier E. 2014. Natural cytotoxicity receptors and their ligands. *Immunol Cell Biol* 92:221–229.

265. Long EO, Kim HS, Liu D, Peterson ME, Rajagopalan S. 2013. Controlling natural killer cell responses: integration of signals for activation and inhibition. *Annu Rev Immunol* 31:227–258.

266. Adib-Conquy M, Scott-Algara D, Cavaillon J-M, Souza-Fonseca-Guimaraes F. 2014. TLR-mediated activation of NK cells and their role in bacterial/viral immune responses in mammals. *Immunol Cell Biol* 92:256–262.

267. Souza-Fonseca-Guimaraes F, Adib-Conquy M, Cavaillon J-M. 2012. Natural killer (NK) cells in antibacterial innate immunity: angels or devils? *Mol Med* 18:270–285.

268. Junqueira-Kipnis AP, Kipnis A, Jamieson A, Juarrero MG, Diefenbach A, Raulet DH, Turner J, Orme IM. 2003. NK cells respond to pulmonary infection with *Mycobacterium tuberculosis*, but play a minimal role in protection. *J Immunol* 171:6039–6045.

269. Feng CG, Kaviratne M, Rothfuchs AG, Cheever A, Hieny S, Young HA, Wynn TA, Sher A. 2006. NK cell-derived IFN-gamma differentially regulates innate resistance and neutrophil response in T cell-deficient hosts infected with *Mycobacterium tuberculosis*. *J Immunol* 177:7086–7093.

270. Vitale M, Della Chiesa M, Carlomagno S, Pende D, Aricò M, Moretta L, Moretta A. 2005. NK-dependent DC maturation is mediated by TNFα and IFNγ released upon engagement of the NKp30 triggering receptor. *Blood* 106:566–571.

271. Schierloh P, Yokobori N, Alemán M, Musella RM, Beigier-Bompadre M, Saab MA, Alves L, Abbate E, de la Barrera SS, Sasiain MC. 2005. Increased susceptibility to apoptosis of CD56^dimCD16^+ NK cells induces the enrichment of IFN-gamma-producing CD56^bright cells in tuberculous pleurisy. *J Immunol* 175:6852–6860.

272. Wu YE, Zhang SW, Peng WG, Li KS, Li K, Jiang JK, Lin JH, Cai YM. 2009. Changes in lymphocyte subsets in the peripheral blood of patients with active pulmonary tuberculosis. *J Int Med Res* 37:1742–1749.

273. Ratcliffe LT, Lukey PT, MacKenzie CR, Ress SR. 1994. Reduced NK activity correlates with active disease in HIV- patients with multidrug-resistant pulmonary tuberculosis. *Clin Exp Immunol* 97:373–379.

274. Ratcliffe LT, Mackenzie CR, Lukey PT, Ress SR. 1992. Reduced natural killer cell activity in multi-drug resistant pulmonary tuberculosis. *Scand J Immunol Suppl* 36(s1):167–170.

275. Wang F, Hou H, Wu S, Tang Q, Huang M, Yin B, Huang J, Liu W, Mao L, Lu Y, Sun Z. 2015. Tim-3 pathway affects NK cell impairment in patients with active tuberculosis. *Cytokine* 76:270–279.

276. Zufferey C, Germano S, Dutta B, Ritz N, Curtis N. 2013. The contribution of non-conventional T cells and NK cells in the mycobacterial-specific IFNγ response in Bacille Calmette-Guérin (BCG)-immunized infants. *PLoS One* 8:e77334.

277. Kleinnijenhuis J, Quintin J, Preijers F, Joosten LAB, Jacobs C, Xavier RJ, van der Meer JWM, van Crevel R, Netea MG. 2014. BCG-induced trained immunity in NK cells: role for non-specific protection to infection. *Clin Immunol* 155:213–219.

278. Kemp K, Hviid L, Kharazmi A, Kemp M. 1997. Interferon-γ production by human T cells and natural killer cells *in vitro* in response to antigens from the two intracellular pathogens *Mycobacterium tuberculosis* and *Leishmania major*. *Scand J Immunol* 46:495–499.

279. Dhiman R, Indramohan M, Barnes PF, Nayak RC, Paidipally P, Rao LVM, Vankayalapati R. 2009. IL-22 produced by human NK cells inhibits growth of *Mycobacterium tuberculosis* by enhancing phagolysosomal fusion. *J Immunol* 183:6639–6645.

280. Denis M. 1994. Interleukin-12 (IL-12) augments cytolytic activity of natural killer cells toward *Mycobacterium tuberculosis*-infected human monocytes. *Cell Immunol* 156:529–536.

281. Katz P, Yeager H Jr, Whalen G, Evans M, Swartz RP, Roecklein J. 1990. Natural killer cell-mediated lysis of *Mycobacterium-avium* complex-infected monocytes. *J Clin Immunol* 10:71–77.

282. Molloy A, Meyn PA, Smith KD, Kaplan G. 1993. Recognition and destruction of Bacillus Calmette-Guerin-infected human monocytes. *J Exp Med* 177:1691–1698.

283. Brill KJ, Li Q, Larkin R, Canaday DH, Kaplan DR, Boom WH, Silver RF. 2001. Human natural killer cells mediate killing of intracellular *Mycobacterium tuberculosis* H37Rv via granule-independent mechanisms. *Infect Immun* 69:1755–1765.

284. Bermudez LE, Wu M, Young LS. 1995. Interleukin-12-stimulated natural killer cells can activate human macrophages to inhibit growth of *Mycobacterium avium*. *Infect Immun* 63:4099–4104.

285. Esin S, Batoni G, Källenius G, Gaines H, Campa M, Svenson SB, Andersson R, Wigzell H. 1996. Proliferation of distinct human T cell subsets in response to live, killed or soluble extracts of *Mycobacterium tuberculosis* and *Myco. avium*. *Clin Exp Immunol* 104:419–425.

286. Esin S, Batoni G, Pardini M, Favilli F, Bottai D, Maisetta G, Florio W, Vanacore R, Wigzell H, Campa M. 2004. Functional characterization of human natural killer cells responding to *Mycobacterium bovis* bacille Calmette-Guérin. *Immunology* 112:143–152.

287. Batoni G, Esin S, Favilli F, Pardini M, Bottai D, Maisetta G, Florio W, Campa M. 2005. Human CD56[bright] and CD56[dim] natural killer cell subsets respond differentially to direct stimulation with Mycobacterium bovis bacillus Calmette-Guérin. *Scand J Immunol* 62:498–506.

288. Portevin D, Young D. 2013. Natural killer cell cytokine response to *M. bovis* BCG is associated with inhibited proliferation, increased apoptosis and ultimate depletion of NKp44(+)CD56(bright) cells. *PLoS One* 8: e68864.

289. Portevin D, Via LE, Eum S, Young D. 2012. Natural killer cells are recruited during pulmonary tuberculosis and their *ex vivo* responses to mycobacteria vary between healthy human donors in association with KIR haplotype. *Cell Microbiol* 14:1734–1744.

290. Sun JC, Lopez-Verges S, Kim CC, DeRisi JL, Lanier LL. 2011. NK cells and immune "memory". *J Immunol* 186:1891–1897.

291. Esin S, Batoni G, Counoupas C, Stringaro A, Brancatisano FL, Colone M, Maisetta G, Florio W, Arancia G, Campa M. 2008. Direct binding of human NK cell natural cytotoxicity receptor NKp44 to the surfaces of mycoacteria and other bacteria. *Infect Immun* 76:1719–1727.

292. Esin S, Counoupas C, Aulicino A, Brancatisano FL, Maisetta G, Bottai D, Di Luca M, Florio W, Campa M, Batoni G. 2013. Interaction of *Mycobacterium tuberculosis* cell wall components with the human natural killer cell receptors NKp44 and Toll-like receptor 2. *Scand J Immunol* 77:460–469.

293. Gerosa F, Baldani-Guerra B, Nisii C, Marchesini V, Carra G, Trinchieri G. 2002. Reciprocal activating interaction between natural killer cells and dendritic cells. *J Exp Med* 195:327–333.

294. Zhang R, Zheng X, Li B, Wei H, Tian Z. 2006. Human NK cells positively regulate gammadelta T cells in response to *Mycobacterium tuberculosis*. *J Immunol* 176: 2610–2616.

295. Boom WH, Balaji KN, Nayak R, Tsukaguchi K, Chervenak KA. 1994. Characterization of a 10- to 14-kilodalton protease-sensitive *Mycobacterium tuberculosis* H37Ra antigen that stimulates human gamma delta T cells. *Infect Immun* 62:5511–5518.

296. Vankayalapati R, Klucar P, Wizel B, Weis SE, Samten B, Safi H, Shams H, Barnes PF. 2004. NK cells regulate CD8+ T cell effector function in response to an intracellular pathogen. *J Immunol* 172:130–137.

297. Roy S, Barnes PF, Garg A, Wu S, Cosman D, Vankayalapati R. 2008. NK cells lyse T regulatory cells that expand in response to an intracellular pathogen. *J Immunol* 180:1729–1736.

298. Barrios-Payán J, Aguilar-León D, Lascurain-Ledezma R, Hernández-Pando R. 2006. Neutrophil participation in early control and immune activation during experimental pulmonary tuberculosis. *Gac Med Mex* 142: 273–281. (In Spanish.)

299. Pedrosa J, Saunders BM, Appelberg R, Orme IM, Silva MT, Cooper AM. 2000. Neutrophils play a protective nonphagocytic role in systemic *Mycobacterium tuberculosis* infection of mice. *Infect Immun* 68:577–583.

300. Fulton SA, Reba SM, Martin TD, Boom WH. 2002. Neutrophil-mediated mycobacteriocidal immunity in the lung during *Mycobacterium bovis* BCG infection in C57BL/6 mice. *Infect Immun* 70:5322–5327.

301. Seiler P, Aichele P, Raupach B, Odermatt B, Steinhoff U, Kaufmann SHE. 2000. Rapid neutrophil response controls fast-replicating intracellular bacteria but not slow-replicating *Mycobacterium tuberculosis*. *J Infect Dis* 181:671–680.

302. Zhang X, Majlessi L, Deriaud E, Leclerc C, Lo-Man R. 2009. Coactivation of Syk kinase and MyD88 adaptor protein pathways by bacteria promotes regulatory properties of neutrophils. *Immunity* 31:761–771.

303. Barnes PF, Leedom JM, Chan LS, Wong SF, Shah J, Vachon LA, Overturf GD, Modlin RL. 1988. Predictors

of short-term prognosis in patients with pulmonary tuberculosis. *J Infect Dis* **158**:366–371.

304. **Antony VB, Sahn SA, Harada RN, Repine JE.** 1983. Lung repair and granuloma formation. Tubercle bacilli stimulated neutrophils release chemotactic factors for monocytes. *Chest* **83**(Suppl):95S–96S.

305. **Abadie V, Badell E, Douillard P, Ensergueix D, Leenen PJM, Tanguy M, Fiette L, Saeland S, Gicquel B, Winter N.** 2005. Neutrophils rapidly migrate via lymphatics after Mycobacterium bovis BCG intradermal vaccination and shuttle live bacilli to the draining lymph nodes. *Blood* **106**:1843–1850.

306. **Silva MT.** 2010. Neutrophils and macrophages work in concert as inducers and effectors of adaptive immunity against extracellular and intracellular microbial pathogens. *J Leukoc Biol* **87**:805–813.

307. **Lemon WS, Feldman WH.** 1943. Experimental tuberculosis pleural effusion. *Am Rev Tuberc* **48**:177–183.

308. **Cruz A, Fraga AG, Fountain JJ, Rangel-Moreno J, Torrado E, Saraiva M, Pereira DR, Randall TD, Pedrosa J, Cooper AM, Castro AG.** 2010. Pathological role of interleukin 17 in mice subjected to repeated BCG vaccination after infection with Mycobacterium tuberculosis. *J Exp Med* **207**:1609–1616.

309. **de Vallière S, Abate G, Blazevic A, Heuertz RM, Hoft DF.** 2005. Enhancement of innate and cell-mediated immunity by antimycobacterial antibodies. *Infect Immun* **73**:6711–6720.

310. **Sugawara I, Udagawa T, Yamada H.** 2004. Rat neutrophils prevent the development of tuberculosis. *Infect Immun* **72**:1804–1806.

311. **Shigenaga T, Dannenberg AM, Lowrie DB, Said W, Urist MJ, Abbey H, Schofield BH, Mounts P, Sugisaki K.** 2001. Immune responses in tuberculosis: antibodies and CD4-CD8 lymphocytes with vascular adhesion molecules and cytokines (chemokines) cause a rapid antigen-specific cell infiltration at sites of bacillus Calmette-Guérin reinfection. *Immunology* **102**:466–479.

312. **Lyons MJ, Yoshimura T, McMurray DN.** 2004. Interleukin (IL)-8 (CXCL8) induces cytokine expression and superoxide formation by guinea pig neutrophils infected with Mycobacterium tuberculosis. *Tuberculosis (Edinb)* **84**:283–292.

313. **Kisich KO, Higgins M, Diamond G, Heifets L.** 2002. Tumor necrosis factor alpha stimulates killing of Mycobacterium tuberculosis by human neutrophils. *Infect Immun* **70**:4591–4599.

314. **Jones GS, Amirault HJ, Andersen BR.** 1990. Killing of Mycobacterium tuberculosis by neutrophils: a nonoxidative process. *J Infect Dis* **162**:700–704.

315. **Denis M.** 1991. Human neutrophils, activated with cytokines or not, do not kill virulent Mycobacterium tuberculosis. *J Infect Dis* **163**:919–920.

316. **Aston C, Rom WN, Talbot AT, Reibman J.** 1998. Early inhibition of mycobacterial growth by human alveolar macrophages is not due to nitric oxide. *Am J Respir Crit Care Med* **157**:1943–1950.

317. **Neufert C, Pai RK, Noss EH, Berger M, Boom WH, Harding CV.** 2001. *Mycobacterium tuberculosis* 19-kDa lipoprotein promotes neutrophil activation. *J Immunol* **167**:1542–1549.

318. **Yang C-T, Cambier CJ, Davis JM, Hall CJ, Crosier PS, Ramakrishnan L.** 2012. Neutrophils exert protection in the early tuberculous granuloma by oxidative killing of mycobacteria phagocytosed from infected macrophages. *Cell Host Microbe* **12**:301–312.

319. **Mattila JT, Maiello P, Sun T, Via LE, Flynn JL.** 2015. Granzyme B-expressing neutrophils correlate with bacteria load in granulomas from *Mycobacterium tuberculosis*-infected cynomolgus macaques. *Cell Microbiol* **17**:1085–1097.

320. **Mantovani A, Cassatella MA, Costantini C, Jaillon S.** 2011. Neutrophils in the activation and regulation of innate and adaptive immunity. *Nat Rev Immunol* **11**: 519–531.

321. **Sawant KV, McMurray DN.** 2007. Guinea pig neutrophils infected with *Mycobacterium tuberculosis* produce cytokines which activate alveolar macrophages in noncontact cultures. *Infect Immun* **75**:1870–1877.

322. **De Santo C, Arscott R, Booth S, Karydis I, Jones M, Asher R, Salio M, Middleton M, Cerundolo V.** 2010. Invariant NKT cells modulate the suppressive activity of IL-10-secreting neutrophils differentiated with serum amyloid A. *Nat Immunol* **11**:1039–1046.

323. **Doz E, Lombard R, Carreras F, Buzoni-Gatel D, Winter N.** 2013. Mycobacteria-infected dendritic cells attract neutrophils that produce IL-10 and specifically shut down Th17 CD4 T cells through their IL-10 receptor. *J Immunol* **191**:3818–3826.

324. **D'Avila H, Roque NR, Cardoso RM, Castro-Faria-Neto HC, Melo RCN, Bozza PT.** 2008. Neutrophils recruited to the site of *Mycobacterium bovis* BCG infection undergo apoptosis and modulate lipid body biogenesis and prostaglandin E production by macrophages. *Cell Microbiol* **10**:2589–2604.

325. **Perskvist N, Long M, Stendahl O, Zheng L.** 2002. *Mycobacterium tuberculosis* promotes apoptosis in human neutrophils by activating caspase-3 and altering expression of Bax/Bcl-xL via an oxygen-dependent pathway. *J Immunol* **168**:6358–6365.

326. **Persson YAZ, Blomgran-Julinder R, Rahman S, Zheng L, Stendahl O.** 2008. *Mycobacterium tuberculosis*-induced apoptotic neutrophils trigger a proinflammatory response in macrophages through release of heat shock protein 72, acting in synergy with the bacteria. *Microbes Infect* **10**:233–240.

327. **Petrofsky M, Bermudez LE.** 1999. Neutrophils from *Mycobacterium avium*-infected mice produce TNF-alpha, IL-12, and IL-1 beta and have a putative role in early host response. *Clin Immunol* **91**:354–358.

328. **Seiler P, Aichele P, Bandermann S, Hauser AE, Lu B, Gerard NP, Gerard C, Ehlers S, Mollenkopf HJ, Kaufmann SHE.** 2003. Early granuloma formation after aerosol *Mycobacterium tuberculosis* infection is regulated by neutrophils via CXCR3-signaling chemokines. *Eur J Immunol* **33**:2676–2686.

329. **Morel C, Badell E, Abadie V, Robledo M, Setterblad N, Gluckman JC, Gicquel B, Boudaly S, Winter N.** 2008. *Mycobacterium bovis* BCG-infected neutrophils

and dendritic cells cooperate to induce specific T cell responses in humans and mice. *Eur J Immunol* **38**: 437–447.

330. Alemán M, de la Barrera S, Schierloh P, Yokobori N, Baldini M, Musella R, Abbate E, Sasiain M. 2007. Spontaneous or *Mycobacterium tuberculosis*-induced apoptotic neutrophils exert opposite effects on the dendritic cell-mediated immune response. *Eur J Immunol* **37**:1524–1537.

331. Blomgran R, Ernst JD. 2011. Lung neutrophils facilitate activation of naive antigen-specific CD4+ T cells during *Mycobacterium tuberculosis* infection. *J Immunol* **186**: 7110–7119.

332. Yang C-W, Strong BSI, Miller MJ, Unanue ER. 2010. Neutrophils influence the level of antigen presentation during the immune response to protein antigens in adjuvants. *J Immunol* **185**:2927–2934.

333. Eum SY, Kong J-H, Hong M-S, Lee Y-J, Kim JH, Hwang S-H, Cho S-N, Via LE, Barry CE III. 2010. Neutrophils are the predominant infected phagocytic cells in the airways of patients with active pulmonary TB. *Chest* **137**:122–128.

334. Condos R, Rom WN, Liu YM, Schluger NW. 1998. Local immune responses correlate with presentation and outcome in tuberculosis. *Am J Respir Crit Care Med* **157**:729–735.

335. Martineau AR, Timms PM, Bothamley GH, Hanifa Y, Islam K, Claxton AP, Packe GE, Moore-Gillon JC, Darmalingam M, Davidson RN, Milburn HJ, Baker LV, Barker RD, Woodward NJ, Venton TR, Barnes KE, Mullett CJ, Coussens AK, Rutterford CM, Mein CA, Davies GR, Wilkinson RJ, Nikolayevskyy V, Drobniewski FA, Eldridge SM, Griffiths CJ. 2011. High-dose vitamin D(3) during intensive-phase antimicrobial treatment of pulmonary tuberculosis: a double-blind randomised controlled trial. *Lancet* **377**: 242–250.

336. Eruslanov EB, Lyadova IV, Kondratieva TK, Majorov KB, Scheglov IV, Orlova MO, Apt AS. 2005. Neutrophil responses to *Mycobacterium tuberculosis* infection in genetically susceptible and resistant mice. *Infect Immun* **73**:1744–1753.

337. Keller C, Hoffmann R, Lang R, Brandau S, Hermann C, Ehlers S. 2006. Genetically determined susceptibility to tuberculosis in mice causally involves accelerated and enhanced recruitment of granulocytes. *Infect Immun* **74**:4295–4309.

338. Ramakrishnan L. 2012. Revisiting the role of the granuloma in tuberculosis. *Nat Rev Immunol* **12**:352–366.

339. Tsai MC, Chakravarty S, Zhu G, Xu J, Tanaka K, Koch C, Tufariello J, Flynn J, Chan J. 2006. Characterization of the tuberculous granuloma in murine and human lungs: cellular composition and relative tissue oxygen tension. *Cell Microbiol* **8**:218–232.

340. Guirado E, Schlesinger LS. 2013. Modeling the *Mycobacterium tuberculosis* granuloma: the critical battlefield in host immunity and disease. *Front Immunol* **4**:98

341. Kaplan G, Post FA, Moreira AL, Wainwright H, Kreiswirth BN, Tanverdi M, Mathema B, Ramaswamy SV, Walther G, Steyn LM, Barry CE III, Bekker L-G. 2003. *Mycobacterium tuberculosis* growth at the cavity surface: a microenvironment with failed immunity. *Infect Immun* **71**:7099–7108.

342. Orme IM, Basaraba RJ. 2014. The formation of the granuloma in tuberculosis infection. *Semin Immunol* **26**:601–609.

343. Russell DG. 2007. Who puts the tubercle in tuberculosis? *Nat Rev Microbiol* **5**:39–47.

344. Silva Miranda M, Breiman A, Allain S, Deknuydt F, Altare F. 2012. The tuberculous granuloma: an unsuccessful host defence mechanism providing a safety shelter for the bacteria? *Clin Dev Immunol* **2012**: 139127.

345. Paige C, Bishai WR. 2010. Penitentiary or penthouse condo: the tuberculous granuloma from the microbe's point of view. *Cell Microbiol* **12**:301–309.

346. Heitmann L, Abad Dar M, Schreiber T, Erdmann H, Behrends J, Mckenzie AN, Brombacher F, Ehlers S, Hölscher C. 2014. The IL-13/IL-4Rα axis is involved in tuberculosis-associated pathology. *J Pathol* **234**: 338–350.

347. Cyktor JC, Carruthers B, Kominsky RA, Beamer GL, Stromberg P, Turner J. 2013. IL-10 inhibits mature fibrotic granuloma formation during *Mycobacterium tuberculosis* infection. *J Immunol* **190**:2778–2790.

348. Pan H, Yan B-S, Rojas M, Shebzukhov YV, Zhou H, Kobzik L, Higgins DE, Daly MJ, Bloom BR, Kramnik I. 2005. Ipr1 gene mediates innate immunity to tuberculosis. *Nature* **434**:767–772.

349. Manabe YC, Kesavan AK, Lopez-Molina J, Hatem CL, Brooks M, Fujiwara R, Hochstein K, Pitt MLM, Tufariello J, Chan J, McMurray DN, Bishai WR, Dannenberg AM Jr, Mendez S. 2008. The aerosol rabbit model of TB latency, reactivation and immune reconstitution inflammatory syndrome. *Tuberculosis (Edinb)* **88**:187–196.

350. Scanga CA, Flynn JL. 2014. Modeling tuberculosis in nonhuman primates. *Cold Spring Harb Perspect Med* **4**: a018564.

351. McMurray D. 1994. Guinea pig model of tuberculosis, p 135–147. *In* Bloom B (ed), *Tuberculosis*. ASM Press, Washington, DC.

352. Guirado E, Mbawuike U, Keiser TL, Arcos J, Azad AK, Wang S-H, Schlesinger LS. 2015. Characterization of host and microbial determinants in individuals with latent tuberculosis infection using a human granuloma model. *MBio* **6**:e02537–14.

353. Puissegur M-P, Botanch C, Duteyrat J-L, Delsol G, Caratero C, Altare F. 2004. An *in vitro* dual model of mycobacterial granulomas to investigate the molecular interactions between mycobacteria and human host cells. *Cell Microbiol* **6**:423–433.

354. Marino S, Linderman JJ, Kirschner DE. 2011. A multifaceted approach to modeling the immune response in tuberculosis. *Wiley Interdisc Rev Syst Biol Med* **3**: 479–489.

355. Marino S, El-Kebir M, Kirschner D. 2011. A hybrid multi-compartment model of granuloma formation and T cell priming in tuberculosis. *J Theor Biol* **280**:50–62.

356. Israel HL, Hetherington HW, Ord JG. 1941. A study of tuberculosis among students of nursing. *JAMA* **117:**839–844.

357. Morrison J, Pai M, Hopewell PC. 2008. Tuberculosis and latent tuberculosis infection in close contacts of people with pulmonary tuberculosis in low-income and middle-income countries: a systematic review and meta-analysis. *Lancet Infect Dis* **8:**359–368.

358. van Crevel R, van der Ven-Jongekrijg J, Netea MG, de Lange W, Kullberg BJ, van der Meer JW. 1999. Disease-specific *ex vivo* stimulation of whole blood for cytokine production: applications in the study of tuberculosis. *J Immunol Methods* **222:**145–153.

359. Wilkinson RJ, Llewelyn M, Toossi Z, Patel P, Pasvol G, Lalvani A, Wright D, Latif M, Davidson RN. 2000. Influence of vitamin D deficiency and vitamin D receptor polymorphisms on tuberculosis among Gujarati Asians in west London: a case-control study. *Lancet* **355:**618–621.

360. Azad AK, Sadee W, Schlesinger LS. 2012. Innate immune gene polymorphisms in tuberculosis. *Infect Immun* **80:**3343–3359.

361. Alemán M, Schierloh P, de la Barrera SS, Musella RM, Saab MA, Baldini M, Abbate E, Sasiain MC. 2004. *Mycobacterium tuberculosis* triggers apoptosis in peripheral neutrophils involving toll-like receptor 2 and p38 mitogen protein kinase in tuberculosis patients. *Infect Immun* **72:**5150–5158.

362. Majeed M, Perskvist N, Ernst JD, Orselius K, Stendahl O. 1998. Roles of calcium and annexins in phagocytosis and elimination of an attenuated strain of *Mycobacterium tuberculosis* in human neutrophils. *Microb Pathog* **24:**309–320.

363. Martineau AR, Newton SM, Wilkinson KA, Kampmann B, Hall BM, Nawroly N, Packe GE, Davidson RN, Griffiths CJ, Wilkinson RJ. 2007. Neutrophil-mediated innate immune resistance to mycobacteria. *J Clin Invest* **117:**1988–1994.

364. Dong Y, Cirimotich CM, Pike A, Chandra R, Dimopoulos G. 2012. Anopheles NF-κB-regulated splicing factors direct pathogen-specific repertoires of the hypervariable pattern recognition receptor AgDscam. *Cell Host Microbe* **12:**521–530.

365. Pham LN, Dionne MS, Shirasu-Hiza M, Schneider DS. 2007. A specific primed immune response in *Drosophila* is dependent on phagocytes. *PLoS Pathog* **3:**e26.

366. Leclerc V, Reichhart J-M. 2004. The immune response of *Drosophila melanogaster*. *Immunol Rev* **198:**59–71.

367. Netea MG. 2013. Training innate immunity: the changing concept of immunological memory in innate host defence. *Eur J Clin Invest* **43:**881–884.

368. Kleinnijenhuis J, Quintin J, Preijers F, Joosten LAB, Ifrim DC, Saeed S, Jacobs C, van Loenhout J, de Jong D, Stunnenberg HG, Xavier RJ, van der Meer JWM, van Crevel R, Netea MG. 2012. Bacille Calmette-Guerin induces NOD2-dependent nonspecific protection from reinfection via epigenetic reprogramming of monocytes. *Proc Natl Acad Sci USA* **109:**17537–17542.

369. Dieli F, Troye-Blomberg M, Ivanyi J, Fournié JJ, Bonneville M, Peyrat MA, Sireci G, Salerno A. 2000. Vgamma9/Vdelta2 T lymphocytes reduce the viability of intracellular *Mycobacterium tuberculosis*. *Eur J Immunol* **30:**1512–1519.

370. Spencer CT, Abate G, Sakala IG, Xia M, Truscott SM, Eickhoff CS, Linn R, Blazevic A, Metkar SS, Peng G, Froelich CJ, Hoft DF. 2013. Granzyme A produced by γ(9)δ(2) T cells induces human macrophages to inhibit growth of an intracellular pathogen. *PLoS Pathog* **9:**e1003119.

Tuberculosis and the Tubercle Bacillus, 2nd ed.
Edited by William R. Jacobs, Jr., Helen McShane, Valerie Mizrahi, and Ian M. Orme
© 2018 American Society for Microbiology, Washington, DC
doi:10.1128/microbiolspec.TBTB2-0018-2016

Cytokines and Chemokines in *Mycobacterium tuberculosis* Infection

2

Racquel Domingo-Gonzalez,[1] Oliver Prince,[1]
Andrea Cooper,[2] and Shabaana A. Khader[1]

INTRODUCTION

Cytokines are soluble, small proteins that are produced by cells and act in a largely paracrine manner to influence the activity of other cells. Currently, the term "cytokine" describes proteins such as the tumor necrosis factor family, the interleukins, and the chemokines. Virtually every nucleated cell can produce and respond to cytokines, placing these molecules at the center of most of the body's homeostatic mechanisms (1). Much of our knowledge of the function of cytokines has been derived from studies wherein homeostasis has been disrupted by infection and the absence of specific cytokines results in a failure to control the disease process. In this context, infection with *Mycobacterium tuberculosis* has proven to be very informative and has highlighted the role of cytokines in controlling infection without promoting uncontrolled and damaging inflammatory responses (2–4). Herein, we focus on the key cytokine and chemokines that have been studied in the context of human TB using experimental medicine as well as *M. tuberculosis* infection of various animal models, including non-human primates (NHPs), mice, and rabbits. Perhaps the most important message of this review is that in a complex disease such as TB the role of any one cytokine cannot be designated either "good" or "bad" but rather that cytokines can elicit both protective and pathologic consequences depending on context.

Why is TB such an informative probe allowing for detailed investigation of the function of cytokines and chemokines in immunity? One recent development in our understanding of TB stems from theories of coevolution between modern humans and *M. tuberculosis*

(5). Evolutionary patterns based on genetic analyses suggest that *M. tuberculosis* and humans coexisted for tens of thousands of years in Africa but that, when humans left Africa and developed a more urban lifestyle, TB developed into a substantial health problem (6). During coevolution between humans and *M. tuberculosis*, *M. tuberculosis* likely evolved tools and stratagems with which to manipulate the human immune response to ensure effective transmission (7); this manipulation has been so successful that it is thought that over one-third of the world's population harbors some form of *M. tuberculosis* infection (8).

Two facts illustrate the focus of *M. tuberculosis* on manipulating the human immune response. First, *M. tuberculosis* is the major active constituent of complete Freund's adjuvant, which has been used for decades to stimulate long-lived cellular immune responses in vertebrate animals. Second, we have exploited the strong and sensitive T-cell-based inflammatory response to *M. tuberculosis* antigens as a skin test to indicate infection with *M. tuberculosis*. Thus, teleologically speaking, we may suggest that *M. tuberculosis* does not fail to induce immunity, it simply manipulates it such that its need to be transmitted is met. This manipulation occurs from the start of the human *M. tuberculosis* interaction when immune surveillance cells of the lung recognize danger through binding of their pattern recognition receptors to exquisitely refined *M. tuberculosis* pathogen-associated molecular molecules. It is this initial interaction that results in production of chemokines and cytokines, which then recruit and activate inflammatory cells (9). Following this initial inter-

[1]Department of Molecular Microbiology, Washington University in St. Louis, St. Louis, MO 63130; [2]Department of Infection, Immunity and Inflammation, University of Leicester, Leicester LE1 7RH, United Kingdom.

action, bacteria migrate to the draining lymph node where they initiate (quite effectively) antigen-specific T cells that differentiate into cytokine-producing cells capable of expressing a variety of chemokine receptors that allow them to traffic away from the lymph node and into sites of tissue inflammation (7, 9). These antigen-specific T cells must then migrate via chemokine gradients, colocate with *M. tuberculosis*-infected phagocytic cells, and release cytokines that activate the infected cells to kill the *M. tuberculosis* (7, 9). If this induction of immunity is not met by *M. tuberculosis*, then the host dies rapidly with no effective transmission of the bacterium to further hosts.

The need for communication between cells both for efficient migration and for specific instruction during expression of immunity is where the critical role of cytokines and chemokines in controlling TB lies. Indeed, for the majority of those infected with *M. tuberculosis*, the efficient expression of immunity via competent cytokine and chemokine expression results in no sign of disease other than an ability to exhibit an inflammatory response to *M. tuberculosis* antigen (i.e., the skin test response). However, for *M. tuberculosis* to be efficiently transmitted, a degraded inflammatory lesion capable of delivering live bacteria to the airways must develop, and it is this evolutionary need that likely drives the development of the disease process in the lung. *M. tuberculosis* expresses molecules that promote inflammatory responses, which then need to be regulated to avoid tissue damage. If the bacterial burden is large or if the bacteria proliferate rapidly, then the coordination between cells mediated by cytokines and chemokines cannot occur quickly enough and immunity cannot be expressed, despite the presence of all of the required components. Understanding the functions and interactions between cytokines and chemokines is therefore critical to our attempts to limit TB. Herein, we discuss the roles of specific cytokines (Table 1) and chemokines (Table 2) in the context of *M. tuberculosis* infection and how they function to stop the development of TB, and also how they might contribute to the progression of disease.

CYTOKINES

Tumor Necrosis Factor Alpha

Tumor necrosis factor alpha (TNFα) is a cytokine that is released following activation of the immune system. Although it is primarily produced by macrophages, TNFα can also be secreted by lymphocytes, mast cells, endothelial cells, and fibroblasts (10). Because most cells exhibit responsiveness to TNFα, it is considered a major proinflammatory mediator. It is produced as a type II transmembrane homotrimeric protein (mTNF) that can become released into the extracellular milieu through the proteolytic action of TNFα-converting enzyme (TACE) (11). Soluble TNF (sTNF) exists as a 51-kDa trimeric protein that is unstable on reaching nanomolar concentrations (12), but which on binding to cognate TNF receptors (TNF-R) induces activation of proinflammatory responses mediated by NFκB, JNK, and p38, as well as promotion of apoptosis (10, 13–16). There are two TNF receptors, TNF-R1 and TNF-R2. Both TNF-R1, also known as CD120a and p55/60, and TNF-R2, also known as CD120b and p75/80, can bind either the membrane or the soluble form of TNFα (17–19). An important regulator of activation is localization of receptor expression, as TNF-R1 is ubiquitously expressed, whereas TNF-R2 expression is restricted to subsets of neuronal cells, T cells, endothelial cells, microglia, oligodendrocytes, cardiac myocytes, thymocytes, and human mesenchymal stem cells (20). Signaling through TNF-R2 can only be activated through mTNF, and not sTNF. This complex interplay between positive and negative regulators of TNF activity reflects the potential disruptive power of TNFα, and this regulation of immunity provides tempting targets for manipulation by *M. tuberculosis*.

Originally described for its ability to promote necrosis of tumors (21), TNFα has since been implicated in proliferation and differentiation of immune cells, as well as multiple inflammatory processes including migration (20) and apoptosis of *M. tuberculosis*-infected cells *in vitro* (22, 23). Upon initial *M. tuberculosis* infection, the interaction between immune surveillance cells such as phagocytes in the lung and the invading *M. tuberculosis* results in the production of multiple proinflammatory cytokines, including TNFα (4) (Fig. 1). Although both virulent and avirulent *M. tuberculosis* are able to induce comparable levels of TNFα by human alveolar macrophages, TNFα produced in response to infection with virulent *M. tuberculosis* strains has less bioactivity (24). This is an example of the ability of the bacterium to manipulate the host response, because the decreased TNFα bioactivity has been attributed to the induction of IL-10 by the virulent strain, which then results in release of soluble TNF-R2 that binds the induced TNFα, thereby inhibiting its function (24). As infection progresses, TNFα plays a role in coordinating the chemokine response within the lung and in facilitating the development of the granuloma; it is also produced by both CD4 and CD8 T cells and plays an important role in optimal macrophage activation (25).

Table 1 The positive and negative roles of cytokines in TB

Cytokine	Receptor/signal	Role in TB
TNFα	TNFR1, TNFR2 JNK, p38, NFκB	Positive: Essential for survival following *M. tuberculosis* infection. Initiation of innate cytokine and chemokine response and phagocyte activation. Negative: Mediator of tissue damage.
IFNγ	IFNGR1, IFNGR2 JAK/STAT	Positive: Essential for survival following *M. tuberculosis* infection. Coordinates and maintains mononuclear inflammation. Expressed by antigen-specific T cells. Negative: Potentially pathogenic.
IFNα/IFNβ	IFNAR1, IFNAR2 JAK, TYK, ISG, ISRE	Positive: Required for initial recruitment of phagocytes to the lung. Negative: Overexpression of IFNα/IFNβ results in recruitment of permissive phagocytes and regulation of T-cell accumulation and function.
IL-6	IL-6R, gp130 JAK, STAT3, MAPK	Positive: Potentiates early immunity – nonessential unless a high-dose infection.
IL-1α/IL-1β	IL-1R1, IL1RAcP MyD88, IRAK4, NFκB	Positive: Essential for survival following *M. tuberculosis* infection. Induction of IL-17. Promotes PGE_2 to limit type I IFN.
IL-18	IL-18Rα, IL-18Rβ MyD88, IRAK, NFκB	Positive: May augment IFNγ – nonessential. Regulator of neutrophil and monocyte accumulation, optimal induction of IFNγ by T cells.
IL-12 p40,p35	12Rβ1, IL-12Rβ2 JAK2, TYK2, STAT4	Positive: IL-12p40 and IL-12p35 essential for survival following *M. tuberculosis* infection. Mediate early T-cell activation, polarization, and survival. Negative: Overexpression of IL-12p70 is toxic during *M. tuberculosis* infection.
IL-23 p40,p19	IL-23R, IL-12Rβ1 JAK2, TYK2, STAT3	Positive: Required for IL-17 and IL-22 expression during *M. tuberculosis* infection. Nonessential in low-dose challenge required for long-term control. Negative: Mediates increased pathology during chronic challenge.
IL-27 EBI3,p28	IL-27Rα, gp130 JAK1/2, TYK2, STAT1/3	Positive: May control inflammation and reduce pathology. Negative: Regulates protective immunity to *M. tuberculosis* infection by limiting the migration and survival of T cells at the inflamed site.
IL-35 p35,EBI3	IL-12Rβ2, gp130 STAT1/4	Positive: Regulate the availability of subunits of IL-12, IL-27. Negative: Potential immunoregulatory role.
IL-17A/F	IL-17RC, IL-17RA	Positive: Essential for survival following infection with some strains of *M. tuberculosis*. Induction and maintenance of chemokine gradients for T-cell migration. Negative: Drives pathology via S100A8/A9 and neutrophils.
IL-22	IL-22R1, IL-10R2 TYK2, JAK1, STAT3	Positive: Induces antimicrobial peptides and promotes epithelial repair, inhibits intracellular growth of *M. tuberculosis* in macrophages.

In *M. tuberculosis* infection models, the importance of TNFα is exemplified by mice deficient in the TNF receptor or following TNF neutralization (26). In these models, TNFα deficiency results in increased susceptibility with mice succumbing to infection within 2 to 3 weeks, while harboring a high bacterial burden (26). Critically, although inflammatory cells accumulate at the site of *M. tuberculosis* infection in TNFα-deficient mice, they do not coalesce to form granulomas (26–29). Granulomas are considered to be a hallmark of TB and are composed of macrophages, multinucleated giants cells, CD4$^+$ and CD8$^+$ T cells, B cells, and neutrophils (30). In one of the earliest studies of the role of TNFα in mycobacterial disease, it was shown that TNFα neutralization following BCG infection led to the loss of granulomas (31). Neutralization of TNFα also leads to decreased expression of key chemokines such as CCL5, CXCL9, and CXCL10. CXCL9 and CXCL10 both bind to the receptor CXCR3 (32, 33),

expressed on activated T cells, while CCR1 and CCR5, expressed on both innate (i.e., macrophages and neutrophils) and adaptive cells (i.e., T and B cells), bind to CCL5 (34). Thus, TNFα sits at the crossroads where innate immunity and acquired immunity, as well as cytokines and chemokines interact. In the absence of TNFα, T cells expressing CXCR3 fail to encounter the ligands CXCL9 and CXCL10 required to recruit these cells into the granuloma. Thus, the required communication between infected phagocytes and the instructive T cells does not occur, resulting in loss of immunity.

The importance of the granuloma in restricting the movement of *M. tuberculosis* to more immunoprivileged sites has long been appreciated (35). Indeed, inhibition of TNFα promotes dissemination of *M. tuberculosis* to sites such as the central nervous system (CNS) (36, 37) wherein adverse events are profound and often irreversible. It is thought that *M. tuberculosis* migrates to the CNS secondarily from a primary site

Table 2 The positive and negative roles of chemokines in TB

Chemokine	Receptor	Role in TB
CCL-3,-4,-5	CCR1	Positive: Upregulated during infection. Nonessential in mouse model
CCL-2,-7,-12	CCR2	Positive: Maximizes and organizes early macrophage and T-cell accumulation in the lung Negative: Mediates recruitment of permissive phagocyte accumulation into the lung
CCL-17,-22	CCR4	Positive: Mediates optimal granuloma formation to mycobacterial antigen Negative: May limit T-cell proliferation via T_{REG}
CCL-3,-4,-5	CCR5	Positive: Regulation of pulmonary infiltrates – nonessential. May mediate early dendritic cell accumulation in the lymph node. May augment macrophage M. tuberculosis killing via CCL5?
CCL-20	CCR6	Positive: Expression of CCR6 on T cells specific for M. tuberculosis antigens Negative: CCL-20 seen at high levels in active TB
CCL-19,-21,	CCR7	Positive: Mediates efficient migration of dendritic cells and M. tuberculosis-specific T-cell activation.
CXCL-1,-2,-3,-5,-6,-7,-8	CXCR1	Positive: Expressed on neutrophils mediates accumulation
	CXCR2	Negative: Absence of CXCR2 or CXCL5 results in improved bacterial control and reduced neutrophil accumulation
CXCL-9, -10,-11	CXCR3	Positive: Required for optimal granuloma formation. Expressed on M. tuberculosis-specific T cells. Use of CXCL9-11 levels to indicate disease level? Required for early recruitment of T cells to lung
CXCL-13	CXCR5	Positive: Required for correct location of T cells within granulomas. Required for B-cell follicle formation in M. tuberculosis-infected lungs. Required for optimal protection.

elsewhere in the host (38, 39), although how it crosses the blood-brain barrier is not clear. Although TNFα is produced in the CNS and is thought to exacerbate progression of TB-related damage in the CNS in a rabbit model (40), use of neuron-specific TNFα-deficient mice has shown that neuron-derived TNFα production is dispensable for protection against CNS-TB (41). These data support the notion that TNFα is critical for the initiation and coordination of cellular responses, but that it has the potential to be pathogenic when expressed in the absence of immunity.

TNFα is required throughout the life of the infected host because reactivation of pulmonary TB occurs in latently infected mice upon neutralization of TNFα (42). Upon neutralization, less defined granuloma formation is seen along with increased bacterial burden in the lung and extrapulmonary sites such as the liver and spleen (42) (Fig. 2). Enhanced histopathology is also observed in TNFα-neutralized mice, supporting the importance of a regulated cellular interaction during M. tuberculosis infection. The protective role of TNFα is further highlighted in those patients with autoimmune and chronic diseases who are undergoing anti-TNFα-neutralizing therapies, including infliximab, adalimumab, and etanercept (43, 44). Although this therapy is successful at treating the autoimmune disease, a significant correlation between reactivation of latent TB in patients undergoing anti-TNFα therapy has been reported (45–52). Patients using infliximab and/or adalimumab have a higher incidence of TB reactivation in extrapulmonary sites compared with etanercept (50). While a mechanism for this has not been determined, mathe-

matical modeling and bioinformatic analysis suggest that reactivation is related to drug tissue penetration, drug half-life, and relative specificity for membrane-bound TNFα or soluble TNFα (53). An intriguing mechanism for the effect of infliximab on immunity to M. tuberculosis infection has been suggested by the observation that this antibody-based drug binds to mTNF expressed on effector memory CD8 T cells, thereby facilitating complement-mediated lysis and likely loss of M. tuberculosis-specific CD8 T cells (54). In a cynomolgus macaque model of TB, latently infected primates were given either soluble TNFα or adalimumab and exhibited increased reactivation and harbored higher bacterial burdens than their latently infected untreated counterparts (55). As would be expected because of the higher bacterial burden and the role of TNFα in limiting bacterial spread, there were more granulomas in the lungs of the treated monkey (26, 55). In the zebrafish model of Mycobacterium marinum infection, TNFα is required for control of mycobacterial growth and to regulate macrophage necrosis (56).

The ability to rapidly diagnose active disease from latent infection would be highly beneficial in identification and prompt treatment of TB. TNFα has recently been proposed as a biomarker to distinguish between active pulmonary disease and latently infected individuals who do not exhibit disease symptoms (57). Using polychromatic flow cytometric analysis, patients with pulmonary TB disease have a higher proportion of single positive TNFα-producing M. tuberculosis-specific CD4+ T cells compared with individuals with latent

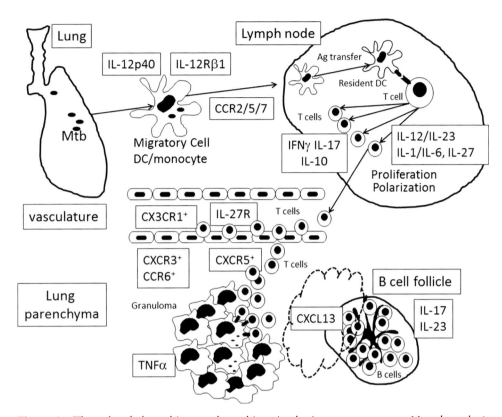

Figure 1   The role of chemokines and cytokines in the innate response to *M. tuberculosis* infection. Upon early infection of the lower airways, *M. tuberculosis* encounters alveolar macrophages and lung epithelial cells. Alveolar macrophages are a major source of proinflammatory cytokines (TNFα), although stromal cells can produce cytokines and chemokines that will also modulate immune responses. During early infection, dendritic cell trafficking from the lungs to the lymph node via CCR7 results in primed naive T cells and initiation of adaptive immune responses. Replicating bacteria generate a fulminant reaction that results in the mobilization and recruitment of both neutrophils and monocytes from the bone marrow via the induction of proinflammatory cytokines and chemokines. Regulation of cellular recruitment occurs via coordinated cytokine and chemokine induction. While initial recruitment of monocytes requires type I IFN, overexpression of this cytokine results in high levels of CCR2-expressing monocytes with limited ability to control bacterial growth. Type II IFN (IFNγ) regulates the recruitment of neutrophils, which is promoted by IL-17. CXCL5 and CXCR2 mediate the recruitment of damaging neutrophils. Mtb, *M. tuberculosis*.

infection (57). This was further confirmed in a blinded study whereby this parameter was the sole diagnostic for pulmonary TB disease (57). TNFα lies at the crux of the TB conundrum. It is critical for control of infection with both phagocyte-activating and granuloma-organizing functions, but too much TNFα can mediate tissue damage and promote transmission (Table 1).

The Interferons

The interferon family demonstrates the potential for similar cytokines to play protective and pathologic roles in TB disease. Based on receptor specificity and sequence homology, the interferons (IFNs) are classified into two

types (58). IFNγ is the only type II interferon and, while structurally related to the type I interferons IFNα and IFNβ, these cytokines use different receptors and have distinct chromosomal locations (58). Unlike type I IFNs that bind to a common heterodimeric receptor composed of IFNAR1 and IFNAR2 chains, IFNγ binds to the IFNγ receptor (IFNGR) which comprises two ligand-binding IFNGR1 chains that associate with two signal-transducing IFNGR2 chains (58). In addition, while IFNγ is essential for survival following *M. tuberculosis* infection the type I IFNs appear to be largely detrimental to the host during TB and may be coopted by the bacterium for its own ends (Table 1).

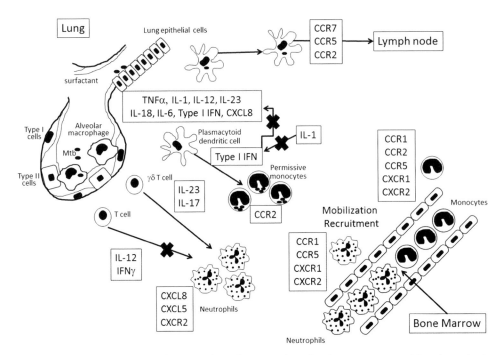

Figure 2 The role of chemokines and cytokines in the adaptive response to *M. tuberculosis* infection. Following *M. tuberculosis* infection of the lung, migratory cells take the bacteria to the draining lymph node likely using both cytokine (IL-12p40) and chemokine (CCR2, CCR7) pathways. Antigen is then transferred to antigen-presenting cells that stimulate naïve T cells via MHC class I and class II. Antigen-presenting cells make cytokines and chemokines to potentiate T-cell proliferation and polarization. Activated T cells migrate from the draining lymph node through the vasculature to the inflamed site. Some T cells remain in the vasculature (CX3CR3$^+$) while others migrate into the parenchyma (CXCR3$^+$CCR6$^+$). Expression of CXCR5 on antigen-specific T cells allows them to respond to IL-23- and IL-17-dependent CXCL13 and locate effectively within the granuloma, where they activate *M. tuberculosis*-infected macrophages. T cells express a variety of cytokines in the lung including IFNγ, TNFα, IL-17, and IL-10 that have both protective and negative effects depending upon the context.

Type II interferon (IFNγ)

IFNγ-IFNGR binding induces signaling within the cell primarily through the Janus kinase/signal transducers and activators of transcription (JAK-STAT) pathways and results in changes in both the migratory and functional capacity of multiple cell types such as macrophages, NK cells, and T cells (59–61). Innate production of IFNγ by phagocytes stimulated through their pattern recognition receptors results in early proinflammatory responses to infection (58, 62) and, unlike TNFα, which is regulated tightly by highly related molecules, production of IFNγ is regulated by cytokines such as IL-12 and IL-18, which are also secreted by immune surveillance cells upon ligation of their pattern recognition receptors (58, 63, 64).

Genetic deficiency in the IFNγ pathway in humans is associated with increased risk for mycobacterial disease and Mendelian susceptibility to mycobacterial disease (MSMD) (65, 66). Autosomal complete recessive IFNγR1-deficient patients exhibit a predisposition for mycobacterial infections manifesting early in life and with poor prognosis (67). IFNγR2 deficiency (either total protein loss or loss of function) has also been observed and results in a similar outcome to IFNγR1 deficiency (68, 69). Similarly, mice that do not express IFNγ because of targeted gene disruption are severely susceptible to both low-dose aerosol (70) and intravenous infection (71, 72) and exhibit poor macrophage activation and exacerbated granulocytic inflammation (70, 71).

The classic function of IFNγ is as a phagocyte-activating cytokine which instructs macrophages and other cells to change function. In particular, in the absence of IFNγ *M. tuberculosis* occupies an intracellular environment wherein there is little reactive radical production; the phagosome does not fuse with lysosomes and remains at neutral pH. There is also an ample supply of iron due to the location of the phagosome in the early endosomal pathway (73). While innate sources of IFNγ can activate macrophages, there is very little control of *M. tuberculosis* growth in the absence of α/β T cells or major histocompatibility complex (MHC) class II following aerosol infection (74), suggesting that both IFNγ and antigen-specific T cells are required for control of this infection. However, whether it is T cells producing IFNγ that are critical has not been definitively demonstrated, but the strongest support of a critical need of CD4+ T cells to make IFNγ is from a transfer model in mice (75). In contrast, memory T cells can mediate protection in the absence of either IFNγ or TNFα, suggesting other functions need to be identified (76). Both CD4+ and CD8+ T cells produce IFNγ and accumulate within the infected lung and, while absence of CD4+ T cells results in rapid susceptibility to *M. tuberculosis* infection, the absence of CD8+ T cells results in susceptibility later in the infection (77). The organization of the granuloma is also disrupted in the absence of CD4+ T cells with predominantly perivascular cuffing of lymphocytes observed (78), suggesting that, in the absence of CD4+ T cells, chemokine gradients are not established for T-cell migration. It is also the case that, while CD8+ T cells can make IFNγ during *M. tuberculosis* infection, they require CD4+ T cells to do so optimally (79).

The induction of IFNγ-producing T cells has been the focus of anti-TB vaccine design but has not been particularly fruitful. It is clear that humans need antigen-specific T-cell responses to control TB (because those with human immunodeficiency virus [HIV]/AIDS develop TB readily) and that absence of IFNγ promotes mycobacterial disease in humans, so why have we not progressed? Again, we come back to the issue of the communication between the T cells and the infected phagocytes. If the T cells are unable to colocate with the phagocytes and/or the phagocytes are unable to respond to the signals delivered by the T cells, then the number of IFNγ-producing T cells circulating throughout the body is meaningless. It is therefore the case that IFNγ production by activated T cells is not a correlate of protection, rather the ability of antigen-specific T cells to penetrate and survive within the infected site may be. In this regard, recent studies demonstrate that not all cytokine-producing antigen-specific T cells are able to penetrate the TB granuloma and some remain in the vasculature or cuff around the vessels and this is related to their expression of transcription factors, chemokine receptors, and differentiation state (80–82); these markers should perhaps be considered as correlates of protection.

IFNγ can act on cells other than macrophages; indeed, its most critical function in TB may not be to activate macrophages but rather to limit polymorphonuclear (PMN) inflammation (Fig. 1). Most susceptible mouse strains exhibit high PMN infiltration in the lungs once infected (83–86), and inhibition of this infiltration improves survival (83). Mice that lack IFNγ exhibit high PMN infiltration as do mice lacking CD4+ T cells (70, 78). Neutrophils that lack the IFNγR fail to undergo apoptosis and accumulate in the lungs of *M. tuberculosis*-infected mice, and their removal improves survival without altering bacterial burden (87). Similarly, chimeric mice lacking IFNγR on their radio-resistant cells overexpress IL-17 and have excessive neutrophil recruitment and reduced survival (88). It is possible that the high IFNγ-producing CD4+ T cells that populate the vasculature (80, 82) are located in such a position to reduce neutrophil accumulation.

Production of IFNγ is a very useful diagnostic tool that has been developed to be more selective than the older skin test assay. In this prominent test for *M. tuberculosis* exposure, *M. tuberculosis* antigens (selected to be unique for *M. tuberculosis* versus other mycobacteria) are used to stimulate IFNγ release (89–91). While this test selects for those who are exposed, it is not optimized to distinguish between those individuals who are infected but healthy and those in the process of developing active disease. Recently, studies have shown that patients that have more IFNγ-producing T cells are actually more likely to progress to active disease, suggesting that this test may be optimized to identify those progressing toward disease (92).

Type I interferon (IFN)

The interferons were first identified more than half a century ago for their antiviral activity (93). Type I IFNs represent the largest group, with at least 13 gene products identified in humans and mice, with IFNα and IFNβ being the best classified and the focus of this section. For clarity, IFNα and IFNβ will be collectively referred to as IFNα/β throughout this section. The innate response to pathogens occurs via Toll-like receptor (TLR) engagement resulting in a complex cytosolic cascade of signal transduction toward IFN-regulatory factor3/7 (IRF3/7)-mediated transcription of IFNα/β genes (94). Secreted IFNα/β engages IFN subunit receptors 1 and 2 (IFNAR1/2) at the cell surface, which then activate dimers of the tyrosine kinases JAK and tyrosine kinase (TYK) (94, 95). The end result is activation of IFN-stimulated gene factor (ISG) that then interacts with IFN-stimulated response elements (ISRE) at the promoters of IFNα/β-regulated genes (94, 95).

The type I IFNs were not thought to play a major role in *M. tuberculosis* infection and indeed infection of IFNAR-deficient mice with a low-dose aerosol of *M. tuberculosis* Erdman strain did not indicate any major impact of the loss of this receptor (96). However, use of strains with increased virulence, such as the W-Beijing strain HN878, has revealed an important strain-dependent outcome in relation to type I IFNs. The pathogenesis of *M. tuberculosis* strain HN878 is associated with IFNα/β-dependent reduction in the activity of the proinflammatory cytokines IFNγ, TNFα, IL-6, and IL-12, as well as in the anti-inflammatory IL-10 (97, 98) (Fig. 1). Intranasal delivery of IFNα/β also results in increased bacterial burden and reduced survival in contrast to IFNγ-treated mice (97). Furthermore, IFNα/β signaling interferes with IFNγ-mediated killing of *M. tuberculosis* (99). One hypothesis regarding the role of type I IFNs during chronic *M. tuberculosis* infection is that the accumulation of plasmacytoid dendritic cells in the lung provides a source of excess type I IFN which then inhibits the accumulation of CD4$^+$ and CD8$^+$ T cells in the lung (98) (Fig. 1). Finally, transcriptional analysis of peripheral blood cells from those exposed to TB shows that both IFNγ and type I IFN signatures occur, but that the type I IFN signature is predominantly associated with neutrophils (100).

In a mechanistic analysis of the function of IFNα/β in TB, polyinosinic-polycytidylic acid and poly-L-lysine and carboxymethylcellulose (poly-IC) were used to induce elevated levels of IFNα/β during *M. tuberculosis* infection (101). This poly-IC treatment results in elevated bacterial burden and increases the recruitment of an apparently permissive CD11b$^+$GR1^{int} cell phenotype recruited via chemokine (C-C motif) ligand 2 (CCL2) and C-C chemokine receptor type 2 (CCR2) (101) (Fig. 1). Similarly, careful analysis of the cells recruited to the lungs of mice lacking either type I or type II IFN receptors demonstrates a protective function for type I IFN signaling in that, in its absence, initial recruitment of target host cells for *M. tuberculosis* does not occur and immunity is compromised (102).

IFNα/β is another perfect example of a "goldilocks" cytokine in TB (Table 1). Just enough is required to initiate recruitment of phagocytes that provide activatable host cells for *M. tuberculosis* to invade; however, production of too much IFNα/β results in large numbers of permissive cells that cannot be effectively activated. Also, too much of this cytokine can limit the activation state of the infected phagocytes and potentially limit the accumulation and function of the T cells required to regulate the mononuclear structure of the granuloma.

Interleukin-6

Interleukin-6 (IL-6) is a pleiotropic cytokine produced in response to inflammatory stimuli (103) and is involved in the essential cellular processes of differentiation, proliferation, and apoptosis. Many cell types express IL-6, including those of lymphoid and nonlymphoid origin (103), and expression can be induced by other cytokines including IL-1, TNFα, and IFNγ (104, 105). IL-6 signals through soluble and membrane-bound IL-6R of which the glycoprotein 130 dimer (gp130) is an essential component (106). Downstream signaling is mediated by a phosphorylation cascade involving JAK, mitogen-activated protein kinase (MAPK), and STAT pathways (106, 107). The pluripotency of IL-6 warrants regulation and this is mediated by suppressor of cytokine signaling (SOCS), which inhibits STAT signaling (106, 107).

The relative importance of IL-6 during TB depends upon the route and dose of infection. As we have discussed, communication between cells is critical for successful expression of immunity and, if the dose is low or bacteria are slow to grow, then the kinetics of the cellular response are not critical. However, if the dose is high and systemic, then the kinetics of the response becomes critical. This concept is illustrated by IL-6, because in its absence (either by antibody treatment or by gene deletion) there is increased susceptibility to intravenous challenge with a large dose of mycobacteria (108, 109). In contrast, in a low-dose aerosol *M. tuberculosis* challenge model, while modestly increased bacterial burden occurs in the lungs of IL-6-deficient mice, the impact is not lethal (110). In both the low- and high-dose challenge models, increased IL-4, as well as reduced or delayed T-cell accumulation and IFNγ expression, is observed, suggesting that IL-6 can act to potentiate IFNγ expression at the site of infection (108, 110). It appears also that IL-6 is required for optimal induction of protective responses during vaccination, because, in its absence, both BCG and a subunit vaccine are less effective (109, 111).

Interpretation of the role of IL-6 in TB is complicated by the fact that the soluble IL-6 receptor can mediate *trans*-signaling and is implicated in inflammatory diseases such as inflammatory bowel disease (112). To address the role of IL-6 further, a gp130 construct capable of sequestering IL-6 in the blood (sgp130FC) was delivered to mice during *M. tuberculosis* infection, but no impact on disease progression was seen. In contrast, when mice are made to overexpress this construct, a temporary but significant increase in bacterial burden occurs during acute infection (113). This observation is consistent with an early role of IL-6 in potentiating immunity during early *M. tuberculosis* infection.

In vivo data support a protective role for IL-6 in the induction of early protective responses mediated through IFNγ (108, 110). Human studies also give us considerable insights into the role of IL-6 during TB. Cavitary TB is the most destructive form of caseous TB whereby necrosis liquefies cellular material and results in compromised lung function. Humans with cavitary TB express lower levels of IL-6 and the chemokine IP-10 in their bronchial alveolar lavage (BAL) fluid in comparison with TB patients without cavitary disease, thereby indicating IL-6 and IP-10 as potential markers of controlled (noncavitary) TB (114). As would be expected, elevated neutrophils were observed in BAL from cavitary TB patients, while noncavitary TB patients presented with elevated alveolar macrophages (114); interestingly, there was no correlation between cytokine expression in BAL fluid and serum cytokine production (114). In contrast, an earlier study identified elevated blood plasma levels of IL-6 from TB patients with developed lung lesions (115). Based on the mechanistic data from animal studies and the human data, IL-6 appears to be associated with effective early expression of immunity in the lung via the combination of regulated mononuclear inflammation and rapid accumulation of lymphocytes. Its effects are modest but may be critical following high-dose exposure or during immunodeficiency.

IL-1 Cytokines

The proinflammatory cytokines IL-1α, IL-1β (collectively called IL-1 here), and IL-18 are members of the IL-1 family (116). IL-1 was first identified in the 1940s as an endogenous pyrogen (117–119). IL-1 and IL-18 as well as their respective receptors (IL-1R1 and IL-18R) are widely expressed by all nucleated cells of the body including endothelial cells, monocytes, macrophages, and neutrophils (116). Expression of IL-1 and IL-18 is mediated in part by the canonical pathway of inflammasome activation, which involves the sensor (e.g., TLR), an adaptor molecule such as myeloid differentiation primary response gene 88 (MyD88), and caspase-1 (120–122). Alternatively, IL-1β and IL-18 can also be induced by the noncanonical inflammasome pathway that is distinguished by the activation of caspase-8 and -11 on the precursor of the cytokines in the cytosol (123, 124). MyD88 is an important cytosolic mediator linking TLR signaling to the transcription of inflammasome components (122).

IL-1α is mostly associated with sterile cell injury (e.g., cigarette smoke), but is also induced during non-sterile cell injury (e.g., bacterial) where it functions locally as an alarmin (125–130). IL-1β is induced during infection and is primarily produced by monocytes, macrophages, and dendritic cells (131–134). IL-1 signals through the IL-1R1 receptor present on a number of cells including endothelial cells, monocytes, macrophages, and T lymphocytes (116, 128, 135, 136). IL-18 is expressed constitutively in the cytosol at low levels as a precursor, which is activated by caspase-1 activity following bacterial stimulation, stimulation by neutrophils or by IL-4 or IFNγ (137–139). IL-18 activity results from colocalization of IL-18 receptor alpha (IL-18Rα) and IL-18 receptor beta (IL-18Rβ) on host cells including monocytes and epithelial cells (140).

IL-1R/IL18R/MyD88

Signaling through MyD88 is shared between TLR, IL-1R, and IL-18R (141–143). MyD88 is an essential component in innate signaling in response to TB, because MyD88 gene-deficient mice exhibit profound susceptibility to *M. tuberculosis* infection (143). Importantly, following mycobacterial stimulation, MyD88 gene-deficient macrophages and dendritic cells exhibit reduced IL-6, TNF, and IL-12p40 production, suggesting a critical role for MyD88 in pattern recognition responses to *M. tuberculosis* infection (143). Aerosol infection results in dramatically increased lung burden coinciding with increased inflammation and accumulation of neutrophils and macrophages (143). Despite the poor innate response to *M. tuberculosis* infection in the MyD88 gene-deficient mice, the accumulation of IFNγ-producing T cells was not affected. It is likely that these antigen-specific cytokine-producing T cells were unable to mediate protection because of failures within the phagocytes accumulating at the site or as a result of being unable to communicate with the infected phagocytes (143). That BCG vaccination results in protection against *M. tuberculosis* infection in MyD88-deficient mice suggests that it is a failure of T cells to accumulate rapidly enough in naive mice that contributes to their susceptibility (143).

What then is MyD88 signaling doing? Comparison of the phenotype of IL-1-deficient mice and MyD88-deficient mice is suggestive in this regard, because both exhibit increased susceptibility with focal necrosis despite generation and accumulation of cytokine-producing T cells (144). These observations suggest that induction of IL-1 is likely Myd88 dependent and that this pathway plays a critical role in protective immunity to TB.

IL-1

IL-1α and IL-1β are interdependent proinflammatory cytokines critical to defense against TB (145–149).

Mice lacking either IL-1α or IL-1β or both are suscepti-ble to acute and chronic infection, respectively, follow-ing challenge with *M. tuberculosis* (145–148). IL-1 α/β double-deficient mice share a similar susceptibility to infection as IL-1R1KO and MyD88KO mice (143, 144, 148, 150). Deficiencies in the IL-1 pathway (IL-1 α/β or IL-1R1) have no impact on the protection against BCG delivered intravenously, suggesting that virulence of the pathogen is a factor in the role of the IL-1 pathway (146). Anti-IL1α and anti-IL-1α/β antibodies delivered subcutaneously to *M. tuberculosis*-infected mice have also been shown to result in loss of body weight and lethality (148). Furthermore, lung sections from anti-IL-1α-treated mice exhibit lung parenchyma consumed by cellular infiltrates (148). During sterile mediated in-flammation, IL-1α appears to be involved in the ex-pression of proinflammatory cytokines such as IL-6 in primary fibroblasts (151), which may be associated with mobilization of neutrophils (152). It has also re-cently been observed that, upon activation of the in-flammasome, IL-1β and IL-18 are capable of inducing expression of the neutrophil-recruiting cytokine IL-17 (153–155). IL-17 responses are essential in the pro-tection against some *M. tuberculosis* strains, such as HN878 and for recall responses to H37Rv (149, 156, 157). Consistent with this, IL-1R1 gene-deficient mice infected with the *M. tuberculosis* strain HN878 pro-duce decreased levels of IL-17 and decreased popula-tions of IL-17-producing cells *in vitro* and *in vivo* (149).

IL-1 is produced by CD11b⁺Ly6G⁻ cells following *M. tuberculosis* infection (145), and rescue of the lethal phenotype in IL-1α mice can be accomplished by di-rected viral expression of IL-1α in CD11c⁺ cells trans-planted in IL-1α gene-deficient mice (147). It would seem, therefore, that a primary function of the IL-1/IL-1R pathway is to mediate the recruitment and coor-dination of cellular responses by the induction of pro-inflammatory cytokines from the stroma (145, 147). One critical aspect of IL-1 function is in promotion of prostaglandin E₂ (PGE₂), which in turn mediates inhi-bition of type I IFN-induced accumulation of permis-sive macrophages at the site of infection (158) (Fig. 1). Prostaglandins such as PGE₂ are produced by the ac-tion of cyclooxygenase (COX) enzymes on arachidonic acid, and, in the absence of inducible COX enzymes, mice are highly susceptible to *M. tuberculosis* infection, and delivery of PGE₂ during *M. tuberculosis* infection results in a partial rescue of the lethal phenotype in IL-1α/β-infected mice (158). Taken together, the underlying function of IL-1 in *M. tuberculosis* appears to be in regulating type I IFN function and helping to maintain the balance between sufficient phagocytes to

mediate control of the intracellular pathogen, while in-hibiting the overrecruitment of permissive macrophages mediated by type I IFN (102).

IL-18

IL-18 is essential for the production of IFNγ from T cells under some conditions (159–163), and, in some instances, its absence can result in increased suscep-tibility to *M. tuberculosis* (150), although, in other con-ditions, increased susceptibility to *M. tuberculosis* infection is not observed (162, 163). Interestingly, when susceptibility is observed, the accumulation of neutro-phils and inflammatory chemokines CXCL1 and CXCL2 is elevated, and depletion of neutrophils and monocytes from the lung results in decreased bacterial burden (150). In *M. tuberculosis*-infected IL-18-deficient mice, an in-creased frequency of IFNγ-producing CD4⁺ and CD8⁺ T cells in the lungs is seen, but total IFNγ production by these T-cell populations is decreased, suggesting that IL-18 could contribute to optimal IFNγ induction dur-ing TB (150, 162, 163). It would appear, therefore, that IL-18 plays a role in inducing high IFNγ production in T cells, but that this is not required for protection, and that its more critical role (perhaps when dose or viru-lence of the *M. tuberculosis* strain is high) is that of reg-ulator of phagocyte accumulation, possibly mirroring the role of IL-1 and MyD88.

Our working model of immunity to TB places the emphasis on rapid and correct accumulation of both phagocytes (macrophages and neutrophils) and T cells to the site of infection. This accumulation is initiated by the innate sensors within the lung and results in the induction of TNF, IFNs, and IL-1 family members. The correct ratio of these cytokines is essential for the bal-ance of permissive and nonpermissive phagocytes and for the development of a granuloma such that infected phagocytes and antigen-specific T cells can communi-cate effectively to stop *M. tuberculosis* growth. How the antigen-specific T cells develop and are regulated is covered below.

IL-12 Cytokine Family

The IL-12 family of cytokines belongs to the IL-6 super-family and is the only family composed of heterodimeric cytokines (164, 165), and this unique feature bestows diverse and pleiotropic functions because of promiscu-ous chain pairing (166). The alpha chains of the IL-12 family (p19, p28, and p35) contain four-helix bundle structures and pair with one of two beta chains (either p40 or Epstein-Barr virus-induced gene 3 [Ebi3]) (164–166). IL-12 is composed of the subunits p35/p40, IL-23 of p19/p40, IL-27 of p28/Ebi3, and IL-35 of p35/

Ebi3 with expression of the distinct subunits being regulated independently (166). In addition, IL-12p40 can also be secreted both as a homodimer (IL-12p80 or IL-12p(40)$_2$) and as a monomer (IL-12p40) (167). Both macrophages and dendritic cells are major producers of IL-12p40, IL-12, IL-23, and IL-27 (168). These cytokines are largely associated with the induction and regulation of cytokine expression within antigen-stimulated T-cell populations.

IL-12

IL-12 plays an important role as a link between innate and adaptive immune responses, and is produced by and influences multiple effector cells (169, 170). Composed of IL-12p35 and IL-12/23p40, IL-12 (IL-12p70) is primarily secreted by macrophages, dendritic cells, and B cells (166, 171, 172). The importance of IL-12 in TB is dramatically illustrated by several experiments of nature wherein humans with IL-12p40 deficiency display an inherent predisposition to *M. tuberculosis* infection (173–178). Furthermore, patients with MSMD harbor deficiencies in IL-12Rβ1, IFNγR1, and IL-12p40, and exhibit susceptibility to *M. tuberculosis* and develop BCGosis following delivery of the BCG vaccine (66, 178–181). Genetic etiology for MSMD is associated with mutations in the autosomal genes *IFNGR1*, *IFNGR2*, *STAT1*, *IL12B*, *IL12BR1*, and X-linked gene *IKKBG*, encoding NF-κB essential modulator (NEMO) (66). All these autosomal genes are associated with IL-12/IFNγ-dependent signaling and the IFNγ-mediated activation of macrophages. Mutations in *IKKBG* impair CD40-dependent IL-12 production in monocytes and dendritic cells, despite normal CD40-mediated induction of costimulatory molecules on dendritic cells (182). These human data highlight the importance of this pathway to TB control.

IL-12 is expressed within the lung at the site of TB (183) and delivery of IL-12 to *M. tuberculosis*-infected mice decreases bacterial burden, while reduction of IL-12 by antibody increases bacterial burden (184). Interestingly, delivery of IL-12 also modestly improves the outcome for mice lacking acquired cellular immunity, suggesting that it can mediate immunity via direct action on innate cells (184). Mice genetically deficient for the IL-12p40 subunit are acutely susceptible to *M. tuberculosis* infection (185, 186), whereas those lacking IL-12p35 exhibit prolonged survival relative to the IL-12p40-deficient mice (186). This, in turn, is dependent on the availability of the IL-23p19 subunit (187). The absence of IL-12p40 results in the substantial loss of antigen-specific IFNγ production (185, 186) (Fig. 2), while the presence of IL-23p19 in the

IL-12p35-deficient mice appears to promote sufficient antigen-specific IFNγ production to increase protection relative to the IL-12p40-deficient mice (187). It also appears that stable and prolonged IL-12 production is required to maintain IFNγ production and to limit bacterial growth long term (188). This requirement for long-term function may also apply in humans, because absence of the IL-12R1 results in poor accumulation of IFNγ-producing memory T cells (189). The innate pattern recognition receptors, TLR2 and TLR9, are necessary for optimal production of IL-12p40 in response to *M. tuberculosis* exposure (190), while the *M. tuberculosis* lipoarabinomannans have been shown to negatively regulate TLR-mediated IL-12 production by inducing an inhibitor of TLR signaling, IRAK-M (191). In contrast, mycobacterial LprA is a TLR2 agonist and promotes IL-12p40 production (192), reflecting the need for *M. tuberculosis* to both induce and regulate IL-12p40 for its own ends.

IL-12 signals through interactions between IL-12/23p40, and IL-12p35 with IL-12Rβ1 and IL-12Rβ2, respectively (193–195), with the IL-12p40 interacting with IL-12Rβ1 on the target cell surface, thereby allowing the IL-12Rβ2 to induce JAK and STAT signaling and activate STAT4 homodimers (166). The homodimer IL-12p40, IL-12(p40)$_2$, antagonizes IL-12-mediated immune responses through competitive binding of IL-12Rβ1 (196–198). However, in TB, it appears that IL-12(p40)$_2$ can also function as an agonist (199), and supports dendritic cell migration to the draining lymph nodes (200, 201), to promote T-cell priming and differentiation (200). Specifically, following *M. tuberculosis* infection, dendritic cells are thought to be the first immune cells to traffic to the draining lymph node (202), and this may occur in an IL-12p40- and IL-12Rβ1-dependent manner (200, 203). Bone marrow-derived dendritic cells from mice deficient in IL-12p40 are unable to activate naive T cells in the draining lymph node following delivery to the lung and fail to confer protective adaptive responses (200). However, treatment of the IL-12p40-deficient dendritic cells with the homodimer IL-12(p40)$_2$ is sufficient to restore migration of the dendritic cells to the draining lymph node and for activation of naive T cells to occur (200). Expression of IL-12Rβ1 is also required to facilitate dendritic cell migration to the draining lymph node (203) and, indeed, CD11c$^+$ cells in the *M. tuberculosis*-infected lung express an alternative splice variant of IL-12Rβ1 that augments IL-12Rβ1-mediated effects (203). In particular, dendritic cells expressing the splice variant exhibit enhanced migration from the infected lung to the draining lymph nodes and supported activation of *M. tuberculosis*-specific T cells (203) (Fig. 2). In an interesting example of cytokine cross talk, mice lacking the p75 receptor for TNF (TNFRp75) exhibit increased IL-12p40 and enhanced IL-12p40-mediated dendritic cell trafficking to draining lymph nodes (204). Thus, IL-12Rβ1 is important for the effector function of IL-12p40 on dendritic cells, as well as mediating recruitment and function of CD4 T cells in response to TB.

IL-23

IL-23 utilizes the p40 beta subunit paired with the alpha chain p19 (205). Before the discovery of IL-23, the interpretation of data from IL-12p40- and IL-12p35-deficient models of disease had been difficult (206). Specifically, studies found that the outcome of IL-12p35 deficiency was not always the same as in IL-12p40-deficient models (207–209). The discovery of IL-23 led to the reassessment of the role of IL-12p40 (205, 206, 208, 209), and disease models previously associated with IL-12 were, in fact, shown to be primarily driven by IL-23 and not IL-12 or they clarified unique disease-driving features of the two cytokines (206, 208–211). Currently, IL-23 and IL-23 pathway antagonists are in phase 2 and phase 3 clinical trials for treating patients with moderate to severe psoriasis (207), making the determination of the role of IL-23 in TB a critical undertaking. IL-23 stabilizes the induction of the T$_H$17 cell subset, which produces IL-17A, IL-17F, and IL-22, and it is also required for the double expression of IL-17 and IFNγ (212). However, IL-23 alone is not sufficient to drive differentiation of T$_H$17 cells, which requires the key cytokines transforming growth factor β (TGFβ) and IL-6 (213). In addition, IL-23 can also induce IFNγ production in human T cells as well as support the proliferation of mouse memory T cells (205, 214). The interaction with its receptor, composed of IL-23R and IL-12Rβ1 subunits, activates the downstream signaling molecules, JAK and STAT, for production of its signature cytokines (166, 205, 214–216). IL-23 primarily signals through STAT3, while IL-12 can signal through STAT1, 3, 5, and 4, but preferentially signals through STAT4 (166). Upon infection with *M. tuberculosis*, lung dendritic cells produce IL-23, likely mediating the induction of IL-17 production (187, 217, 218).

Although IL-23 is important for generation of *M. tuberculosis*-specific IL-17-producing T cells (Fig. 2), mice deficient in IL-23p19 control *M. tuberculosis* effectively for up to 90 days whereupon bacterial growth increases relative to intact mice (187, 219). In addition, treatment of *M. tuberculosis*-infected mice with adenovirus-expressing IL-23 reduces *M. tuberculosis*

burden and increases cellular responses (220). In the absence of IL-23p19, *M. tuberculosis*-infected mice did not develop well-organized B-cell follicles, and this was associated with a complete absence of IL-17 and IL-22 in the lung. In addition, there was very little expression of the B-cell follicle-associated chemokine CXCL13 resulting in increased accumulation of lymphocytes around the vessels rather than within the granulomatous regions (219) (Fig. 2). Thus, in support of our working model, coordinated communication between lymphocytes and infected macrophages is inefficient in the absence of specific cytokines/chemokines (in this case, IL-23-dependent CXCL13) and bacterial growth occurs in the absence of this efficient communication.

IL-23 also plays a chemokine-dependent role in the efficient expression of vaccine-induced mucosal immunity. This role was first highlighted in mice subcutaneously vaccinated with an adjuvant-paired I-A^b-restricted ESAT6$_{(1-20)}$ peptide, which induces both IFNγ- and IL-17-producing antigen-specific CD4$^+$ T cell responses (157). Critically, the improved kinetics of the vaccine-induced IFNγ-producing T cells is lost in the absence of IL-23, because this cytokine is required for the generation of lung resident IL-17 producing CD4$^+$ memory T cells that generate a chemokine gradient facilitating the accelerated IFNγ response. In the absence of IL-23, vaccine-induced protection to *M. tuberculosis* challenge is lost (157). Coimmunization of mice with a DNA vaccine composed of *M. tuberculosis* antigen 85B (Ag85B) and an IL-23-expressing plasmid also confers enhanced protection through the induction of augmented T-cell proliferation and IFNγ production in comparison with Ag85B alone (217). Other studies also support an important role for IL-17-producing CD4$^+$ T-cell subsets in mediating mucosal vaccine-driven protection (156, 221–223). Specifically, adoptive transfer of *M. tuberculosis*-specific IL-17-producing T cells into unchallenged mice confers protection following exposure to *M. tuberculosis* (156). Furthermore, use of adjuvants capable of driving lung-resident IL-17-producing cells is able to initiate early CXCL13 expression, thereby promoting appropriate accumulation of CXCR5$^+$ T cells within the *M. tuberculosis*-induced inflammatory site (221). These IL-17-producing T cells are long lived (222) and are associated with improved protection when recombinant BCG vaccines are used (223).

IL-27

IL-12 and IL-23 are proinflammatory cytokines with the capacity to drive cytokine production in T cells (168, 224, 225). In contrast to this clear role for IL-12 and IL-23, IL-27 is pluripotent and has a complex and sometimes apparently contradictory capacity to influence inflammation and lymphocyte function (166, 226–228), indicating a pleiotropic nature for IL-27. IL-27 is composed of the p28 alpha and Ebi3 beta chains, and signals through the IL-27Rα (WSX-1 or TCCR) and gp130 receptor subunits (166, 229, 230). IL-27 can mediate suppression of IL-17-production by T cells (231) via STAT1 signaling to promote IL-10-producing Tr1cell-like regulatory populations (232). It also promotes proliferation (229) and polarization via T-bet (233) in naive T cells (Fig. 2).

In the context of *M. tuberculosis* infection, IL-27R-deficient mice challenged with *M. tuberculosis* exhibit lower bacterial burden in the lungs and increased granuloma-localized lymphocytes (234, 235), but these mice succumb to disease earlier than control animals (235). Thus, while IL-27R activity appears to limit expression of immunity locally, it may actually protect from undue pathologic damage. Because of the pleiotropic nature of IL-27 it is very difficult to dissect out its specific function in TB. The absence of the gp130 component of the IL-27R on phagocytes during *M. tuberculosis* infection results in loss of the increased inflammatory consequences of IL-27R deficiency but does not impact the reduced bacterial burden seen in mice lacking IL-27R on all cells, suggesting that these two aspects of IL-27R deficiency are independent (236). In contrast, mice lacking IL-27R only on T cells exhibit the improved ability to control bacterial burden over the long term (82). This improvement was associated with enhanced localization and reduced differentiation (i.e., reduced T-bet expression) of IL-27R-deficient CD4+ T cells within the infected lung parenchyma. *M. tuberculosis*-specific CD4+ T cells lacking IL-27R are also intrinsically fitter than IL-27R-sufficient CD4+ T cells in mice within the same environment (82) (Fig. 2). The importance of IL-27 is further confirmed in human patients, wherein IL-27 is significantly increased in patients with active TB compared with latently infected individuals (82). In our working model of TB immunity, IL-27 appears to play the role of mediator of increased inflammation within the phagocyte population while also serving to limit the efficacy of the T-cell population by driving them to a state of differentiation that limits their ability to locate to, and persist within, the inflamed granuloma.

IL-35

IL-35, a dimeric protein encoded by IL-12α and IL-27β chains, has been shown to suppress CD4+ T-cell responses (237). It is thought to be primarily expressed by regulatory T (T$_{REG}$) cells (238) and is required for

optimal function both *in vivo* and *in vitro* (239). IL-35 is important for the generation of human and mouse T$_{REG}$ cells, termed iT$_R$35 cells (239), which function independently of IL-10 and TGFβ. While a specific function for IL-35 in *M. tuberculosis* infection has not been directly addressed, the relative availability of IL-35 in the presence and absence of the other IL-12 family subunits makes consideration of this cytokine an important part of any interpretation of outcome in mice or humans lacking IL-12 family subunits.

IL-23-Dependent Cytokines

IL-17

The IL-17 cytokine family is composed of six members, IL-17A to IL-17F, with IL-17A and IL-17F being the most studied. Production of IL-17 is conventionally attributed to T cells, but other lymphocytes as well as innate immune cells can produce this cytokine (240). IL-17 cytokines are proinflammatory and can be protective or pathogenic depending on the nature of the challenge faced by the host (241, 242). It is at mucosal sites that IL-17 plays its most important regulatory and protective role against invading pathogens.

Following mycobacterial infection, lung-resident γδ T cells are a primary source of early IL-17 (218), and likely support early neutrophil accumulation (243) (Fig. 1). Following BCG infection, IL-17 expression can be detected as early as day 1 postinfection and is dependent on IL-23 expression (243). One recently identified capacity of IL-17 is to regulate mycobacterially induced IL-10 (244). Following vaccination with BCG, dendritic cells produce PGE$_2$, which is required for the induction of both IL-10 and IL-23 with the IL-23 being required for IL-17 production (244). This IL-17 is then thought to downregulate IL-10 production, thereby allowing increased IL-12 that subsequently promotes IFNγ production. In the absence of IL-10, the IL-23-mediated IL-17 is not required and, in the absence of IL-23, BCG fails to effectively induce protective IFNγ-producing T cells (244). This study was the first to show that PGE$_2$ induction of IL-17 was sufficient to overcome the inhibitory effects of IL-10 and support the generation of antigen-specific and cytokine-producing T cells during mycobacterial vaccination and challenge.

As with IL-23, low-dose challenge with some strains of IL-17A (i.e., H37Rv and CDC1551) in the absence of IL-17 results in no obvious phenotype (149, 187, 245) until late in disease (219). In contrast, following infection with the W-Beijing strain HN878 of *M. tuberculosis*, IL-17R expression on radio-resistant cells (likely fibroblasts) of the lung is required to coordinate the rapid accumulation of cells within the lung via the induction of CXCL13 and recruitment of CXCR5+ T cells to lymphoid follicles within the tissue (149) (Fig. 2). Importantly, the W-Beijing HN878 *M. tuberculosis* strain induces high levels of IL-1β and IL-17 relative to other *M. tuberculosis* strains (149) and also induces excess type I IFN (97), which is capable of bringing in permissive macrophages in a CCR2-dependent manner (101) (Fig. 1). HN878 induces an environment that is highly permissive for its growth, and it is this environment that results in the need for the optimum expression of immunity wherein IL-17 promotes rapid accumulation and the correct localization of the T cells needed to change the permissive macrophages to ones that limit bacterial growth (149).

The role of IL-17 in initiating early coordination of cellular responses in naive mice is apparent when the challenge is significant as in the case of HN878; however, the concept of IL-17 as a coordinator of early mucosal responses in TB actually stems from vaccine work. Initial studies using a defined subunit vaccine determined that lung-resident IL-17-producing cells induced by vaccination are vital for the induction of the chemokines (CXCL9, CXCL10, and CXCL11) required for the accumulation of IFNγ-producing memory T cells (157). Further studies have shown that adoptive transfer of *M. tuberculosis*-specific IL-17-producing T cells into naive mice is able to mediate protection in an aerosol challenge model, thereby identifying these types of cells as valid targets for vaccine-mediated induction (156). Finally, mucosal immunization with *M. tuberculosis* antigens induces potent IL-17 responses that improve upon BCG vaccine-induced protection in mice (221). Interestingly, in mucosal vaccine models, IL-17 rather than IFNγ appears to be most important for vaccine-induced protection against *M. tuberculosis*, providing support for the model that it is the coordination of the cellular response that is the determining factor in the success of vaccination (221, 246). Critically, antigen-specific IL-17-producing memory T cells are induced by vaccination and respond up to 2 years postvaccination (222). These memory T cells appear to be metastable and become IFNγ producers within the lung (222), probably as a result of the action of IL-23 (212). In fact, pluripotent memory T cells capable of producing not only IL-17 but also TNF and IL-2 may be the most appropriate target T cells for vaccination (247). Manipulation of BCG can also result in increased induction of IL-17-producing memory cells, and this is associated with improved protection as in the case of the recombinant BCG strain rBCGΔureC:Hly (223).

Thus, IL-17 drives the induction of CXCL9-11 to recruit protective antigen-specific T cells, as well as CXCL-13 to localize CXCR5+ cytokine-producing T cells within TB granulomas. Despite the protective outcome of IL-17 discussed above, IL-23-dependent IL-17 production is also associated with damaging neutrophil accumulation during a chronic restimulation model of TB (248). Indeed, exacerbated production of IL-17 appears to drive pathology by inducing S100A8/A9 proteins that recruit neutrophils into the lung (249). Thus, IL-17 also fits the bill as a "goldilocks" cytokine in TB (Table 1).

IL-22
IL-22 is primarily produced by CD4+ T cells as well as γδ T cells, natural killer (NK) cells, and innate lymphoid cells following exposure to innate or infectious stimuli (250). IL-22 can have dual effects in the context of inflammation, and this has been attributed to its coexpression along with IL-17 (250, 251). The major functions of IL-22 are the regeneration and survival of the intestinal, airway, and external epithelium, as well as stimulating the secretion of antimicrobial peptides such as lipocalin and β-defensin (245, 250, 252). In the context of *M. tuberculosis*, IL-22 is expressed at higher levels than IL-17 at the site of infection and within granulomas from TB patients and NHP models (253, 254). Furthermore, in NHPs infected with *M. tuberculosis*, CD4+ T cells expressing membrane-bound IL-22 limit *M. tuberculosis* intracellular growth in macrophages (255). IL-22 can also inhibit intracellular growth of *M. tuberculosis* in human monocyte-derived macrophages by promoting phagolysosomal fusion and induction of Calgranulin A, a heterodimer of S100A8 and S100A9 proteins (256). Moreover, human NK cells cultured with *M. tuberculosis*-infected macrophages produce IL-22 and mediate macrophage activation (257). Finally, IL-22 increases as patients receive anti-TB treatment, and this has been associated with a decrease in a regulatory B-cell population (CD19+CD1d+ CD5+ B cell), the *in vitro* depletion of which results in enhanced IL-22 production by T cells (258).

Animal studies using low-dose aerosol challenge indicate that, in uncomplicated infection models, IL-22-producing T cells accumulate in the lung and express IFNγ (259). In the absence of this cytokine, however, there appear to be no significant consequences (260). However, in a BCG vaccine model, NK1.1+ cells appear to make IL-22, which contributes to protection by regulating T_REG cells (261). Taken together, the current data suggest a protective role for IL-22 in TB disease progression, possibly via antimicrobial peptide production, cellular function, and promotion of epithelial repair.

Regulatory Cytokines

IL-4, IL-5, IL-13

IL-4 was first described as a product of CD4$^+$ T lymphocytes that are now known as T$_H$2 T cells (262, 263). T$_H$2 responses inhibit T$_H$1 responses (264–266). IL-4, IL-5, and IL-13 are the signature cytokines associated with T$_H$2 responses; they are induced in response to helminth infections and contribute to diseases such as asthma and allergy (267–270); they mediate expulsion of multicellular parasites occupying mucosal tissues. IL-4R signaling requires heterodimerization of IL-4Rα (shared with IL-13) and the common gamma chain (shared with IL-2) (271). The IL-4 receptor (IL-4R) is the primary mediator of action, and ligation of IL-4R results in signal transduction via STAT-6 and subsequent GATA-3 transcription (272–275). Both STAT-6 and GATA-3 distinguish T$_H$2 cells from other T$_H$ cells, including T$_H$1 and T$_H$17 (270). IL-4 expression is, in part, regulated by IL-2 and is associated with the differentiation of T$_H$2 cells, which then express and maintain IL-4 and IL-5 in a positive feedback loop (276, 277). IL-4R is expressed on many cell types, including lymphocytes, epithelial cells, and fibroblasts (278, 279). IL-5 is primarily associated with recruitment of eosinophils (280) and basophils (281) and the development of antibody-producing B cells (282, 283). The IL-5 receptor comes in both low- and high-affinity forms whose activity is context dependent when expressed on the surface of lymphocytes, eosinophils, and basophils (284).

During TB, IL-4 levels are quite variable, with mRNA detectable in peripheral blood mononuclear cells (285) and IL-4-producing T cells isolatable from TB patients (286); however, peripheral blood mononuclear cells from active, *M. tuberculosis* culture-positive patients show decreased IL-4 expression (287–289). While a significant increase in IL-4 is observed in the plasma of TB patients compared with household contacts (290), IL-4 plasma levels are not different between HIV patients and non-HIV patients with TB (290, 291), and anti-TB treatment is associated with decreased plasma IL-4 levels (290). IL-4 mRNA has been shown to be upregulated in the necrotic areas in the lungs of HIV$^+$ patients with pleural TB (292) and is consistent with increased CD4$^+$ cells expressing IL-4 in TB patients exhibiting cavitary disease (293). In an NHP model, IL-4-expressing T cells are increased transiently at week 6 post-*M. tuberculosis* infection; however, this population is not sustained (294). One reason for the variable association of IL-4 expression with disease profile may lie in the fact that infection with

M. tuberculosis is associated with expression of the IL-4 antagonist IL-4δ2, and it may be the relative levels of IL-4 and its splice variant that define the impact of the cytokine on disease outcome (295–297).

Aerosol *M. tuberculosis* infection of mice deficient in IL-4, IL-4/IL-13, IL-4Rα, or STAT-6 fails to result in early differences in bacterial burden (298, 299) despite increased levels of IFNγ (110); however, during chronic infection, bacterial burden increases in IL-4Rα and STAT-6 gene-deficient mice (298). IL-4 can influence *M. tuberculosis*-induced granulomas, because overexpression of this cytokine by adenovirus results in increased accumulation of monocytes and eosinophils within the granuloma (300). This demonstrates that IL-4 has the potential to deviate the *M. tuberculosis*-induced granuloma from its mononuclear to a more granulocytic characteristic (35, 301), but that its impact on disease is not strong.

Information regarding the role of IL-5 in TB is limited; however, following intranasal infection of IL-4- or IL-5-deficient mice with BCG effective clearance is observed with no differences in bacterial burden or lung pathology among IL-4- and IL-5-deficient mice (302). One area where this cytokine may play a role, however, is in HIV coinfection, because IL-5 is not observed in NHP monocytes infected with *M. tuberculosis*, but, during coinfection with simian immunodeficiency virus (SIV), IL-5 and IL-13 are increased (303). NHP models coinfected with SIV and *M. tuberculosis* show disrupted CD4$^+$ T-cell levels (303), and the mechanism of loss appears to be related to monocyte-derived IL-5 that was induced following SIV infection (303).

IL-13 was originally described as a T-cell-derived cytokine capable of inhibiting proinflammatory cytokine production (304, 305); IL-13 function has since been extended to include regulating airway restriction and antihelminth responses (306–308). Furthermore, IL-13 is not only produced by T$_H$2 cells, but can also be generated by invariant NK T cells (iNKT), granulocytes (e.g., basophils, eosinophils, and mast cell), murine group 2 innate lymphoid cells (ILC2s), and human "chemoattractant receptor-homologous molecule expressed on T$_H$2 lymphocytes" (CRTH2)-type 2 ILCs (309–313). It is structurally similar to IL-4 and signals through cell surface receptor heterodimers composed of IL-4Rα and IL-13Rα1 subunits to activate STAT6 (313).

Although not much is known regarding IL-13 in *M. tuberculosis* infection, whole blood mRNA from latently infected children shows increased IL-13 compared with uninfected controls (314), although IL-13 levels are not different between actively and latently infected children (314). IL-13 may play a modulatory role in autophagy, which is an important homeostatic mechanism for intracellular degradation and has a protective function during mycobacterial infection (315–317). Indeed, in both murine and human macrophages, IL-13 and IL-4 are independently capable of inhibiting autophagy as well as IFNγ-induced autophagy-mediated killing of *M. tuberculosis* (317). Transgenic mice overexpressing IL-13 succumb to infection with *M. tuberculosis* sooner than control mice and have more necrotic granulomas within the lung (318), and this is associated with delayed expression of IFNγ and IL-17-producing CD4+ T cells and increased arginase production by macrophages within the necrotic granulomas (318). While this overexpression of IL-13 represents an artificial situation, it highlights the potential for disruption of the T-cell response to have a profound effect on TB development. Studies utilizing IL-13 gene-deficient mice are necessary to truly uncover the distinct role for IL-13 in TB.

Transforming Growth Factor β

TGFβ is a pleiotropic cytokine and regulates hundreds of genes (319–322) to modulate inflammation, cell proliferation, and differentiation, as well as cell migration (323–325). TGFβ can be made by various cell types, including all leukocytes (e.g., lymphocytes, macrophages, monocytes, dendritic cells) (325, 326). Not surprisingly, the impact of TGFβ on disease outcomes is dependent on cell type and stage of cellular differentiation, as well as the cytokine milieu (327).

TGFβ levels are increased in blood monocytes isolated from TB patients compared with uninfected individuals (328), and TGFβ localizes primarily to multinucleated Langhans giant cells within the granulomas of TB patients (328). TGFβ is induced in human blood monocytes by *M. tuberculosis* lipoarabinomannans (329), and human monocytes treated with TGFβ allow for increased intracellular *M. tuberculosis* survival, suggesting that TGFβ can play a regulatory role and potentially negative role in the context of *M. tuberculosis* infection (330). T cells and monocytes from TB patients cocultured with natural inhibitors of TGFβ, such as decorin and latency-associated peptide, exhibit restored T-cell proliferation and monocytic control of *M. tuberculosis*, again suggesting that TGFβ is a regulatory inhibitor of both T-cell responses and antibacterial activity (331). TGFβ is also able to induce IL-10 and to synergize with this cytokine to suppress IFNγ production (332). The contribution of TGFβ polymorphisms to TB susceptibility is not clear (333, 334). The polymorphism +869T/C does not correlate with increased

susceptibility in a Chinese population (334), whereas the same polymorphism in an Indian population reveals a significant susceptibility to *M. tuberculosis* in patients harboring this polymorphism. Our knowledge of the importance of context in the function of TGFβ suggests that other genetic or indeed cultural differences may mask the contribution of this polymorphism. Taken together, the data suggest that TGFβ plays an inhibitory role in host responses to *M. tuberculosis* infection.

IL-10

IL-10 was initially identified as a "cytokine synthesis inhibitory factor" produced by Th2 cells (335). However, IL-10 can be produced by other T-cell subsets including T_H1 and T_H17 cells, macrophages, some dendritic cell subsets, myeloid-derived suppressor cells, B cells, and neutrophils (336). In addition, T_{REG} cells are also a major source of IL-10 and serve to limit potentially pathogenic immune responses (336). IL-10 signals through the IL-10R, which comprises IL-10R1 and IL-10R2 (337). IL-10R1 is induced on hematopoietic cells, while IL-10R2 is expressed constitutively on most tissues and immune cells (336). In myeloid cells, IL-10 production can occur via TLR-MyD88-dependent pathways (338), as well as TLR-independent C-type lectin receptor engagement (339).

In the context of TB, meta-analyses suggest that polymorphisms in the IL-10 gene, specifically −1082G/A polymorphisms in Europeans and −592A/C polymorphisms in Asians, are significantly associated with TB risk (340). Furthermore, antigen-specific IL-10 production is found in pulmonary TB patients (341, 342) and, along with TNFα production, can be used to reliably distinguish between latent TB and pulmonary TB (342). In addition, increased accumulation of T_{REG} cells expressing IL-10 correlates with increased bacterial burden and more severe TB in an Indian population (343, 344), and a high level of IL-10 at the end of treatment in pulmonary TB patients is associated with TB recurrence (345). Finally, infection with helminths in TB patients results in decreased antigen-specific IFNγ and IL-17 responses, which are dependent on IL-10, because IL-10 blockade significantly increases frequencies of IFNγ-producing cells (346, 347).

Following mycobacterial stimulation, dendritic cells and macrophages both produce IL-10 (338, 348). In macrophages, IL-10 can block phagosome maturation and macrophage activation in a STAT3-dependent manner, thus allowing a niche for *M. tuberculosis* to replicate and survive within the phagosome (349). In addition, IL-10 can inhibit aspects of IFNγ-mediated macrophage activation (350). In dendritic cells, mycobacterially induced IL-10 production can inhibit antigen presentation through the downregulation of MHC class II molecules, decreased IL-12 production, and inhibition of dendritic cell trafficking to the lymph nodes for T-cell priming (351, 352). In keeping with this regulatory role for IL-10, studies have shown that IL-10 gene-deficient mice infected with *M. tuberculosis* exhibit increased T_H1 and T_H17 responses, and this coincides with improved *M. tuberculosis* control during chronic infection (336) (Fig. 2). The effect is not dramatic and indeed some challenge models fail to show an impact of IL-10 gene deficiency (299, 353, 354). Interestingly, CBA mice generate significant early macrophage IL-10 production correlating with increased susceptibility to *M. tuberculosis* infection (355). This increased susceptibility also coincides with reduced expression of TNFα and IFNγ in T cells and can be reversed by blocking IL-10R signaling very early in infection (355). In CBA IL-10 gene-deficient mice, *M. tuberculosis* infection results in development of fibrotic granulomas with similarity to lesions seen in humans (356). In vaccine models, blocking IL-10 at the time of BCG vaccination (336), or using IL-10 gene-deficient mice in BCG vaccination and *M. tuberculosis* challenge experiments (244), demonstrates that IL-10 limits IFNγ and IL-17 responses during priming and decreases vaccine-induced protection against *M. tuberculosis* challenge. Computational modeling also highlights the pleiotropic role for IL-10 (357). Importantly, there are differences in the role of specific cytokines depending on the nature of the *M. tuberculosis* strains being examined. Indeed, the W-Beijing HN878 strain induces robust IL-10 production to inhibit the induction of a Th1 response (98). In the future, therefore, addressing the role for IL-10 in the context of infection, a variety of *M. tuberculosis* strains will likely provide novel insights into the function of IL-10 in TB.

THE CHEMOKINES

Limiting bacterial spread and containment of inflammation within discrete sites are hallmarks of disease control in TB and dovetail with the establishment of the TB granuloma. The TB granuloma is a multicellular immune bolus consisting of a number of cell types including macrophages, neutrophils, lymphocytes, and B cells, among others (358). Formation of the TB granuloma is governed by coordinated expression of the chemotactic cytokines referred to as chemokines. Chemokine expression establishes a chemical gradient that

drives mobilization and recruitment of cells from peripheral organs to the site of infection and within the granuloma. The importance of this coordination has recently emerged to be critical in disease control with proper localization of CD4 T cells in the lung parenchyma being paramount (80–82).

Since the discovery of the first chemokine, now known as CXCL8 (i.e., IL-8), numerous chemokines have been identified, resulting in the need for a uniform nomenclature currently based on primary sequences of chemokine ligands (359–361). These chemokine ligands modulate biological processes through interactions with seven transmembrane G protein-coupled receptors (360, 362). Chemokines are divided into four families (C, CC, CXC, CX3C) based on the presence of cysteine(s) and the presence or absence of nonconserved amino acids between those cysteines (360, 361). The CC chemokine receptors (CCR) are involved in the recruitment of monocytes, neutrophils, lymphocytes, and macrophages (34). During bacterial infection, signaling via pattern recognition receptors drives the expression of CC chemokine ligands (CCL) and the development of gradients that are responded to by specific cell surface chemokine receptors (34) with functional recruitment involving monomeric or dimeric forms in the respective chemokine ligands (363). CXC chemokine ligands, denoted as CXCL, contain a nonconserved amino acid between the two cysteines, unlike CCL chemokines (360, 361). The number of chemokine ligands outnumbers the chemokine receptors, suggesting redundant or highly refined roles for the receptors as in the case for CCR4 expression mediating the migration of both T_H1 and T_H2 responses (363). This is further exemplified by CXC receptors (CXCR), which are capable of binding multiple CXCLs to promote the migration of specific cells along a chemokine gradient (360). Because development of the granuloma and communication between the cells within the granuloma are so critical for control of disease, this section will explore the roles chemokines play in modulating TB disease outcome. In accordance with the most recent chemokine nomenclature, CCRs and CCLs as well as CXCRs and their ligands, CXCLs, are numbered (e.g., CCR2, CCL2) in a manner that avoids the previous random naming system (364) (Table 2).

CC Receptors and Their Ligands
CCR1
CCR1 is expressed by T lymphocytes, neutrophils, dendritic cells, monocytes, and macrophages (365–369). Under normal conditions, CCR1 is constitutively expressed

at low levels, but it is upregulated during stimulation of neutrophils with granulocyte-macrophage colony-stimulating factor (GM-CSF) and during the differentiation of monocytes to macrophages (369, 370).

In TB patients, CD4$^+$ T lymphocytes expressing CCR1 are elevated in the pleural fluid (371), and, in the blood, increased levels of CCR1$^+$ T lymphocytes, natural killer (NK) cells, and neutrophils are seen (372). *In vitro*, human neutrophils express both CCR1 and produce CCL3 upon infection with *M. tuberculosis* (373). Infection with *M. tuberculosis* induces the expression of the CCR1 ligands CCL3, CCL4, and CCL5 in the lung (374, 375); however, CCR1 deficiency in mice does not impact control or disease progression following *M. tuberculosis* infection (35). Thus, it is likely that, while CCR1 correlates with cellular activation during TB, it does not appear to play a strong role in protection.

CCR2

CCR2 has a similar distribution pattern as CCR1 on hematopoietic cells (376, 377). Expression of CCR2 on monocytes and its interaction with CCL2 and CCL7 are essential for mobilization of monocytes from the bone marrow into the circulation and into sites of inflammation (378). Increased levels of CCL2 in the serum of pulmonary TB and TB patients with disseminated disease have been reported (379) and are associated with the damaging influx of inflammatory cells during TB pleurisy (371, 372). At a minimum, the presence of CCR2 and its ligands is a potential indicator of disease severity in TB patients.

Low-dose aerosol *M. tuberculosis* infection of mice elicits increased expression of CCL2, CCL7, and CCL12 in the lung during the acute stages of *M. tuberculosis* infection (380). Accordingly, mice deficient in CCR2 or CCL2 are defective in macrophage and T-lymphocyte recruitment following *M. tuberculosis* infection (380–383) (Fig. 1). Consistent with defects in recruitment of immune cells, granuloma formation in CCR2 gene-deficient mice is delayed, and is associated with peri-vascular cuffing and loosely formed granulomas (380). Similarly, *M. tuberculosis*-infected CCL2 gene-deficient mice also exhibit decreased granulomatous inflammation in *M. tuberculosis*-infected lungs (382, 383), despite these innate and adaptive immune defects, CCR2 gene-deficient mice are not more susceptible to low-dose *M. tuberculosis* infection using either the aerosol or intravenous route (380). When taken in the context of the role of the type I IFNs in recruiting just enough (102) but not too many phagocytes (101), it may be that using a simple gene deficiency model to dissect the role of each chemokine or chemokine receptor will not be informative (Fig. 1).

CCR4

CCR4 is expressed on T-cell subsets including T$_H$17, T$_H$2, and T$_{REG}$ cells that mediate allergic responses and protection against extracellular pathogens (384–386). T lymphocytes expressing CCR4 are mobilized via a chemokine gradient established by dendritic cells in the context of both allergic and parasite-induced inflammation (387–392). In the context of *M. tuberculosis* infection, T$_{REG}$ cells are increased in the peripheral blood of TB patients and inhibit production of IFNγ by *M. tuberculosis*-specific CD4$^+$ T cells (393, 394), and CCR4 antagonists promote proliferation of T cells during MVA85A vaccination (395). The ligand for CCR4, CCL17, but not CCL22 has also been shown to be elevated in the serum of active TB patients (396). These data suggest that CCR4-mediated regulation of T-cell responses to *M. tuberculosis* antigens may occur during TB and that antagonism of CCR4 maybe a target for therapeutic use or as an adjuvant during vaccination. Mechanistic analysis of CCR4 function during mycobacterially induced granuloma responses demonstrates that, despite delivery of mycobacterial and helminth antigens inducing both CCL17 and CCL22 in mouse lungs, the absence of CCR4 results in reduced granuloma formation in following mycobacterial but not helminth antigen challenge (397). Further investigation of the role of CCR4 in the development of immunity and immunopathology is likely warranted.

CCR5

CCR5 is expressed on monocytes, macrophages, T lymphocytes, neutrophils, and dendritic cells (34, 376, 377, 398) and responds to CCL3, CCL4, and CCL5 (374, 375). CCR5 is most notable in the study of HIV infection, where CCR5 facilitates viral entry into T lymphocytes and macrophages (398, 399). HIV infection dramatically compromises immunity to TB, and this is thought to be largely as a result of compromised T-cell function; however, blocking CCL5 in cultures of *M. tuberculosis*-infected alveolar macrophages from HIV patients results in enhanced *M. tuberculosis* growth (374), suggesting that CCL5 can directly promote bacterial killing by *M. tuberculosis*-infected macrophages. Interestingly, analysis of single-nucleotide polymorphisms in *CCL5* has identified two risk haplotypes, A-C-T and G-C-C, that are associated with susceptibility to TB (400). What remains unclear is whether this haplotype is associated with increased or decreased CCL5 production.

In the mouse model of *M. tuberculosis* infection, all three CCR5 ligands are upregulated in the lungs, with CCL5 being induced to the highest level (375, 401). Upon *M. tuberculosis* infection, CCL5 gene-deficient mice exhibit transient early impairment in granuloma formation and delayed T-cell recruitment (401), while CCR5 deficiency results in increased inflammation in the lung (375) (Fig. 1). The observed delayed T-cell recruitment into the lungs of CCL5-deficient mice (401) is not entirely surprising, because CCR5-CCL5 are important for dendritic cell trafficking to the lymph nodes, facilitating T-cell activation and accumulation during TB (375, 401). The difference between the outcome for the CCR5- and CCL5-deficient mice in terms of inflammatory outcome may reflect the action of other CCR5 ligands acting in the absence of CCL5. The increased accumulation of CD4$^+$ and CD8$^+$ T lymphocytes, myeloid cells, neutrophils, and macrophages in the lungs of chronically infected CCR5-deficient mice suggests, however, that any compensating ligand is not optimal at limiting pathologic consequences (375). Whether the models are showing true redundancy in the chemokine or our failure to appreciate the subtle nature of the function of each chemokine is still an issue for debate (402).

CCR6

CCR6 has only one known ligand, CCL20 (403), and is expressed on effector and memory T cells, myeloid dendritic cells, and B cells. CCR6 is important for the recruitment of CCR6-expressing cells to mucosal surfaces and their localization at sites of inflammation in epithelial tissues (403, 404). While CCR6 plays a vital role under both homeostatic and inflammatory conditions, it has been implicated in pathologic conditions, particularly in cancer and rheumatoid arthritis models (405, 406). Although few studies have investigated the role of CCR6 in *M. tuberculosis* infections, emerging data support a protective role for CCR6 (407). Specifically, memory CD4$^+$ T cells specific for *M. tuberculosis* antigens coexpress CXCR3 and CCR6 and these CXCR3$^+$CCR6$^+$ CD4$^+$ T cells are associated with an IFNγ response (386). Following *ex vivo* expansion, those CD4$^+$ T cells that produced IL-17A in response to *M. tuberculosis* coexpressed CXCR3 and CCR6 (408). In a detailed analysis of reactivity to mycobacterial antigens it was found that CXCR3$^+$CCR6$^+$ IFNγ-producing CD4$^+$ T cells from latently *M. tuberculosis*-infected individuals responded to three immunodominant antigenic islands within the *M. tuberculosis* genome that were all associated with bacterial secretion systems (409) (Fig. 2). The CCR6 ligand, CCL20, appears at high levels in peripheral blood mononuclear cells, myeloid-derived macrophages, and bronchoalveolar lavage samples from TB patients (410, 411) and increased CCL20 mRNA is seen in murine and NHP lung (412, 413). It is likely therefore that CCR6 mediates the localization of memory cells to sites of *M. tuberculosis*-induced inflammation. Mouse studies have identified a critical role for CCR6 in the innate immune-mediated control following acute BCG infection (407). Innate cell types, such as CD1b-restricted iNKT cells, are impacted by the absence of CCR6, in that they fail to accumulate effectively in the lung, and this is associated with poor bacterial control and increased susceptibility to *M. tuberculosis* infection (407). Collectively, the current literature suggests that there is a correlation between CCR6 expression and bacterial control; however, mechanistic studies investigating the function of CCR6 in innate immune responses as well as its role in directing memory T-cell migration are required.

CCR7

Correct localization of dendritic cells and T and B cells is critical for the function of secondary lymphoid tissues (414). CCR7 ligation by CCL19 and CCL21 is vital for the positioning of T cells and dendritic cells in the paracortical region of these secondary lymphoid organs (SLO) (415) (Figs. 1 and 2). CCL19 and CCL21 are constitutively expressed by SLO stromal cells, while CCL21, but not CCL19, is expressed on lymphatic endothelial and high endothelial venules (415–418). CCR7 has also been implicated in thymic function and development, as well as homeostatic and inflammation-induced migration of dendritic cells to draining lymph nodes via the afferent lymphatics. In *M. tuberculosis* infections, it is thought to be necessary for dendritic cells from the lungs to relocate in the SLOs, activate naive T cells, and elicit recruitment of T cells into the site of infection for bacterial control. Early migration of mature dendritic cells to the mediastinal lymph node is supported by CCR7 (419), and CCR7-deficient mice exhibit impaired dendritic cell migration to this node (420) (Fig. 2). Similarly, *plt* mutant mice, which lack expression of CCL19 and CCL21-Ser in SLO, also have poor dendritic cell migration (421), and proliferation of adoptively transferred *M. tuberculosis*-specific CD4$^+$ T cells is delayed in mice deficient of CCR7 (420) and *plt* mice (422). Interestingly, the CCR7 chemokine ligand, CCL19, is present within granulomas containing B-cell aggregates that resemble lymphoid structures, and in the absence of CCR7 these B-cell follicles are also absent (416). While these mice display disorganized B-cell aggregation, the enhanced lymphocytic infiltrations observed in the lungs of CCR7 gene-deficient mice are sufficient to control *M. tuberculosis* to levels comparable to CCR7-sufficient mice (416). Similarly to CCR7-deficient mice, *plt* mutant mice fail to develop B-cell follicles and have disorganized granulomas (422). However, unlike CCR7-deficient mice, *plt* mutant mice also have delayed accumulation of IFNγ-producing T cells and maintain higher bacterial burden (422). Thus, it seems that CCR7 plays an important role in the proper migration of dendritic cells to the draining lymph node for priming and activation of T cells, as well as the migration of CD4⁺ T cells into lymphoid follicles following *M. tuberculosis* infection.

CXC Receptors and Their Ligands

CXCR1 and CXCR2

CXCR1 and CXCR2 share the binding partners, CXCL6 and CXCL8, while CXCR2 can exclusively bind to CXCL1-3, CXCL5, and CXCL7 (423). All these CXCLs contain the ELR motif, corresponding to a Glu-Leu-Arg tripeptide motif at the amino terminus region, adjacent to their CXC sequence. The functional role of this ELR motif is to confer angiogenic activity to the ELR-containing chemokine (424) and this motif is important for ligand-receptor binding interactions on neutrophils (425, 426). Ligand binding to CXCR1 and CXCR2 causes degranulation, intracellular calcium mobilization, and phosphorylation of MAPK (427).

Although most notably expressed on neutrophils in TB patients, both CXCR1 and CXCR2 can also be expressed on NK cells, T cells, and monocytes (423, 428). Comparison of CXCR1 expression on peripheral blood from TB patients shows that individuals with pulmonary TB have increased CXCR1, whereas latent TB patients have increased CXCR2 in whole blood (429). Moreover, increased CXCR1 correlates with impaired oxidative function in leukocytes, suggesting a possible regulatory role for CXCR1 on oxidative stress (429). CXCR2-deficient mice infected intraperitoneally with *Mycobacterium avium* have decreased neutrophil accumulation and increased bacterial burden (430). However, following pulmonary infection with *M. avium*, no difference in cellular infiltrate or bacterial burden is observed, which highlights the importance of route and dose on identifying the function of the highly redundant chemokines.

CXCL8 has been the most studied CXCR1/2 ligand in the context of TB and this important neutrophil chemoattractant is expressed by multiple cell types, including alveolar epithelial cells, monocytes, macrophages, and fibroblasts upon *M. tuberculosis* infection *in vitro*

(431–434) (Fig. 1). Following *in vivo M. tuberculosis* infection, pulmonary granulomas containing fibroblasts are also capable of secreting CXCL8 (431), and TB sputum samples contain elevated CXCL8 levels (435). CXCL8 is present at high levels at positive tuberculin skin reaction sites and is associated with high levels of neutrophils at this site (436). Furthermore, neutrophils isolated from pulmonary TB patients have increased expression of CXCL8, which is further increased following *ex vivo* infection with H37Rv but not the clinical strains, S7 and S10, suggesting strain-specific regulation of CXCL8 production in neutrophils (373). Whether CXCL8 is associated with a protective or pathologic response remains controversial (437, 438). Serum CXCL8 levels from pulmonary TB patients following treatment with antibiotics decreased, suggesting that CXCL8 could be a marker for treatment efficacy (439). Whether disease improvement is directly correlated to reduced CXCL8 levels or simply a reflection of reduced neutrophil accumulation is unclear (Fig. 1).

CXCL5, which is also a CXCR2 ligand, plays an important role in host responses against *M. tuberculosis* (440), because both CXCR2 and CXCL5 gene-deficient mice display lower bacterial burden following *M. tuberculosis* infection, which correlates with reduced neutrophil accumulation to the lung (440). In this model, alveolar epithelial secretion of CXCL5, mediating the recruitment of neutrophils, is dependent on TLR2 engagement with *M. tuberculosis* and blocking of neutrophil recruitment improves outcome in the lung (440) (Fig. 1). It appears that CXCR2 plays an important role in the pathologic granulomatous response during TB, and this could be an important target for host-directed therapy.

CXCR3

CXCR3 binds to its chemokine ligand partners, CXCL9, CXCL10, and CXCL11, also known as MIG, IP-10, and I-TAC, respectively (428, 441). It is expressed primarily by activated CD4⁺ and CD8⁺ T cells, and is detected on B cells and innate lymphocytes such as NK cells and NKT cells (428). CXCR3 expression is associated with supporting localization of cells to the site of infection (442, 443). Most notably, CXCR3 expression on effector T cells plays an important role in the migration of T cells both *in vitro* and *in vivo* (33, 441, 444–446) and the transcription factor T-bet transactivates CXCR3 on T cells to promote this migration (441) (Fig. 2). It is characterized as an inflammatory chemokine receptor on T cells and is significantly enhanced on T cells from inflamed tissues in human inflammatory reactions and has been implicated in various human and murine disease models, including idiopathic pulmonary fibrosis and asthma (441, 443, 447).

In response to *M. tuberculosis* infection, CXCR3-expressing T cells are found in the caseous, necrotic granulomas, and bronchoalveolar lavage in the NHP model, as well as in the lungs of infected mice (428). The presence of these cells correlates with elevated expression of CXCL9, CXCL10, and CXCL11 localized within granulomas (428), but CXCR3-deficient mice do not exhibit differences in bacterial burden following low-dose aerosol infection with *M. tuberculosis* (448, 449). Despite the absence of a bacterial phenotype, CXCR3-deficient mice do develop fewer granulomas of decreased size (448, 449), suggesting that CXCR3 is important for granuloma formation. The coexpression of CXCR3 with CCR6 on memory T cells in latently infected humans supports the importance of this receptor on the migration and function of human T cells during TB, but the precise role is not clear (Fig. 2). Human data support a protective role for CXCR3-binding chemokines because CXCL9 levels correlate with disease severity (379, 450), although the role of CXCL10 is unclear. CXCL10 has been proposed as a biomarker for improvement, because reduction of this chemokine in the serum relative to levels at recruitment is observed following TB treatment, and nonresponders do not show the same decrease (439, 451). Unfortunately, CXCL10 levels cannot distinguish between active and latent TB in children (452).

The mechanistic basis for CXCL10 activity in TB is not fully defined. In some cases, active TB can result in destruction of the lung parenchyma, leading to cavities. In AIDS-associated TB, increased CXCL10 is associated with noncavitary TB, whereas cavitary TB is associated with increased GM-CSF (114, 453). CXCL10 is important for modulating CXCL9 and CCL2, which promote disease, while CXCL10 is significantly increased in patients with active pulmonary tuberculosis (100), and there may be a genetic association between a single-nucleotide polymorphism within the CXCL-10 promoter (135G/A) and TB susceptibility (454).

Additional studies are needed to confirm whether CXCR3 and its ligands are protective or harmful to disease outcome. It is also unclear how CXCL9-11 is induced and whether its induction is a direct result of *M. tuberculosis* infection or whether upregulated expression results from expression of cytokines capable of inducing CXCL9-11 expression (455–458). Still, animal models support CXCR3 and expression of its ligands as important regulators for granuloma formation (449, 459) (Fig. 2).

CXCR5

The B-cell chemoattractant, CXCL13, is the only known ligand for CXCR5. It is preferentially produced in B-cell follicles and, through its binding with CXCR5, is important for the development of lymphoid follicles. In lymphoid organs, the main source for CXCL13 is the follicular dendritic cell (460). However, IL-17-producing T cells have also been shown to express CXCL13 in a *Candida albicans* infection model as well as in synovial fluid from patients with rheumatoid arthritis (461). CXCL13 expression recruits CXCR5-expressing B cells and coordinates the correct position of these cells within SLO (462). A similar role has also been highlighted during *M. tuberculosis* infections. *M. tuberculosis* granulomas contain B cells, follicular dendritic cells, and high endothelial venules and thus provide important points of entry for trafficking lymphocytes (4, 428). CXCL13 is also elevated in *M. tuberculosis*-infected mice and is important for the localization of CXCR5$^+$ T cells to the lung parenchyma as well as the activation of phagocytes and control of bacterial growth (422, 459) (Fig. 2). With the use of NHP and mouse models of *M. tuberculosis*, CXCR5$^+$ T cells have been shown to traffic toward ectopic lymphoid follicles (bronchus-associated lymphoid tissues [iBALT]), adjacent to granulomas where CXCL13 is localized. In the absence of CXCR5, mice fail to develop iBALT and are more susceptible *M. tuberculosis* (459) with the impaired response being rescued through the adoptive transfer of CXCR5-sufficient T cells, suggesting that CXCR5 expression on T cells is important for both protection and the development of B-cell follicles. Furthermore, CXCR5 is required for the maintenance of *M. tuberculosis*-specific CD4$^+$ T cells during chronic infection (81). B cells from *M. tuberculosis*-infected murine lungs are also able to migrate along a CXCL13 chemotactic gradient *in vitro* via their expression of CXCR5 (463). IL-23- and IL-17R-dependent induction of CXCL13 within the *M. tuberculosis*-infected lungs appears to be important for control of this infection, and CXCL-13- and CXCR5-deficient mice are the only chemokine-deficient mice that show increased susceptibility upon *M. tuberculosis* infection, suggesting that this cytokine/chemokine axis is nonredundant in *M. tuberculosis* infection (Fig. 2).

CONCLUSION

Chemokines and cytokines are critical for initiating and coordinating the organized and sequential recruitment and activation of cells into *M. tuberculosis*-infected lungs (Figs. 1 and 2). Correct mononuclear cellular recruitment and localization are essential to ensure control of bacterial growth without the development of diffuse and damaging granulocytic inflammation. An important block to our understanding of TB pathogenesis lies in dissecting the critical aspects of the cytokine/chemokine interplay in light of the conditional role these molecules play throughout infection and disease development (Tables 1 and 2). Much of the data highlighted in this review appear at first glance to be contradictory, but it is the balance between the cytokines and chemokines that is critical, and the "goldilocks" (not too much and not too little) phenomenon is paramount in any discussion of the role of these molecules in TB. Determination of how the key chemokines/cytokines and their receptors are balanced and how the loss of that balance can promote disease is vital to understanding TB pathogenesis and to identifying novel therapies for effective eradication of this disease.

Citation. Domingo-Gonzalez R, Prince O, Cooper A, Khader S. 2016. Cytokines and chemokines in *Mycobacterium tuberculosis* infection. Microbiol Spectrum 4(5):TBTB2-0018-2016.

References

1. Dinarello CA. 2007. Historical insights into cytokines. *Eur J Immunol* 37(Suppl 1):S34–S45.

2. Cooper AM. 2009. Cell-mediated immune responses in tuberculosis. *Annu Rev Immunol* 27:393–422.

3. Flynn JL, Chan J. 2003. Immune evasion by *Mycobacterium tuberculosis*: living with the enemy. *Curr Opin Immunol* 15:450–455.

4. Flynn JL, Chan J. 2001. Immunology of tuberculosis. *Annu Rev Immunol* 19:93–129.

5. Brites D, Gagneux S. 2015. Co-evolution of *Mycobacterium tuberculosis* and *Homo sapiens*. *Immunol Rev* 264:6–24.

6. Comas I, Coscolla M, Luo T, Borrell S, Holt KE, Kato-Maeda M, Parkhill J, Malla B, Berg S, Thwaites G, Yeboah-Manu D, Bothamley G, Mei J, Wei L, Bentley S, Harris SR, Niemann S, Diel R, Aseffa A, Gao Q, Young D, Gagneux S. 2013. Out-of-Africa migration and Neolithic coexpansion of *Mycobacterium tuberculosis* with modern humans. *Nat Genet* 45:1176–1182.

7. Orme IM, Robinson RT, Cooper AM. 2015. The balance between protective and pathogenic immune responses in the TB-infected lung. *Nat Immunol* 16:57–63.

8. Dye C, Glaziou P, Floyd K, Raviglione M. 2013. Prospects for tuberculosis elimination. *Annu Rev Public Health* 34:271–286.

9. Robinson RT, Orme IM, Cooper AM. 2015. The onset of adaptive immunity in the mouse model of tuberculosis and the factors that compromise its expression. *Immunol Rev* 264:46–59.

10. Wajant H, Pfizenmaier K, Scheurich P. 2003. Tumor necrosis factor signaling. *Cell Death Differ* 10:45–65.

11. Black RA, Rauch CT, Kozlosky CJ, Peschon JJ, Slack JL, Wolfson MF, Castner BJ, Stocking KL, Reddy P, Srinivasan S, Nelson N, Boiani N, Schooley KA, Gerhart M, Davis R, Fitzner JN, Johnson RS, Paxton RJ, March CJ, Cerretti DP. 1997. A metalloproteinase disintegrin that releases tumour-necrosis factor-alpha from cells. *Nature* 385:729–733.

12. Bazan JF. 1993. Emerging families of cytokines and receptors. *Curr Biol* 3:603–606.

13. Devin A, Lin Y, Yamaoka S, Li Z, Karin M, Liu Zg. 2001. The alpha and beta subunits of IkappaB kinase (IKK) mediate TRAF2-dependent IKK recruitment to tumor necrosis factor (TNF) receptor 1 in response to TNF. *Mol Cell Biol* 21:3986–3994.

14. Hsu H, Huang J, Shu HB, Baichwal V, Goeddel DV. 1996. TNF-dependent recruitment of the protein kinase RIP to the TNF receptor-1 signaling complex. *Immunity* 4:387–396.

15. Hsu H, Xiong J, Goeddel DV. 1995. The TNF receptor 1-associated protein TRADD signals cell death and NF-kappa B activation. *Cell* 81:495–504.

16. Jiang Y, Woronicz JD, Liu W, Goeddel DV. 1999. Prevention of constitutive TNF receptor 1 signaling by silencer of death domains. *Science* 283:543–546.

17. Naismith JH, Sprang SR. 1998. Modularity in the TNF-receptor family. *Trends Biochem Sci* 23:74–79.

18. Banner DW, D'Arcy A, Janes W, Gentz R, Schoenfeld HJ, Broger C, Loetscher H, Lesslauer W. 1993. Crystal structure of the soluble human 55 kd TNF receptor-human TNF beta complex: implications for TNF receptor activation. *Cell* 73:431–445.

19. Chan FK, Chun HJ, Zheng L, Siegel RM, Bui KL, Lenardo MJ. 2000. A domain in TNF receptors that mediates ligand-independent receptor assembly and signaling. *Science* 288:2351–2354.

20. Faustman DL, Davis M. 2013. TNF Receptor 2 and Disease: Autoimmunity and Regenerative Medicine. *Front Immunol* 4:478

21. Carswell EA, Old LJ, Kassel RL, Green S, Fiore N, Williamson B. 1975. An endotoxin-induced serum factor that causes necrosis of tumors. *Proc Natl Acad Sci USA* 72:3666–3670.

22. Keane J, Balcewicz-Sablinska MK, Remold HG, Chupp GL, Meek BB, Fenton MJ, Kornfeld H. 1997. Infection by *Mycobacterium tuberculosis* promotes human alveolar macrophage apoptosis. *Infect Immun* 65:298–304.

23. Keane J, Remold HG, Kornfeld H. 2000. Virulent *Mycobacterium tuberculosis* strains evade apoptosis of infected alveolar macrophages. *J Immunol* 164:2016–2020.

24. Balcewicz-Sablinska MK, Keane J, Kornfeld H, Remold HG. 1998. Pathogenic *Mycobacterium tuberculosis* evades apoptosis of host macrophages by release of TNF-R2, resulting in inactivation of TNF-alpha. *J Immunol* 161:2636–2641.

25. Serbina NV, Flynn JL. 1999. Early emergence of CD8(+) T cells primed for production of type 1 cytokines in the lungs of *Mycobacterium tuberculosis*-infected mice. *Infect Immun* 67:3980–3988.

26. Flynn JL, Goldstein MM, Chan J, Triebold KJ, Pfeffer K, Lowenstein CJ, Schreiber R, Mak TW, Bloom BR. 1995. Tumor necrosis factor-alpha is required in the protective immune response against *Mycobacterium tuberculosis* in mice. *Immunity* 2:561–572.

27. Algood HM, Lin PL, Flynn JL. 2005. Tumor necrosis factor and chemokine interactions in the formation and maintenance of granulomas in tuberculosis. *Clin Infect Dis* 41(Suppl 3):S189–S193.

28. Roach DR, Bean AG, Demangel C, France MP, Briscoe H, Britton WJ. 2002. TNF regulates chemokine induction essential for cell recruitment, granuloma formation, and clearance of mycobacterial infection. *J Immunol* 168:4620–4627.

29. Bean AG, Roach DR, Briscoe H, France MP, Korner H, Sedgwick JD, Britton WJ. 1999. Structural deficiencies in granuloma formation in TNF gene-targeted mice underlie the heightened susceptibility to aerosol *Mycobacterium tuberculosis* infection, which is not compensated for by lymphotoxin. *J Immunol* 162:3504–3511.

30. Lin PL, Plessner HL, Voitenok NN, Flynn JL. 2007. Tumor necrosis factor and tuberculosis. *J Investig Dermatol Symp Proc* 12:22–25.

31. Kindler V, Sappino AP, Grau GE, Piguet PF, Vassalli P. 1989. The inducing role of tumor necrosis factor in the development of bactericidal granulomas during BCG infection. *Cell* 56:731–740.

32. Farber JM. 1997. Mig and IP-10: CXC chemokines that target lymphocytes. *J Leukoc Biol* 61:246–257.

33. Cole KE, Strick CA, Paradis TJ, Ogborne KT, Loetscher M, Gladue RP, Lin W, Boyd JG, Moser B, Wood DE, Sahagan BG, Neote K. 1998. Interferon-inducible T cell alpha chemoattractant (I-TAC): a novel non-ELR CXC chemokine with potent activity on activated T cells through selective high affinity binding to CXCR3. *J Exp Med* 187:2009–2021.

34. Griffith JW, Sokol CL, Luster AD. 2014. Chemokines and chemokine receptors: positioning cells for host defense and immunity. *Annu Rev Immunol* 32:659–702.

35. Saunders BM, Britton WJ. 2007. Life and death in the granuloma: immunopathology of tuberculosis. *Immunol Cell Biol* 85:103–111.

36. Lynch K, Farrell M. 2010. Cerebral tuberculoma in a patient receiving anti-TNF alpha (adalimumab) treatment. *Clin Rheumatol* 29:1201–1204.

37. Seong SS, Choi CB, Woo JH, Bae KW, Joung CL, Uhm WS, Kim TH, Jun JB, Yoo DH, Lee JT, Bae SC. 2007. Incidence of tuberculosis in Korean patients with rheumatoid arthritis (RA): effects of RA itself and of tumor necrosis factor blockers. *J Rheumatol* 34:706–711.

38. Be NA, Kim KS, Bishai WR, Jain SK. 2009. Pathogenesis of central nervous system tuberculosis. *Curr Mol Med* 9:94–99.

39. Leonard JM, Des Prez RM. 1990. Tuberculous meningitis. *Infect Dis Clin North Am* 4:769–787.

40. Tsenova L, Bergtold A, Freedman VH, Young RA, Kaplan G. 1999. Tumor necrosis factor alpha is a determinant of pathogenesis and disease progression in mycobacterial infection in the central nervous system. *Proc Natl Acad Sci USA* 96:5657–5662.

41. Francisco NM, Hsu NJ, Keeton R, Randall P, Sebesho B, Allie N, Govender D, Quesniaux V, Ryffel B, Kellaway L, Jacobs M. 2015. TNF-dependent regulation and activation of innate immune cells are essential for host protection against cerebral tuberculosis. *J Neuroinflammation* 12:125.

42. Mohan VP, Scanga CA, Yu K, Scott HM, Tanaka KE, Tsang E, Tsai MM, Flynn JL, Chan J. 2001. Effects of tumor necrosis factor alpha on host immune response in chronic persistent tuberculosis: possible role for limiting pathology. *Infect Immun* 69:1847–1855.

43. Feldmann M. 2002. Development of anti-TNF therapy for rheumatoid arthritis. *Nat Rev Immunol* 2:364–371.

44. Peyrin-Biroulet L. 2010. Anti-TNF therapy in inflammatory bowel diseases: a huge review. *Minerva Gastroenterol Dietol* 56:233–243.

45. Shaikha SA, Mansour K, Riad H. 2012. Reactivation of tuberculosis in three cases of psoriasis after initiation of anti-TNF therapy. *Case Rep Dermatol* 4:41–46.

46. Keane J, Gershon S, Wise RP, Mirabile-Levens E, Kasznica J, Schwieterman WD, Siegel JN, Braun MM. 2001. Tuberculosis associated with infliximab, a tumor necrosis factor alpha-neutralizing agent. *N Engl J Med* 345:1098–1104.

47. Keane J. 2005. TNF-blocking agents and tuberculosis: new drugs illuminate an old topic. *Rheumatology (Oxford)* 44:714–720.

48. Raval A, Akhavan-Toyserkani G, Brinker A, Avigan M. 2007. Brief communication: characteristics of spontaneous cases of tuberculosis associated with infliximab. *Ann Intern Med* 147:699–702

49. Gómez-Reino JJ, Carmona L, Valverde VR, Mola EM, Montero MD, BIOBADASER Group. 2003. Treatment of rheumatoid arthritis with tumor necrosis factor inhibitors may predispose to significant increase in tuberculosis risk: a multicenter active-surveillance report. *Arthritis Rheum* 48:2122–2127.

50. Dixon WG, Watson K, Lunt M, Hyrich KL, Silman AJ, Symmons DP, British Society for Rheumatology Biologics Register. 2006. Rates of serious infection, including site-specific and bacterial intracellular infection, in rheumatoid arthritis patients receiving anti-tumor necrosis factor therapy: results from the British Society for Rheumatology Biologics Register. *Arthritis Rheum* 54:2368–2376.

51. Askling J, Fored CM, Brandt L, Baecklund E, Bertilsson L, Cöster L, Geborek P, Jacobsson LT, Lindblad S, Lysholm J, Rantapää-Dahlqvist S, Saxne T, Romanus V, Klareskog L, Feltelius N. 2005. Risk and case characteristics of tuberculosis in rheumatoid arthritis associated with tumor necrosis factor antagonists in Sweden. *Arthritis Rheum* 52:1986–1992.

52. Tubach F, Salmon D, Ravaud P, Allanore Y, Goupille P, Bréban M, Pallot-Prades B, Pouplin S, Sacchi A, Chichemanian RM, Bretagne S, Emilie D, Lemann M, Lortholary O, Mariette X; Research Axed on Tolerance of Biotherapies Group. 2009. Risk of tuberculosis is higher with anti-tumor necrosis factor monoclonal

antibody therapy than with soluble tumor necrosis factor receptor therapy: the three-year prospective French Research Axed on Tolerance of Biotherapies registry. *Arthritis Rheum* **60**:1884–1894. (Erratum **60**:2540.)

53. Fallahi-Sichani M, Flynn JL, Linderman JJ, Kirschner DE. 2012. Differential risk of tuberculosis reactivation among anti-TNF therapies is due to drug binding kinetics and permeability. *J Immunol* **188**:3169–3178.

54. Bruns H, Meinken C, Schauenberg P, Härter G, Kern P, Modlin RL, Antoni C, Stenger S. 2009. Anti-TNF immunotherapy reduces CD8+ T cell-mediated antimicrobial activity against *Mycobacterium tuberculosis* in humans. *J Clin Invest* **119**:1167–1177.

55. Lin PL, Myers A, Smith LK, Bigbee C, Bigbee M, Fuhrman C, Grieser H, Chiosea I, Voitenek NN, Capuano SV, Klein E, Flynn JL. 2010. Tumor necrosis factor neutralization results in disseminated disease in acute and latent *Mycobacterium tuberculosis* infection with normal granuloma structure in a cynomolgus macaque model. *Arthritis Rheum* **62**:340–350.

56. Clay H, Volkman HE, Ramakrishnan L. 2008. Tumor necrosis factor signaling mediates resistance to mycobacteria by inhibiting bacterial growth and macrophage death. *Immunity* **29**:283–294.

57. Harari A, Rozot V, Bellutti Enders F, Perreau M, Stalder JM, Nicod LP, Cavassini M, Calandra T, Blanchet CL, Jaton K, Faouzi M, Day CL, Hanekom WA, Bart PA, Pantaleo G. 2011. Dominant TNF-α+ *Mycobacterium tuberculosis*-specific CD4+ T cell responses discriminate between latent infection and active disease. *Nat Med* **17**:372–376.

58. Schroder K, Hertzog PJ, Ravasi T, Hume DA. 2004. Interferon-gamma: an overview of signals, mechanisms and functions. *J Leukoc Biol* **75**:163–189.

59. Greenlund AC, Farrar MA, Viviano BL, Schreiber RD. 1994. Ligand-induced IFN gamma receptor tyrosine phosphorylation couples the receptor to its signal transduction system (p91). *EMBO J* **13**:1591–1600.

60. Kovarik P, Stoiber D, Novy M, Decker T. 1998. Stat1 combines signals derived from IFN-gamma and LPS receptors during macrophage activation. *EMBO J* **17**:3660–3668.

61. Frucht DM, Fukao T, Bogdan C, Schindler H, O'Shea JJ, Koyasu S. 2001. IFN-gamma production by antigen-presenting cells: mechanisms emerge. *Trends Immunol* **22**:556–560.

62. Reed JM, Branigan PJ, Bamezai A. 2008. Interferon gamma enhances clonal expansion and survival of CD4+ T cells. *J Interferon Cytokine Res* **28**:611–622.

63. Munder M, Mallo M, Eichmann K, Modolell M. 1998. Murine macrophages secrete interferon gamma upon combined stimulation with interleukin (IL)-12 and IL-18: a novel pathway of autocrine macrophage activation. *J Exp Med* **187**:2103–2108.

64. Otani T, Nakamura S, Toki M, Motoda R, Kurimoto M, Orita K. 1999. Identification of IFN-gamma-producing cells in IL-12/IL-18-treated mice. *Cell Immunol* **198**:111–119.

65. Zhang SY, Boisson-Dupuis S, Chapgier A, Yang K, Bustamante J, Puel A, Picard C, Abel L, Jouanguy E,

Casanova JL. 2008. Inborn errors of interferon (IFN)-mediated immunity in humans: insights into the respective roles of IFN-alpha/beta, IFN-gamma, and IFN-lambda in host defense. *Immunol Rev* **226**:29–40.

66. Filipe-Santos O, Bustamante J, Chapgier A, Vogt G, de Beaucoudrey L, Feinberg J, Jouanguy E, Boisson-Dupuis S, Fieschi C, Picard C, Casanova JL. 2006. Inborn errors of IL-12/23- and IFN-gamma-mediated immunity: molecular, cellular, and clinical features. *Semin Immunol* **18**:347–361.

67. Sologuren I, Boisson-Dupuis S, Pestano J, Vincent QB, Fernández-Pérez L, Chapgier A, Cárdenes M, Feinberg J, García-Laorden MI, Picard C, Santiago E, Kong X, Jannière L, Colino E, Herrera-Ramos E, Francés A, Navarrete C, Blanche S, Faria E, Remiszewski P, Cordeiro A, Freeman A, Holland S, Abarca K, Valerón-Lemaur M, Gonçalo-Marques J, Silveira L, García-Castellano J, Caminero J, Pérez-Arellano JL, Bustamante J, Abel L, Casanova J-L, Rodríguez-Gallego C. 2011. Partial recessive IFN-γR1 deficiency: genetic, immunological and clinical features of 14 patients from 11 kindreds. *Hum Mol Genet* **20**:1509–1523.

68. Vogt G, Chapgier A, Yang K, Chuzhanova N, Feinberg J, Fieschi C, Boisson-Dupuis S, Alcais A, Filipe-Santos O, Bustamante J, de Beaucoudrey L, Al-Mohsen I, Al-Hajjar S, Al-Ghonaium A, Adimi P, Mirsaeidi M, Khalilzadeh S, Rosenzweig S, de la Calle Martin O, Bauer TR, Puck JM, Ochs HD, Furthner D, Engelhorn C, Belohradsky B, Mansouri D, Holland SM, Schreiber RD, Abel L, Cooper DN, Soudais C, Casanova JL. 2005. Gains of glycosylation comprise an unexpectedly large group of pathogenic mutations. *Nat Genet* **37**:692–700.

69. Dorman SE, Holland SM. 1998. Mutation in the signal-transducing chain of the interferon-gamma receptor and susceptibility to mycobacterial infection. *J Clin Invest* **101**:2364–2369.

70. Cooper AM, Dalton DK, Stewart TA, Griffin JP, Russell DG, Orme IM. 1993. Disseminated tuberculosis in interferon gamma gene-disrupted mice. *J Exp Med* **178**:2243–2247.

71. Flynn JL, Chan J, Triebold KJ, Dalton DK, Stewart TA, Bloom BR. 1993. An essential role for interferon gamma in resistance to *Mycobacterium tuberculosis* infection. *J Exp Med* **178**:2249–2254.

72. Dalton DK, Pitts-Meek S, Keshav S, Figari IS, Bradley A, Stewart TA. 1993. Multiple defects of immune cell function in mice with disrupted interferon-gamma genes. *Science* **259**:1739–1742.

73. Russell DG. 2001. *Mycobacterium tuberculosis*: here today, and here tomorrow. *Nat Rev Mol Cell Biol* **2**:569–586.

74. Mogues T, Goodrich ME, Ryan L, LaCourse R, North RJ. 2001. The relative importance of T cell subsets in immunity and immunopathology of airborne *Mycobacterium tuberculosis* infection in mice. *J Exp Med* **193**:271–280.

75. Green AM, Difazio R, Flynn JL. 2013. IFN-γ from CD4 T cells is essential for host survival and enhances CD8 T cell function during Mycobacterium tuberculosis infection. *J Immunol* **190**:270–277.

76. Gallegos AM, van Heijst JW, Samstein M, Su X, Pamer EG, Glickman MS. 2011. A gamma interferon independent mechanism of CD4 T cell mediated control of *M. tuberculosis* infection in vivo. *PLoS Pathog* 7: e1002052.

77. Caruso AM, Serbina N, Klein E, Triebold K, Bloom BR, Flynn JL. 1999. Mice deficient in CD4 T cells have only transiently diminished levels of IFN-gamma, yet succumb to tuberculosis. *J Immunol* 162:5407–5416.

78. Saunders BM, Frank AA, Orme IM, Cooper AM. 2002. CD4 is required for the development of a protective granulomatous response to pulmonary tuberculosis. *Cell Immunol* 216:65–72.

79. Serbina NV, Lazarevic V, Flynn JL. 2001. CD4(+) T cells are required for the development of cytotoxic CD8(+) T cells during *Mycobacterium tuberculosis* infection. *J Immunol* 167:6991–7000.

80. Sakai S, Kauffman KD, Schenkel JM, McBerry CC, Mayer-Barber KD, Masopust D, Barber DL. 2014. Cutting edge: control of *Mycobacterium tuberculosis* infection by a subset of lung parenchyma-homing CD4 T cells. *J Immunol* 192:2965–2969.

81. Moguche AO, Shafiani S, Clemons C, Larson RP, Dinh C, Higdon LE, Cambier CJ, Sissons JR, Gallegos AM, Fink PJ, Urdahl KB. 2015. ICOS and Bcl6-dependent pathways maintain a CD4 T cell population with memory-like properties during tuberculosis. *J Exp Med* 212:715–728.

82. Torrado E, Fountain JJ, Liao M, Tighe M, Reiley WW, Lai RP, Meintjes G, Pearl JE, Chen X, Zak DE, Thompson EG, Aderem A, Ghilardi N, Solache A, McKinstry KK, Strutt TM, Wilkinson RJ, Swain SL, Cooper AM. 2015. Interleukin 27R regulates CD4+ T cell phenotype and impacts protective immunity during *Mycobacterium tuberculosis* infection. *J Exp Med* 212:1449–1463.

83. Keller C, Hoffmann R, Lang R, Brandau S, Hermann C, Ehlers S. 2006. Genetically determined susceptibility to tuberculosis in mice causally involves accelerated and enhanced recruitment of granulocytes. *Infect Immun* 74:4295–4309.

84. Eruslanov EB, Lyadova IV, Kondratieva TK, Majorov KB, Scheglov IV, Orlova MO, Apt AS. 2005. Neutrophil responses to *Mycobacterium tuberculosis* infection in genetically susceptible and resistant mice. *Infect Immun* 73:1744–1753.

85. Majorov KB, Eruslanov EB, Rubakova EI, Kondratieva TK, Apt AS. 2005. Analysis of cellular phenotypes that mediate genetic resistance to tuberculosis using a radiation bone marrow chimera approach. *Infect Immun* 73:6174–6178.

86. Mitsos LM, Cardon LR, Fortin A, Ryan L, LaCourse R, North RJ, Gros P. 2000. Genetic control of susceptibility to infection with *Mycobacterium tuberculosis* in mice. *Genes Immun* 1:467–477.

87. Nandi B, Behar SM. 2011. Regulation of neutrophils by interferon-γ limits lung inflammation during tuberculosis infection. *J Exp Med* 208:2251–2262.

88. Desvignes L, Ernst JD. 2009. Interferon-γ-responsive nonhematopoietic cells regulate the immune response to *Mycobacterium tuberculosis*. *Immunity* 31:974–985.

89. Stefan DC, Dippenaar A, Detjen AK, Schaaf HS, Marais BJ, Kriel B, Loebenberg L, Walzl G, Hesseling AC. 2010. Interferon-gamma release assays for the detection of *Mycobacterium tuberculosis* infection in children with cancer. *Int J Tuberc Lung Dis* 14:689–694.

90. Abu-Taleb AM, El-Sokkary RH, El Tarhouny SA. 2011. Interferon-gamma release assay for detection of latent tuberculosis infection in casual and close contacts of tuberculosis cases. *East Mediterr Health J* 17:749–753.

91. Ferrara G, Losi M, D'Amico R, Cagarelli R, Pezzi AM, Meacci M, Meccugni B, Marchetti Dori I, Rumpianesi F, Roversi P, Casali L, Fabbri LM, Richeldi L. 2009. Interferon-gamma-release assays detect recent tuberculosis re-infection in elderly contacts. *Int J Immunopathol Pharmacol* 22:669–677.

92. Diel R, Loddenkemper R, Niemann S, Meywald-Walter K, Nienhaus A. 2011. Negative and positive predictive value of a whole-blood interferon-γ release assay for developing active tuberculosis: an update. *Am J Respir Crit Care Med* 183:88–95.

93. Isaacs A, Lindenmann J. 1957. Virus interference. I. The interferon. *Proc R Soc Lond B Biol Sci* 147:258–267.

94. McNab F, Mayer-Barber K, Sher A, Wack A, O'Garra A. 2015. Type I interferons in infectious disease. *Nat Rev Immunol* 15:87–103.

95. Honda K, Takaoka A, Taniguchi T. 2006. Type I interferon [corrected] gene induction by the interferon regulatory factor family of transcription factors. *Immunity* 25:349–360

96. Cooper AM, Pearl JE, Brooks JV, Ehlers S, Orme IM. 2000. Expression of the nitric oxide synthase 2 gene is not essential for early control of *Mycobacterium tuberculosis* in the murine lung. *Infect Immun* 68:6879–6882.

97. Manca C, Tsenova L, Bergtold A, Freeman S, Tovey M, Musser JM, Barry CE III, Freedman VH, Kaplan G. 2001. Virulence of a *Mycobacterium tuberculosis* clinical isolate in mice is determined by failure to induce Th1 type immunity and is associated with induction of IFN-alpha/beta. *Proc Natl Acad Sci USA* 98:5752–5757.

98. Ordway D, Henao-Tamayo M, Harton M, Palanisamy G, Troudt J, Shanley C, Basaraba RJ, Orme IM. 2007. The hypervirulent *Mycobacterium tuberculosis* strain HN878 induces a potent TH1 response followed by rapid down-regulation. *J Immunol* 179:522–531.

99. McNab FW, Ewbank J, Howes A, Moreira-Teixeira L, Martirosyan A, Ghilardi N, Saraiva M, O'Garra A. 2014. Type I IFN induces IL-10 production in an IL-27-independent manner and blocks responsiveness to IFN-γ for production of IL-12 and bacterial killing in *Mycobacterium tuberculosis*-infected macrophages. *J Immunol* 193:3600–3612.

100. Berry MP, Graham CM, McNab FW, Xu Z, Bloch SA, Oni T, Wilkinson KA, Banchereau R, Skinner J, Wilkinson RJ, Quinn C, Blankenship D, Dhawan R, Cush JJ, Mejias A, Ramilo O, Kon OM, Pascual V, Banchereau J, Chaussabel D, O'Garra A. 2010. An interferon-inducible neutrophil-driven blood transcriptional signature in human tuberculosis. *Nature* 466:973–977.

101. Antonelli LR, Gigliotti Rothfuchs A, Gonçalves R, Roffê E, Cheever AW, Bafica A, Salazar AM, Feng CG, Sher A. 2010. Intranasal Poly-IC treatment exacerbates tuberculosis in mice through the pulmonary recruitment of a pathogen-permissive monocyte/macrophage population. *J Clin Invest* 120:1674–1682.

102. Desvignes L, Wolf AJ, Ernst JD. 2012. Dynamic roles of type I and type II IFNs in early infection with *Mycobacterium tuberculosis*. *J Immunol* 188:6205–6215.

103. Van Snick J. 1990. Interleukin-6: an overview. *Annu Rev Immunol* 8:253–278.

104. Shalaby MR, Waage A, Espevik T. 1989. Cytokine regulation of interleukin 6 production by human endothelial cells. *Cell Immunol* 121:372–382.

105. Sanceau J, Beranger F, Gaudelet C, Wietzerbin J. 1989. IFN-gamma is an essential cosignal for triggering IFN-beta 2/BSF-2/IL-6 gene expression in human monocytic cell lines. *Ann N Y Acad Sci* 557:130–143, discussion 141–143.

106. Heinrich PC, Behrmann I, Haan S, Hermanns HM, Müller-Newen G, Schaper F. 2003. Principles of interleukin (IL)-6-type cytokine signalling and its regulation. *Biochem J* 374:1–20.

107. Heinrich PC, Behrmann I, Müller-Newen G, Schaper F, Graeve L. 1998. Interleukin-6-type cytokine signalling through the gp130/Jak/STAT pathway. *Biochem J* 334: 297–314.

108. Ladel CH, Blum C, Dreher A, Reifenberg K, Kopf M, Kaufmann SH. 1997. Lethal tuberculosis in interleukin-6-deficient mutant mice. *Infect Immun* 65:4843–4849.

109. Appelberg R, Castro AG, Pedrosa J, Minóprio P. 1994. Role of interleukin-6 in the induction of protective T cells during mycobacterial infections in mice. *Immunology* 82:361–364.

110. Saunders BM, Frank AA, Orme IM, Cooper AM. 2000. Interleukin-6 induces early gamma interferon production in the infected lung but is not required for generation of specific immunity to *Mycobacterium tuberculosis* infection. *Infect Immun* 68:3322–3326.

111. Leal IS, Smedegârd B, Andersen P, Appelberg R. 1999. Interleukin-6 and interleukin-12 participate in induction of a type 1 protective T-cell response during vaccination with a tuberculosis subunit vaccine. *Infect Immun* 67: 5747–5754.

112. Atreya R, Neurath MF. 2005. Involvement of IL-6 in the pathogenesis of inflammatory bowel disease and colon cancer. *Clin Rev Allergy Immunol* 28:187–196.

113. Sodenkamp J, Waetzig GH, Scheller J, Seegert D, Grötzinger J, Rose-John S, Ehlers S, Hölscher C. 2012. Therapeutic targeting of interleukin-6 trans-signaling does not affect the outcome of experimental tuberculosis. *Immunobiology* 217:996–1004.

114. Nolan A, Condos R, Huie ML, Dawson R, Dheda K, Bateman E, Rom WN, Weiden MD. 2013. Elevated IP-10 and IL-6 from bronchoalveolar lavage cells are biomarkers of non-cavitary tuberculosis. *Int J Tuberc Lung Dis* 17:922–927.

115. el-Ahmady O, Mansour M, Zoeir H, Mansour O. 1997. Elevated concentrations of interleukins and leukotriene in response to *Mycobacterium tuberculosis* infection. *Ann Clin Biochem* 34:160–164.

116. Dinarello CA. 1991. Interleukin-1 and interleukin-1 antagonism. *Blood* 77:1627–1652.

117. Menkin V. 1943. The effect of the leukocytosis-promoting factor on the growth of cells in the bone marrow. *Am J Pathol* 19:1021–1029.

118. Menkin V. 1943. Studies on the isolation of the factor responsible for tissue injury in inflammation. *Science* 97:165–167.

119. Menkin V. 1944. Chemical basis of fever. *Science* 100: 337–338.

120. Gross O, Yazdi AS, Thomas CJ, Masin M, Heinz LX, Guarda G, Quadroni M, Drexler SK, Tschopp J. 2012. Inflammasome activators induce interleukin-1α secretion via distinct pathways with differential requirement for the protease function of caspase-1. *Immunity* 36:388–400.

121. Sansonetti PJ, Phalipon A, Arondel J, Thirumalai K, Banerjee S, Akira S, Takeda K, Zychlinsky A. 2000. Caspase-1 activation of IL-1beta and IL-18 are essential for Shigella flexneri-induced inflammation. *Immunity* 12:581–590.

122. Latz E, Xiao TS, Stutz A. 2013. Activation and regulation of the inflammasomes. *Nat Rev Immunol* 13: 397–411.

123. Kayagaki N, Warming S, Lamkanfi M, Vande Walle L, Louie S, Dong J, Newton K, Qu Y, Liu J, Heldens S, Zhang J, Lee WP, Roose-Girma M, Dixit VM. 2011. Non-canonical inflammasome activation targets caspase-11. *Nature* 479:117–121.

124. Bossaller L, Chiang PI, Schmidt-Lauber C, Ganesan S, Kaiser WJ, Rathinam VA, Mocarski ES, Subramanian D, Green DR, Silverman N, Fitzgerald KA, Marshak-Rothstein A, Latz E. 2012. Cutting edge: FAS (CD95) mediates noncanonical IL-1β and IL-18 maturation via caspase-8 in an RIP3-independent manner. *J Immunol* 189:5508–5512.

125. Chen CJ, Kono H, Golenbock D, Reed G, Akira S, Rock KL. 2007. Identification of a key pathway required for the sterile inflammatory response triggered by dying cells. *Nat Med* 13:851–856.

126. Rider P, Carmi Y, Guttman O, Braiman A, Cohen I, Voronov E, White MR, Dinarello CA, Apte RN. 2011. IL-1α and IL-1β recruit different myeloid cells and promote different stages of sterile inflammation. *J Immunol* 187:4835–4843.

127. Berda-Haddad Y, Robert S, Salers P, Zekraoui L, Farnarier C, Dinarello CA, Dignat-George F, Kaplanski G. 2011. Sterile inflammation of endothelial cell-derived apoptotic bodies is mediated by interleukin-1α. *Proc Natl Acad Sci USA* 108:20684–20689.

128. Botelho FM, Bauer CM, Finch D, Nikota JK, Zavitz CC, Kelly A, Lambert KN, Piper S, Foster ML, Goldring JJ, Wedzicha JA, Bassett J, Bramson J, Iwakura Y, Sleeman M, Kolbeck R, Coyle AJ, Humbles AA, Stämpfli MR. 2011. IL-1α/IL-1R1 expression in chronic obstructive pulmonary disease and mechanistic relevance to smoke-induced neutrophilia in mice. *PLoS One* 6:e28457.

129. Freigang S, Ampenberger F, Weiss A, Kanneganti T-D, Iwakura Y, Hersberger M, Kopf M. 2013. Fatty acid-induced mitochondrial uncoupling elicits inflammasome-independent IL-1α and sterile vascular inflammation in atherosclerosis. *Nat Immunol* 14:1045–1053.

130. Barry KC, Fontana MF, Portman JL, Dugan AS, Vance RE. 2013. IL-1α signaling initiates the inflammatory response to virulent Legionella pneumophila in vivo. *J Immunol* 190:6329–6339.

131. Biondo C, Mancuso G, Midiri A, Signorino G, Domina M, Lanza Cariccio V, Mohammadi N, Venza M, Venza I, Teti G, Beninati C. 2014. The interleukin-1β/CXCL1/2/neutrophil axis mediates host protection against group B streptococcal infection. *Infect Immun* 82:4508–4517.

132. Guo H, Gao J, Taxman DJ, Ting JP, Su L. 2014. HIV-1 infection induces interleukin-1β production via TLR8 protein-dependent and NLRP3 inflammasome mechanisms in human monocytes. *J Biol Chem* 289:21716–21726.

133. Rynko AE, Fryer AD, Jacoby DB. 2014. Interleukin-1β mediates virus-induced m2 muscarinic receptor dysfunction and airway hyperreactivity. *Am J Respir Cell Mol Biol* 51:494–501.

134. Shigematsu Y, Niwa T, Rehnberg E, Toyoda T, Yoshida S, Mori A, Wakabayashi M, Iwakura Y, Ichinose M, Kim YJ, Ushijima T. 2013. Interleukin-1β induced by *Helicobacter pylori* infection enhances mouse gastric carcinogenesis. *Cancer Lett* 340:141–147.

135. Dinarello CA. 2011. Interleukin-1 in the pathogenesis and treatment of inflammatory diseases. *Blood* 117:3720–3732.

136. Konsman JP, Vigues S, Mackerlova L, Bristow A, Blomqvist A. 2004. Rat brain vascular distribution of interleukin-1 type-1 receptor immunoreactivity: relationship to patterns of inducible cyclooxygenase expression by peripheral inflammatory stimuli. *J Comp Neurol* 472:113–129.

137. Marshall JD, Aste-Amézaga M, Chehimi SS, Murphy M, Olsen H, Trinchieri G. 1999. Regulation of human IL-18 mRNA expression. *Clin Immunol* 90:15–21.

138. Puren AJ, Fantuzzi G, Dinarello CA. 1999. Gene expression, synthesis, and secretion of interleukin 18 and interleukin 1beta are differentially regulated in human blood mononuclear cells and mouse spleen cells. *Proc Natl Acad Sci USA* 96:2256–2261.

139. Sugawara S, Uehara A, Nochi T, Yamaguchi T, Ueda H, Sugiyama A, Hanzawa K, Kumagai K, Okamura H, Takada H. 2001. Neutrophil proteinase 3-mediated induction of bioactive IL-18 secretion by human oral epithelial cells. *J Immunol* 167:6568–6575.

140. Dinarello CA, Novick D, Kim S, Kaplanski G. 2013. Interleukin-18 and IL-18 binding protein. *Front Immunol* 4:289.

141. Hölscher C, Reiling N, Schaible UE, Hölscher A, Bathmann C, Korbel D, Lenz I, Sonntag T, Kröger S, Akira S, Mossmann H, Kirschning CJ, Wagner H, Freudenberg M, Ehlers S. 2008. Containment of aerogenic *Mycobacterium tuberculosis* infection in mice does not require MyD88 adaptor function for TLR2, -4 and -9. *Eur J Immunol* 38:680–694.

142. O'Neill LA, Bowie AG. 2007. The family of five: TIR-domain-containing adaptors in Toll-like receptor signalling. *Nat Rev Immunol* 7:353–364.

143. Fremond CM, Yeremeev V, Nicolle DM, Jacobs M, Quesniaux VF, Ryffel B. 2004. Fatal *Mycobacterium tuberculosis* infection despite adaptive immune response in the absence of MyD88. *J Clin Invest* 114:1790–1799.

144. Fremond CM, Togbe D, Doz E, Rose S, Vasseur V, Maillet I, Jacobs M, Ryffel B, Quesniaux VF. 2007. IL-1 receptor-mediated signal is an essential component of MyD88-dependent innate response to *Mycobacterium tuberculosis* infection. *J Immunol* 179:1178–1189.

145. Mayer-Barber KD, Andrade BB, Barber DL, Hieny S, Feng CG, Caspar P, Oland S, Gordon S, Sher A. 2011. Innate and adaptive interferons suppress IL-1α and IL-1β production by distinct pulmonary myeloid subsets during *Mycobacterium tuberculosis* infection. *Immunity* 35:1023–1034.

146. Bourigault ML, Segueni N, Rose S, Court N, Vacher R, Vasseur V, Erard F, Le Bert M, Garcia I, Iwakura Y, Jacobs M, Ryffel B, Quesniaux VF. 2013. Relative contribution of IL-1α, IL-1β and TNF to the host response to *Mycobacterium tuberculosis* and attenuated *M. bovis* BCG. *Immun Inflamm Dis* 1:47–62.

147. Di Paolo NC, Shafiani S, Day T, Papayannopoulou T, Russell DW, Iwakura Y, Sherman D, Urdahl K, Shayakhmetov DM. 2015. Interdependence between interleukin-1 and tumor necrosis factor regulates TNF-dependent control of *Mycobacterium tuberculosis* infection. *Immunity* 43:1125–1136. (Erratum: 44:438.)

148. Guler R, Parihar SP, Spohn G, Johansen P, Brombacher F, Bachmann MF. 2011. Blocking IL-1α but not IL-1β increases susceptibility to chronic *Mycobacterium tuberculosis* infection in mice. *Vaccine* 29:1339–1346.

149. Gopal R, Monin L, Slight S, Uche U, Blanchard E, Fallert Junecko BA, Ramos-Payan R, Stallings CL, Reinhart TA, Kolls JK, Kaushal D, Nagarajan U, Rangel-Moreno J, Khader SA. 2014. Unexpected role for IL-17 in protective immunity against hypervirulent *Mycobacterium tuberculosis* HN878 infection. *PLoS Pathog* 10:e1004099.

150. Schneider BE, Korbel D, Hagens K, Koch M, Raupach B, Enders J, Kaufmann SH, Mittrücker HW, Schaible UE. 2010. A role for IL-18 in protective immunity against *Mycobacterium tuberculosis*. *Eur J Immunol* 40:396–405.

151. Suwara MI, Green NJ, Borthwick LA, Mann J, Mayer-Barber KD, Barron L, Corris PA, Farrow SN, Wynn TA, Fisher AJ, Mann DA. 2014. IL-1α released from damaged epithelial cells is sufficient and essential to trigger inflammatory responses in human lung fibroblasts. *Mucosal Immunol* 7:684–693.

152. Fielding CA, McLoughlin RM, McLeod L, Colmont CS, Najdovska M, Grail D, Ernst M, Jones SA, Topley N, Jenkins BJ. 2008. IL-6 regulates neutrophil trafficking during acute inflammation via STAT3. *J Immunol* 181:2189–2195.

153. Lalor SJ, Dungan LS, Sutton CE, Basdeo SA, Fletcher JM, Mills KH. 2011. Caspase-1-processed cytokines IL-1beta and IL-18 promote IL-17 production by

gammadelta and CD4 T cells that mediate autoimmunity. *J Immunol* **186**:5738–5748.

154. Dunne A, Ross PJ, Pospisilova E, Masin J, Meaney A, Sutton CE, Iwakura Y, Tschopp J, Sebo P, Mills KH. 2010. Inflammasome activation by adenylate cyclase toxin directs Th17 responses and protection against *Bordetella pertussis*. *J Immunol* **185**:1711–1719.

155. Chung Y, Chang SH, Martinez GJ, Yang XO, Nurieva R, Kang HS, Ma L, Watowich SS, Jetten AM, Tian Q, Dong C. 2009. Critical regulation of early Th17 cell differentiation by interleukin-1 signaling. *Immunity* **30**:576–587.

156. Monin L, Griffiths KL, Slight S, Lin Y, Rangel-Moreno J, Khader SA. 2015. Immune requirements for protective Th17 recall responses to *Mycobacterium tuberculosis* challenge. *Mucosal Immunol* **8**:1099–1109.

157. Khader SA, Bell GK, Pearl JE, Fountain JJ, Rangel-Moreno J, Cilley GE, Shen F, Eaton SM, Gaffen SL, Swain SL, Locksley RM, Haynes L, Randall TD, Cooper AM. 2007. IL-23 and IL-17 in the establishment of protective pulmonary CD4+ T cell responses after vaccination and during *Mycobacterium tuberculosis* challenge. *Nat Immunol* **8**:369–377.

158. Mayer-Barber KD, Andrade BB, Oland SD, Amaral EP, Barber DL, Gonzales J, Derrick SC, Shi R, Kumar NP, Wei W, Yuan X, Zhang G, Cai Y, Babu S, Catalfamo M, Salazar AM, Via LE, Barry CE III, Sher A. 2014. Host-directed therapy of tuberculosis based on interleukin-1 and type I interferon crosstalk. *Nature* **511**:99–103.

159. Tominaga K, Yoshimoto T, Torigoe K, Kurimoto M, Matsui K, Hada T, Okamura H, Nakanishi K. 2000. IL-12 synergizes with IL-18 or IL-1beta for IFN-gamma production from human T cells. *Int Immunol* **12**:151–160.

160. Okamura H, Kashiwamura S, Tsutsui H, Yoshimoto T, Nakanishi K. 1998. Regulation of interferon-gamma production by IL-12 and IL-18. *Curr Opin Immunol* **10**:259–264.

161. Bohn E, Sing A, Zumbihl R, Bielfeldt C, Okamura H, Kurimoto M, Heesemann J, Autenrieth IB. 1998. IL-18 (IFN-gamma-inducing factor) regulates early cytokine production in, and promotes resolution of, bacterial infection in mice. *J Immunol* **160**:299–307.

162. Sugawara I, Yamada H, Kaneko H, Mizuno S, Takeda K, Akira S. 1999. Role of interleukin-18 (IL-18) in mycobacterial infection in IL-18-gene-disrupted mice. *Infect Immun* **67**:2585–2589.

163. Kinjo Y, Kawakami K, Uezu K, Yara S, Miyagi K, Koguchi Y, Hoshino T, Okamoto M, Kawase Y, Yokota K, Yoshino K, Takeda K, Akira S, Saito A. 2002. Contribution of IL-18 to Th1 response and host defense against infection by *Mycobacterium tuberculosis*: a comparative study with IL-12p40. *J Immunol* **169**:323–329.

164. Jones LL, Vignali DA. 2011. Molecular interactions within the IL-6/IL-12 cytokine/receptor superfamily. *Immunol Res* **51**:5–14.

165. Collison LW, Vignali DA. 2008. Interleukin-35: odd one out or part of the family? *Immunol Rev* **226**:248–262

166. Vignali DA, Kuchroo VK. 2012. IL-12 family cytokines: immunological playmakers. *Nat Immunol* **13**:722–728.

167. Méndez-Samperio P. 2010. Role of interleukin-12 family cytokines in the cellular response to mycobacterial disease. *Int J Infect Dis* **14**:e366–e371.

168. Hunter CA. 2005. New IL-12-family members: IL-23 and IL-27, cytokines with divergent functions. *Nat Rev Immunol* **5**:521–531.

169. Kobayashi M, Fitz L, Ryan M, Hewick RM, Clark SC, Chan S, Loudon R, Sherman F, Perussia B, Trinchieri G. 1989. Identification and purification of natural killer cell stimulatory factor (NKSF), a cytokine with multiple biologic effects on human lymphocytes. *J Exp Med* **170**:827–845.

170. Gately MK, et al. 1991. Regulation of human lymphocyte proliferation by a heterodimeric cytokine, IL-12 (cytotoxic lymphocyte maturation factor). *J Immunol* **147**:874–882.

171. Ma X, Trinchieri G. 2001. Regulation of interleukin-12 production in antigen-presenting cells. *Adv Immunol* **79**:55–92.

172. O'Shea JJ, Paul WE. 2002. Regulation of T(H)1 differentiation–controlling the controllers. *Nat Immunol* **3**:506–508.

173. Ozbek N, Fieschi C, Yilmaz BT, de Beaucoudrey L, Demirhan B, Feinberg J, Bikmaz YE, Casanova JL. 2005. Interleukin-12 receptor beta 1 chain deficiency in a child with disseminated tuberculosis. *Clin Infect Dis* **40**:e55–e58.

174. Dorman SE, Holland SM. 2000. Interferon-gamma and interleukin-12 pathway defects and human disease. *Cytokine Growth Factor Rev* **11**:321–333.

175. Picard C, Fieschi C, Altare F, Al-Jumaah S, Al-Hajjar S, Feinberg J, Dupuis S, Soudais C, Al-Mohsen IZ, Génin E, Lammas D, Kumararatne DS, Leclerc T, Rafii A, Frayha H, Murugasu B, Wah LB, Sinniah R, Loubser M, Okamoto E, Al-Ghonaium A, Tufenkeji H, Abel L, Casanova JL. 2002. Inherited interleukin-12 deficiency: IL12B genotype and clinical phenotype of 13 patients from six kindreds. *Am J Hum Genet* **70**:336–348.

176. Altare F, Ensser A, Breiman A, Reichenbach J, Baghdadi JE, Fischer A, Emile JF, Gaillard JL, Meinl E, Casanova JL. 2001. Interleukin-12 receptor beta1 deficiency in a patient with abdominal tuberculosis. *J Infect Dis* **184**:231–236.

177. Caragol I, Raspall M, Fieschi C, Feinberg J, Larrosa MN, Hernández M, Figueras C, Bertrán JM, Casanova JL, Español T. 2003. Clinical tuberculosis in 2 of 3 siblings with interleukin-12 receptor beta1 deficiency. *Clin Infect Dis* **37**:302–306.

178. Casanova JL, Abel L. 2002. Genetic dissection of immunity to mycobacteria: the human model. *Annu Rev Immunol* **20**:581–620.

179. Bogunovic D, Byun M, Durfee LA, Abhyankar A, Sanal O, Mansouri D, Salem S, Radovanovic I, Grant AV, Adimi P, Mansouri N, Okada S, Bryant VL, Kong XF, Kreins A, Velez MM, Boisson B, Khalilzadeh S, Ozcelik U, Darazam IA, Schoggins JW, Rice CM, Al-Muhsen S, Behr M, Vogt G, Puel A, Bustamante J, Gros P, Huibregtse JM, Abel L, Boisson-Dupuis S, Casanova JL. 2012. Mycobacterial disease and impaired IFN-γ immunity in humans with inherited ISG15 deficiency. *Science* **337**:1684–1688.

180. Bustamante J, Arias AA, Vogt G, Picard C, Galicia LB, Prando C, Grant AV, Marchal CC, Hubeau M, Chapgier A, de Beaucoudrey L, Puel A, Feinberg J, Valinetz E, Jannière L, Besse C, Boland A, Brisseau JM, Blanche S, Lortholary O, Fieschi C, Emile JF, Boisson-Dupuis S, Al-Muhsen S, Woda B, Newburger PE, Condino-Neto A, Dinauer MC, Abel L, Casanova JL. 2011. Germline CYBB mutations that selectively affect macrophages in kindreds with X-linked predisposition to tuberculous mycobacterial disease. *Nat Immunol* 12:213–221.

181. Bustamante J, Picard C, Boisson-Dupuis S, Abel L, Casanova J-L. 2011. Genetic lessons learned from X-linked Mendelian susceptibility to mycobacterial diseases. *Ann N Y Acad Sci* 1246:92–101.

182. Filipe-Santos O, Bustamante J, Haverkamp MH, Vinolo E, Ku CL, Puel A, Frucht DM, Christel K, von Bernuth H, Jouanguy E, Feinberg J, Durandy A, Senechal B, Chapgier A, Vogt G, de Beaucoudrey L, Fieschi C, Picard C, Garfa M, Chemli J, Bejaoui M, Tsolia MN, Kutukculer N, Plebani A, Notarangelo L, Bodemer C, Geissmann F, Israël A, Véron M, Knackstedt M, Barbouche R, Abel L, Magdorf K, Gendrel D, Agou F, Holland SM, Casanova JL. 2006. X-linked susceptibility to mycobacteria is caused by mutations in NEMO impairing CD40-dependent IL-12 production. *J Exp Med* 203:1745–1759.

183. Zhang M, Gately MK, Wang E, Gong J, Wolf SF, Lu S, Modlin RL, Barnes PF. 1994. Interleukin 12 at the site of disease in tuberculosis. *J Clin Invest* 93:1733–1739.

184. Cooper AM, Roberts AD, Rhoades ER, Callahan JE, Getzy DM, Orme IM. 1995. The role of interleukin-12 in acquired immunity to Mycobacterium tuberculosis infection. *Immunology* 84:423–432.

185. Cooper AM, Magram J, Ferrante J, Orme IM. 1997. Interleukin 12 (IL-12) is crucial to the development of protective immunity in mice intravenously infected with mycobacterium tuberculosis. *J Exp Med* 186:39–45.

186. Cooper AM, Kipnis A, Turner J, Magram J, Ferrante J, Orme IM. 2002. Mice lacking bioactive IL-12 can generate protective, antigen-specific cellular responses to mycobacterial infection only if the IL-12 p40 subunit is present. *J Immunol* 168:1322–1327.

187. Khader SA, Pearl JE, Sakamoto K, Gilmartin L, Bell GK, Jelley-Gibbs DM, Ghilardi N, deSauvage F, Cooper AM. 2005. IL-23 compensates for the absence of IL-12p70 and is essential for the IL-17 response during tuberculosis but is dispensable for protection and antigen-specific IFN-gamma responses if IL-12p70 is available. *J Immunol* 175:788–795.

188. Feng CG, Jankovic D, Kullberg M, Cheever A, Scanga CA, Hieny S, Caspar P, Yap GS, Sher A. 2005. Maintenance of pulmonary Th1 effector function in chronic tuberculosis requires persistent IL-12 production. *J Immunol* 174:4185–4192.

189. Cleary AM, Tu W, Enright A, Giffon T, Dewaal-Malefyt R, Gutierrez K, Lewis DB. 2003. Impaired accumulation and function of memory CD4 T cells in human IL-12 receptor beta 1 deficiency. *J Immunol* 170:597–603.

190. Bafica A, Scanga CA, Feng CG, Leifer C, Cheever A, Sher A. 2005. TLR9 regulates Th1 responses and cooperates with TLR2 in mediating optimal resistance to *Mycobacterium tuberculosis*. *J Exp Med* 202:1715–1724.

191. Pathak SK, Basu S, Bhattacharyya A, Pathak S, Kundu M, Basu J. 2005. *Mycobacterium tuberculosis* lipoarabinomannan-mediated IRAK-M induction negatively regulates Toll-like receptor-dependent interleukin-12 p40 production in macrophages. *J Biol Chem* 280:42794–42800.

192. Pecora ND, Gehring AJ, Canaday DH, Boom WH, Harding CV. 2006. *Mycobacterium tuberculosis* LprA is a lipoprotein agonist of TLR2 that regulates innate immunity and APC function. *J Immunol* 177:422–429.

193. Presky DH, Yang H, Minetti LJ, Chua AO, Nabavi N, Wu CY, Gately MK, Gubler U. 1996. A functional interleukin 12 receptor complex is composed of two beta-type cytokine receptor subunits. *Proc Natl Acad Sci USA* 93:14002–14007.

194. Chua AO, et al. 1994. Expression cloning of a human IL-12 receptor component. A new member of the cytokine receptor superfamily with strong homology to gp130. *J Immunol* 153:128–136.

195. Chua AO, Wilkinson VL, Presky DH, Gubler U. 1995. Cloning and characterization of a mouse IL-12 receptor-beta component. *J Immunol* 155:4286–4294.

196. Gillessen S, Carvajal D, Ling P, Podlaski FJ, Stremlo DL, Familletti PC, Gubler U, Presky DH, Stern AS, Gately MK. 1995. Mouse interleukin-12 (IL-12) p40 homodimer: a potent IL-12 antagonist. *Eur J Immunol* 25:200–206.

197. Gately MK, Carvajal DM, Connaughton SE, Gillessen S, Warrier RR, Kolinsky KD, Wilkinson VL, Dwyer CM, Higgins GF Jr, Podlaski FJ, Faherty DA, Familletti PC, Stern AS, Presky DH. 1996. Interleukin-12 antagonist activity of mouse interleukin-12 p40 homodimer in vitro and in vivo. *Ann N Y Acad Sci* 795(1 Interleukin 1):1–12.

198. Mattner F, Fischer S, Guckes S, Jin S, Kaulen H, Schmitt E, Rüde E, Germann T. 1993. The interleukin-12 subunit p40 specifically inhibits effects of the interleukin-12 heterodimer. *Eur J Immunol* 23:2202–2208.

199. Hölscher C, Atkinson RA, Arendse B, Brown N, Myburgh E, Alber G, Brombacher F. 2001. A protective and agonistic function of IL-12p40 in mycobacterial infection. *J Immunol* 167:6957–6966.

200. Khader SA, Partida-Sanchez S, Bell G, Jelley-Gibbs DM, Swain S, Pearl JE, Ghilardi N, Desauvage FJ, Lund FE, Cooper AM. 2006. Interleukin 12p40 is required for dendritic cell migration and T cell priming after *Mycobacterium tuberculosis* infection. *J Exp Med* 203:1805–1815.

201. Reinhardt RL, Hong S, Kang SJ, Wang ZE, Locksley RM. 2006. Visualization of IL-12/23p40 in vivo reveals immunostimulatory dendritic cell migrants that promote Th1 differentiation. *J Immunol* 177:1618–1627.

202. Wolf AJ, Desvignes L, Linas B, Banaiee N, Tamura T, Takatsu K, Ernst JD. 2008. Initiation of the adaptive immune response to *Mycobacterium tuberculosis* depends on antigen production in the local lymph node, not the lungs. *J Exp Med* 205:105–115.

203. Robinson RT, Khader SA, Martino CA, Fountain JJ, Teixeira-Coelho M, Pearl JE, Smiley ST, Winslow GM, Woodland DL, Walter MJ, Conejo-Garcia JR, Gubler U, Cooper AM. 2010. *Mycobacterium tuberculosis* infection induces il12rb1 splicing to generate a novel IL-12Rbeta1 isoform that enhances DC migration. *J Exp Med* 207:591–605. (Erratum: 207:897.)

204. Keeton R, Allie N, Dambuza I, Abel B, Hsu NJ, Sebesho B, Randall P, Burger P, Fick E, Quesniaux VF, Ryffel B, Jacobs M. 2014. Soluble TNFRp75 regulates host protective immunity against *Mycobacterium tuberculosis*. *J Clin Invest* 124:1537–1551.

205. Oppmann B, Lesley R, Blom B, Timans JC, Xu Y, Hunte B, Vega F, Yu N, Wang J, Singh K, Zonin F, Vaisberg E, Churakova T, Liu M, Gorman D, Wagner J, Zurawski S, Liu Y, Abrams JS, Moore KW, Rennick D, de Waal-Malefyt R, Hannum C, Bazan JF, Kastelein RA. 2000. Novel p19 protein engages IL-12p40 to form a cytokine, IL-23, with biological activities similar as well as distinct from IL-12. *Immunity* 13:715–725.

206. Uhlig HH, McKenzie BS, Hue S, Thompson C, Joyce-Shaikh B, Stepankova R, Robinson N, Buonocore S, Tlaskalova-Hogenova H, Cua DJ, Powrie F. 2006. Differential activity of IL-12 and IL-23 in mucosal and systemic innate immune pathology. *Immunity* 25:309–318.

207. Teng MW, Bowman EP, McElwee JJ, Smyth MJ, Casanova JL, Cooper AM, Cua DJ. 2015. IL-12 and IL-23 cytokines: from discovery to targeted therapies for immune-mediated inflammatory diseases. *Nat Med* 21:719–729.

208. Cua DJ, Sherlock J, Chen Y, Murphy CA, Joyce B, Seymour B, Lucian L, To W, Kwan S, Churakova T, Zurawski S, Wiekowski M, Lira SA, Gorman D, Kastelein RA, Sedgwick JD. 2003. Interleukin-23 rather than interleukin-12 is the critical cytokine for autoimmune inflammation of the brain. *Nature* 421:744–748.

209. Murphy CA, Langrish CL, Chen Y, Blumenschein W, McClanahan T, Kastelein RA, Sedgwick JD, Cua DJ. 2003. Divergent pro- and antiinflammatory roles for IL-23 and IL-12 in joint autoimmune inflammation. *J Exp Med* 198:1951–1957.

210. Kroenke MA, Carlson TJ, Andjelkovic AV, Segal BM. 2008. IL-12- and IL-23-modulated T cells induce distinct types of EAE based on histology, CNS chemokine profile, and response to cytokine inhibition. *J Exp Med* 205:1535–1541.

211. Ivanov II, McKenzie BS, Zhou L, Tadokoro CE, Lepelley A, Lafaille JJ, Cua DJ, Littman DR. 2006. The orphan nuclear receptor RORgammat directs the differentiation program of proinflammatory IL-17+ T helper cells. *Cell* 126:1121–1133.

212. Hirota K, Duarte JH, Veldhoen M, Hornsby E, Li Y, Cua DJ, Ahlfors H, Wilhelm C, Tolaini M, Menzel U, Garefalaki A, Potocnik AJ, Stockinger B. 2011. Fate mapping of IL-17-producing T cells in inflammatory responses. *Nat Immunol* 12:255–263.

213. Weaver CT, Hatton RD, Mangan PR, Harrington LE. 2007. IL-17 family cytokines and the expanding diversity of effector T cell lineages. *Annu Rev Immunol* 25:821–852.

214. Parham C, Chirica M, Timans J, Vaisberg E, Travis M, Cheung J, Pflanz S, Zhang R, Singh KP, Vega F, To W, Wagner J, O'Farrell AM, McClanahan T, Zurawski S, Hannum C, Gorman D, Rennick DM, Kastelein RA, de Waal Malefyt R, Moore KW. 2002. A receptor for the heterodimeric cytokine IL-23 is composed of IL-12Rbeta1 and a novel cytokine receptor subunit, IL-23R. *J Immunol* 168:5699–5708.

215. Watford WT, Hissong BD, Bream JH, Kanno Y, Muul L, O'Shea JJ. 2004. Signaling by IL-12 and IL-23 and the immunoregulatory roles of STAT4. *Immunol Rev* 202:139–156.

216. Trinchieri G. 2003. Interleukin-12 and the regulation of innate resistance and adaptive immunity. *Nat Rev Immunol* 3:133–146.

217. Wozniak TM, Ryan AA, Triccas JA, Britton WJ. 2006. Plasmid interleukin-23 (IL-23), but not plasmid IL-27, enhances the protective efficacy of a DNA vaccine against *Mycobacterium tuberculosis* infection. *Infect Immun* 74:557–565.

218. Lockhart E, Green AM, Flynn JL. 2006. IL-17 production is dominated by gammadelta T cells rather than CD4 T cells during *Mycobacterium tuberculosis* infection. *J Immunol* 177:4662–4669.

219. Khader SA, Guglani L, Rangel-Moreno J, Gopal R, Junecko BA, Fountain JJ, Martino C, Pearl JE, Tighe M, Lin YY, Slight S, Kolls JK, Reinhart TA, Randall TD, Cooper AM. 2011. IL-23 is required for long-term control of *Mycobacterium tuberculosis* and B cell follicle formation in the infected lung. *J Immunol* 187:5402–5407.

220. Happel KI, Lockhart EA, Mason CM, Porretta E, Keoshkerian E, Odden AR, Nelson S, Ramsay AJ. 2005. Pulmonary interleukin-23 gene delivery increases local T-cell immunity and controls growth of *Mycobacterium tuberculosis* in the lungs. *Infect Immun* 73:5782–5788.

221. Gopal R, Rangel-Moreno J, Slight S, Lin Y, Nawar HF, Fallert Junecko BA, Reinhart TA, Kolls J, Randall TD, Connell TD, Khader SA. 2013. Interleukin-17-dependent CXCL13 mediates mucosal vaccine-induced immunity against tuberculosis. *Mucosal Immunol* 6:972–984.

222. Lindenstrøm T, Woodworth J, Dietrich J, Aagaard C, Andersen P, Agger EM. 2012. Vaccine-induced th17 cells are maintained long-term postvaccination as a distinct and phenotypically stable memory subset. *Infect Immun* 80:3533–3544.

223. Desel C, Dorhoi A, Bandermann S, Grode L, Eisele B, Kaufmann SH. 2011. Recombinant BCG ΔureC hly+ induces superior protection over parental BCG by stimulating a balanced combination of type 1 and type 17 cytokine responses. *J Infect Dis* 204:1573–1584.

224. Kastelein RA, Hunter CA, Cua DJ. 2007. Discovery and biology of IL-23 and IL-27: related but functionally distinct regulators of inflammation. *Annu Rev Immunol* 25:221–242.

225. Langrish CL, McKenzie BS, Wilson NJ, de Waal Malefyt R, Kastelein RA, Cua DJ. 2004. IL-12 and IL-23: master regulators of innate and adaptive immunity. *Immunol Rev* 202:96–105.

226. Cox JH, Kljavin NM, Ramamoorthi N, Diehl L, Batten M, Ghilardi N. 2011. IL-27 promotes T cell-dependent colitis through multiple mechanisms. *J Exp Med* 208: 115–123.

227. Shimizu S, Sugiyama N, Masutani K, Sadanaga A, Miyazaki Y, Inoue Y, Akahoshi M, Katafuchi R, Hirakata H, Harada M, Hamano S, Nakashima H, Yoshida H. 2005. Membranous glomerulonephritis development with Th2-type immune deviations in MRL/lpr mice deficient for IL-27 receptor (WSX-1). *J Immunol* 175:7185–7192.

228. Cao Y, Doodes PD, Glant TT, Finnegan A. 2008. IL-27 induces a Th1 immune response and susceptibility to experimental arthritis. *J Immunol* 180:922–930.

229. Pflanz S, Timans JC, Cheung J, Rosales R, Kanzler H, Gilbert J, Hibbert L, Churakova T, Travis M, Vaisberg E, Blumenschein WM, Mattson JD, Wagner JL, To W, Zurawski S, McClanahan TK, Gorman DM, Bazan JF, de Waal Malefyt R, Rennick D, Kastelein RA. 2002. IL-27, a heterodimeric cytokine composed of EBI3 and p28 protein, induces proliferation of naive CD4+ T cells. *Immunity* 16:779–790.

230. Pflanz S, Hibbert L, Mattson J, Rosales R, Vaisberg E, Bazan JF, Phillips JH, McClanahan TK, de Waal Malefyt R, Kastelein RA. 2004. WSX-1 and glycoprotein 130 constitute a signal-transducing receptor for IL-27. *J Immunol* 172:2225–2231.

231. Batten M, Li J, Yi S, Kljavin NM, Danilenko DM, Lucas S, Lee J, de Sauvage FJ, Ghilardi N. 2006. Interleukin 27 limits autoimmune encephalomyelitis by suppressing the development of interleukin 17-producing T cells. *Nat Immunol* 7:929–936.

232. Neufert C, Becker C, Wirtz S, Fantini MC, Weigmann B, Galle PR, Neurath MF. 2007. IL-27 controls the development of inducible regulatory T cells and Th17 cells via differential effects on STAT1. *Eur J Immunol* 37:1809–1816.

233. Takeda A, Hamano S, Yamanaka A, Hanada T, Ishibashi T, Mak TW, Yoshimura A, Yoshida H. 2003. Cutting edge: role of IL-27/WSX-1 signaling for induction of T-bet through activation of STAT1 during initial Th1 commitment. *J Immunol* 170:4886–4890.

234. Pearl JE, Khader SA, Solache A, Gilmartin L, Ghilardi N, deSauvage F, Cooper AM. 2004. IL-27 signaling compromises control of bacterial growth in mycobacteria-infected mice. *J Immunol* 173:7490–7496.

235. Hölscher C, Hölscher A, Rückerl D, Yoshimoto T, Yoshida H, Mak T, Saris C, Ehlers S. 2005. The IL-27 receptor chain WSX-1 differentially regulates anti-bacterial immunity and survival during experimental tuberculosis. *J Immunol* 174:3534–3544.

236. Sodenkamp J, Behrends J, Förster I, Müller W, Ehlers S, Hölscher C. 2011. gp130 on macrophages/granulocytes modulates inflammation during experimental tuberculosis. *Eur J Cell Biol* 90:505–514.

237. Neurath MF. 2008. IL-12 family members in experimental colitis. *Mucosal Immunol* 1(Suppl 1):S28–S30.

238. Vignali DA, Collison LW, Workman CJ. 2008. How regulatory T cells work. *Nat Rev Immunol* 8:523–532.

239. Collison LW, Workman CJ, Kuo TT, Boyd K, Wang Y, Vignali KM, Cross R, Sehy D, Blumberg RS, Vignali DA. 2007. The inhibitory cytokine IL-35 contributes to regulatory T-cell function. *Nature* 450:566–569.

240. Jin W, Dong C. 2013. IL-17 cytokines in immunity and inflammation. *Emerg Microbes Infect* 2:e60.

241. Ishigame H, Kakuta S, Nagai T, Kadoki M, Nambu A, Komiyama Y, Fujikado N, Tanahashi Y, Akitsu A, Kotaki H, Sudo K, Nakae S, Sasakawa C, Iwakura Y. 2009. Differential roles of interleukin-17A and -17F in host defense against mucoepithelial bacterial infection and allergic responses. *Immunity* 30:108–119.

242. Yang XO, Chang SH, Park H, Nurieva R, Shah B, Acero L, Wang YH, Schluns KS, Broaddus RR, Zhu Z, Dong C. 2008. Regulation of inflammatory responses by IL-17F. *J Exp Med* 205:1063–1075.

243. Umemura M, Yahagi A, Hamada S, Begum MD, Watanabe H, Kawakami K, Suda T, Sudo K, Nakae S, Iwakura Y, Matsuzaki G. 2007. IL-17-mediated regulation of innate and acquired immune response against pulmonary *Mycobacterium bovis* bacille Calmette-Guerin infection. *J Immunol* 178:3786–3796.

244. Gopal R, Lin Y, Obermajer N, Slight S, Nuthalapati N, Ahmed M, Kalinski P, Khader SA. 2012. IL-23-dependent IL-17 drives Th1-cell responses following *Mycobacterium bovis* BCG vaccination. *Eur J Immunol* 42:364–373.

245. Aujla SJ, Chan YR, Zheng M, Fei M, Askew DJ, Pociask DA, Reinhart TA, McAllister F, Edeal J, Gaus K, Husain S, Kreindler JL, Dubin PJ, Pilewski JM, Myerburg MM, Mason CA, Iwakura Y, Kolls JK. 2008. IL-22 mediates mucosal host defense against Gram-negative bacterial pneumonia. *Nat Med* 14:275–281.

246. Aguilo N, Alvarez-Arguedas S, Uranga S, Marinova D, Monzón M, Badiola J, Martin C. 2016. Pulmonary but not subcutaneous delivery of BCG vaccine confers protection to tuberculosis-susceptible mice by an interleukin 17-dependent mechanism. *J Infect Dis* 213:831–839.

247. Cruz A, Torrado E, Carmona J, Fraga AG, Costa P, Rodrigues F, Appelberg R, Correia-Neves M, Cooper AM, Saraiva M, Pedrosa J, Castro AG. 2015. BCG vaccination-induced long-lasting control of *Mycobacterium tuberculosis* correlates with the accumulation of a novel population of CD4⁺IL-17⁺TNF⁺IL-2⁺ T cells. *Vaccine* 33:85–91.

248. Cruz A, Fraga AG, Fountain JJ, Rangel-Moreno J, Torrado E, Saraiva M, Pereira DR, Randall TD, Pedrosa J, Cooper AM, Castro AG. 2010. Pathological role of interleukin 17 in mice subjected to repeated BCG vaccination after infection with *Mycobacterium tuberculosis*. *J Exp Med* 207:1609–1616.

249. Gopal R, Monin L, Torres D, Slight S, Mehra S, McKenna KC, Fallert Junecko BA, Reinhart TA, Kolls J, Báez-Saldaña R, Cruz-Lagunas A, Rodríguez-Reyna TS, Kumar NP, Tessier P, Roth J, Selman M, Becerril-Villanueva E, Baquera-Heredia J, Cumming B, Kasprowicz VO, Steyn AJ, Babu S, Kaushal D, Zúñiga J, Vogl T, Rangel-Moreno J, Khader SA. 2013. S100A8/A9 proteins mediate neutrophilic inflammation and lung pathology during tuberculosis. *Am J Respir Crit Care Med* 188:1137–1146.

250. McAleer JP, Kolls JK. 2014. Directing traffic: IL-17 and IL-22 coordinate pulmonary immune defense. *Immunol Rev* 260:129–144.

251. Sonnenberg GF, Nair MG, Kirn TJ, Zaph C, Fouser LA, Artis D. 2010. Pathological versus protective functions of IL-22 in airway inflammation are regulated by IL-17A. *J Exp Med* 207:1293–1305.

252. Kolls JK, McCray PB Jr, Chan YR. 2008. Cytokine-mediated regulation of antimicrobial proteins. *Nat Rev Immunol* 8:829–835.

253. Matthews K, Wilkinson KA, Kalsdorf B, Roberts T, Diacon A, Walzl G, Wolske J, Ntsekhe M, Syed F, Russell J, Mayosi BM, Dawson R, Dheda K, Wilkinson RJ, Hanekom WA, Scriba TJ. 2011. Predominance of interleukin-22 over interleukin-17 at the site of disease in human tuberculosis. *Tuberculosis (Edinb)* 91:587–593.

254. Yao S, Huang D, Chen CY, Halliday L, Zeng G, Wang RC, Chen ZW. 2010. Differentiation, distribution and gammadelta T cell-driven regulation of IL-22-producing T cells in tuberculosis. *PLoS Pathog* 6:e1000789.

255. Zeng G, Chen CY, Huang D, Yao S, Wang RC, Chen ZW. 2011. Membrane-bound IL-22 after de novo production in tuberculosis and anti-*Mycobacterium tuberculosis* effector function of IL-22+ CD4+ T cells. *J Immunol* 187:190–199.

256. Dhiman R, Venkatasubramanian S, Paidipally P, Barnes PF, Tvinnereim A, Vankayalapati R. 2014. Interleukin 22 inhibits intracellular growth of *Mycobacterium tuberculosis* by enhancing calgranulin A expression. *J Infect Dis* 209:578–587.

257. Dhiman R, Indramohan M, Barnes PF, Nayak RC, Paidipally P, Rao LV, Vankayalapati R. 2009. IL-22 produced by human NK cells inhibits growth of *Mycobacterium tuberculosis* by enhancing phagolysosomal fusion. *J Immunol* 183:6639–6645.

258. Zhang M, Zeng G, Yang Q, Zhang J, Zhu X, Chen Q, Suthakaran P, Zhang Y, Deng Q, Liu H, Zhou B, Chen X. 2014. Anti-tuberculosis treatment enhances the production of IL-22 through reducing the frequencies of regulatory B cell. *Tuberculosis (Edinb)* 94:238–244.

259. Behrends J, Renauld JC, Ehlers S, Hölscher C. 2013. IL-22 is mainly produced by IFNγ-secreting cells but is dispensable for host protection against *Mycobacterium tuberculosis* infection. *PLoS One* 8:e57379.

260. Wilson MS, Feng CG, Barber DL, Yarovinsky F, Cheever AW, Sher A, Grigg M, Collins M, Fouser L, Wynn TA. 2010. Redundant and pathogenic roles for IL-22 in mycobacterial, protozoan, and helminth infections. *J Immunol* 184:4378–4390.

261. Dhiman R, Periasamy S, Barnes PF, Jaiswal AG, Paidipally P, Barnes AB, Tvinnereim A, Vankayalapati R. 2012. NK1.1+ cells and IL-22 regulate vaccine-induced protective immunity against challenge with *Mycobacterium tuberculosis*. *J Immunol* 189:897–905.

262. Mosmann TR, Cherwinski H, Bond MW, Giedlin MA, Coffman RL. 1986. Two types of murine helper T cell clone. I. Definition according to profiles of lymphokine activities and secreted proteins. *J Immunol* 136:2348–2357.

263. Killar L, MacDonald G, West J, Woods A, Bottomly K. 1987. Cloned, Ia-restricted T cells that do not produce interleukin 4(IL 4)/B cell stimulatory factor 1(BSF-1) fail to help antigen-specific B cells. *J Immunol* 138:1674–1679.

264. Powrie F, Menon S, Coffman RL. 1993. Interleukin-4 and interleukin-10 synergize to inhibit cell-mediated immunity in vivo. *Eur J Immunol* 23:3043–3049.

265. Appelberg R, Orme IM, Pinto de Sousa MI, Silva MT. 1992. In vitro effects of interleukin-4 on interferon-gamma-induced macrophage activation. *Immunology* 76:553–559.

266. Ferber IA, Lee HJ, Zonin F, Heath V, Mui A, Arai N, O'Garra A. 1999. GATA-3 significantly downregulates IFN-gamma production from developing Th1 cells in addition to inducing IL-4 and IL-5 levels. *Clin Immunol* 91:134–144.

267. Steinke JW, Borish L. 2001. Th2 cytokines and asthma. Interleukin-4: its role in the pathogenesis of asthma, and targeting it for asthma treatment with interleukin-4 receptor antagonists. *Respir Res* 2:66–70.

268. Stone KD, Prussin C, Metcalfe DD. 2010. IgE, mast cells, basophils, and eosinophils. *J Allergy Clin Immunol* 125(Suppl 2):S73–S80.

269. MacDonald AS, Araujo MI, Pearce EJ. 2002. Immunology of parasitic helminth infections. *Infect Immun* 70:427–433.

270. Zhu J, Paul WE. 2008. CD4 T cells: fates, functions, and faults. *Blood* 112:1557–1569.

271. Nelms K, Keegan AD, Zamorano J, Ryan JJ, Paul WE. 1999. The IL-4 receptor: signaling mechanisms and biologic functions. *Annu Rev Immunol* 17:701–738.

272. Zheng W, Flavell RA. 1997. The transcription factor GATA-3 is necessary and sufficient for Th2 cytokine gene expression in CD4 T cells. *Cell* 89:587–596.

273. Zhang DH, Cohn L, Ray P, Bottomly K, Ray A. 1997. Transcription factor GATA-3 is differentially expressed in murine Th1 and Th2 cells and controls Th2-specific expression of the interleukin-5 gene. *J Biol Chem* 272:21597–21603.

274. Kaplan MH, Schindler U, Smiley ST, Grusby MJ. 1996. Stat6 is required for mediating responses to IL-4 and for development of Th2 cells. *Immunity* 4:313–319.

275. Shimoda K, van Deursent J, Sangster MY, Sarawar SR, Carson RT, Tripp RA, Chu C, Quelle FW, Nosaka T, Vignali DA, Doherty PC, Grosveld G, Paul WE, Ihle JN. 1996. Lack of IL-4-induced Th2 response and IgE class switching in mice with disrupted Stat6 gene. *Nature* 380:630–633.

276. Swain SL, Weinberg AD, English M, Huston G. 1990. IL-4 directs the development of Th2-like helper effectors. *J Immunol* 145:3796–3806.

277. Le Gros G, Ben-Sasson SZ, Seder R, Finkelman FD, Paul WE. 1990. Generation of interleukin 4 (IL-4)-producing cells in vivo and in vitro: IL-2 and IL-4 are required for in vitro generation of IL-4-producing cells. *J Exp Med* 172:921–929.

278. Lowenthal JW, Castle BE, Christiansen J, Schreurs J, Rennick D, Arai N, Hoy P, Takebe Y, Howard M.

1988. Expression of high affinity receptors for murine interleukin 4 (BSF-1) on hemopoietic and nonhemopoietic cells. *J Immunol* 140:456–464.

279. Ohara J, Paul WE. 1987. Receptors for B-cell stimulatory factor-1 expressed on cells of haematopoietic lineage. *Nature* 325:537–540.

280. Coffman RL, Seymour BW, Hudak S, Jackson J, Rennick D. 1989. Antibody to interleukin-5 inhibits helminth-induced eosinophilia in mice. *Science* 245:308–310.

281. Phillips C, Coward WR, Pritchard DI, Hewitt CR. 2003. Basophils express a type 2 cytokine profile on exposure to proteases from helminths and house dust mites. *J Leukoc Biol* 73:165–171.

282. Hitoshi Y, Yamaguchi N, Mita S, Sonoda E, Takaki S, Tominaga A, Takatsu K. 1990. Distribution of IL-5 receptor-positive B cells. Expression of IL-5 receptor on Ly-1(CD5)+ B cells. *J Immunol* 144:4218–4225.

283. Rolink AG, Thalmann P, Kikuchi Y, Erdei A. 1990. Characterization of the interleukin 5-reactive splenic B cell population. *Eur J Immunol* 20:1949–1956.

284. Takatsu K. 2011. Interleukin-5 and IL-5 receptor in health and diseases. *Proc Jpn Acad, Ser B, Phys Biol Sci* 87:463–485.

285. Schauf V, Rom WN, Smith KA, Sampaio EP, Meyn PA, Tramontana JM, Cohn ZA, Kaplan G. 1993. Cytokine gene activation and modified responsiveness to interleukin-2 in the blood of tuberculosis patients. *J Infect Dis* 168:1056–1059.

286. Surcel HM, Troye-Blomberg M, Paulie S, Andersson G, Moreno C, Pasvol G, Ivanyi J. 1994. Th1/Th2 profiles in tuberculosis, based on the proliferation and cytokine response of blood lymphocytes to mycobacterial antigens. *Immunology* 81:171–176.

287. Zhang M, Gong J, Iyer DV, Jones BE, Modlin RL, Barnes PF. 1994. T cell cytokine responses in persons with tuberculosis and human immunodeficiency virus infection. *J Clin Invest* 94:2435–2442.

288. Lin Y, Zhang M, Hofman FM, Gong J, Barnes PF. 1996. Absence of a prominent Th2 cytokine response in human tuberculosis. *Infect Immun* 64:1351–1356.

289. Lai CK, Ho S, Chan CH, Chan J, Choy D, Leung R, Lai KN. 1997. Cytokine gene expression profile of circulating CD4+ T cells in active pulmonary tuberculosis. *Chest* 111:606–611.

290. Mihret A, Bekele Y, Bobosha K, Kidd M, Aseffa A, Howe R, Walzl G. 2013. Plasma cytokines and chemokines differentiate between active disease and non-active tuberculosis infection. *J Infect* 66:357–365.

291. Mihret A, Abebe M, Bekele Y, Aseffa A, Walzl G, Howe R. 2014. Impact of HIV co-infection on plasma level of cytokines and chemokines of pulmonary tuberculosis patients. *BMC Infect Dis* 14:125.

292. Bezuidenhout J, Roberts T, Muller L, van Helden P, Walzl G. 2009. Pleural tuberculosis in patients with early HIV infection is associated with increased TNF-alpha expression and necrosis in granulomas. *PLoS One* 4:e4228.

293. Mazzarella G, Bianco A, Perna F, D'Auria D, Grella E, Moscariello E, Sanduzzi A. 2003. T lymphocyte pheno-

typic profile in lung segments affected by cavitary and non-cavitary tuberculosis. *Clin Exp Immunol* 132:283–288.

294. Mattila JT, Diedrich CR, Lin PL, Phuah J, Flynn JL. 2011. Simian immunodeficiency virus-induced changes in T cell cytokine responses in cynomolgus macaques with latent *Mycobacterium tuberculosis* infection are associated with timing of reactivation. *J Immunol* 186:3527–3537.

295. Wassie L, Demissie A, Aseffa A, Abebe M, Yamuah L, Tilahun H, Petros B, Rook G, Zumla A, Andersen P, Doherty TM. 2008. Ex vivo cytokine mRNA levels correlate with changing clinical status of ethiopian TB patients and their contacts over time. *PLoS One* 3:e1522.

296. Fletcher HA, Owiafe P, Jeffries D, Hill P, Rook GA, Zumla A, Doherty TM, Brookes RH, Vacsel Study Group. 2004. Increased expression of mRNA encoding interleukin (IL)-4 and its splice variant IL-4delta2 in cells from contacts of *Mycobacterium tuberculosis*, in the absence of in vitro stimulation. *Immunology* 112:669–673.

297. Demissie A, Abebe M, Aseffa A, Rook G, Fletcher H, Zumla A, Weldingh K, Brock I, Andersen P, Doherty TM, VACSEL Study Group. 2004. Healthy individuals that control a latent infection with *Mycobacterium tuberculosis* express high levels of Th1 cytokines and the IL-4 antagonist IL-4delta2. *J Immunol* 172:6938–6943.

298. Jung YJ, LaCourse R, Ryan L, North RJ. 2002. Evidence inconsistent with a negative influence of T helper 2 cells on protection afforded by a dominant T helper 1 response against *Mycobacterium tuberculosis* lung infection in mice. *Infect Immun* 70:6436–6443.

299. North RJ. 1998. Mice incapable of making IL-4 or IL-10 display normal resistance to infection with *Mycobacterium tuberculosis*. *Clin Exp Immunol* 113:55–58.

300. Lukacs NW, Addison CL, Gauldie J, Graham F, Simpson K, Strieter RM, Warmington K, Chensue SW, Kunkel SL. 1997. Transgene-induced production of IL-4 alters the development and collagen expression of T helper cell 1-type pulmonary granulomas. *J Immunol* 158:4478–4484.

301. Ramakrishnan L. 2012. Revisiting the role of the granuloma in tuberculosis. *Nat Rev Immunol* 12:352–366.

302. Erb KJ, Kirman J, Delahunt B, Chen W, Le Gros G. 1998. IL-4, IL-5 and IL-10 are not required for the control of M. bovis-BCG infection in mice. *Immunol Cell Biol* 76:41–46.

303. Diedrich CR, Mattila JT, Flynn JL. 2013. Monocyte-derived IL-5 reduces TNF production by *Mycobacterium tuberculosis*-specific CD4 T cells during SIV/M. tuberculosis coinfection. *J Immunol* 190:6320–6328.

304. Minty A, Chalon P, Derocq J-M, Dumont X, Guillemot J-C, Kaghad M, Labit C, Leplatois P, Liauzun P, Miloux B, Minty C, Casellas P, Loison G, Lupker J, Shire D, Ferrara P, Caput D. 1993. Interleukin-13 is a new human lymphokine regulating inflammatory and immune responses. *Nature* 362:248–250.

305. McKenzie AN, Culpepper JA, de Waal Malefyt R, Briere F, Punnonen J, Aversa G, Sato A, Dang W, Cocks

BG, Menon S. 1993. Interleukin 13, a T-cell-derived cytokine that regulates human monocyte and B-cell function. *Proc Natl Acad Sci USA* **90**:3735–3739.

306. Wynn TA. 2003. IL-13 effector functions. *Annu Rev Immunol* **21**:425–456.

307. Zhu Z, Homer RJ, Wang Z, Chen Q, Geba GP, Wang J, Zhang Y, Elias JA. 1999. Pulmonary expression of interleukin-13 causes inflammation, mucus hypersecretion, subepithelial fibrosis, physiologic abnormalities, and eotaxin production. *J Clin Invest* **103**:779–788.

308. Wynn TA, Eltoum I, Oswald IP, Cheever AW, Sher A. 1994. Endogenous interleukin 12 (IL-12) regulates granuloma formation induced by eggs of *Schistosoma mansoni* and exogenous IL-12 both inhibits and prophylactically immunizes against egg pathology. *J Exp Med* **179**:1551–1561.

309. Gessner A, Mohrs K, Mohrs M. 2005. Mast cells, basophils, and eosinophils acquire constitutive IL-4 and IL-13 transcripts during lineage differentiation that are sufficient for rapid cytokine production. *J Immunol* **174**:1063–1072.

310. Ying S, Humbert M, Barkans J, Corrigan CJ, Pfister R, Menz G, Larché M, Robinson DS, Durham SR, Kay AB. 1997. Expression of IL-4 and IL-5 mRNA and protein product by CD4+ and CD8+ T cells, eosinophils, and mast cells in bronchial biopsies obtained from atopic and nonatopic (intrinsic) asthmatics. *J Immunol* **158**:3539–3544.

311. O'Brien TF, Bao K, Dell'Aringa M, Ang WX, Abraham S, Reinhardt RL. 2016. Cytokine expression by invariant natural killer T cells is tightly regulated throughout development and settings of type-2 inflammation. *Mucosal Immunol* **9**:597–609.

312. Bao K, Reinhardt RL. 2015. The differential expression of IL-4 and IL-13 and its impact on type-2 immunity. *Cytokine* **75**:25–37.

313. McCormick SM, Heller NM. 2015. Commentary: IL-4 and IL-13 receptors and signaling. *Cytokine* **75**:38–50.

314. Dhanasekaran S, Jenum S, Stavrum R, Ritz C, Faurholt-Jepsen D, Kenneth J, Vaz M, Grewal HM, Doherty TM, Doherty M, Grewal HMS, Hesseling AC, Jacob A, Jahnsen F, Kenneth J, Kurpad AV, Lindtjorn B, Macaden R, Nelson J, Sumithra S, Vaz M, Walker R, TB Trials Study Group. 2013. Identification of biomarkers for *Mycobacterium tuberculosis* infection and disease in BCG-vaccinated young children in Southern India. *Genes Immun* **14**:356–364.

315. Gutierrez MG, Master SS, Singh SB, Taylor GA, Colombo MI, Deretic V. 2004. Autophagy is a defense mechanism inhibiting BCG and *Mycobacterium tuberculosis* survival in infected macrophages. *Cell* **119**:753–766.

316. Singh SB, Davis AS, Taylor GA, Deretic V. 2006. Human IRGM induces autophagy to eliminate intracellular mycobacteria. *Science* **313**:1438–1441.

317. Harris J, De Haro SA, Master SS, Keane J, Roberts EA, Delgado M, Deretic V. 2007. T helper 2 cytokines inhibit autophagic control of intracellular *Mycobacterium tuberculosis*. *Immunity* **27**:505–517.

318. Heitmann L, Abad Dar M, Schreiber T, Erdmann H, Behrends J, Mckenzie ANJ, Brombacher F, Ehlers S, Hölscher C. 2014. The IL-13/IL-4Rα axis is involved in tuberculosis-associated pathology. *J Pathol* **234**:338–350.

319. Massagué J. 2012. TGFβ signalling in context. *Nat Rev Mol Cell Biol* **13**:616–630.

320. Feng XH, Derynck R. 2005. Specificity and versatility in TGF-β signaling through Smads. *Annu Rev Cell Dev Biol* **21**:659–693.

321. Massagué J, Seoane J, Wotton D. 2005. Smad transcription factors. *Genes Dev* **19**:2783–2810.

322. Trompouki E, Bowman TV, Lawton LN, Fan ZP, Wu DC, DiBiase A, Martin CS, Cech JN, Sessa AK, Leblanc JL, Li P, Durand EM, Mosimann C, Heffner GC, Daley GQ, Paulson RF, Young RA, Zon LI. 2011. Lineage regulators direct BMP and Wnt pathways to cell-specific programs during differentiation and regeneration. *Cell* **147**:577–589.

323. Taylor AW. 2009. Review of the activation of TGF-beta in immunity. *J Leukoc Biol* **85**:29–33.

324. Roberts AB, Sporn MB. 1988. Transforming growth factor beta. *Adv Cancer Res* **51**:107–145.

325. Massagué J. 1990. The transforming growth factor-beta family. *Annu Rev Cell Biol* **6**:597–641.

326. Letterio JJ, Roberts AB. 1998. Regulation of immune responses by TGF-beta. *Annu Rev Immunol* **16**:137–161.

327. Sporn MB, Roberts AB. 1992. Autocrine secretion–10 years later. *Ann Intern Med* **117**:408–414.

328. Toossi Z, Gogate P, Shiratsuchi H, Young T, Ellner JJ. 1995. Enhanced production of TGF-beta by blood monocytes from patients with active tuberculosis and presence of TGF-beta in tuberculous granulomatous lung lesions. *J Immunol* **154**:465–473.

329. Dahl KE, Shiratsuchi H, Hamilton BD, Ellner JJ, Toossi Z. 1996. Selective induction of transforming growth factor beta in human monocytes by lipoarabinomannan of *Mycobacterium tuberculosis*. *Infect Immun* **64**:399–405.

330. Hirsch CS, Yoneda T, Averill L, Ellner JJ, Toossi Z. 1994. Enhancement of intracellular growth of *Mycobacterium tuberculosis* in human monocytes by transforming growth factor-beta 1. *J Infect Dis* **170**:1229–1237.

331. Hirsch CS, Ellner JJ, Blinkhorn R, Toossi Z. 1997. In vitro restoration of T cell responses in tuberculosis and augmentation of monocyte effector function against *Mycobacterium tuberculosis* by natural inhibitors of transforming growth factor beta. *Proc Natl Acad Sci USA* **94**:3926–3931.

332. Othieno C, Hirsch CS, Hamilton BD, Wilkinson K, Ellner JJ, Toossi Z. 1999. Interaction of *Mycobacterium tuberculosis*-induced transforming growth factor beta1 and interleukin-10. *Infect Immun* **67**:5730–5735.

333. Sivangala R, Ponnana M, Thada S, Joshi L, Ansari S, Hussain H, Valluri V, Gaddam S. 2014. Association of cytokine gene polymorphisms in patients with tuberculosis and their household contacts. *Scand J Immunol* **79**:197–205.

334. Mak JC, Leung HC, Sham AS, Mok TY, Poon YN, Ling SO, Wong KC, Chan-Yeung M. 2007. Genetic polymorphisms and plasma levels of transforming growth factor-beta(1) in Chinese patients with tuberculosis in Hong Kong. *Cytokine* **40**:177–182.

335. Vieira P, de Waal-Malefyt R, Dang MN, Johnson KE, Kastelein R, Fiorentino DF, deVries JE, Roncarolo MG, Mosmann TR, Moore KW. 1991. Isolation and expression of human cytokine synthesis inhibitory factor cDNA clones: homology to Epstein-Barr virus open reading frame BCRFI. *Proc Natl Acad Sci USA* **88**: 1172–1176.

336. Redford PS, Murray PJ, O'Garra A. 2011. The role of IL-10 in immune regulation during *M. tuberculosis* infection. *Mucosal Immunol* **4**:261–270.

337. Liu Y, Wei SH, Ho AS, de Waal Malefyt R, Moore KW. 1994. Expression cloning and characterization of a human IL-10 receptor. *J Immunol* **152**:1821–1829.

338. Jang S, Uematsu S, Akira S, Salgame P. 2004. IL-6 and IL-10 induction from dendritic cells in response to *Mycobacterium tuberculosis* is predominantly dependent on TLR2-mediated recognition. *J Immunol* **173**: 3392–3397.

339. Rogers NC, Slack EC, Edwards AD, Nolte MA, Schulz O, Schweighoffer E, Williams DL, Gordon S, Tybulewicz VL, Brown GD, Reis e Sousa C. 2005. Syk-dependent cytokine induction by Dectin-1 reveals a novel pattern recognition pathway for C type lectins. *Immunity* **22**:507–517.

340. Ke Z, Yuan L, Ma J, Zhang X, Guo Y, Xiong H. 2015. IL-10 polymorphisms and tuberculosis susceptibility: an updated meta-analysis. *Yonsei Med J* **56**:1274–1287.

341. Jeong YH, Hur YG, Lee H, Kim S, Cho JE, Chang J, Shin SJ, Lee H, Kang YA, Cho SN, Ha SJ. 2015. Discrimination between active and latent tuberculosis based on ratio of antigen-specific to mitogen-induced IP-10 production. *J Clin Microbiol* **53**:504–510.

342. Tebruegge M, Dutta B, Donath S, Ritz N, Forbes B, Camacho-Badilla K, Clifford V, Zufferey C, Robins-Browne R, Hanekom W, Graham SM, Connell T, Curtis N. 2015. Mycobacteria-specific cytokine responses detect tuberculosis infection and distinguish latent from active tuberculosis. *Am J Respir Crit Care Med* **192**: 485–499

343. Kumar NP, Moideen K, Banurekha VV, Nair D, Sridhar R, Nutman TB, Babu S. 2015. IL-27 and TGFβ mediated expansion of Th1 and adaptive regulatory T cells expressing IL-10 correlates with bacterial burden and disease severity in pulmonary tuberculosis. *Immun Inflamm Dis* **3**:289–299.

344. Eum SY, Jeon BY, Min JH, Kim SC, Cho S, Park SK, Cho SN. 2008. Tumor necrosis factor-alpha and interleukin-10 in whole blood is associated with disease progression in pulmonary multidrug-resistant tuberculosis patients. *Respiration* **76**:331–337.

345. Lago PM, Boéchat N, Migueis DP, Almeida AS, Lazzarini LC, Saldanha MM, Kritski AL, Ho JL, Lapa e Silva JR. 2012. Interleukin-10 and interferon-gamma patterns during tuberculosis treatment: possible association with recurrence. *Int J Tuberc Lung Dis* **16**:656–659.

346. George PJ, Pavan Kumar N, Jaganathan J, Dolla C, Kumaran P, Nair D, Banurekha VV, Shen K, Nutman TB, Babu S. 2015. Modulation of pro- and anti-inflammatory cytokines in active and latent tuberculosis by coexistent *Strongyloides stercoralis* infection. *Tuberculosis (Edinb)* **95**:822–828.

347. George PJ, Anuradha R, Kumar NP, Sridhar R, Banurekha VV, Nutman TB, Babu S. 2014. Helminth infections coincident with active pulmonary tuberculosis inhibit mono- and multifunctional CD4+ and CD8+ T cell responses in a process dependent on IL-10. *PLoS Pathog* **10**:e1004375

348. Verreck FA, de Boer T, Langenberg DM, Hoeve MA, Kramer M, Vaisberg E, Kastelein R, Kolk A, de Waal-Malefyt R, Ottenhoff TH. 2004. Human IL-23-producing type 1 macrophages promote but IL-10-producing type 2 macrophages subvert immunity to (myco)bacteria. *Proc Natl Acad Sci USA* **101**:4560–4565.

349. O'Leary S, O'Sullivan MP, Keane J. 2011. IL-10 blocks phagosome maturation in *mycobacterium tuberculosis*-infected human macrophages. *Am J Respir Cell Mol Biol* **45**:172–180.

350. Oswald IP, Wynn TA, Sher A, James SL. 1992. Interleukin 10 inhibits macrophage microbicidal activity by blocking the endogenous production of tumor necrosis factor alpha required as a costimulatory factor for interferon gamma-induced activation. *Proc Natl Acad Sci USA* **89**:8676–8680.

351. Moore KW, de Waal Malefyt R, Coffman RL, O'Garra A. 2001. Interleukin-10 and the interleukin-10 receptor. *Annu Rev Immunol* **19**:683–765.

352. Richardson ET, Shukla S, Sweet DR, Wearsch PA, Tsichlis PN, Boom WH, Harding CV. 2015. Toll-like receptor 2-dependent extracellular signal-regulated kinase signaling in *Mycobacterium tuberculosis*-infected macrophages drives anti-inflammatory responses and inhibits Th1 polarization of responding T cells. *Infect Immun* **83**:2242–2254.

353. Jung YJ, Ryan L, LaCourse R, North RJ. 2003. Increased interleukin-10 expression is not responsible for failure of T helper 1 immunity to resolve airborne *Mycobacterium tuberculosis* infection in mice. *Immunology* **109**:295–299.

354. Higgins DM, Sanchez-Campillo J, Rosas-Taraco AG, Lee EJ, Orme IM, Gonzalez-Juarrero M. 2009. Lack of IL-10 alters inflammatory and immune responses during pulmonary *Mycobacterium tuberculosis* infection. *Tuberculosis (Edinb)* **89**:149–157.

355. Beamer GL, Flaherty DK, Assogba BD, Stromberg P, Gonzalez-Juarrero M, de Waal Malefyt R, Vesosky B, Turner J. 2008. Interleukin-10 promotes *Mycobacterium tuberculosis* disease progression in CBA/J mice. *J Immunol* **181**:5545–5550.

356. Cyktor JC, Carruthers B, Kominsky RA, Beamer GL, Stromberg P, Turner J. 2013. IL-10 inhibits mature fibrotic granuloma formation during *Mycobacterium tuberculosis* infection. *J Immunol* **190**:2778–2790.

357. Cilfone NA, Ford CB, Marino S, Mattila JT, Gideon HP, Flynn JL, Kirschner DE, Linderman JJ. 2015. Com-

putational modeling predicts IL-10 control of lesion sterilization by balancing early host immunity-mediated antimicrobial responses with caseation during *Mycobacterium tuberculosis* infection. *J Immunol* **194**:664–677.

358. **Dorhoi A, Kaufmann SH.** 2016. Pathology and immune reactivity: understanding multidimensionality in pulmonary tuberculosis. *Semin Immunopathol* **38**:153–166.

359. **Yoshimura T.** 2015. Discovery of IL-8/CXCL8 (The Story from Frederick). *Front Immunol* **6**:278.

360. **Murphy PM, Baggiolini M, Charo IF, Hébert CA, Horuk R, Matsushima K, Miller LH, Oppenheim JJ, Power CA.** 2000. International union of pharmacology. XXII. Nomenclature for chemokine receptors. *Pharmacol Rev* **52**:145–176.

361. **Murphy PM.** 2002. International Union of Pharmacology. XXX. Update on chemokine receptor nomenclature. *Pharmacol Rev* **54**:227–229.

362. **Bacon K, Baggiolini M, Broxmeyer H, Horuk R, Lindley I, Mantovani A, Maysushima K, Murphy P, Nomiyama H, Oppenheim J, Rot A, Schall T, Tsang M, Thorpe R, Van Damme J, Wadhwa M, Yoshie O, Zlotnik A, Zoon K, IUIS/WHO Subcommittee on Chemokine Nomenclature.** 2002. Chemokine/chemokine receptor nomenclature. *J Interferon Cytokine Res* **22**:1067–1068.

363. **Zlotnik A, Yoshie O.** 2012. The chemokine superfamily revisited. *Immunity* **36**:705–716.

364. **Zlotnik A, Yoshie O.** 2000. Chemokines: a new classification system and their role in immunity. *Immunity* **12**:121–127.

365. **Su SB, Mukaida N, Wang J, Nomura H, Matsushima K.** 1996. Preparation of specific polyclonal antibodies to a C-C chemokine receptor, CCR1, and determination of CCR1 expression on various types of leukocytes. *J Leukoc Biol* **60**:658–666.

366. **Neote K, DiGregorio D, Mak JY, Horuk R, Schall TJ.** 1993. Molecular cloning, functional expression, and signaling characteristics of a C-C chemokine receptor. *Cell* **72**:415–425.

367. **Gao JL, Kuhns DB, Tiffany HL, McDermott D, Li X, Francke U, Murphy PM.** 1993. Structure and functional expression of the human macrophage inflammatory protein 1 alpha/RANTES receptor. *J Exp Med* **177**:1421–1427.

368. **Gao JL, Murphy PM.** 1995. Cloning and differential tissue-specific expression of three mouse beta chemokine receptor-like genes, including the gene for a functional macrophage inflammatory protein-1 alpha receptor. *J Biol Chem* **270**:17494–17501.

369. **Kaufmann A, Salentin R, Gemsa D, Sprenger H.** 2001. Increase of CCR1 and CCR5 expression and enhanced functional response to MIP-1 alpha during differentiation of human monocytes to macrophages. *J Leukoc Biol* **69**:248–252.

370. **Cheng SS, Lai JJ, Lukacs NW, Kunkel SL.** 2001. Granulocyte-macrophage colony stimulating factor up-regulates CCR1 in human neutrophils. *J Immunol* **166**:1178–1184.

371. **Pokkali S, Das SD, Logamurthy R.** 2008. Expression of CXC and CC type of chemokines and its receptors in tuberculous and non-tuberculous effusions. *Cytokine* **41**:307–314

372. **Pokkali S, Das SD.** 2009. Augmented chemokine levels and chemokine receptor expression on immune cells during pulmonary tuberculosis. *Hum Immunol* **70**:110–115.

373. **Hilda JN, Narasimhan M, Das SD.** 2014. Neutrophils from pulmonary tuberculosis patients show augmented levels of chemokines MIP-1α, IL-8 and MCP-1 which further increase upon in vitro infection with mycobacterial strains. *Hum Immunol* **75**:914–922.

374. **Saukkonen JJ, Bazydlo B, Thomas M, Strieter RM, Keane J, Kornfeld H.** 2002. Beta-chemokines are induced by *Mycobacterium tuberculosis* and inhibit its growth. *Infect Immun* **70**:1684–1693.

375. **Algood HM, Flynn JL.** 2004. CCR5-deficient mice control *Mycobacterium tuberculosis* infection despite increased pulmonary lymphocytic infiltration. *J Immunol* **173**:3287–3296.

376. **Randolph GJ, Ochando J, Partida-Sánchez S.** 2008. Migration of dendritic cell subsets and their precursors. *Annu Rev Immunol* **26**:293–316.

377. **Glatzel A, Wesch D, Schiemann F, Brandt E, Janssen O, Kabelitz D.** 2002. Patterns of chemokine receptor expression on peripheral blood gamma delta T lymphocytes: strong expression of CCR5 is a selective feature of V delta 2/V gamma 9 gamma delta T cells. *J Immunol* **168**:4920–4929.

378. **Tsou CL, Peters W, Si Y, Slaymaker S, Aslanian AM, Weisberg SP, Mack M, Charo IF.** 2007. Critical roles for CCR2 and MCP-3 in monocyte mobilization from bone marrow and recruitment to inflammatory sites. *J Clin Invest* **117**:902–909.

379. **Hasan Z, Jamil B, Khan J, Ali R, Khan MA, Nasir N, Yusuf MS, Jamil S, Irfan M, Hussain R.** 2009. Relationship between circulating levels of IFN-gamma, IL-10, CXCL9 and CCL2 in pulmonary and extrapulmonary tuberculosis is dependent on disease severity. *Scand J Immunol* **69**:259–267.

380. **Scott HM, Flynn JL.** 2002. *Mycobacterium tuberculosis* in chemokine receptor 2-deficient mice: influence of dose on disease progression. *Infect Immun* **70**:5946–5954.

381. **Peters W, Scott HM, Chambers HF, Flynn JL, Charo IF, Ernst JD.** 2001. Chemokine receptor 2 serves an early and essential role in resistance to *Mycobacterium tuberculosis*. *Proc Natl Acad Sci USA* **98**:7958–7963.

382. **Lu B, Rutledge BJ, Gu L, Fiorillo J, Lukacs NW, Kunkel SL, North R, Gerard C, Rollins BJ.** 1998. Abnormalities in monocyte recruitment and cytokine expression in monocyte chemoattractant protein 1-deficient mice. *J Exp Med* **187**:601–608.

383. **Kipnis A, Basaraba RJ, Orme IM, Cooper AM.** 2003. Role of chemokine ligand 2 in the protective response to early murine pulmonary tuberculosis. *Immunology* **109**:547–551.

384. **Iellem A, Mariani M, Lang R, Recalde H, Panina-Bordignon P, Sinigaglia F, D'Ambrosio D.** 2001. Unique chemotactic response profile and specific expression of chemokine receptors CCR4 and CCR8 by CD4(+)CD25(+) regulatory T cells. *J Exp Med* **194**:847–854.

385. Curiel TJ, Coukos G, Zou L, Alvarez X, Cheng P, Mottram P, Evdemon-Hogan M, Conejo-Garcia JR, Zhang L, Burow M, Zhu Y, Wei S, Kryczek I, Daniel B, Gordon A, Myers L, Lackner A, Disis ML, Knutson KL, Chen L, Zou W. 2004. Specific recruitment of regulatory T cells in ovarian carcinoma fosters immune privilege and predicts reduced survival. *Nat Med* 10:942–949.

386. Acosta-Rodriguez EV, Rivino L, Geginat J, Jarrossay D, Gattorno M, Lanzavecchia A, Sallusto F, Napolitani G. 2007. Surface phenotype and antigenic specificity of human interleukin 17-producing T helper memory cells. *Nat Immunol* 8:639–646.

387. Kunkel EJ, Boisvert J, Murphy K, Vierra MA, Genovese MC, Wardlaw AJ, Greenberg HB, Hodge MR, Wu L, Butcher EC, Campbell JJ. 2002. Expression of the chemokine receptors CCR4, CCR5, and CXCR3 by human tissue-infiltrating lymphocytes. *Am J Pathol* 160:347–355.

388. Hu Z, Lancaster JN, Sasiponganan C, Ehrlich LI. 2015. CCR4 promotes medullary entry and thymocyte-dendritic cell interactions required for central tolerance. *J Exp Med* 212:1947–1965.

389. Cowan JE, McCarthy NI, Parnell SM, White AJ, Bacon A, Serge A, Irla M, Lane PJ, Jenkinson EJ, Jenkinson WE, Anderson G. 2014. Differential requirement for CCR4 and CCR7 during the development of innate and adaptive αβT cells in the adult thymus. *J Immunol* 193:1204–1212.

390. Andrew DP, Ruffing N, Kim CH, Miao W, Heath H, Li Y, Murphy K, Campbell JJ, Butcher EC, Wu L. 2001. C-C chemokine receptor 4 expression defines a major subset of circulating nonintestinal memory T cells of both Th1 and Th2 potential. *J Immunol* 166:103–111.

391. Paul WE, Zhu J. 2010. How are T(H)2-type immune responses initiated and amplified? *Nat Rev Immunol* 10:225–235.

392. Oliphant CJ, Barlow JL, McKenzie AN. 2011. Insights into the initiation of type 2 immune responses. *Immunology* 134:378–385.

393. Li L, Lao SH, Wu CY. 2007. Increased frequency of CD4(+)CD25(high) Treg cells inhibit BCG-specific induction of IFN-gamma by CD4(+) T cells from TB patients. *Tuberculosis (Edinb)* 87:526–534.

394. Roberts T, Beyers N, Aguirre A, Walzl G. 2007. Immunosuppression during active tuberculosis is characterized by decreased interferon- gamma production and CD25 expression with elevated forkhead box P3, transforming growth factor- beta, and interleukin-4 mRNA levels. *J Infect Dis* 195:870–878.

395. Bayry J, Tchilian EZ, Davies MN, Forbes EK, Draper SJ, Kaveri SV, Hill AV, Kazatchkine MD, Beverley PC, Flower DR, Tough DF. 2008. In silico identified CCR4 antagonists target regulatory T cells and exert adjuvant activity in vaccination. *Proc Natl Acad Sci USA* 105:10221–10226.

396. Feng Y, Yin H, Mai G, Mao L, Yue J, Xiao H, Hu Z. 2011. Elevated serum levels of CCL17 correlate with increased peripheral blood platelet count in patients with active tuberculosis in China. *Clin Vaccine Immunol* 18:629–632.

397. Freeman CM, Stolberg VR, Chiu BC, Lukacs NW, Kunkel SL, Chensue SW. 2006. CCR4 participation in Th type 1 (mycobacterial) and Th type 2 (schistosomal) anamnestic pulmonary granulomatous responses. *J Immunol* 177:4149–4158.

398. Dragic T, Litwin V, Allaway GP, Martin SR, Huang Y, Nagashima KA, Cayanan C, Maddon PJ, Koup RA, Moore JP, Paxton WA. 1996. HIV-1 entry into CD4+ cells is mediated by the chemokine receptor CC-CKR-5. *Nature* 381:667–673.

399. Deng H, Liu R, Ellmeier W, Choe S, Unutmaz D, Burkhart M, Di Marzio P, Marmon S, Sutton RE, Hill CM, Davis CB, Peiper SC, Schall TJ, Littman DR, Landau NR. 1996. Identification of a major co-receptor for primary isolates of HIV-1. *Nature* 381:661–666.

400. Chu SF, Tam CM, Wong HS, Kam KM, Lau YL, Chiang AK. 2007. Association between RANTES functional polymorphisms and tuberculosis in Hong Kong Chinese. *Genes Immun* 8:475–479.

401. Vesosky B, Rottinghaus EK, Stromberg P, Turner J, Beamer G. 2010. CCL5 participates in early protection against *Mycobacterium tuberculosis*. *J Leukoc Biol* 87:1153–1165.

402. Mantovani A. 1999. The chemokine system: redundancy for robust outputs. *Immunol Today* 20:254–257.

403. Schutyser E, Struyf S, Van Damme J. 2003. The CC chemokine CCL20 and its receptor CCR6. *Cytokine Growth Factor Rev* 14:409–426.

404. Ito T, Carson WF 4th, Cavassani KA, Connett JM, Kunkel SL. 2011. CCR6 as a mediator of immunity in the lung and gut. *Exp Cell Res* 317:613–619.

405. Nandi B, Pai C, Huang Q, Prabhala RH, Munshi NC, Gold JS. 2014. CCR6, the sole receptor for the chemokine CCL20, promotes spontaneous intestinal tumorigenesis. *PLoS One* 9:e97566.

406. Lee AY, Körner H. 2014. CCR6 and CCL20: emerging players in the pathogenesis of rheumatoid arthritis. *Immunol Cell Biol* 92:354–358.

407. Stolberg VR, Chiu BC, Martin BE, Shah SA, Sandor M, Chensue SW. 2011. Cysteine-cysteinyl chemokine receptor 6 mediates invariant natural killer T cell airway recruitment and innate stage resistance during mycobacterial infection. *J Innate Immun* 3:99–108.

408. Perreau M, Rozot V, Welles HC, Belluti-Enders F, Vigano S, Maillard M, Dorta G, Mazza-Stalder J, Bart PA, Roger T, Calandra T, Nicod L, Harari A. 2013. Lack of *Mycobacterium tuberculosis*-specific interleukin-17A-producing CD4+ T cells in active disease. *Eur J Immunol* 43:939–948.

409. Lindestam Arlehamn CS, Gerasimova A, Mele F, Henderson R, Swann J, Greenbaum JA, Kim Y, Sidney J, James EA, Taplitz R, McKinney DM, Kwok WW, Grey H, Sallusto F, Peters B, Sette A. 2013. Memory T cells in latent *Mycobacterium tuberculosis* infection are directed against three antigenic islands and largely contained in a CXCR3+CCR6+ Th1 subset. *PLoS Pathog* 9:e1003130.

410. Rivero-Lezcano OM, González-Cortés C, Reyes-Ruvalcaba D, Diez-Tascón C. 2010. CCL20 is overexpressed in *Mycobacterium tuberculosis*-infected monocytes and

inhibits the production of reactive oxygen species (ROS). *Clin Exp Immunol* 162:289–297.

411. Lee JS, Lee JY, Son JW, Oh JH, Shin DM, Yuk JM, Song CH, Paik TH, Jo EK. 2008. Expression and regulation of the CC-chemokine ligand 20 during human tuberculosis. *Scand J Immunol* 67:77–85.

412. Kang DD, Lin Y, Moreno JR, Randall TD, Khader SA. 2011. Profiling early lung immune responses in the mouse model of tuberculosis. *PLoS One* 6:e16161

413. Mehra S, Pahar B, Dutta NK, Conerly CN, Philippi-Falkenstein K, Alvarez X, Kaushal D. 2010. Transcriptional reprogramming in nonhuman primate (rhesus macaque) tuberculosis granulomas. *PLoS One* 5:e12266

414. Förster R, Davalos-Misslitz AC, Rot A. 2008. CCR7 and its ligands: balancing immunity and tolerance. *Nat Rev Immunol* 8:362–371.

415. Gunn MD, Kyuwa S, Tam C, Kakiuchi T, Matsuzawa A, Williams LT, Nakano H. 1999. Mice lacking expression of secondary lymphoid organ chemokine have defects in lymphocyte homing and dendritic cell localization. *J Exp Med* 189:451–460.

416. Kahnert A, Höpken UE, Stein M, Bandermann S, Lipp M, Kaufmann SH. 2007. *Mycobacterium tuberculosis* triggers formation of lymphoid structure in murine lungs. *J Infect Dis* 195:46–54.

417. Gunn MD, Tangemann K, Tam C, Cyster JG, Rosen SD, Williams LT. 1998. A chemokine expressed in lymphoid high endothelial venules promotes the adhesion and chemotaxis of naive T lymphocytes. *Proc Natl Acad Sci USA* 95:258–263.

418. Saeki H, Moore AM, Brown MJ, Hwang ST. 1999. Cutting edge: secondary lymphoid-tissue chemokine (SLC) and CC chemokine receptor 7 (CCR7) participate in the emigration pathway of mature dendritic cells from the skin to regional lymph nodes. *J Immunol* 162:2472–2475.

419. Bhatt K, Hickman SP, Salgame P. 2004. Cutting edge: a new approach to modeling early lung immunity in murine tuberculosis. *J Immunol* 172:2748–2751.

420. Olmos S, Stukes S, Ernst JD. 2010. Ectopic activation of *Mycobacterium tuberculosis*-specific CD4+ T cells in lungs of CCR7-/- mice. *J Immunol* 184:895–901.

421. Nakano H, Gunn MD. 2001. Gene duplications at the chemokine locus on mouse chromosome 4: multiple strain-specific haplotypes and the deletion of secondary lymphoid-organ chemokine and EBI-1 ligand chemokine genes in the plt mutation. *J Immunol* 166:361–369.

422. Khader SA, Rangel-Moreno J, Fountain JJ, Martino CA, Reiley WW, Pearl JE, Winslow GM, Woodland DL, Randall TD, Cooper AM. 2009. In a murine tuberculosis model, the absence of homeostatic chemokines delays granuloma formation and protective immunity. *J Immunol* 183:8004–8014.

423. Allen SJ, Crown SE, Handel TM. 2007. Chemokine: receptor structure, interactions, and antagonism. *Annu Rev Immunol* 25:787–820.

424. Strieter RM, Polverini PJ, Kunkel SL, Arenberg DA, Burdick MD, Kasper J, Dzuiba J, Van Damme J, Walz A, Marriott D, Chan S-Y, Roczniak S, Shanafelt AB. 1995. The functional role of the ELR motif in CXC chemokine-mediated angiogenesis. *J Biol Chem* 270:27348–27357.

425. Hébert CA, Vitangcol RV, Baker JB. 1991. Scanning mutagenesis of interleukin-8 identifies a cluster of residues required for receptor binding. *J Biol Chem* 266:18989–18994.

426. Clark-Lewis I, Dewald B, Geiser T, Moser B, Baggiolini M. 1993. Platelet factor 4 binds to interleukin 8 receptors and activates neutrophils when its N terminus is modified with Glu-Leu-Arg. *Proc Natl Acad Sci USA* 90:3574–3577.

427. Jones SA, Moser B, Thelen M. 1995. A comparison of post-receptor signal transduction events in Jurkat cells transfected with either IL-8R1 or IL-8R2. Chemokine mediated activation of p42/p44 MAP-kinase (ERK-2). *FEBS Lett* 364:211–214.

428. Slight SR, Khader SA. 2013. Chemokines shape the immune responses to tuberculosis. *Cytokine Growth Factor Rev* 24:105–113.

429. Alaridah N, Winqvist N, Håkansson G, Tenland E, Rönnholm A, Sturegård E, Björkman P, Godaly G. 2015. Impaired CXCR1-dependent oxidative defence in active tuberculosis patients. *Tuberculosis (Edinb)* 95:744–750.

430. Gonçalves AS, Appelberg R. 2002. The involvement of the chemokine receptor CXCR2 in neutrophil recruitment in LPS-induced inflammation and in *Mycobacterium avium* infection. *Scand J Immunol* 55:585–591.

431. O'Kane CM, Boyle JJ, Horncastle DE, Elkington PT, Friedland JS. 2007. Monocyte-dependent fibroblast CXCL8 secretion occurs in tuberculosis and limits survival of mycobacteria within macrophages. *J Immunol* 178:3767–3776.

432. Friedland JS, Remick DG, Shattock R, Griffin GE. 1992. Secretion of interleukin-8 following phagocytosis of *Mycobacterium tuberculosis* by human monocyte cell lines. *Eur J Immunol* 22:1373–1378.

433. Zhang Y, Broser M, Cohen H, Bodkin M, Law K, Reibman J, Rom WN. 1995. Enhanced interleukin-8 release and gene expression in macrophages after exposure to *Mycobacterium tuberculosis* and its components. *J Clin Invest* 95:586–592.

434. Lin Y, Zhang M, Barnes PF. 1998. Chemokine production by a human alveolar epithelial cell line in response to *Mycobacterium tuberculosis*. *Infect Immun* 66:1121–1126.

435. Kurashima K, Mukaida N, Fujimura M, Yasui M, Nakazumi Y, Matsuda T, Matsushima K. 1997. Elevated chemokine levels in bronchoalveolar lavage fluid of tuberculosis patients. *Am J Respir Crit Care Med* 155:1474–1477.

436. Larsen CG, et al. 1995. The delayed-type hypersensitivity reaction is dependent on IL-8. Inhibition of a tuberculin skin reaction by an anti-IL-8 monoclonal antibody. *J Immunol* 155:2151–2157.

437. Ma X, Reich RA, Wright JA, Tooker HR, Teeter LD, Musser JM, Graviss EA. 2003. Association between

interleukin-8 gene alleles and human susceptibility to tuberculosis disease. *J Infect Dis* 188:349–355.

438. Cooke GS, Campbell SJ, Fielding K, Sillah J, Manneh K, Sirugo G, Bennett S, McAdam KP, Lienhardt C, Hill AV. 2004. Interleukin-8 polymorphism is not associated with pulmonary tuberculosis in the gambia. *J Infect Dis* 189:1545–1546, author reply 1546.

439. Almeida CS, Abramo C, Alves CC, Mazzoccoli L, Ferreira AP, Teixeira HC. 2009. Anti-mycobacterial treatment reduces high plasma levels of CXC-chemokines detected in active tuberculosis by cytometric bead array. *Mem Inst Oswaldo Cruz* 104:1039–1041.

440. Nouailles G, Dorhoi A, Koch M, Zerrahn J, Weiner J III, Faé KC, Arrey F, Kuhlmann S, Bandermann S, Loewe D, Mollenkopf HJ, Vogelzang A, Meyer-Schwesinger C, Mittrücker HW, McEwen G, Kaufmann SH. 2014. CXCL5-secreting pulmonary epithelial cells drive destructive neutrophilic inflammation in tuberculosis. *J Clin Invest* 124:1268–1282.

441. Groom JR, Luster AD. 2011. CXCR3 in T cell function. *Exp Cell Res* 317:620–631.

442. Thomas SY, Hou R, Boyson JE, Means TK, Hess C, Olson DP, Strominger JL, Brenner MB, Gumperz JE, Wilson SB, Luster AD. 2003. CD1d-restricted NKT cells express a chemokine receptor profile indicative of Th1-type inflammatory homing cells. *J Immunol* 171: 2571–2580.

443. Qin S, Rottman JB, Myers P, Kassam N, Weinblatt M, Loetscher M, Koch AE, Moser B, Mackay CR. 1998. The chemokine receptors CXCR3 and CCR5 mark subsets of T cells associated with certain inflammatory reactions. *J Clin Invest* 101:746–754.

444. Lu B, Humbles A, Bota D, Gerard C, Moser B, Soler D, Luster AD, Gerard NP. 1999. Structure and function of the murine chemokine receptor CXCR3. *Eur J Immunol* 29:3804–3812.

445. Campanella GS, Grimm J, Manice LA, Colvin RA, Medoff BD, Wojtkiewicz GR, Weissleder R, Luster AD. 2006. Oligomerization of CXCL10 is necessary for endothelial cell presentation and in vivo activity. *J Immunol* 177:6991–6998.

446. Loetscher M, Loetscher P, Brass N, Meese E, Moser B. 1998. Lymphocyte-specific chemokine receptor CXCR3: regulation, chemokine binding and gene localization. *Eur J Immunol* 28:3696–3705.

447. Shields PL, Morland CM, Salmon M, Qin S, Hubscher SG, Adams DH. 1999. Chemokine and chemokine receptor interactions provide a mechanism for selective T cell recruitment to specific liver compartments within hepatitis C-infected liver. *J Immunol* 163:6236–6243.

448. Seiler P, Aichele P, Bandermann S, Hauser AE, Lu B, Gerard NP, Gerard C, Ehlers S, Mollenkopf HJ, Kaufmann SH. 2003. Early granuloma formation after aerosol *Mycobacterium tuberculosis* infection is regulated by neutrophils via CXCR3-signaling chemokines. *Eur J Immunol* 33:2676–2686.

449. Chakravarty SD, Xu J, Lu B, Gerard C, Flynn J, Chan J. 2007. The chemokine receptor CXCR3 attenuates the control of chronic *Mycobacterium tuberculosis* infection in BALB/c mice. *J Immunol* 178:1723–1735.

450. Hasan Z, Jamil B, Ashraf M, Islam M, Dojki M, Irfan M, Hussain R. 2009. Differential live *Mycobacterium tuberculosis*-, *M. bovis* BCG-, recombinant ESAT6-, and culture filtrate protein 10-induced immunity in tuberculosis. *Clin Vaccine Immunol* 16:991–998.

451. Azzurri A, Sow OY, Amedei A, Bah B, Diallo S, Peri G, Benagiano M, D'Elios MM, Mantovani A, Del Prete G. 2005. IFN-gamma-inducible protein 10 and pentraxin 3 plasma levels are tools for monitoring inflammation and disease activity in *Mycobacterium tuberculosis* infection. *Microbes Infect* 7:1–8.

452. Whittaker E, Gordon A, Kampmann B. 2008. Is IP-10 a better biomarker for active and latent tuberculosis in children than IFNgamma? *PLoS One* 3:e3901.

453. Kibiki GS, Myers LC, Kalambo CF, Hoang SB, Stoler MH, Stroup SE, Houpt ER. 2007. Bronchoalveolar neutrophils, interferon gamma-inducible protein 10 and interleukin-7 in AIDS-associated tuberculosis. *Clin Exp Immunol* 148:254–259.

454. Tang NL, Fan HP, Chang KC, Ching JK, Kong KP, Yew WW, Kam KM, Leung CC, Tam CM, Blackwell J, Chan CY. 2009. Genetic association between a chemokine gene CXCL-10 (IP-10, interferon gamma inducible protein 10) and susceptibility to tuberculosis. *Clin Chim Acta* 406: 98–102.

455. Loos T, Dekeyzer L, Struyf S, Schutyser E, Gijsbers K, Gouwy M, Fraeyman A, Put W, Ronsse I, Grillet B, Opdenakker G, Van Damme J, Proost P. 2006. TLR ligands and cytokines induce CXCR3 ligands in endothelial cells: enhanced CXCL9 in autoimmune arthritis. *Lab Invest* 86:902–916.

456. Kanda N, Shimizu T, Tada Y, Watanabe S. 2007. IL-18 enhances IFN-gamma-induced production of CXCL9, CXCL10, and CXCL11 in human keratinocytes. *Eur J Immunol* 37:338–350.

457. Basset L, Chevalier S, Danger Y, Arshad MI, Piquet-Pellorce C, Gascan H, Samson M. 2015. Interleukin-27 and IFNγ regulate the expression of CXCL9, CXCL10, and CXCL11 in hepatitis. *J Mol Med (Berl)* 93:1355–1367.

458. Oo YH, Banz V, Kavanagh D, Liaskou E, Withers DR, Humphreys E, Reynolds GM, Lee-Turner L, Kalia N, Hubscher SG, Klenerman P, Eksteen B, Adams DH. 2012. CXCR3-dependent recruitment and CCR6-mediated positioning of Th-17 cells in the inflamed liver. *J Hepatol* 57:1044–1051.

459. Slight SR, Rangel-Moreno J, Gopal R, Lin Y, Fallert Junecko BA, Mehra S, Selman M, Becerril-Villanueva E, Baquera-Heredia J, Pavon L, Kaushal D, Reinhart TA, Randall TD, Khader SA. 2013. CXCR5+ T helper cells mediate protective immunity against tuberculosis. *J Clin Invest* 123:712–726.

460. Vermi W, Lonardi S, Bosisio D, Uguccioni M, Danelon G, Pileri S, Fletcher C, Sozzani S, Zorzi F, Arrigoni G, Doglioni C, Ponzoni M, Facchetti F. 2008. Identification of CXCL13 as a new marker for follicular dendritic cell sarcoma. *J Pathol* 216:356–364.

461. Takagi R, Higashi T, Hashimoto K, Nakano K, Mizuno Y, Okazaki Y, Matsushita S. 2008. B cell chemoattractant CXCL13 is preferentially expressed by human Th17 cell clones. *J Immunol* 181:186–189.

462. Gunn MD, Ngo VN, Ansel KM, Ekland EH, Cyster JG, Williams LT. 1998. A B-cell-homing chemokine made in lymphoid follicles activates Burkitt's lymphoma receptor-1. *Nature* **391**:799–803.

463. Maglione PJ, Xu J, Chan J. 2007. B cells moderate inflammatory progression and enhance bacterial containment upon pulmonary challenge with *Mycobacterium tuberculosis*. *J Immunol* **178**:7222–7234.

Tuberculosis and the Tubercle Bacillus, 2nd ed.
Edited by William R. Jacobs, Jr., Helen McShane, Valerie Mizrahi, and Ian M. Orme
© 2018 American Society for Microbiology, Washington, DC
doi:10.1128/microbiolspec.TBTB2-0006-2016

Regulation of Immunity to Tuberculosis

3

Susanna Brighenti[1] and Diane J. Ordway[2]

REGULATORY CELLS IN IMMUNE HOMEOSTASIS AND SUPPRESSION

Homeostasis in the immune system has the essential function to minimize deleterious immune-mediated inflammation caused by commensal microorganisms, immune responses against self and environmental antigens, as well as metabolic inflammatory conditions. Homeostatic regulation is enabled by regulatory T (Treg) cells that mediate immune suppression as a vital mechanism of negative regulation. Treg cells have the capacity to prevent not only potentially damaging autoimmune responses, but also protective immunity, and thus the number of Treg cells is a crucial determinant of the regulatory burden on the immune system. The presence of low numbers of Treg cells can trigger fatal autoimmunity, whereas having high numbers can cause overt immunosuppression. Specifically, this means that the combination of the overall number and specific subsets of regulatory cells maintains the order in the immune system by a process of imposing negative regulation on other cells in the immune system. In this review, we will discuss the role of the distinct regulatory immune cell subsets in the development of tuberculosis (TB).

Regulatory T Cells

In recent years, many insights into the process of immune homeostasis have been gained, leading to the understanding that Treg cells are fundamental to immune regulation and the establishment of immune homeostasis. Treg can basically be defined as T cells with specific suppressive abilities, mediated by downregulation of proliferation and effector functions of different types of immune cells.

Naturally occurring and induced Treg cells

Nowadays, it is generally accepted that naturally occurring Treg cells regulate peripheral tolerance, control autoimmune diseases, and restrict chronic inflammation to prevent immunopathology. The finding that Treg cells were required for prevention of autoimmune disease occurred when neonatal thymectomized mice developed an autoimmune disease that was prevented by transferring T cells from adult mice (1, 2). However, it was the discovery that the subset of T cells responsible for suppression of autoimmunity expressed high levels of CD25 (the high-affinity interleukin-2 [IL-2] receptor α) and the transcription factor forkhead box P3 (Foxp3+) as the "master control gene" that defined this subset as a distinct T cell lineage (3–6). Foxp3 acts as a transcriptional regulator because it can bind to the promoters for genes involved in Treg cell function and, in that way, suppress the transcription of key genes following stimulation of T cell receptors (7). A suppressive role for Foxp3 expression was further identified as the genetic defect underlying a lethal inflammatory autoimmunity in scurfy mice (8, 9). Importantly, the autoimmune phenotype in the scurfy mouse could be reversed by transfer of CD4+ T cells but not CD8+ T cells (10, 11), confirming a dominant suppressive role for CD4+ Foxp3+ cells (12). The lack of Foxp3+ T cells due to mutations in their Foxp3 locus is also found in human disease and results in IPEX syndrome (immune dysregulation, polyendocrinopathy, enteropathy, X-linked syndrome) and XLAAD (X-linked autoimmunity allergic dysregulation syndrome), emphasizing the importance of Treg cells in the maintenance of normal immune homeostasis (13). Without bone marrow transplantation, the IPEX and XLAAD

[1]Center for Infectious Medicine (CIM), F59, Department of Medicine, Karolinska Institutet, Karolinska University Hospital Huddinge, Stockholm, Sweden; [2]Mycobacteria Research Laboratories, Department of Microbiology, Immunology and Pathology, Colorado State University, Fort Collins, CO 80523.

(14) syndromes result in a lethal disease showing the requirement of Foxp3 for immune homeostasis in humans (12). Patients with a CD25 deficiency develop a similar IPEX-like syndrome caused by a defective production of the anti-inflammatory cytokine IL-10 (15).

Treg cells can exert a suppressive function on immune responses for a short or long duration. Treg populations are normally characterized based on their site of development, phenotype, and function (16). Thus, these cells are developmentally classified into natural Tregs (nTregs) or induced Tregs (iTregs) as well as adaptive Tregs. Natural Tregs develop in the thymus by a process of major histocompatibility complex (MHC) class II T cell receptor (TCR)-dependent interactions with self-antigens resulting in high avidity selection (4, 6). Naturally occurring CD4+ CD25+ Foxp3+ Tregs typically constitute 2 to 3% of peripheral blood (17) and this population can be expanded and recirculated in the body upon antigen stimulation. It has also been recognized that Foxp3+ Tregs can be generated from mature conventional CD4+ T cells outside the thymus by many conditions such as chronic antigen stimulation, limited costimulation, and the presence of the anti-inflammatory cytokine transforming growth factor β (TGF-β) (18) or IL-10 (19). Importantly, true Tregs are mostly identified by coexpression of CD25 and Foxp3 since both these markers are also expressed by recently activated conventional T cells and are thus not specific to Tregs (20). Expression of other surface markers has been exploited to improve identification of distinct Treg populations. For instance, coexpression with CTLA-4 and/or GITR or downregulation of certain receptors on Tregs such as CD127 and CD49d are believed to represent better signatures of true Tregs. However, we currently lack identification of a single marker that is specific to Tregs and that is not upregulated upon activation of conventional CD4+ T cells.

Mechanisms of Treg suppression

The suppressive functions of both nTregs and iTregs depend on their individual antigen-specific TCRs. Since the pathways of development of nTregs and iTregs are different, these cells have nonoverlapping specificities resulting in immune suppression in different tissue immune sites and target cells. The specific mechanisms of Treg suppression and how these cells affect disease outcome remain poorly understood. Tregs have been emphasized mostly because of their versatility of suppression through multiple mechanisms including both soluble factors and cell-contact-dependent receptor-ligand interactions. Accordingly, mechanisms that con-

tribute to immune suppression involve (i) secretion of suppressive cytokines such as IL-10, TGF-β, and IL-35 (21) that can directly inhibit the function of responder T cells and myeloid cells (22) or secretion of other factors that affect amino acid availability and energy metabolism, as well as (ii) cell membrane-bound receptors such as the high-affinity TCR and other molecules with regulatory properties including CTLA-4, GITR, LAG3, CD39, PD-1, and Nrp1 (18). Typical negative effects of Tregs are suppression of cell growth, cytolytic activity, and reduced production of inflammatory cytokines. Impaired production of Th1 (IL-2, gamma interferon [IFN-γ]) and Th17 cytokines (IL-17) leads to decreased proliferation and defective induction of antimicrobial effector functions. Treg cells that express high levels of the IL-2Rα chain (CD25) have the capacity to compete with effector T cells for IL-2, resulting in cytokine-mediated deprivation of the effector cells and Bim-mediated apoptosis (22). In addition, the function of antigen-presenting cells (APCs) can be inhibited by downregulation of costimulatory molecules such as CD80/CD86 that result in an inability of APCs to stimulate proinflammatory responses (23). Lately, it has also been suggested that iTreg cells can kill APCs through a granzyme B-dependent mechanism (24). Thus, activated Treg cells may function to directly kill effector cells in a manner similar to CD8+ cytolytic T cells (22). Stimulated Treg cells may also express known receptors (e.g., galectin-1) on their cell surface that can interact with receptors on effector T cells, resulting in cell cycle arrest (22). Examples of suppressive mechanisms that are mediated by cell membrane-bound receptors on the Treg cells to inhibit the function of APCs or other cells of the innate immune system are further presented in Fig. 1 (22).

Treg CELL RESPONSES IN HUMAN TB

While enhanced Treg responses are desirable in autoimmune conditions and organ transplantations, increased Tregs in different forms of cancer as well as several infectious diseases has been associated with poor prognosis. In contrast to some acute viral infections where Treg cells may play a beneficial role, pathogen-specific Treg cells suppress Th1 immunity and may be expanded and overexpressed at the site of infection during chronic intracellular infections including TB (25, 26). There is probably a functional plasticity in Treg cell suppression that may shift following infection with different types of pathogens. Below we will discuss the relevance of different immunoregulatory pathways in human TB with a focus on Treg cells.

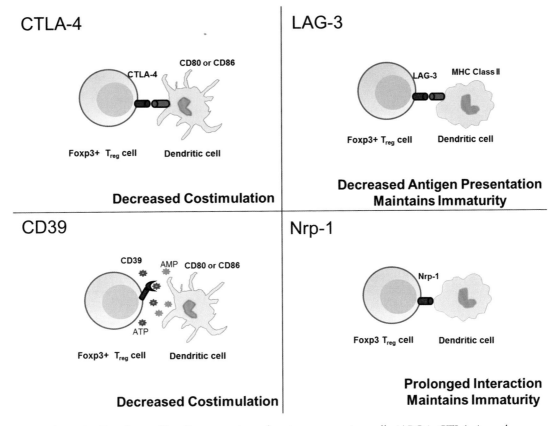

Figure 1 Regulatory T cell suppression of antigen-presenting cells (APCs). CTLA-4 on the surface of Treg cells can prevent or depress the upregulation of CD80 and CD86, the major costimulatory molecules on APC. LAG-3 on Treg cells can interact with MHC class II on APCs, by binding of LAG-3 to MHC class II molecules on immature DCs, causing an inhibitory signal that suppresses DC maturation and immaturity. Tissue destruction results in extracellular ATP that functions as an indicator and exerts inflammatory effects on DCs. Catalytic inactivation of extracellular ATP by CD39 represents an anti-inflammatory mechanism that may be used by Treg cells to prevent the deleterious effects of ATP on antigen-presenting cell function. In contrast, Nrp-1 (neuropilin) promotes extended interactions between Treg cells and immature DCs and limits access of the effector cells to APCs.

Treg-Mediated Manipulation of Immune Cell Activation in Human TB

Growing evidence suggests that a Th1/Th2/Treg balance is crucial to control progression of active TB disease (27–30). *M. tuberculosis*-specific Th1 (IL-12, IFN-γ, tumor necrosis factor alpha [TNF-α]) and Th17 (IL-17, IL-22) cells promote inflammation and activate antimicrobial effector functions in infected macrophages as well as in *M. tuberculosis*-specific cytotoxic T lymphocytes (CTLs) to enhance bacterial killing and containment of *M. tuberculosis* infection through granuloma formation (31, 32). Instead, development of a Th2 (IL-4, IL-13) or Treg (IL-10, TGF-β) response efficiently antagonizes protective cellular immunity, which could result in loss of TB control (33, 34). In humans, the onset of adaptive immune responses in TB

is considerably delayed compared with responses to other pathogens (35). Instead, excess Treg cell activity and production of anti-inflammatory mediators early in TB infection may promote mycobacterial growth and survival. Here, growing evidence from both humans and experimental animal models suggests that *M. tuberculosis* can induce Treg cells with immunosuppressive functions that interfere with protective responses in TB. In 2006, a number of studies reported that CD25+ and Foxp3+ nTreg cells were elevated in the circulation and at the site of infection in patients with active pulmonary TB (36, 37). CD4+ CD25+ Foxp3+ Treg cells isolated from blood of patients with active TB efficiently suppressed the proliferation and IFN-γ production by CD4+ CD25– responder T cells in an *in vitro* coculture system (38). Conversely, *in vitro* depletion of

CD25^{hi} Treg cells from peripheral blood mononuclear cells (PBMCs) obtained from patients with active TB could rescue antigen-specific IFN-γ production to levels comparable to latent TB controls (39). Similarly, vaccination with the novel BCG-booster vaccine, MVA85A, resulted in reduced levels of CD4+ CD25^{hi} Foxp3+ Treg cells in peripheral blood from immunized study subjects, which correlated to increased IFN-γ but reduced TGF-β expression in PBMCs and serum samples (40). Other studies have confirmed these findings and determined that CD4+ CD25+ Treg cells in active TB coexpressed Foxp3, CTLA-4, GITR, PD-1, and CD39 at the protein level (41–43) and also higher levels of CD45RO and HLA-DR together with lower levels of CD127 (44) and CD45RA compared with CD4+ CD25– T cells (41). These reports were followed by a number of studies describing the balance of effector cell to Treg cell responses in TB patients (45). While conventional αβ effector T cells are important in TB defense, γδ T cells that recognize lipid- and phosphoantigens can be induced in response to *M. tuberculosis* and complement the protective functions of CD4+ and CD8+ T cells. Here, it has been shown that Treg cells can also suppress the function of Vdelta2 T cells (46) that express both IFN-γ and the antimicrobial peptide granulysin, which are instrumental in killing of *M. tuberculosis*-infected macrophages (47). Importantly, CD4+ CD25+ Foxp3+ Treg cells from blood of patients with active TB diminished the ability of both alveolar and monocyte-derived macrophages to inhibit intracellular *M. tuberculosis* growth in the presence of CD4+ effector cells, which supports the notion that Tregs actively subvert antimycobacterial immunity in human TB (48).

However, Treg activity is also required to some extent to control pathological inflammation. Accordingly, Foxp3+ Treg cells expressing CTLA-4 have been associated with significantly decreased levels of the Th17 cytokines IL-17 and IL-23 in individuals with positive tuberculin skin tests who have latent TB (49). Similarly, the frequency of *M. tuberculosis*-specific IFN-γ producing CD4+ T cells has been shown to be significantly higher in HIV patients with TB-associated immune reconstitution inflammatory syndrome (TB-IRIS) compared with non-IRIS patients whereas the proportion of CD4+ Foxp3+ Treg cells was low in both groups, indicating that the severe inflammation could be caused by defective immune regulation (50). Furthermore, the risk of TB is increased three times in patients with diabetes mellitus (DM) and TB/DM patients have been shown to possess elevated frequencies of *M. tuberculosis*-specific CD4+ Th1 cells and also Th17 cells but decreased

baseline levels of CD4+ CD25+ Foxp3+ CD127^{dim} Treg cells that could contribute to increased immunopathology and comorbidity in TB/DM disease (51). The importance of a balanced immune response in TB disease is illustrated in Fig. 2.

In vitro expansion of mycobacteria-specific Treg cells

Mycobacteria-specific CD4+ CD25^{hi} Foxp3+ Treg cells obtained from PBMCs of latently infected individuals can be expanded *in vitro* in the presence of *Mycobacterium bovis* BCG and TGF-β (44) or by stimulation with *M. tuberculosis*-specific antigens ESAT-6 and Ag85B (52). Such Tregs express CTLA-4, GITR, and OX40, but low levels of CD127 and efficiently suppress responder T cell proliferation (44). It has also been demonstrated that *M. tuberculosis*-specific antigens can induce an expansion of different IL-10-producing subsets including both natural CD4+ CD25+ Foxp3+ and induced CD4+ CD25– Foxp3-Treg subsets in whole blood samples from patients with pulmonary TB (53). In line with these findings, the cell wall component of virulent *M. tuberculosis*, ManLAM (mannose-capped lipoarabinomannan), induced an expansion of human Treg cells *in vitro* in a prostaglandin E2-dependent manner (54), which suggests that *M. tuberculosis*-infected macrophages producing ManLAM as well as prostaglandin E2 may inhibit proper Th1 cell activation by the expansion of Treg cells. *M. tuberculosis* could also modulate dendritic cells (DCs) to express programmed death 1 (PD1) and expand CD4+ CD25+ Foxp3+ Tregs via the PD1-PD ligand 1 pathway (42, 55). Apparently, this Treg expansion occurred mainly from a CD4+ CCR4+ T cell subset (42). This is interesting, since CCR4 is the receptor for CCL4, CCL17, and CCL22, which are chemokines shown to be involved in the recruitment of Treg cells and subsequent progression of active TB (56). As such, CCR4– antagonists have been shown to block CCL22- and CCL17-mediated recruitment of human Tregs and Th2 cells and, instead, promote DC-mediated proliferation of human CD4+ T cells (57).

Th2 cells producing IL-4 and IL-13 have been shown to be detrimental in the control of intracellular *M. tuberculosis* infection, because these Th2 cytokines suppress IFN-γ production by Th1 cells and IFN-γ-mediated effects including M1 macrophage activation (33, 58). Th2 cytokines can also inhibit Th1-induced autophagy and thus reduce the intracellular degradation of *M. tuberculosis* bacteria (59). Th2 responses with increased production of IL-4 in patients with active TB may antagonize the host defense and lead to

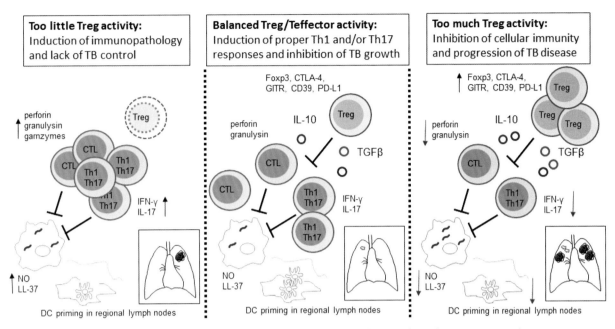

Figure 2 A combination of host immune factors and *M. tuberculosis* strain virulence can result in a distinctive host immunophenotype over time, resulting in multiple outcomes. During infection too little Treg activity can lead to a greater Th1 immune response, resulting in tissue damage and bacterial growth. A balance of both Th1 and Treg immunity can result in proper antibacterial immunity, leading to reduced TB growth. Excessive Treg activity results in a counterregulatory Treg response that ultimately impairs host immunity against the tubercle bacillus, allowing disease progression.

induction of fibrosis and cavitation (60, 61), which compromise lung function in TB patients. It has also been demonstrated that IL-4 can induce development and expansion of CD25+ Tregs from human naive CD4+ CD25− T cells that show an anergic phenotype and prevent proliferation of CD4+ CD25− responder T cells comparable to nCD4+ CD25+ Treg cells (62). IL-4-induced Tregs resemble nTregs including high expression of Foxp3, CTLA-4, and GITR (62).

In vitro expanded, but not freshly isolated Treg cells can be lysed by activated human NK cells via the activating NK cell receptors NKG2D and NKp46 (63). Thus, in individuals with latent TB who manage to control the infection, *in vivo* activated NK cells may kill *M. tuberculosis*-infected macrophages (64) but also certain Treg populations, which could result in an inhibited Treg expansion and instead promote the development of a proper Th1 response (63). Conversely, an early, local expansion of Treg cells in patients with active TB disease could be explained by decreased NK cell activity and increased Treg numbers in TB (54, 64).

CD39+ Treg cell subsets in human TB

It has previously been proposed that Tregs in human TB are phenotypically characterized by surface expres-

sion of CD39, an ectonucleotidase that metabolizes proinflammatory extracellular ATP (43). CD39 hydrolyzes extracellular ATP to generate adenosine, which binds to adenosine receptors and inhibits T cell and NK cell responses (65, 66). Thus, adenosine suppresses the immune system by increasing the expansion and regulatory activity of Treg cells and simultaneously decreasing effector T cell functions. Antigen-specific CD4+ T cells expressing CD39 are more abundant in active than in latent TB and correlate with the production of IL-10 (67). It is not clear if and how this Treg subset differs from the naturally occurring CD4+ CD25+ Foxp3+ Treg cells, but perhaps the CD4+ CD39+ Treg cells are induced as a consequence of the immunosuppressive environment in progressive TB disease. Peripheral CD4+ CD25+ CD39[hi] Treg cells have previously been shown to decrease in number in healthy volunteers who were vaccinated with the novel TB vaccine candidate, MVA85A (68). However, study subjects with a preexisting immunity to mycobacteria were associated with higher numbers of CD4+ CD25[hi] CD39+ T cells in the periphery and a reduced capacity to produce IL-17A following MVA85A immunization, suggesting that Tregs in TB could also suppress Th17 proinflammatory responses (68). Consumption of extracellular ATP by PBMCs from MVA85A-vaccinated subjects drops 2 weeks postvaccination, corresponding to a drop in CD4+ CD25+ CD39+ Treg cells and a concomitant rise in CD4+ T cells coexpressing IL-17 and IFN-γ (69). These findings suggest that CD39+ Tregs are partly responsible for ATP consumption and that a decline in Treg cells may liberate proinflammatory extracellular ATP that help to drive the development of IL17+/IFN-γ+ effector T cells that could have an instrumental role in vaccine-induced protection in human TB. While the numbers of both Th17 cells and CD39+ Tregs were both shown to increase in TB pleural effusions compared with blood, Th17 cell numbers inversely correlated with Tregs in pleural fluid but not in blood (70). Coculture of naive CD4+ T cells together with CD39+ Tregs resulted in diminished numbers of Th17 cells. These numbers were restored upon inhibition of Treg activity (70). These studies suggest that pleural CD39+ Tregs could inhibit generation and differentiation of Th17 cells. The immunosuppressive properties of CD39 have also been demonstrated in the context of *M. tuberculosis*-activated human CD8+ CD39+ Treg cells that coexpressed the Treg markers CD25, Foxp3, LAG-3, and CCL4 and suppressed the proliferation of CD4+ Th1 responder cells (71).

Human Treg cells and clinical *M. tuberculosis* strains

Whereas it is clear that immunosuppressive Treg cells are induced in patients with active TB, it was not clear how Treg frequency or function could be affected by different clinical strains of *M. tuberculosis*. Interestingly, some strains of the highly virulent W-Beijing family can modulate the cytokine expression in human monocytes (72). Here, enhanced *M. tuberculosis* growth in human macrophages was shown to be a specific trait of strain 210 that is consistent with an enhanced persistence and frequency of outbreaks of this strain (73). Likewise, *in vitro* infection of human monocytes with *M. tuberculosis* strain HN878 and related W-Beijing isolates preferentially induced a Th2-polarized immune response characterized by IL-4 and IL-13 production (74). Another *M. tuberculosis* strain, the multidrug-resistant (MDR)-TB outbreak strain M of the Haarlem lineage, was shown to induce lower amounts of IFN-γ but higher levels of IL-4 in CD4+ and CD8+ T cells in comparison with the laboratory H37Rv strain and also lower CTL activity assessed as low expression of the degranulation marker CD107 (75). PBMCs from MDR-TB patients had an increased proportion of Foxp3+ Treg cells compared with patients with drug-susceptible TB or healthy controls, and, although

in vitro depletion of CD25-positive Treg cells increased both IFN-γ expression and CTL activity in TB patients, CTL responses remained relatively low in PBMC samples from MDR-TB patients stimulated with the M outbreak strains (75). These results suggest that the virulence of different *M. tuberculosis* strains could have a significant impact on the Th1/Th2/Treg cell balance in human TB disease that can lead to an impairment of the CTL response required to kill *M. tuberculosis*-infected cells at the site of infection. The M strain has also been shown to stimulate IL-17 production upon exposure to PBMCs, which is consistent with excess amounts of IL-17 in MDR-TB patients that could shift the immunological balance and promote inflammation and tissue pathology in the TB-infected lung (76).

Human Treg cells and anti-TB treatment

In active TB, an increase in both activated CD38+ HLA-DR+ effector T cells as well as CD4+ CD25+ CD127− Treg cells has previously been shown to associate with a higher bacterial burden (77). Consistent with this finding, CD4+ Foxp3+ Treg cells were detected at a higher frequency in patients with sputum-smear-positive TB compared with sputum-smear-negative TB (78). Whereas CD25+ CD127− Treg cell frequency was primarily elevated in active TB, enhanced levels of Tregs were also found in patients with latent TB compared with healthy controls, suggesting that Treg cell activity is also present in individuals who control TB infection (77). Interestingly, while individuals with latent TB maintained elevated CD4+ CD25+ CD127− Treg levels after 3 months of preventive therapy, there was a significant increase in the fraction of CD4+ CD24+ Foxp3+ Tregs posttreatment (77). Possibly, different Treg subsets may have different functions at different stages of TB infection that emerge to balance effector T cell responses and immune-mediated pathology. Another study reported that an increase in CD4+ CD25+ Foxp3+ Treg cells and increased levels of IL-10 in active TB gradually declined upon successful anti-TB chemotherapy, while production of IFN-γ was elevated (79). Treg-mediated suppression of protective immunity was dependent on the PD1-PD-1L pathway, and the persistence of Treg cells was significant in patients with MDR-TB who did not respond to standard chemotherapy (52, 79). However, CD4+ CD25+ Foxp3+ Treg numbers were reduced in MDR-TB patients after surgical removal of pathological lesions of the Mtb-infected lung (80). Consistent with these data, it was found that Foxp3, TGF-β, and IL-4 mRNA expression was increased in patients with active TB compared with patients who had been treated with chemotherapy for 6 months or individuals with latent TB upon *in vitro* stimulation of whole blood samples with *M. bovis* BCG (81). A lower T-bet to GATA-3 ratio in patients with active TB may also imply a shift of the immune response from a Th1 toward a Th2 profile (81). This is supported by the finding that successful anti-TB treatment raises the IFN-γ/IL-4 ratio (79).

Treg Responses at the Local Site of *M. tuberculosis* Infection

While most studies on immune cells involved in human TB are based on blood samples, the immune response detected and monitored in the peripheral circulation may not provide a proper reflection of the specific host-pathogen interactions that occur at the site of infection. Accordingly, most reports that have compared effector as well as regulatory responses in peripheral blood with sites of TB disease (60, 82, 83) conclude that there is an accumulation of *M. tuberculosis*-specific immune cells at the site of infection, which highlights the importance to study *M. tuberculosis*-specific immune responses at the local site. Local pathogenesis of TB infection in humans remains elusive in many aspects, including the complex network of cells that comprise the TB granuloma, but also the local microenvironment that surrounds the granulomas. The TB granuloma is a dynamic structure and thus the cellular composition and the function of the granuloma may vary depending on the phase of TB infection (84, 85). The balance of local immune responses in the granuloma will finally dictate bacterial control versus pathology. Selected inflammatory mediators and immunoregulatory pathways can limit or facilitate TB depending on their temporal and tissue dynamics.

Treg responses in tissue

We have previously shown that CD8+ CTLs are scanty and have an impaired expression of the cytolytic and antimicrobial effector molecules perforin and granulysin in granulomatous lesions both in lung (86) and lymph nodes (87) from patients with active pulmonary TB or local TB lymphadenitis, respectively. While the CTL response in the TB granuloma was diminished, our *in situ* findings suggest that lymph node granulomas contained increased numbers of CD4+ Foxp3+ Treg cells compared with tissue sites outside the granulomas (87). In addition, coexpression of the Treg cell markers, CTLA-4 and GITR as well as TGF-β, was particularly high inside the granulomas (87), which supports the conclusion that functional Treg cells are accumulated at the site of bacterial persistence. Thus, *M. tuberculosis* may induce local expansion of Treg

cells and use Treg cell-mediated immunosuppression to sustain bacterial replication at the site of infection (88). Compartmentalization of local immune responses may also result in impaired antimicrobial effector T cell responses and thus reduce contact-dependent killing of *M. tuberculosis*-infected cells inside the granuloma (89). Recently, mRNA and *in situ* analysis of *M. tuberculosis*-infected lung tissue from patients with chronic incurable TB revealed that both perforin and granulysin were low despite an upregulation of CD3+ T cell expression (90). Instead, we found significantly elevated levels of CD20+ IgG+ B cells and Foxp3+ Treg cells in the TB lesions in comparison with distal lung parenchyma (90). It would be interesting to study whether such B cells are merely antibody-secreting B cells that emerge as a consequence of tissue damage and progressive TB disease or if these B cells have a regulatory function that may also support the maintenance of Foxp3+ Tregs at the site of *M. tuberculosis* infection.

Treg responses in cell and fluid samples from sites of active TB disease

In parallel to studies in tissue, bronchoalveolar lavage (BAL) and pleural fluid samples obtained from the lung and pleura of patients with pulmonary or pleural TB can be used to study local *M. tuberculosis* immune responses. As such, CD4+ CD25+ Foxp3+ Treg cells and Foxp3-mRNA expression have been shown to be significantly higher at the site of *M. tuberculosis* infection in the lung compared with the peripheral blood (37, 91). Here, Foxp3+ Treg cells obtained from the BAL of patients with pulmonary TB predominantly produced IL-10 and suppressed *M. tuberculosis*-specific proliferation of autologous T cells (91). An increased frequency of CD4+ CD25+ CD127− Treg cells has also been found in BAL samples compared with blood from individuals with latent TB (92). Results from TB/DM patients confirm that CD4+ CD25+ CD127− Treg frequencies as well as IL-10 expression were significantly higher in BAL than in peripheral blood, while IFN-γ expression was significantly lower (93). Moreover, it was determined that the frequency of CD4+ CD25 Foxp3+ Tregs was significantly higher in pleural effusions compared with blood from patients with TB pleuritic, but also compared with patients with lung malignancies (94). Macrophages and T cells in the pleural fluid expressed high concentrations CCL22, which was chemotactic for CD4+ CD25hi T cells *in vitro*, and anti-CCL22 antibody partly inhibited this chemotactic activity (56). Thus, CCL22 may be responsible for the infiltration of CD4+ CD25hi Treg cells into the pleural space. Similarly, a high proportion of CD4+ CD25hi

Foxp3+ Tregs and also CD4+ CD107+ and CD8+ CD107+ effector T cells were detected in pleural fluid compared with blood samples from patients with TB pleuritis (95). Treg numbers were higher in TB patients with a combined pleural and pulmonary disease than in pleural TB only (95). Subsequent Treg depletion enhanced Mtb-induced IFN-γ and CD4+ and CD8+ degranulation responses in vitro and decreased CD4+ IL-10+ cells in pleural fluid (95). These results are consistent with our findings from tissue that an impaired CTL response is associated with an enhanced Treg activity in active TB. Altogether, the findings from tissue and other clinical samples obtained from the site of TB disease suggest that Treg cells redistribute from the blood to the lungs and draining lymph nodes upon TB infection, where they are retained within the granulomatous lesions together with effector T cells. An imbalance between effector T cells and Treg cells at pathological sites may be associated with impaired cellular immunity and clinical manifestations in human TB.

Treg CELL RESPONSES IN EXPERIMENTAL ANIMAL MODELS OF TB

A wide variety of experimental animal models have been used to dissect the immune response to M. tuberculosis (96–98). Mice are the most widely used small-animal model because of the relatively low cost, extensive availability of immunological reagents, and the availability of inbred and genetically engineered strains with characterized genotypes. Thus, it is not surprising that Treg cells were first observed in a C57BL/6 mouse model of M. tuberculosis (99). The mouse model has been widely used to understand the function of these cells during TB infection and disease progression. The one notable disadvantage of C57BL/6 mice and the majority of mouse models is that the pulmonary and extrapulmonary pathology following aerosol challenge with M. tuberculosis lacks important morphologic features, such as the development of necrotic granulomas that are commonly present upon infection of humans (100). This deficit is a major drawback because different host responses reflected in the histopathology of the lesions are predicted to present different immune microenvironments impacting the state of the bacilli, thus resulting in diverse outcomes of infection and disease. The process of development of granulomatous necrosis in human TB involves the presence of robust inflammation that in turn requires immune regulation by Tregs.

A superior model to evaluate the development of immunoregulation in response to the expansion of pulmonary granulomatous necrosis is the guinea pig low-dose aerosol infection model, which shares many of these clinical features with human TB disease (101, 102). The weakness of the guinea pig model has always been the lack of molecular and immunological reagents. This has improved over the years and has enabled studies of Treg cells, not only in the context of immunity, but also bacterial strain virulence (103–105), vaccination (106, 107), and drug treatment (105, 108).

Non-human primates (NHPs) are used to model human TB disease because of their remarkably similar genomes, physiology, and immune systems. The advantages of the NHP model are a high susceptibility to infection with M. tuberculosis, generating the full spectrum of disease states, including acute TB, latent infection, and chronic progressive disease (109). The obvious weaknesses of the NHP model are the required biosafety containment and the cost of conducting the animal studies (110, 111).

Large differences in the immunology, pathology, and spectrum of TB disease exist between the mouse model and the NHP model. However, despite these differences, many of the earlier observations of suppressor function of Tregs present in small-animal models have been confirmed in subsequent NHP studies. For instance, cynomolgus macaques infected with M. tuberculosis presenting with primary TB demonstrated the presence of suppressor Tregs in active disease. Moreover, this study supported that Treg suppression occurred as a result of an indirect response to inflammation, instead of as a causative factor in progression to active disease (112) as previously noted in murine models (113).

M. tuberculosis induces a remarkably different spectrum of disease and immunopathology based on strain virulence, host genetics, and a variety of complex environmental factors. Animal models cannot completely mimic human TB disease. But human-like necrotic and non-necrotic granulomas can develop in novel mouse models, guinea pigs, and NHPs, which facilitates in vivo studies on the cellular dynamics present in the TB granuloma. Most likely, the balance of these granuloma types has an impact on the clinical outcome. Diverse experimental animal models, through their different microenvironments and immune regulation, could reveal under what circumstances Treg cell function may impact TB disease progression versus resolution. This will be discussed later in this review.

Treg Cells in Mouse Models of TB

The mouse model has been essential in understanding regulatory immunity primarily because of the wealth of immunological reagents. Foxp3 subcellular localization limits, to some extent, the ability to study Treg function in humans, NHPs, and guinea pigs. This is because the Foxp3 receptor cannot be bound by an external antibody, allowing it to be studied by using cell sorting and adoptive transfer techniques that can only be achieved by using genetically engineered reporter mice. Despite these drawbacks in the mouse model to study Treg cells is the development of genetically engineered Foxp3 GFP+ transgenic mice that express Foxp3 green fluorescent protein (GFP). Advances enable the use of reporter mice expressing fluorescent GFP Foxp3, permitting cell sorting and adoptive transfer into recipient mice (114). Other mouse models available to study Foxp3+ cells utilize antibodies to deplete specific cell types, such as transgenic mice having T cells with a single specificity and conditional knockout mice with specific targeted genes of Foxp3+ cells (88). The combination of the reagents and the multiple genetically engineered mouse models ultimately facilitates the discovery of Treg cell function in the mouse model of TB.

Treg cells in early TB infection

The mouse model does reflect some aspects of human TB disease. Primarily, after a low-dose *M. tuberculosis* aerosol exposure in mice (as with infection in humans), the arrival of CD4+ T cells produces IFN-γ in the lungs (115). Ultimately, this delayed arrival of protective CD4+ Th1 cells to the site of infection permits the bacilli to replicate within the pulmonary cavity with only resident cell immune control. Obviously, this armors *M. tuberculosis* with the advantage to establish a productive infection in the lungs before the acquired immune response can be expressed. Another similarity between mouse and human TB is that after *M. tuberculosis* exposure, Tregs increase in numbers, and highly activated cells are present at the sites of infection. The initial studies that aimed to understand the function of Tregs in mice focused on removal of Tregs by targeting the CD25 receptor using anti-CD25 antibody treatment, which resulted in contradictory information. Most likely, this method of Treg removal resulted in incomplete elimination of true Treg cells, because CD25 is expressed at different levels on Foxp3+ Treg cells, as well as non-Foxp3+ T cells following T cell activation (99). Initial studies employing the CD25-antibody treatment method (99) prior to infection with *M. bovis* or *M. tuberculosis* demonstrated increased Th1 effector cells and cytokines, although no differences were detected in bacterial organ burden or pulmonary pathology. Other, contradictory studies (116) used adoptive transfer experiments to transfer sorted populations of CD4+ CD25– (non-Treg effector cells) with and without CD4+ CD25+ (Tregs) into recipient RAG knockout mice before exposure to *M. tuberculosis* infection. The animals receiving the mixture of effector and Treg cells compared with CD4+ CD25– effector cells alone demonstrated increased bacterial burdens, which indicated that CD4+ CD25+ Tregs were responsible for suppression of antimycobacterial immunity.

Since all activated effector cells express transient and high levels of CD25, elimination of all Foxp3+ Treg cells based on removal of CD25-expressing cells was not an efficient method. Thus, advances toward a different approach were needed. A new method attempted to eliminate all Foxp3+ cells by generating mixed bone marrow chimeras using Foxp3 sufficient and deficient bone marrow. Antibodies toward a congenic marker (Thy1.1) were utilized to deplete all Foxp3+ T cells (114) before infection with *M. tuberculosis* H37Rv, resulting in a 1.0 Log10 bacterial reduction in the lungs. These investigations once again supported the notion that removal of suppressor cells enhanced host protection and bacterial clearance. However, after complete removal of Foxp3+ Treg cells, these mice rapidly developed multiorgan autoimmunity. Importantly, these studies illustrated that complete removal of different populations of Tregs during TB infection or disease would be ineffective as a treatment approach. Recent studies addressed the possible risk of removal of Foxp3+ Treg cells after TB infection and increased tissue injury (117). These studies showed that after *M. tuberculosis* exposure of mice and removal of Foxp3+ Treg cells during acquired immunity, a temporary reduction in bacterial burden occurred but ultimately resulted in reduced animal survival (118, 119). Correspondingly, studies evaluating the early effects of Tregs in mice infected with a highly virulent W-Beijing clinical strain HN878 showed a rise in Treg frequencies after 2 weeks that were higher than the laboratory strain H37Rv (118). These studies, summarized in Table 1, suggested that increased Treg frequencies during TB result in a worse clinical outcome. Although removal of Tregs results in temporary enhanced protective immunity, driving down the bacterial burden, the resultant autoimmunity or increased inflammation and tissue damage adversely impact TB outcome.

During homeostasis, induced Tregs specific for antigens derived from commensal bacteria can reside in the regional lymph nodes of the gastrointestinal tract (120, 121). Thus, it was unclear if the proliferation of Tregs was in response to mounting TB-derived inflammation and self-antigens or if Tregs recognize and expand specifically to *M. tuberculosis*-derived antigens. Identification of a dual delay in the expansion of not only

Table 1   Impacts of Foxp3+ on host defense against *M. tuberculosis*

Bacterial strain	Disease impact	Outcome of cell manipulation of Foxp3+ on host defense	Caveats
M. bovis BCG *M. tuberculosis* Erdman	None	CD25+ antibody depletion before infection in C57BL/6 mice increased Th1 cytokines but no change in lung bacterial burden/pathology (1).	CD25+ expressed at different level on Tregs and non-Tregs.
M. tuberculosis H37Rv	Detrimental	Adoptive transfer of CD4+ CD25– and CD4+ CD25+ into RAG$^{-/-}$ increased bacterial burden (38).	Cell sorting based on CD25 includes Tregs and non-Tregs.
M. tuberculosis H37Rv	Protective	Selective depletion of Foxp3+ cells in mixed chimera mice enhanced bacterial clearance (35).	Depletion of Foxp3+ cells results in autoimmunity.
M. tuberculosis HN878	Detrimental	CD25+ antibody depletion after TB exposure during acquired immunity led to a temporary reduction in bacterial burden but reduced animal survival (22).	CD25+ expressed at a different level on Tregs and non-Tregs.

effector T cells, but also Tregs 2 weeks after TB infection, indicated that early inflammation alone was inadequate to trigger Treg cell expansion (122). Nevertheless, after DCs carry *M. tuberculosis* to the draining lymph nodes, expansion of both effector and Treg cells populations occurs (122). Cell transfer studies employing Tregs derived from T cell receptor transgenic mice specific for *M. tuberculosis* Ag85B$_{240-254}$:I-A^b demonstrated proliferation of these cells only in wild-type infected mice compared with an *M. tuberculosis* strain devoid of Ag85B (122). These results support the notion that during infection with TB, Treg priming and preferential expansion are caused by specific Tregs recognizing *M. tuberculosis*-specific antigens. Ancillary studies demonstrated that activated Tregs were capable of inhibiting antigen presentation by DCs in the lymph node via downregulation of CD80/86 that impaired the costimulatory signal required for priming of naïve T cells (123, 124), which ultimately delayed effector T cell migration back to the lung. Although support for the presence of pathogen-specific Tregs has been reported in numerous infections, including *Leishmania major* (125, 126), several other infections such as *Listeria monocytogenes* (127) and retroviral infections (128) show no evidence of pathogen-specific Tregs. This has been confirmed by screening major histocompatibility complex class II tetramers containing epitopes recognized by effector T cells that failed to identify Foxp3+ Treg cells. These studies indicate a need for further investigations using multiple model systems and different clinical strains of pathogens to confirm the existence of pathogen-specific Tregs.

Treg cells in chronic TB infection
Treg cells recruited during inflammation accumulate over time and persist even after inflammation has resolved. The recognition that distinct populations of

mouse Treg cells express these and other inflammatory homing receptors raised the likelihood that specialized populations of Treg cells are recruited to different types of inflammatory responses, and that these may share molecular characteristics with proinflammatory T cell populations. In fact, several recent studies have established that regulation of Th1, Th2, and Th17 responses by Treg cells has separate molecular requirements (129–132). Accordingly, specialization of the Treg response may occur during TB. Treg cells that express the Th1-type transcriptional factor T-bet can survive in hostile, inflammatory environments (133). These Treg cells expressing both T-bet and Foxp3+ are not capable of producing IFN-γ. However, upregulation of the chemokine receptor CXCR3 permits these cells to migrate to inflammatory sites of *M. tuberculosis* infection and exert local immunosuppression. T-bet expression in Tregs also enables these cells to proliferate and avoid cell death during TB (125, 130). Recent studies provide strong evidence that the main function of Foxp3 is to act as a transcriptional repressor. Foxp3 binding alone was not sufficient to establish suppression in resting Treg cells, where Foxp3-bound regulatory elements are only poised for repression. Moreover, an inflammatory stimulus was subsequently required to incorporate the polycomb group histone methyltransferase Ezh2 into the complex and deposit repressive chromatin modifications at Foxp3-bound loci (134). This approach used systemic inflammation caused by Treg cell depletion as inflammatory stimulus. More research is required to identify the specific inflammatory signals that were sensed and led to chromatin remodeling. Additional studies assayed wild-type C57BL/6 mice infected with *M. tuberculosis* Erdman and mice that do not express TLR2 (TLR2KO), which leads to increased inflammation in the lung and uncontrolled bacterial growth (135). The increased inflammation present in the lungs of *M. tuberculosis*-infected TLR2KO mice was due to the diminished ability of Tregs to accumulate in the lungs. Moreover, the ability to recruit Tregs to the lungs was restored in TLR2KO mice if they were adoptively transferred with macrophages from wild-type mice. These studies support a role for TLR2 in protection against chronic *M. tuberculosis* infection by controlling Treg accumulation in the lung that could limit inflammation-induced tissue damage. Other findings show that both Foxp3+ Tregs and TGF-β-producing CD103+ DCs were diminished in the lungs of highly susceptible DBA/2 mice compared with resistant mice during chronic infection, while Treg numbers were maintained in the lymph nodes of DBA/2 mice (136). Despite reduced Treg cell numbers in the lung, bacterial loads remained high at the site of infection (136). Together, these studies highlight the complexity of the Treg response and the need for further research teasing apart *M. tuberculosis* Treg specificity and function as well as molecular inflammatory requirements in the lung and lymph node microenvironment using different model systems.

Treg cells and clinical *M. tuberculosis* strains

The majority of TB research focused on understanding Th1, Th2, and Th17 effector cells in the mouse model supports the notion that different *M. tuberculosis* strains are capable of modulating these immune responses. Thus, it is understandable that different *M. tuberculosis* strains most likely will also influence our understanding of Treg cells. The majority of studies on Tregs in TB used laboratory-adapted *M. tuberculosis* strains such as H37Rv and Erdman. Studies evaluating the early and late effects of Tregs in mice infected with the highly virulent W-Beijing clinical strain HN878 demonstrated that, after 2 weeks, Tregs began to increase in frequency during the chronic phase of the disease and were associated with a decline in Th1 immunity, increased bacterial burden and granuloma lesion scores, and reduced animal survival (113). In additional studies, C3Heb/FeJ mice that are capable of forming necrotic tubercle granulomas in contrast to resistant C3H/HeOuJ mice were infected with the W-Beijing clinical strain SA161 and, 25 days after the infection, the percentage of CD4+ Foxp3+ cells in both models remained similar (137). However, as the C3Heb/FeJ mice progressed into chronic disease, the frequency of CD4+ Foxp3+ Tregs declined and was associated with deteriorating Th17 and Th1 immunity. As the C3H/HeOuJ mice developed chronic disease, Treg frequency increased concomitant with an increase in Th17 and a decline in Th1 immunity. Ancillary stud-

ies in human TB suggest that IL-32 is a host-protective cytokine and likewise, in transgenic mice expressing the human IL-32γ gene, protects mice against *M. tuberculosis* HN878 infection by inducing an increase in the numbers of IFN-γ+ and TNF-α+ T cells in the lungs and lymph nodes that correlated with decreased Foxp3+ Treg cells in the lymph node (138). Together, these studies highlight the importance of Tregs on the lymph node microenvironment and the subsequent induction of immunity that dictates the development of pulmonary granulomas.

Treg cells and TB vaccination

In early life, Treg and other regulatory immune responses may be induced that can potentially impact vaccine efficacy (139). The only licensed vaccine against TB is the BCG vaccine (a live attenuated vaccine) administered to infants in the first few days of life (140). BCG induces the expansion of effective T cell responses and is protective in infants against meningeal TB (141). Despite this, BCG also induces Treg expansion (118) that could limit its ability to induce long-lived optimal protective immunity against TB. In fact, BCG vaccine-induced efficacy against TB wanes during the adolescent and adult years (142).

It has recently been hypothesized that this lack of long-lived protection by BCG originates from induction of Tregs through vaccination. Vaccines for TB are usually tested against the laboratory strains H37Rv or Erdman. Mice vaccinated with BCG and then challenged with *M. tuberculosis* H37Rv are significantly protected, denoted by a 1.0 to 1.5 log reduction in organ bacterial burden, and this protection is sustained during early and chronic disease (143). There is very limited information as to whether the existing BCG vaccine, or any of the new vaccine candidates in the current pipeline, will be effective against the newly emerging clinical strains of *M. tuberculosis*, many of which appear to be highly virulent (113). We have previously shown that highly virulent W-Beijing strains can potently induce the emergence of CD4+ Foxp3+ Treg cells that is associated to a significant ablation of the protective effect of BCG vaccination, thus causing progressive, fatal disease in the mouse model (143). Our studies showed that when BCG-vaccinated mice were infected with the HN878 and SA161 strains, the mice were initially protected against the two W-Beijing strains up to 30 days (143). However, this protection waned during chronic infection, and the animals exhibited increasingly severe lung pathology associated with a strong early effector T cell response, which then declined and was replaced by the steady influx of

Foxp3+ Treg cells into the lungs (143). These studies support the notion that Treg-mediated downregulation of effector cell responses may be a serious impediment to the efficacy of BCG-based vaccines.

Additional studies focused on evaluating if the success of BCG vaccination was dependent on the type of granulomas formed in the lung such as the presence of necrotic or nonnecrotic granulomas. In these studies, the impact of prior BCG vaccination of C3Heb/FeJ (forms necrotic granulomas) and C3H/HeOuJ mice (forms nonnecrotic granulomas) infected with a W-Beijing strain SA161 demonstrated that BCG reduced bacterial loads in both mouse strains 25 days after infection compared with controls (137). However, during chronic infection, vaccine efficacy waned in C3H/HeOuJ but not in C3Heb/FeJ mice. Protection in vaccinated C3Heb/FeJ mice was associated with reduced numbers of CD11b+Gr1+ cells, increased numbers of effector and memory T cells, and an absence of necrotic granulomas. BCG vaccine efficacy waned in C3H/HeOuJ mice, as indicated by reduced expression of IFN-γ and increased expressions of IL-17, IL-10, and Foxp3 by T cells, compared with C3Heb/FeJ mice. These studies support the theory that one role of the BCG vaccine efficacy is to delay the development of primary granuloma necrosis, which is consistent with a reduction in Gr1+ neutrophils that is the cell type responsible for this necrosis.

Further studies were conducted to understand if TB infection and the ensuing Treg response could control inflammation or directly dampen the acquired immune response. It is plausible that subpopulations may exist within the pathogen-specific Treg cell population that differ in their functional properties. Recently, we provided evidence, using both cell depletion and adoptive transfer strategies, that Treg cells can have either property dependent on the type of stimulus. Cell depletion resulted in a rapid but transient drop in the lung bacterial load, suggesting enhancement or temporary reexpansion of effector immunity (118). Transfer of Treg cells into Rag$^{-/-}$ or marked congenic mice worsened the course of TB disease and the depressed cellular influx of effector T cells into the lungs (118). Interestingly, such cells from *M. tuberculosis*-infected donors seemed to preferentially depress the inflammatory response and neutrophil influx, whereas such cells from BCG-vaccinated and then *M. tuberculosis*-challenged donors seemed focused on more severe depression of protective acquired immunity as shown in Fig. 3. Collectively, these qualitative differences possibly relate to the growing knowledge reflecting the plasticity of the Treg cell response.

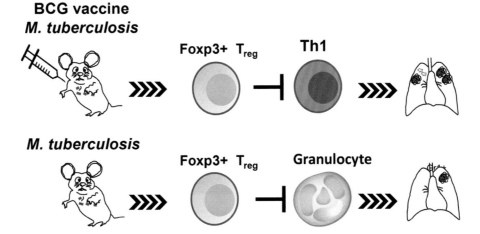

Figure 3 Model of proposed regulatory T cell suppression in mice BCG vaccinated and exposed to clinical *M. tuberculosis* and clinical *M. tuberculosis* alone. (**Top**) The initial BCG vaccination results in bacterial lymph node persistence in the animal TB model that leads to the presence of Treg and Th17 cells. Upon a subsequent infection with *M. tuberculosis* Th1 and Th17 cells expand at a high rate, causing GR1+ influx and pulmonary tissue damage. In an attempt to limit this damage Tregs expand with Th1 immunity and produce IL-10 and CTLA4 binds to CD80/CD86 costimulatory molecules to limit effector T cell expansion. The abundance of Th17 cells can also have a negative regulatory feedback on Th1 effector cells. (**Bottom**)*M. tuberculosis* infection in mice results in expansion of Th1 IFN-γ effector cells capable of limiting further expansion of Th17 cells producing IL-17 induction of GR1+ cells and pulmonary pathology. Treg cells will expand with the Th1 effector immunity limiting Th17 cells through IL-2 consumption with CD25 or IL-10 production.

Treg cells and anti-TB treatment

Surrogate biomarkers for detection of bacterial clearance are required for evaluation of treatment efficacy and as readouts in clinical trials evaluating new TB treatment modalities. Nonetheless, the dynamics of Tregs during treatment of TB is still not fully understood. Despite this, studies by ourselves and others have shown reduced numbers of Tregs during TB treatment (144). We demonstrated that mice that cleared infection with the virulent W-Beijing *M. tuberculosis* strain HN878 after chemotherapy were initially highly resistant to rechallenge with the same organism (145). Even 20 to 30 days after the reinfection, there was no evidence of a Treg cell response in these mice, but the memory T cell response steadily contracted. Interestingly, T cells harvested from the lungs showed evidence of increased PD-1 expression, indicating exhaustion. These data indicated that when a primary *M. tuberculosis* infection is successfully treated with standard anti-TB drugs, upon subsequent *M. tuberculosis* exposures, the memory T cell response is not long lived because of exhaustion. What they show, in this model, is there is not a "memory Treg response."

Treg Cells in the Guinea Pig Model of TB

Low-dose aerosol infection with *M. tuberculosis* in the guinea pig model produces a well-characterized disease that shares important morphologic and clinical features with human TB (100). This is in contrast to the mouse model that has a significant disadvantage, because the pulmonary and extrapulmonary pathology following aerosol challenge with *M. tuberculosis* lacks important morphologic features that are commonly present in guinea pigs, NHPs, and humans. Still, mice are the most widely used small-animal model because of the broader availability of immunological reagents, and of inbred and genetically engineered strains with well-defined genotypes. In the past, the primary drawback of the guinea pig model was a relative lack of specific immunological reagents that could be used to monitor the emerging acquired immune response in TB-infected animals. For example, intracellular flow cytometric staining of cells in this model is currently technologically not possible. However, this situation is gradually improving with the availability of flow cytometric reagents and the development of PCR-based techniques to measure key cytokines, chemokines, and Foxp3+ Treg cells (146).

Initial studies in the guinea pig model (100) showed that the responding T cells are mostly CD4+ T cells and that, after day 30 of *M. tuberculosis* infection, the number of these cells in the lungs drops dramatically.

This drop in CD4+ T cells appears to be replaced by a steady increase in B cells and granulocytes that were associated with a worsened lung pathology. The development of PCR-based techniques to measure key cytokines and Foxp3+ Treg cells led to a deeper understanding of the regulation of immunity in this model (146). Studies infecting guinea pigs with two highly virulent W-Beijing strains resulted in severe lung pathology, associated with large influxes of activated CD4+ and CD8+ T cells into the lungs (146). A progressive increase in neutrophils was also present, combined with early enhanced mRNA levels for Th1 cytokines that later declined and were replaced by increasing levels of message encoding for Foxp3, IL-10, and TGF-β. These observations support the hypothesis that W-Beijing strains are potent inducers of Treg cells that may be trying to protect the animal by suppressing inflammation, but, by dampening effect or immunity, lung damage continues, which in humans would potentially aid transmission of the infection. Additional research has detected differences between the abilities of four of the Beijing *M. tuberculosis* sublineages to grow in the lungs of guinea pigs and found that members of one Beijing subfamily (RD207) were significantly more pathogenic, resulting in severe lung damage (104). The RD207 strains also induced much higher levels of markers associated with Treg cells and showed a significant loss of activated T cells in the lungs over the course of the infections (104). Based on these data, we hypothesize that the sublineages of *M. tuberculosis* are associated with distinct pathological and clinical phenotypes and that these differences influence the transmissibility of particular *M. tuberculosis* strains in human populations.

Research focused on studying the comorbidity of TB and type 2 diabetes mellitus (147) demonstrated that *M. tuberculosis* infection of diabetic guinea pigs resulted in severe and rapidly progressive TB with a shortened survival interval, more severe pulmonary and extrapulmonary pathology, and a higher bacterial burden compared with glucose-intolerant and nondiabetic controls (147). Compared with nondiabetics, diabetic guinea pigs with TB had an exacerbated proinflammatory response with more severe granulocytic inflammation and higher gene expression of the cytokines/chemokines IFN-γ, IL-17A, IL-8, and Treg-associated IL-10 in the lung and of IFN-γ, TNF-α, IL-8, and monocyte chemoattractant protein-1 in the spleen, especially in the chronic phase of TB infection. Thus, progression of TB disease in guinea pigs with impaired glucose tolerance is associated with increased inflammation and bacterial burden that may trigger an enhanced Treg response.

Treg cells in BCG vaccination and anti-TB treatment

In guinea pigs, BCG vaccination slows the progression of TB disease and reduces the severity of necrotic granulomas, which have been shown to harbor a population of drug-tolerant bacilli (105). Thus, BCG vaccination may be used as a strategy to reduce TB disease severity in guinea pigs to enhance the efficacy of treatment with a combination of anti-TB drugs (105). Here, it was found that BCG combined with rifampin, isoniazid, and pyrizinamide (RHZ) prevented a spike in both activated CD4+ CD45^{hi} T cells and CD4+/CD8+ T cell expressing the homing receptor CT4 until late TB infection. In contrast, the BCG-alone group had histological evidence of active TB disease associated with significantly increased numbers of MHC class II+ macrophages, B cells, and neutrophils in the peripheral circulation. Thus, the combination of BCG vaccination and drug therapy was more effective at resolving TB granulomas such that fewer animals had evidence of residual lesions in the lung and thus less reactivation disease at 500 days after *M. tuberculosis* infection. Additional studies have evaluated the efficacy of a regimen combining bedaquiline with rifampin and pyrazinamide (108). This drug regimen effectively reduced mycobacterial loads in the lungs to undetectable levels after 8 weeks of treatment. Clinical recovery was associated with a substantial improvement in lung pathology and a reduction in all immune cell subsets, including activated CD4+/CD8+ T cells, macrophages, B cells, and neutrophils. Together these data indicate that Treg cells in the guinea pig model can be reduced with BCG vaccination and/or antimycobacterial drug treatment.

Treg Cells in Non-Human Primate Models of TB

The NHP model has also been used for research studying the immune response and host-pathogen interactions in TB. It is clear that a low-dose challenge with virulent *M. tuberculosis* strains in NHPs can result in the full clinical spectrum seen in humans, including latent and active TB infection (112, 148). One advantage of the NHP model is that human reagents are usually cross-reactive with macaques, further enabling the use of this model system to study TB. Importantly, the complete spectrum of primary and secondary stages of granuloma development that are present in humans can be detected in *M. tuberculosis*-infected NHPs, which allows tracking inflammatory and regulatory cells in both necrotic and nonnecrotic granulomas (148, 149). Last, a critical advantage of the NHP TB model is the ability to generate clinical correlates of infection by utilizing blood complete blood cell counts and chemistries, serum C-reactive protein, and differential centrifugation values, thoracic X rays, tuberculin skin tests, and IFN-γ release assays, which are also methods used to monitor TB disease in humans (150).

A central and challenging question, regardless of the TB model used, has been to address whether increased Tregs predispose the host to develop active TB or if increased Treg frequencies occur in response to inflammation in active TB disease. After low-dose *M. tuberculosis* infection of cynomolgus macaques, the frequency of CD4+ Foxp3+ cells in peripheral blood rapidly decreased and simultaneously increased in the airways regardless of whether the animals had primary or latent TB, suggesting that Tregs were redistributed to the site of infection (112). Interestingly, latently infected monkeys had a significantly higher frequency of Tregs in peripheral blood prior to infection and during early infection compared with those that developed active disease (112). Moreover, it was evident that monkeys with active disease had increased peripheral Tregs because they developed TB disease, and, 16 weeks postinfection, both Foxp3+ Tregs and total CD4+ T cells also increased in the airways (112). Similar to human TB, CD3+ Foxp3+ Treg cells were mainly located inside TB granulomas in involved lung and lymph node tissues (112), which suggested that Tregs accumulate together with effector cells at the local site of TB infection. Additional studies in rhesus macaques discovered that lymphocyte-activation gene 3 (LAG3), which is mainly expressed by Tregs, is highly expressed in the lungs and particularly in the granulomatous lesions of animals with active TB (151). Interestingly, LAG3 was not expressed in the lungs or in the lung granulomas of animals exhibiting latent TB, which highlights that LAG3 expression on Tregs coincides with high bacterial burdens and changes in the host Th1 response (151). Simian immunodeficiency virus-induced reactivation of latent TB caused an increased expression of LAG3 in the lungs, and this response was not observed in NHPs infected with non-MTB bacterial pathogens (151). These studies suggest that increased levels of Treg cells in active TB disease arise in response to increased inflammation, instead of being the causative factor for progression of active disease.

A genome-wide systems biology approach employing specific whole-genome microarrays has been used in rhesus macaques to specifically study host gene expression in TB lesions obtained from the lungs of infected animals during early and late stages of infection, respectively (150). Together these results indicated that *M. tuberculosis* infection and TB disease progression modulate the granuloma microenvironment from an initial induction of a Th1 gene expression profile that is subsequently repressed and exchanged by anti-inflammatory gene expression markers in late granulomas (152). It has also been described that IL-2 treatment early after *M. tuberculosis* infection of macaques induced simultaneous expansion of CD4+ CD25+ Foxp3+ Tregs as well as effector T cells producing IFN-γ and perforin (153). Interestingly, this dual expansion of Tregs and effector T cell populations resulted in IL-2-induced resistance to form TB lesions in the lung, and *in vitro* depletion of both Tregs and effector cells significantly reduced the ability to induce immune protection (153). According to this study, both activated Foxp3+ Tregs and effector T cells are required to confer resistance to severe TB without enhancing *M. tuberculosis* infection. In line with these findings, recent studies using cynomolgus macaques showed that few multifunctional and few Mtb-specific T cells making any cytokines were present in the granulomas. Instead the granulomas appeared to be multifunctional in the sense that different combinations of T cells producing single cytokines IFN-γ, IL-2, TNF, or IL-17 were present in separate TB lesions that existed in the infected animals (154). Furthermore, sterile granulomas had higher frequencies of T cells making IL-17, TNF, and Th1 cytokines (IFN-γ, IL-2, or TNF) and/or Th17 (IL-17) compared with nonsterile granulomas (154). More importantly, a combinatorial analysis of pairwise cytokine responses showed that granulomas with T cells producing both proinflammatory (IL-17 or TNF) and anti-inflammatory (IL-10) cytokines were associated with *M. tuberculosis* sterilization (154). Altogether, combined inflammatory and Treg cell responses may contribute to *M. tuberculosis* killing at the local site of infection (153, 154). These studies also illustrate that a balance between proinflammatory and anti-inflammatory responses is required for reduced pathology and control of bacterial burden.

CONCLUDING REMARKS

Studies on the phenotype, frequency, and function of both natural and induced subsets of Treg cells have been conducted in both humans and experimental animal models, including mice, guinea pigs, and NHPs. These studies illustrate that it is very challenging to study the clinical relevance of Tregs and how these cells contribute to immunopathogenesis and/or immune protection in the development of TB disease in humans. However, additional clinical and animal studies are required to uncover the Treg pathogen-specific subpopulations likely involved in both protection and immunopathology. Additional detailed analysis to describe the Treg cell dynamics in the granulomatous lesions throughout the course of TB infection may shed light on their contribution to protective and/or harmful clinical outcomes. Therefore, we need to study regulatory cells and their functions in both patients and animal models to obtain new and complementary knowledge that could give us valuable information regarding specific Treg cell subsets. A better understanding of the mechanisms by which Treg cells counteract protective immune responses in TB could support the design of new therapeutic approaches aimed at inducing highly efficient T cell responses with simultaneous generation of targeted Treg cell populations capable of inflammatory control and lack of protective immunosuppression.

Citation. Brighenti S, Ordway DJ. 2016. Regulation of immunity to tuberculosis. Microbiol Spectrum 4(6):TBTB2-0006-2016.

References

1. **Sakaguchi S, Takahashi T, Nishizuka Y.** 1982. Study on cellular events in postthymectomy autoimmune oophoritis in mice. I. Requirement of Lyt-1 effector cells for oocytes damage after adoptive transfer. *J Exp Med* **156:**1565–1576.

2. **Asano M, Toda M, Sakaguchi N, Sakaguchi S.** 1996. Autoimmune disease as a consequence of developmental abnormality of a T cell subpopulation. *J Exp Med* **184:**387–396.

3. **Sakaguchi S, Sakaguchi N, Asano M, Itoh M, Toda M.** 1995. Immunologic self-tolerance maintained by activated T cells expressing IL-2 receptor alpha-chains (CD25). Breakdown of a single mechanism of self-tolerance causes various autoimmune diseases. *J Immunol* **155:**1151–1164.

4. **Hori S, Nomura T, Sakaguchi S.** 2003. Control of regulatory T cell development by the transcription factor Foxp3. *Science* **299:**1057–1061.

5. **Khattri R, Cox T, Yasayko SA, Ramsdell F.** 2003. An essential role for Scurfin in CD4+CD25+ T regulatory cells. *Nat Immunol* **4:**337–342.

6. **Fontenot JD, Gavin MA, Rudensky AY.** 2003. Foxp3 programs the development and function of CD4+ CD25+ regulatory T cells. *Nat Immunol* **4:**330–336..

7. **Marson A, Kretschmer K, Frampton GM, Jacobsen ES, Polansky JK, MacIsaac KD, Levine SS, Fraenkel E, von Boehmer H, Young RA.** 2007. Foxp3 occupancy and regulation of key target genes during T-cell stimulation. *Nature* **445:**931–935.

8. **Sharma R, Jarjour WN, Zheng L, Gaskin F, Fu SM, Ju ST.** 2007. Large functional repertoire of regulatory T-cell suppressible autoimmune T cells in scurfy mice. *J Autoimmun* **29:**10–19.

9. **Ochs HD, Gambineri E, Torgerson TR.** 2007. IPEX, FOXP3 and regulatory T-cells: a model for autoimmunity. *Immunol Res* **38:**112–121.

10. Mayer CT, Tian L, Hesse C, Kühl AA, Swallow M, Kruse F, Thiele M, Gershwin ME, Liston A, Sparwasser T. 2014. Anti-CD4 treatment inhibits autoimmunity in scurfy mice through the attenuation of co-stimulatory signals. *J Autoimmun* 50:23–32.

11. Torgerson TR, Ochs HD. 2002. Immune dysregulation, polyendocrinopathy, enteropathy, X-linked syndrome: a model of immune dysregulation. *Curr Opin Allergy Clin Immunol* 2:481–487.

12. Brunkow ME, Jeffery EW, Hjerrild KA, Paeper B, Clark LB, Yasayko SA, Wilkinson JE, Galas D, Ziegler SF, Ramsdell F. 2001. Disruption of a new forkhead/winged-helix protein, scurfin, results in the fatal lymphoproliferative disorder of the scurfy mouse. *Nat Genet* 27:68–73.

13. Bennett CL, Ochs HD. 2001. IPEX is a unique X-linked syndrome characterized by immune dysfunction, polyendocrinopathy, enteropathy, and a variety of autoimmune phenomena. *Curr Opin Pediatr* 13:533–538.

14. Li B, Samanta A, Song X, Iacono KT, Brennan P, Chatila TA, Roncador G, Banham AH, Riley JL, Wang Q, Shen Y, Saouaf SJ, Greene MI. 2007. FOXP3 is a homo-oligomer and a component of a supramolecular regulatory complex disabled in the human XLAAD/IPEX autoimmune disease. *Int Immunol* 19:825–835.

15. Caudy AA, Reddy ST, Chatila T, Atkinson JP, Verbsky JW. 2007. CD25 deficiency causes an immune dysregulation, polyendocrinopathy, enteropathy, X-linked-like syndrome, and defective IL-10 expression from CD4 lymphocytes. *J Allergy Clin Immunol* 119:482–487.

16. Josefowicz SZ, Lu LF, Rudensky AY. 2012. Regulatory T cells: mechanisms of differentiation and function. *Annu Rev Immunol* 30:531–564.

17. Kang SM, Tang Q, Bluestone JA. 2007. CD4+CD25+ regulatory T cells in transplantation: progress, challenges and prospects. *Am J Transplant* 7:1457–1463.

18. Curotto de Lafaille MA, Lafaille JJ. 2009. Natural and adaptive foxp3+ regulatory T cells: more of the same or a division of labor? *Immunity* 30:626–635.

19. Groux H, O'Garra A, Bigler M, Rouleau M, Antonenko S, de Vries JE, Roncarolo MG. 1997. A CD4+ T-cell subset inhibits antigen-specific T-cell responses and prevents colitis. *Nature* 389:737–742.

20. Sakaguchi S. 2004. Naturally arising CD4+ regulatory t cells for immunologic self-tolerance and negative control of immune responses. *Annu Rev Immunol* 22:531–562.

21. Collison LW, Workman CJ, Kuo TT, Boyd K, Wang Y, Vignali KM, Cross R, Sehy D, Blumberg RS, Vignali DA. 2007. The inhibitory cytokine IL-35 contributes to regulatory T-cell function. *Nature* 450:566–569.

22. Shevach EM. 2009. Mechanisms of foxp3+ T regulatory cell-mediated suppression. *Immunity* 30:636–645.

23. Wood KJ, Bushell A, Hester J. 2012. Regulatory immune cells in transplantation. *Nat Rev Immunol* 12:417–430.

24. Magnani CF, Alberigo G, Bacchetta R, Serafini G, Andreani M, Roncarolo MG, Gregori S. 2011. Killing of myeloid APCs via HLA class I, CD2 and CD226

25. defines a novel mechanism of suppression by human Tr1 cells. *Eur J Immunol* 41:1652–1662.

26. Rowe JH, Ertelt JM, Way SS. 2012. Foxp3(+) regulatory T cells, immune stimulation and host defence against infection. *Immunology* 136:1–10.

27. Belkaid Y, Piccirillo CA, Mendez S, Shevach EM, Sacks DL. 2002. CD4+CD25+ regulatory T cells control Leishmania major persistence and immunity. *Nature* 420:502–507.

28. Herrera MT, Torres M, Nevels D, Perez-Redondo CN, Ellner JJ, Sada E, Schwander SK. 2009. Compartmentalized bronchoalveolar IFN-gamma and IL-12 response in human pulmonary tuberculosis. *Tuberculosis (Edinb)* 89:38–47.

29. Gerosa F, Nisii C, Righetti S, Micciolo R, Marchesini M, Cazzadori A, Trinchieri G. 1999. CD4(+) T cell clones producing both interferon-gamma and interleukin-10 predominate in bronchoalveolar lavages of active pulmonary tuberculosis patients. *Clin Immunol* 92:224–234.

30. Lienhardt C, Azzurri A, Amedei A, Fielding K, Sillah J, Sow OY, Bah B, Benagiano M, Diallo A, Manetti R, Manneh K, Gustafson P, Bennett S, D'Elios MM, McAdam K, Del Prete G. 2002. Active tuberculosis in Africa is associated with reduced Th1 and increased Th2 activity in vivo. *Eur J Immunol* 32:1605–1613.

31. Sharma SK, Mitra DK, Balamurugan A, Pandey RM, Mehra NK. 2002. Cytokine polarization in miliary and pleural tuberculosis. *J Clin Immunol* 22:345–352.

32. Kaufmann SH. 2002. Protection against tuberculosis: cytokines, T cells, and macrophages. *Ann Rheum Dis* 61(Suppl 2):ii54–ii58.

33. Munk ME, Emoto M. 1995. Functions of T-cell subsets and cytokines in mycobacterial infections. *Eur Respir J Suppl* 20:668s–675s.

34. Rook GA. 2007. Th2 cytokines in susceptibility to tuberculosis. *Curr Mol Med* 7:327–337.

35. Newcomb DC, Zhou W, Moore ML, Goleniewska K, Hershey GK, Kolls JK, Peebles RS Jr. 2009. A functional IL-13 receptor is expressed on polarized murine CD4+ Th17 cells and IL-13 signaling attenuates Th17 cytokine production. *J Immunol* 182:5317–5321.

36. Miller JD, van der Most RG, Akondy RS, Glidewell JT, Albott S, Masopust D, Murali-Krishna K, Mahar PL, Edupuganti S, Lalor S, Germon S, Del Rio C, Mulligan MJ, Staprans SI, Altman JD, Feinberg MB, Ahmed R. 2008. Human effector and memory CD8+ T cell responses to smallpox and yellow fever vaccines. *Immunity* 28:710–722.

37. Ribeiro-Rodrigues R, Resende Co T, Rojas R, Toossi Z, Dietze R, Boom WH, Maciel E, Hirsch CS. 2006. A role for CD4+CD25+ T cells in regulation of the immune response during human tuberculosis. *Clin Exp Immunol* 144:25–34.

38. Guyot-Revol V, Innes JA, Hackforth S, Hinks T, Lalvani A. 2006. Regulatory T cells are expanded in blood and disease sites in patients with tuberculosis. *Am J Respir Crit Care Med* 173:803–810.

39. Chen X, Zhou B, Li M, Deng Q, Wu X, Le X, Wu C, Larmonier N, Zhang W, Zhang H, Wang H, Katsanis E.

2007. CD4(+)CD25(+)FoxP3(+) regulatory T cells suppress Mycobacterium tuberculosis immunity in patients with active disease. *Clin Immunol* **123**:50–59.

39. Hougardy JM, Place S, Hildebrand M, Drowart A, Debrie AS, Locht C, Mascart F. 2007. Regulatory T cells depress immune responses to protective antigens in active tuberculosis. *Am J Respir Crit Care Med* **176**: 409–416.

40. Fletcher HA, Pathan AA, Berthoud TK, Dunachie SJ, Whelan KT, Alder NC, Sander CR, Hill AV, McShane H. 2008. Boosting BCG vaccination with MVA85A downregulates the immunoregulatory cytokine TGF-beta1. *Vaccine* **26**:5269–5275.

41. Li L, Lao SH, Wu CY. 2007. Increased frequency of CD4(+)CD25(high) Treg cells inhibit BCG-specific induction of IFN-gamma by CD4(+) T cells from TB patients. *Tuberculosis (Edinb)* **87**:526–534.

42. Periasamy S, Dhiman R, Barnes PF, Paidipally P, Tvinnereim A, Bandaru A, Valluri VL, Vankayalapati R. 2011. Programmed death 1 and cytokine inducible SH2-containing protein dependent expansion of regulatory T cells upon stimulation with Mycobacterium tuberculosis. *J Infect Dis* **203**:1256–1263.

43. Chiacchio T, Casetti R, Butera O, Vanini V, Carrara S, Girardi E, Di Mitri D, Battistini L, Martini F, Borsellino G, Goletti D. 2009. Characterization of regulatory T cells identified as CD4(+)CD25(high)CD39(+) in patients with active tuberculosis. *Clin Exp Immunol* **156**:463–470.

44. Hougardy JM, Verscheure V, Locht C, Mascart F. 2007. In vitro expansion of CD4+CD25highFOXP3+ CD127low/- regulatory T cells from peripheral blood lymphocytes of healthy Mycobacterium tuberculosis-infected humans. *Microbes Infect* **9**:1325–1332.

45. He XY, Xiao L, Chen HB, Hao J, Li J, Wang YJ, He K, Gao Y, Shi BY. 2010. T regulatory cells and Th1/Th2 cytokines in peripheral blood from tuberculosis patients. *Eur J Clin Microbiol Infect Dis* **29**:643–650.

46. Mahan CS, Thomas JJ, Boom WH, Rojas RE. 2009. CD4+ CD25(high) Foxp3+ regulatory T cells downregulate human Vdelta2+ T-lymphocyte function triggered by anti-CD3 or phosphoantigen. *Immunology* **127**:398–407.

47. Dieli F, Troye-Blomberg M, Ivanyi J, Fournié JJ, Krensky AM, Bonneville M, Peyrat MA, Caccamo N, Sireci G, Salerno A. 2001. Granulysin-dependent killing of intracellular and extracellular Mycobacterium tuberculosis by Vgamma9/Vdelta2 T lymphocytes. *J Infect Dis* **184**:1082–1085.

48. Semple PL, Binder AB, Davids M, Maredza A, van Zyl-Smit RN, Dheda K. 2013. Regulatory T cells attenuate mycobacterial stasis in alveolar and blood-derived macrophages from patients with tuberculosis. *Am J Respir Crit Care Med* **187**:1249–1258.

49. Babu S, Bhat SQ, Kumar NP, Kumaraswami V, Nutman TB. 2010. Regulatory T cells modulate Th17 responses in patients with positive tuberculin skin test results. *J Infect Dis* **201**:20–31.

50. Meintjes G, Wilkinson KA, Rangaka MX, Skolimowska K, van Veen K, Abrahams M, Seldon R, Pepper DJ, Rebe K, Mouton P, van Cutsem G, Nicol MP, Maartens G, Wilkinson RJ. 2008. Type 1 helper T cells and FoxP3-positive T cells in HIV-tuberculosis-associated immune reconstitution inflammatory syndrome. *Am J Respir Crit Care Med* **178**:1083–1089.

51. Kumar NP, Sridhar R, Banurekha VV, Jawahar MS, Nutman TB, Babu S. 2013. Expansion of pathogen-specific T-helper 1 and T-helper 17 cells in pulmonary tuberculosis with coincident type 2 diabetes mellitus. *J Infect Dis* **208**:739–748.

52. Wu YE, Du ZR, Cai YM, Peng WG, Zheng GZ, Zheng GL, Wu LB, Li K. 2015. Effective expansion of forkhead box P3? regulatory T cells via early secreted antigenic target 6 and antigen 85 complex B from Mycobacterium tuberculosis. *Mol Med Rep* **11**:3134–3142.

53. Kumar NP, Moideen K, Banurekha VV, Nair D, Sridhar R, Nutman TB, Babu S. 2015. IL-27 and TGFβ mediated expansion of Th1 and adaptive regulatory T cells expressing IL-10 correlates with bacterial burden and disease severity in pulmonary tuberculosis. *Immun Inflamm Dis* **3**:289–299.

54. Garg A, Barnes PF, Roy S, Quiroga MF, Wu S, García VE, Krutzik SR, Weis SE, Vankayalapati R. 2008. Mannose-capped lipoarabinomannan- and prostaglandin E2-dependent expansion of regulatory T cells in human *Mycobacterium tuberculosis* infection. *Eur J Immunol* **38**:459–469.

55. Trinath J, Maddur MS, Kaveri SV, Balaji KN, Bayry J. 2012. *Mycobacterium tuberculosis* promotes regulatory T-cell expansion via induction of programmed death-1 ligand 1 (PD-L1, CD274) on dendritic cells. *J Infect Dis* **205**:694–696.

56. Wu C, Zhou Q, Qin XJ, Qin SM, Shi HZ. 2010. CCL22 is involved in the recruitment of CD4+CD25 high T cells into tuberculous pleural effusions. *Respirology* **15**:522–529.

57. Bayry J, Tchilian EZ, Davies MN, Forbes EK, Draper SJ, Kaveri SV, Hill AV, Kazatchkine MD, Beverley PC, Flower DR, Tough DF. 2008. In silico identified CCR4 antagonists target regulatory T cells and exert adjuvant activity in vaccination. *Proc Natl Acad Sci USA* **105**: 10221–10226.

58. Gordon S. 2003. Alternative activation of macrophages. *Nat Rev Immunol* **3**:23–35.

59. Harris J, De Haro SA, Master SS, Keane J, Roberts EA, Delgado M, Deretic V. 2007. T helper 2 cytokines inhibit autophagic control of intracellular Mycobacterium tuberculosis. *Immunity* **27**:505–517.

60. Ashenafi S, Aderaye G, Bekele A, Zewdie M, Aseffa G, Hoang AT, Carow B, Habtamu M, Wijkander M, Rottenberg M, Aseffa A, Andersson J, Svensson M, Brighenti S. 2014. Progression of clinical tuberculosis is associated with a Th2 immune response signature in combination with elevated levels of SOCS3. *Clin Immunol* **151**:84–99.

61. van Crevel R, Karyadi E, Preyers F, Leenders M, Kullberg BJ, Nelwan RH, van der Meer JW. 2000. Increased production of interleukin 4 by CD4+ and CD8+ T cells from patients with tuberculosis is related to the presence of pulmonary cavities. *J Infect Dis* **181**: 1194–1197.

62. Skapenko A, Kalden JR, Lipsky PE, Schulze-Koops H. 2005. The IL-4 receptor alpha-chain-binding cytokines, IL-4 and IL-13, induce forkhead box P3-expressing CD25+CD4+ regulatory T cells from CD25-CD4+ precursors. *J Immunol* **175**:6107–6116.

63. Roy S, Barnes PF, Garg A, Wu S, Cosman D, Vankayalapati R. 2008. NK cells lyse T regulatory cells that expand in response to an intracellular pathogen. *J Immunol* **180**:1729–1736.

64. Vankayalapati R, Wizel B, Weis SE, Safi H, Lakey DL, Mandelboim O, Samten B, Porgador A, Barnes PF. 2002. The NKp46 receptor contributes to NK cell lysis of mononuclear phagocytes infected with an intracellular bacterium. *J Immunol* **168**:3451–3457.

65. Borsellino G, Kleinewietfeld M, Di Mitri D, Sternjak A, Diamantini A, Giometto R, Höpner S, Centonze D, Bernardi G, Dell'Acqua ML, Rossini PM, Battistini L, Rötzschke O, Falk K. 2007. Expression of ectonucleoidase CD39 by Foxp3+ Treg cells: hydrolysis of extracellular ATP and immune suppression. *Blood* **110**: 1225–1232.

66. Lokshin A, Raskovalova T, Huang X, Zacharia LC, Jackson EK, Gorelik E. 2006. Adenosine-mediated inhibition of the cytotoxic activity and cytokine production by activated natural killer cells. *Cancer Res* **66**:7758–7765.

67. Kim K, Perera R, Tan DB, Fernandez S, Seddiki N, Waring J, French MA. 2014. Circulating mycobacterial-reactive CD4+ T cells with an immunosuppressive phenotype are higher in active tuberculosis than latent tuberculosis infection. *Tuberculosis (Edinb)* **94**:494–501.

68. de Cassan SC, Pathan AA, Sander CR, Minassian A, Rowland R, Hill AV, McShane H, Fletcher HA. 2010. Investigating the induction of vaccine-induced Th17 and regulatory T cells in healthy, *Mycobacterium bovis* BCG-immunized adults vaccinated with a new tuberculosis vaccine, MVA85A. *Clin Vaccine Immunol* **17**: 1066–1073.

69. Griffiths KL, Pathan AA, Minassian AM, Sander CR, Beveridge NE, Hill AV, Fletcher HA, McShane H. 2011. Th1/Th17 cell induction and corresponding reduction in ATP consumption following vaccination with the novel *Mycobacterium tuberculosis* vaccine MVA85A. *PLoS One* **6**:e23463.

70. Ye ZJ, Zhou Q, Du RH, Li X, Huang B, Shi HZ. 2011. Imbalance of Th17 cells and regulatory T cells in tuberculous pleural effusion. *Clin Vaccine Immunol* **18**: 1608–1615.

71. Boer MC, van Meijgaarden KE, Bastid J, Ottenhoff TH, Joosten SA. 2013. CD39 is involved in mediating suppression by *Mycobacterium bovis* BCG-activated human CD8(+) CD39(+) regulatory T cells. *Eur J Immunol* **43**:1925–1932.

72. Sinsimer D, Huet G, Manca C, Tsenova L, Koo MS, Kurepina N, Kana B, Mathema B, Marras SA, Kreiswirth BN, Guilhot C, Kaplan G. 2008. The phenolic glycolipid of Mycobacterium tuberculosis differentially modulates the early host cytokine response but does not in itself confer hypervirulence. *Infect Immun* **76**:3027–3036.

73. Theus S, Eisenach K, Fomukong N, Silver RF, Cave MD. 2007. Beijing family *Mycobacterium tuberculosis* strains differ in their intracellular growth in THP-1 macrophages. *Int J Tuberc Lung Dis* **11**:1087–1093.

74. Manca C, Reed MB, Freeman S, Mathema B, Kreiswirth B, Barry CE III, Kaplan G. 2004. Differential monocyte activation underlies strain-specific *Mycobacterium tuberculosis* pathogenesis. *Infect Immun* **72**:5511–5514.

75. Geffner L, Yokobori N, Basile J, Schierloh P, Balboa L, Romero MM, Ritacco V, Vescovo M, González Montaner P, Lopez B, Barrera L, Alemán M, Abatte E, Sasiain MC, de la Barrera S. 2009. Patients with multidrug-resistant tuberculosis display impaired Th1 responses and enhanced regulatory T-cell levels in response to an outbreak of multidrug-resistant *Mycobacterium tuberculosis* M and Ra strains. *Infect Immun* **77**:5025–5034.

76. Basile JI, Geffner LJ, Romero MM, Balboa L, Sabio Y García C, Ritacco V, García A, Cuffré M, Abbate E, López B, Barrera L, Ambroggi M, Alemán M, Sasiain MC, de la Barrera SS. 2011. Outbreaks of mycobacterium tuberculosis MDR strains induce high IL-17 T-cell response in patients with MDR tuberculosis that is closely associated with high antigen load. *J Infect Dis* **204**:1054–1064.

77. Wergeland I, Assmus J, Dyrhol-Riise AM. 2011. T regulatory cells and immune activation in *Mycobacterium tuberculosis* infection and the effect of preventive therapy. *Scand J Immunol* **73**:234–242.

78. Lim HJ, Park JS, Cho YJ, Yoon HI, Park KU, Lee CT, Lee JH. 2013. CD4(+)FoxP3(+) T regulatory cells in drug-susceptible and multidrug-resistant tuberculosis. *Tuberculosis (Edinb)* **93**:523–528.

79. Singh A, Dey AB, Mohan A, Sharma PK, Mitra DK. 2012. Foxp3+ regulatory T cells among tuberculosis patients: impact on prognosis and restoration of antigen specific IFN-γ producing T cells. *PLoS One* **7**:e44728.

80. Wu YE, Peng WG, Cai YM, Zheng GZ, Zheng GL, Lin JH, Zhang SW, Li K. 2010. Decrease in CD4+CD25+ FoxP3+ Treg cells after pulmonary resection in the treatment of cavity multidrug-resistant tuberculosis. *Int J Infect Dis* **14**:e815–e822.

81. Roberts T, Beyers N, Aguirre A, Walzl G. 2007. Immunosuppression during active tuberculosis is characterized by decreased interferon- gamma production and CD25 expression with elevated forkhead box P3, transforming growth factor- beta, and interleukin-4 mRNA levels. *J Infect Dis* **195**:870–878.

82. Nemeth J, Winkler HM, Zwick RH, Rumetshofer R, Schenk P, Burghuber OC, Graninger W, Ramharter M, Winkler S. 2009. Recruitment of *Mycobacterium tuberculosis* specific CD4+ T cells to the site of infection for diagnosis of active tuberculosis. *J Intern Med* **265**: 163–168.

83. Barnes PF, Mistry SD, Cooper CL, Pirmez C, Rea TH, Modlin RL. 1989. Compartmentalization of a CD4+ T lymphocyte subpopulation in tuberculous pleuritis. *J Immunol* **142**:1114–1119.

84. Brighenti S, Andersson J. 2012. Local immune responses in human tuberculosis: learning from the site of infection. *J Infect Dis* **205**(Suppl 2):S316–S324.

85. Flynn JL, Chan J, Lin PL. 2011. Macrophages and control of granulomatous inflammation in tuberculosis. *Mucosal Immunol* 4:271–278.

86. Andersson J, Samarina A, Fink J, Rahman S, Grundström S. 2007. Impaired expression of perforin and granulysin in CD8+ T cells at the site of infection in human chronic pulmonary tuberculosis. *Infect Immun* 75:5210–5222.

87. Rahman S, Gudetta B, Fink J, Granath A, Ashenafi S, Aseffa A, Derbew M, Svensson M, Andersson J, Brighenti SG. 2009. Compartmentalization of immune responses in human tuberculosis: few CD8+ effector T cells but elevated levels of FoxP3+ regulatory t cells in the granulomatous lesions. *Am J Pathol* 174:2211–2224.

88. Larson RP, Shafiani S, Urdahl KB. 2013. Foxp3(+) regulatory T cells in tuberculosis. *Adv Exp Med Biol* 783:165–180.

89. Kaplan G, Post FA, Moreira AL, Wainwright H, Kreiswirth BN, Tanverdi M, Mathema B, Ramaswamy SV, Walther G, Steyn LM, Barry CE III, Bekker LG. 2003. *Mycobacterium tuberculosis* growth at the cavity surface: a microenvironment with failed immunity. *Infect Immun* 71:7099–7108.

90. Rahman S, Rehn A, Rahman J, Andersson J, Svensson M, Brighenti S. 2015. Pulmonary tuberculosis patients with a vitamin D deficiency demonstrate low local expression of the antimicrobial peptide LL-37 but enhanced FoxP3+ regulatory T cells and IgG-secreting cells. *Clin Immunol* 156:85–97.

91. Sharma PK, Saha PK, Singh A, Sharma SK, Ghosh B, Mitra DK. 2009. FoxP3+ regulatory T cells suppress effector T-cell function at pathologic site in miliary tuberculosis. *Am J Respir Crit Care Med* 179:1061–1070.

92. Herzmann C, Ernst M, Ehlers S, Stenger S, Maertzdorf J, Sotgiu G, Lange C. 2012. Increased frequencies of pulmonary regulatory T-cells in latent Mycobacterium tuberculosis infection. *Eur Respir J* 40:1450–1457.

93. Sun Q, Zhang Q, Xiao H, Cui H, Su B. 2012. Significance of the frequency of CD4+CD25+CD127- T-cells in patients with pulmonary tuberculosis and diabetes mellitus. *Respirology* 17:876–882.

94. Ibrahim L, Salah M, Abd El Rahman A, Zeidan A, Ragb M. 2013. Crucial role of CD4+CD 25+ FOXP3+ T regulatory cell, interferon-γ and interleukin-16 in malignant and tuberculous pleural effusions. *Immunol Invest* 42:122–136.

95. Geffner L, Basile JI, Yokobori N, Sabio Y García C, Musella R, Castagnino J, Sasiain MC, de la Barrera S. 2014. CD4(+) CD25(high) forkhead box protein 3(+) regulatory T lymphocytes suppress interferon-γ and CD107 expression in CD4(+) and CD8(+) T cells from tuberculous pleural effusions. *Clin Exp Immunol* 175: 235–245.

96. Orme IM. 2005. Mouse and guinea pig models for testing new tuberculosis vaccines. *Tuberculosis (Edinb)* 85:13–17.

97. Lenaerts A, Barry CE III, Dartois V. 2015. Heterogeneity in tuberculosis pathology, microenvironments and therapeutic responses. *Immunol Rev* 264:288–307.

98. Sharpe SA, Eschelbach E, Basaraba RJ, Gleeson F, Hall GA, McIntyre A, Williams A, Kraft SL, Clark S, Gooch K, Hatch G, Orme IM, Marsh PD, Dennis MJ. 2009. Determination of lesion volume by MRI and stereology in a macaque model of tuberculosis. *Tuberculosis (Edinb)* 89:405–416.

99. Quinn KM, McHugh RS, Rich FJ, Goldsack LM, de Lisle GW, Buddle BM, Delahunt B, Kirman JR. 2006. Inactivation of CD4+ CD25+ regulatory T cells during early mycobacterial infection increases cytokine production but does not affect pathogen load. *Immunol Cell Biol* 84:467–474.

100. Ordway D, Palanisamy G, Henao-Tamayo M, Smith EE, Shanley C, Orme IM, Basaraba RJ. 2007. The cellular immune response to Mycobacterium tuberculosis infection in the guinea pig. *J Immunol* 179:2532–2541.

101. McMurray DN. 2003. Hematogenous reseeding of the lung in low-dose, aerosol-infected guinea pigs: unique features of the host-pathogen interface in secondary tubercles. *Tuberculosis (Edinb)* 83:131–134.

102. Turner OC, Basaraba RJ, Orme IM. 2003. Immunopathogenesis of pulmonary granulomas in the guinea pig after infection with Mycobacterium tuberculosis. *Infect Immun* 71:864–871.

103. Somashekar BS, Amin AG, Tripathi P, MacKinnon N, Rithner CD, Shanley CA, Basaraba R, Henao-Tamayo M, Kato-Maeda M, Ramamoorthy A, Orme IM, Ordway DJ, Chatterjee D. 2012. Metabolomic signatures in guinea pigs infected with epidemic-associated W-Beijing strains of Mycobacterium tuberculosis. *J Proteome Res* 11:4873–4884.

104. Kato-Maeda M, Shanley CA, Ackart D, Jarlsberg LG, Shang S, Obregon-Henao A, Harton M, Basaraba RJ, Henao-Tamayo M, Barrozo JC, Rose J, Kawamura LM, Coscolla M, Fofanov VY, Koshinsky H, Gagneux S, Hopewell PC, Ordway DJ, Orme IM. 2012. Beijing sublineages of Mycobacterium tuberculosis differ in pathogenicity in the guinea pig. *Clin Vaccine Immunol* 19:1227–1237.

105. Shang S, Shanley CA, Caraway ML, Orme EA, Henao-Tamayo M, Hascall-Dove L, Ackart D, Orme IM, Ordway DJ, Basaraba RJ. 2012. Drug treatment combined with BCG vaccination reduces disease reactivation in guinea pigs infected with Mycobacterium tuberculosis. *Vaccine* 30:1572–1582.

106. Ordway D, Henao-Tamayo M, Shanley C, Smith EE, Palanisamy G, Wang B, Basaraba RJ, Orme IM. 2008. Influence of *Mycobacterium bovis* BCG vaccination on cellular immune response of guinea pigs challenged with *Mycobacterium tuberculosis*. *Clin Vaccine Immunol* 15:1248–1258.

107. Bertholet S, Ireton GC, Ordway DJ, Windish HP, Pine SO, Kahn M, Phan T, Orme IM, Vedvick TS, Baldwin SL, Coler RN, Reed SG. 2010. A defined tuberculosis vaccine candidate boosts BCG and protects against multidrug-resistant *Mycobacterium tuberculosis*. *Sci Transl Med* 2:53ra74.

108. Shang S, Shanley CA, Caraway ML, Orme EA, Henao-Tamayo M, Hascall-Dove L, Ackart D, Lenaerts AJ, Basaraba RJ, Orme IM, Ordway DJ. 2011. Activities of

TMC207, rifampin, and pyrazinamide against *Myco-bacterium tuberculosis* infection in guinea pigs. *Anti-microb Agents Chemother* 55:124–131.

109. Flynn JL, Gideon HP, Mattila JT, Lin PL. 2015. Immunology studies in non-human primate models of tuberculosis. *Immunol Rev* 264:60–73.

110. Sharpe SA, McShane H, Dennis MJ, Basaraba RJ, Gleeson F, Hall G, McIntyre A, Gooch K, Clark S, Beveridge NE, Nuth E, White A, Marriott A, Dowall S, Hill AV, Williams A, Marsh PD. 2010. Establishment of an aerosol challenge model of tuberculosis in rhesus macaques and an evaluation of endpoints for vaccine testing. *Clin Vaccine Immunol* 17:1170–1182.

111. Flynn JL, Capuano SV, Croix D, Pawar S, Myers A, Zinovik A, Klein E. 2003. Non-human primates: a model for tuberculosis research. *Tuberculosis (Edinb)* 83:116–118.

112. Green AM, Mattila JT, Bigbee CL, Bongers KS, Lin PL, Flynn JL. 2010. CD4(+) regulatory T cells in a cyno-molgus macaque model of *Mycobacterium tuberculosis* infection. *J Infect Dis* 202:533–541.

113. Ordway D, Henao-Tamayo M, Harton M, Palanisamy G, Troudt J, Shanley C, Basaraba RJ, Orme IM. 2007. The hypervirulent *Mycobacterium tuberculosis* strain HN878 induces a potent TH1 response followed by rapid down-regulation. *J Immunol* 179:522–531.

114. Scott-Browne JP, Shafiani S, Tucker-Heard G, Ishida-Tsubota K, Fontenot JD, Rudensky AY, Bevan MJ, Urdahl KB. 2007. Expansion and function of Foxp3-expressing T regulatory cells during tuberculosis. *J Exp Med* 204:2159–2169.

115. Cooper AM. 2009. Cell-mediated immune responses in tuberculosis. *Annu Rev Immunol* 27:393–422.

116. Kursar M, Koch M, Mittrücker HW, Nouailles G, Bonhagen K, Kamradt T, Kaufmann SH. 2007. Cutting Edge: regulatory T cells prevent efficient clearance of *Mycobacterium tuberculosis*. *J Immunol* 178:2661–2665.

117. Nunes-Alves C, Booty MG, Carpenter SM, Jayaraman P, Rothchild AC, Behar SM. 2014. In search of a new paradigm for protective immunity to TB. *Nat Rev Microbiol* 12:289–299.

118. Henao-Tamayo MI, Obregon-Henao A, Arnett K, Shanley CA, Podell B, Orme IM, Ordway D. 2016. Effect of BCG vaccination on CD4+Foxp3+ T cells during the acquired immune response to *Mycobacterium tuberculosis* infection. *J Leukoc Biol* 99:605–617.

119. Orme IM, Robinson RT, Cooper AM. 2015. The balance between protective and pathogenic immune responses in the TB-infected lung. *Nat Immunol* 16:57–63.

120. Lathrop SK, Bloom SM, Rao SM, Nutsch K, Lio CW, Santacruz N, Peterson DA, Stappenbeck TS, Hsieh CS. 2011. Peripheral education of the immune system by colonic commensal microbiota. *Nature* 478:250–254.

121. Kuhn KA, Stappenbeck TS. 2013. Peripheral education of the immune system by the colonic microbiota. *Semin Immunol* 25:364–369.

122. Shafiani S, Tucker-Heard G, Kariyone A, Takatsu K, Urdahl KB. 2010. Pathogen-specific regulatory T cells

123. Wing K, Onishi Y, Prieto-Martin P, Yamaguchi T, Miyara M, Fehervari Z, Nomura T, Sakaguchi S. 2008. CTLA-4 control over Foxp3+ regulatory T cell function. *Science* 322:271–275.

124. Onishi Y, Fehervari Z, Yamaguchi T, Sakaguchi S. 2008. Foxp3+ natural regulatory T cells preferentially form aggregates on dendritic cells in vitro and actively inhibit their maturation. *Proc Natl Acad Sci USA* 105:10113–10118.

125. Urdahl KB, Shafiani S, Ernst JD. 2011. Initiation and regulation of T-cell responses in tuberculosis. *Mucosal Immunol* 4:288–293.

126. Belkaid Y, Tarbell K. 2009. Regulatory T cells in the control of host-microorganism interactions (*). *Annu Rev Immunol* 27:551–589.

127. Ertelt JM, Rowe JH, Johanns TM, Lai JC, McLachlan JB, Way SS. 2009. Selective priming and expansion of antigen-specific Foxp3- CD4+ T cells during Listeria monocytogenes infection. *J Immunol* 182:3032–3038.

128. Antunes I, Tolaini M, Kissenpfennig A, Iwashiro M, Kuribayashi K, Malissen B, Hasenkrug K, Kassiotis G. 2008. Retrovirus-specificity of regulatory T cells is neither present nor required in preventing retrovirus-induced bone marrow immune pathology. *Immunity* 29:782–794.

129. Gratz IK, Campbell DJ. 2014. Organ-specific and memory treg cells: specificity, development, function, and maintenance. *Front Immunol* 5:333.

130. Koch MA, Tucker-Heard G, Perdue NR, Killebrew JR, Urdahl KB, Campbell DJ. 2009. The transcription factor T-bet controls regulatory T cell homeostasis and function during type 1 inflammation. *Nat Immunol* 10:595–602.

131. Chaudhry A, Rudra D, Treuting P, Samstein RM, Liang Y, Kas A, Rudensky AY. 2009. CD4+ regulatory T cells control TH17 responses in a Stat3-dependent manner. *Science* 326:986–991.

132. Zheng Y, Chaudhry A, Kas A, deRoos P, Kim JM, Chu TT, Corcoran L, Treuting P, Klein U, Rudensky AY. 2009. Regulatory T-cell suppressor program co-opts transcription factor IRF4 to control T(H)2 responses. *Nature* 458:351–356.

133. Campbell DJ, Koch MA. 2011. Phenotypical and functional specialization of FOXP3+ regulatory T cells. *Nat Rev Immunol* 11:119–130.

134. Arvey A, van der Veeken J, Samstein RM, Feng Y, Stamatoyannopoulos JA, Rudensky AY. 2014. Inflammation-induced repression of chromatin bound by the transcription factor Foxp3 in regulatory T cells. *Nat Immunol* 15:580–587.

135. McBride A, Konowich J, Salgame P. 2013. Host defense and recruitment of Foxp3? T regulatory cells to the lungs in chronic *Mycobacterium tuberculosis* infection requires toll-like receptor 2. *PLoS Pathog* 9:e1003397.

136. Leepiyasakulchai C, Ignatowicz L, Pawlowski A, Källenius G, Sköld M. 2012. Failure to recruit anti-inflammatory CD103+ dendritic cells and a diminished

CD4+ Foxp3+ regulatory T cell pool in mice that display excessive lung inflammation and increased susceptibility to *Mycobacterium tuberculosis*. *Infect Immun* 80:1128–1139.

137. Henao-Tamayo M, Obregón-Henao A, Creissen E, Shanley C, Orme I, Ordway DJ. 2015. Differential *Mycobacterium bovis* BCG vaccine-derived efficacy in C3Heb/FeJ and C3H/HeOuJ mice exposed to a clinical strain of *Mycobacterium tuberculosis*. *Clin Vaccine Immunol* 22:91–98.

138. Bai X, Shang S, Henao-Tamayo M, Basaraba RJ, Ovrutsky AR, Matsuda JL, Takeda K, Chan MM, Dakhama A, Kinney WH, Trostel J, Bai A, Honda JR, Achcar R, Hartney J, Joosten LA, Kim SH, Orme I, Dinarello CA, Ordway DJ, Chan ED. 2015. Human IL-32 expression protects mice against a hypervirulent strain of Mycobacterium tuberculosis. *Proc Natl Acad Sci USA* 112:5111–5116.

139. Ndure J, Flanagan KL. 2014. Targeting regulatory T cells to improve vaccine immunogenicity in early life. *Front Microbiol* 5:477.

140. Fine PE. 1995. Variation in protection by BCG: implications of and for heterologous immunity. *Lancet* 346:1339–1345.

141. Pitt JM, Blankley S, McShane H, O'Garra A. 2013. Vaccination against tuberculosis: how can we better BCG? *Microb Pathog* 58:2–16.

142. Orme IM. 2013. Vaccine development for tuberculosis: current progress. *Drugs* 73:1015–1024.

143. Ordway DJ, Shang S, Henao-Tamayo M, Obregon-Henao A, Nold L, Caraway M, Shanley CA, Basaraba RJ, Duncan CG, Orme IM. 2011. Mycobacterium bovis BCG-mediated protection against W-Beijing strains of *Mycobacterium tuberculosis* is diminished concomitant with the emergence of regulatory T cells. *Clin Vaccine Immunol* 18:1527–1535.

144. Feruglio SL, Tonby K, Kvale D, Dyrhol-Riise AM. 2015. Early dynamics of T helper cell cytokines and T regulatory cells in response to treatment of active *Mycobacterium tuberculosis* infection. *Clin Exp Immunol* 179:454–465.

145. Henao-Tamayo M, Obregón-Henao A, Ordway DJ, Shang S, Duncan CG, Orme IM. 2012. A mouse model of tuberculosis reinfection. *Tuberculosis (Edinb)* 92:211–217.

146. Shang S, Harton M, Tamayo MH, Shanley C, Palanisamy GS, Caraway M, Chan ED, Basaraba RJ, Orme IM, Ordway DJ. 2011. Increased Foxp3 expression in guinea pigs infected with W-Beijing strains of *M. tuberculosis*. *Tuberculosis (Edinb)* 91:378–385.

147. Podell BK, Ackart DF, Obregon-Henao A, Eck SP, Henao-Tamayo M, Richardson M, Orme IM, Ordway DJ, Basaraba RJ. 2014. Increased severity of tuberculosis in Guinea pigs with type 2 diabetes: a model of diabetes-tuberculosis comorbidity. *Am J Pathol* 184:1104–1118.

148. Capuano SV III, Croix DA, Pawar S, Zinovik A, Myers A, Lin PL, Bissel S, Fuhrman C, Klein E, Flynn JL. 2003. Experimental *Mycobacterium tuberculosis* infection of cynomolgus macaques closely resembles the various manifestations of human M. *tuberculosis* infection. *Infect Immun* 71:5831–5844.

149. Lin PL, Rodgers M, Smith L, Bigbee M, Myers A, Bigbee C, Chiosea I, Capuano SV, Fuhrman C, Klein E, Flynn JL. 2009. Quantitative comparison of active and latent tuberculosis in the cynomolgus macaque model. *Infect Immun* 77:4631–4642.

150. Kaushal D, Mehra S, Didier PJ, Lackner AA. 2012. The non-human primate model of tuberculosis. *J Med Primatol* 41:191–201.

151. Phillips BL, Mehra S, Ahsan MH, Selman M, Khader SA, Kaushal D. 2015. LAG3 expression in active *Mycobacterium tuberculosis* infections. *Am J Pathol* 185:820–833.

152. Mehra S, Pahar B, Dutta NK, Conerly CN, Philippi-Falkenstein K, Alvarez X, Kaushal D. 2010. Transcriptional reprogramming in nonhuman primate (rhesus macaque) tuberculosis granulomas. *PLoS One* 5:e12266.

153. Chen CY, Huang D, Yao S, Halliday L, Zeng G, Wang RC, Chen ZW. 2012. IL-2 simultaneously expands Foxp3+ T regulatory and T effector cells and confers resistance to severe tuberculosis (TB): implicative Treg-T effector cooperation in immunity to TB. *J Immunol* 188:4278–4288.

154. Gideon HP, Phuah J, Myers AJ, Bryson BD, Rodgers MA, Coleman MT, Maiello P, Rutledge T, Marino S, Fortune SM, Kirschner DE, Lin PL, Flynn JL. 2015. Variability in tuberculosis granuloma T cell responses exists, but a balance of pro- and anti-inflammatory cytokines is associated with sterilization. *PLoS Pathog* 11:e1004603.

Tuberculosis and the Tubercle Bacillus, 2nd ed.
Edited by William R. Jacobs, Jr., Helen McShane, Valerie Mizrahi, and Ian M. Orme
© 2018 American Society for Microbiology, Washington, DC
doi:10.1128/microbiolspec.TBTB2-0009-2016

The Memory Immune Response to Tuberculosis

4

Joanna R. Kirman[1], Marcela I. Henao-Tamayo[2], and Else Marie Agger[3]

INTRODUCTION

Mycobacterium tuberculosis is one of the most successful pathogens with approximately 30% of the world's population harboring the bacterium. Although some highly exposed individuals appear resistant to infection with *M. tuberculosis* (1), once an individual is infected, there is little evidence that the ensuing immune response leads to sterilizing immunity (2). Instead, the majority of individuals infected with *M. tuberculosis* (>90%) develop an asymptomatic chronic tuberculosis (TB) infection known as latent TB. During latent infection, activated host immune cells result in arrest of mycobacterial growth and control of disease progression. Active disease can develop from latent infection if the immune response is sufficiently suppressed, and, over their lifetime, this will occur in 5 to 10% of the latently infected individuals (3).

The immune system is compartmentalized into innate and adaptive arms. The innate immune system is considered a nonspecific, fast-acting first line of defense against invading microorganisms. By contrast, the adaptive immune system has evolved to be capable of generating vast antigen receptor diversity, so it is highly specific but much slower to respond than the innate immune response. A hallmark of the adaptive immune system is its ability to "remember." When memory T and B cells recognize antigen, they generate effector responses that are quantitatively and qualitatively superior to those of antigen-inexperienced (naive) T or B cells.

Memory immune responses also occur more rapidly than naive responses, resulting in efficient reduction or prevention of disease upon a subsequent exposure to a pathogen. Vaccination is thought to rely mainly on adaptive immunological memory. To that end, considerable efforts have been devoted toward understanding the immune responses to mycobacteria and, in particular, the memory immune responses with the ultimate aim of identifying key protective mechanisms that can be translated into new and better TB vaccines and therapeutic interventions.

The current vaccine against TB, an attenuated form of *Mycobacterium bovis* named bacillus Calmette-Guérin (BCG), has been in use since 1921 and is the most widely used of all vaccines (100 million doses administered annually). BCG is given to more than 80% of all neonates and infants, particularly in countries with middle and high endemicity, where it is a part of the national immunization program (4). Although BCG is protective against systemic forms of TB disease that are common during childhood, the ability of BCG to protect adults against pulmonary TB disease is more questionable, with efficacy rates ranging from 80% down to no effect in the large Chingleput trial in India (4–6). Since almost 90% of new TB cases are in adults (154), an effective vaccine against adult pulmonary TB is urgently required. Therefore, it is imperative that the requirements for the generation and maintenance of protective immune memory to TB be characterized and understood.

CD4 T cells and in particular T helper (Th) 1 cells, characterized by their secretion of interferon-γ (IFN-γ), are known to play an essential role in immune control of primary TB infection. This is supported by a number of observations including impaired immunity to mycobacterial disease in mice and humans with inborn genetic defects in the IFN-γ pathway (7, 8). In addition, there is increased prevalence of TB in human immuno-

[1]Department of Microbiology and Immunology, University of Otago, Dunedin, New Zealand; [2]Department of Microbiology, Immunology and Pathology, Mycobacteria Research Laboratory, Colorado State University, Fort Collins, CO 80523; [3]Department of Infectious Disease Immunology, Statens Serum Institut, Artillerivej 5, 2300 Copenhagen S, Denmark.

deficiency virus (HIV) patients with low CD4 T cell counts (9) and heightened susceptibility to TB in T cell-deficient mice. The importance of CD4 T cells to the memory immune response was first illustrated by classical adoptive transfer studies in mice that showed that memory CD4 T cells afforded enhanced protection to *M. tuberculosis* challenge compared with naive T cells (10). By contrast, memory CD8 T cells and memory B cells are thought to play less significant roles in protection against TB.

Based on this dogma, for many years TB vaccine research has focused on identifying the most vigorous Th1-inducing antigens and vaccine constructs, using the ability to secrete IFN-γ as a marker of success. The first novel TB vaccine to reach clinical efficacy testing, modified vaccinia virus Ankara (MVA) expressing antigen 85A from *M. tuberculosis* (MVA85), was found to induce 5 to 30 times more IFN-γ-producing CD4 T cells at 24 weeks postvaccination in BCG-vaccinated humans compared with those receiving BCG alone, a profile that was assumed to be a good memory response and led to substantial support for further clinical testing (11). The vaccine, designed to boost BCG, failed to enhance protection against TB disease and infection (12).

Scientists have yet to determine the T cell memory subsets that lead to immune protection against TB. Compared with the previous focus on CD4 T cells and IFN-γ, it is clear today that memory responses to TB are much more complex and probably involve several T cell subsets and potentially innate cell subsets. In the past decade, multifunctional CD4 T cells that secrete IFN-γ, interleukin-2 (IL-2), and tumor necrosis factor α (TNF-α) simultaneously have gained significant interest as a correlate of long-term memory. This has resulted in extensive monitoring of T cells that co-secrete cytokines in preclinical and clinical vaccine tests; however, it is still not clear if these cells are important components of a protective memory response to *M. tuberculosis* (13). It is crucial that we understand fundamental memory immunity to successfully transform this into a novel TB vaccine where the ultimate aim is to establish long-lived protective memory (14).

This review describes the key adaptive and innate immune cells involved in the memory response in humans infected with *M. tuberculosis* and from various animal models that we rely on in our efforts to identify successful protective immunity. Last, with several novel TB vaccines in clinical testing, we describe recent developments on how to monitor vaccine memory in clinical trials.

PROTECTIVE MEMORY AGAINST TB

In the mid-1970s, Lefford performed an adoptive transfer study in mice that provided the first evidence that T cells were mediators of protective memory immunity (15). Lymphoid cells were harvested from BCG-vaccinated donor mice and transferred into sublethally irradiated recipient mice, and adoptive immunity was measured after recipient mice received an intravenous challenge with BCG or *M. tuberculosis*. Lefford made two important observations. First, he found that the transferred protective immunity was not sterilizing immunity, nor did it prevent early bacterial replication, but rather the transferred protection manifested as a 5- to 10-fold reduction in spleen bacterial counts after 2 weeks of infection. Second, Lefford observed that little or no adoptive transfer of immunity could be detected in normal recipient mice that had not been irradiated. These two features of the mouse model of adoptive immunity to TB, that hold true even when the more realistic low-dose aerosol challenge model is used, have perplexed and challenged immunologists over the following decades. First, the early bacterial replication that proceeds unchecked even in the presence of protective memory T cells presents a major challenge to those developing new TB vaccines, since it appears that, even in the presence of protective memory immune cells, the infection is still able to establish. Second, the need to use irradiated or T cell-deficient recipient mice to observe transferred protection has presented a major obstacle to identifying protective memory subsets (described in "Memory T Cell Heterogeneity," below). Only recently, by using T cell receptor (TCR) transgenic (Tg) donor mice that have T cells specific for a single TB antigen, has protective cellular immunity been successfully transferred into non-irradiated immunocompetent recipient mice (16, 17).

A decade after the studies by Lefford that pinpointed T cells, rather than immune serum, as the key mediator of protection, Orme made the pivotal discovery that CD4 T cells mediated adoptively transferred protection to TB (10). Orme used antibiotic-treated *M. tuberculosis*-infected mice ("immune" mice) as donors, and, at a point when the bacterial load was undetectable, transferred T cell-enriched spleen cells from the "immune" mice into irradiated recipients. The recipient mice were then challenged intravenously with *M. tuberculosis*. Importantly, these passive cell transfer studies demonstrated that immunity was mediated by CD4 T cells and not CD8 T cells. Furthermore, Orme found that the cell populations isolated from actively infected mice differed from those of "immune" mice. If the challenge was delayed up to 20 days after transfer, the cells from actively infected mice lost their protective activity whereas cells from the antibiotic-treated immune mice remained active. Exposure of the "immune" donor mice to cyclophosphamide or irradiation prior to transfer did not abrogate protection, indicating that memory cells at the time of harvest were not in a state of division. Based on these studies it was concluded that the protective memory immune subset was composed of long-lived non-dividing CD4 T cells.

The North laboratory conducted a careful study comparing the immune response of antibiotic cured "immune" mice to the response of naive mice upon low-dose aerosol *M. tuberculosis* reinfection (18). As many other researchers have found, the shortened period of progressive bacterial replication in "immune" mice (15 days compared with 20 days in naive mice), resulted in a 10-fold reduction in lung bacterial burden that persisted until day 50 after infection. Of note, it was found that, although the "immune" mice had a faster Th1 immune response with an earlier accumulation of TB-specific cells in the lung, there was no evidence that the secondary response was improved qualitatively or quantitatively compared with the response of naive mice. It was suggested that this earlier induction of immunity in the lung led to earlier immune control, and therefore a reduced bacterial burden; however, for the same reasons that the primary infection fails to clear the infection, the secondary response also does not lead to cure.

Based on these studies in mice, it seemed logical to surmise that people who had been successfully treated for TB would be more resistant to reinfection than uninfected individuals. Therefore, it was surprising when Verver et al. reported that the incidence rate of TB reinfection in previously treated TB patients from a region of high endemicity was four times higher than the rate of TB infection in previously uninfected individuals (19). A further study found that reinfection became more common than relapse after 1 year posttreatment for TB (20).

These studies would imply that long-term protective immunity does not exist in humans; however, there are alternative explanations for the discrepancy between the findings in mice and those in humans. First, the mouse study was conducted in inbred and therefore genetically identical animals, each with the same level of innate resistance to infection. Given the high variability in susceptibility between different inbred mouse strains to TB, it is clear that genetic factors play a key role in resistance to TB. In an outbred human population, individuals with high susceptibility to TB will exist, and T cell-mediated immunity may fail to counteract this

exquisite susceptibility. Second, a reinfection study of "immune" mice found that, although there was a rapid memory T cell response that led to initial protection, over time the immune response contracted and bacterial numbers increased. The reinfected mice eventually died of progressive disease (21). Both explanations have serious ramifications for vaccine development; it is not yet known if vaccination can overcome genetic susceptibility to infection and the protective effects of a vaccine can be sustained after reinfection.

GENERATION OF MEMORY T CELLS

Following infection or immunization, an adaptive effector immune response develops and then resolves, leaving behind a pool of long-lived antigen-specific lymphocytes that can mediate heightened resistance to infection. These long-lived cells, known as memory lymphocytes, form a heterogeneous population that is both numerically and functionally superior to antigen-inexperienced cells. Subsets of memory cells are strategically located in anatomical sites that are most likely to be exposed to infection, which, in the case of TB, is the lung. Memory cells are able to respond quickly and produce appropriate effector molecules upon reinfection. Their superior function is due in part to epigenetic reprogramming of the memory cell that prepares specific gene loci for accelerated transcription of effector molecules.

It is important to note that much of what is known of memory immune responses is based on mouse studies of memory CD8 T cell generation and maintenance in the context of responses to virus infection. Far less is understood about memory CD4 T cells and their role in protection, especially in the context of TB. Although CD4 T cells outnumber CD8 T cells in the body (22), in most acute viral models of infection the CD4 T cell response is much lower in magnitude than the CD8 T cell response, making CD4 T cells more challenging to study. Moreover, major histocompatibility complex (MHC) class I multimers that can be used to detect antigen-specific CD8 T cells by flow cytometry have been far more accessible than MHC class II multimers to detect CD4 T cells.

The requirements for memory development as well as survival are known to differ between CD4 and CD8 T cells (23). For example, the common γ chain cytokines IL-7 and IL-15 are both required to regulate homeostasis of the CD8 memory T cell pool; whereas memory CD4 T cells are more reliant on IL-7 than IL-15 (24). Therefore, caution must be taken when extrapolating findings from studies of CD8 T cells to CD4 T cells.

Development of Memory T Cells after TB Infection or Vaccination

The lung is the most common site of initial TB infection. Here, local antigen-presenting cells (APCs) such as dendritic cells (DCs) take up the mycobacterium and its antigens and subsequently migrate to the lung-draining lymph nodes (25). In the lymph node, DCs present antigens to naive T cells, which then become activated and differentiate into populations of effector cells with multiple functions. Following vaccination, similar steps occur that result in activation of effector T cells; however, different APC subsets may be involved depending on the route of vaccination.

After eradication of a pathogen or in the case of vaccination following clearance of antigen, the immune response contracts and most effector T cells die (up to 95%) (26). Several thousand cells survive beyond the contraction of the effector response, and these are known as memory T cells. The size of the surviving cell pool may rely on the initial clonal burst size (27), which again is determined by the T cell precursor frequency, extent of proliferation during the effector stage, as well as the degree of cell death during the contraction phase (28).

Since *M. tuberculosis* is a chronic infection and the live organisms in the BCG vaccine persist for months or even years, in both situations there is prolonged antigen exposure and chronic inflammation. This type of microenvironment can lead to immune exhaustion and cell death, and may drive generation of exhausted or dysfunctional effector T cells rather than memory T cells (29). However, insufficient antigen exposure, such as from suboptimal vaccination, may generate a very small clonal burst and thereby fail to generate sufficient numbers of memory cells. Therefore, when attempting to generate effective immunological memory against TB through vaccination, it is important to consider the mechanisms that influence clonal burst size and cell death during the contraction phase.

Models of T Cell Fate

The factors that determine whether a T cell becomes a terminally differentiated effector cell that dies upon antigen clearance or whether it develops into a long-lived memory T cell that survives are not yet fully known. Several models have been proposed to describe how the fate of an individual T cell is determined (Fig. 1).

The simplest model, the linear differentiation model, suggests that memory T cells are generated directly from differentiated effector cells. This model is supported by data from adoptive transfer studies of both effector CD4 and CD8 T cells, and these studies show

that the memory populations retain functional polarization similar to the effector cells from which they developed (30).

By contrast to the linear differentiation model, the progressive differentiation model states that the degree of activation of a naive cell dictates the outcome (i.e., effector versus memory). In this model effector cells are highly activated terminally differentiated cells that eventually die, whereas less activated cells become memory cells that have self-renewal capacity and the ability to further differentiate (31). This model is supported by analysis of transcriptional profiles of naive, memory, and effector CD8 T cells generated after vaccination, which suggested cumulative antigen stimulation drove naive T cells to differentiate into memory T cells and then into terminally differentiated effector T cells (32).

Alternatively, the divergent model suggests that T cells become destined to an effector or memory lineage early after activation. A significant body of experimental data suggests that, when T cells undergo division, they can give rise to phenotypically and functionally distinct progeny. This process, first described by the Reiner laboratory in 2007, is known as asymmetric cell division and results from the polarity that develops in the cell due to immune synapse formation (32). The immunological synapse leads to proteins and receptors clustering on the cell membrane at the area of contact between the T cell and the APC, and cytoplasmic contents also become unevenly distributed. As a result of this asymmetry, when the cell divides, one daughter cell acquires properties that lead it to develop into a terminally differentiated effector cell that can mediate acute effector functions and then dies. The remaining daughter cell acquires properties that promote its development into a self-renewing memory cell capable of persisting beyond the contraction of the effector response. It is thought that this distinction in fate can occur as early as the first cell division; however, the ultimate destiny of the cell is determined by a combination of cell-intrinsic signals and cues derived from the microenvironment during maturation (33).

Although these models appear very disparate, it is very likely that multiple pathways operate simultaneously that lead to development of a heterogeneous memory T cell pool. The pathways involved are likely to vary between CD4 and CD8 T cells, between the different T helper subsets, and between the different memory T cell subsets (described in "Memory T Cell Heterogeneity") given that the factors that support generation, survival, and persistence of each subset may be quite different. Since the development of immunological memory is fundamental to effective TB vaccination,

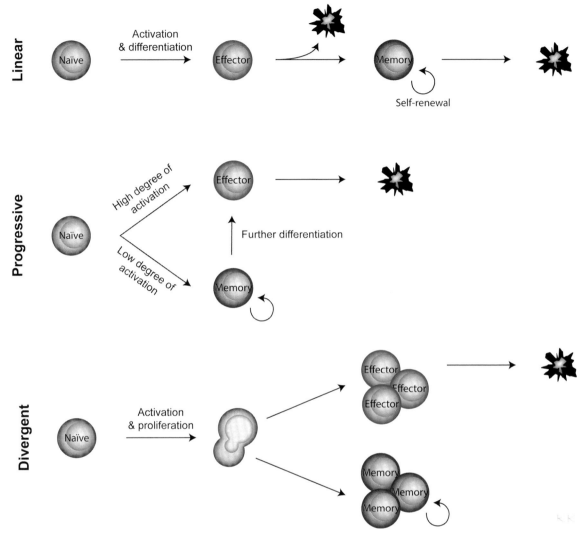

Figure 1   Three proposed models for memory T cell differentiation. In the linear differentiation model, self-renewing memory T cells differentiate directly from effector T cells. In the progressive differentiation model, the degree of activation dictates the outcome, with highly activated cells developing into terminally differentiated effector cells and moderately activated cells developing into memory T cells with the capacity to differentiate into effector cells upon further stimulation. In the divergent model, T cell fate is determined through asymmetric cell division resulting in daughter cells that are destined to become either effector or memory T cells. These methods of T cell differentiation may coexist.

the processes best capable of generating long-lived protective memory T cells need to be better understood.

MEMORY T CELL HETEROGENEITY

Central Memory and Effector Memory T Cell Subsets

In 1999 a seminal study by Sallusto et al. redefined our understanding of memory immunity by revealing that

there were in fact two memory T cell compartments that could be defined based on their effector function, ability to proliferate, and anatomical location (34) (Fig. 2). One T cell subset predominated in the secondary lymphoid organs and was termed central memory (T_{CM}). Similar to naive T cells, T_{CM} expressed CCR7 and CD62L, but also produced IL-2 and proliferated extensively. By contrast, the second subset, designated effector memory cells (T_{EM}), was found mainly in peripheral sites including the lungs (35, 36). T_{EM}, defined

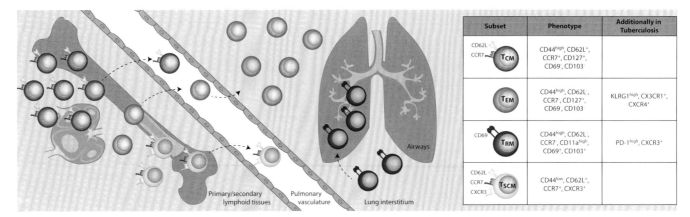

Subset	Phenotype	Additionally in Tuberculosis
T$_{CM}$	CD44^{high}, CD62L$^+$, CCR7$^+$, CD127$^+$, CD69$^-$, CD103$^-$	
T$_{EM}$	CD44^{high}, CD62L$^-$, CCR7$^-$, CD127$^+$, CD69$^-$, CD103$^-$	KLRG1^{high}, CX3CR1$^+$, CXCR4$^+$
T$_{RM}$	CD44^{high}, CD62L$^-$, CCR7$^-$, CD11a^{high}, CD69$^+$, CD103$^+$	PD-1^{high}, CXCR3$^+$
T$_{SCM}$	CD44^{low}, CD62L$^+$, CCR7$^+$, CXCR3$^+$	

Figure 2 T cell memory phenotypes. After effector immunity is established, several memory populations are generated. T$_{CM}$ cells, which are CD62L^{hi} and CCR7^{hi}, reside predominantly in the lymphoid organs. T$_{EM}$, CD62L^{lo}, and CCR7^{lo} are found mostly in peripheral tissues, including the lung, and can recirculate. T$_{RM}$ cells are CD69^{hi}, CD62L^{lo}, and CCR7^{lo} and are found permanently in the lung. Finally, more recently, T$_{SCM}$ cells have been described; they are CD62L^{hi} and CXCR3^{hi}. Other cell markers have been associated with some phenotypes specifically in tuberculosis infection; these are described in the table inset.

by their lack of expression of the lymph-node-homing molecules CCR7 and CD62L, are able to recirculate through different peripheral anatomical sites, depending on their expression of specific tissue-homing receptors such as selectin ligands, integrins, and addressins (37). T$_{EM}$ have been shown to be capable of producing a range of effector cytokines, including IFN-γ, IL-2, IL-17, and TNF-α. In this regard, the T$_{EM}$ population is very heterogeneous, because it includes cells that have differing migratory phenotypes and effector functions.

BCG vaccination in animals and humans has been shown to induce multifunctional CD4 T$_{EM}$-like cells, and, after mucosal BCG delivery, these T$_{EM}$-like cells can be found in appreciable numbers in the lung and bronchoalveolar lavage fluid (38–42). The relative importance of the T$_{CM}$ and T$_{EM}$ CD4 subsets to protective memory immunity against TB has been subject to intense investigation. Based on the adoptive transfer model of Lefford, in which T cells from "immune" or vaccinated mice are transferred into immunodeficient recipient mice, two studies found that central memory-like CD4 T cells (CD62L^{hi}) rather than effector memory T cells (CD62L^{lo}) mediated protection against TB (43, 44). However, using Lefford's model in this context was problematic, since the transfer of CD62L^{hi} cells into a lymphopenic mouse can lead to development of colitis and systemic inflammation (45). Recently, a similar study was conducted using adoptive transfer of memory subsets of TCR Tg CD4 T cells into naive, immunocompetent recipient mice, that were

then subject to a low-dose aerosol *M. tuberculosis* challenge (17). This study from the Kaufmann laboratory showed that T$_{CM}$ cells, but not T$_{EM}$, could transfer protection to the recipient mice. Although the observed enhanced protection following adoptive transfer could be due to a greater proliferative capacity of T$_{CM}$ population compared with T$_{EM}$ (46), there is increasing evidence that T$_{CM}$ play an important protective role during *M. tuberculosis* infection. In particular, the protective ability of TB vaccines has been correlated with their ability to induce high levels of T$_{CM}$.

Orme has proposed that the failure of the BCG vaccine to protect adults against pulmonary TB is due to its propensity to induce T$_{EM}$ rather than T$_{CM}$ (47). Orme suggests that, since T$_{EM}$ are shorter lived than T$_{CM}$, this could account for the effectiveness of BCG during childhood and its waning efficacy in adults. Boosting BCG with an adjuvanted subunit vaccine increased the numbers of IL-2 producing CD62L high CD4 T cells and this was accompanied with a better control of the bacterial infection at the later stage of infection (48). Subcutaneous delivery of the BCG vaccine in mice establishes much higher numbers of T$_{EM}$ in the lungs, spleen, and lymph nodes than T$_{CM}$ (49). By contrast, aerosol delivery of BCG to rhesus macaques led to expansion of CD4 T$_{CM}$ in peripheral blood, implying that route of antigen exposure may also be one factor that is important in determining which memory subsets develop (40). Together this suggests that new TB vaccines and immunization strategies should be tested for their ability to generate a robust population of T_{CM} that are maintained efficiently even in the face of a chronic *M. tuberculosis* infection.

Resident Memory T Cells

Recently, it has been established that additional memory T cell populations exist, beyond T_{EM} and T_{CM}. This includes a population of T cells that, distinct from circulating populations of memory cells, permanently resides in peripheral tissues after an infection is cleared. This population, first described in the skin after herpes simplex virus infection by the Carbone laboratory in 2009, was termed tissue-resident memory (T_{RM}) (50). Like T_{EM}, T_{RM} cells lack CD62L and CCR7 and are found in peripheral tissues, particularly the skin and the mucosae; however, distinct from the T_{EM} subset, T_{RM} do not circulate in the blood. T_{RM} were initially described as a subset of antigen-experienced CD8 T cells that expressed the adhesion molecule CD103; however, CD4 T_{RM} have also been identified, although their expression of CD103 is low or undetectable (51).

While it appears that CD4 T_{RM} share similar tissue distribution profiles to CD8 T_{RM}, their specific patterns of localization may be different. Importantly, CD4 T_{RM} have been identified in mouse lungs. A notable study in a mouse parabiosis model demonstrated that a noncirculating population of memory CD4 T cells persisted in the lungs after influenza infection (52). This population of cells expressed elevated CD69 and CD11a, and was shown to be protective against influenza, whereas memory cells from the spleen were less protective, even though they were able to migrate to the lung. This study suggested that the tissue localization is a critical factor for inducing protective immunity against lung infection, and generating tissue-resident memory populations should be an important consideration for TB vaccine design. BCG vaccination is more protective against aerosol *M. tuberculosis* challenge than parenteral delivery, in support of the concept that generating memory populations in the lung is important for protection (53–55). Furthermore, BCG-vaccinated mice have been found to be protected when fingolimod, a molecule that prevents egress of effector and memory lymphocytes from secondary lymphoid organs, was given during an infectious lung challenge, suggesting that memory lymphocytes that are present in the lung following vaccination are sufficient for protection (56). However, relatively few TB vaccines delivered through the mucosal surfaces have shown a clear protective advantage compared with conventional parenteral vaccines, and there is a need for focusing on how to successfully exploit the protective potential of pulmonary Th1 cells and/or T_{RM} by means of vaccination.

Two distinct populations of pulmonary Th1 cells have been shown to develop during the effector phase of the immune response to aerosol *M. tuberculosis* infection and remained stable for up to 6 months postinfection (57). In this study, fluorochrome-labeled antibody against CD45 was injected intravenously, where it bound to cells in the vasculature, but not cells in lung tissue. One CD4 population, which was unlabeled by the intravenous anti-CD45 antibody and populated the lung parenchyma, was CXCR3^{hi}; the second CXCR1^{hi}KLRG1^{hi} population was retained within the lung vasculature. Although the parenchymal Th1 cells produced less IFN-γ than the vasculature Th1 cells at 30 days after infection, when the sorted populations were adoptively transferred into lymphopenic recipients, the parenchymal Th1 cells were found to provide superior protection against *M. tuberculosis* infection. It is possible that the parenchymal CXCR3^{hi} Th1 cells go on to develop into T_{RM} during the contraction stage of the immune response, or if the infection is cleared by antibiotic treatment. Nonetheless, this study leads to the important conclusion that IFN-γ production alone without the ability to gain access to the lung parenchyma leads to inefficient protection and again highlights the point that location is key for protective immune responses.

A recent study by Moguche et al. provided further evidence of a protective role for lung parenchymal Th1 cells (58). A subset of CD4 T cells that expressed Programmed Cell Death Protein-1 (PD-1) was maintained in the lung parenchyma of mice during chronic TB infection. To determine whether this subset survived following antigen withdrawal, the mark of a memory response, polyclonal PD-1$^+$ cells from the lung were sorted and then transferred into uninfected animals. The PD-1$^+$ cells persisted in recipient mice for the duration of the 28-day experiment; however, their survival was dependent on Inducible Costimulator ligand (ICOSL). Upon adoptive transfer into lymphopenic recipient mice, sorted polyclonal PD-1$^+$ cells were found to provide better protection against *M. tuberculosis* challenge than the terminally differentiated Th1 cells that predominantly resided within the vasculature.

Similar to T_{RM}, PD-1+ parenchymal Th1 cells expressed low levels of CD62L and high levels of CD69. However, the PD-1+ parenchymal Th1 cells were also found to share many features in common with the T follicular helper (T_{FH}) cell CD4 cell subset, which serves to support B cell activation and maturation. T_{FH} differentiation requires expression of the master regulator transcription factor B cell lymphoma (Bcl)6, which is induced by ICOS and cytokines including

IL-6 and IL-21. By generating bone marrow chimeras, Moguche et al. showed that Bcl6 was required for the generation of both PD-1⁺ cells and terminally differentiated Th1 cells, suggesting that fully differentiated Th1 cells originated from the Bcl6-dependent parenchymal PD-1⁺ cells. This previously unappreciated pathway for inducing a protective Th1 effector response provides exciting new possibilities for TB vaccine design.

Stem Cell-Like Memory T Cells

A further recently defined memory T cell subset is T stem cell-like memory (T$_{SCM}$). This subset comprises early stage multipotential memory CD4 and CD8 T cells that have stem cell-like properties, including self-renewal capability and the capacity to produce more highly differentiated daughter cells (59, 60). T$_{SCM}$ express many cell surface markers at levels similar to naive T cells and, in that regard, are CD44^{low}CD62L^{high} in mice and CD45RO⁻, CD45RA⁺, CD62L⁺ in humans (61). Despite this, T$_{SCM}$ express many markers in common with memory T cells and share many of the heightened functional attributes of memory T cells. The phenotype of T$_{SCM}$ is defined as positive for Bcl-2, the β chain of the IL-2 and IL-15 receptor (IL-2Rβ), and the chemokine (C-X-C motif) receptor CXCR3.

A recent series of particularly heroic experiments from the Busch laboratory, which incorporated trigenerational serial single-cell adoptive transfers of TCR Tg CD8 T cells into naive mice followed by infection with *Listeria monocytogenes*, demonstrated that individual T$_{CM}$ cells can act as stem cells (62). In this study, in addition to naive T cells, both primary and secondary T$_{CM}$ cells were capable of generating phenotypically diverse progeny as well as maintaining self-renewal capacity. Of note, in this study, CD44^{low} memory T cells were undetectable, meaning that this subset differed from the phenotype of T$_{SCM}$, detailed in the work of others.

The role of T$_{SCM}$ in protection against TB is at present unexplored. However, there are clear opportunities for improving TB vaccination through the identification and targeting of memory cells that have the capacity to self-renew, are protective, and can produce highly differentiated progeny.

CD4 Th1 MEMORY IMMUNITY

Th1 Cell Activation and Function

CD4 T cells are primed in secondary lymphoid organs by DC that process and present *M. tuberculosis* antigen on major histocompatibility complex (MHC) class II

molecules as well as providing sufficient co-stimulatory signals to result in T cell activation. TCRs on the surface of CD4 T cells recognize the antigen and activate a signaling cascade that leads to gene transcription that promotes T cell expansion and differentiation into effector cells. The cytokine milieu at the time of T cell activation directs CD4 T cells to differentiate into distinct effector subsets by inducing master transcription factors that drive subset specification (Fig. 3). The resulting T helper subsets retain some plasticity since the expression of the master transcription factors is not necessarily stable. Despite this, cytokine memory does occur and is thought to do so through epigenetic imprinting as histone architecture is modified during T cell differentiation.

Th1 differentiation depends on the presence of IL-12 during T cell activation. During TB infection, it is thought that DCs are a major source of this Th1-inducing cytokine, although macrophages can produce IL-12 albeit at much lower levels (63). IL-12 induces expression of the transcription factor Tbet, the master regulator that is necessary and sufficient for IFN-γ production and Th1 lineage commitment.

How Th1 memory cells develop has been the subject of much debate. Wu et al. demonstrated that IFN-γ-producing memory CD4 T cells developed from cells that had been activated under Th1 conditions and expressed Tbet, but did not secrete IFN-γ upon restimulation *in vitro* (64). In this study, IFN-γ-producing effector cells did not give rise to memory T cells. These data are congruent with both the progressive differentiation model and divergent model of memory T cell generation. By contrast, a separate study using cytokine reporter mice led to the opposite conclusion that IFN-γ-producing effector CD4 T cells developed into memory Th1 cells, supporting a linear model of memory Th1 development (65). It is not clear which pathway of memory Th1 generation occurs after *M. tuberculosis* infection or vaccination; however, it is a critical point to understand. If IFN-γ-producing effector cells do not develop into memory cells, along with the IFN-γ-independent protection against TB discussed below, this may explain why IFN-γ production by CD4 T cells is a poor correlate of vaccine-induced protection.

IFN-γ-Independent Protection Against TB by Memory Th1 Cells

Multiple lines of evidence, from animal models and human studies, point toward the crucial role that Th1 cells play in the control of a primary *M. tuberculosis* infection. The essential role of CD4 T cells during primary infection was demonstrated by CD4 T cell de-

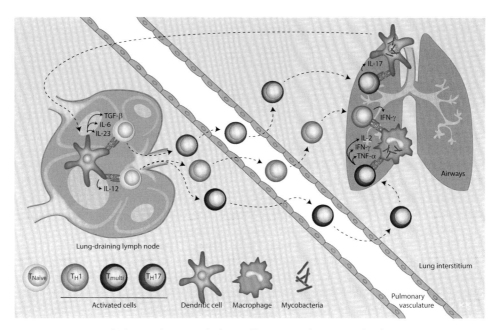

Figure 3 CD4 T helper subsets and their effector cytokines involved in immune protection against *M. tuberculosis*. After exposure to *M. tuberculosis* in the lung, dendritic cells bearing antigen stimulate naive CD4 T cells in the draining lymph nodes. Activated T cells differentiate in single- or multicytokine-producing cells, depending on the cytokine milieu at the time of activation. Effector cells migrate through the pulmonary vasculature into the lung where they produce effector cytokines that promote the antimycobacterial activity of infected cells. Multicytokine-producing CD4 T cells are thought to be more potent producers of cytokine than single-cytokine-producing cells.

pletion studies in mice, experiments that resulted in increased severity of infection and shortened survival (66–68). Subsequently, it was discovered that mice and humans deficient in the genes important for IFN-γ production and signaling were exceptionally susceptible to mycobacterial infection (8, 69–71).

Given the importance of Th1 cells in protection against primary disease (72), it was presumed that they would also be critical in mediating memory immunity against *M. tuberculosis* infection. Indeed, in a series of adoptive transfer studies, Orme showed that CD4 T cells isolated from the spleen of *M. tuberculosis*-infected then antibiotic-treated immune mice were able to protect naive irradiated recipient mice from TB challenge (10). Yet, despite the mountain of data suggesting IFN-γ-producing Th1 cells are essential for protection against primary TB infection, over the past decades there has been increasing evidence that suggests the IFN-γ-signaling pathway is not essential for CD4 T cell-mediated protective memory immunity against TB.

The first hints that IFN-γ-independent mechanisms may exist came from the repeated failure of researchers to correlate the ability of a vaccine to induce IFN-γ-producing Th1 cells with protection against TB challenge, in both mouse and human studies (73–77). In 2003, Cowley and Elkins vaccinated IFN-γ-deficient mice with BCG, and convincingly demonstrated the existence of a CD4-dependent, but IFN-γ-independent, mechanism of protection against TB (78). More recently, elegant adoptive transfer studies using cells from *M. tuberculosis*-specific CD4 TCR Tg mice activated under Th1-priming conditions demonstrated an IFN-γ-independent mechanism of protection against TB (16). Gallegos et al. discovered that Th1-primed TCR Tg cells from IFN-γ-deficient donors, as well as cells from IFN-γ and TNF-α-double-deficient donors, could protect recipient mice from *M. tuberculosis* almost as well as Th1-primed TCR Tg cells from wild-type donors. These data suggest that Th1-primed CD4 TCR Tg cells have a mechanism for protection against *M. tuberculosis* that is independent of IFN-γ and TNF-α. Moreover, Th1-primed CD4 TCR Tg cells from mice deficient in the Th1-inducing master regulator transcription factor, Tbet, were also found to be effective in protecting recipient mice, and recipient mice deficient in the IFN-γ-induced effector molecule nitric oxide were protected too. Together, these studies imply that these IFN-γ-dependent pathways of controlling infection might be redundant in the context of memory immunity against TB.

Compared with studies in inbred rodents, it is far more challenging to study the role of memory Th1 cells in humans; however, a recent efficacy trial of the most advanced TB vaccine candidate, modified vaccinia Ankara virus expressing antigen 85A from *M. tuberculosis* (MVA85A), confirmed that the induction of IFN-γ-producing Th1 memory cells through vaccination does not correlate with protection against disease (12, 79, 80). This was further supported by the finding of a study of more than 5,000 South African infants, in which investigators reported that the frequency of *M. tuberculosis*-specific CD4 T cells and their cytokine profile, including IFN-γ production, did not correlate with protection against TB (77).

Therefore, although IFN-γ is essential for control of TB infection, the mechanism by which CD4 T cells protect against TB appears to be independent of their ability to produce this cytokine. This has major implications for vaccine design, since IFN-γ has long been used as a measure of immunogenicity. More intricate assessments of cytokine production, such as measuring multicytokine-producing CD4 T cells, garnered significant interest as a correlate of long-term memory after they were first reported by the Seder laboratory in 2003 (13). These cells, which produce three or more cytokines simultaneously and are designated multifunctional, produced higher levels of each cytokine per cell than single-cytokine-producing cells, suggesting they were qualitatively superior; nonetheless, their induction by vaccination does not always correlate with protection against TB (77, 81). The critical question remains: which cytokines or mechanisms employed by memory CD4 T cells mediate protection against TB? To date the answer remains elusive.

CD4 Th17 MEMORY IMMUNITY

IL-17 can be produced by CD4 Th17 αβ T cells as well as γδ T cells, and both T cell subsets have been identified in TB patients and in animal models of *M. tuberculosis* infection (82, 83); however, the contribution of the relatively newly discovered Th17 lineage to protection against TB is still under debate.

Differentiation of CD4 T cells into Th17 cells requires the influence of the polarizing cytokines transforming growth factor-β (TGF-β), IL-6, and IL-23, which induce expression of the transcription factors RORγt and RORα (84, 85). The Th17 CD4 subset, characterized by the production of IL-17A and IL-17F

as signature cytokines, was first described in 1993 as having a key role against extracellular pathogens and in the pathogenesis of autoimmune diseases (86, 87). More recently, it has been shown that the Th17 pathway also is induced in humans during infection with intracellular microorganisms such as *M. tuberculosis*, and therefore could play a role in protective immunity against these pathogens. Conversely, a detrimental role for Th17 CD4 T cells leading to exacerbated mucosal pathology has also been suggested (88).

In mice already harboring an *M. tuberculosis* infection, repeated BCG vaccinations resulted in an increased number of neutrophils and IL-17 producing cells in the lungs accompanied by enhanced lung pathology, an effect that was abrogated by administering anti-IL-17 antibodies (89). It was suggested that this inflammatory response, known as the Koch phenomenon, occurs because of dysregulated IL-17 responses and that vaccine strategies that activated the Th17 T cell subset should be considered with caution. However, in mice vaccination using recombinant BCG that induces elevated IL-17 levels, intranasal BCG administration that leads to enhanced IL-17 secretion, or adjuvants selectively known to induce strong IL-17 responses, no associated pathology has been observed even when given as postexposure vaccines (90–92).

A number of studies have assessed the induction of IL-17 and the Th17-associated cytokines IL-21 and IL-22 in human blood samples obtained from patients with different TB exposure categories and upon stimulation with different mycobacterial antigens. Although some studies have failed to demonstrate Th17 responses as an inherent component of the memory response to mycobacterial antigen (93, 94), the majority of studies have shown IL-17 production by infected individuals and, in particular, elevated levels in latently *M. tuberculosis*-infected individuals compared with patients with active TB (95–100). The South African Tuberculosis Vaccine Initiative (SATVI) laboratory showed that IL-17-producing CD4 T cells constituted almost 10% of the overall cytokine response in mycobacteria-exposed healthy donors, a significantly higher level than in patients with active TB disease (101). This does not seem to be correlated with the recruitment of these cells to the disease sites, because Th17 CD4 T cells appear to be absent from bronchoalveolar lavage (BAL) and pericardial fluid of TB patients (96, 102).

From animal studies, Th17 responses are mainly thought to have a role during the early stages of infection where they precede the Th1 response and induce chemokines that facilitate the recruitment of protective CD4 T cells into the lungs (103). Whether the same early role also applies to Th17 responses in humans remains unexplored, but it could explain why limited IL-17 production is seen in TB patients that must have harbored the pathogen for an extended period. BCG vaccination in humans seems to induce only negligible levels of IL-17, particularly in settings with low mycobacterial exposure such as the United Kingdom. By contrast, responses to a range of cytokines including IL-17 were higher postvaccination in more high-endemicity settings such as Malawi and South Africa (77, 104, 105). The SATVI laboratory attempted to correlate frequencies, cytokine profiles, and patterns of mycobacteria-specific T cells to protection against TB in a study of >5,000 BCG-vaccinated infants, but IL-17 signatures were not identified as a correlate of protection by BCG (77).

There are a number of possible explanations for the difficulties faced when exploring the role of the Th17 subset. The levels of soluble IL-17 and numbers of IL-17-secreting CD4 T cells are relatively low in comparison with IFN-γ responses, and it is possible that these are below detection levels for standard assays. It is also possible that the antigen of choice for restimulation dictates the cytokine pattern because certain antigens seem to selectively induce IL-17-positive CD4 T cells, for example, the heparin-binding hemagglutinin protein, HBHA (97, 106). As a further technical explanation for the lack of IL-17 responses, the majority of human studies have been performed using incubation times optimized for measuring IFN-γ responses, whereas optimal IL-17 detection seems to require a longer antigen exposure and expansion period (96). Adding to the controversy and complexity of Th17 responses, it is possible that different mycobacterial strains induce different levels of IL-17 response with a stronger induction by more virulent and drug-resistant strains (107). In this regard, Khader's laboratory recently reported that whereas IL-17 is dispensable for achieving protection against laboratory-adapted mycobacterial strains, highly virulent M. tuberculosis strains require production of IL-17 for optimal protective immunity in mice (108).

M. tuberculosis infection studies in IL-17-deficient mice show that this cytokine is not essential for controlling mycobacterial growth during the early phase of primary infection (109); however, a number of vaccine studies have quite convincingly demonstrated a protective role for memory Th17 cells in mice. Khader and Cooper induced IL-17-producing CD4 T cells by subunit vaccination and showed that this population triggered the early induction of CXCR-3-ligating chemokines at the site of infection where they were responsible for accelerated recruitment of protective memory CD4 T cells producing IFN-γ (103, 110). In addition, vaccine-induced Th17 responses have also been associated with the generation of well-organized lymphoid structures where T cells are optimally localized to activate infected macrophages (111).

The Britton laboratory reported that BCG vaccination of IL-12p40-deficient mice induced a robust Th17 response (112). Following an *in vitro* expansion step, it was found that adoptive transfer of these BCG-specific IL-17-secreting CD4 T cells into lymphopenic hosts conferred protection against M. tuberculosis infection, even though IFN-γ production by the IL-12p40-deficient cells was decreased enormously compared with the level produced by CD4 T cells from wild-type mice. Together, these data suggest a critical role for Th17 cells in vaccine-induced memory immune responses and that vaccine strategies that activate Th17 cells deserve specific focus. In this regard, it has recently become clear how to selectively induce Th17 responses either by vaccination through mucosal routes (90) or by the use of distinct immunomodulators such as ligands for the C-type lectin receptor Mincle (113).

Using subunit vaccination based on a cationic liposome adjuvant, the Agger laboratory induced a highly stable Th17 memory population that maintained its functionality and phenotype for almost 2 years postvaccination (114). The memory Th17 cells were recruited from the lymph nodes into the lung upon M. tuberculosis challenge, and the Th17 cells demonstrated functional plasticity as they acquired the ability to produce IFN-γ and IL-17 simultaneously. Although most vaccine studies support a role for the Th17 subset, a recent publication showed that, despite induction of long-lived IL-17-producing CD4 T cells in the lungs of mice vaccinated intranasally with a fusion protein subunit vaccine delivered in adjuvant (an oil-in-water stable nanoemulsion designated GLA-SE), protection was independent of the IL-17 receptor (115). All these findings clearly illustrate that there is a need for further exploring the possible role of Th17 responses in humans as well as in murine infection and vaccine studies.

ALTERNATIVE MEDIATORS OF MEMORY IMMUNITY

CD8 T Cells

Early adoptive transfer studies suggest conventional memory CD8 T cells play a lesser role than memory CD4 T cells in the protective recall response to TB (10). Nevertheless, memory CD8 T cells have the ability to elicit potentially protective effector functions such as cytokine production, production of cytotoxic molecules such as perforin, granzyme, and granulysin that can either lyse TB-infected cells or directly kill *M. tuberculosis* (116, 117).

CD8 T cells are activated by TCR recognition of antigenic peptides on MHC class I, either by conventional proteasomal processing of cytoplasmic antigens, cross-presentation of exogenous antigens taken up through phagocytosis, or by cross-dressing where preformed MHC class I and peptide complexes are transferred directly from the surface of one cell to an APC (118–120). After infection, *M. tuberculosis* is taken up by DCs and macrophages and is thought to reside within the phagosome. However, there is good evidence that TB antigens can be processed onto MHC class I through the cytosolic pathway, as well as through cross-presentation, and mycobacterial escape from the phagosome into the cytosol does not appear to be a requirement for MHC class I presentation (119). Autophagy, the process of proteolytic degradation of cytosolic components such as aggregated proteins or damaged organelles by the lysosome, could also result in processing and loading of TB antigen onto MHC class I (121).

It is clear that CD8 T cells can be activated by *M. tuberculosis* infection and by some vaccines against TB, including BCG. The importance of memory CD8 T cells for protection against TB is less clear; however, several studies have shown that memory CD8 T cells can be protective against TB (122–124).

Experiments conducted in BCG-vaccinated CD4-deficient mice revealed that these mice developed activated CD8 T cells, and were protected against intranasal *M. tuberculosis* infection (~100-fold reduction in lung bacterial burden compared with unvaccinated controls) (123). Although this protection was delayed by 6 and 12 weeks after challenge, the level of protection was equivalent to that of BCG-vaccinated intact mice. Depletion of the CD8 T cells in CD4-deficient mice partially abrogated these protective effects (~60% reduction in protection), implying that the CD8 T cells generated by BCG vaccination contributed to this protection in the absence of CD4 T cells.

CD8 T cell memory has also been shown to develop after *M. tuberculosis* infection in mice (125). During chronic infection, the CD8 T cells had a T_{EM} phenotype; however, following antibiotic treatment, the proportion of CD8 T cells with a T_{CM} phenotype increased. Moreover, the CD8 memory T cells were observed to expand rapidly following rechallenge, implying that they had features consistent with functional memory cells. In a separate study of antibiotic-treated

M. tuberculosis-infected mice, memory CD8 T cells were observed to produce IFN-γ early after rechallenge, indicating their heightened functional capacity compared with naive CD8 T cells (126). A recent study from the Behar laboratory challenges the current dogma, that memory CD8 T cells will outperform naive cells. Using a subunit vaccine, a robust memory CD8 T cell response could be generated; however, upon *M. tuberculosis* challenge, naive T cells were able to outcompete the vaccine-induced memory T cells, unless the memory T cells had a higher-affinity TCR than the naive cells. This study implies that generating memory T cells with high-affinity TCRs is an additional important consideration for vaccine design (127).

New TB vaccines have been designed to target the development of CD8 memory T cells. These include recombinant BCG vaccines designed to improve access of mycobacterial antigens to the MHC class I cytosolic presentation pathway (128, 129). Viral vectors are also potent inducers of CD8 T cell memory, and intranasal immunization of mice with a recombinant adenoviral vaccine induced *M. tuberculosis* antigen-specific CD8 T cells with activated effector memory phenotype in the airway lumen (124). Vaccinated mice were protected from an intranasal *M. tuberculosis* infection even when CD4 T cells were depleted prior to challenge. DNA vaccines against TB have also been shown to elicit protective memory CD8 T cells (130), but overall studies on the role of CD8 T cells have been performed in mice whereas data supporting a role of CD8 T cells in more advanced animal models including non-human primates are still relatively scarce.

γδ T Cells

Phosphoantigen-specific γδ T cells expand in number and mount multifunctional responses during *M. tuberculosis* infection in humans or non-human primates. A very recent study adoptively transferred *ex vivo* expanded autologous phosphoantigen-specific Vγ2Vδ2 into *M. tuberculosis*-infected cynomolgus macaques. Transfer of these memory-phenotype γδ T cells reduced bacterial burdens in the lungs, liver, and spleen, suggesting that this cell subset merits consideration for rational TB vaccine design (155).

Innate Memory

The existence of heterologous protection afforded by BCG vaccination of animals and humans has been well known for many decades (131–136). Recently, the immunological mechanisms for these broadly protective effects were described, and some were found to be independent of T and B cells. The discovery that the immunological memory of a pathogen encounter is not restricted to the adaptive arm of the immune system can be game changing. The term "trained immunity" has been coined to describe the phenomenon by which the innate immune system mediates protection to secondary pathogen exposures (137). Because of the lack of specific antigen receptors on most innate cells, the protective effects are unspecific, and "trained" innate cells are able to mediate protection against an extremely diverse range of pathogenic organisms.

Trained Immunity in Monocytes

The Netea laboratory discovered that the molecular mechanisms that underpin trained immunity in monocytes following BCG exposure involve a shift in glucose metabolism toward glycolysis leading to epigenetic reprogramming (137, 156). Promoter regions of genes encoding cytokines and pattern recognition receptors (PRRs) had methylation states characteristic of transcriptionally active genes. These changes led to improved pathogen recognition by PRR on the trained monocytes as well as enhanced proinflammatory cytokine production. The development of trained monocytes required the PRR NOD2, because they did not develop in its absence (138). Intriguingly, although some effects of BCG on monocytes waned after 3 months, the expression of some PPRs and activation markers remained elevated for up to 1 year after BCG vaccination, suggesting that some BCG-induced changes in monocytes are short-lived, while others are sustained (139).

NK Cell Memory

Like T and B cells, NK cells develop from a common lymphoid progenitor; however, they have been considered innate cells because they express germline-encoded activating receptors and can respond rapidly to pathogens. Recently, with the use of a mouse model of cytomegalovirus infection, it was discovered that NK cells share certain features of adaptive immune cells, including the ability to develop into long-lived memory cells with self-renewal capabilities and functional recall responses (140). Although little is known about these cells in the context of protection against TB, NK cells with a memory-like phenotype have been detected in patients with TB pleurisy, and these cells were found to respond more rapidly to IL-12 stimulation than other NK cells (141). Whether targeting the NK memory compartment through vaccination enhances protection against TB remains to be answered; however, the stimulation of innate cells through vaccination is certainly a new and interesting avenue worthy of pursuing.

T CELL MEMORY AND TB VACCINATION

Can BCG Induce Durable and Protective Responses?

Several hypotheses have been proposed to explain the variable efficacy of BCG in adults against pulmonary TB, including differences in BCG strains, varying degrees of exposure to environmental mycobacteria, and genetic differences of both the human host and the pathogen (142, 143). Adding to this, it has been proposed that BCG is incapable of providing long-lived protection, a hypothesis supported by the fact that incidence rates of TB increase dramatically in early adulthood when the BCG vaccination supposedly took place more than 10 years earlier. Ideally, a vaccine should provide life-long protection, and it has been a common belief that live vaccines such as BCG lead to the generation and maintenance of a good memory response. Although a few studies have demonstrated persistence of BCG efficacy for up to 60 years (144, 145), a comprehensive systemic review of 132 BCG trials supports efficacy up to 10 years but also that protection appears to decline after this time point (146).

Data from animal models have recently suggested that BCG may in fact induce the "wrong" kind of memory T cell response, and this could be an underlying explanation for the waning of BCG efficacy (47). In mice, parenteral BCG vaccination preferentially induces T_{EM} that have a good immediate effect but, over time, are believed to be more prone to exhaustion imposed by a chronic infection or continuous mycobacterial exposure (49). Boosting BCG with a subunit vaccine directing the memory response toward a higher proportion of T_{CM} is correlated with better long-term protection (48). Recent adoptive transfer experiments showed that protection afforded by the recombinant BCG expressing listerolysin ($\Delta ureC::hly$ vaccine) could be ascribed in part to T_{CM} (17). Because the novel TB vaccine candidates are either BCG booster vaccines or live mycobacterial vaccines that may have the same inherent problem with preferential induction of T_{EM}, continued research into mycobacterial memory immunity is certainly warranted.

Memory Immunity Induced by Novel TB Vaccines

More than 20 novel TB vaccines have been tested in clinical trials over the past decade and evaluated for their ability to evoke primarily T cell responses. Obviously, given the logistic challenges and often limited funding available for these trials, the detailed study of more long-lived (greater than 6 months postvaccination) vaccine-induced memory immunity has been limited to just a few vaccine candidates. The most advanced new TB vaccine and the first to enter efficacy testing since the large-scale trials of BCG, MVA85A, was found to induce durable Th1 responses measured as a significant number of Ag85A-specific IFN-γ-producing cells more than 3 years after vaccination compared with a placebo group (147). The response was dominated by CD4 T cells coexpressing IFN-γ/TNF-α/IL-2, but also cells secreting IFN-γ alone and with both profiles consistent with both T$_{EM}$ (CCR7$^-$CD45RA$^-$) and T$_{CM}$ (CCR7$^+$CD45RA$^-$) phenotypes. Interestingly, the T cell profiles were more biased toward T$_{EM}$ in infants, the trial population in which MVA85A failed to provide improved protection (12). It has been hypothesized that viral vectored vaccines may induce immune responses that are too biased toward T$_{EM}$ responses and that the attrition of memory T cell responses can explain the lack of protection of the MVA85A vaccine. So far, this remains speculative, and comparisons of the long-term quality of T cell responses induced by different types of vaccines have only been conducted in mice (148).

Although we do not yet know the implications, the kinetics of T cell responses over time after vaccination with viral vectored vaccines and adjuvanted subunit vaccines are clearly different. Vaccination with MVA85A induced very strong IFN-γ responses (often more than 1,000 spot-forming cells per million peripheral blood mononuclear cells) at the peak of response 7 days postvaccination after which there was a marked contraction of the T cell responses (11). The kinetics after vaccination with the fusion protein H1 in the adjuvants IC31 or CAF01 followed a different pattern with peak IFN-γ responses 6 weeks after the second vaccination (14 weeks after the first vaccination) and reaching overall lower levels that remained at a relatively constant level until the end of trials 2 to 3 years after vaccination (149, 150). Using flow cytometry, the responding T cells were mostly found residing among the IFN-γ/IL-2/TNF-α and TNF-α/IL-2 coproducing CD4 T cells with no contribution of IFN-γ single producers (151).

In a recent trial with the H56 vaccine using the adjuvant IC31, the TNF-α/IL-2 coproducing CD4 T cells were found to be mainly T$_{CM}$ (CCR7+ CD45RA–) (152). The M72 vaccine in the liposomal adjuvant AS01 induced a similar response, with the main CD4 T cell populations cosecreting IL-2/TNF-α/IFN-γ or TNF-α/IL-2 (153). This vaccine is currently in efficacy testing and may help to clarify whether there is a link between the ability of a vaccine to induce T$_{CM}$ and protection in humans.

Far less encouraging is the finding that vaccine-induced memory T cells are under profound pressure when vaccinating individuals already harboring mycobacteria. In Quantiferon-positive individuals vaccinated with H56/IC31, IFN-γ single producing CD4 T cells emerged over time, whereas the number of IL-2/TNF-α CD4 T cells decreased (152). Such data clearly emphasize that we need not only to address the ability of a vaccine to provide short-term memory and protection, but also to monitor long-term protective efficacy in different settings with different levels of exposure to TB.

Acknowledgments. We thank Karen S. Korsholm (Statens Serum Institut) for preparing the illustrations.

Citation. Kirman JR, Henao-Tamayo MI, Agger EM. 2016. The memory immune response to tuberculosis. Microbiol Spectrum 4(6):TBTB2-0009-2016.

References

1. **Verrall AJ, Netea MG, Alisjahbana B, Hill PC, van Crevel R.** 2014. Early clearance of *Mycobacterium tuberculosis*: a new frontier in prevention. *Immunology* **141:**506–513.

2. **Huynh KK, Joshi SA, Brown EJ.** 2011. A delicate dance: host response to mycobacteria. *Curr Opin Immunol* **23:**464–472.

3. **Comstock GW, Livesay VT, Woolpert SF.** 1974. The prognosis of a positive tuberculin reaction in childhood and adolescence. *Am J Epidemiol* **99:**131–138.

4. **Trunz BB, Fine P, Dye C.** 2006. Effect of BCG vaccination on childhood tuberculous meningitis and miliary tuberculosis worldwide: a meta-analysis and assessment of cost-effectiveness. *Lancet* **367:**1173–1180.

5. **Anonymous.** 1999. Fifteen year follow up of trial of BCG vaccines in south India for tuberculosis prevention. Tuberculosis Research Centre (ICMR), Chennai. *Indian J Med Res* **110:**56–69.

6. **Colditz GA, Berkey CS, Mosteller F, Brewer TF, Wilson ME, Burdick E, Fineberg HV.** 1995. The efficacy of bacillus Calmette-Guérin vaccination of newborns and infants in the prevention of tuberculosis: meta-analyses of the published literature. *Pediatrics* **96:**29–35.

7. **Bogunovic D, Byun M, Durfee LA, Abhyankar A, Sanal O, Mansouri D, Salem S, Radovanovic I, Grant AV, Adimi P, Mansouri N, Okada S, Bryant VL, Kong XF, Kreins A, Velez MM, Boisson B, Khalilzadeh S, Ozcelik U, Darazam IA, Schoggins JW, Rice CM, Al-Muhsen S, Behr M, Vogt G, Puel A, Bustamante J, Gros P, Huibregtse JM, Abel L, Boisson-Dupuis S, Casanova JL.** 2012. Mycobacterial disease and impaired IFN-γ immunity in humans with inherited ISG15 deficiency. *Science* **337:**1684–1688.

8. **Flynn JL, Chan J, Triebold KJ, Dalton DK, Stewart TA, Bloom BR.** 1993. An essential role for interferon gamma in resistance to *Mycobacterium tuberculosis* infection. *J Exp Med* **178:**2249–2254.

9. **Pape JW, Liautaud B, Thomas F, Mathurin JR, St Amand MM, Boncy M, Pean V, Pamphile M, Laroche AC,**

Johnson WD Jr. 1983. Characteristics of the acquired immunodeficiency syndrome (AIDS) in Haiti. *N Engl J Med* 309:945–950.

10. Orme IM. 1988. Characteristics and specificity of acquired immunologic memory to *Mycobacterium tuberculosis* infection. *J Immunol* 140:3589–3593.

11. McShane H, Pathan AA, Sander CR, Keating SM, Gilbert SC, Huygen K, Fletcher HA, Hill AV. 2004. Recombinant modified vaccinia virus Ankara expressing antigen 85A boosts BCG-primed and naturally acquired antimycobacterial immunity in humans. *Nat Med* 10:1240–1244.

12. Tameris MD, Hatherill M, Landry BS, Scriba TJ, Snowden MA, Lockhart S, Shea JE, McClain JB, Hussey GD, Hanekom WA, Mahomed H, McShane H, MVA85A 020 Trial Study Team. 2013. Safety and efficacy of MVA85A, a new tuberculosis vaccine, in infants previously vaccinated with BCG: a randomised, placebo-controlled phase 2b trial. *Lancet* 381:1021–1028.

13. Darrah PA, Patel DT, De Luca PM, Lindsay RW, Davey DF, Flynn BJ, Hoff ST, Andersen P, Reed SG, Morris SL, Roederer M, Seder RA. 2007. Multifunctional TH1 cells define a correlate of vaccine-mediated protection against *Leishmania major*. *Nat Med* 13:843–850.

14. Henao-Tamayo M, Ordway DJ, Orme IM. 2014. Memory T cell subsets in tuberculosis: what should we be targeting? *Tuberculosis (Edinb)* 94:455–461.

15. Lefford MJ. 1975. Transfer of adoptive immunity to tuberculosis in mice. *Infect Immun* 11:1174–1181.

16. Gallegos AM, van Heijst JW, Samstein M, Su X, Pamer EG, Glickman MS. 2011. A gamma interferon independent mechanism of CD4 T cell mediated control of *M. tuberculosis* infection in vivo. *PLoS Pathog* 7:e1002052.

17. Vogelzang A, Perdomo C, Zedler U, Kuhlmann S, Hurwitz R, Gengenbacher M, Kaufmann SH. 2014. Central memory CD4+ T cells are responsible for the recombinant Bacillus Calmette-Guérin ΔureC::hly vaccine's superior protection against tuberculosis. *J Infect Dis* 210:1928–1937.

18. Jung YJ, Ryan L, LaCourse R, North RJ. 2005. Properties and protective value of the secondary versus primary T helper type 1 response to airborne *Mycobacterium tuberculosis* infection in mice. *J Exp Med* 201:1915–1924.

19. Verver S, Warren RM, Beyers N, Richardson M, van der Spuy GD, Borgdorff MW, Enarson DA, Behr MA, van Helden PD. 2005. Rate of reinfection tuberculosis after successful treatment is higher than rate of new tuberculosis. *Am J Respir Crit Care Med* 171:1430–1435.

20. Marx FM, Dunbar R, Enarson DA, Williams BG, Warren RM, van der Spuy GD, van Helden PD, Beyers N. 2014. The temporal dynamics of relapse and reinfection tuberculosis after successful treatment: a retrospective cohort study. *Clin Infect Dis* 58:1676–1683.

21. Henao-Tamayo M, Obregón-Henao A, Ordway DJ, Shang S, Duncan CG, Orme IM. 2012. A mouse model of tuberculosis reinfection. *Tuberculosis (Edinb)* 92:211–217.

22. Neuenhahn M, Busch DH. 2013. Whole-body anatomy of human T cells. *Immunity* 38:10–12.

23. Seder RA, Ahmed R. 2003. Similarities and differences in CD4+ and CD8+ effector and memory T cell generation. *Nat Immunol* 4:835–842.

24. van Leeuwen EM, Sprent J, Surh CD. 2009. Generation and maintenance of memory CD4(+) T Cells. *Curr Opin Immunol* 21:167–172.

25. Wolf AJ, Desvignes L, Linas B, Banaiee N, Tamura T, Takatsu K, Ernst JD. 2008. Initiation of the adaptive immune response to *Mycobacterium tuberculosis* depends on antigen production in the local lymph node, not the lungs. *J Exp Med* 205:105–115.

26. Hand TW, Kaech SM. 2009. Intrinsic and extrinsic control of effector T cell survival and memory T cell development. *Immunol Res* 45:46–61.

27. Hou S, Hyland L, Ryan KW, Portner A, Doherty PC. 1994. Virus-specific CD8+ T-cell memory determined by clonal burst size. *Nature* 369:652–654.

28. Welsh RM, Selin LK, Razvi ES. 1995. Role of apoptosis in the regulation of virus-induced T cell responses, immune suppression, and memory. *J Cell Biochem* 59:135–142.

29. Behar SM, Carpenter SM, Booty MG, Barber DL, Jayaraman P. 2014. Orchestration of pulmonary T cell immunity during *Mycobacterium tuberculosis* infection: immunity interruptus. *Semin Immunol* 26:559–577.

30. Löhning M, Hegazy AN, Pinschewer DD, Busse D, Lang KS, Höfer T, Radbruch A, Zinkernagel RM, Hengartner H. 2008. Long-lived virus-reactive memory T cells generated from purified cytokine-secreting T helper type 1 and type 2 effectors. *J Exp Med* 205:53–61.

31. Ahmed R, Bevan MJ, Reiner SL, Fearon DT. 2009. The precursors of memory: models and controversies. *Nat Rev Immunol* 9:662–668.

32. Roychoudhuri R, Lefebvre F, Honda M, Pan L, Ji Y, Klebanoff CA, Nichols CN, Fourati S, Hegazy AN, Goulet JP, Gattinoni L, Nabel GJ, Gilliet M, Cameron M, Restifo NP, Sékaly RP, Flatz L. 2015. Transcriptional profiles reveal a stepwise developmental program of memory CD8(+) T cell differentiation. *Vaccine* 33:914–923.

33. Arsenio J, Metz PJ, Chang JT. 2015. Asymmetric cell division in T lymphocyte fate diversification. *Trends Immunol* 36:670–683.

34. Sallusto F, Lenig D, Förster R, Lipp M, Lanzavecchia A. 1999. Two subsets of memory T lymphocytes with distinct homing potentials and effector functions. *Nature* 401:708–712.

35. Masopust D, Vezys V, Marzo AL, Lefrançois L. 2001. Preferential localization of effector memory cells in non-lymphoid tissue. *Science* 291:2413–2417.

36. Reinhardt RL, Khoruts A, Merica R, Zell T, Jenkins MK. 2001. Visualizing the generation of memory CD4 T cells in the whole body. *Nature* 410:101–105.

37. Ebert LM, Schaerli P, Moser B. 2005. Chemokine-mediated control of T cell traffic in lymphoid and peripheral tissues. *Mol Immunol* 42:799–809.

38. Cruz A, Torrado E, Carmona J, Fraga AG, Costa P, Rodrigues F, Appelberg R, Correia-Neves M, Cooper AM, Saraiva M, Pedrosa J, Castro AG. 2015. BCG vaccination-induced long-lasting control of *Mycobacterium tuberculosis* correlates with the accumulation of a novel population of CD4⁺IL-17⁺TNF⁺IL-2⁺ T cells. *Vaccine* 33:85–91.

39. Ancelet LR, Aldwell FE, Rich FJ, Kirman JR. 2012. Oral vaccination with lipid-formulated BCG induces a long-lived, multifunctional CD4(+) T cell memory immune response. *PLoS One* 7:e45888.

40. White AD, Sarfas C, West K, Sibley LS, Wareham AS, Clark S, Dennis MJ, Williams A, Marsh PD, Sharpe SA. 2015. Evaluation of the immunogenicity of *Mycobacterium bovis* BCG delivered by aerosol to the lungs of macaques. *Clin Vaccine Immunol* 22:992–1003.

41. Soares AP, Kwong Chung CK, Choice T, Hughes EJ, Jacobs G, van Rensburg EJ, Khomba G, de Kock M, Lerumo L, Makhethe L, Maneli MH, Pienaar B, Smit E, Tena-Coki NG, van Wyk L, Boom WH, Kaplan G, Scriba TJ, Hanekom WA. 2013. Longitudinal changes in CD4(+) T-cell memory responses induced by BCG vaccination of newborns. *J Infect Dis* 207:1084–1094.

42. Tena-Coki NG, Scriba TJ, Peteni N, Eley B, Wilkinson RJ, Andersen P, Hanekom WA, Kampmann B. 2010. CD4 and CD8 T-cell responses to mycobacterial antigens in African children. *Am J Respir Crit Care Med* 182:120–129.

43. Andersen P, Smedegaard B. 2000. CD4(+) T-cell subsets that mediate immunological memory to *Mycobacterium tuberculosis* infection in mice. *Infect Immun* 68:621–629.

44. Kipnis A, Irwin S, Izzo AA, Basaraba RJ, Orme IM. 2005. Memory T lymphocytes generated by *Mycobacterium bovis* BCG vaccination reside within a CD4 CD44lo CD62 ligand(hi) population. *Infect Immun* 73:7759–7764.

45. Ancelet L, Rich FJ, Delahunt B, Kirman JR. 2012. Dissecting memory T cell responses to TB: concerns using adoptive transfer into immunodeficient mice. *Tuberculosis (Edinb)* 92:422–433.

46. Wherry EJ, Teichgräber V, Becker TC, Masopust D, Kaech SM, Antia R, von Andrian UH, Ahmed R. 2003. Lineage relationship and protective immunity of memory CD8 T cell subsets. *Nat Immunol* 4:225–234.

47. Orme IM. 2010. The Achilles heel of BCG. *Tuberculosis (Edinb)* 90:329–332.

48. Lindenstrøm T, Knudsen NP, Agger EM, Andersen P. 2013. Control of chronic mycobacterium tuberculosis infection by CD4 KLRG1- IL-2-secreting central memory cells. *J Immunol* 190:6311–6319.

49. Henao-Tamayo MI, Ordway DJ, Irwin SM, Shang S, Shanley C, Orme IM. 2010. Phenotypic definition of effector and memory T-lymphocyte subsets in mice chronically infected with *Mycobacterium tuberculosis*. *Clin Vaccine Immunol* 17:618–625.

50. Gebhardt T, Wakim LM, Eidsmo L, Reading PC, Heath WR, Carbone FR. 2009. Memory T cells in nonlymphoid tissue that provide enhanced local immunity during infection with herpes simplex virus. *Nat Immunol* 10:524–530.

51. Glennie ND, Yeramilli VA, Beiting DP, Volk SW, Weaver CT, Scott P. 2015. Skin-resident memory CD4+ T cells enhance protection against *Leishmania major* infection. *J Exp Med* 212:1405–1414.

52. Teijaro JR, Turner D, Pham Q, Wherry EJ, Lefrançois L, Farber DL. 2011. Cutting edge: tissue-retentive lung memory CD4 T cells mediate optimal protection to respiratory virus infection. *J Immunol* 187:5510–5514.

53. Giri PK, Verma I, Khuller GK. 2006. Protective efficacy of intranasal vaccination with *Mycobacterium bovis* BCG against airway *Mycobacterium tuberculosis* challenge in mice. *J Infect* 53:350–356.

54. Derrick SC, Kolibab K, Yang A, Morris SL. 2014. Intranasal administration of *Mycobacterium bovis* BCG induces superior protection against aerosol infection with *Mycobacterium tuberculosis* in mice. *Clin Vaccine Immunol* 21:1443–1451.

55. Barclay WR, Busey WM, Dalgard DW, Good RC, Janicki BW, Kasik JE, Ribi E, Ulrich CE, Wolinsky E. 1973. Protection of monkeys against airborne tuberculosis by aerosol vaccination with bacillus Calmette-Guerin. *Am Rev Respir Dis* 107:351–358.

56. Connor LM, Harvie MC, Rich FJ, Quinn KM, Brinkmann V, Le Gros G, Kirman JR. 2010. A key role for lung-resident memory lymphocytes in protective immune responses after BCG vaccination. *Eur J Immunol* 40:2482–2492.

57. Sakai S, Kauffman KD, Schenkel JM, McBerry CC, Mayer-Barber KD, Masopust D, Barber DL. 2014. Cutting edge: control of *Mycobacterium tuberculosis* infection by a subset of lung parenchyma-homing CD4 T cells. *J Immunol* 192:2965–2969.

58. Moguche AO, Shafiani S, Clemons C, Larson RP, Dinh C, Higdon LE, Cambier CJ, Sissons JR, Gallegos AM, Fink PJ, Urdahl KB. 2015. ICOS and Bcl6-dependent pathways maintain a CD4 T cell population with memory-like properties during tuberculosis. *J Exp Med* 212:715–728.

59. Gattinoni L, Lugli E, Ji Y, Pos Z, Paulos CM, Quigley MF, Almeida JR, Gostick E, Yu Z, Carpenito C, Wang E, Douek DC, Price DA, June CH, Marincola FM, Roederer M, Restifo NP. 2011. A human memory T cell subset with stem cell-like properties. *Nat Med* 17:1290–1297.

60. Stemberger C, Neuenhahn M, Gebhardt FE, Schiemann M, Buchholz VR, Busch DH. 2009. Stem cell-like plasticity of naïve and distinct memory CD8+ T cell subsets. *Semin Immunol* 21:62–68.

61. Gattinoni L, Zhong XS, Palmer DC, Ji Y, Hinrichs CS, Yu Z, Wrzesinski C, Boni A, Cassard L, Garvin LM, Paulos CM, Muranski P, Restifo NP. 2009. Wnt signaling arrests effector T cell differentiation and generates CD8+ memory stem cells. *Nat Med* 15:808–813.

62. Graef P, Buchholz VR, Stemberger C, Flossdorf M, Henkel L, Schiemann M, Drexler I, Höfer T, Riddell SR, Busch DH. 2014. Serial transfer of single-cell-derived immunocompetence reveals stemness of CD8(+) central memory T cells. *Immunity* 41:116–126.

63. Pompei L, Jang S, Zamlynny B, Ravikumar S, McBride A, Hickman SP, Salgame P. 2007. Disparity in IL-12 release in dendritic cells and macrophages in response

to Mycobacterium tuberculosis is due to use of distinct TLRs. *J Immunol* 178:5192–5199.

64. Wu CY, Kirman JR, Rotte MJ, Davey DF, Perfetto SP, Rhee EG, Freidag BL, Hill BJ, Douek DC, Seder RA. 2002. Distinct lineages of T(H)1 cells have differential capacities for memory cell generation in vivo. *Nat Immunol* 3:852–858.

65. Harrington LE, Janowski KM, Oliver JR, Zajac AJ, Weaver CT. 2008. Memory CD4 T cells emerge from effector T-cell progenitors. *Nature* 452:356–360.

66. Leveton C, Barnass S, Champion B, Lucas S, De Souza B, Nicol M, Banerjee D, Rook G. 1989. T-cell-mediated protection of mice against virulent *Mycobacterium tuberculosis. Infect Immun* 57:390–395.

67. Flory CM, Hubbard RD, Collins FM. 1992. Effects of in vivo T lymphocyte subset depletion on mycobacterial infections in mice. *J Leukoc Biol* 51:225–229.

68. Müller I, Cobbold SP, Waldmann H, Kaufmann SH. 1987. Impaired resistance to *Mycobacterium tuberculosis* infection after selective in vivo depletion of L3T4+ and Lyt-2+ T cells. *Infect Immun* 55:2037–2041.

69. Cooper AM, Dalton DK, Stewart TA, Griffin JP, Russell DG, Orme IM. 1993. Disseminated tuberculosis in interferon gamma gene-disrupted mice. *J Exp Med* 178:2243–2247.

70. Jouanguy E, Altare F, Lamhamedi S, Revy P, Emile JF, Newport M, Levin M, Blanche S, Seboun E, Fischer A, Casanova JL. 1996. Interferon-gamma-receptor deficiency in an infant with fatal bacille Calmette-Guérin infection. *N Engl J Med* 335:1956–1961.

71. Jouanguy E, Lamhamedi-Cherradi S, Altare F, Fondanèche MC, Tuerlinckx D, Blanche S, Emile JF, Gaillard JL, Schreiber R, Levin M, Fischer A, Hivroz C, Casanova JL. 1997. Partial interferon-gamma receptor 1 deficiency in a child with tuberculoid bacillus Calmette-Guérin infection and a sibling with clinical tuberculosis. *J Clin Invest* 100:2658–2664.

72. Green AM, Difazio R, Flynn JL. 2013. IFN-γ from CD4 T cells is essential for host survival and enhances CD8 T cell function during *Mycobacterium tuberculosis* infection. *J Immunol* 190:270–277.

73. Leal IS, Smedegård B, Andersen P, Appelberg R. 2001. Failure to induce enhanced protection against tuberculosis by increasing T-cell-dependent interferon-gamma generation. *Immunology* 104:157–161.

74. Mittrücker HW, Steinhoff U, Köhler A, Krause M, Lazar D, Mex P, Miekley D, Kaufmann SH. 2007. Poor correlation between BCG vaccination-induced T cell responses and protection against tuberculosis. *Proc Natl Acad Sci USA* 104:12434–12439.

75. Elias D, Akuffo H, Britton S. 2005. PPD induced in vitro interferon gamma production is not a reliable correlate of protection against *Mycobacterium tuberculosis. Trans R Soc Trop Med Hyg* 99:363–368.

76. Majlessi L, Simsova M, Jarvis Z, Brodin P, Rojas MJ, Bauche C, Nouzé C, Ladant D, Cole ST, Sebo P, Leclerc C. 2006. An increase in antimycobacterial Th1-cell responses by prime-boost protocols of immunization does not enhance protection against tuberculosis. *Infect Immun* 74:2128–2137.

77. Kagina BM, Abel B, Scriba TJ, Hughes EJ, Keyser A, Soares A, Gamieldien H, Sidibana M, Hatherill M, Gelderbloem S, Mahomed H, Hawkridge A, Hussey G, Kaplan G, Hanekom WA; other members of the South African Tuberculosis Vaccine Initiative. 2010. Specific T cell frequency and cytokine expression profile do not correlate with protection against tuberculosis after bacillus Calmette-Guérin vaccination of newborns. *Am J Respir Crit Care Med* 182:1073–1079.

78. Cowley SC, Elkins KL. 2003. CD4+ T cells mediate IFN-gamma-independent control of *Mycobacterium tuberculosis* infection both in vitro and in vivo. *J Immunol* 171:4689–4699.

79. Scriba TJ, Tameris M, Mansoor N, Smit E, van der Merwe L, Isaacs F, Keyser A, Moyo S, Brittain N, Lawrie A, Gelderbloem S, Veldsman A, Hatherill M, Hawkridge A, Hill AV, Hussey GD, Mahomed H, McShane H, Hanekom WA. 2010. Modified vaccinia Ankara-expressing Ag85A, a novel tuberculosis vaccine, is safe in adolescents and children, and induces polyfunctional CD4+ T cells. *Eur J Immunol* 40:279–290.

80. Hawkridge T, Scriba TJ, Gelderbloem S, Smit E, Tameris M, Moyo S, Lang T, Veldsman A, Hatherill M, Merwe L, Fletcher HA, Mahomed H, Hill AV, Hanekom WA, Hussey GD, McShane H. 2008. Safety and immunogenicity of a new tuberculosis vaccine, MVA85A, in healthy adults in South Africa. *J Infect Dis* 198:544–552.

81. Darrah PA, Bolton DL, Lackner AA, Kaushal D, Aye PP, Mehra S, Blanchard JL, Didier PJ, Roy CJ, Rao SS, Hokey DA, Scanga CA, Sizemore DR, Sadoff JC, Roederer M, Seder RA. 2014. Aerosol vaccination with AERAS-402 elicits robust cellular immune responses in the lungs of rhesus macaques but fails to protect against high-dose *Mycobacterium tuberculosis* challenge. *J Immunol* 193:1799–1811.

82. Peng MY, Wang ZH, Yao CY, Jiang LN, Jin QL, Wang J, Li BQ. 2008. Interleukin 17-producing gamma delta T cells increased in patients with active pulmonary tuberculosis. *Cell Mol Immunol* 5:203–208.

83. Lockhart E, Green AM, Flynn JL. 2006. IL-17 production is dominated by gammadelta T cells rather than CD4 T cells during *Mycobacterium tuberculosis* infection. *J Immunol* 177:4662–4669.

84. Bettelli E, Carrier Y, Gao W, Korn T, Strom TB, Oukka M, Weiner HL, Kuchroo VK. 2006. Reciprocal developmental pathways for the generation of pathogenic effector TH17 and regulatory T cells. *Nature* 441:235–238.

85. Yang XO, Pappu BP, Nurieva R, Akimzhanov A, Kang HS, Chung Y, Ma L, Shah B, Panopoulos AD, Schluns KS, Watowich SS, Tian Q, Jetten AM, Dong C. 2008. T helper 17 lineage differentiation is programmed by orphan nuclear receptors ROR alpha and ROR gamma. *Immunity* 28:29–39.

86. Rouvier E, Luciani MF, Mattéi MG, Denizot F, Golstein P. 1993. CTLA-8, cloned from an activated T cell, bearing AU-rich messenger RNA instability sequences, and homologous to a herpesvirus saimiri gene. *J Immunol* 150:5445–5456.

87. Ye P, Rodriguez FH, Kanaly S, Stocking KL, Schurr J, Schwarzenberger P, Oliver P, Huang W, Zhang P, Zhang J, Shellito JE, Bagby GJ, Nelson S, Charrier K, Peschon JJ, Kolls JK. 2001. Requirement of interleukin 17 receptor signaling for lung CXC chemokine and granulocyte colony-stimulating factor expression, neutrophil recruitment, and host defense. *J Exp Med* **194:** 519–527.

88. Guglani L, Khader SA. 2010. Th17 cytokines in mucosal immunity and inflammation. *Curr Opin HIV AIDS* **5:**120–127.

89. Cruz A, Fraga AG, Fountain JJ, Rangel-Moreno J, Torrado E, Saraiva M, Pereira DR, Randall TD, Pedrosa J, Cooper AM, Castro AG. 2010. Pathological role of interleukin 17 in mice subjected to repeated BCG vaccination after infection with *Mycobacterium tuberculosis*. *J Exp Med* **207:**1609–1616.

90. Griffiths KL, Stylianou E, Poyntz HC, Betts GJ, Fletcher HA, McShane H. 2013. Cholera toxin enhances vaccine-induced protection against *Mycobacterium tuberculosis* challenge in mice. *PLoS One* **8:**e78312.

91. Aagaard C, Hoang T, Dietrich J, Cardona PJ, Izzo A, Dolganov G, Schoolnik GK, Cassidy JP, Billeskov R, Andersen P. 2011. A multistage tuberculosis vaccine that confers efficient protection before and after exposure. *Nat Med* **17:**189–194.

92. Desel C, Dorhoi A, Bandermann S, Grode L, Eisele B, Kaufmann SH. 2011. Recombinant BCG ΔureC hly+ induces superior protection over parental BCG by stimulating a balanced combination of type 1 and type 17 cytokine responses. *J Infect Dis* **204:**1573–1584.

93. Acosta-Rodriguez EV, Rivino L, Geginat J, Jarrossay D, Gattorno M, Lanzavecchia A, Sallusto F, Napolitani G. 2007. Surface phenotype and antigenic specificity of human interleukin 17-producing T helper memory cells. *Nat Immunol* **8:**639–646.

94. Marín ND, París SC, Rojas M, García LF. 2012. Reduced frequency of memory T cells and increased Th17 responses in patients with active tuberculosis. *Clin Vaccine Immunol* **19:**1667–1676.

95. Nunnari G, Pinzone MR, Vancheri C, Palermo F, Cacopardo B. 2013. Interferon-γ and interleukin-17 production from PPD-stimulated PBMCss of patients with pulmonary tuberculosis. *Clin Invest Med* **36:**E64–E71.

96. Perreau M, Rozot V, Welles HC, Belluti-Enders F, Vigano S, Maillard M, Dorta G, Mazza-Stalder J, Bart PA, Roger T, Calandra T, Nicod L, Harari A. 2013. Lack of *Mycobacterium tuberculosis*-specific interleukin-17A-producing CD4+ T cells in active disease. *Eur J Immunol* **43:**939–948.

97. Loxton AG, Black GF, Stanley K, Walzl G. 2012. Heparin-binding hemagglutinin induces IFN-γ(+) IL-2(+) IL-17(+) multifunctional CD4(+) T cells during latent but not active tuberculosis disease. *Clin Vaccine Immunol* **19:**746–751.

98. Kumar NP, Anuradha R, Suresh R, Ganesh R, Shankar J, Kumaraswami V, Nutman TB, Babu S. 2011. Suppressed type 1, type 2, and type 17 cytokine responses in active tuberculosis in children. *Clin Vaccine Immunol* **18:**1856–1864.

99. Chen X, Zhang M, Liao M, Graner MW, Wu C, Yang Q, Liu H, Zhou B. 2010. Reduced Th17 response in patients with tuberculosis correlates with IL-6R expression on CD4+ T Cells. *Am J Respir Crit Care Med* **181:**734–742.

100. Sutherland JS, Adetifa IM, Hill PC, Adegbola RA, Ota MO. 2009. Pattern and diversity of cytokine production differentiates between *Mycobacterium tuberculosis* infection and disease. *Eur J Immunol* **39:**723–729.

101. Scriba TJ, Kalsdorf B, Abrahams DA, Isaacs F, Hofmeister J, Black G, Hassan HY, Wilkinson RJ, Walzl G, Gelderbloem SJ, Mahomed H, Hussey GD, Hanekom WA. 2008. Distinct, specific IL-17- and IL-22-producing CD4+ T cell subsets contribute to the human anti-mycobacterial immune response. *J Immunol* **180:**1962–1970.

102. Matthews K, Wilkinson KA, Kalsdorf B, Roberts T, Diacon A, Walzl G, Wolske J, Ntsekhe M, Syed F, Russell J, Mayosi BM, Dawson R, Dheda K, Wilkinson RJ, Hanekom WA, Scriba TJ. 2011. Predominance of interleukin-22 over interleukin-17 at the site of disease in human tuberculosis. *Tuberculosis (Edinb)* **91:**587–593.

103. Khader SA, Bell GK, Pearl JE, Fountain JJ, Rangel-Moreno J, Cilley GE, Shen F, Eaton SM, Gaffen SL, Swain SL, Locksley RM, Haynes L, Randall TD, Cooper AM. 2007. IL-23 and IL-17 in the establishment of protective pulmonary CD4+ T cell responses after vaccination and during *Mycobacterium tuberculosis* challenge. *Nat Immunol* **8:**369–377.

104. Lalor MK, Floyd S, Gorak-Stolinska P, Ben-Smith A, Weir RE, Smith SG, Newport MJ, Blitz R, Mvula H, Branson K, McGrath N, Crampin AC, Fine PE, Dockrell HM. 2011. BCG vaccination induces different cytokine profiles following infant BCG vaccination in the UK and Malawi. *J Infect Dis* **204:**1075–1085.

105. Smith SG, Lalor MK, Gorak-Stolinska P, Blitz R, Beveridge NE, Worth A, McShane H, Dockrell HM. 2010. *Mycobacterium tuberculosis* PPD-induced immune biomarkers measurable in vitro following BCG vaccination of UK adolescents by multiplex bead array and intracellular cytokine staining. *BMC Immunol* **11:**35.

106. Kassa D, Ran L, Geberemeskel W, Tebeje M, Alemu A, Selase A, Tegbaru B, Franken KL, Friggen AH, van Meijgaarden KE, Ottenhoff TH, Wolday D, Messele T, van Baarle D. 2012. Analysis of immune responses against a wide range of *Mycobacterium tuberculosis* antigens in patients with active pulmonary tuberculosis. *Clin Vaccine Immunol* **19:**1907–1915.

107. Basile JI, Geffner LJ, Romero MM, Balboa L, Sabio Y García C, Ritacco V, García A, Cuffré M, Abbate E, López B, Barrera L, Ambroggi M, Alemán M, Sasiain MC, de la Barrera SS. 2011. Outbreaks of mycobacterium tuberculosis MDR strains induce high IL-17 T-cell response inpatients with MDR tuberculosis that is closely associated with high antigen load. *J Infect Dis* **204:**1054–1064.

108. Gopal R, Monin L, Slight S, Uche U, Blanchard E, Fallert Junecko BA, Ramos-Payan R, Stallings CL, Reinhart TA, Kolls JK, Kaushal D, Nagarajan U,

Rangel-Moreno J, Khader SA. 2014. Unexpected role for IL-17 in protective immunity against hypervirulent *Mycobacterium tuberculosis* HN878 infection. *PLoS Pathog* 10:e1004099.

109. Khader SA, Pearl JE, Sakamoto K, Gilmartin L, Bell GK, Jelley-Gibbs DM, Ghilardi N, deSauvage F, Cooper AM. 2005. IL-23 compensates for the absence of IL-12p70 and is essential for the IL-17 response during tuberculosis but is dispensable for protection and antigen-specific IFN-gamma responses if IL-12p70 is available. *J Immunol* 175:788–795.

110. Cooper AM, Khader SA. 2008. The role of cytokines in the initiation, expansion, and control of cellular immunity to tuberculosis. *Immunol Rev* 226:191–204.

111. Gopal R, Rangel-Moreno J, Slight S, Lin Y, Nawar HF, Fallert Junecko BA, Reinhart TA, Kolls J, Randall TD, Connell TD, Khader SA. 2013. Interleukin-17-dependent CXCL13 mediates mucosal vaccine-induced immunity against tuberculosis. *Mucosal Immunol* 6:972–984.

112. Wozniak TM, Saunders BM, Ryan AA, Britton WJ. 2010. Mycobacterium bovis BCG-specific Th17 cells confer partial protection against *Mycobacterium tuberculosis* infection in the absence of gamma interferon. *Infect Immun* 78:4187–4194.

113. Werninghaus K, Babiak A, Gross O, Hölscher C, Dietrich H, Agger EM, Mages J, Mocsai A, Schoenen H, Finger K, Nimmerjahn F, Brown GD, Kirschning C, Heit A, Andersen P, Wagner H, Ruland J, Lang R. 2009. Adjuvanticity of a synthetic cord factor analogue for subunit *Mycobacterium tuberculosis* vaccination requires FcRgamma-Syk-Card9-dependent innate immune activation. *J Exp Med* 206:89–97.

114. Lindenstrøm T, Woodworth J, Dietrich J, Aagaard C, Andersen P, Agger EM. 2012. Vaccine-induced th17 cells are maintained long-term postvaccination as a distinct and phenotypically stable memory subset. *Infect Immun* 80:3533–3544.

115. Orr MT, Beebe EA, Hudson TE, Argilla D, Huang PW, Reese VA, Fox CB, Reed SG, Coler RN. 2015. Mucosal delivery switches the response to an adjuvanted tuberculosis vaccine from systemic TH1 to tissue-resident TH17 responses without impacting the protective efficacy. *Vaccine* 33:6570–6578.

116. Stenger S, Hanson DA, Teitelbaum R, Dewan P, Niazi KR, Froelich CJ, Ganz T, Thoma-Uszynski S, Melián A, Bogdan C, Porcelli SA, Bloom BR, Krensky AM, Modlin RL. 1998. An antimicrobial activity of cytolytic T cells mediated by granulysin. *Science* 282:121–125.

117. Lu CC, Wu TS, Hsu YJ, Chang CJ, Lin CS, Chia JH, Wu TL, Huang TT, Martel J, Ojcius DM, Young JD, Lai HC. 2014. NK cells kill mycobacteria directly by releasing perforin and granulysin. *J Leukoc Biol* 96:1119–1129.

118. Tzelepis F, Verway M, Daoud J, Gillard J, Hassani-Ardakani K, Dunn J, Downey J, Gentile ME, Jaworska J, Sanchez AM, Nédélec Y, Vali H, Tabrizian M, Kristof AS, King IL, Barreiro LB, Divangahi M. 2015. Annexin1 regulates DC efferocytosis and cross-presentation during *Mycobacterium tuberculosis* infection. *J Clin Invest* 125:752–768.

119. Harriff MJ, Purdy GE, Lewinsohn DM. 2012. Escape from the phagosome: the explanation for MHC-I processing of mycobacterial antigens? *Front Immunol* 3:40.

120. Leavy O. 2011. Antigen presentation: cross-dress to impress. *Nat Rev Immunol* 11:302–303.

121. Behar SM, Baehrecke EH. 2015. Tuberculosis: autophagy is not the answer. *Nature* 528:482–483.

122. Silva CL, Bonato VL, Lima VM, Faccioli LH, Leão SC. 1999. Characterization of the memory/activated T cells that mediate the long-lived host response against tuberculosis after bacillus Calmette-Guérin or DNA vaccination. *Immunology* 97:573–581.

123. Wang J, Santosuosso M, Ngai P, Zganiacz A, Xing Z. 2004. Activation of CD8 T cells by mycobacterial vaccination protects against pulmonary tuberculosis in the absence of CD4 T cells. *J Immunol* 173:4590–4597.

124. Jeyanathan M, Mu J, McCormick S, Damjanovic D, Small CL, Shaler CR, Kugathasan K, Xing Z. 2010. Murine airway luminal antituberculosis memory CD8 T cells by mucosal immunization are maintained via antigen-driven in situ proliferation, independent of peripheral T cell recruitment. *Am J Respir Crit Care Med* 181:862–872.

125. Kamath A, Woodworth JS, Behar SM. 2006. Antigen-specific CD8+ T cells and the development of central memory during *Mycobacterium tuberculosis* infection. *J Immunol* 177:6361–6369.

126. Serbina NV, Flynn JL. 2001. CD8(+) T cells participate in the memory immune response to *Mycobacterium tuberculosis*. *Infect Immun* 69:4320–4328.

127. Carpenter SM, Nunes-Alves C, Booty MG, Way SS, Behar SM. 2016. A higher activation threshold of memory CD8+ T cells has a fitness cost that is modified by TCR affinity during tuberculosis. *PLoS Pathog* 12:e1005380.

128. Hess J, Miko D, Catic A, Lehmensiek V, Russell DG, Kaufmann SH. 1998. *Mycobacterium bovis* Bacille Calmette-Guérin strains secreting listeriolysin of *Listeria monocytogenes*. *Proc Natl Acad Sci USA* 95:5299–5304.

129. Sun R, Skeiky YA, Izzo A, Dheenadhayalan V, Imam Z, Penn E, Stagliano K, Haddock S, Mueller S, Fulkerson J, Scanga C, Grover A, Derrick SC, Morris S, Hone DM, Horwitz MA, Kaufmann SH, Sadoff JC. 2009. Novel recombinant BCG expressing perfringolysin O and the over-expression of key immunodominant antigens; pre-clinical characterization, safety and protection against challenge with *Mycobacterium tuberculosis*. *Vaccine* 27:4412–4423.

130. Derrick SC, Repique C, Snoy P, Yang AL, Morris S. 2004. Immunization with a DNA vaccine cocktail protects mice lacking CD4 cells against an aerogenic infection with *Mycobacterium tuberculosis*. *Infect Immun* 72:1685–1692.

131. Coppel S, Youmans GP. 1969. Specificity of acquired resistance produced by immunization with mycobacterial cells and mycobacterial fractions. *J Bacteriol* 97:114–120.

132. Smrkovski LL, Larson CL. 1977. Effect of treatment with BCG on the course of visceral leishmaniasis in BALB/c mice. *Infect Immun* 16:249–257.

133. Ghadirian E, Kongshavn PA. 1986. Protection of mice against intestinal amoebiasis with BCG, *Corynebacterium parvum* and *Listeria monocytogenes*. *Parasite Immunol* **8**:663–667.

134. de Castro MJ, Pardo-Seco J, Martinón-Torres F. 2015. Nonspecific (heterologous) protection of neonatal BCG vaccination against hospitalization due to respiratory infection and sepsis. *Clin Infect Dis* **60**:1611–1619.

135. Jensen KJ, Larsen N, Biering-Sørensen S, Andersen A, Eriksen HB, Monteiro I, Hougaard D, Aaby P, Netea MG, Flanagan KL, Benn CS. 2015. Heterologous immunological effects of early BCG vaccination in low-birth-weight infants in Guinea-Bissau: a randomized-controlled trial. *J Infect Dis* **211**:956–967.

136. Ritz N, Mui M, Balloch A, Curtis N. 2013. Non-specific effect of Bacille Calmette-Guérin vaccine on the immune response to routine immunisations. *Vaccine* **31**:3098–3103.

137. Netea MG, Quintin J, van der Meer JW. 2011. Trained immunity: a memory for innate host defense. *Cell Host Microbe* **9**:355–361.

138. Kleinnijenhuis J, Quintin J, Preijers F, Joosten LA, Ifrim DC, Saeed S, Jacobs C, van Loenhout J, de Jong D, Stunnenberg HG, Xavier RJ, van der Meer JW, van Crevel R, Netea MG. 2012. Bacille Calmette-Guerin induces NOD2-dependent nonspecific protection from reinfection via epigenetic reprogramming of monocytes. *Proc Natl Acad Sci USA* **109**:17537–17542.

139. Kleinnijenhuis J, Quintin J, Preijers F, Benn CS, Joosten LA, Jacobs C, van Loenhout J, Xavier RJ, Aaby P, van der Meer JW, van Crevel R, Netea MG. 2014. Long-lasting effects of BCG vaccination on both heterologous Th1/Th17 responses and innate trained immunity. *J Innate Immun* **6**:152–158.

140. Sun JC, Beilke JN, Lanier LL. 2009. Adaptive immune features of natural killer cells. *Nature* **457**:557–561.

141. Fu X, Liu Y, Li L, Li Q, Qiao D, Wang H, Lao S, Fan Y, Wu C. 2011. Human natural killer cells expressing the memory-associated marker CD45RO from tuberculous pleurisy respond more strongly and rapidly than CD45RO- natural killer cells following stimulation with interleukin-12. *Immunology* **134**:41–49.

142. Davids V, Hanekom WA, Mansoor N, Gamieldien H, Gelderbloem SJ, Hawkridge A, Hussey GD, Hughes EJ, Soler J, Murray RA, Ress SR, Kaplan G. 2006. The effect of bacille Calmette-Guérin vaccine strain and route of administration on induced immune responses in vaccinated infants. *J Infect Dis* **193**:531–536.

143. Fine PE. 1995. Variation in protection by BCG: implications of and for heterologous immunity. *Lancet* **346**: 1339–1345.

144. Aronson NE, Santosham M, Comstock GW, Howard RS, Moulton LH, Rhoades ER, Harrison LH. 2004. Long-term efficacy of BCG vaccine in American Indians and Alaska Natives: a 60-year follow-up study. *JAMA* **291**:2086–2091.

145. Barreto ML, Rodrigues LC, Cunha SS, Pereira S, Hijjar MA, Ichihara MY, de Brito SC, Dourado I. 2002. Design of the Brazilian BCG-REVAC trial against tuberculosis: a large, simple randomized community trial to evaluate the impact on tuberculosis of BCG revaccination at school age. *Control Clin Trials* **23**:540–553.

146. Abubakar I, Pimpin L, Ariti C, Beynon R, Mangtani P, Sterne JA, Fine PE, Smith PG, Lipman M, Elliman D, Watson JM, Drumright LN, Whiting PF, Vynnycky E, Rodrigues LC. 2013. Systematic review and meta-analysis of the current evidence on the duration of protection by bacillus Calmette-Guérin vaccination against tuberculosis. *Health Technol Assess* **17**:1–372, v–vi.

147. Tameris M, Geldenhuys H, Luabeya AK, Smit E, Hughes JE, Vermaak S, Hanekom WA, Hatherill M, Mahomed H, McShane H, Scriba TJ. 2014. The candidate TB vaccine, MVA85A, induces highly durable Th1 responses. *PLoS One* **9**:e87340.

148. Billeskov R, Christensen JP, Aagaard C, Andersen P, Dietrich J. 2013. Comparing adjuvanted H28 and modified vaccinia virus ankara expressingH28 in a mouse and a non-human primate tuberculosis model. *PLoS One* **8**:e72185.

149. van Dissel JT, Arend SM, Prins C, Bang P, Tingskov PN, Lingnau K, Nouta J, Klein MR, Rosenkrands I, Ottenhoff TH, Kromann I, Doherty TM, Andersen P. 2010. Ag85B-ESAT-6 adjuvanted with IC31 promotes strong and long-lived *Mycobacterium tuberculosis* specific T cell responses in naïve human volunteers. *Vaccine* **28**:3571–3581.

150. van Dissel JT, Joosten SA, Hoff ST, Soonawala D, Prins C, Hokey DA, O'Dee DM, Graves A, Thierry-Carstensen B, Andreasen LV, Ruhwald M, de Visser AW, Agger EM, Ottenhoff TH, Kromann I, Andersen P. 2014. A novel liposomal adjuvant system, CAF01, promotes long-lived *Mycobacterium tuberculosis*-specific T-cell responses in human. *Vaccine* **32**:7098–7107.

151. Reither K, Katsoulis L, Beattie T, Gardiner N, Lenz N, Said K, Mfinanga E, Pohl C, Fielding KL, Jeffery H, Kagina BM, Hughes EJ, Scriba TJ, Hanekom WA, Hoff ST, Bang P, Kromann I, Daubenberger C, Andersen P, Churchyard GJ. 2014. Safety and immunogenicity of H1/IC31, an adjuvanted TB subunit vaccine, in HIV-infected adults with CD4+ lymphocyte counts greater than 350 cells/mm3: a phase II, multi-centre, double-blind, randomized, placebo-controlled trial. *PLoS One* **9**:e114602.

152. Luabeya AK, Kagina BM, Tameris MD, Geldenhuys H, Hoff ST, Shi Z, Kromann I, Hatherill M, Mahomed H, Hanekom WA, Andersen P, Scriba TJ, Schoeman E, Krohn C, Day CL, Africa H, Makhethe L, Smit E, Brown Y, Suliman S, Hughes EJ, Bang P, Snowden MA, McClain B, Hussey GD, Hussey GD. 2015. First-in-human trial of the post-exposure tuberculosis vaccine H56:IC31 in *Mycobacterium tuberculosis* infected and non-infected healthy adults. *Vaccine* **33**:4130–4140.

153. Montoya J, Solon JA, Cunanan SR, Acosta L, Bollaerts A, Moris P, Janssens M, Jongert E, Demoitié MA, Mettens P, Gatchalian S, Vinals C, Cohen J, Ofori-Anyinam O. 2013. A randomized, controlled dose-finding Phase II study of the M72/AS01 candidate tuberculosis vaccine in healthy PPD-positive adults. *J Clin Immunol* **33**:1360–1375.

154. World Health Organization. 2015. *Global Tuberculosis Report 2015*. WHO Press, Geneva, Switzerland.

155. Qaqish A, Huang D, Chen CY, Zhang Z, Wang R, Li S, Yang E, Lu Y, Larsen MH, Jacobs WR Jr, Qian L, Frencher J, Shen L, Chen ZW. 2017. Adoptive transfer of phosphoantigen-specific γδ T cell subset attenuates *Mycobacterium tuberculosis* infection in nonhuman primates. *J Immunol* **198:**4753–4763.

156. Arts RJ, Carvalho A, La Rocca C, Palma C, Rodrigues F, Silvestre R, Kleinnijenhuis J, Lachmandas E, Gonçalves LG, Belinha A, Cunha C, Oosting M, Joosten LA, Matarese G, van Crevel R, Netea MG. 2016. Immunometabolic pathways in BCG-induced trained immunity. *Cell Rep* **17:**2562–2571.

Tuberculosis and the Tubercle Bacillus, 2nd ed.
Edited by William R. Jacobs, Jr., Helen McShane, Valerie Mizrahi, and Ian M. Orme
© 2018 American Society for Microbiology, Washington, DC
doi:10.1128/microbiolspec.TBTB2-0029-2016

Pathology of Tuberculosis: How the Pathology of Human Tuberculosis Informs and Directs Animal Models

5

Randall J. Basaraba[1] and Robert L. Hunter[2]

INTRODUCTION

Progress toward developing new strategies to control the spread of *Mycobacterium tuberculosis* is limited by a poor understanding of the basic pathogenesis of post-primary tuberculosis (TB). Progress is being made in developing more rapid diagnostic assays and implementing new anti-TB drug combinations, but we are failing to answer key scientific questions that will further advance the development of new treatment and prevention strategies. In a recent statement, Dr. Anthony Fauci, head of the National Institute of Allergy and Infectious Diseases, said, "We need to better understand the delicate balance between the host and pathogen in the context of the entire biological system and this requires a radical and transformational approach." *M. tuberculosis* has coevolved with its human host for centuries. The more recent emergence of antimicrobial drug-resistant strains represents an additional challenge to controlling the global spread of TB. No new TB vaccines have been shown to be more effective than the original bacillus Calmette-Guérin (BCG) developed over 100 years ago. The development of new anti-TB drugs lags far behind the need, and prospects for host-directed therapies have validated neither targets nor biomarkers.

In nature, *M. tuberculosis* is a human, obligate, intracellular bacterial pathogen. While it can infect nearly any warm-blooded animal, the majority of experimentally infected laboratory animals cannot easily transmit the infection through aerosol exposure. In addition, while *M. tuberculosis* infections in small animal models consistently develop the acute stages of primary TB dis-

ease, they fail to develop the late stages of post-primary disease. Post-primary TB accounts for 80% of clinical disease and nearly 100% of transmission of infection in humans, yet very little is known about the pathogenesis. Gross and histopathological examination of tissues from human patients was central to the study of TB for 150 years, from 1800 until 1950. However, the use of pathology to study TB fell out of favor as a consequence of scientific advances and changing attitudes. First, the discovery of antibiotics that were effective against *M. tuberculosis* led many to believe that TB and other bacterial diseases would soon be eradicated and therefore not in need of further study. Second, the advances in the fields of immunology, molecular biology, and genetics in the second half of the 20th century replaced morphologic pathology as a cutting-edge science. Finally, fewer routine autopsies were performed on patients that died of TB or other diseases, which significantly decreased the availability of tissue samples to study early-stage disease. Lung samples from TB patients are still occasionally available following surgical excision as an adjunct to antimicrobial therapy, but these represent the most chronic stages of active TB disease and have limited value as a research resource.

As a consequence, when the value of the pathology of human and animal TB was again realized in the 1980s, appropriate tissue samples were seldom available. As a surrogate, a variety of animal models were used to help advance the basic understanding of TB pathology and pathogenesis as well as to better understand the impact vaccination and antimicrobial drug treatment have on the progression of active TB disease.

[1]Department of Microbiology, Immunology, and Pathology, College of Veterinary Medicine and Biomedical Sciences, Colorado State University, Fort Collins, CO 80524; [2]Department of Pathology and Laboratory Medicine, McGovern Medical School, University of Texas Health Science Center at Houston, Houston, TX 77030.

117

However, it became increasingly obvious that there were limitations to the use of animal models to study the basic pathogenesis of human pulmonary and extrapulmonary TB.

Many model species develop early lesions that resemble primary TB in humans (Fig. 1). However, with the possible exception of non-human primates, few animals develop the full spectrum of disease and, in particular, post-primary TB. One of the most important manifestations of post-primary TB is the development of thin-walled cavities that support proliferation of massive numbers of extracellular *M. tuberculosis* (Fig. 2,

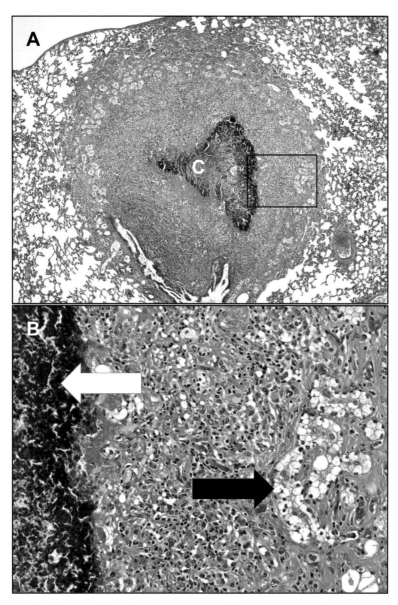

Figure 1   Well-delineated foci of granulomatous inflammation (granuloma) within the lung is a common manifestation of primary tuberculosis in humans and many laboratory animals. (**A**) A low-magnification view of a primary lung granuloma from an *M. tuberculosis*-infected guinea pig has an area of central necrosis that is partially calcified (**C**). (**B**) The wall of the lesion contains active lymphocytic and histiocytic inflammation and is well delineated from the surrounding normal lung parenchyma by a fibrous capsule that contains regenerative airway epithelium (black arrow). A higher-magnification view of the central dystrophic calcification (white arrow) shows residual tissue necrosis that harbors extracellular bacilli. Hematoxylin and eosin (H&E) stain.

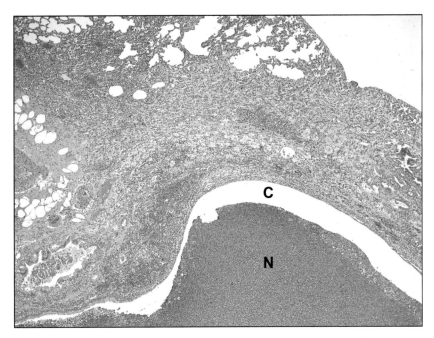

Figure 2 An important manifestation of post-primary TB in humans that is not seen in many small animal models is the formation of thin wall cavities. Cavity formation (C) represents one of the most destructive manifestations of active tuberculosis in humans and nonhuman primates. The lung parenchyma is replaced by an open space that often contains necrotic cellular debris (N) and myriads of extracellular and intracellular bacilli that can be transmitted between individuals though aerosol spread. The wall of the cavity consists of mixed inflammation similar to primary granulomas and similarly is delineated from the more normal parenchyma by a fibrous capsule that impairs the penetration of antimicrobial drugs. H&E stain.

Fig. 3), which increases the likelihood of transmission between individuals through aerosols. To survive and spread within the human population, *M. tuberculosis* induces a nonprotective immune response in some individuals that leads to extensive tissue damage and high bacterial burden, which if left untreated will result in death of the host. Some individuals, however, either clear the infection or remain healthy but harbor small numbers of bacilli that contribute to the development of reactivation disease later in life. In this way, *M. tuberculosis* persists within the population and serves as a reservoir of infection, thus maintaining the transmission cycle. Therefore, the coevolution of *M. tuberculosis* with humans has resulted in a complex, multifaceted host response such that individuals that develop active TB transmit soon after exposure, while those that remain asymptomatic have the potential to spread disease following the development of post-primary TB (2). Many attempts to identify the specific immune responses that determine whether the host response will be protective or result in active TB disease have been unsuccessful. What remains the fundamental, unanswered question is a poor understanding of how the

tubercle bacillus survives in the face of an aggressive immune response, thus creating a microenvironment that favors *M. tuberculosis* persistence (2).

Due to the relative lack of tissues from *M. tuberculosis*-infected patients, the current literature pertaining to TB pathology and pathogenesis is based almost entirely on animal studies using models that do not necessarily mimic all the important features of naturally occurring human disease (3–5). Stimulated by inconsistencies in the recent literature, we attempted to understand the pathology of human post-primary TB from studies published during the preantibiotic era as well as through the study of autopsy tissue samples obtained from untreated patients. Many of the books describing human TB pathology are either out of print or use unfamiliar nomenclature. More importantly, gross and histopathological images or illustrations from this literature are either nonexistent or of poor quality and therefore not suitable for primary reexamination. We were fortunate to acquire tissues from untreated TB from medical examiners, historic collections, and international collaborators. Comprehensive study of these samples enabled us to reevaluate and reinterpret find-

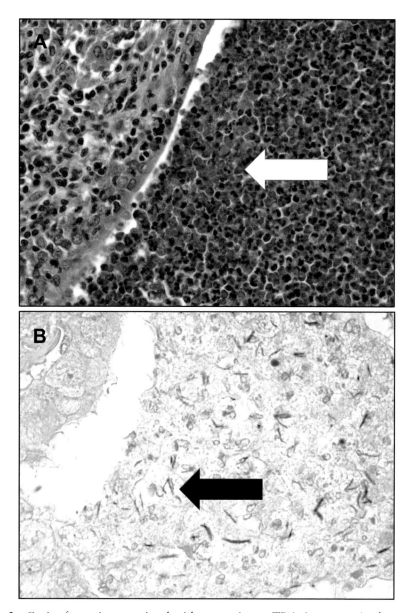

Figure 3 Cavity formation associated with post-primary TB is important in the transmission of bacilli between individuals due to the large numbers of extracellular and intracellular bacilli. (**A**) High-magnification images of a cavitary lung lesion shown filling the lumen with necrotic cellular debris (white arrow). (**B**) An acid-fast stain shows that bacilli within the necrotic debris are arranged in small clusters or as individuals (black arrow) and are mostly extracellular. The high numbers of bacilli within these lesions are important in the transmission of *M. tuberculosis* between individuals, especially when cavities communicate with lung airways. H&E stain.

ings reported in the older literature and to develop a comprehensive model explaining the pathogenesis of post-primary TB (6).

Specifically, we reexamined the paradigm that the host responses resulting in the formation of caseous granulomas represent the early stages of both primary and post-primary TB as suggested by animal studies

of the late 20th century. We concluded that this interpretation is not supported by the data or generated by pathologists or radiologists who extensively studied the pathology of human pulmonary TB in the preantibiotic era (7–23). The current paradigm is that caseous granulomas are the origin of both primary and post-primary TB and that cavities arise from erosion of necrotic granulomas into bronchi, which is not supported by the literature or our studies. Moreover, the use of mice and other small animal models to study the basic *in vivo* pathogenesis and immunological response of *M. tuberculosis* infection has further complicated our understanding of TB disease progression. Through extensive review of the literature and re-examination of tissues from untreated human TB patients, we have concluded that post-primary TB develops as an obstructive lobular pneumonia that spreads asymptomatically via bronchi within individuals with a high degree of *M. tuberculosis*-specific immunity (Fig. 4) (3, 6). This revised description of the pathology is supported by hundreds of publications from Rene Laënnec using gross pathology as early as 1804 through more recent histological studies and advanced imaging techniques such as high-resolution magnetic resonance imaging and computed tomography (24).

The revised interpretation based on more recent examination of tissue sections from untreated human patients is also supported by two other observations, which explains the pathogenesis of post-primary TB (25). Post-primary TB is consistently associated with bronchial obstruction from any number of causes, resulting in a postobstructive lipid pneumonia that progresses to cavitary lesions (26). Moreover, in the early stages of post-primary TB, lipid pneumonia is in part due to intracellular and extracellular accumulation of secreted mycobacterial antigens as well as excess host lipids in asymptomatic patients. These observations led to the formulation of a new model of TB pathogenesis using the metaphor of a three-act play. The critical new component is act 2, or what we refer to as the sneak attack. This is the process in which accumulation of mycobacterial antigens and host lipids ultimately trigger a massive necrotizing reaction that leads to cavitary lesions that communicate with conducting airways. As a consequence, the rapid proliferation and accumulation of infectious bacilli overwhelm host defenses and contribute to efficient transmission of the organism to new hosts.

The dictionary defines paradigm as "a framework containing the basic assumptions, ways of thinking, and methodology that are commonly accepted by members of the scientific community." Accordingly, a new paradigm calls for new experimental approaches and validation. This article attempts to briefly summarize our current understanding of human post-primary TB. It will then describe how different animal models have or can be used to specifically address the knowledge gaps that continue to slow progress toward preventing, diagnosing, and effectively treating human TB.

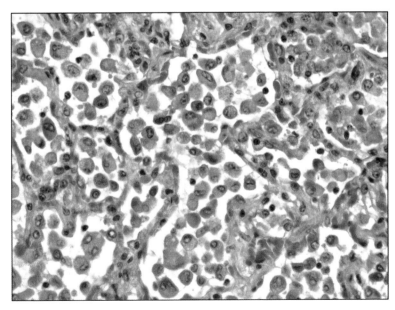

Figure 4 Intrapulmonary spread of mixed inflammatory cells within the lung parenchyma results in an obstructive lobar pneumonia and is involved in the early pathogenesis of post-primary TB. In contrast to primary lesions, the filling of alveoli with mixed inflammatory cells, including foamy macrophages, in the absence of necrosis contributes to airway obstruction and the development of post-primary TB. H&E stain.

TB DISEASE PROGRESSION
IN ANIMAL MODELS

The host response to *M. tuberculosis* infection in all mammalian species is almost universally characterized as granulomatous inflammation. The timeline of the basic host response to experimental *M. tuberculosis* infection in the various animal models has been reviewed (27, 28). It is widely accepted that progressive *M. tuberculosis* infection in mice, rabbits, guinea pigs, and non-human primates as well as humans is somewhat limited in the early stages of infection by an adaptive immune response that has a characteristic histological appearance. However, there is increasing evidence to suggest that *M. tuberculosis* simultaneously adapts to a changing microenvironment as a consequence of the changing host immune responses. The adaptations of *M. tuberculosis* to immune pressure results in the selection of small populations of nonreplicating, drug-tolerant bacilli that are able to persist for months or years in asymptomatic hosts. These bacteria maintain a low metabolic state, and the persistence of secreted and nonsecreted antigens is able to continually manipulate the host's response. In both untreated adult humans and animals, death in the late stages of disease is due to progressive pulmonary and extrapulmonary inflammation and, ultimately, multiorgan failure. Several lines of evidence, especially the observation that bacterial numbers may not increase significantly even in the late stages of disease, suggest that the tissue damage is due largely to ongoing responses to accumulated mycobacterial antigens (Fig. 5). What accounts for the disconnect between bacterial numbers and lesion severity in animal models compared to humans is likely the result of an unnaturally high challenge dose combined with the ongoing bacterial replication in species with minimal resistance combined with the persistence of *M. tuberculosis* antigens. According to North, "a central problem in tuberculosis research is the inability to explain why immunity to infection does not enable mice, guinea pigs, rabbits or susceptible humans to resolve lung infection and thereby stop development of disease" (28).

THE PRIMARY HOST RESPONSE TO
M. TUBERCULOSIS INFECTION

After decades of animal experimentation, it has become clear that no one animal model adequately mimics all the complexities of human TB. Animal models are not only limited by the differences in the inherent host response to experimental *M. tuberculosis* infection but are also subject to experimental differences in challenge strain, dose, and route of infection. In addition, the choice of animal model is heavily influenced by practi-

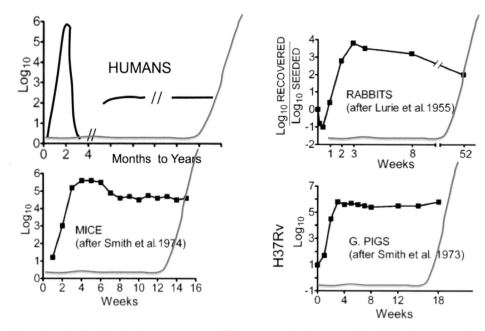

Figure 5 Similarities in the time course of humans and animal models of TB demonstrating that pathology does not correlate with increased numbers of bacteria. A central problem in TB research is to explain why immunity to infection does not enable mice, guinea pigs, rabbits, or susceptible humans to resolve lung infection and thereby stop the development of disease.

cal considerations given the cost of maintaining certain species in specialized, biocontainment facilities that are not readily available to most investigators. Accepting the experimental variables that influence the host responses to *M. tuberculosis* infection, investigators involved in anti-TB drug research and development have attempted to standardize animal model protocols to increase the reproducibility of data between laboratories and institutions (29). While this has helped to ensure that drug treatment responses in mice are reproducible, the use of models that better mimic the naturally occurring disease in humans continues to be overlooked. With improved knowledge of the pathology of human TB, it is increasingly recognized that all model species have advantages and disadvantages and can be experimentally manipulated to answer specific questions. However, what remains imperative is that data from animal models be interpreted in the context of naturally occurring TB in humans. "One should never forget the limitations of experimental studies in animals. They provide useful hypotheses and certain facts not observable in man, but in no case can they replace observations in man for ultimate understanding of the disease in human beings" (21).

We argue here that the foundation by which to compare data derived from TB animal models be based on our fundamental understanding of human TB, particularly in patients in which the clinical course has not been altered by antimicrobial drug treatment. Due to obvious ethical considerations, the availability of samples that meet this criteria are limited to postmortem cases from patients that have died from either progressive TB or unrelated accidents or diseases. In a series of recently published studies, Hunter et al. outlined how the primary literature describing the pathology of human TB patients combined with more contemporary approaches including advanced imaging to redefine the relationship, or lack thereof, between primary and post-primary TB disease (3, 4, 6). The challenge is to determine how to apply the technological advances we now have available in combination with what we have learned from studying TB animal models to fill the critical knowledge gaps.

Each of the animal strains or species used for TB research has unique characteristics, and none fully reproduce the human disease, especially the late disease that produces most adult disease and nearly all transmission of infection. However, as pointed out by North, many share common characteristics with the human disease. In particular, mice, rabbits, guinea pigs, and humans all develop immunity sufficient to limit proliferation of organisms in a few weeks but are unable to eliminate all organisms (Fig. 1). The infection then persists asymptomatically for months before the animals rapidly develop inflammation and disease and die, frequently with little or no increase in numbers of viable *M. tuberculosis* organisms (2, 30). The tissue damage is thought to be an immunopathology somehow triggered by mycobacterial antigens, not by live *M. tuberculosis* itself. A better understanding of the commonalities of how *M. tuberculosis* produces disease without increasing in number in quite different histologic lesions would be a major advance.

Briefly, the characteristic response to primary infection with *M. tuberculosis* in humans and most animal models involves the localized accumulation of mixed inflammatory and immune cells into a discrete nodular mass referred to as a granuloma. "Granulomatous inflammation" is a broadly used term to describe an infiltrate of primarily mononuclear cells composed mostly of macrophages and lymphocytes. Granulomatous inflammation is not a unique response to mycobacterial infections but can be seen in fungal infections as well as in response to foreign bodies (31). In addition, multinucleated giant cells are a frequent feature of TB granulomas, but they too are not unique to *M. tuberculosis* infection. The primary TB granuloma in humans does have important morphological characteristics that are shared with some commonly used animal models. Specifically, the distribution of different mononuclear cell populations combined with the development of central caseous necrosis, fibrous encapsulation, and dystrophic calcification are features seen in immunologically naive non-human primates and guinea pigs and less often in certain strains of mice and rabbits. Developing post-primary TB in humans has a different pathology that is an asymptomatic obstructive lobular pneumonia that progresses to cavity formation in the most aggressive response or serves as a focus of limited granuloma formation (3). As reported in detail by Canetti and others, granulomas in post-primary TB arise only in response to caseation necrosis and are never the cause of it (19, 21, 32). Nevertheless, the disease in humans and many animals shares the common feature of a prolonged asymptomatic period before development of clinical disease that is frequently not accompanied by a large increase in bacterial load.

HYPERSENSITIVITY IN THE PATHOGENESIS OF POST-PRIMARY TB

An important contribution to the pathogenesis of human post-primary TB involves hypersensitivity to mycobacterial antigens (33, 34). Guinea pigs are among the model species that develop the most robust hypersensitivity responses to *M. tuberculosis* infection. Studies by McMurray et al. showed that the morphological features of experimental *M. tuberculosis* infection in guinea pigs differed depending on whether animals were immunologically naive or vaccinated with BCG prior to aerosol exposure (35). In nonvaccinated guinea pigs, the primary response was that of the prototypical TB granuloma that frequently developed central necrosis (36). The similarity between TB granulomas in humans and guinea pigs compared to other model species has been recognized for many decades, which explains why it remains a mainstay in TB research. McMurray showed, however, that the initial response to aerosol infection of BCG-vaccinated guinea pigs differed in that the granulomatous response at the site of infection in the lung was composed primarily of mature lymphocytes which failed to organize into discrete granulomatous masses and rarely developed central necrosis. Moreover, the investigators equated the primary response in BCG-vaccinated animals to secondary lesions resulting from endogenous reinfection of the lung following dissemination of bacilli in naive guinea pigs (35). They further concluded that the differences in lesion morphology were a consequence of the combined effects of hematogenous dissemination of bacilli to extrapulmonary sites including peripheral lymphoid tissues. In the case of guinea pigs, sensitization with BCG prior to *M. tuberculosis* infection provided partial protection resulting in delayed progression of active disease and a less destructive inflammatory response.

In contrast, immunologically naive rabbits are relatively resistant to infection with less virulent laboratory strains of *M. tuberculosis* but are more susceptible to *Mycobacterium bovis* (37). Unlike guinea pigs, a more aggressive proinflammatoy response develops in rabbits that are first sensitized by repeated BCG vaccination (38). The resulting lesions more closely resemble TB abscesses and occasionally form cavitary lesions when lesions communicate with conducting airways. Due to the potential for TB lesions in rabbits to cavitate, this animal model has been used in an attempt to link initial granuloma formation to the development of post-primary TB pathogenesis in humans (39). This overlooks the fact that the pathology produced by *M. bovis* is different from that of *M. tuberculosis* (3). Moreover, this model has been used recently to study the impact lesion morphology, specifically abscesses or cavitary lesions, has on TB drug penetration (40–45). These studies have been facilitated by the discovery that rabbits are susceptible to more virulent *M. tuberculosis* challenge strains including human clinical strains (39, 46). Studies from rabbits support the hypothesis

that in humans, cavity formation is linked to an aggressive proinflammatory response, which can be triggered in individuals first sensitized with *M. tuberculosis* or nontuberculous mycobacterium. However, these data fail to support the direct relationship between the primary granulomas and post-primary TB disease.

Post-Primary Lung Reinfection

The term "post-primary TB" denotes an infection that begins after a primary infection. This host response in previously infected and immunized individuals accounts for 80% of all clinical human pulmonary TB. Consequently, studies of infection of previously sensitized hosts are important to understanding human TB but are rarely conducted. The pathology of developing human post-primary TB has been unequivocally established by scores of papers by dozens of authors, each of whom had personally studied hundreds of cases from a period of nearly 200 years (47). In our proposed pathogenesis of human post-primary TB, intrabronchial spread of infection and airway obstruction factors prominently in the pathogenesis of post-primary cavity formation. Reinfection of the lung following hematogenous dissemination of bacilli has been studied in both guinea pig and mouse TB models, where lung infection can spread through intrabronchiolar and lymphatic routes. The role of intrapulmonary lymphatic spread of *M. tuberculosis* has been best characterized in guinea pigs. Guinea pigs and non-human primates, like humans, have prominent peribronchial and perivascular connective tissue that supports well-developed and inducible bronchus-associated lymphoid tissue as well as an extensive network of intrapulmonary lymphatics (48–50). The intralymphatic spread of *M. tuberculosis* from a primary lung infection was first described in guinea pigs in the mid to late 19th century (51, 52). Studies by Klein showed that following experimental infection of guinea pigs with exudate obtained from human TB patients, spread along lymphatic vasculature was among the earliest manifestations of *M. tuberculosis* infection (48, 51). More recent studies have confirmed that granulomatous lymphangitis is also an early manifestation following low-dose aerosol exposure of guinea pigs and non-human primates to *M. tuberculosis* (49, 50). With the progression of lymphangiocentric lesions, vascular obstruction is followed by granuloma expansion, which accounts for the consistent perivascular and peribronchial distribution of primary granulomas in animals and humans.

Little is known about the significance of lymphangiocentric lesions in the pathogenesis of post-primary TB in humans. The close association with pulmonary arteries, veins, and airways raises the possibility that the expansion of these lesions may be among the first to communicate with conducting airways and predispose to cavity formation. The reason why cavitary disease is not a consistent finding in *M. tuberculosis*-infected guinea pigs in contrast to primates may be related to the well-developed connective tissue stroma that supports airways as well as blood and lymphatic vasculature (53). Another pathway to direct airway involvement that may predispose to cavity formation is endobronchial TB, which is a rare manifestation of experimental *M. tuberculosis* infections in animals but is universally found in developing human post-primary TB (54). The potential role of *M. tuberculosis*-induced pulmonary lymphangitis may be an early manifestation of post-primary TB in humans but requires further investigation.

In the proposed pathogenesis of human post-primary TB, bronchial obstruction and endobronchial TB factor significantly in the development of endogenous lipid pneumonia and, subsequently, lesion cavitation. Based on extensive review of the human pathology literature and more recent histopathological examination of human lung lesions, airway obstruction contributes to the localized accumulation of foamy macrophages, which are a consistent feature of *M. tuberculosis* infection in animals and humans (55, 56). Foam cell formation is not unique to TB but is a morphological feature of cellular degeneration. Foam cells are a prominent feature of atherosclerosis and are an important component of intravascular plaque formation in patients with peripheral and coronary vascular disease. The foamy appearance of macrophages can be due to swollen cytoplasmic organelles as a result of dysregulated fluid homeostasis (hydropic degeneration). In addition, an imbalance between lipid accumulation and efflux can also account for cytoplasmic vacuolization and foam cell formation (57). Whereas foam cell formation has been directly linked to obstructed airways in human TB, foamy macrophage accumulation within primary granulomas is a consistent finding in animals even in the absence of airway obstruction (58, 59). Moreover, in model species that fail to develop granuloma necrosis, foam cells that contain intracellular bacilli are a prominent histological feature (58, 60–63). These data suggest that while endogenous lipid pneumonia may contribute to the pathogenesis of post-primary TB in humans, there remains a knowledge gap linking foam cell formation with the proinflammatory response that progresses to cavitary disease (55, 64).

A potential cause of airway obstruction that is shared by humans and animals with TB is the migration and accumulation of mixed inflammatory cells within airway lumens. Processes associated with lesion resolution or healing accompany the progression of inflammation. As mentioned previously, the proliferation of fibroblasts and the deposition of extracellular matrix proteins as well as the deposition of dystrophic calcification is obvious evidence of lesion resolution. An important step in the resolution of inflammation is the elimination of senescent inflammatory cells as they approach the end of their functional life span. Neutrophils are among the first cells to respond to *M. tuberculosis* and other bacterial infections but also have one of the shortest life spans of all white blood cells (65–67). Senescent neutrophils and other inflammatory cells migrate and are eliminated from the body through mucosal surfaces including airways. Leukocytes near the end of their lifespan are eliminated by transepithelial migration into the lumens of mucosal surfaces including the lung (65, 68–70). In TB patients and animal models, infected and noninfected senescent leukocytes accumulate within airway lumens and reach the oropharynx through mucociliary clearance and contribute to the formation of sputum to be swallowed or expectorated. The accumulation of mixed inflammatory cells within the lumens of small airways is a consistent histological finding in *M. tuberculosis*-infected animals but may not necessarily represent functional obstruction (58, 61). These findings suggest that the accumulation and potential obstruction of small airways in animal models of *M. tuberculosis* infection is a common feature across species and therefore does not fully explain the development of human post-primary TB.

DISCUSSION AND CONCLUSIONS

Much has been learned from studying the basic pathogenesis and immune response to *M. tuberculosis* infection in animals. However, one of the major differences is that none of the commonly used animal models mimic the natural transition from primary to post-primary disease seen in humans. Post-primary TB is arguably the most important stage of active TB disease, yet very little is known about the factors that determine whether *M. tuberculosis* exposure results in an established infection and disease. Extensive study of human TB pathology combined with review of the literature from the preantibiotic era has suggested hypotheses about the factors that contribute to post-primary disease that can be tested in animal models. Collectively, studies in animals demonstrate the patterns of disease that contribute to post-primary TB, yet no one animal model recapitulates the naturally occurring disease in humans.

The possibility exists that experimental manipulation of individual or a combination of different animal models can be used to systematically fill the knowledge gaps pertaining to post-primary TB. Gaining a better understanding of the factors that promote or limit TB progression through the combined study of human and animal TB will contribute significantly to development of new diagnostics and means of prevention and treatment of TB.

It has long been recognized that the immune response in tuberculosis can both provide protection and contribute to tissue damage. Many attempts to identify the specific immune responses responsible for these opposing responses have been unsuccessful. The new paradigm provides an explanation of how the same immune responses can be responsible for both. Protection is provided when isolated mycobacteria are engulfed and killed by macrophages in an immune individual. The tissue damaging response occurs upon release of secreted antigens that have been stored within alveolar macrophages in asymptomatic patients. The sudden release of these antigens in sensitized people produces massive reactions (otherwise known as the Koch phenomena) and may represent the early manifestations of post-primary cavity formation.

In studying TB further, we believe that it would be profitable to focus on the commonalities of different models rather than their differences. Our hypothesis to explain the common course of disease in these various species in spite of markedly different pathologies is as follows. In humans mycobacterial antigens are sequestered within alveolar microphages until they are released to produce caseous pneumonia. We believe a key to understanding TB is an understanding of how *M. tuberculosis* stores and then releases the antigens to produce a massive necrotizing reaction. In mice a similar type of obstructive alveolar pneumonia is observed with accumulation of antigen, but it leads to a progressive fibrosis rather than caseous necrosis. Since certain immunocompetent mice are able to produce caseating granulomas when challenged appropriately, we believe their failure to do so following low-dose infection may be due to a lack of an antigen load sufficient to promote a proinflammatory response (71). Rabbits and guinea pigs, however, do develop progressive caseating granulomas in their lungs rather than the alveolar pneumonia (2). These slowly progress until the animals die, even though the numbers of viable *M. tuberculosis* organisms do not markedly increase. We hypothesize that this may be explained by the inability of the macrophages in these animals to limit the production of mycobacterial antigens and to keep that production

retained within macrophages. Consequently, there is a continual release of the antigens, which drives the progressive granulomas even though the number of organisms is not changing. The key question again, as stated by North, is "to explain why immunity to infection does not enable mice, guinea pigs, rabbits or susceptible humans to resolve lung infection and thereby stop development of disease" (28). How do small numbers of *M. tuberculosis* organisms persist in all of these models in spite of different pathologies and produce the conditions for massive clinical disease?

There are many impediments to progress in understanding the pathogenesis of post-primary tuberculosis. Many investigators have studied granulomas following the first infection, trying to extrapolate that through the entire process. However, it has been clear for over a century that the most important parameter determining the course of infection is the existence of previous infection. Post-primary tuberculosis is thus named because it occurs after the primary disease. It is characterized by much greater necrosis development of cavities and transmission. The belief that granulomas are the characteristic lesion of both primary and post-primary tuberculosis has encouraged investigators to concentrate only on early lesions that are inappropriate for post-primary TB.

A second element that has impeded progress is the insistence on infecting animals with a low-dose aerosol of *M. tuberculosis* to simulate the natural infection. While this provides some standardization and facilitates comparison among studies, there has been no explanation of why the route of infection should be the major determining factor in a disease that occurs 10 to 30 years after infection. Even reinfection tuberculosis develops 1 to 2 years after infection. A better approach is to attempt to reproduce in animals the conditions that occur in humans at particular times of infection. For example, we read that caseous granulomas occur when large numbers of organisms are found in localized areas of immunized individuals. Simulating this in mice by injecting large numbers of organisms into a sensitized animal produced classic caseating granulomas (71). This demonstrated that the inability of mice to produce caseous granulomas following low-dose aerosol infection is due not to their inability to develop appropriate immune responses, but rather to accumulating sufficient proinflammatory antigens at a particular site. In another example, injection of viable *M. tuberculosis* into sensitized animals stimulates accumulation of foamy macrophages in alveoli within 24 hours (1). Study of the pathology of human TB suggests numerous other areas where animal models can be developed to simulate and study individual phases of the human disease.

We have recently reported that the pathology of post-primary TB in the human lung is quite different from that in animal models and that tissues demonstrating such lesions are exceedingly scarce. While the difficulties in obtaining tissue are immense, the benefits and potential are substantial. Most importantly, TB is the human disease and autopsies are the only place where it can be seen in its developing untreated form. Surgical resections, with very few exceptions, are for chronic TB that has been treated and no longer shows the characteristic lesions of developing post-primary TB. Second, modern technology has produced means of identifying and quantitatively measuring parameters on tissue sections that were not possible a few years ago. We can measure DNA sequences, RNA expression, proteins, cytokines, and cells to better understand the changing microenvironment at various stages of *M. tuberculosis* infection. In the case of TB, more focused studies of human tissues is essential for directing, focusing, and correlating studies on animal models. Consequently, it will be important to develop tissue banks of such tissues. It is also necessary to develop new animal models that can be used in conjunction with a more accurate version of human pathology to finally answer major questions about this disease.

Citation. Basaraba RJ, Hunter RL. 2017. Pathology of Tuberculosis: how the pathology of human tuberculosis informs and directs animal models. Microbiol Spectrum 5(3):TBTB2-0029-2016.

References

1. **Nuermberger EL, Yoshimatsu T, Tyagi S, Bishai WR, Grosset JH.** 2004. Paucibacillary tuberculosis in mice after prior aerosol immunization with *Mycobacterium bovis* BCG. *Infect Immun* 72:1065–1071.

2. **Dannenberg AM Jr.** 2006. *Pathogenesis of Human Pulmonary Tuberculosis: Insights from the Rabbit Model*, p 453. ASM Press, Washington, DC.

3. **Hunter RL.** 2011. Pathology of post primary tuberculosis of the lung: an illustrated critical review. *Tuberculosis (Edinb)* 91:497–509.

4. **Hunter RL, Actor JK, Hwang SA, Karev V, Jagannath C.** 2014. Pathogenesis of post primary tuberculosis: immunity and hypersensitivity in the development of cavities. *Ann Clin Lab Sci* 44:365–387.

5. **Hunter RL, Jagannath C, Actor JK.** 2007. Pathology of postprimary tuberculosis in humans and mice: contradiction of long-held beliefs. *Tuberculosis (Edinb)* 87:267–278.

6. **Hunter RL.** 2016. Tuberculosis as a three-act play: a new paradigm for the pathogenesis of pulmonary tuberculosis. *Tuberculosis (Edinb)* 97:8–17.

7. **Laennec R.** 1821. *A Treatise on Diseases of the Chest in Which They Are Described According to Their Anatomical Characters, and Their Diagnosis Established on a New Principle by Means of Acoustick Instruments*, p 437. T&G Underwood, London, United Kingdom (reprinted 1979 by The Classics of Medicine Library, Birmingham, AL).

8. **Dubos R, Dubos G.** 1987. *The White Plague. Tuberculosis, Man, and Society*. Rutgers Univesity Press, New Brunswick, NJ.

9. **Bennett JH.** 1854. *The Pathology and Treatment of Pulmonary Tuberculosis*, p 180. Blanchard and Lea, Philadelphia, PA.

10. **Virchow R.** 1860. *Cellular Pathology as Based upon Physiological and Pathological Histology*, 2nd ed. John Churchill, London, United Kingdom (reprinted 1978 by The Classics of Medicine Library, Birmingham, AL).

11. **Powell RD.** 1876. *On Consumption and on Certain Diseases of Lungs and Pleura, chapter 2*, p 291. H.K. Lewis, London, United Kingdom.

12. **Tyndale J.** 1878. *The Present Status of the Pathology of Consumption and Tuberculosis*. Trow's Printing and Bookbinding Co, New York, NY.

13. **Cornil V, Ranvier L.** 1880. Pathological histology of the respiratory apparatus, part III, section I, chapter II, p 394–445. *In A Manual of Pathological Histology, Translated with Notes and Additions by EO Shakespeare and JHC Simms*. Henry C Lea, Philadephia, PA.

14. **Hamilton JD.** 1883. *On the Pathology of Bronchitis, Catarrhal Pneumonia. Tubercle and Allied Lesions of the Human Lung*. Macmillan and Co, London, United Kingdom.

15. **Hektoen L, Reisman D.** 1901. *A Text-Book of Pathology for the Use of Students and Practitoners of Medicine and Surgery*, **vol 2**. W.B. Saunders & Company, London, United Kingdom.

16. **Osler W, McCrae T.** 1921. *The Principles and Practice of Medicine*, p 184–255. D. Appleton and Company, New York, NY.

17. **Opie E, Aronson J.** 1927. Tubercle bacilli in latent tuberculous lesions and in lung tissue without tuberculous lesions. *Arch Pathol Lab Med* 4:1–21.

18. **Kayne GG, Pagel W, O'Shaughenessy L.** 1939. *Pulmonary Tuberculosis, Pathology, Diagnosis and Management*. Oxford University Press, London, United Kingdom.

19. **Rich A.** 1951. The factors responsible for the characteristics of tuberculous lesions and symptoms, p 713. *In The Pathogenesis of Tuberculosis*, 2nd ed. Charles C Thomas, Springfield, IL.

20. **Medlar EM.** 1950. Pathogenetic concepts of tuberculosis. *Am J Med* 9:611–622.

21. **Canetti G.** 1955. *The Tubercle Bacillus in the Pulmonary Lesion of Man. Histobacteriology and Its Bearing on the Therapy of Pulmonary Tuberculosis*, p 226. Springer Publishing, New York, NY.

22. **Gunn FD.** 1961. Tuberculosis, p 243–263. *In Anderson WAD (ed), Pathology*, 4th ed. C.V. Mosby Company, St Louis, MO.

23. **Pagel W.** 1964. The morbid anatomy and histology of tuberculosis: an introduction in simple terms, p 36–63. *In Pulmonary Tuberculosis, Bacteriology, Pathology, Diagnosis, Management, Epidemiology and Prevention*. Oxford University Press, London, United Kingdom.

24. Aaron L, Saadoun D, Calatroni I, Launay O, Mémain N, Vincent V, Marchal G, Dupont B, Bouchaud O, Valeyre D, Lortholary O. 2004. Tuberculosis in HIV-infected patients: a comprehensive review. *Clin Microbiol Infect* **10**: 388–398.

25. Mustafa T, Leversen NA, Sviland L, Wiker HG. 2014. Differential *in vivo* expression of mycobacterial antigens in *Mycobacterium tuberculosis* infected lungs and lymph node tissues. *BMC Infect Dis* **14**:535.

26. Hunter RL. 2011. On the pathogenesis of post primary tuberculosis: the role of bronchial obstruction in the pathogenesis of cavities. *Tuberculosis (Edinb)* **91**(Suppl 1): S6–S10.

27. Sanders BM, Orme IM, Basaraba RJ. 2008. Immunopathology of tuberculosis. *In* Kaufmann SHE, Britton WJ (ed), *Handbook of Tuberculosis: Immunology and Cell Biology*. Wiley-VCH Verlag, Weinheim, Germany.

28. North RJ, Jung YJ. 2004. Immunity to tuberculosis. *Annu Rev Immunol* **22**:599–623.

29. Franzblau SG, DeGroote MA, Cho SH, Andries K, Nuermberger E, Orme IM, Mdluli K, Angulo-Barturen I, Dick T, Dartois V, Lenaerts AJ. 2012. Comprehensive analysis of methods used for the evaluation of compounds against *Mycobacterium tuberculosis*. *Tuberculosis (Edinb)* **92**:453–488.

30. Dannenberg AM Jr, Collins FM. 2001. Progressive pulmonary tuberculosis is not due to increasing numbers of viable bacilli in rabbits, mice and guinea pigs, but is due to a continuous host response to mycobacterial products. *Tuberculosis (Edinb)* **81**:229–242.

31. Molina-Ruiz AM, Requena L. 2015. Foreign body granulomas. *Dermatol Clin* **33**:497–523.

32. Medlar EM. 1955. The behavior of pulmonary tuberculous lesions: a pathological study. *Am Rev Tuberc* **71**: 1–244.

33. Dannenberg AM Jr. 1991. Delayed-type hypersensitivity and cell-mediated immunity in the pathogenesis of tuberculosis. *Immunol Today* **12**:228–233.

34. Dannenberg AM Jr, Higuchi S. 1979. Chronic inflammation involving cellular hypersensitivity. *Chest* **75**(Suppl): 265–266.

35. McMurray DN. 2003. Hematogenous reseeding of the lung in low-dose, aerosol-infected guinea pigs: unique features of the host-pathogen interface in secondary tubercles. *Tuberculosis (Edinb)* **83**:131–134.

36. McMurray DN. 2001. Disease model: pulmonary tuberculosis. *Trends Mol Med* **7**:135–137.

37. Converse PJ, Dannenberg AM Jr, Shigenaga T, McMurray DN, Phalen SW, Stanford JL, Rook GA, Koru-Sengul T, Abbey H, Estep JE, Pitt ML. 1998. Pulmonary bovine-type tuberculosis in rabbits: bacillary virulence, inhaled dose effects, tuberculin sensitivity, and *Mycobacterium vaccae* immunotherapy. *Clin Diagn Lab Immunol* **5**: 871–881.

38. Dannenberg AM Jr. 2009. Liquefaction and cavity formation in pulmonary TB: a simple method in rabbit skin to test inhibitors. *Tuberculosis (Edinb)* **89**:243–247.

39. Converse PJ, Dannenberg AM Jr, Estep JE, Sugisaki K, Abe Y, Schofield BH, Pitt ML. 1996. Cavitary tuberculosis produced in rabbits by aerosolized virulent tubercle bacilli. *Infect Immun* **64**:4776–4787.

40. Barclay WR, Ebert RH, Le Roy GV, Manthei RW, Roth LJ. 1953. Distribution and excretion of radioactive isoniazid in tuberculous patients. *J Am Med Assoc* **151**: 1384–1388.

41. Barclay WR, Ebert RH, Manthei RW, Roth LJ. 1953. Distribution of C14 labeled isoniazid in sensitive and resistant tubercle bacilli and in infected and uninfected tissues in tuberculous patients. *Trans Annu Meet Natl Tuberc Assoc* **49**:192–195.

42. Coleman MT, Chen RY, Lee M, Lin PL, Dodd LE, Maiello P, Via LE, Kim Y, Marriner G, Dartois V, Scanga C, Janssen C, Wang J, Klein E, Cho SN, Barry CE III, Flynn JL. 2014. PET/CT imaging reveals a therapeutic response to oxazolidinones in macaques and humans with tuberculosis. *Sci Transl Med* **6**:265ra167.

43. Dartois V. 2014. The path of anti-tuberculosis drugs: from blood to lesions to mycobacterial cells. *Nat Rev Microbiol* **12**:159–167.

44. Prideaux B, ElNaggar MS, Zimmerman M, Wiseman JM, Li X, Dartois V. 2015. Mass spectrometry imaging of levofloxacin distribution in TB-infected pulmonary lesions by MALDI-MSI and continuous liquid micro-junction surface sampling. *Int J Mass Spectrom* **377**: 699–708.

45. Prideaux B, Via LE, Zimmerman MD, Eum S, Sarathy J, O'Brien P, Chen C, Kaya F, Weiner DM, Chen PY, Song T, Lee M, Shim TS, Cho JS, Kim W, Cho SN, Olivier KN, Barry CE III, Dartois V. 2015. The association between sterilizing activity and drug distribution into tuberculosis lesions. *Nat Med* **21**:1223–1227.

46. Subbian S, Tsenova L, Yang G, O'Brien P, Parsons S, Peixoto B, Taylor L, Fallows D, Kaplan G. 2011. Chronic pulmonary cavitary tuberculosis in rabbits: a failed host immune response. *Open Biol* **1**:110016.

47. Hunter WA, Cundy T, Rabone D, Hofman PL, Harris M, Regan F, Robinson E, Cutfield WS. 2004. Insulin sensitivity in the offspring of women with type 1 and type 2 diabetes. *Diabetes Care* **27**:1148–1152.

48. Klein EE. 1875. *The Anatomy of the Lymphatic System. The Lung*, **vol 2**. Smith, Elder and Co., London, United Kingdom.

49. Basaraba RJ, Smith EE, Shanley CA, Orme IM. 2006. Pulmonary lymphatics are primary sites of *Mycobacterium tuberculosis* infection in guinea pigs infected by aerosol. *Infect Immun* **74**:5397–5401.

50. Rayner EL, Pearson GR, Hall GA, Basaraba RJ, Gleeson F, McIntyre A, Clark S, Williams A, Dennis MJ, Sharpe SA. 2013. Early lesions following aerosol infection of rhesus macaques (*Macaca mulatta*) with *Mycobacterium tuberculosis* strain H37RV. *J Comp Pathol* **149**:475–485.

51. Klein EE. 1873. Contributions to the normal and pathological anatomy of the lymphatic system of the lungs. *Proc R Soc Lond* **22**:133–145.

52. Sanderson JB. 1867. *Communicability of Tubercle by Innoculation*. Report of the Medical Officer of the Privy Council. London, United Kingdom.

53. Basaraba RJ, Dailey DD, McFarland CT, Shanley CA, Smith EE, McMurray DN, Orme IM. 2006. Lymphadenitis as a major element of disease in the guinea pig model of tuberculosis. *Tuberculosis (Edinb)* **86**:386–394.

54. Lee P. 2015. Endobronchial tuberculosis. *Indian J Tuberc* **62**:7–12.

55. Peyron P, Vaubourgeix J, Poquet Y, Levillain F, Botanch C, Bardou F, Daffé M, Emile JF, Marchou B, Cardona PJ, de Chastellier C, Altare F. 2008. Foamy macrophages from tuberculous patients' granulomas constitute a nutrient-rich reservoir for *M. tuberculosis* persistence. *PLoS Pathog* **4**:e1000204.

56. Russell DG, Cardona PJ, Kim MJ, Allain S, Altare F. 2009. Foamy macrophages and the progression of the human tuberculosis granuloma. *Nat Immunol* **10**:943–948.

57. Mallat Z. 2014. Macrophages. *Arterioscler Thromb Vasc Biol* **34**:2509–2519.

58. Basaraba RJ. 2008. Experimental tuberculosis: the role of comparative pathology in the discovery of improved tuberculosis treatment strategies. *Tuberculosis (Edinb)* **88** (Suppl 1):S35–S47.

59. Irwin SM, Driver E, Lyon E, Schrupp C, Ryan G, Gonzalez-Juarrero M, Basaraba RJ, Nuermberger EL, Lenaerts AJ. 2015. Presence of multiple lesion types with vastly different microenvironments in C3HeB/FeJ mice following aerosol infection with *Mycobacterium tuberculosis*. *Dis Model Mech* **8**:591–602.

60. Canetti G. 1956. Dynamic aspects of the pathology and bacteriology of tuberculous lesions. *Am Rev Tuberc* **74**:13–21, discussion, 22–27.

61. Saunders BM. 2008. Immunopathology of tuberculosis, p 245–278. *In* Kaufmann SHE, Britton WJ (ed), *Handbook of Tuberculosis: Immunology and Cell Biology*. Wiley-VCH Verlag, Weinheim, Germany.

62. Ryan GJ, Hoff DR, Driver ER, Voskuil MI, Gonzalez-Juarrero M, Basaraba RJ, Crick DC, Spencer JS, Lenaerts AJ. 2010. Multiple *M. tuberculosis* phenotypes in mouse and guinea pig lung tissue revealed by a dual-staining approach. *PLoS One* **5**:e11108.

63. Ryan GJ, Shapiro HM, Lenaerts AJ. 2014. Improving acid-fast fluorescent staining for the detection of mycobacteria using a new nucleic acid staining approach. *Tuberculosis (Edinb)* **94**:511–518.

64. Bozza PT, Melo RCN, Bandeira-Melo C. 2007. Leukocyte lipid bodies regulation and function: contribution to allergy and host defense. *Pharmacol Ther* **113**:30–49.

65. Kipnis A, Basaraba RJ, Turner J, Orme IM. 2003. Increased neutrophil influx but no impairment of protective immunity to tuberculosis in mice lacking the CD44 molecule. *J Leukoc Biol* **74**:992–997.

66. Ordway D, Palanisamy G, Henao-Tamayo M, Smith EE, Shanley C, Orme IM, Basaraba RJ. 2007. The cellular immune response to *Mycobacterium tuberculosis* infection in the guinea pig. *J Immunol* **179**:2532–2541.

67. Tsai MC, Chakravarty S, Zhu G, Xu J, Tanaka K, Koch C, Tufariello J, Flynn J, Chan J. 2006. Characterization of the tuberculous granuloma in murine and human lungs: cellular composition and relative tissue oxygen tension. *Cell Microbiol* **8**:218–232.

68. Guo RF, Ward PA. 2002. Mediators and regulation of neutrophil accumulation in inflammatory responses in lung: insights from the IgG immune complex model. *Free Radic Biol Med* **33**:303–310.

69. Hu M, Miller EJ, Lin X, Simms HH. 2004. Transmigration across a lung epithelial monolayer delays apoptosis of polymorphonuclear leukocytes. *Surgery* **135**:87–98.

70. Zemans RL, Colgan SP, Downey GP. 2009. Transepithelial migration of neutrophils: mechanisms and implications for acute lung injury. *Am J Respir Cell Mol Biol* **40**:519–535.

71. Hunter RL, Olsen M, Jagannath C, Actor JK. 2006. Trehalose 6,6′-dimycolate and lipid in the pathogenesis of caseating granulomas of tuberculosis in mice. *Am J Pathol* **168**:1249–1261.

Tuberculosis and the Tubercle Bacillus, 2nd ed.
Edited by William R. Jacobs, Jr., Helen McShane, Valerie Mizrahi, and Ian M. Orme
© 2018 American Society for Microbiology, Washington, DC
doi:10.1128/microbiolspec.TBTB2-0004-2015

B. ANIMAL MODELS

Animal Models of Tuberculosis: An Overview

6

Ann Williams[1] and Ian M. Orme[2]

Animal models are an integral part of the scientific process, reflecting the physiological and anatomical similarities between many animal species and human beings. In the context of infectious diseases, multiple animal models have been used to extend our understanding of their pathophysiology and the host response to them. This is the backbone also of vaccine research, producing vaccines against once-dreaded multiple diseases that in previous centuries claimed the lives of many millions of people. Animal models are also invaluable in designing therapies, particularly drugs, with which to combat these diseases.

It is important to consider, however, that animals are *not* humans, even when the species used is genetically very close to *Homo sapiens*. Accordingly, care has to be used in interpreting data from a specific animal model and it cannot be absolutely guaranteed that the specific observation—for instance, disease pathology or a T-cell subset response—is identical to events happening in an infected human. In other words, while animal models can collectively provide a massive amount of information, not all of it will apply to human disease, and the true art of animal modeling is to understand what information is useful and pertinent, and what may be less useful and even potentially misleading.

Scientists who use animal models are acutely aware of the ethical issues in using other creatures that share our planet. Regulations and an ethical code of conduct ensure that suffering is avoided completely or at least kept to a minimum, and, in the case of chronic diseases such as tuberculosis, animals are carefully monitored and euthanized when they start to show clinical signs (such as weight loss) that are predictive of severe disease. Alternatively, disease burden can be measured at a fixed time point prior to the development of clinical signs. In addition, there is a consensus that, wherever possible, a minimum number of animals are used that can still provide a statistically valid result. These considerations have resulted in the current concept of "replacement, reduction, and refinement" for animal usage, first suggested in 1959 (1).

MAJOR ANIMAL MODELS OF TUBERCULOSIS

The use of animal models in tuberculosis research extends back to the 19th century when the identity of the tuberculosis bacillus—and the idea that tuberculosis just "ran in families" was incorrect and, instead, that the disease had an infectious origin—were only just being realized. Koch, after his seminal discovery, soon found that if he injected cultures of the *Mycobacterium tuberculosis* bacilli into mice, they developed lesions not unlike those seen in the lungs of patients, and it was soon discovered that the organism could also cause disease in multiple animals, including rabbits, guinea pigs, and rats. It became apparent that there were differences in apparent susceptibility between the species, with infected mice often outliving guinea pigs as an example, and that, in addition, the environment also played a role. The latter idea was first tested by E. L. Trudeau, who showed that rabbits kept in an environment that included sunlight and good nutrition (on "Rabbit Island") lived longer than rabbits kept in a basement laboratory with poor nutrition.

[1]Health UK, Porton Down SP4 0JG, United Kingdom; [2]Colorado State University, Fort Collins, CO 80523.

Mice

As described elsewhere (77), studies in animal models, particularly the mouse, have provided a wealth of information about the functions of the immune response against *M. tuberculosis*. Early studies, including observations in athymic mice and cell transfer studies (2–5), first pointed to the central role of T lymphocytes in protective immunity, and over the past 3 decades or so have blossomed into a progressively deeper understanding of the complex immune response this organism elicits. This has happened in concert with refinement of the mouse model. An initial movement from the use of wild mice to inbred strains of mice can be traced back to the first MHC studies by Gorer, and these inbred strains started in appear in the tuberculosis field about 40 years ago. Advances in mainstream immunology have subsequently generated transgenic mice that have a variety of uses, as well as congenic lines (CD45, for example) that can be used to track cells of host origin after cell transfer. Mutations arising in inbred strains have also been useful; as an example. the FeJ mutant on the C3H background develops severely necrotic tuberculous lesions not seen in other inbred strains (6).

Perhaps the most important advance in the mouse model was the development of technology that allowed targeted disruption of individual genes in this animal, providing "gene knockout mice." This provided a wealth of information regarding the role of various molecules in host immune systems that substantially advanced our knowledge of these. This included the central role of gamma interferon, long suspected but definitively proven in IFNγ-KO mice (7, 8), and the pleiotropic roles of tumor necrosis factor alpha (9). Mice lacking CD4 cells lost their ability to resist infection (10), whereas this was less pronounced in CD8-deficient mice until well into the chronic phase of the disease (11). In addition, the relative roles of myriad cytokines and chemokines were revealed by this new technology. In fact, given that disruption of many different genes mostly resulted in loss of resistance in mice to tuberculosis, either completely or temporarily, directly illustrated the highly complex and integrated nature of the overall host response.

Guinea Pigs

Guinea pigs are an extremely useful model of tuberculosis because they exhibit multiple similarities to human disease, especially lung necrosis, lymphadenopathy, and disease dissemination (12, 13). For this reason, they have been generally regarded as the gold standard for testing vaccine efficacy, their primary

use in the field for decades (14, 15). A limitation of the model for many years was the lack of immunologic reagents that could be used to measure their immune response, but this situation has recently changed, principally because of the efforts of McMurray, who painstakingly developed assays for guinea pig cytokines and chemokines, and Ordway, who solved the serious problem of autofluorescence, allowing the application of flow cytometry to immune cells in this model.

In fact, early studies in tuberculosis primarily used the guinea pig model, both for vaccine testing and for developing skin test diagnostic reagents. This popularity reflected the susceptibility of this animal to tuberculosis, in contrast to other models such as the mouse and rat. This is not absolutely the case, however, and the general consensus—based on the use of laboratory strains—that "mice are resistant, guinea pigs are susceptible" has been recently challenged (16, 17), reflecting newer information arising from the study of clinical strains. In these newer studies, it has been observed that, first, certain newly emerging clinical isolates can grow even better in mice than in guinea pigs, and, second, guinea pigs can live for a significant period of time *despite* bearing large necrotic lesions in their lungs (18, 19).

In contrast to vaccines, the use of the guinea pig to test drugs against tuberculosis has been much more limited and confined mainly to the classical literature. This situation has undergone a renaissance recently, however, with the development of humane methods to administer drugs over extended periods of therapy (20), with an important outcome of this being the first demonstration that an experimental new drug, bedaquiline, substantially reduced the duration of therapy when given with conventional drugs (21).

Non-Human Primates

Over the past decade or so, considerable effort has been put into the development of non-human primate (NHP) models of tuberculosis, and there are now several world-class facilities with this capability. The most commonly used NHP for tuberculosis (TB) studies is the macaque species (rhesus and cynomolgus), and several reviews have been written describing *M. tuberculosis* infection in these species (22–24). Because of genetic similarities with humans, reflected in our similar immune systems, there is general agreement that NHPs are the most important "gateway" for progression to efficacy testing in humans. Currently, there are various permutations of the macaque model with regard to species, route of challenge, and the primary readout of disease burden that is used to demonstrate vaccine efficacy. Considerable efforts are currently under way to better understand the impact of these different variables with the goal of more standardized models to allow reproducible vaccine efficacy testing. This will enable critically important studies where candidate vaccines are tested for efficacy in NHPs in study designs that bridge to early clinical studies of the same vaccines.

OTHER ANIMAL MODELS

Zebrafish

The zebrafish is a (very) small animal model of tuberculosis that has contributed useful information in terms of the pathogenesis of the disease. It has various advantages, including ease of use, and optical transparency in its larval stage, making it very amenable to imaging techniques (25).

The zebrafish cannot be infected with *M. tuberculosis* because of its much lower body temperature, but it can be productively infected with *Mycobacterium marinum*, a genetically related mycobacterium that can infect cold-blooded aquatic animals such as fish and frogs.

Like *M. tuberculosis*, *M. marinum* can be genetically manipulated, allowing the generation of mutant and transgenic strains. Zebrafish develop granulomatous-like structures when infected with *M. marinum*, which, as in many other animal models, can degenerate and become necrotic (26). As in mice and guinea pigs, the early granulomatous response is insufficient to contain the infection initially, and bacilli disseminate to other organs. In addition, the zebrafish expresses multiple elements of both innate and acquired immunity. In this model, however, acquired immunity takes several weeks to develop (27), whereas in mammals this occurs much faster.

A major strength of the model is that larval zebrafish are optically transparent and this allows serial observations using high-resolution microscopy (28). In addition, the animal can easily be modified genetically, and the effects of inactivation of genes using antisense oligonucleotides can persist for several days (29). A further useful property is that larval zebrafish have no phagocytes in their hindbrain cavity (HBC) and so, if bacilli are injected here, the kinetics of ingress of macrophages and neutrophils can be measured. If the bacilli are injected via the caudal vein, they encounter such cells straight away. If the HBC route is used, it can also be used to show cellular accumulations if host molecules are injected into this site, such as interleukin-

8, CCL2, or leukotriene B4 (30). This is a unique and useful aspect of this model.

The zebrafish model provides data suggesting avoidance by *M. marinum* of the influx of neutrophils into lesions (30). This is different from observations in mice and in guinea pigs where early neutrophil influx has been implicated in early lesion necrosis (12, 31). Observations in humans (32, 33) do not support this either, suggesting a different mechanism of pathogenesis between *M. marinum* and *M. tuberculosis*, and draws into question interpretations drawn in fish (29) versus hosts possessing lungs (34).

Rabbits

Rabbits were used by Trudeau as a disease model at the end of the 19th century, but the model came to prominence in the 1930s because of the seminal studies by Lurie who described the disease process and developed inbred lines of rabbits of differing susceptibility (35, 36). This was followed by further studies performed in conjunction with Dannenberg that started to provide a framework for the first important models of the pathogenesis of the disease (37), as well as a distinction between protective cellular immunity, and potentially damaging mechanisms of "delayed type hypersensitivity" (38–40).

Rabbits can be infected with the laboratory strains H37Rv and Erdman, but they are quite resistant to these strains and, as a result, a larger dose of viable bacilli ($>10^3$) is often needed to establish a productive infection (41). In contrast, infection of these animals with the Ravenel strain of *Mycobacterium bovis* causes a rapid and severe disease process in which large areas of the lung become necrotic and then liquefy (42). This event has been regarded as a model of human disease cavity formation, but not everyone agrees (43), and it may reflect a different mechanism of pathogenesis separate from that caused by *M. tuberculosis*.

Although there may be useful attributes of the model, the larger size of rabbits makes the model more expensive and less tractable than mice or guinea pigs and it has never been seriously developed for vaccine or drug testing. Where it has provided some useful information is as a model of cerebral tuberculosis (44), although, here again, virulent *M. bovis* is needed to effectively establish this.

Rats

The rat model was first described in detail in seminal articles by Gray in the late 1950s in studies in which he compared the outcomes of infection in rats and mice (45–47). Thereafter, the literature on this model is very sparse until two 1973 studies by Lefford in which he demonstrated that thoracic duct lymphocytes (but not serum) conferred protection to recipient rats challenged with *M. tuberculosis* H37Rv, thus providing the first clues that immunity to tuberculosis was mediated by lymphocytes (48, 49). In recent years, however, very little has been done with this model, except as a potential diabetes/tuberculosis model (50).

Cattle

Cattle are natural hosts of *M. bovis* and are one of the target species (alongside wildlife reservoirs) for interventions aimed at controlling bovine TB. Highly relevant host-pathogen interaction studies can therefore be performed by experimental infection of cattle. The close similarity of *M. bovis* to *M. tuberculosis* means that there is potential synergy in the efforts to find a vaccine to control human and bovine TB. An example of this is studies where vaccines that have been developed for use in humans have been evaluated in the cattle *M. bovis* model and demonstrated efficacy (51). The relatively large size of these animals presents challenges in terms of housing at biosafety level 3 containment and quantities of drug or vaccine needed but there are advantages similar to those of the non-human primates in terms of frequent and sequential sample collection. A major advantage of the cattle model of *M. bovis* is the ability to conduct field trials, including natural transmission studies, where it is possible to evaluate the ability of a vaccine to prevent disease caused by a naturally acquired infection.

Mini Pigs

A mini pig model of *M. tuberculosis* infection has been described (52) as an alternative means of studying latent TB infection and the impact of treatments on lung lesion development. A key advantage of this model is related to the anatomy of the lungs which, because of the large size of these animals, and like humans, have intralobular septae that influence the development of granulomatous pathology. Similar to the cattle model for bovine TB, there are considerable practical and cost implications that prevent this model from being applied widely.

PRACTICAL APPLICATIONS OF ANIMAL MODELS

Host Response and Pathogenesis

For several decades, animal models have been used to try to predict the human immune response to tubercu-

losis infection, with the aim to improve the design of vaccines and diagnostic approaches. This basic research in animal models has provided fundamental information, the most important being that vaccines against TB have to induce protective T cells, rather than establish antibody responses as many other vaccines do. We now know that a favorable host response is driven by recognition systems, principally Toll-like receptors, which has helped in the development of new adjuvant formulations designed to maximize the T helper 1 (TH1) response, particularly to protein-based vaccine candidates. Animal studies have illustrated that the TH1 mechanism is not exclusive, however, and that, even within the CD4 subset, there are additional types of cells (interleukin-17-secreting cells, Foxp3+ regulatory T cells) that are clearly part of the overall equation, and that, moreover, additional subsets including NK, NKT cells, and CD8+ MAIT cells may be playing a contributory role (53, 54).

Animal models have also provided information about other aspects that could not be obtained by simply observing humans. One important example is the nature of the memory T-cell response (55), which is of course the primary target of new vaccines, discussed further below. Despite this, the field is still having difficulty on occasion in translating information from animals to humans, the most notorious being the search for "correlates of protection" (56). It would be invaluable to have biomarkers indicating that a response to a given vaccine gave very high confidence that the individual was likely to be completely protected, or that a drug regimen was completely sterilizing, but this has not been achieved. The most famous example was the concept that if an interferon gamma (IFNγ) response was present, this indicated protection, which has not turned out to be useful.

All the animal models studied to date develop granulomatous inflammation resulting in the formation of a wall of tissue called a granuloma, which is designed to try to contain the infection (57). Our ability to form these structures probably arose from more primitive responses to particles, which gradually evolved into a more complex response centrally controlled by chemokines released by host immunity. The fine structure of the granuloma differs considerably between different animal models, ranging from relatively acellular granulomas in zebrafish to highly calcified lesions in cattle. Mice and guinea pigs differ considerably as well, and, while many reviews describe the mouse granuloma as disorganized and those in guinea pigs as organized, in fact the reverse is true (57). In mice, there are highly organized foci of CD4 cells as well as some small follicles of B cells, surrounded on the perimeter by CD8 cells. This type of pattern can be seen in human lungs, as well. In guinea pigs, however, the center of the granuloma becomes necrotic, as in humans, and this compresses the cellular response, leading to a disorganized cuff of randomly mixed CD4 and CD8 T cells.

Non-necrotic secondary lesions are a facet of the guinea pig model, and these tend to be pleural, supporting the idea that they get established by bacilli escaping from primary lesions and being carried down the peripheral lymphatics, an idea that challenges the classical view that secondary sites of infection are established by blood-borne bacteria. A further element of this is a cellular response in the lymphatic vessels themselves—lymphangitis—clearly visible in this animal model (58).

In all the models, there is clear evidence that granulomas are dynamic. Some become necrotic, whereas others show evidence of wound healing and/or fibrosis. Granuloma formation in zebrafish (29) can be observed after only a few days, whereas this takes much longer in mammals. This leads some (16) to suggest that the response in zebrafish is more akin to a primitive particle response rather than a true granuloma. While both zebrafish and mammalian models quickly develop an "epithelioid macrophage" field of cells, major aggregates of lymphocytes, seen in larger animal models, are less developed.

These differences may explain why macrophages in zebrafish entering sites of infection then leave and disseminate disease (59). Because this happens in a hemocoel, this is inevitable and is probably different from events in the lungs of larger models in which dendritic cells pick up bacilli in the interstitium and then enter lymphatic capillaries to carry them to draining lymph nodes, an essential event in triggering acquired immunity (60).

Animal models are invaluable for the study of pathological changes in response to infection because the kinetics and dynamics of the response can be described in relation to a single infection event. It could be argued, however, that this is not relevant for human TB infection, which occurs in the context of multiple exposures. More complex animal models are being considered or used that involve repeated exposure and exposure to natural aerosols. In the latter case, where guinea pigs were exposed to natural aerosols from TB patients, an unexpected spectrum of disease pathology was revealed that did not match the classical pattern of disease described following experimental infection (61). Although this altered pathology could have been explained by the differences in the *M. tuberculosis* strain that caused infection, such studies serve to illustrate

that the findings from experimental studies should be interpreted with caution and should, wherever possible, be corroborated by findings in humans rather than become the accepted dogma.

Assessment of Vaccines

Vaccines have been tested in animal models for many decades and have enabled the progression of several candidates through to efficacy testing in humans. Despite some promising candidates being identified during the preclinical stages of testing, a new candidate that can facilitate the current BCG vaccine, or even replace it, has not been identified. Ongoing efficacy trials may yet yield a superior vaccine but, in the meantime, the research and development activities continue.

Process and Capacity

In a perfect world, a new candidate would be tested in a minimum of two different animal species, by at least two separate laboratories that themselves have no vested interest, using adequate vaccination to challenge intervals, with sufficient animals in each group to provide statistical power, and with relevant clinical isolates as the challenge inoculum. Once a reasonable number of vaccines have been identified as "active," then head-to-head evaluations would help prioritize the candidates for final testing in NHPs.

A lack of resources and a limited degree of global cooperation have, until now, prevented this. A large number of candidates have been tested in mice, reflecting the fact that many laboratories have that capability but, frequently, the candidate does not progress to being tested in more advanced or stringent models. There is a variety of reasons for this, but cost and capacity are the main ones. Even at the guinea pig level, very few facilities are equipped (and have the experience) to conduct appropriately controlled and powered efficacy testing using this model. The costs associated with caging or feed are much higher than studies in mice, and so the cost of even a relatively small study can become prohibitive. One solution to this is for vaccine developers to apply for their candidates to be tested by independent laboratories that have expertise in the animal models rather than in vaccine development. Such facilities are supported by NIH funding in the United States and by the European Union. These facilities provide increased capacity, an independent evaluation of efficacy, and the capability to conduct comparative evaluations where the efficacy of one candidate can be compared directly with another. Given the advantages of independent testing facilities, it would be beneficial to the field to mobilize resources to increase the capacity in terms of including more laboratories and extending the models that are offered, beyond mice and guinea pigs.

Mechanism of Protection

BCG is invariably used as a positive control in evaluating new candidates, but this imprints a built-in bias (62). It assumes that a new candidate will induce protective mechanisms that have similar kinetics to BCG, and will result in at least a minimum of 0.5 to 0.7 $\log_{10}$ reduction in lung CFU levels after low-dose aerosol infection. If the new candidate works differently, such as needing a finite time as well as boosting to achieve a stable, long-lived memory T-cell response, or, alternatively, if it does not reduce the bacterial load but still can establish granulomas that are highly stable and bacteriostatic, then, in our current screening protocols, it would be rejected as inactive (63). There is therefore a risk that new candidates or novel mechanisms of action have been lost because of this assumption. In this regard, a vaccine that induces an immune response but completely fails to provide any signal of efficacy can provide extremely useful information about mechanisms of protection. Unfortunately, such information is often not accessible because of the tendency for reporting only positive efficacy data. The importance of negative data is recognized by most researchers, yet it remains extremely difficult to get these data published and made available to others.

Vaccine Testing Protocols

Many factors must be considered when constructing models for vaccine testing. The first major consideration is the vaccine to challenge interval; in many protocols, the challenge infection is given at the peak of the effector T-cell response to the (positive control) BCG vaccine. Although a candidate may demonstrate protective immunity (assuming it has similar kinetics to BCG) under such a protocol, no information will be obtained about the induction of adequate memory immunity. For example, BCG establishes memory immune T cells in the lungs in about 10 to 15 weeks, but, in some protocols, the challenge infection is given only 6 to 8 weeks post-BCG.

The other key consideration is the infectious challenge, since the strain of *M. tuberculosis* used, the route, and dose of challenge can all have an impact on the vaccine-induced host response. This could be termed "bacterial immunogenicity," which is the speed with which host immunity recognizes the presence of the challenge infection. It is probably related to the kinetics of bacterial production of immunodominant antigens such as ESAT6. Most laboratories rely on challenge studies that use either H37Rv or Erdman as the infectious agent, since these strains replicate well in most of the animal models, they are drug-sensitive, and they allow direct comparisons of data between laboratories. However, there is a growing concern that they do not reflect reality, given the increasing frequency of newly emerging clinical isolates that are more virulent and induce much broader T-cell responses (64).

There is evidence that strain fitness is an important consideration, and this has recently been proposed (18) as a factor in the failure of the MVA85A vaccine to boost BCG in a phase IIb efficacy trial. This arose from the observation that, while highly virulent Beijing strains from the United States and the Western Cape (where the trial was conducted) grew equally well in unvaccinated guinea pigs, BCG strongly inhibited strains from the Cape, whereas its activity against the U.S. strains was far more variable. This suggested the possibility (yet to be proven) that, while the Western Cape strains were highly virulent, they were also of relatively low fitness and it was not possible to see the effect of the MVA85A boost above that afforded by BCG alone (65). This is supported by data that suggest that host recognition of these infections is rapidly leading to more effective control by BCG (18).

The impact of vaccine on challenge interval and challenge strain is illustrated in Fig. 1. Following introduction of a vaccine, there is an effector immune response, which eventually contracts and is replaced by an emerging memory immune response. This takes a finite time, and, in many protocols, boosting vaccines are given before memory has had a chance to become fully established (explaining why many boosting candidates fail). After the challenge infection is given, the speed of recognition of the infection depends on its native immunogenicity, coupled with its ability to grow, with "ΔCFU with time" reflecting its intrinsic virulence. Finally, what is not always taken into account is that an isolate can be virulent, but also vary in fitness, with high-fitness strains more likely to be only transiently affected by the immunity the vaccine has generated.

Assessment of New Drugs

Animal models have played a significant role in the assessment of new drugs against tuberculosis, beginning with the testing of streptomycin in guinea pigs by Feldman in the mid-1950s, followed by seminal studies in various animal species pioneered by Mitchison, Grosset, and others since then. In general, drugs found to be effective in these models tend to be equally effective in humans. In fact, most of the conventional drug

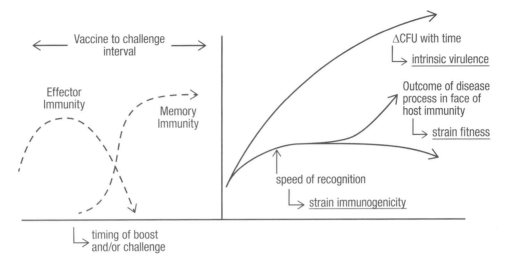

Figure 1 The theoretical relationship among virulence, immunogenicity, and fitness, and its importance in the assessment of vaccine efficacy. In assessing whether a vaccine is active, the vaccine to challenge (or boost) interval is critical. In most protocols, this interval is relatively short, and so a boosting candidate, or the challenge infection itself, is given before the effector immune response has completely contracted and the subsequent memory immune response (the true target) has become fully established. After challenge, the change in CFU levels versus time indicates the intrinsic virulence of the strain used. If the vaccine has induced memory immunity, the growth of the challenge infection is slowed, but the rapidity with which this happens also depends on the immunogenicity of the organism. Finally, recent studies (see reference 18, for example) indicate that certain clinical strains, despite high virulence, are very effectively controlled by BCG vaccination, suggesting low fitness, whereas others are transiently inhibited but after a while continue to grow progressively.

regimens in use today were thoroughly tested in mice and other models.

Basic parameters needed to advance a potential tuberculosis drug are obtained from such models, including safety, maximum tolerated dose, and pharmacokinetic and pharmacodynamic determinations. This remains useful today, because the emergence of drug resistance has spurred the continued development of new drugs for tuberculosis.

The mouse models continue to advance and undergo refinements. The availability of IFNγ gene-disrupted mice provided a rapidly progressive infection model (66), which had the benefit of substantially reducing the amount of compound needed for evaluation, as well as a rapid readout of effectiveness. Similarly, the highly reproducible reactivation of disease seen in granulocyte-macrophage colony-stimulating factor knockout mice allowed the screening of compounds to prevent this (67). More recently, the C3HeB/FeJ mutant mouse model has been used to evaluate drugs in a model of severe lung necrosis (68).

As with certain vaccine candidates, some studies in different laboratories have yielded different results. One such example is metronidazole, which had some activity in a rabbit model, but consistently failed to

have any activity in several other models (69–71). A subsequent reevaluation of the mouse model (72, 73) led to the conclusion that laboratory strains should not be used just by themselves, and that there was variability even between the H37Rv strains kept in different laboratories, emphasizing the point (also made above in the context of vaccines) that the efficacy of new drug regimens needs to tested and reproduced by more than one laboratory before moving to clinical trials. A positive outcome of these problems was that they resulted in a collective discussion between the major screening laboratory groups, with an agreement to cooperate and converge toward a rationally derived set of standardized assays and protocols to use to evaluate compounds in the future.

LIMITATIONS

To What Extent Are Animal Models Predictive?

This question is particularly relevant, given the recent failure of the MVA85A trial in South Africa (74). The vaccine candidate had undergone extensive testing, showing activity in mice, guinea pigs, and NHP, as well as being safe and immunogenic in early clinical studies, and thus many were quick to conclude that the animal models are by definition "not predictive." This was followed by a period of considerable introspection, particularly by those reflecting on the ongoing development of alternative vaccine candidates that have progressed to the clinic following testing in the same or similar animal models as MVA85A.

The outcome of such reflection, inevitably, is that there is clearly room for improvement and refinement of the animal models and the criteria that are used to prioritize the most promising vaccines. As recently discussed (75), MVA85A was tested in multiple models but always against laboratory strains, and not against more virulent Beijing strains. MVA85A was tested in infants, whereas the animal studies used adults with fully developed immune systems. The infant trial was additionally powered to observe a much greater improvement in efficacy over BCG alone than was detected in the animal studies where the difference between BCG boosted with MVA85A and BCG alone was only ever a small improvement. In an experimental setting where many variables are controlled, small improvements in efficacy can be observed with relatively small and tractable experiments. Prior to the trial, there was no benchmark against which to evaluate the performance of the animal models, and we did not know whether the small but significant improvements in efficacy in animals had any relevance to efficacy in humans. It appears, in retrospect, that a much stronger efficacy signal may be needed in animals. This could be a greater effect in the existing models or demonstration of efficacy in more complex and stringent animal models.

A commonly used protocol to measure whether a vaccine can boost BCG in animals is to demonstrate further reduction in CFU in the organs (compared with BCG alone) at an early time point postchallenge. This protocol has high statistical power to detect small differences and is therefore useful in screening and in comparing vaccines head-to-head. It could be argued that a more relevant and therefore predictive approach is the demonstration of increased long-term survival (Kaplan-Meier analysis). This is a much more stringent test of efficacy because the difference in mean survival times between the BCG and BCG-boost vaccine needs to be substantial. This is due to the low statistical power of TB vaccine survival studies, which, as discussed previously (62), require either very large group sizes or highly potent vaccines that induce close to 100% survival.

As discussed above, a parameter that has received very little attention is the fitness of the local strains against which the vaccine is being tested. Thus, we assume that if vaccine X works against H37Rv, then it will naturally work in the field. This could be a serious flaw since strain fitness could be an important variable. If it is low (circulating in a region with malnutrition and high rates of HIV) and BCG strongly protects against it, then the boost vaccine would be expected to offer only a small improvement. It would be impossible to observe a small, statistically significant boosting effect in a trial powered to observe a 60% improvement over BCG. In other words, it is feasible that the MVA85A candidate was tested in a boosting situation where boosting was not achievable. This argues strongly for a consideration of the target population for the vaccine when designing animal studies and this includes incorporation of relevant *M. tuberculosis* strains.

The complexity of human TB disease and the many variables that will influence the potency of a vaccine in different populations or environments can never be fully replicated in animal models. Different animal models can recapitulate certain features and be used to test hypotheses and make decisions in vaccine development, but it is important to not to assume that all information gleaned from animal models is predictive. Human lungs develop necrosis similarly to guinea pigs, but, in terms of cellular organization, they are more similar to that seen in mice (76). NHPs are considered the closest to humans, but there are differences in their lung anatomy—the human lung, being much larger, has secondary lobes held together by intralobular septae, which are absent in the lungs of much smaller NHP. Having recognized the limitations in terms of predicting outcomes in humans, it is imperative that, moving forward, animal models are improved wherever possible and that there is greater scrutiny and stringency when evaluating whether a candidate vaccine shows protection in animals that could translate to efficacy in humans.

Ethical and Husbandry Issues

Animal studies, even those conducted with small animals, bear a cost that is both financial and ethical. The facilities needed to conduct these studies require a high level of sophistication, particularly when operating at biosafety level 3, which involves complex engineering and equipment to maintain operator protection. There are stringent rules and regulations covering both the animal welfare and biosafety aspects that must be considered in the logistics of the experiment design and conduct.

It can be difficult to achieve the level of funding that will cover the purchase of sufficient animals combined with their facility per diem costs, and this can lead to compromise in study design, for example, using shorter vaccine-to-challenge or vaccine-to-boost intervals than is ideal. While applying the principles of "replacement, reduction, and refinement" in animal studies, it is essential that this be balanced against the need to have sufficient statistical power (63). Experiments that cannot be interpreted are not ethically justified and there may be a case for increasing the number of animals to perform a robust study that has a high benefit to (ethical) cost ratio.

Most regulatory bodies (in the United States, the U.S. Department of Agriculture) have strict rules for the use of animals in research. This includes having predetermined endpoints for humane euthanasia. Tuberculosis is a progressive disease in most animal models, and so considerable care has to be taken (both by the scientific staff and the laboratory animal facility staff) to avoid, as much as possible, stress to the animal, to use care in terms of handling or restraint, and to monitor continuously for suffering. As an example, in the context of tuberculosis in guinea pigs, measurement of weight, observation of eye color (changes from bright pink to dark pink/red as the animal sickens), and measurement (using a pulse-Ox device) of arterial oxygen tension have proven useful to some degree, whereas measurement of body temperature is not (complicated by the body's natural diurnal rhythm).

Animal husbandry issues are themselves important. Mice are usually housed in groups of five, and where possible this should be done for guinea pigs as well, given their highly social interactions. Enrichment is important as well (as an example, mice have hours of fun shredding used toilet rolls and making nests from them). Above all, the husbandry staff needs to be aware of the risks: some species such as NHPs are dangerous and can bite, whereas others, such as rabbits, have the potential to shed bacilli in their urine.

Concluding Remarks

Animal models have underpinned TB research historically and continue to provide essential information to identify antigen targets and vaccination strategies through pathogenesis and host-response studies. Various animal models have been used to establish proof of concept for vaccine immunogenicity, safety and efficacy (and therapeutic effect of drugs) and, in conjunction with human studies, have enabled progression of several candidates to clinical trials. Animal studies should always be justifiable and appropriately designed to obtain maximum benefit from the results, and there should be a greater commitment to sharing results, par-

ticularly negative data. As clinical trial data emerge, we are learning more about the predictive value of the animal models, and it is clear that improvements can be made, particularly with regard to consideration of the target human population for the vaccines.

Citation. Williams A, Orme IM. 2016. Animal models of tuberculosis: an overview. Microbiol Spectrum 4(4):TBTB2-0004-2015.

References

1. **Russell WMS, Burch RL.** 1959. *The Principles of Humane Experimental Technique*. Methuen, London, United Kingdom.
2. **Lefford MJ.** 1975. Transfer of adoptive immunity to tuberculosis in mice. *Infect Immun* 11:1174–1181.
3. **North RJ.** 1973. Importance of thymus-derived lymphocytes in cell-mediated immunity to infection. *Cell Immunol* 7:166–176.
4. **Orme IM.** 1987. The kinetics of emergence and loss of mediator T lymphocytes acquired in response to infection with *Mycobacterium tuberculosis*. *J Immunol* 138:293–298.
5. **Orme IM, Collins FM.** 1983. Protection against *Mycobacterium tuberculosis* infection by adoptive immunotherapy. Requirement for T cell-deficient recipients. *J Exp Med* 158:74–83.
6. **Driver ER, Ryan GJ, Hoff DR, Irwin SM, Basaraba RJ, Kramnik I, Lenaerts AJ.** 2012. Evaluation of a mouse model of necrotic granuloma formation using C3HeB/FeJ mice for testing of drugs against *Mycobacterium tuberculosis*. *Antimicrob Agents Chemother* 56:3181–3195.
7. **Cooper AM, Dalton DK, Stewart TA, Griffin JP, Russell DG, Orme IM.** 1993. Disseminated tuberculosis in interferon gamma gene-disrupted mice. *J Exp Med* 178:2243–2247.
8. **Flynn JL, Chan J, Triebold KJ, Dalton DK, Stewart TA, Bloom BR.** 1993. An essential role for interferon gamma in resistance to *Mycobacterium tuberculosis* infection. *J Exp Med* 178:2249–2254.
9. **Flynn JL, Goldstein MM, Chan J, Triebold KJ, Pfeffer K, Lowenstein CJ, Schreiber R, Mak TW, Bloom BR.** 1995. Tumor necrosis factor-alpha is required in the protective immune response against *Mycobacterium tuberculosis* in mice. *Immunity* 2:561–572.
10. **Saunders BM, Frank AA, Orme IM, Cooper AM.** 2002. CD4 is required for the development of a protective granulomatous response to pulmonary tuberculosis. *Cell Immunol* 216:65–72.
11. **Turner J, D'Souza CD, Pearl JE, Marietta P, Noel M, Frank AA, Appelberg R, Orme IM, Cooper AM.** 2001. CD8- and CD95/95L-dependent mechanisms of resistance in mice with chronic pulmonary tuberculosis. *Am J Respir Cell Mol Biol* 24:203–209.
12. **Basaraba RJ.** 2008. Experimental tuberculosis: the role of comparative pathology in the discovery of improved tuberculosis treatment strategies. *Tuberculosis (Edinb)* 88(Suppl 1):S35–S47.

13. McMurray DN, Collins FM, Dannenberg AM Jr, Smith DW. 1996. Pathogenesis of experimental tuberculosis in animal models. *Curr Top Microbiol Immunol* **215:**157–179.

14. McMurray DN. 2001. A coordinated strategy for evaluating new vaccines for human and animal tuberculosis. *Tuberculosis (Edinb)* **81:**141–146.

15. McMurray DN. 2001. Determinants of vaccine-induced resistance in animal models of pulmonary tuberculosis. *Scand J Infect Dis* **33:**175–178.

16. Orme IM. 2011. Development of new vaccines and drugs for TB: limitations and potential strategic errors. *Future Microbiol* **6:**161–177.

17. Orme IM. 2013. Vaccine development for tuberculosis: current progress. *Drugs* **73:**1015–1024.

18. Henao-Tamayo M, Shanley CA, Verma D, Zilavy A, Stapleton MC, Furney SK, Podell B, Orme IM. 2015. The efficacy of the BCG vaccine against newly emerging clinical strains of *Mycobacterium tuberculosis*. *PLoS One* **10:**e0136500.

19. Shanley CA, Streicher EM, Warren RM, Victor TC, Orme IM. 2013. Characterization of W-Beijing isolates of *Mycobacterium tuberculosis* from the Western Cape. *Vaccine* **31:**5934–5939.

20. Ordway DJ, Shanley CA, Caraway ML, Orme EA, Bucy DS, Hascall-Dove L, Henao-Tamayo M, Harton MR, Shang S, Ackart D, Kraft SL, Lenaerts AJ, Basaraba RJ, Orme IM. 2010. Evaluation of standard chemotherapy in the guinea pig model of tuberculosis. *Antimicrob Agents Chemother* **54:**1820–1833.

21. Shang S, Shanley CA, Caraway ML, Orme EA, Henao-Tamayo M, Hascall-Dove L, Ackart D, Lenaerts AJ, Basaraba RJ, Orme IM, Ordway DJ. 2011. Activities of TMC207, rifampin, and pyrazinamide against *Mycobacterium tuberculosis* infection in guinea pigs. *Antimicrob Agents Chemother* **55:**124–131.

22. Peña JC, Ho WZ. 2015. Monkey models of tuberculosis: lessons learned. *Infect Immun* **83:**852–862.

23. Flynn JL, Gideon HP, Mattila JT, Lin PL. 2015. Immunology studies in non-human primate models of tuberculosis. *Immunol Rev* **264:**60–73.

24. Scanga CA, Flynn JL. 2014. Modeling tuberculosis in nonhuman primates. *Cold Spring Harb Perspect Med* **4:**a018564.

25. Takaki K, Davis JM, Winglee K, Ramakrishnan L. 2013. Evaluation of the pathogenesis and treatment of *Mycobacterium marinum* infection in zebrafish. *Nat Protoc* **8:**1114–1124.

26. Swaim LE, Connolly LE, Volkman HE, Humbert O, Born DE, Ramakrishnan L. 2006. *Mycobacterium marinum* infection of adult zebrafish causes caseating granulomatous tuberculosis and is moderated by adaptive immunity. *Infect Immun* **74:**6108–6117.

27. Davis JM, Clay H, Lewis JL, Ghori N, Herbomel P, Ramakrishnan L. 2002. Real-time visualization of mycobacterium-macrophage interactions leading to initiation of granuloma formation in zebrafish embryos. *Immunity* **17:**693–702.

28. Cosma CL, Swaim LE, Volkman H, Ramakrishnan L, Davis JM. 2006. Zebrafish and frog models of Mycobac-

terium marinum infection. *Curr Protoc Immunol* Chapter 10:Unit 10B. 2.

29. Ramakrishnan L. 2013. The zebrafish guide to tuberculosis immunity and treatment. *Cold Spring Harb Symp Quant Biol* **78:**179–192.

30. Yang CT, Cambier CJ, Davis JM, Hall CJ, Crosier PS, Ramakrishnan L. 2012. Neutrophils exert protection in the early tuberculous granuloma by oxidative killing of mycobacteria phagocytosed from infected macrophages. *Cell Host Microbe* **12:**301–312.

31. Turner OC, Basaraba RJ, Frank AA, Orme IM. 2003. Granuloma formation in mouse and guinea pig models of experimental tuberculosis, p 65–84. *In* Boros DL (ed), *Granulomatous Infections and Inflammation: Cellular and Molecular Mechanisms.* ASM Press, Washington, DC.

32. Berry MP, Graham CM, McNab FW, Xu Z, Bloch SA, Oni T, Wilkinson KA, Banchereau R, Skinner J, Wilkinson RJ, Quinn C, Blankenship D, Dhawan R, Cush JJ, Mejias A, Ramilo O, Kon OM, Pascual V, Banchereau J, Chaussabel D, O'Garra A. 2010. An interferon-inducible neutrophil-driven blood transcriptional signature in human tuberculosis. *Nature* **466:**973–977.

33. Eum SY, Kong JH, Hong MS, Lee YJ, Kim JH, Hwang SH, Cho SN, Via LE, Barry CE III. 2010. Neutrophils are the predominant infected phagocytic cells in the airways of patients with active pulmonary TB. *Chest* **137:**122–128.

34. Orme IM. 2014. A new unifying theory of the pathogenesis of tuberculosis. *Tuberculosis (Edinb)* **94:**8–14.

35. Lurie MB. 1939. Studies on the mechanism of immunity in tuberculosis: the mobilization of mononuclear phagocytes in normal and immunized animals and their relative capacities for division and phagocytosis. *J Exp Med* **69:**579–599.

36. Lurie MB. 1939. Studies on the mechanism of immunity in tuberculosis: the role of extracellular factors and local immunity in the fixation and inhibition of growth of tubercle bacilli. *J Exp Med* **69:**555–578.

37. Lurie MB, Zappasodi P, Cardona-Lynch E, Dannenberg AM Jr. 1952. The response to the intracutaneous inoculation of BCG as an index of native resistance to tuberculosis. *J Immunol* **68:**369–387.

38. Dannenberg AM Jr. 1968. Cellular hypersensitivity and cellular immunity in the pathogensis of tuberculosis: specificity, systemic and local nature, and associated macrophage enzymes. *Bacteriol Rev* **32:**85–102.

39. Dannenberg AM Jr. 1970. Pathogenesis of tuberculosis: local and systemic immunity and cellular hypersensitivity. *Bull Int Union Tuberc* **43:**177–178.

40. Dannenberg AM Jr. 1991. Delayed-type hypersensitivity and cell-mediated immunity in the pathogenesis of tuberculosis. *Immunol Today* **12:**228–233.

41. Manabe YC, Dannenberg AM Jr, Tyagi SK, Hatem CL, Yoder M, Woolwine SC, Zook BC, Pitt ML, Bishai WR. 2003. Different strains of *Mycobacterium tuberculosis* cause various spectrums of disease in the rabbit model of tuberculosis. *Infect Immun* **71:**6004–6011.

42. Nedeltchev GG, Raghunand TR, Jassal MS, Lun S, Cheng QJ, Bishai WR. 2009. Extrapulmonary dissemina-

tion of *Mycobacterium bovis* but not *Mycobacterium tuberculosis* in a bronchoscopic rabbit model of cavitary tuberculosis. *Infect Immun* **77**:598–603.

43. Hunter RL, Jagannath C, Actor JK. 2007. Pathology of postprimary tuberculosis in humans and mice: contradiction of long-held beliefs. *Tuberculosis (Edinb)* **87**: 267–278.

44. Tsenova L, Ellison E, Harbacheuski R, Moreira AL, Kurepina N, Reed MB, Mathema B, Barry CE III, Kaplan G. 2005. Virulence of selected *Mycobacterium tuberculosis* clinical isolates in the rabbit model of meningitis is dependent on phenolic glycolipid produced by the bacilli. *J Infect Dis* **192**:98–106.

45. Gray DF, Noble JL, O'Hara M. 1961. Allergy in experimental rat tuberculosis. *J Hyg (Lond)* **59**:427–436.

46. Gray DF. 1961. The relative natural resistance of rats and mice to experimental pulmonary tuberculosis. *J Hyg (Lond)* **59**:471–477.

47. Gray DF, Graham-Smith H, Noble JL. 1960. Variations in natural resistance to tuberculosis. *J Hyg (Lond)* **58**: 215–227.

48. Lefford MJ, McGregor DD, Mackaness GB. 1973. Properties of lymphocytes which confer adoptive immunity to tuberculosis in rats. *Immunology* **25**:703–715.

49. Lefford MJ, McGregor DD, Mackaness GB. 1973. Immune response to *Mycobacterium tuberculosis* in rats. *Infect Immun* **8**:182–189.

50. Sugawara I, Mizuno S. 2008. Higher susceptibility of type 1 diabetic rats to *Mycobacterium tuberculosis* infection. *Tohoku J Exp Med* **216**:363–370.

51. Vordermeier HM, Villarreal-Ramos B, Cockle PJ, McAulay M, Rhodes SG, Thacker T, Gilbert SC, McShane H, Hill AV, Xing Z, Hewinson RG. 2009. Viral booster vaccines improve *Mycobacterium bovis* BCG-induced protection against bovine tuberculosis. *Infect Immun* **77**:3364–3373.

52. Gil O, Díaz I, Vilaplana C, Tapia G, Díaz J, Fort M, Cáceres N, Pinto S, Caylà J, Corner L, Domingo M, Cardona PJ. 2010. Granuloma encapsulation is a key factor for containing tuberculosis infection in minipigs. *PLoS One* **5**:e10030.

53. Margulies DH. 2014. The in-betweeners: MAIT cells join the innate-like lymphocytes gang. *J Exp Med* **211**: 1501–1502.

54. Cowley SC. 2014. MAIT cells and pathogen defense. *Cell Mol Life Sci* **71**:4831–4840.

55. Henao-Tamayo M, Ordway DJ, Orme IM. 2014. Memory T cell subsets in tuberculosis: what should we be targeting? *Tuberculosis (Edinb)* **94**:455–461.

56. Fletcher HA. 2007. Correlates of immune protection from tuberculosis. *Curr Mol Med* **7**:319–325.

57. Orme IM, Basaraba RJ. 2014. The formation of the granuloma in tuberculosis infection. *Semin Immunol* **26**: 601–609.

58. Basaraba RJ, Smith EE, Shanley CA, Orme IM. 2006. Pulmonary lymphatics are primary sites of *Mycobacterium tuberculosis* infection in guinea pigs infected by aerosol. *Infect Immun* **74**:5397–5401.

59. Davis JM, Ramakrishnan L. 2009. The role of the granuloma in expansion and dissemination of early tuberculous infection. *Cell* **136**:37–49.

60. Urdahl KB, Shafiani S, Ernst JD. 2011. Initiation and regulation of T-cell responses in tuberculosis. *Mucosal Immunol* **4**:288–293.

61. Dharmadhikari AS, Basaraba RJ, Van Der Walt ML, Weyer K, Mphahlele M, Venter K, Jensen PA, First MW, Parsons S, McMurray DN, Orme IM, Nardell EA. 2011. Natural infection of guinea pigs exposed to patients with highly drug-resistant tuberculosis. *Tuberculosis (Edinb)* **91**:329–338.

62. McShane H, Jacobs WR, Fine PE, Reed SG, McMurray DN, Behr M, Williams A, Orme IM. 2012. BCG: myths, realities, and the need for alternative vaccine strategies. *Tuberculosis (Edinb)* **92**:283–288.

63. Williams A, Hall Y, Orme IM. 2009. Evaluation of new vaccines for tuberculosis in the guinea pig model. *Tuberculosis (Edinb)* **89**:389–397.

64. Orme IM. 2015. Tuberculosis vaccine types and timings. *Clin Vaccine Immunol* **22**:249–257.

65. Orme I. 2014. Letter to the editor. *Tuberculosis (Edinb)* **94**:717.

66. Lenaerts AJ, Gruppo V, Brooks JV, Orme IM. 2003. Rapid in vivo screening of experimental drugs for tuberculosis using gamma interferon gene-disrupted mice. *Antimicrob Agents Chemother* **47**:783–785.

67. Woolhiser LK, Hoff DR, Marietta KS, Orme IM, Lenaerts AJ. 2009. Testing of experimental compounds in a relapse model of tuberculosis using granulocyte-macrophage colony-stimulating factor gene-disrupted mice. *Antimicrob Agents Chemother* **53**:306–308.

68. Lanoix JP, Lenaerts AJ, Nuermberger EL. 2015. Heterogeneous disease progression and treatment response in a C3HeB/FeJ mouse model of tuberculosis. *Dis Model Mech* **8**:603–610.

69. Brooks JV, Furney SK, Orme IM. 1999. Metronidazole therapy in mice infected with tuberculosis. *Antimicrob Agents Chemother* **43**:1285–1288.

70. Hoff DR, Caraway ML, Brooks EJ, Driver ER, Ryan GJ, Peloquin CA, Orme IM, Basaraba RJ, Lenaerts AJ. 2008. Metronidazole lacks antibacterial activity in guinea pigs infected with *Mycobacterium tuberculosis*. *Antimicrob Agents Chemother* **52**:4137–4140.

71. Klinkenberg LG, Sutherland LA, Bishai WR, Karakousis PC. 2008. Metronidazole lacks activity against *Mycobacterium tuberculosis* in an in vivo hypoxic granuloma model of latency. *J Infect Dis* **198**:275–283.

72. De Groote MA, Gilliland JC, Wells CL, Brooks EJ, Woolhiser LK, Gruppo V, Peloquin CA, Orme IM, Lenaerts AJ. 2011. Comparative studies evaluating mouse models used for efficacy testing of experimental drugs against *Mycobacterium tuberculosis*. *Antimicrob Agents Chemother* **55**:1237–1247.

73. De Groote MA, Gruppo V, Woolhiser LK, Orme IM, Gilliland JC, Lenaerts AJ. 2012. Importance of confirming data on the in vivo efficacy of novel antibacterial drug regimens against various strains of *Mycobacterium tuberculosis*. *Antimicrob Agents Chemother* **56**:731–738.

74. Tameris MD, Hatherill M, Landry BS, Scriba TJ, Snowden MA, Lockhart S, Shea JE, McClain JB, Hussey GD, Hanekom WA, Mahomed H, McShane H; MVA85A 020 Trial Study Team. 2013. Safety and efficacy of MVA85A, a new tuberculosis vaccine, in infants previously vacci-

nated with BCG: a randomised, placebo-controlled phase
2b trial. *Lancet* **381:**1021–1028.

75. **McShane H, Williams A.** 2014. A review of preclinical animal models utilised for TB vaccine evaluation in the context of recent human efficacy data. *Tuberculosis (Edinb)*
94:105–110.

76. **Brighenti S, Andersson J.** 2012. Local immune responses
in human tuberculosis: learning from the site of infection.
J Infect Dis **205**(Suppl 2)**:**S316–S324.

77. **Jacobs WR Jr, McShane H, Mizrahi V, Orme IM (ed).**
Tuberculosis and the Tubercle Bacillus, 2nd ed. ASM
Press, Washington, DC, in press.

Tuberculosis and the Tubercle Bacillus, 2nd ed.
Edited by William R. Jacobs, Jr., Helen McShane, Valerie Mizrahi, and Ian M. Orme
© 2018 American Society for Microbiology, Washington, DC
doi:10.1128/microbiolspec.TBTB2-0002-2015

Mouse and Guinea Pig Models of Tuberculosis

7

Ian M. Orme and Diane J. Ordway

Small-animal models have provided a vast amount of useful information about the nature of tuberculosis infection and its pathogenesis, the host response to it, and the activity of potential new vaccines and drugs. While it is possible that central mechanisms would have been eventually discovered directly in humans, there is no doubt that much of what we know about the immune response to the disease was substantially accelerated by studies in the mouse model, which took direct advantage of the literal explosion in the availability of reagents developed by the mainstream immunology field over the past 3 or so decades. These advances have allowed us to define in great detail the nature of the T-cell response to *Mycobacterium tuberculosis* and its various elements, including control of activation and cellular recruitment by cytokines and chemokines, as well as more practical applications in the form of using this inexpensive model to test vaccines and drugs.

Far fewer laboratories have used the more difficult and more expensive guinea pig model, but it has one great advantage in that it demonstrates many elements of immunopathology that are very similar to that seen in infected human beings, particularly the development of primary lesion necrosis (until recently missing in most mouse models). In addition, partly because of this facet, it has proven to be very important for vaccine testing, and many agree it is a vital gateway prior to final evaluations in non-human primates.

In this article we provide an overview of important observations made in these models and their usages. More specific details, particularly regarding the innate and acquired immune responses, are covered in more detail elsewhere (178).

THE MOUSE MODEL

As noted elsewhere (178), soon after Koch discovered the tuberculosis bacterium, he found that the organism could readily infect mice, and this model has been a mainstay of research ever since. In particular, much of what we presently know about the immune response to the disease has been determined in this species.

In the 1920s the great geneticist Clarence Little began to develop "inbred" strains of mice in an effort to understand the genetic basis of tumor rejection. This impressed the British scientist Haldane, who obtained three lines of mice and asked his student, Gorer, to use them in his studies. This work, of course, paved the way to our current understanding of histocompatibility molecules and their key role in the presentation of antigens, and their central role in mechanisms of tissue rejection. By the late 1970s, commercial breeders had produced many inbred strains of mice (and their F1s), and these were almost universally used in studies of the immune response, including the response to tuberculosis.

Much of the early work in the mouse model concerned the relationship between "cellular immunity" and "delayed-type hypersensitivity" (measured as a skin response to tuberculin/purified protein derivative and thought to be a reflection of damaging pathology in the lungs) (1, 2), as well as simple but fundamental studies into the effects of culture conditions, routes and timings of infections, and so forth. In the 1980s, work took a more specific turn, with the first observations that thymus-derived "T cells" mediated immunity to tuberculosis (3), followed thereafter by the first distinction between the effects of CD4 and CD8 cells (4) (at the time, the latter were regarded as "suppressor T cells" and so the demonstration they could prolong survival

Colorado State University, Fort Collins, CO 80523.

after adoptive transfer was a shock), as well as studies demonstrating the induction of memory T cells (5, 6).

The 1990s saw a rejuvenation of the mouse model because of increasing concerns about the spread of tuberculosis globally and a concomitant rise in funding. A major breakthrough regarded the development of "gene disrupted" (gene knockout) mice, which opened the floodgates of our understanding of the relative importance of many molecules involved in the host immune response. This period also saw the development of multiple innovative vaccines and vaccine types that were tested in the mouse model, as were many new potential chemotherapies (the mouse is still today the initial screening point for new vaccines and drugs).

With the major components of immunity to tuberculosis mostly identified, the past 15 years have seen a continuing refinement in knowledge in terms of more precise detail. We now appreciate that both cytokines (interleukin [IL]-10, IL-12 for example) and chemokines exist as families of proteins directing immunity to tuberculosis, or related mechanisms, such as the correct recruitment of needed cell types to sites of infection. This refinement has been driven by the availability of a huge range of reagents, both at the mouse level (gene knockout, transgenic, congenic strains) and immunological (recognition of a vast number of cell markers [CD antigens] and monoclonal antibodies to them), which has specifically facilitated the application of flow cytometry. In addition, the mouse has helped us recognize the potential importance of multiple other cell types that were not initially recognized, including γδTCR T cells, NK cells, iNKT cells, as well as newly discovered cells such MAIT cells.

Gene-Disrupted Mice

Studies in gene knockout mice quickly confirmed the prevailing hypothesis that TH1 responses were centrally important to protective immunity. Mice in which the gene for gamma interferon (IFN-γ) was disrupted and then infected either by low-dose aerosol (7) or intravenously (8) completely lost their resistance to the infection, demonstrating the crucial participation of this cytokine. Soon after, a further study showed that mice lacking the tumor necrosis factor alpha (TNF-α) p55-receptor rapidly died after intravenous high-dose inoculation (9), indicating the equally important and vital contribution of TNF-α. In addition, it is now known that the TH1 response depends on T-bet expression, and mice lacking this transcription factor have decreased resistance (10).

The IFN-γ response is controlled by the IL-12 family of cytokines. Mice lacking the ability to synthesize this cytokine have no resistance to tuberculosis (11, 12), but

various peptide chains belonging to the IL-12 family can compensate, as elegantly shown in a series of further studies by Cooper et al. (13).

Other studies quickly followed. Mice lacking B cells, IL-4, or IL-10 did not show initial loss of resistance to infection, demonstrating the lack of importance of antibodies or TH2 responses, whereas mice lacking IL-6, or phoX (the animal cannot make a respiratory burst) only showed transient loss of resistance. Mice lacking γδTCR were not less resistant (14), but their granulomatous response in the lungs was more disorganized and contained many neutrophils (15), consistent with knowledge that they can secrete cytokines including IL-17 that control cell influx (16). Disruption of other genes controlling influx, such as CCR2, its ligand CCL2, CXCR3, and CCR5, all influence the capacity of the mouse to control the disease (17).

Mice lacking granulocyte-macrophage colony-stimulating factor (GM-CSF) die rapidly of tuberculosis, and the absence of this cytokine negatively influences levels of other molecules, including TNF-α, lymphotactin (XCL1), RANTES (CCL5), and MIP-1α/β. If the mice are "rescued" by drug treatment, they still reactivate soon afterward, a useful model for testing new drugs designed to prevent this (18). Studies in 2007 showed that lymphotactin secretion by activated CD8 cells helped drive the protective CD4 response and contributed to the stabilization of the granulomatous response (19).

There has recently been renewed interest in the role of the type I interferons in tuberculosis (20). It was earlier shown (21) that mice infected with a virulent strain of *M. tuberculosis* produced more IFN-αβ, and subsequent work in knockout mice lacking these cytokines demonstrated increased resistance (22). Increased IFN-αβ production by the host seems to be driven by the ESX-1 virulence factor of the bacterium (23), and this may be linked to excessive prostaglandin production (20). Gene disruption of the receptor for IFN-I protects mice from lethal infection (24). In contrast, however, another study (25) suggested a protective role for type I cytokines.

Results using gene knockout mice are not always consistent. For instance, mice lacking the β2-microglobulin molecule, essential to recognition of antigen by CD8 T cells, were rapidly killed by high-dose intravenous infection (26), but mice lacking the CD8 molecule itself showed no differences in response to low-dose aerosol infection in wild-type C57BL/6 mice until well into the chronic phase of the infection, at which point the disease grew progressively (27). The latter observation should be regarded in the context of a further study (28) showing that CD8 cells in mouse granulomas seem to be preferentially distributed on the edges of granulomas, perhaps suggesting that one of their roles might be to trap macrophages containing disseminating bacilli trying to move out of granulomatous lesions as they gradually break down.

Immunodeficient, Transgenic, and Congenic Mice

One of the first indications that T cells were involved in resistance to tuberculosis was the observation that mice on the BALB/c background lacking a thymus gland (called "nude mice" because they were also hairless) were highly susceptible to the infection (29). Subsequently, the actual genetic basis of this was found to be a disruption of the Foxn1 gene or the HNF-3/forkhead homolog 11 gene. This was more recently followed by the development of mice with severe combined immunodeficiency ("SCID mice") which have a deficiency in the enzyme Prkdc ("protein kinase, DNA activated, catalytic polypeptide"), which in turn does not allow V/D/J recombination to occur, preventing the maturity of both cellular and humoral immunity (30). These mice are highly susceptible to *M. tuberculosis* infection and die quickly, and one application of this is safety tests; for instance, if a new *M. tuberculosis* mutant is generated as a potential vaccine candidate, then it is usually tested in SCID mice to ensure that it is safe.

More recently, mice have become available that are deficient in the RAG-1 and RAG-2 genes ("Rag-knockout" mice). These genes encode enzymes that play an important role in the rearrangement and recombination of the genes of immunoglobulin and T-cell receptor molecules during the process of VDJ recombination, and as a result lack a functional T-cell response (31). As a result, they are very useful both for safety testing, as noted above, and for T cell adoptive transfer studies.

Transgene mice have proven useful in a variety of ways. For instance, transgenic mice have been used to reveal the relative effects of oxygen and nitrogen antimicrobial radicals (32). In another study, infection of mice possessing transgenic expression of T cells specific for ovalbumin were still able to express some limited early resistance to *M. tuberculosis* infection (33), and this was found subsequently to be due to TLR2 triggering by the Rv1411 cell wall lipoprotein of the bacillus. A further important advance was the development of "humanized" transgenic mice expressing human HLA major histocompatibility complex (MHC) molecules (34, 35) to give a clearer picture of specific epitopes that would be presented by these molecules. Transgenic

mice have also been generated that have a restricted T-cell receptor (TCR) repertoire (such as to ESAT-6), which allows these cells to be tracked over the course of the infection after adoptive transfer (36).

Congenic mice were not developed for tuberculosis research *per se*, but have proved useful in adoptive transfer studies to delineate by flow cytometric analysis between recipient host responses and those mediated by the transferred donor cells. Examples of congenic markers include CD45.1/CD45.2, and Thy-1.1/Thy-1.2.

Innate Immunity

Research into innate immunity in mice has revealed that they possess complex and redundant mechanisms designed to detect "danger signals," including the complex "Toll-like" receptors (TLR), of which now over a dozen have been found. TLRs are type I membrane proteins containing an extracellular domain with leucine-rich repeats and a cytoplasmic portion with homology to the IL-1 receptor (IL-1R) family, the triggering of which is transmitted into the cytoplasm by the protein MyD88. The relative importance of various receptors has been controversial. Most agree that TLR2 seems to be the predominant recognition receptor for mycobacterial products (37) driving the IL-12 response, and loss of TLR2, but not TLR4, increases susceptibility to *M. tuberculosis* infection (38–42). TLR2 and TLR9 appear to synergize in this respect (43), although TLR2 is not essential in the case of secondary reexposure to the disease (44). Not everybody agrees, however, with two studies claiming an important role for TLR4 (45, 46).

A major target of TLR2 is the 19-kDa lipoprotein of *M. tuberculosis* (47, 48), but it is also known that, if macrophages undergo prolonged exposure, this inhibits antigen processing (49); TLR2-independent mechanisms also exist (50). Another mycobacterial virulence factor, ESAT-6, can also bind TLR2 and diminish cell signaling (51) via interaction with extracellular kinases (52). Because TLR2 signaling leads to IL-12 production and TH1 immunity, this has been exploited as a vaccine strategy (53).

Other "pattern recognition" systems may also be involved. For instance, nucleotide-binding oligomerization domain 2 (NOD2) transfected cells recognize *M. tuberculosis* (54, 55) and NOD2 gene knockout mice are more susceptible to infection (56). NOD2 appears to be triggered by muramyl dipeptide motifs in the peptidoglycan cell wall of the bacillus (57, 58).

Genetic Studies in Mice

With the wide availability of multiple inbred strains of mice, it was inevitable that these would be used to try to understand the genetic basis of susceptibility to tuberculosis infection. In fact, it was long known that certain inbred strains, such as C57BL/6 and BALB/c mice, coped much better with high-dose challenge infections compared with other inbred strains such as CBA, DBA, and mice on the C3H background (59–61). Various theories were proposed to explain this, including rates of dissemination of bacteria from the lungs (62), and the poor expression of integrin molecules by T cells in "susceptible" strains (63).

By the 1980s it was recognized that resistance to certain infections (*Salmonella*, *Leishmania*) could be mapped to a certain gene (*Ity*, *Lsh*), and Turcotte and his colleagues discovered a homologous gene based on the behavior of BCG infections in different mouse strains, which they designated *Bcg*. In 1993, this gene was cloned and found to code for the now designated "natural resistance-associated macrophage protein" or *Nramp* (also called "solute carrier" Slc-11). These are proteins defined by a conserved hydrophobic core of 10 to 12 transmembrane domains, and function as transporters of divalent metal ions, particularly iron (64, 65).

For a time, it was thought that *Bcg/Nramp* could be a centrally important marker of resistance or susceptibility, not just to BCG, but tuberculosis as well (66, 67). However, it was soon discovered that, while this gene played a role in resistance to BCG infection, the designation of whether a mouse was Bcg^s or Bcg^r depended on its response to the Montreal strain of BCG, whereas virtually all other strains of BCG did not allow this distinction (68). In addition, further studies (69) showed that this trait was expressed by the progeny of hemopoietic precursor cells, but that subsequent backcross analysis revealed data suggesting that this resistance was controlled by more than one gene. Statistical analysis of the data by the maximum likelihood method suggested polygenic control, although the probability values suggested control by a major gene, presumably *Bcg*, influenced by modifier genes. Multiple studies a decade later addressed this directly, showing that different levels of resistance to *M. tuberculosis* infection in different mouse strains were also unrelated to their *Bcg* phenotype (70) and, in fact, segregated independently (71). Subsequent studies, in which B10 mice were backcrossed onto the C3H background, further confirmed that susceptibility was a multigenic trait (72).

The latter approach was then used to identify a new gene locus (like *Nramp*, on chromosome 1), designated *sst1*, that had a strong influence on susceptibility to tuberculosis, with congenic *sst1*-susceptible mice exhibiting poor immunity and severe lung damage (73); in addition, these mice responded poorly to BCG vaccination (74) and developed lung necrosis (75), which is unusual in mice. Further evidence for multigenic control was then provided by Apt and his colleagues using two strains of mice his team had developed: I/St mice that were highly susceptible, and A/Sn mice that were resistant (76), with the susceptibility of the I/St mice attributed to poor bactericidal activity of lung macrophages in these mice (77). A differential response by granulocytes has also been implicated (78).

A new and potentially important resource that should be mentioned are "diversity outbred mice" which are designed to permit the analysis of multiple complex genetic traits. These consist of heterogeneous stocks of mice derived from multiple inbred founder strains and maintained as outbreeding populations so as to increase mapping precision and introduce additional genetic diversity. Currently, these exist as a heterogeneous stock derived from eight inbred founder strains and maintained by randomized breeding among 175 mating pairs (79). Hopefully, application of this resource to the tuberculosis research field will occur in the near future.

The Mouse Response to Infection

Many of the earliest studies in the mouse gave the *M. tuberculosis* infection, often in very high doses, via a lateral tail vein or by injection into the peritoneum. As the field evolved, delivery via the nose or directly into the trachea was also used, so that much of the inoculum was deposited in the upper respiratory tract, with a small percentage surviving the mucosal surfaces and penetrating the tidal air volume sufficiently to reach the alveolus. Even today, these approaches are still used, but over the past 25 years or so many laboratories have tended to move toward the much more realistic low-dose aerosol model. By taking advantage of nebulizer delivery into contained animal caging, such as the widely used Glas-Col device, 50 to 200 or so viable bacilli can be deposited in the mouse lung in a reproducible manner (80–82). Larger instruments are needed for guinea pigs (Fig. 1).

As noted above, in many studies, mice on the C57 background tend to be used the most often. The uptake in the lungs can be determined by agar plating (usually 24 h or so after exposure) and the growth of the infection can be monitored against time thereafter by this method. Initial growth of *M. tuberculosis* strains is progressive, but as the immune response begins to recognize the presence of the infection, the increase in the numbers of bacteria (CFU) begins to slow down and flatten off (Fig. 2A). As described in detail elsewhere (178), this slowing reflects the activity of both innate

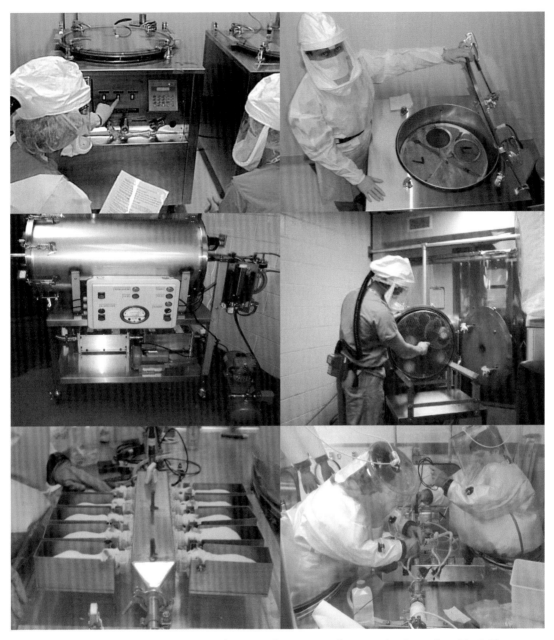

Figure 1 Commonly used devices for aerosol exposure of mice and guinea pigs. (**Top**) Glas-Col aerosol exposure device. The exposure cage is placed into the central chamber of the machine and closed from above by a tight gasket; this cage can hold approximately 100 mice at a time. (**Center**) The famous "Madison Chamber" first designed at the University of Wisconsin. The central chamber holds up to 18 guinea pigs at a time. (**Bottom panels**) The Henderson apparatus, which is a "nose-only" aerosol exposure device. This system can be readily used for infections of both mice and guinea pigs. (Photo courtesy of Ann Williams, with permission.)

and acquired immune mechanisms. In our working model (83), the ability of the bacteria to reach the lung interstitium is a key event in establishing a site of infection, from which it is then carried to draining lymph nodes and presented to T cells (84). This takes a finite time to occur, giving the infection enough time to become established and grow unrestrained, at least for a while.

Protective T cells (most of which are CD4+) can be detected in 7 to 10 days or so and they continue to

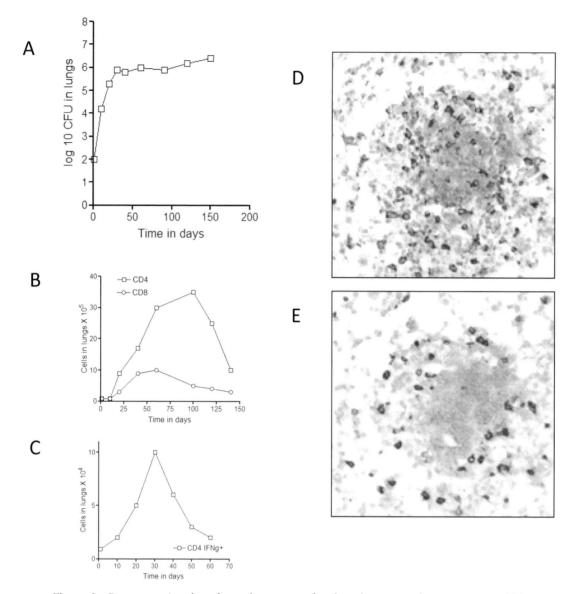

Figure 2 Representative data from the mouse after low-dose aerosol exposure to ~100 *M. tuberculosis* (in these examples, H37Rv). (**A**) After about 30 days of progressive growth the infection is controlled and contained. There follows what many regard as a "chronic phase" during which some animals may start to die of lung damage. (**B, C**) Influx of CD4 cells, which comprise the bulk of the T-cell response, and CD8 cells. A fraction of the total CD4 cell numbers stain positive for IFN-γ, and the numbers of these steadily contract after day 30 as the course of the infection is controlled. (**D, E**) Immunohistochemical identification of CD4 and CD8 cells in lung granulomatous tissue. CD4 cells tend to spread evenly across the lesions, whereas CD8 cells take up a more peripheral position. (Photos courtesy of O. Turner, with permission.)

expand in numbers and enter sites of infection in the mouse lung (Fig. 2B and C). Macrophages in the lesion become activated and release multiple antimicrobial products, and more are recruited in from the blood, thus forming the characteristic granuloma structure (85). Thus, these mechanisms first *control* and then *contain* the tuberculosis infection. However, because protection is not that rapidly established, bacilli escape from primary lesions in the lungs and disseminate in the blood to the spleen (and potentially other organs).

After 30 to 40 days or so, many studies describe the gradual establishment of "chronic disease" (even "latent" tuberculosis [86]) as the CFU values flatten. This is, in fact, not the case, because a closer evaluation often shows that the lung burden is actually increasing, albeit very slowly. At the same time, the effector immune response contracts, and after ~100 days or so, most T cells remaining in the lungs express markers suggesting they fall into the category of effector memory T cells (87).

As the infection continues, the granulomas in the lungs begin to degenerate (85), but initially, contrary to many reviews on this topic (see reference 88) that describe mouse granulomas as "disorganized," these structures in fact show evidence of considerable organization. This is discussed elsewhere, but the general argument that guinea pig granulomas are organized in spherical structures, whereas mouse granulomas are more disorganized and consist of cell aggregates, may be in need of reevaluation. It can be argued that guinea pig lesions (and those in humans) are not spherical because they are organized in that manner, but because the developing central caseum physically compresses the cells in the structure into this shape. Moreover, lymphocyte subsets are not organized in these compressed cellular rims, but instead are scattered, and this contrasts strongly with (what appear to be) organized aggregates of CD4 cells and B cells/plasma cells, surrounded by more peripheral cuffs of CD8 cells in the mouse granuloma (89) (Fig. 2D and E and 3). In this

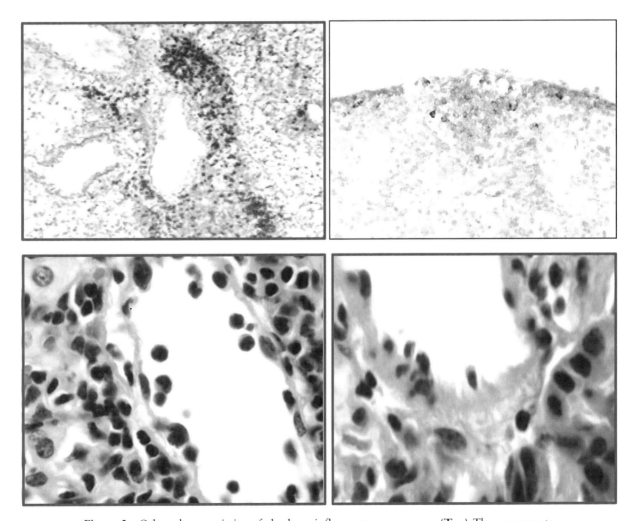

Figure 3 Other characteristics of the lung inflammatory response. (**Top**) The response to low-dose aerosol infection also includes the influx of aggregates of B cells (left) and small numbers of γδ+ T cells (right). (**Bottom**) Early during the course of the infection, cells can be seen interacting or adhering to the airway epithelial surface (left), but, as the disease process continues, this surface swells and degenerates (right). (Photos courtesy of O. Turner and M. Gonzalez-Juarrero, with permission.)

regard, a recent careful immunochemical analysis of human lung granulomas (90) in fact demonstrates that this structure also contains large aggregates of CD4 cells lying within sheets of macrophages, much lower numbers of CD8 distributed mainly on the lesion periphery, and scattered clumps of B cells; in other words, organized very similarly to our observations in the mouse model.

Mice eventually succumb to infection over time as granulomatous lesions gradually degenerate, although the actual kinetics of this event differs between inbred mouse strains (91). Degeneration seems linked to IL-10 production (92, 93), although the possibility that this cytokine is produced to dampen the inflammation in the lungs this process causes, but accidentally interferes with any residual T-cell immunity, has yet to be resolved (94). More recently, it has been shown (95) that blockade of the IL-10 receptor can improve protection against *M. tuberculosis* and that IL-10 may be directly interfering with the integrity of the lesion fibrosis process (96) and, in addition to CD4 cells and macrophages, may also be produced by CD8 cells (97).

For many years, the obvious focus of research into these processes was the activity of effector T-cell populations, especially those that were actively secreting IFN-γ. More recently, however, the field is facing the realization that the overall T-cell response is in fact very complex (17, 84, 98). The effector T cell clearly contracts and is replaced by effector memory T cells (in the lungs) and smaller numbers of central memory T cells in more central lymphoid tissues (87). This distribution pattern is also elicited by BCG vaccination in mice (87, 99), allowing speculation (100) that an inability of the vaccine to induce a more balanced response might be a factor in its loss of efficacy beyond childhood. This is further supported by the fact that

potent new vaccines appear to be better at inducing this specific memory T-cell subset (101). It is also very unclear what happens to the memory T-cell response after it is triggered, and recent disturbing data suggest that it is in fact far from stable (102), supporting the viewpoint that much is still to be learned (and needed if we are going to develop truly effective new vaccines) (103).

Adding to this complexity is the further realization that previously unrecognized T-cell subsets are also potentially key players in the overall response, notably CD4 Foxp3+ "regulatory T cells" and CD4 cells secreting the IL-17 family of cytokines (see reference 178). Regulatory T cells were initially observed due to their high expression of CD25 and mRNA encoding Foxp3, and their depletion increased IFN-γ responses *in vitro* (104). Expression of Foxp3 is a key marker allowing analysis (Fig. 4). Two studies published in 2007 provided the first demonstrations *in vivo* that regulatory T cells were involved in the immune response in mice; the first showed the ability of virulent clinical strains of *M. tuberculosis* to induce this subset (22), and a second published soon afterward showed the kinetics of accumulation of these cells into the lungs (105). Similarly, there is now considerable evidence that "TH17" are important in the overall response and are generally thought to be specifically directing cellular traffic into infected lesions (106–108), as well as potentially having some direct protective properties of their own (109).

THE GUINEA PIG

Progressive disease in the guinea pig, and multiple similarities to the disease in humans in terms of immunopathology make this species an ideal model of tuberculosis. In contrast to the mouse, however, the overall literature

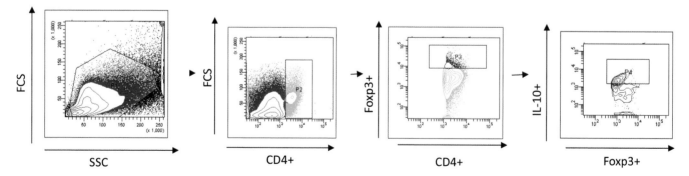

Figure 4 Some newly emerging strains of *M. tuberculosis* induce the appearance of regulatory T cells in the lungs. These can be identified and gated using flow cytometry because of their intracellular expression of the Foxp3 marker. Usually, approximately 50% of these cells are capable of secreting the cytokine IL-10.

on this animal model is far sparser. This reflects multiple issues, including the availability of level III animal holding capacities, animal husbandry expertise, and the availability of devices needed for aerosol exposure ("Madison chambers" and Henderson devices being the instruments of choice; see Fig. 1). In addition, the sheer expense of the model has become a major limitation (>$150 per animal from a major supplier, with animal per diem costs $2 to $3 per day or more for what are often very lengthy experiments). Accordingly, despite the overall attraction of the model, progress in developing it has moved much more slowly than with the mouse model.

Pioneering studies on the model began to emerge in the 1950s by Middlebrook and Dubos and their colleagues, followed by seminal work on the model by Smith and his colleagues at the University of Wisconsin, who produced many important papers for nearly the next 4 decades (facilitated by the development of the "Madison aerosol chamber" by their Department of Engineering) and focused on studies looking at the pathogenesis of the disease in the lungs, bacterial dissemination from this site, and various attempts to standardize the model in terms of testing BCG vaccines (110–114). In contrast, probably reflecting the almost complete lack of reagents, aspects regarding the lung pathology and the T-cell response were essentially unaddressed.

An important spin-off from the development of this model included the impact of malnutrition/calorific restriction on the course of the disease (115–117), as well as some limited attempts to test chemotherapy in these animals (118). By the early 1990s, however, the emphasis changed (119–121), and the guinea pig reemerged as a major model for vaccine testing, driven initially by Horwitz's laboratory showing that major secreted proteins of the bacillus could immunize the animal (122), followed later by the first demonstration that DNA-based vaccines could also work in this species (123). The following decade saw the first constructions of recombinant BCG vaccines (124) that could outperform regular BCG (125), the first successful testing of auxotrophic mutants as vaccines (126), as well as gene-deleted mutants such as ΔsecA2 (127) and SO2 (128), and new fusion protein candidates including an Ag85/ESAT-6 fusion (129) and a fusion (M72) that was both protective (130) and BCG boosting (131).

The same decade saw the first detailed description of the pathologic process in guinea pigs infected by low-dose aerosol (132), summarized in Fig. 5 in the context of our newly proposed model of pathogenesis, as well as the role of individual molecules including TGFβ (133), IL-8 (134), CCL5 (135), and TNF (136).

The field also saw some technical advances, including the application of magnetic resonance imaging (137), laser capture analysis (138), and the first testing of a new device for airborne sampling ("cough machine") that was then applied to clinical studies (139).

Reinforcing the similarities between pathology in the guinea pig and humans, studies at this time showed the generation of severe lymphadenopathy, lymphangitis (blockage of lymphatic vessels), and considerable accumulation of ferric ions in areas of necrosis occupied by the "necrosis-associated extracellular clusters" (NECs) (140–142). Copper accumulation mechanisms may also be involved (143).

A further advance has been the application of flow cytometry to this model. This was initially very hard to achieve, mainly because of a big signal background (autofluorescence). The culprit here were the granulocytes, but studies by Ordway (144) found that if this was gated out by using a specific antibody (MIL4), then mononuclear populations could be clearly seen (Fig. 6). Only a few additional antibodies are available at this time, but they are sufficient to measure the major subsets including CD4 cells, CD8 cells, B cells, and activated macrophages. The first studies using this approach revealed a strong cellular response involving mostly CD4 cells, but, after 30 days of the infection, the numbers of these cells in the lungs dropped significantly and were replaced by a steady increase in B cells and granulocytes (Fig. 7) (144). At this time, the lung pathology worsened considerably. This model is still very limited, however; nobody as yet has been able to measure intracellular markers such as IFN-γ or Foxp3 (although these can be detected by reverse transcriptase PCR), nor are there antibodies to surface markers such as CD44 or CCR7. Unfortunately, CD62L, which is so useful in the mouse model, is not present in the guinea pig.

The field at this time also saw a return of the use of the model to test new drugs. One such study, in 2007, was designed to test a new compound (R207910, now bedaquiline) but in the process made what could turn out to be a major discovery (145). For many years it was unclear why, despite extensive and apparently completely successful chemotherapy (both in animals and humans), some bacilli still survived and gave rise to reactivation disease. The prevailing idea was that these bacilli were in a state of latency, as well as acquiring drug resistance or tolerance somehow (146). However, this study revealed clumps or clusters of bacilli in lesion necrosis, and subsequent studies by Lenaerts and her team, in which they developed new advanced staining techniques (147, 148) to better detect these clusters, revealed the presence of large numbers of these structures

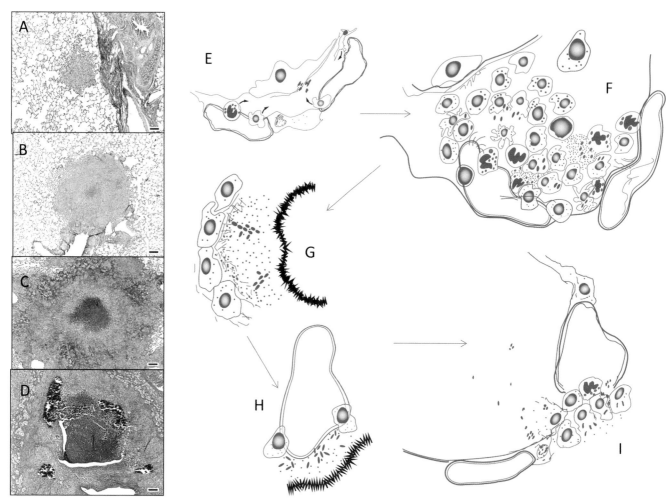

Figure 5 Immunopathology of the guinea pig model. (**A–D**) After 5 to 10 days after aerosol infection, small lesions appear, usually near larger airways. These consist mostly of macrophages, with a few lymphocytes and neutrophils beginning to arrive. By day 15 to 20 the lesion has become much larger (**B**) and the first signs of central necrosis are visible. By day 30 to 40 the lesion has the appearance of the "classical granuloma," with a large central area of necrosis obvious and with host cells remaining viable being compressed outward. Thereafter, the lesion becomes very large (**D**) and is dominated by a process of central dystrophic calcification (this entire process is described in greater detail in reference 88). (Photos courtesy of O. Turner.) More recently, we have attempted to explain this process in a "unifying theory" to relate it to reactivation disease (see reference 83). In our current working model, the infecting bacilli use their ESX proteins to escape the alveolar macrophage that engulfed them and reach the interstitium, which swells with tissue fluid due to the inflammation (**E**). Macrophages, dendritic cells, lymphocytes, and neutrophils accumulate at this new site of infection (**F**). The dendritic cells carry bacilli (or antigen secreted by them) off to the draining lymph node (a crucial event in generating acquired immunity), while (we propose) the local neutrophils degenerate and hence trigger the beginnings of the development of necrosis. Gradually, the lesion takes on its characteristic appearance, as the central lesion first starts to calcify (**G**). By now, many bacteria are extracellular, and some (we now believe based on recent new evidence) survive by becoming nonplanktonic and acid-fast-negative small communities. As the lesion calcifies, some of these communities get physically forced back toward normoxic tissue (**H**), where they may be recognized by host cells and trigger memory immunity. If this is not successfully dealt with, reactivation disease ensues, with the potential that some bacilli escape into the airway and can be potentially transmitted (**I**). (Photos in panels A to D courtesy of O. Turner, reprinted from reference 89. Panels E to I adapted from reference 83.)

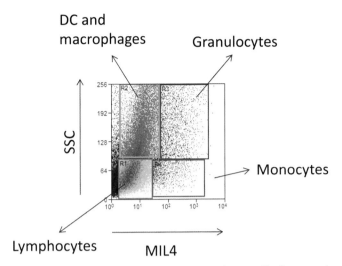

Figure 6 A new approach to gating host cells harvested from the guinea pig lung. The major impediment caused by severe autofluorescence in this model can be subverted by gating side scatter against the antibody MIL4. This reveals otherwise "hidden" lymphocytes, macrophages, and monocytes, while still allowing enumeration of the granulocyte response. DC, dendritic cells; SSC, side scatter.

remaining in necrosis that were invisible by acid-fast staining.

At much the same time, another group made the (at the time very surprising) observation that cultures of *M. tuberculosis* could form biofilms (149), thus providing a completely different explanation for bacterial persistence instead of latency, as well as explaining their apparent drug resistance. Based on these observations, collectively, we have proposed (83) an entirely new model of the pathogenesis of the disease, in which we propose that these NECs are in fact some form of biofilm-like communities that are drug tolerant as a result (and recent *in vitro* studies also strongly support this idea [150, 151]). As for the possibility of latency, two separate studies addressed whether the drug metronidazole (which targets bacilli under very low oxygen tension conditions, a primary facet of the "latency hypothesis") could possibly help remove these putative organisms; both studies showed no effect (152, 153).

Prolonged drug testing in guinea pigs presents some practical difficulties, mostly reflecting the responsiveness of the animal to stress. This was solved by developing a completely stress-free feeding method that allowed long-term studies and that resulted in a thorough analysis of the host response in the animal as the infection was steadily cleared, including the first use of magnetic resonance imaging to follow the resolution of lesions (154) (Fig. 8). This also revealed that even apparently successful chemotherapy still left be-

hind some residual lesion necrosis, as well as incomplete resolution of lymphoid vessel lymphangitis, which implicates these sites as the sources of reactivation disease. Subsequent studies then showed that combining BCG vaccination prior to challenge facilitates subsequent chemotherapy (155) and further reduces relapse rates in guinea pigs, but in nonvaccinated animals even highly effective bedaquiline-containing regimens still relapse at a similar rate to that seen with conventional chemotherapy (156).

In a fascinating new approach, recent studies have attempted to model direct human-to-guinea pig transmission, first performed in the classic studies by Riley and Wells 60 years ago. In the first new study, in 2008 in Peru, guinea pigs were infected by exposure to exhaled air from patients with multidrug-resistant tuberculosis (157), and it was subsequently shown that the frequency of guinea pig infection could be reduced by exposing the air to UV radiation (158). A more recent study, in South Africa, had a similar outcome if guinea pigs were exposed to multidrug-resistant patients, but it was also noted that as soon as patients began to respond to treatment, their infectiousness dropped rapidly (159). This in itself was an important observation.

New vaccines continue to be tested in this model, including the new fusion H1 (160), the fusion ID93 (161), alpha-crystallin (162), RUTI (163), and MTBVAC (164), as well as potential new postexposure vaccine candidates (165, 166). The model is also proving useful in defining the virulence of clinical strains (167, 168) and its possible relation to regulatory T-cell induction (169), as well as the transmission patterns of these organisms (170), their metabolomics signatures (171, 172), and whole genomic responses (173). Finally, a new and potentially very important application is to use the guinea pig to study diabetes mellitus and tuberculosis comorbidity (174) (an accidental observation made at Colorado State University when guinea pigs were fed drugs spiked in large amounts of sucrose).

As the reader would be aware, a major event in our field recently was the first large-scale phase IIb efficacy trial (in over 40 years) conducted in South Africa, in which the MVA85A vaccine was tested for its ability to boost BCG in infants and potentially reduce the number of children subsequently developing tuberculosis (175). While numbers did decline, they were insufficient to result in a statistically significant difference. This was disappointing (176), but even more disappointing was the questioning by multiple agencies, as well as the clinical tuberculosis research side of the field, of the entire usefulness of animal models—the idea being that since MVA85A worked in mice, guinea pigs, and macaques,

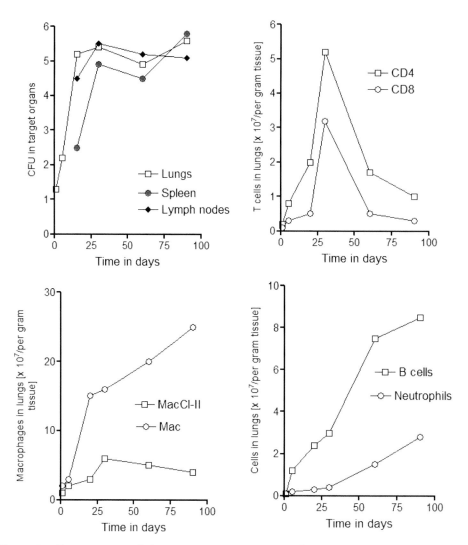

Figure 7 Characteristics of the guinea pig response to infection. After exposure to 10 to 20 bacilli, between 5-log and 6-log can be detected in all three major target organs after a month. There are strong CD4 and CD8 responses initially, but these then contract after ~30 days. There is a strong and progressive influx of macrophages into the lungs, but only a small percentage of these appear to be activated (class II MHC[hi]). After day 30 or so, significant numbers of B cells begin to arrive, as do neutrophils, presumably responding to the lung damage. (Adapted from reference 144.)

but then did not work in the South Africa trial, these models are invalid as vaccine predictors.

Proponents of this argument do have a case, at least to an extent. Clearly, efficacy studies in various animals and in humans are different. Humans are given BCG as infants, when their immune system is not fully matured. In various parts of the world, they are then continuously exposed to environmental mycobacteria. When they do contract tuberculosis, it is due to exposure to a clinical strain, not a half-century-old laboratory-adapted strain.

Returning to the MVA85A trial issue, completely lost in the argument at the time was the actual virulence/

fitness of the strains prevalent in the trial site area. A very recent study (177) addressed this and made the observation that clinical isolates from that area of the Western Cape were consistently *highly inhibited* in the guinea pig model by BCG vaccination. This result was interpreted as suggesting that strains in this area are of low fitness (transmitted in an area where there is both poor nutrition and very high rates of HIV infection), and furthermore that because of this, BCG by itself would be very effective, and therefore it would be virtually impossible to demonstrate any statistically significant boosting effect by a second vaccination. At this

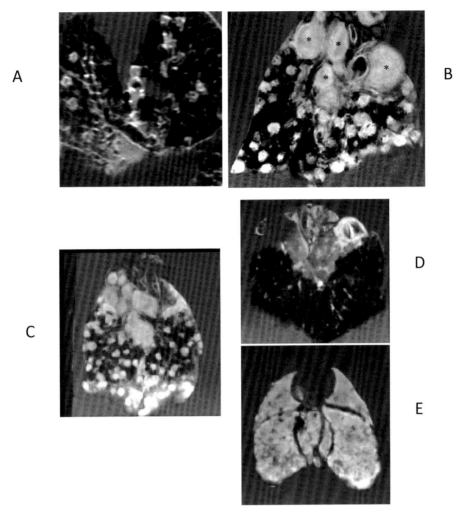

Figure 8 Magnetic resonance imaging of infected guinea pig lungs. (**A**) A day-30 image showing obvious lesions with transparent central necrosis ("doughnut appearance"; not obvious using other imaging methods). (**B**) Severe lymphadenopathy, which occurs rapidly, is readily seen by MRI. (**C**) Day-30 imaging prior to treatment for the next 4 months with chemotherapy, resolving most of the lesions (**D**), in comparison with untreated animals in which the lungs eventually become almost completely consolidated (**E**). (Photos courtesy of Susan Kraft. Adapted from reference 154.)

time, however, given the continued emphasis of the field on the laboratory-adapted strains (H37Rv, Erdman), the role of clinical isolate bacterial fitness has essentially been ignored to date.

Citation. Orme IM, Ordway DJ. 2016. Mouse and guinea pig models of tuberculosis. Microbiol Spectrum 4(4):TBTB2-0002-2015.

References

1. **Mackaness GB.** 1964. The immunological basis of acquired cellular resistance. *J Exp Med* **120**:105–120.
2. **Mackaness GB.** 1967. The relationship of delayed hypersensitivity to acquired cellular resistance. *Br Med Bull* **23**:52–54.
3. **Orme IM, Collins FM.** 1983. Protection against *Mycobacterium tuberculosis* infection by adoptive immunotherapy. Requirement for T cell-deficient recipients. *J Exp Med* **158**:74–83.
4. **Orme IM.** 1987. The kinetics of emergence and loss of mediator T lymphocytes acquired in response to infection with *Mycobacterium tuberculosis*. *J Immunol* **138**:293–298.
5. **Orme IM.** 1988. Characteristics and specificity of acquired immunologic memory to *Mycobacterium tuberculosis* infection. *J Immunol* **140**:3589–3593.
6. **Andersen P, Heron I.** 1993. Specificity of a protective memory immune response against *Mycobacterium tuberculosis*. *Infect Immun* **61**:844–851.
7. **Cooper AM, Dalton DK, Stewart TA, Griffin JP, Russell DG, Orme IM.** 1993. Disseminated tuberculosis

in interferon gamma gene-disrupted mice. *J Exp Med* **178**:2243–2247.

8. Flynn JL, Chan J, Triebold KJ, Dalton DK, Stewart TA, Bloom BR. 1993. An essential role for interferon gamma in resistance to *Mycobacterium tuberculosis* infection. *J Exp Med* **178**:2249–2254.

9. Flynn JL, Goldstein MM, Chan J, Triebold KJ, Pfeffer K, Lowenstein CJ, Schreiber R, Mak TW, Bloom BR. 1995. Tumor necrosis factor-alpha is required in the protective immune response against *Mycobacterium tuberculosis* in mice. *Immunity* **2**:561–572.

10. Lord GM, Rao RM, Choe H, Sullivan BM, Lichtman AH, Luscinskas FW, Glimcher LH. 2005. T-bet is required for optimal proinflammatory CD4+ T-cell trafficking. *Blood* **106**:3432–3439.

11. Cooper AM, Magram J, Ferrante J, Orme IM. 1997. Interleukin 12 (IL-12) is crucial to the development of protective immunity in mice intravenously infected with *Mycobacterium tuberculosis*. *J Exp Med* **186**:39–45.

12. Cooper AM, Roberts AD, Rhoades ER, Callahan JE, Getzy DM, Orme IM. 1995. The role of interleukin-12 in acquired immunity to *Mycobacterium tuberculosis* infection. *Immunology* **84**:423–432.

13. Cooper AM, Solache A, Khader SA. 2007. Interleukin-12 and tuberculosis: an old story revisited. *Curr Opin Immunol* **19**:441–447.

14. Ladel CH, Hess J, Daugelat S, Mombaerts P, Tonegawa S, Kaufmann SH. 1995. Contribution of alpha/beta and gamma/delta T lymphocytes to immunity against *Mycobacterium bovis* bacillus Calmette Guérin: studies with T cell receptor-deficient mutant mice. *Eur J Immunol* **25**:838–846.

15. D'Souza CD, Cooper AM, Frank AA, Mazzaccaro RJ, Bloom BR, Orme IM. 1997. An anti-inflammatory role for gamma delta T lymphocytes in acquired immunity to *Mycobacterium tuberculosis*. *J Immunol* **158**:1217–1221.

16. Lockhart E, Green AM, Flynn JL. 2006. IL-17 production is dominated by gammadelta T cells rather than CD4 T cells during *Mycobacterium tuberculosis* infection. *J Immunol* **177**:4662–4669.

17. Orme IM, Robinson RT, Cooper AM. 2015. The balance between protective and pathogenic immune responses in the TB-infected lung. *Nat Immunol* **16**:57–63.

18. Gonzalez-Juarrero M, Hattle JM, Izzo A, Junqueira-Kipnis AP, Shim TS, Trapnell BC, Cooper AM, Orme IM. 2005. Disruption of granulocyte macrophage-colony stimulating factor production in the lungs severely affects the ability of mice to control *Mycobacterium tuberculosis* infection. *J Leukoc Biol* **77**:914–922.

19. Ordway D, Higgins DM, Sanchez-Campillo J, Spencer JS, Henao-Tamayo M, Harton M, Orme IM, Gonzalez Juarrero M. 2007. XCL1 (lymphotactin) chemokine produced by activated CD8 T cells during the chronic stage of infection with *Mycobacterium tuberculosis* negatively affects production of IFN-gamma by CD4 T cells and participates in granuloma stability. *J Leukoc Biol* **82**:1221–1229.

20. Mayer-Barber KD, Andrade BB, Oland SD, Amaral EP, Barber DL, Gonzales J, Derrick SC, Shi R, Kumar NP, Wei W, Yuan X, Zhang G, Cai Y, Babu S, Catalfamo M, Salazar AM, Via LE, Barry CE III, Sher A. 2014. Host-directed therapy of tuberculosis based on interleukin-1 and type I interferon crosstalk. *Nature* **511**:99–103.

21. Manca C, Tsenova L, Freeman S, Barczak AK, Tovey M, Murray PJ, Barry C III, Kaplan G. 2005. Hypervirulent *M. tuberculosis* W/Beijing strains upregulate type I IFNs and increase expression of negative regulators of the Jak-Stat pathway. *J Interferon Cytokine Res* **25**:694–701.

22. Ordway D, Henao-Tamayo M, Harton M, Palanisamy G, Troudt J, Shanley C, Basaraba RJ, Orme IM. 2007. The hypervirulent *Mycobacterium tuberculosis* strain HN878 induces a potent TH1 response followed by rapid down-regulation. *J Immunol* **179**:522–531.

23. Stanley SA, Johndrow JE, Manzanillo P, Cox JS. 2007. The type I IFN response to infection with *Mycobacterium tuberculosis* requires ESX-1-mediated secretion and contributes to pathogenesis. *J Immunol* **178**:3143–3152.

24. Dorhoi A, Yeremeev V, Nouailles G, Weiner J III, Jörg S, Heinemann E, Oberbeck-Müller D, Knaul JK, Vogelzang A, Reece ST, Hahnke K, Mollenkopf HJ, Brinkmann V, Kaufmann SH. 2014. Type I IFN signaling triggers immunopathology in tuberculosis-susceptible mice by modulating lung phagocyte dynamics. *Eur J Immunol* **44**:2380–2393.

25. Desvignes L, Wolf AJ, Ernst JD. 2012. Dynamic roles of type I and type II IFNs in early infection with *Mycobacterium tuberculosis*. *J Immunol* **188**:6205–6215.

26. Flynn JL, Goldstein MM, Triebold KJ, Koller B, Bloom BR. 1992. Major histocompatibility complex class I-restricted T cells are required for resistance to *Mycobacterium tuberculosis* infection. *Proc Natl Acad Sci USA* **89**:12013–12017.

27. Turner J, D'Souza CD, Pearl JE, Marietta P, Noel M, Frank AA, Appelberg R, Orme IM, Cooper AM. 2001. CD8- and CD95/95L-dependent mechanisms of resistance in mice with chronic pulmonary tuberculosis. *Am J Respir Cell Mol Biol* **24**:203–209.

28. Gonzalez-Juarrero M, Turner OC, Turner J, Marietta P, Brooks JV, Orme IM. 2001. Temporal and spatial arrangement of lymphocytes within lung granulomas induced by aerosol infection with *Mycobacterium tuberculosis*. *Infect Immun* **69**:1722–1728.

29. North RJ. 1973. Importance of thymus-derived lymphocytes in cell-mediated immunity to infection. *Cell Immunol* **7**:166–176.

30. Bosma GC, Custer RP, Bosma MJ. 1983. A severe combined immunodeficiency mutation in the mouse. *Nature* **301**:527–530.

31. Shinkai Y, et al. 1992. RAG-2-deficient mice lack mature lymphocytes owing to inability to initiate V(D)J rearrangement. *Cell* **68**:855–867.

32. Adams LB, Dinauer MC, Morgenstern DE, Krahenbuhl JL. 1997. Comparison of the roles of reactive oxygen and nitrogen intermediates in the host response to *Mycobacterium tuberculosis* using transgenic mice. *Tuber Lung Dis* **78**:237–246.

33. Turner J, Dobos KM, Keen MA, Frank AA, Ehlers S, Orme IM, Belisle JT, Cooper AM. 2004. A limited antigen-specific cellular response is sufficient for the early control of *Mycobacterium tuberculosis* in the lung but is insufficient for long-term survival. *Infect Immun* 72:3759–3768.

34. Geluk A, Taneja V, van Meijgaarden KE, Zanelli E, Abou-Zeid C, Thole JE, de Vries RR, David CS, Ottenhoff TH. 1998. Identification of HLA class II-restricted determinants of *Mycobacterium tuberculosis*-derived proteins by using HLA-transgenic, class II-deficient mice. *Proc Natl Acad Sci USA* 95:10797–10802.

35. Geluk A, van Meijgaarden KE, Franken KL, Drijfhout JW, D'Souza S, Necker A, Huygen K, Ottenhoff TH. 2000. Identification of major epitopes of *Mycobacterium tuberculosis* AG85B that are recognized by HLA-A*0201-restricted CD8+ T cells in HLA-transgenic mice and humans. *J Immunol* 165:6463–6471.

36. Reiley WW, Calayag MD, Wittmer ST, Huntington JL, Pearl JE, Fountain JJ, Martino CA, Roberts AD, Cooper AM, Winslow GM, Woodland DL. 2008. ESAT-6-specific CD4 T cell responses to aerosol *Mycobacterium tuberculosis* infection are initiated in the mediastinal lymph nodes. *Proc Natl Acad Sci USA* 105:10961–10966.

37. Stenger S, Modlin RL. 2002. Control of *Mycobacterium tuberculosis* through mammalian Toll-like receptors. *Curr Opin Immunol* 14:452–457

38. Chackerian AA, Perera TV, Behar SM. 2001. Gamma interferon-producing CD4+ T lymphocytes in the lung correlate with resistance to infection with *Mycobacterium tuberculosis*. *Infect Immun* 69:2666–2674.

39. Reiling N, Hölscher C, Fehrenbach A, Kröger S, Kirschning CJ, Goyert S, Ehlers S. 2002. Cutting edge: toll-like receptor (TLR)2- and TLR4-mediated pathogen recognition in resistance to airborne infection with *Mycobacterium tuberculosis*. *J Immunol* 169:3480–3484.

40. Kamath AB, Alt J, Debbabi H, Behar SM. 2003. Toll-like receptor 4-defective C3H/HeJ mice are not more susceptible than other C3H substrains to infection with *Mycobacterium tuberculosis*. *Infect Immun* 71:4112–4118.

41. Shim TS, Turner OC, Orme IM. 2003. Toll-like receptor 4 plays no role in susceptibility of mice to *Mycobacterium tuberculosis* infection. *Tuberculosis (Edinb)* 83:367–371.

42. Drennan MB, Nicolle D, Quesniaux VJ, Jacobs M, Allie N, Mpagi J, Frémond C, Wagner H, Kirschning C, Ryffel B. 2004. Toll-like receptor 2-deficient mice succumb to *Mycobacterium tuberculosis* infection. *Am J Pathol* 164:49–57.

43. Bafica A, Scanga CA, Feng CG, Leifer C, Cheever A, Sher A. 2005. TLR9 regulates Th1 responses and cooperates with TLR2 in mediating optimal resistance to *Mycobacterium tuberculosis*. *J Exp Med* 202:1715–1724.

44. McBride A, Bhatt K, Salgame P. 2011. Development of a secondary immune response to *Mycobacterium tuberculosis* is independent of Toll-like receptor 2. *Infect Immun* 79:1118–1123.

45. Abel B, Thieblemont N, Quesniaux VJ, Brown N, Mpagi J, Miyake K, Bihl F, Ryffel B. 2002. Toll-like receptor 4 expression is required to control chronic *Mycobacterium tuberculosis* infection in mice. *J Immunol* 169:3155–3162.

46. Branger J, Leemans JC, Florquin S, Weijer S, Speelman P, Van Der Poll T. 2004. Toll-like receptor 4 plays a protective role in pulmonary tuberculosis in mice. *Int Immunol* 16:509–516.

47. Brightbill HD, Libraty DH, Krutzik SR, Yang RB, Belisle JT, Bleharski JR, Maitland M, Norgard MV, Plevy SE, Smale ST, Brennan PJ, Bloom BR, Godowski PJ, Modlin RL. 1999. Host defense mechanisms triggered by microbial lipoproteins through toll-like receptors. *Science* 285:732–736.

48. Tobian AA, Potter NS, Ramachandra L, Pai RK, Convery M, Boom WH, Harding CV. 2003. Alternate class I MHC antigen processing is inhibited by Toll-like receptor signaling pathogen-associated molecular patterns: *Mycobacterium tuberculosis* 19-kDa lipoprotein, CpG DNA, and lipopolysaccharide. *J Immunol* 171:1413–1422.

49. Noss EH, Pai RK, Sellati TJ, Radolf JD, Belisle J, Golenbock DT, Boom WH, Harding CV. 2001. Toll-like receptor 2-dependent inhibition of macrophage class II MHC expression and antigen processing by 19-kDa lipoprotein of *Mycobacterium tuberculosis*. *J Immunol* 167:910–918.

50. Kincaid EZ, Wolf AJ, Desvignes L, Mahapatra S, Crick DC, Brennan PJ, Pavelka MS Jr, Ernst JD. 2007. Codominance of TLR2-dependent and TLR2-independent modulation of MHC class II in *Mycobacterium tuberculosis* infection in vivo. *J Immunol* 179:3187–3195.

51. Pathak SK, Basu S, Basu KK, Banerjee A, Pathak S, Bhattacharyya A, Kaisho T, Kundu M, Basu J. 2007. Direct extracellular interaction between the early secreted antigen ESAT-6 of *Mycobacterium tuberculosis* and TLR2 inhibits TLR signaling in macrophages. *Nat Immunol* 8:610–618.

52. Richardson ET, Shukla S, Sweet DR, Wearsch PA, Tsichlis PN, Boom WH, Harding CV. 2015. Toll-like receptor 2-dependent extracellular signal-regulated kinase signaling in *Mycobacterium tuberculosis*-infected macrophages drives anti-inflammatory responses and inhibits Th1 polarization of responding T cells. *Infect Immun* 83:2242–2254.

53. Wang B, Henao-Tamayo M, Harton M, Ordway D, Shanley C, Basaraba RJ, Orme IM. 2007. A Toll-like receptor-2-directed fusion protein vaccine against tuberculosis. *Clin Vaccine Immunol* 14:902–906.

54. Ferwerda G, Girardin SE, Kullberg BJ, Le Bourhis L, de Jong DJ, Langenberg DM, van Crevel R, Adema GJ, Ottenhoff TH, Van der Meer JW, Netea MG. 2005. NOD2 and toll-like receptors are nonredundant recognition systems of *Mycobacterium tuberculosis*. *PLoS Pathog* 1:e74.

55. Ferwerda G, Kullberg BJ, de Jong DJ, Girardin SE, Langenberg DM, van Crevel R, Ottenhoff TH, Van der Meer JW, Netea MG. 2007. *Mycobacterium paratuberculosis* is recognized by Toll-like receptors and NOD2. *J Leukoc Biol* 82:1011–1018.

56. Divangahi M, Mostowy S, Coulombe F, Kozak R, Guillot L, Veyrier F, Kobayashi KS, Flavell RA, Gros P, Behr MA. 2008. NOD2-deficient mice have impaired resistance to *Mycobacterium tuberculosis* infection through defective innate and adaptive immunity. *J Immunol* **181**:7157–7165.

57. Gandotra S, Jang S, Murray PJ, Salgame P, Ehrt S. 2007. Nucleotide-binding oligomerization domain protein 2-deficient mice control infection with *Mycobacterium tuberculosis*. *Infect Immun* **75**:5127–5134.

58. Pandey AK, Yang Y, Jiang Z, Fortune SM, Coulombe F, Behr MA, Fitzgerald KA, Sassetti CM, Kelliher MA. 2009. NOD2, RIP2 and IRF5 play a critical role in the type I interferon response to *Mycobacterium tuberculosis*. *PLoS Pathog* **5**:e1000500.

59. Chackerian AA, Behar SM. 2003. Susceptibility to *Mycobacterium tuberculosis*: lessons from inbred strains of mice. *Tuberculosis (Edinb)* **83**:279–285.

60. Gupta UD, Katoch VM. 2005. Animal models of tuberculosis. *Tuberculosis (Edinb)* **85**:277–293.

61. Beamer GL, Turner J. 2005. Murine models of susceptibility to tuberculosis. *Arch Immunol Ther Exp (Warsz)* **53**:469–483.

62. Chackerian AA, Alt JM, Perera TV, Dascher CC, Behar SM. 2002. Dissemination of *Mycobacterium tuberculosis* is influenced by host factors and precedes the initiation of T-cell immunity. *Infect Immun* **70**:4501–4509.

63. Gruppo V, Turner OC, Orme IM, Turner J. 2002. Reduced up-regulation of memory and adhesion/integrin molecules in susceptible mice and poor expression of immunity to pulmonary tuberculosis. *Microbiology* **148**:2959–2966.

64. Buu N, Sánchez F, Schurr E. 2000. The Bcg host-resistance gene. *Clin Infect Dis* **31**(Suppl 3):S81–S85.

65. Vidal S, Tremblay ML, Govoni G, Gauthier S, Sebastiani G, Malo D, Skamene E, Olivier M, Jothy S, Gros P. 1995. The Ity/Lsh/Bcg locus: natural resistance to infection with intracellular parasites is abrogated by disruption of the Nramp1 gene. *J Exp Med* **182**:655–666.

66. Skamene E, Gros P, Forget A, Kongshavn PA, St Charles C, Taylor BA. 1982. Genetic regulation of resistance to intracellular pathogens. *Nature* **297**:506–509.

67. Skamene E. 1994. The Bcg gene story. *Immunobiology* **191**:451–460

68. Orme IM, Stokes RW, Collins FM. 1985. Only two out of fifteen BCG strains follow the Bcg pattern, p 285–289. *In* Skamene E (ed), *Genetic Control of Host Resistance to Infection and Malignancy*. Alan R. Liss, New York.

69. Orme IM, Stokes RW, Collins FM. 1986. Genetic control of natural resistance to nontuberculous mycobacterial infections in mice. *Infect Immun* **54**:56–62.

70. North RJ, Medina E. 1996. Significance of the antimicrobial resistance gene, Nramp1, in resistance to virulent *Mycobacterium tuberculosis* infection. *Res Immunol* **147**:493–499.

71. Medina E, Rogerson BJ, North RJ. 1996. The Nramp1 antimicrobial resistance gene segregates independently

72. Kramnik I, Demant P, Bloom BB. 1998. Susceptibility to tuberculosis as a complex genetic trait: analysis using recombinant congenic strains of mice. *Novartis Foundation Symp* **217**:120–137.

73. Kramnik I, Dietrich WF, Demant P, Bloom BR. 2000. Genetic control of resistance to experimental infection with virulent *Mycobacterium tuberculosis*. *Proc Natl Acad Sci USA* **97**:8560–8565.

74. Yan BS, Pichugin AV, Jobe O, Helming L, Eruslanov EB, Gutiérrez-Pabello JA, Rojas M, Shebzukhov YV, Kobzik L, Kramnik I. 2007. Progression of pulmonary tuberculosis and efficiency of bacillus Calmette-Guérin vaccination are genetically controlled via a common sst1-mediated mechanism of innate immunity. *J Immunol* **179**:6919–6932.

75. Pichugin AV, Yan BS, Sloutsky A, Kobzik L, Kramnik I. 2009. Dominant role of the sst1 locus in pathogenesis of necrotizing lung granulomas during chronic tuberculosis infection and reactivation in genetically resistant hosts. *Am J Pathol* **174**:2190–2201.

76. Sánchez F, Radaeva TV, Nikonenko BV, Persson AS, Sengul S, Schalling M, Schurr E, Apt AS, Lavebratt C. 2003. Multigenic control of disease severity after virulent *Mycobacterium tuberculosis* infection in mice. *Infect Immun* **71**:126–131.

77. Majorov KB, Lyadova IV, Kondratieva TK, Eruslanov EB, Rubakova EI, Orlova MO, Mischenko VV, Apt AS. 2003. Different innate ability of I/St and A/Sn mice to combat virulent *Mycobacterium tuberculosis*: phenotypes expressed in lung and extrapulmonary macrophages. *Infect Immun* **71**:697–707.

78. Keller C, Hoffmann R, Lang R, Brandau S, Hermann C, Ehlers S. 2006. Genetically determined susceptibility to tuberculosis in mice causally involves accelerated and enhanced recruitment of granulocytes. *Infect Immun* **74**:4295–4309.

79. Churchill GA, Gatti DM, Munger SC, Svenson KL. 2012. The Diversity Outbred mouse population. *Mamm Genome* **23**:713–718.

80. Kelly BP, Furney SK, Jessen MT, Orme IM. 1996. Low-dose aerosol infection model for testing drugs for efficacy against *Mycobacterium tuberculosis*. *Antimicrob Agents Chemother* **40**:2809–2812.

81. Ordway DJ, Orme IM. 2010. Murine and guinea pig models of tuberculosis, p 271–306. *In* Kaufmann SHE, Kabelitz D (ed), *Methods in Microbiology*. Academic Press, San Diego, CA.

82. Ordway DJ, Orme IM. 2011. Animal models of mycobacteria infection. *Curr Protoc Immunol* **Chapter 19**: Unit19.15.

83. Orme IM. 2014. A new unifying theory of the pathogenesis of tuberculosis. *Tuberculosis (Edinb)* **94**:8–14.

84. Ernst JD. 2012. The immunological life cycle of tuberculosis. *Nat Rev Immunol* **12**:581–591.

85. Rhoades ER, Frank AA, Orme IM. 1997. Progression of chronic pulmonary tuberculosis in mice aerogenically infected with virulent *Mycobacterium tuberculosis*. *Tuber Lung Dis* **78**:57–66.

86. Flynn JL, Scanga CA, Tanaka KE, Chan J. 1998. Effects of aminoguanidine on latent murine tuberculosis. *J Immunol* 160:1796–1803.

87. Henao-Tamayo MI, Ordway DJ, Irwin SM, Shang S, Shanley C, Orme IM. 2010. Phenotypic definition of effector and memory T-lymphocyte subsets in mice chronically infected with *Mycobacterium tuberculosis*. *Clin Vaccine Immunol* 17:618–625.

88. Orme IM, Basaraba RJ. 2014. The formation of the granuloma in tuberculosis infection. *Semin Immunol* 26:601–609

89. Turner OC, Basaraba RJ, Frank AA, Orme IM. 2003. Granuloma formation in mouse and guinea pig models of experimental tuberculosis, p 65–84. *In* Boros DL (ed), *Granulomatous Infections and Inflammation: Cellular and Molecular Mechanisms*. ASM Press, Washington, DC.

90. Brighenti S, Andersson J. 2012. Local immune responses in human tuberculosis: learning from the site of infection. *J Infect Dis* 205(Suppl 2):S316–S324.

91. Turner J, Gonzalez-Juarrero M, Saunders BM, Brooks JV, Marietta P, Ellis DL, Frank AA, Cooper AM, Orme IM. 2001. Immunological basis for reactivation of tuberculosis in mice. *Infect Immun* 69:3264–3270.

92. Turner J, Gonzalez-Juarrero M, Ellis DL, Basaraba RJ, Kipnis A, Orme IM, Cooper AM. 2002. In vivo IL-10 production reactivates chronic pulmonary tuberculosis in C57BL/6 mice. *J Immunol* 169:6343–6351.

93. Beamer GL, Flaherty DK, Assogba BD, Stromberg P, Gonzalez-Juarrero M, de Waal Malefyt R, Vesosky B, Turner J. 2008. Interleukin-10 promotes *Mycobacterium tuberculosis* disease progression in CBA/J mice. *J Immunol* 181:5545–5550.

94. Higgins DM, Sanchez-Campillo J, Rosas-Taraco AG, Lee EJ, Orme IM, Gonzalez-Juarrero M. 2009. Lack of IL-10 alters inflammatory and immune responses during pulmonary *Mycobacterium tuberculosis* infection. *Tuberculosis (Edinb)* 89:149–157.

95. Pitt JM, Stavropoulos E, Redford PS, Beebe AM, Bancroft GJ, Young DB, O'Garra A. 2012. Blockade of IL-10 signaling during bacillus Calmette-Guérin vaccination enhances and sustains Th1, Th17, and innate lymphoid IFN-γ and IL-17 responses and increases protection to *Mycobacterium tuberculosis* infection. *J Immunol* 189:4079–4087.

96. Cyktor JC, Carruthers B, Kominsky RA, Beamer GL, Stromberg P, Turner J. 2013. IL-10 inhibits mature fibrotic granuloma formation during *Mycobacterium tuberculosis* infection. *J Immunol* 190:2778–2790.

97. Cyktor JC, Carruthers B, Beamer GL, Turner J. 2013. Clonal expansions of CD8+ T cells with IL-10 secreting capacity occur during chronic *Mycobacterium tuberculosis* infection. *PLoS One* 8:e58612

98. Behar SM, Carpenter SM, Booty MG, Barber DL, Jayaraman P. 2014. Orchestration of pulmonary T cell immunity during *Mycobacterium tuberculosis* infection: immunity interruptus. *Semin Immunol* 26:559–577.

99. Kaveh DA, Carmen Garcia-Pelayo M, Hogarth PJ. 2014. Persistent BCG bacilli perpetuate CD4 T effector memory and optimal protection against tuberculosis. *Vaccine* 32:6911–6918.

100. Orme IM. 2010. The Achilles heel of BCG. *Tuberculosis (Edinb)* 90:329–332.

101. Vogelzang A, Perdomo C, Zedler U, Kuhlmann S, Hurwitz R, Gengenbacher M, Kaufmann SH. 2014. Central memory CD4+ T cells are responsible for the recombinant Bacillus Calmette-Guérin ΔureC:hly vaccine's superior protection against tuberculosis. *J Infect Dis* 210:1928–1937.

102. Henao-Tamayo M, Obregón-Henao A, Ordway DJ, Shang S, Duncan CG, Orme IM. 2012. A mouse model of tuberculosis reinfection. *Tuberculosis (Edinb)* 92:211–217.

103. Henao-Tamayo M, Ordway DJ, Orme IM. 2014. Memory T cell subsets in tuberculosis: what should we be targeting? *Tuberculosis (Edinb)* 94:455–461.

104. Guyot-Revol V, Innes JA, Hackforth S, Hinks T, Lalvani A. 2006. Regulatory T cells are expanded in blood and disease sites in patients with tuberculosis. *Am J Respir Crit Care Med* 173:803–810.

105. Scott-Browne JP, Shafiani S, Tucker-Heard G, Ishida-Tsubota K, Fontenot JD, Rudensky AY, Bevan MJ, Urdahl KB. 2007. Expansion and function of Foxp3-expressing T regulatory cells during tuberculosis. *J Exp Med* 204:2159–2169.

106. Khader SA. 2010. Th17 cytokines: the good, the bad, and the unknown. *Cytokine Growth Factor Rev* 21:403–404

107. Khader SA, Bell GK, Pearl JE, Fountain JJ, Rangel-Moreno J, Cilley GE, Shen F, Eaton SM, Gaffen SL, Swain SL, Locksley RM, Haynes L, Randall TD, Cooper AM. 2007. IL-23 and IL-17 in the establishment of protective pulmonary CD4+ T cell responses after vaccination and during *Mycobacterium tuberculosis* challenge. *Nat Immunol* 8:369–377.

108. Khader SA, Cooper AM. 2008. IL-23 and IL-17 in tuberculosis. *Cytokine* 41:79–83.

109. Wozniak TM, Saunders BM, Ryan AA, Britton WJ. 2010. *Mycobacterium bovis* BCG-specific Th17 cells confer partial protection against *Mycobacterium tuberculosis* infection in the absence of gamma interferon. *Infect Immun* 78:4187–4194.

110. Smith DW, Fok JS, Ho RS, Harding GE, Wiegeshaus E, Arora PK. 1975. Influence of BCG vaccination on the pathogenesis of experimental airborne tuberculosis. *J Hyg Epidemiol Microbiol Immunol* 19:407–417.

111. Smith DW, Harding GE. 1977. Animal model of human disease. Pulmonary tuberculosis. Animal model: experimental airborne tuberculosis in the guinea pig. *Am J Pathol* 89:273–276.

112. Smith DW, McMurray DN, Wiegeshaus EH, Grover AA, Harding GE. 1970. Host-parasite relationships in experimental airborne tuberculosis. IV. Early events in the course of infection in vaccinated and nonvaccinated guinea pigs. *Am Rev Respir Dis* 102:937–949.

113. Smith DW, Wiegeshaus E, Navalkar R, Grover AA. 1966. Host-parasite relationships in experimental airborne tuberculosis. I. Preliminary studies in BCG-vaccinated and nonvaccinated animals. *J Bacteriol* 91:718–724.

114. Smith DW, Wiegeshaus EH. 1989. What animal models can teach us about the pathogenesis of tuberculosis in humans. *Rev Infect Dis* 11(Suppl 2):S385–S393.

115. McMurray DN, Carlomagno MA, Mintzer CL, Tetzlaff CL. 1985. *Mycobacterium bovis* BCG vaccine fails to protect protein-deficient guinea pigs against respiratory challenge with virulent *Mycobacterium tuberculosis*. *Infect Immun* 50:555–559.

116. McMurray DN, Kimball MS, Tetzlaff CL, Mintzer CL. 1986. Effects of protein deprivation and BCG vaccination on alveolar macrophage function in pulmonary tuberculosis. *Am Rev Respir Dis* 133:1081–1085.

117. McMurray DN, Mintzer CL, Tetzlaff CL, Carlomagno MA. 1986. The influence of dietary protein on the protective effect of BCG in guinea pigs. *Tubercle* 67:31–39.

118. Grosset J. 1980. Bacteriologic basis of short-course chemotherapy for tuberculosis. *Clin Chest Med* 1:231–241.

119. McMurray DN. 2001. A coordinated strategy for evaluating new vaccines for human and animal tuberculosis. *Tuberculosis (Edinb)* 81:141–146.

120. McMurray DN. 2001. Determinants of vaccine-induced resistance in animal models of pulmonary tuberculosis. *Scand J Infect Dis* 33:175–178.

121. McMurray DN, Dai G, Phalen S. 1999. Mechanisms of vaccine-induced resistance in a guinea pig model of pulmonary tuberculosis. *Tuber Lung Dis* 79:261–266.

122. Pal PG, Horwitz MA. 1992. Immunization with extracellular proteins of *Mycobacterium tuberculosis* induces cell-mediated immune responses and substantial protective immunity in a guinea pig model of pulmonary tuberculosis. *Infect Immun* 60:4781–4792.

123. Horwitz MA, Lee BW, Dillon BJ, Harth G. 1995. Protective immunity against tuberculosis induced by vaccination with major extracellular proteins of *Mycobacterium tuberculosis*. *Proc Natl Acad Sci USA* 92:1530–1534.

124. Horwitz MA, Harth G, Dillon BJ, Maslesa-Galic' S. 2000. Recombinant bacillus calmette-guerin (BCG) vaccines expressing the *Mycobacterium tuberculosis* 30-kDa major secretory protein induce greater protective immunity against tuberculosis than conventional BCG vaccines in a highly susceptible animal model. *Proc Natl Acad Sci USA* 97:13853–13858.

125. Horwitz MA, Harth G. 2003. A new vaccine against tuberculosis affords greater survival after challenge than the current vaccine in the guinea pig model of pulmonary tuberculosis. *Infect Immun* 71:1672–1679.

126. Sampson SL, Dascher CC, Sambandamurthy VK, Russell RG, Jacobs WR Jr, Bloom BR, Hondalus MK. 2004. Protection elicited by a double leucine and pantothenate auxotroph of *Mycobacterium tuberculosis* in guinea pigs. *Infect Immun* 72:3031–3037.

127. Hinchey J, Lee S, Jeon BY, Basaraba RJ, Venkataswamy MM, Chen B, Chan J, Braunstein M, Orme IM, Derrick SC, Morris SL, Jacobs WR Jr, Porcelli SA. 2007. Enhanced priming of adaptive immunity by a proapoptotic mutant of *Mycobacterium tuberculosis*. *J Clin Invest* 117:2279–2288.

128. Cardona PJ, Asensio JG, Arbués A, Otal I, Lafoz C, Gil O, Caceres N, Ausina V, Gicquel B, Martin C. 2009. Extended safety studies of the attenuated live tuberculosis vaccine SO2 based on phoP mutant. *Vaccine* 27:2499–2505.

129. Olsen AW, Williams A, Okkels LM, Hatch G, Andersen P. 2004. Protective effect of a tuberculosis subunit vaccine based on a fusion of antigen 85B and ESAT-6 in the aerosol guinea pig model. *Infect Immun* 72:6148–6150

130. Skeiky YA, Alderson MR, Ovendale PJ, Guderian JA, Brandt L, Dillon DC, Campos-Neto A, Lobet Y, Dalemans W, Orme IM, Reed SG. 2004. Differential immune responses and protective efficacy induced by components of a tuberculosis polyprotein vaccine, Mtb72F, delivered as naked DNA or recombinant protein. *J Immunol* 172:7618–7628.

131. Brandt L, Skeiky YA, Alderson MR, Lobet Y, Dalemans W, Turner OC, Basaraba RJ, Izzo AA, Lasco TM, Chapman PL, Reed SG, Orme IM. 2004. The protective effect of the *Mycobacterium bovis* BCG vaccine is increased by coadministration with the *Mycobacterium tuberculosis* 72-kilodalton fusion polyprotein Mtb72F in *M. tuberculosis*-infected guinea pigs. *Infect Immun* 72:6622–6632.

132. Turner OC, Basaraba RJ, Orme IM. 2003. Immunopathogenesis of pulmonary granulomas in the guinea pig after infection with *Mycobacterium tuberculosis*. *Infect Immun* 71:864–871.

133. Allen SS, Cassone L, Lasco TM, McMurray DN. 2004. Effect of neutralizing transforming growth factor beta1 on the immune response against *Mycobacterium tuberculosis* in guinea pigs. *Infect Immun* 72:1358–1363.

134. Lyons MJ, Yoshimura T, McMurray DN. 2004. Interleukin (IL)-8 (CXCL8) induces cytokine expression and superoxide formation by guinea pig neutrophils infected with *Mycobacterium tuberculosis*. *Tuberculosis (Edinb)* 84:283–292

135. Skwor TA, Cho H, Cassidy C, Yoshimura T, McMurray DN. 2004. Recombinant guinea pig CCL5 (RANTES) differentially modulates cytokine production in alveolar and peritoneal macrophages. *J Leukoc Biol* 76:1229–1239.

136. Yamamoto T, Lasco TM, Uchida K, Goto Y, Jeevan A, McFarland C, Ly L, Yamamoto S, McMurray DN. 2007. *Mycobacterium bovis* BCG vaccination modulates TNF-alpha production after pulmonary challenge with virulent *Mycobacterium tuberculosis* in guinea pigs. *Tuberculosis (Edinb)* 87:155–165.

137. Kraft SL, Dailey D, Kovach M, Stasiak KL, Bennett J, McFarland CT, McMurray DN, Izzo AA, Orme IM, Basaraba RJ. 2004. Magnetic resonance imaging of pulmonary lesions in guinea pigs infected with *Mycobacterium tuberculosis*. *Infect Immun* 72:5963–5971.

138. Ly LH, Russell MI, McMurray DN. 2008. Cytokine profiles in primary and secondary pulmonary granulomas of Guinea pigs with tuberculosis. *Am J Respir Cell Mol Biol* 38:455–462.

139. Fennelly KP. 2007. Variability of airborne transmission of *Mycobacterium tuberculosis*: implications for control of tuberculosis in the HIV era. *Clin Infect Dis* 44:1358–1360.

140. Basaraba RJ, Bielefeldt-Ohmann H, Eschelbach EK, Reisenhauer C, Tolnay AE, Taraba LC, Shanley CA, Smith EA, Bedwell CL, Chlipala EA, Orme IM. 2008. Increased expression of host iron-binding proteins precedes iron accumulation and calcification of primary lung lesions in experimental tuberculosis in the guinea pig. *Tuberculosis (Edinb)* 88:69–79.

141. Basaraba RJ, Dailey DD, McFarland CT, Shanley CA, Smith EE, McMurray DN, Orme IM. 2006. Lymphadenitis as a major element of disease in the guinea pig model of tuberculosis. *Tuberculosis (Edinb)* 86:386–394.

142. Basaraba RJ, Smith EE, Shanley CA, Orme IM. 2006. Pulmonary lymphatics are primary sites of Mycobacterium tuberculosis infection in guinea pigs infected by aerosol. *Infect Immun* 74:5397–5401.

143. Ward SK, Abomoelak B, Hoye EA, Steinberg H, Talaat AM. 2010. CtpV: a putative copper exporter required for full virulence of *Mycobacterium tuberculosis*. *Mol Microbiol* 77:1096–1110.

144. Ordway D, Palanisamy G, Henao-Tamayo M, Smith EE, Shanley C, Orme IM, Basaraba RJ. 2007. The cellular immune response to *Mycobacterium tuberculosis* infection in the guinea pig. *J Immunol* 179:2532–2541.

145. Lenaerts AJ, Hoff D, Aly S, Ehlers S, Andries K, Cantarero L, Orme IM, Basaraba RJ. 2007. Location of persisting mycobacteria in a Guinea pig model of tuberculosis revealed by r207910. *Antimicrob Agents Chemother* 51:3338–3345

146. Barry CE III, Boshoff HI, Dartois V, Dick T, Ehrt S, Flynn J, Schnappinger D, Wilkinson RJ, Young D. 2009. The spectrum of latent tuberculosis: rethinking the biology and intervention strategies. *Nat Rev Microbiol* 7:845–855.

147. Hoff DR, Ryan GJ, Driver ER, Ssemakulu CC, De Groote MA, Basaraba RJ, Lenaerts AJ. 2011. Location of intra- and extracellular M. tuberculosis populations in lungs of mice and guinea pigs during disease progression and after drug treatment. *PLoS One* 6:e17550

148. Ryan GJ, Hoff DR, Driver ER, Voskuil MI, Gonzalez-Juarrero M, Basaraba RJ, Crick DC, Spencer JS, Lenaerts AJ. 2010. Multiple M. tuberculosis phenotypes in mouse and guinea pig lung tissue revealed by a dual-staining approach. *PLoS One* 5:e11108

149. Ojha AK, Baughn AD, Sambandan D, Hsu T, Trivelli X, Guerardel Y, Alahari A, Kremer L, Jacobs WR Jr, Hatfull GF. 2008. Growth of *Mycobacterium tuberculosis* biofilms containing free mycolic acids and harbouring drug-tolerant bacteria. *Mol Microbiol* 69:164–174.

150. Ackart DF, Hascall-Dove L, Caceres SM, Kirk NM, Podell BK, Melander C, Orme IM, Leid JG, Nick JA, Basaraba RJ. 2014. Expression of antimicrobial drug tolerance by attached communities of *Mycobacterium tuberculosis*. *Pathog Dis* 70:359–369.

151. Ackart DF, Lindsey EA, Podell BK, Melander RJ, Basaraba RJ, Melander C. 2014. Reversal of *Mycobacterium tuberculosis* phenotypic drug resistance by 2-aminoimidazole-based small molecules. *Pathog Dis* 70:370–378.

152. Hoff DR, Caraway ML, Brooks EJ, Driver ER, Ryan GJ, Peloquin CA, Orme IM, Basaraba RJ, Lenaerts AJ. 2008. Metronidazole lacks antibacterial activity in guinea pigs infected with *Mycobacterium tuberculosis*. *Antimicrob Agents Chemother* 52:4137–4140.

153. Klinkenberg LG, Sutherland LA, Bishai WR, Karakousis PC. 2008. Metronidazole lacks activity against *Mycobacterium tuberculosis* in an in vivo hypoxic granuloma model of latency. *J Infect Dis* 198:275–283.

154. Ordway DJ, Shanley CA, Caraway ML, Orme EA, Bucy DS, Hascall-Dove L, Henao-Tamayo M, Harton MR, Shang S, Ackart D, Kraft SL, Lenaerts AJ, Basaraba RJ, Orme IM. 2010. Evaluation of standard chemotherapy in the guinea pig model of tuberculosis. *Antimicrob Agents Chemother* 54:1820–1833.

155. Shang S, Shanley CA, Caraway ML, Orme EA, Henao-Tamayo M, Hascall-Dove L, Ackart D, Orme IM, Ordway DJ, Basaraba RJ. 2012. Drug treatment combined with BCG vaccination reduces disease reactivation in guinea pigs infected with *Mycobacterium tuberculosis*. *Vaccine* 30:1572–1582.

156. Shang S, Shanley CA, Caraway ML, Orme EA, Henao-Tamayo M, Hascall-Dove L, Ackart D, Lenaerts AJ, Basaraba RJ, Orme IM, Ordway DJ. 2011. Activities of TMC207, rifampin, and pyrazinamide against *Mycobacterium tuberculosis* infection in guinea pigs. *Antimicrob Agents Chemother* 55:124–131.

157. Escombe AR, Moore DA, Gilman RH, Pan W, Navincopa M, Ticona E, Martínez C, Caviedes L, Sheen P, Gonzalez A, Noakes CJ, Friedland JS, Evans CA. 2008. The infectiousness of tuberculosis patients coinfected with HIV. *PLoS Med* 5:e188

158. Escombe AR, Moore DA, Gilman RH, Navincopa M, Ticona E, Mitchell B, Noakes C, Martínez C, Sheen P, Ramirez R, Quino W, Gonzalez A, Friedland JS, Evans CA. 2009. Upper-room ultraviolet light and negative air ionization to prevent tuberculosis transmission. *PLoS Med* 6:e1000043

159. Dharmadhikari AS, Basaraba RJ, Van Der Walt ML, Weyer K, Mphahlele M, Venter K, Jensen PA, First MW, Parsons S, McMurray DN, Orme IM, Nardell EA. 2011. Natural infection of guinea pigs exposed to patients with highly drug-resistant tuberculosis. *Tuberculosis (Edinb)* 91:329–338.

160. Ottenhoff TH, Doherty TM, van Dissel JT, Bang P, Lingnau K, Kromann I, Andersen P. 2010. First in humans: a new molecularly defined vaccine shows excellent safety and strong induction of long-lived *Mycobacterium tuberculosis*-specific Th1-cell like responses. *Hum Vaccin* 6:1007–1015.

161. Bertholet S, Ireton GC, Ordway DJ, Windish HP, Pine SO, Kahn M, Phan T, Orme IM, Vedvick TS, Baldwin SL, Coler RN, Reed SG. 2010. A defined tuberculosis vaccine candidate boosts BCG and protects against multidrug-resistant *Mycobacterium tuberculosis*. *Sci Transl Med* 2:53ra74

162. Dey B, Jain R, Khera A, Gupta UD, Katoch VM, Ramanathan VD, Tyagi AK. 2011. Latency antigen α-crystallin based vaccination imparts a robust protection against TB by modulating the dynamics of pulmonary cytokines. *PLoS One* 6:e18773

163. Vilaplana C, Gil O, Cáceres N, Pinto S, Díaz J, Cardona PJ. 2011. Prophylactic effect of a therapeutic vaccine against TB based on fragments of *Mycobacterium tuberculosis*. *PLoS One* 6:e20404.

164. Arbues A, Aguilo JI, Gonzalo-Asensio J, Marinova D, Uranga S, Puentes E, Fernandez C, Parra A, Cardona PJ, Vilaplana C, Ausina V, Williams A, Clark S, Malaga W, Guilhot C, Gicquel B, Martin C. 2013. Construction, characterization and preclinical evaluation of MTBVAC, the first live-attenuated *M. tuberculosis*-based vaccine to enter clinical trials. *Vaccine* 31:4867–4873.

165. Henao-Tamayo M, Palaniswamy GS, Smith EE, Shanley CA, Wang B, Orme IM, Basaraba RJ, DuTeau NM, Ordway D. 2009. Post-exposure vaccination against *Mycobacterium tuberculosis*. *Tuberculosis (Edinb)* 89: 142–148.

166. Shanley CA, Ireton GC, Baldwin SL, Coler RN, Reed SG, Basaraba RJ, Orme IM. 2014. Therapeutic vaccination against relevant high virulence clinical isolates of *Mycobacterium tuberculosis*. *Tuberculosis (Edinb)* 94: 140–147.

167. Palanisamy GS, DuTeau N, Eisenach KD, Cave DM, Theus SA, Kreiswirth BN, Basaraba RJ, Orme IM. 2009. Clinical strains of *Mycobacterium tuberculosis* display a wide range of virulence in guinea pigs. *Tuberculosis (Edinb)* 89:203–209.

168. Palanisamy GS, Smith EE, Shanley CA, Ordway DJ, Orme IM, Basaraba RJ. 2008. Disseminated disease severity as a measure of virulence of *Mycobacterium tuberculosis* in the guinea pig model. *Tuberculosis (Edinb)* 88:295–306.

169. Shang S, Harton M, Tamayo MH, Shanley C, Palanisamy GS, Caraway M, Chan ED, Basaraba RJ, Orme IM, Ordway DJ. 2011. Increased Foxp3 expression in guinea pigs infected with W-Beijing strains of *M. tuberculosis*. *Tuberculosis (Edinb)* 91:378–385.

170. Kato-Maeda M, Shanley CA, Ackart D, Jarlsberg LG, Shang S, Obregon-Henao A, Harton M, Basaraba RJ, Henao-Tamayo M, Barrozo JC, Rose J, Kawamura LM, Coscolla M, Fofanov VY, Koshinsky H, Gagneux S, Hopewell PC, Ordway DJ, Orme IM. 2012. Beijing sublineages of *Mycobacterium tuberculosis* differ in pathogenicity in the guinea pig. *Clin Vaccine Immunol* 19:1227–1237.

171. Somashekar BS, Amin AG, Rithner CD, Troudt J, Basaraba R, Izzo A, Crick DC, Chatterjee D. 2011. Metabolic profiling of lung granuloma in *Mycobacterium tuberculosis* infected guinea pigs: ex vivo 1H magic angle spinning NMR studies. *J Proteome Res* 10: 4186–4195.

172. Somashekar BS, Amin AG, Tripathi P, MacKinnon N, Rithner CD, Shanley CA, Basaraba R, Henao-Tamayo M, Kato-Maeda M, Ramamoorthy A, Orme IM, Ordway DJ, Chatterjee D. 2012. Metabolomic signatures in guinea pigs infected with epidemic-associated W-Beijing strains of *Mycobacterium tuberculosis*. *J Proteome Res* 11: 4873–4884.

173. Aiyaz M, Bipin C, Pantulwar V, Mugasimangalam R, Shanley CA, Ordway DJ, Orme IM. 2014. Whole genome response in guinea pigs infected with the high virulence strain Mycobacterium tuberculosis TT372. *Tuberculosis (Edinb)* 94:606–615.

174. Podell BK, Ackart DF, Obregon-Henao A, Eck SP, Henao-Tamayo M, Richardson M, Orme IM, Ordway DJ, Basaraba RJ. 2014. Increased severity of tuberculosis in Guinea pigs with type 2 diabetes: a model of diabetes-tuberculosis comorbidity. *Am J Pathol* 184:1104–1118.

175. Tameris MD, Hatherill M, Landry BS, Scriba TJ, Snowden MA, Lockhart S, Shea JE, McClain JB, Hussey GD, Hanekom WA, Mahomed H, McShane H, MVA85A 020 Trial Study Team. 2013. Safety and efficacy of MVA85A, a new tuberculosis vaccine, in infants previously vaccinated with BCG: a randomised, placebo-controlled phase 2b trial. *Lancet* 381:1021–1028.

176. McShane H, Williams A. 2014. A review of preclinical animal models utilised for TB vaccine evaluation in the context of recent human efficacy data. *Tuberculosis (Edinb)* 94:105–110.

177. Henao-Tamayo M, Shanley CA, Verma D, Zilavy A, Stapleton MC, Furney SK, Podell B, Orme IM. 2015. The efficacy of the BCG Vaccine Against Newly Emerging Clinical Strains of *Mycobacterium tuberculosis*. *PLoS One* 10:e0136500.

178. Jacobs WR Jr, McShane H, Mizrahi V, Orme IM (ed). *Tuberculosis and the Tubercle Bacillus*, 2nd ed. ASM Press, Washington, DC, in press.

Tuberculosis and the Tubercle Bacillus, 2nd ed.
Edited by William R. Jacobs, Jr., Helen McShane, Valerie Mizrahi, and Ian M. Orme
© 2018 American Society for Microbiology, Washington, DC
doi:10.1128/microbiolspec.TBTB2-0007-2016

Non-Human Primate Models of Tuberculosis

8

Juliet C. Peña[1] and Wen-Zhe Ho[1,2]

INTRODUCTION

Among the animal models of tuberculosis (TB), the non-human primates (NHPs), particularly rhesus macaques (*Macaca fascicularis*) and cynomolgus macaques (*Macaca mulatta*), share the greatest anatomical and physiological similarities with humans. Macaques are highly susceptible to *Mycobacterium tuberculosis* infection and manifest the complete spectrum of clinical and pathological manifestations of TB as seen in humans. Therefore, the macaque models have been used extensively for investigating the pathogenesis of *M. tuberculosis* infection and for preclinical testing of drugs and vaccines against TB. This review focuses on published major studies that exemplify how the rhesus and cynomolgus macaques have enhanced and may continue to advance global efforts in TB research.

Validation of Macaques in TB Research

The macaques have proven to be a suitable model for understanding human TB, because they exhibit remarkable similarities to humans in virtually every aspect of their anatomy and physiology (1–3). As such, macaques respond likewise to many human immunologic, pathological, and drug agents, providing a tremendous advantage over other animal models (4, 5, 73). The macaques appear naturally susceptible to *M. tuberculosis* infection and can display all features of human TB disease, ranging from acute and active infection to asymptomatic and latent infection. The literature shows that macaques and humans share extensive clinical manifestations of TB, including pulmonary and extrapulmonary signs and symptoms (4, 5). Researchers can monitor the disease course of *M. tuberculosis* infection in macaques by measuring nearly identical parameters as tested in humans, ranging from skin and blood tests to radiographic im-

aging and body fluid samples (Table 1). In addition, multidrug chemotherapy for TB provides effective treatment in both humans and macaques (6, 7). Furthermore, similarly as in humans, bacillus Calmette-Guérin (BCG) vaccination exhibits variable efficacy in macaques of even the same species (8–10). Table 1 outlines the similarities and differences in *M. tuberculosis* infection between humans and the rhesus macaques (RMs) and cynomolgus macaques (CMs).

Historical Use of Macaque Models

The use of macaque models for TB studies traces back to published literature from the 1960s. This "Golden Age" of TB research using macaque models through the 1970s generated valuable data on the evolving BCG vaccine (11), as well as one report on the TB drug efficacy of ethambutol and isoniazid (7). The majority of these early studies focused on the BCG-induced immune reactions and vaccine efficacy (12–18). All pertinent studies published during this era used Indian RM models, which underwent intrabronchial, intratracheal, or aerosol infection with *M. tuberculosis*. The estimated mycobacterial retention rate in mammalian lungs after aerosol exposure had derived from prior animal models, including macaques exposed to anthrax spores, as well as guinea pigs and mice infected with *M. tuberculosis* (19). Figure 1 recaps the major published articles of macaque models with experimental *M. tuberculosis* infection during this time period (7, 12–18).

Nearly 2 decades after the Golden Age, another study using macaques experimentally infected with *M. tuberculosis* was published (20). This large research gap in using macaque models for TB studies could be due to several factors, including the high maintenance

---

[1]Department of Pathology and Laboratory Medicine, Temple University Lewis Katz School of Medicine, Philadelphia, PA 19140; [2]Animal Biosafety Level III Laboratory at the Center for Animal Experiment, State Key Laboratory of Virology, Wuhan University, Wuhan, China.

Table 1   Comparison of TB in humans versus rhesus and cynomolgus macaques[a]

Parameter	Humans	Rhesus macaques	Cynomolgus macaques
Clinical manifestations			
Disease progression	Acute << Latent	Acute >> Latent	Acute > Latent
Acute: weeks to months	(10%) (90%)	(90%) (10%)	(60%) (40%)
Latent: months to years			
Active/chronic infection			
• Cough	+	+	+
• Bloody sputum	+	+	+
• Increased body temperature	+	+	+
• Weight loss	+	+	+
Latent infection			
• No clinical signs	+	+	+
• Activated by coinfection (HIV or SIV)	+	+	+
Clinical tests			
• Skin tests:	+	+	+
PPD	+	+	+
Old tuberculin	+	+	+
• Blood tests:	+	+	+
ELISA, ELISpot	–	+	+
Quantiferon-TB Gold	+	+	+
Primagram	+	+	+
CBC, ESR, CRP, LT	+	+	+
• Imaging:			
Chest X-ray, MRI, PET-CT			
• Fluid sampling:			
BAL, gastric aspirate			
Pathology			
• Caseous granulomas	+	+	+
• Calcification	+/–	+/–	+/–
• Fibrous capsule	+/–	+/–	+/–
• Pulmonary cavities	+	+	+
• Disseminated lesions	+/–	+/–	+/–

[a]The majority of macaques, particularly the rhesus species, develop acute or active TB after artificial infection, whereas 90% of infected humans have latent TB. Chronic infection is defined as persistent signs of active disease, radiographic involvement, or culture positivity. Although the PPD and OT skin tests are used in both humans and macaques, these diagnostic examinations are less reliable in macaques than in humans (72). Also, macaques exhibit a more random than apical distribution of pulmonary cavities. BAL, bronchoalveolar lavage; CBC, complete blood count; CRP, C-reactive protein; CT, computed tomography; ELISA, enzyme-linked immunosorbent assay; ELISpot, enzyme-linked immunosorbent spot assay; ESR, erythrocyte sedimentation rate; LT, lymphocyte transformation; MRI, magnetic resonance imaging; PPD, purified protein derivative; PET, positron emission tomography; rBCG, recombinant bacillus Calmette-Guérin; SIV, simian immunodeficiency virus; TB, tuberculosis. (+) indicates a present finding or functional modality; (–) means an absent finding or unused modality; (+/–) represents a variable finding; (%) refers to the global percentage infected with *M. tuberculosis*.

costs and necessary space and equipment for biocontainment to properly conduct such experiments (5). Additionally, the limited animal availability, handling difficulties, and adverse public opinions have discouraged TB research with NHPs. However, with greater research funding and the emergence of compatible reagents for macaques, further investigations on *M. tuberculosis* infection using NHP models had regained momentum (4). Especially amid the expansion of the National Primate Research Centers (NPRCs), TB in-

vestigators revisited the macaque model of experimental *M. tuberculosis* inoculation with a renewed enthusiasm. A series of proceeding investigations dedicated their macaque research to assessing novel TB vaccines and drugs, as well as understanding the pathogenesis of *M. tuberculosis* infection and reactivation. Figure 2 abridges the RM (8, 21–41, 74–77) and CM (4, 10, 20, 37, 38, 42–58, 74, 78–80) models of experimental *M. tuberculosis* infection after the Golden Age, from 1996 to 2017.

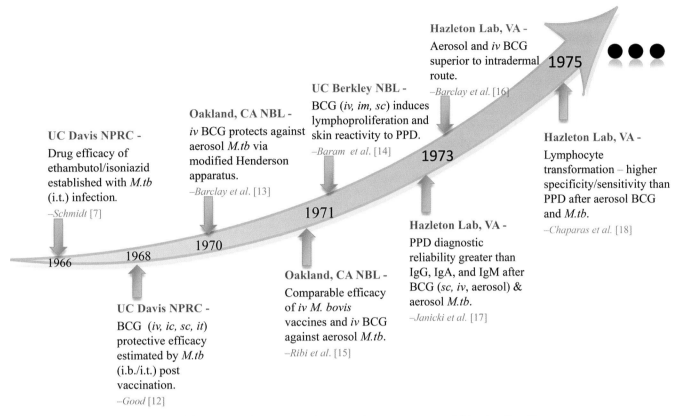

Figure 1 "Golden Age" of TB research using rhesus macaques. This timeline illustrates major studies of experimental *M. tuberculosis* infection in Indian rhesus macaques during the so-called "Golden Age" from the 1960s to 1970s (7, 12–18). Events are organized chronologically by year of publication. Thus, the 10-year study by Good et al. (12) actually began before the first reported investigation in 1966. The location of the experiments (in red) and the first/corresponding author (in blue) are indicated as well. BCG, bacillus Calmette-Guérin; BPRC, Biomedical Primate Research Center; Hazleton Laboratories (former organization purchased by Covance Inc.); ic, intracutaneous; im, intramuscular; it, intratracheal; iv, intravenous; M.tb, Mycobacterium tuberculosis; NBL, Naval Biological Laboratories; NPRC, National Primate Research Center; PPD, purified protein derivative; sc, subcutaneous; UC, University of California.

Rhesus macaques of Indian origin have often been used as NHP models because they are the primary species provided by the breeding facilities in the United States. However, at least seven studies have been reported as using Chinese RM in Wuhan, China (29, 30, 76), Solna, Sweden (23, 24), and Rijswijk, the Netherlands (25, 77). So far, within the scientific literature illustrating macaque models of *M. tuberculosis* infection, the routes of inoculation have included intrabronchial instillation, as well as intratracheal, aerosol, and intranasal infection. More recently, RM infected with *M. tuberculosis* via aerosol or intrabronchial instillation have shown similar TB disease outcomes regardless of variations in pulmonary pathology (41). Although zoonotic TB outbreaks have revealed horizontal transmission of *M. tuberculosis*,

an experimental macaque model of natural *M. tuberculosis* infection has not been reported. Tables 2 to 4 state the route, dose, and *M. tuberculosis* strain of infection in each study design along with the major findings of the listed articles.

A COMPARISON OF RHESUS AND CYNOMOLGUS MACAQUE MODELS OF TB

Both RM and CM models have served to evaluate the efficacy of TB vaccines and drugs, as well as improve our understanding of the immunopathogenesis of *M. tuberculosis* infection and reactivation. However, the two species have differences worth noting. For example, one investigation revealed that BCG provides

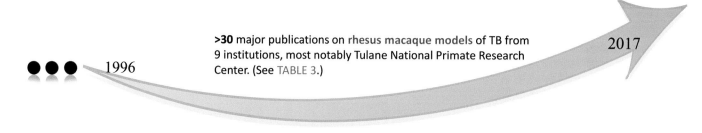

> **>30** major publications on rhesus macaque models of TB from 9 institutions, most notably Tulane National Primate Research Center. (See TABLE 3.)

2017

1996

> **>30** major publications on cynomolgus macaque models of TB from 10 institutions, most notably University of Pittsburg. (See TABLE 4.)

Figure 2 Twenty-first century TB research using rhesus and cynomolgus macaques. This is a summary timeline of important studies of experimental *M. tuberculosis* infection in rhesus and cynomolgus macaques from 1996 to 2017. Only one study (20) was published before 2001.

greater protective efficacy in CM than in RM against *M. tuberculosis* infection (37). Later investigations exploring ultra-low-dose aerosol challenge and stereological techniques for measuring bacterial burden showed that RMs are more susceptible than CMs are to *M. tuberculosis* infection (59, 60). As a result, RMs are more often used for the study of active TB, whereas CMs provide better models of latent or chronic TB (4). In further comparative studies, Mauritian CMs showed higher susceptibility to *M. tuberculosis* infection and more rapid disease progression than Indian RMs and Chinese CMs. However, Mauritian CMs exhibited less variation in pulmonary disease burden and total gross pathology scores, suggesting this type of macaque may be an appropriate model for studying TB transmission (74, 79). Depending on the route and dose of *M. tuberculosis* infection, as well as the *M. tuberculosis* strain of inoculum, either CMs or RMs can develop acute, chronic, or latent TB. Therefore, several research endeavors have employed both species for developing and determining the efficacy of TB-screening immunoassays (61–64) (Table 2).

Rhesus Macaques

The RMs have been used extensively to study TB (Table 3). The early investigations during the Golden Age (16–20) specifically showed that *M. tuberculosis* infection in RMs progresses rapidly within 8 to 9 weeks after aerosol inhalation of the attenuated H37Rv strain at low doses of up to 62 CFU. In 2004, the Tulane NPRC established a model of asymptomatic, or latent, *M. tuberculosis* infection of RMs (21). The investigators revealed that the RMs are a good model for not only active TB, but also asymptomatic TB, using lower doses (30 CFU) of H37Rv strain. In addi-

tion to RMs of Indian origin, Chinese RMs could also be used as a viable model of acute TB (29). Chinese RMs are highly susceptible to *M. tuberculosis* infection and develop active TB regardless of the dose of H37Rv strain used (29). In an attempt to improve the methods to monitor the progression of TB disease, Helke et al. (22) from the Oregon NPRC showed that using high-resolution radiographic and fine immunologic studies can help define the disease status in RMs as in humans. Namely, computed tomography evaluation and *M. tuberculosis*-specific T cell frequencies measured by enzyme-linked immunosorbent spot (ELISpot) assays correlated tightly with the bacterial burden and severity of disease (22).

Cynomolgus Macaques

In addition to the RMs, the CMs have contributed as animal models in the study of TB (Table 4), particularly after the so-called Golden Age (11). The first published CM investigation of controlled *M. tuberculosis* infection stemmed from the work of Walsh et al. (20) in the Philippines, in collaboration with the University of California Los Angeles School of Medicine. In this project, the Philippine CM was found to be an excellent model of not only acute TB but also chronic TB. This research pioneered the intratracheal *M. tuberculosis* infection of Philippine CM. Capuano et al. (4) from the University of Pittsburgh later developed a CM model representing the full spectrum of human *M. tuberculosis* infection by infecting the macaques after intrabronchial inoculation with a low dose (25 CFU) of the Erdman strain. Interestingly, this low dose of inoculum precipitated various reactions in the CMs, ranging from latent TB to active-chronic and even rapidly progressive TB. The pulmonary as well as extrapulmonary

Table 2 TB studies using both rhesus macaques and cynomolgus macaques[a]

No. of macaques	M. tuberculosis strain (inoculation route), dose(s) (CFU)	Major findings	Reference(s)
6 RM 6 CM	Erdman (i.t.), 3,000	BCG provides greater protective efficacy against TB in CM than in RM.	37[b]
8 RM 15 CM	Erdman (i.t.), 1,000–3,000	In vitro IFN-γ assays provide reproducible, reliable results while causing less stress than the PPD skin test.	61
5 RM 4 CM[c]	Erdman (i.t.), 100	Synthetic peptides may be used in lieu of the full-length ESAT-6 protein in TB diagnostic antibody detection assays.	62
26 RM 4 RM 3 RM 16 CM	Erdman (i.t.), 30–1,000 H37Rv (i.t.), 210 Beijing (i.t.), 1,000 Erdman (i.t.), 100–1,000[d]	The highest rate of TB detection is achieved when the skin test is combined with the PrimaTB STAT-PAK immunoassay.	63
4 RM 6 CM	H37Rv (i.b.), 1,000 Erdman (i.b.), 25	The multiplex microbead immunoassay profiles M. tuberculosis antibodies at multiple stages of infection/disease.	64
9 RM 21 CM	Erdman K01 (a.), 30–500	MR stereology provides the most accurate, quantifiable measurement of TB disease burden. RMs exhibit higher susceptibility to M. tuberculosis than CMs.	60
6 RM 4 RM 14 CM	Erdman (i.b.), 500 H37Rv (i.b.), 1,000 Erdman (i.b.), 25	M. tuberculosis antibody profiles depend on the NHP species and infecting M. tuberculosis strain but do not significantly change with TB disease progression.	38
8 RM 8 CM	Erdman K01 (a.), 21–28	Ultra-low-dose aerosol challenge with M. tuberculosis leads to higher TB disease burden in RMs than in CMs.	59
18 CM 9 RM	Erdman K01 (a.) 150–1,650	Mauritian CMs show less variation in TB pulmonary disease burden and pathology than Indian RMs or Chinese CMs within M. tuberculosis exposure dose groups.	74, 79

[a]Table 2 displays the experimental designs and major conclusions drawn from TB studies using both rhesus and cynomolgus macaques. All studies (37, 60–64) used Indian RM models. a., aerosol; BCG, bacillus Calmette-Guérin; CM, cynomolgus macaques; Erdman, ATCC 35801 strain unless indicated as K01 strain; i.b., intrabronchial; IFN-γ, gamma interferon; i.t., intratracheal; MR, magnetic resonance; PPD, purified protein derivative; RM, rhesus macaques; TB, tuberculosis.
[b]TB vaccine-related study.
[c]Studies (62, 63) also used African green monkeys.
[d]Additional RM/CM/African green monkey groups were inoculated with mycobacteria M. kansaii and M. avium (63).

manifestations of M. tuberculosis-infected CMs at different stages of infection closely resembled the pathological and clinical findings of TB in humans, as evidenced by the standard laboratory examinations (4) (Table 1). Many of the proceeding publications on CM models of M. tuberculosis infection were similarly published by researchers at the University of Pittsburgh (45–48, 50, 54, 55). Hence, CM models have more recently been used for evaluating drugs and vaccines against TB (37, 44, 50).

UNIQUE MACAQUE MODELS OF TB

Macaque Models for TB Vaccine Evaluation
Using the RM model, researchers from the Swedish Institute of Infectious Disease Control strived to amplify and extend immune protection against M. tuberculosis. They showed that a recombinant BCG (AFRO-1) could induce strong antigen-specific T cell responses when combined with the TB vaccine vector rAD35 (23, 24). The Biomedical Primate Research Center in Rijswijk, the Netherlands, aimed to develop a model to test TB vaccines before progressing to human clinical trials (25). By using an RM model inoculated intratracheally with the Erdman strain of M. tuberculosis, the study revealed that prior immunization with the MVA.85-boosted BCG and an attenuated, phoP-deficient TB vaccine provided effective protection against M. tuberculosis infection. A novel aerosol challenge model achieved by Sharpe et al. (26) helped to assess the endpoints for testing the BCG/MVA.85 vaccine. This NHP model used a three-jet Collision nebulizer in addition to the modified Henderson apparatus, as described by Barclay et al. (13), in a head-out plethysmography chamber. The findings from these studies indicated that the gamma-interferon indices—ELISpot and enzyme-linked immunosorbent assay (ELISA)—do not relate to the protection against TB; only the magnetic resonance imaging readouts offered a reliable correlate, using

Table 3 TB studies using rhesus macaques[a]

No. of RM	*M. tuberculosis* strain (inoculation route), dose(s) (CFU)	Major findings	Reference(s)
	Experimental design		
8	Erdman (i.b.), 10–150	RMs are a good model for latent TB, using low doses of H37Rv.	21
12	H37Rv (i.b.), 30–6,000,000		
4	H37Rv (i.b.), 1,000	High-resolution radiographic and fine immunologic studies provide definition of TB disease progression.	22
18	Erdman (i.t.), 500	Recombinant BCG (AFRO-1) induces strong antigen-specific T cell responses with TB vaccine vector (rAD35).	23, 24[b]
24	Erdman (i.t.), 1,000	MVA.85 boosting of BCG and an attenuated, *phoP*-deficient TB vaccine shows protective efficacy against TB.	25[b]
16	Erdman K01 (a.), 40–65	RM may be used as models of *M. tuberculosis* aerosol challenge. IFN-γ (ELISpot, ELISA) does not correlate with protection against TB; only magnetic resonance imaging offers a reliable correlate.	26
NP	NP	Early TB lesions have a highly proinflammatory environment, expressing IFN-γ, TNF-α, JAK, STAT and C-C/C-X-C chemokines. In contrast, late TB lesions have a silenced inflammatory response.	27
12	326 CDC1551 Himar 1 mutants (i.n.), 100,000	Virulence mechanisms of *M. tuberculosis* include transport of lipid virulence factors; biosynthesis of cell-wall arabinan and peptidoglycan; DNA repair; sterol metabolism; and lung cell entry.	28
9	H37Rv (i.b.), 50–3,000	Chinese RMs are highly susceptible to *M. tuberculosis* infection and develop active TB regardless of the doses of H37Rv or Erdman strain used.	29, 30
24	Erdman (i.b.), 25–500		
16	CDC1551 (i.n.), 50	RMs are an excellent model of TB/HIV coinfection and can be used to study TB latency and reactivation.	31
6	Erdman K01 (i.b.), 500	Stereological analysis provides quantitative data showing a strong correlation between bacterial load and lung granulomas.	32
13	CDC1551 (i.n.), 5,000	The *M. tuberculosis* stress response factor *sigH* is required for *M. tuberculosis* replication in mammalian lungs.	33
3	Erdman (i.b./i.n.), 5–50	Newborn macaques infected with aerosolized *M. tuberculosis* develop human-like immunologic responses and make a good model for pediatric TB/HIV.	35
32	Erdman K01 (i.b.), 275	RM aerosol vaccination with AERAS-402 elicits transient cellular immune responses in the blood and robust, sustained immune responses in bronchoalveolar lavage, but does not protect against high-dose *M. tuberculosis*.	8[b]
17	CDC1551 (a.), 100	Clinical profiles vary considerably among RMs infected with *M. tuberculosis* but can help identify predictive biomarkers for TB susceptibility along with gene expression profiles.	36
6	H37Rv (a.), 50–100	The DosR regulon modulates host T-cell responses against *M. tuberculosis*, allowing *M. tuberculosis* to persist.	40
21	DosR mutants (a.), 50–100		
5	DosR-complemented strain (a.), 50–100		
22[c]	CDC1551 (a.), 50	Lymphocyte-activation gene 3 is expressed primarily on CD4 T-cells of lung granulomas of *M. tuberculosis*-infected and SIV-coinfected RMs, coinciding with high bacterial burdens and changes in the host type 1 helper T cell response.	39
10	CDC1551 (a.), 1,000		
2	Erdman K01 (a.), 35	*M. tuberculosis* challenge via aerosol or intrabronchial instillation leads to similar TB disease outcomes although different distributions of pulmonary pathology in RMs.	41
2	Erdman K01 (i.b.), 35		
24	Erdman K01 (a.), 100	Intravenous BCG induces greater protection than other routes of BCG administration (i.d. +/− i.t., a.) while correlating with higher antigen-specific CD4 effector memory T-cell populations in RMs.	75[b]
9c	H37Rv (i.b.), 34	Chinese RMs coinfected with SIV and *M. tuberculosis* exhibit more progressive TB disease than RMs mono-infected with *M. tuberculosis*.	76
36	Erdman K01 (i.b.), 500	Pulmonary mucosal BCG provides protection against TB in RMs that are not responsive to BCG (i.d.).	77[b]

[a]Table 3 outlines the study designs and major findings of TB investigations using rhesus macaques. All studies, except for those reported in references 28 to 30 and 33, used Indian rhesus macaques. a., aerosol; BCG, bacillus Calmette-Guérin; ELISA, enzyme-linked immunosorbent assay; ELISpot, enzyme-linked immunosorbent spot assay; Erdman, ATCC35801 strain unless indicated as K01 strain; i.b., intrabronchial; i.d., intradermal; INF-γ, gamma interferon; i.n., intranasal; i.t., intratracheal; NP, the information is not provided in the paper; RM, rhesus macaques; SIV, simian immunodeficiency virus; TB, tuberculosis; TNF-α, tumor necrosis factor alpha.
[b]TB vaccine-related studies.
[c]One subgroup of macaques was coinfected with *M. tuberculosis* and SIV.

Table 4 TB studies using cynomolgus macaques[a]

No. of CM	*M. tuberculosis* strain (inoculation route), dose(s) (CFU)	Major findings	Reference(s)
	Experimental design		
28	Erdman (i.t.), 10–100,000	The Philippine CM provides an excellent model of chronic TB.	20
17	Erdman (i.b.), 25	Low-dose infection of CM represents the full spectrum of human *M. tuberculosis* infection and provides a model to study latent, as well as active-chronic and rapidly progressive, TB.	4
16	Erdman (i.t.), 500	CM vaccination with 72f rBCG vaccine provides better protective efficacy than BCG.	42[b]
44	Erdman (i.t.), 500	CM vaccination with HSP65 + IL-12/HVJ vaccine provides better protective efficacy than BCG.	42, 43[b]
15	Erdman (i.t.), dose not reported	CM vaccination with Mtb72F/AS02A provides greater protective efficacy than BCG alone.	44[b]
24	Erdman (i.b.), 1,000	CM vaccination with mc²6020 or mc²6030 provides less protection than BCG.	10[b]
25	Erdman (i.b.), 25	At necropsy, CMs with active TB have more lung T cells and more IFN-γ from PBMC, BAL, and mediastinal lymph nodes than CMs with latent TB.	45
24	Erdman (i.b.), 25	Neutralization of tumor necrosis factor results in disseminated disease in acute and latent TB infection with normal granuloma structure in a CM model.	46
41	Erdman (i.b.), 25	Regulatory T cells in active TB occur in response to increased inflammation, not as a causal factor of disease progression.	47
15	Erdman (i.b.), 25	Reactivation of latent TB with SIV is associated with early T cell depletion and not virus load.	48
7[c]	Erdman (i.b.), 25	*M. tuberculosis*-specific multifunctional T cells are better correlates of antigen load and disease status than of protection.	49
5	Erdman (i.b.), 200		
33	Erdman (i.t.), 25–500	The multistage vaccine H56 boosts the effects of BCG to protect CM against active TB and reactivation of latent TB.	50
14	Erdman (i.b.), 25–200	The CM model of *M. tuberculosis* infection mimics human TB, particularly in granuloma type and structure.	51
8	Erdman (i.t.), 250	*M. tuberculosis* may modulate protective immune responses via the use of indoleamine 2,3-dioxygenase (immunosuppressant) found in nonlymphocytic regions of TB granulomas.	9[b]
9	Erdman (i.b.), 25	Experimental and epidemiologic estimates of the *M. tuberculosis* mutation rate are comparable.	52
27	Erdman (i.b.), 500	Early expansion/differentiation of Vγ2Vδ2 T effector cells during *M. tuberculosis* infection increases resistance to TB.	53
26	Erdman (i.b.), 25–400	TB granulomas evolve and resolve independently within a single host; individual lesions respond differently to different drugs. Overall PET and CT signals can predict successful TB drug treatment.	54
12	Erdman (i.b.), 1,000	Compared with nonvaccinated CMs, BCG-vaccinated CMs exhibit higher expression of TNF-α, IL-10, IL-1b, TLR-4, IL-17, IL-6, IL-12, and iNOS in the lungs.	56[b]
39	Erdman (i.b.), 25	The sterilization of TB granulomas occurs in both active and latent TB amidst the differential killing of *M. tuberculosis* within a single host.	55
2	SNP strains (i.b.), 34		
8	Erdman (i.b.), 240–500	CM vaccination with BCG transiently increases levels of macrophages and lymphocytes in the blood with later recruitment in the lungs; however, *M. tuberculosis* continues to replicate in the lungs.	57[b]
NP	Erdman (i.b.), 25	NF-κB signaling in TB granulomas is a marker of macrophage polarization early during *M. tuberculosis* infection and predictive of granuloma outcome.	58
30	Erdman (i.t.), 500–1,000	Boosting BCG with H56 in adjuvants (CAF01/04/05) results in better survival rates compared to BCG alone. However, the level of vaccine-specific IFN-γ production does not correlate with or predict disease outcome in CMs.	78[b]
6	Erdman (i.b.), 38–60	In CMs, TB granulomas have higher [⁶⁴Cu]-LLP2A uptake than uninfected tissues and show significant correlations between LLP2A signal and macrophage and T-cell numbers.	80

[a]Table 4 outlines the study designs and major findings of TB investigations that used cynomolgus macaques. BAL, bronchoalveolar lavage; BCG, bacillus Calmette-Guérin; CM, cynomolgus macaques; CT, computed tomography; Erdman, ATCC 35801 strain; i.b., intrabronchial; IL, interleukin; i.t., intratracheal; IFN-γ, gamma interferon; iNOS, inducible nitric oxide synthase; NP, the information is not provided in the paper; PBMC, peripheral blood mononuclear cells; PET, positron emission tomography; rBCG, recombinant BCG; SIV, simian immunodeficiency virus; SNP, *M. tuberculosis* strains with single-nucleotide polymorphism; TB, tuberculosis; TNF-α, tumor necrosis factor alpha.
[b]TB vaccine-related studies.
[c]One subgroup of macaques was coinfected with *M. tuberculosis* and SIV (49).

ex vivo lung samples removed at necropsy (13, 26). Another way to objectively measure the efficacy of TB vaccines and drugs was later developed by Luciw et al. (32) at the California NPRC. The conclusions drawn from these studies showed that stereological analysis from magnetic resonance imaging could provide quantitative data, revealing a significant correlation between bacterial load and lung granulomas.

More recent studies using RMs have explored how different routes of BCG vaccination can alter protection against *M. tuberculosis* infection. Intravenous BCG induced greater protection than other routes of BCG administration while inducing higher antigen-specific CD4 effector memory T-cell populations in RMs (75). For RMs that were not responsive to intradermal BCG, pulmonary mucosal BCG vaccination reduced local pathology and improved hematological and immunological parameters after *M. tuberculosis* infection (77). Unveiling the most efficacious route(s) of administration is one necessary component in developing a reliable TB vaccine.

CM models were used much later than RM models for testing TB vaccines. Between 2005 and 2012, three studies using CM models evaluated the efficacy of TB vaccines that had been tested previously with small-animal models, including guinea pigs and mice (42, 43). The first project evaluated the efficacy of the 72f recombinant BCG vaccine and HASP65 + IL-12/HVJ vaccine (42), which another team of investigators also tested later in Osaka, Japan (43). Both research investigations showed that the recombinant BCG vaccines were more effective than BCG alone. Soon after, the multistage vaccine H56 was found to increase the effects of BCG to protect CM against active TB and the reactivation of latent TB (50). Boosting BCG with H56 in adjuvants (CAF01/04/05) also resulted in better survival rates compared to BCG alone (78). Ultimately, the macaque models have presented the potential to help evaluate preventative methods and interventions before reaching human clinical trials, particularly for TB vaccines (65). Table 5 provides further details on the vaccine dosages and routes of inoculation used in these studies.

Macaque Models for TB Drug Evaluation

Another recent investigation of experimental *M. tuberculosis* infection in a CM model also came from the

Table 5 Novel TB vaccine models using macaques[a]

	Experimental design			
No. of macaques	*M. tuberculosis* strain (inoculation route), dose(s) (CFU)	Vaccine(s)	(inoculation route), dose(s)	Reference(s)
15 RM	Erdman (i.t.), 500	AFRO-1/rAD35-TBS	(i.d.) 2×10^5 CFU (i.m.) 2×10^{11} v.p.	23, 24
24 RM	Erdman (i.d.), 1,000	BCG/MVA.85A	(i.d.) 5×10^5 CFU (i.d.) 5×10^8 PFU;	25
		SO2	(i.d.) 5×10^5 CFU	
24 CM	Erdman (i.b.), 1,000	mc^{2}6020 or mc^{2}6030	(i.d.) 9×10^6 CFU (i.d.) 9×10^6 CFU	10
16 CM	Erdman (i.t.), 500	72f rBCG	(i.d.) 10^6 CFU	42
44 CM	Erdman (i.t.), 500	HSP65 + IL-12/HVJ	(i.m.) 400 µg	42, 43
15 CM	Erdman (i.t.), dose not reported	Mtb72F/AS02A	(i.m.) 40 µg/500 µl	44
32 RM	Erdman K01 (i.b.), 275	BCG and/or rAD35-TBS	(i.d.) 5×10^5 CFU (a.) 3×10^{10} v.p.	8
30 CM	Erdman (i.t.), 500–1,000	BCG+/– H56/(CAF01/04/05)	(i.d.) $2–8\times10^5$ CFU (i.m.) 50 µg/500 µl	78
36 RM	Erdman K01 (i.b.), 500	BCG	(i.d. and/or e.b.) 5×10^5 CFU	77

[a]Table 5 highlights novel TB vaccine models that used macaques from 2008 through 2017. In all vaccine studies listed, the novel inoculum was more efficacious than BCG alone. Parameters used to determine greater vaccine efficacy compared with BCG alone included a local increase in CD8+ cytolytic T cells, reduced expression of the *M. tuberculosis*-specific antigen, and prolonged survival after the challenge. Other considerations involved increased induction of specific IFN-γ responses, reduced pathology and chest X-ray scores, and decreased average lung bacterial counts upon infectious challenge. Reduction in C-reactive protein levels, body weight loss, and decrease of erythrocyte-associated hematologic parameters as markers of inflammatory infection were also taken into account. a., aerosol; AFRO-1, a recombinant BCG expressing perfringolysin and overexpressing *M. tuberculosis* antigens Ag85A, Ag85B, and TB10.4; BCG, bacillus Calmette-Guérin (Tokyo or Danish strain 1331); CM, cynomolgus macaques; e.b., endobronchial; HSP65, mycobacterial heat shock protein; HVJ, hemagglutinating virus of Japan liposome; i.b., intrabronchial; i.d., intradermal; IL-12, interleukin-12; i.m., intramuscular; i.t., intratracheal; mc^{2}6020 (H37Rv lysA panCD) and mc^{2}6030 (H37Rv RD1 panCD), live attenuated *M. tuberculosis* double-deletion vaccine strains; Mtb72f/AS02A, fusion protein of *M. tuberculosis* virulence factors Mtb32 and Mtb39 in AS02A adjuvant; MVA.85A, modified vaccinia virus Ankara expressing antigen 85A; rAD35-TBS, replication-deficient adenovirus serotype 35 vector expressing synthetic scrambled *M. tuberculosis* antigens Ag85A, Ag85B, and TB10.4 (AERAS-402); RM, rhesus macaques; SO2, attenuated, *phoP*-deficient *M. tuberculosis*; v.p., viral particles.

University of Pittsburgh School of Medicine (54, 55). The objective was to determine potential alternative markers for evaluating the efficacy of TB drugs. The studies compared the overall metabolic and radiographic changes, as well as the variations within individual granulomas, in CMs infected with *M. tuberculosis*. Results from the studies revealed that TB granulomas evolve and resolve independently within a single host and that individual lesions respond variably to different drugs (54). Furthermore, the clinical findings concluded that the overall positron emission tomography (PET) and computed tomography (CT) signals could be used as prognostic markers to predict successful TB drug therapies. However, the overall metabolic and radiographic changes were nonspecific indicators of metabolic activity, measured from ^{18}F-fluorodeoxyglucose-radiolabeled glucose in PET/CT imaging data (54). One way to address this ambiguity is to use another PET probe, such as [^{64}Cu]-LLP2A, to identify recruitment and differentiation of unique cell populations in granulomas (80). Using a combination of probes may help to advance TB diagnosis and treatment.

Macaque Models for the Study of TB Pathogenesis

By gaining a better understanding of the pathogenesis of *M. tuberculosis* infection and reactivation of latent TB, researchers can further develop and improve treatment strategies. As such, investigators at the Tulane NPRC profiled the TB granuloma transcriptome in an RM model to identify key immune signaling pathways that are activated during *M. tuberculosis* infection (27). Previously, scientists from the Chicago Center for Biomedical Research characterized gene networks in RMs after only BCG vaccination/infection (66). Mechanistic studies of *M. tuberculosis* pathogenesis defined more specific factors employed by *M. tuberculosis* to successfully infect and persist in mammalian lungs (28). The identification of a potential therapeutic target sparked from the discovery of the *M. tuberculosis* stress response factor sigH as an important player in the growth/replication of *M. tuberculosis* (33, 34).

Lin et al. (45) characterized the clinical manifestations of TB disease within the three stages: latent, active-chronic, and rapidly progressive TB. The results of these studies showed that at necropsy, the CMs with active TB had more CD4+ and CD8+ T cells in the lungs and more gamma-interferon from peripheral blood mononuclear cells, bronchoalveolar lavage, and mediastinal lymph nodes than CMs with latent TB (45). The same research group also showed that tumor necrosis factor neutralization resulted in disseminated

disease in both acute and latent TB with normal granulomatous structures (46). Another CM study examined the role of CD4+ regulatory T cells in active TB, which occurred in response to increased inflammation rather than acting as a causative factor in the progression to active disease (47).

The pathological hallmark of *M. tuberculosis* infection of lung tissue is granuloma formation (67). In light of the discovery that TB granulomas change uniquely within a host (54), an investigation by Lin et al. (55) aimed to define how these structures vary between CMs with latent and active TB. Interestingly, the sterilization of the granulomas occurred in both stages of TB, regardless of the differential killing of bacteria within a single host (55). Moreover, TB vaccine-related studies have exposed possible genetic mechanisms of host resistance to *M. tuberculosis* after immunization (56), as well as immunosuppressant mechanisms of *M. tuberculosis* virulence (57). While adding insight into the molecular and pathological pathways of TB progression, these findings may also help to evaluate the disease status as well as incentivize the development of novel therapeutic targets. For example, recent studies (58) show that the dynamics of NF-κB signaling in TB granulomas is a viable therapeutic target to promote macrophage polarization early during infection and to improve outcome. Further evidence of the DosR regulon as a modulator of host T cell responses against *M. tuberculosis*, allowing mycobacterial persistence (40), may similarly help develop potential therapeutic targets.

M. tuberculosis/Simian Immunodeficiency Virus Coinfection Macaque Models

Macaques also serve as an excellent model of coinfection with simian immunodeficiency virus (SIV), the counterpart of HIV, which is of importance to understand TB latency and reactivation (31, 68). Upon inoculation with high-dose BCG (31, 69, 70), low-dose Erdman strain (48), or CDC1551 clinical isolate (39), latently infected RMs and CMs had reactivated TB when coinfected with SIV. Pathogenic SIV-BCG interactions facilitated the development of TB-like disease (70), while antiretroviral agents restored *M. tuberculosis*-specific T cell immune responses (31). The reactivation of latent TB in CM infected with SIV was associated with early T cell depletion and not the virus load (48). Recent reports by Guo et al. (68, 76) showed that SIV infection facilitated *M. tuberculosis* dissemination in coinfected RMs. The researchers demonstrated that SIV-*M. tuberculosis*-coinfected animals had significantly lower levels of TB-specific biomarkers, gamma interferon (IFN-γ) and interleukin-22 (IL-22), than monoinfected animals (68). Coinfected RMs also had higher bacterial counts and more prevalent lesions on chest X-rays and necropsy (76). Another particularly innovative RM model of TB was established at the Southwest NPRC (35). The purpose of this study was to institute an NHP model for pediatric TB/HIV coinfection. Newborn macaques were infected with *M. tuberculosis* Erdman strain intrabronchially or via the aerosol route, using an ultrasonic nebulizer specifically adapted for the newborn macaque nose. Investigators confirmed *M. tuberculosis* infection by various methods, including chest X rays, ELISpot, bronchoalveolar and gastric lavages, and necropsy. Because people with HIV/AIDS carry a high risk of *M. tuberculosis* infection and disease severity, it is clinically significant to have an NHP model that mimics coinfection. Understanding the pathogenesis of *M. tuberculosis*/SIV coinfection in macaque models can lead to better management and control of the human TB epidemic.

KEY POINTS AND FUTURE RESEARCH STRATEGIES

Overall, the literature on macaque models of TB has shared four important issues and opportunities for improvement. First, scientists must address the biosafety requirements, cost of equipment and maintenance, and animal availability when considering the use of NHP models in TB research. One alternative is to experiment with smaller genera and species of NHPs that still recapitulate human TB, such as the common marmoset (*Callithrix jacchus*) model. The marmosets' much higher susceptibility to *M. tuberculosis* infection and aggressive TB disease progression compared with other NHPs, however, may limit the smaller model's use in long-term studies of immunological response or detecting subtle differences in the virulence of mutant *M. tuberculosis* strains (71). Second, the reviewed literature shows that different animal species, individually and as a whole, respond differently when exposed to *M. tuberculosis* in terms of immunopathogenesis of the TB disease (38, 64) (Table 2). Therefore, investigators must define the purpose of the study for the appropriate selection of NHP species. Third, the strain of *M. tuberculosis* used for inoculation can significantly impact the disease outcome. Instead of employing merely laboratory-adopted Erdman or H37Rv strains, study designs should include clinical isolates of *M. tuberculosis*. Although this approach may introduce more variability into the NHP studies of TB while making studies performed at different sites more difficult to compare, the findings would

likely further mimic human TB disease and add valuable knowledge for the clinical situation. Last, most of the macaque studies so far have shown only acute TB, which is much less prevalent than latent TB in humans. Hence, it is necessary to establish clinically more relevant NHP models that resemble human passive airway transmission. By creating an NHP model of natural *M. tuberculosis* infection under experimental conditions, researchers would be able to test novel and current TB vaccines/drugs for protection against *M. tuberculosis* infection.

CONCLUDING REMARKS

The NHP models have served as a valuable tool in TB research over the past several decades. As illustrated in the literature, the CM and RM TB models have clinically revealed similar manifestations of TB disease or latency through multiple diagnostic and prognostic parameters. Even the variability in immune responses to *M. tuberculosis* infection imitates the diverse human host reactions to the pathogen (36). Although some studies on TB vaccine evaluation have been conducted by using experimentally infected macaques, the majority of these studies hardly showed the reduction of TB disease progression by BCG-based vaccines. Therefore, a pressing need prevails to establish NHP models that can demonstrate BCG-mediated protection against *M. tuberculosis* infection besides TB disease progression. Even with this shortcoming, however, NHP models that broadly recapitulate many aspects of human TB disease have significant advantages over other (lower vertebrate) animals. Especially in the realm of translational research, the preclinical usage of NHP models for advancing treatments and prevention of *M. tuberculosis* infection is noteworthy.

GLOSSARY

Cynomolgus macaque (CM) *Macaca fascicularis*, also called long-tailed macaques, a species of Old World monkeys native to Southeast Asia.

CDC 1551 A clinical isolate of *M. tuberculosis*, exhibiting a similar degree of virulence as the Erdman strain.

Erdman strain A virulent subset of *M. tuberculosis* existing in two forms, including the laboratory ATCC35801 and the clinically isolated K01 strains; most commonly used to study acute tuberculosis.

H37Rv An attenuated laboratory strain of *M. tuberculosis* typically used to study latent infection.

Modified Henderson apparatus A device for studying the infectivity and virulence of microorganisms in small air droplets; the three components include a continuous aerosol-generating unit (Collision spray), exposure unit, and sampling unit.

Rhesus macaque (RM) *Macaca mulatta*, a species of Old World monkeys native to Asia; RMs of Indian origin are the most frequently used RM species in tuberculosis research.

Acknowledgments. J.C.P. and W.H. were the sole contributors to the literature analysis and written work. Graphic illustrations were developed by J.C.P and W.H.

Citation. Peña JC, Ho W-Z. 2016. Non-human primate models of tuberculosis. Microbiol Spectrum 4(4):TBTB2-0007-2016.

References

1. Ackermann RR (ed). 2003. *A comparative primate dissection guide, version 1.0.* See more at http://www.archaeology.uct.ac.za/age/faculty-and-staff/rebecca-rogers-ackermann#sthash.M7Y7sPzv.dpuf.

2. Carlsson HE, Schapiro SJ, Farah I, Hau J. 2004. Use of primates in research: a global overview. *Am J Primatol* 63:225–237.

3. O'Neil RM, Ashack RJ, Goodman FR. 1981. A comparative study of the respiratory responses to bronchoactive agents in rhesus and cynomolgus monkeys. *J Pharmacol Methods* 5:267–273.

4. Capuano SV III, Croix DA, Pawar S, Zinovik A, Myers A, Lin PL, Bissel S, Fuhrman C, Klein E, Flynn JL. 2003. Experimental *Mycobacterium tuberculosis* infection of cynomolgus macaques closely resembles the various manifestations of human *M. tuberculosis* infection. *Infect Immun* 71:5831–5844.

5. Flynn JL. 2006. Lessons from experimental *Mycobacterium tuberculosis* infections. *Microbes Infect* 8:1179–1188.

6. Wolf RH, Gibson SV, Watson EA, Baskin GB. 1988. Multidrug chemotherapy of tuberculosis in rhesus monkeys. *Lab Anim Sci* 38:25–33.

7. Schmidt LH. 1966. Studies on the antituberculous activity of ethambutol in monkeys. *Ann N Y Acad Sci* 135(2 New Antituber):747–758.

8. Darrah PA, Bolton DL, Lackner AA, Kaushal D, Aye PP, Mehra S, Blanchard JL, Didier PJ, Roy CJ, Rao SS, Hokey DA, Scanga CA, Sizemore DR, Sadoff JC, Roederer M, Seder RA. 2014. Aerosol vaccination with AERAS-402 elicits robust cellular immune responses in the lungs of rhesus macaques but fails to protect against high-dose *Mycobacterium tuberculosis* challenge. *J Immunol* 193:1799–1811.

9. Mehra S, Alvarez X, Didier PJ, Doyle LA, Blanchard JL, Lackner AA, Kaushal D. 2013. Granuloma correlates of protection against tuberculosis and mechanisms of immune modulation by *Mycobacterium tuberculosis*. *J Infect Dis* 207:1115–1127.

10. Larsen MH, Biermann K, Chen B, Hsu T, Sambandamurthy VK, Lackner AA, Aye PP, Didier P, Huang D, Shao L, Wei H, Letvin NL, Frothingham R, Haynes BF, Chen ZW, Jacobs WR Jr. 2009. Efficacy and safety of live attenuated persistent and rapidly cleared *Mycobacterium tuberculosis* vaccine candidates in nonhuman primates. *Vaccine* 27:4709–4717.

11. McMurray DN. 2000. A nonhuman primate model for preclinical testing of new tuberculosis vaccines. *Clin Infect Dis* 30(Suppl 3):S210–S212.

12. Good RC. 1968. Biology of the mycobacterioses. Simian tuberculosis: immunologic aspects. *Ann N Y Acad Sci* 154(1 Biology of My):200–213.

13. Barclay WR, Anacker RL, Brehmer W, Leif W, Ribi E. 1970. Aerosol-induced tuberculosis in subhuman primates and the course of the disease after intravenous BCG vaccination. *Infect Immun* 2:574–582.

14. Baram P, Soltysik L, Condoulis W. 1971. The in vitro assay of tuberculin hypersensitivity in *Macaca mulatta* sensitized with bacille Calmette Guerin cell wall vaccine and-or infected with virulent *Mycobacterium tuberculosis*. *Lab Anim Sci* 21:727–733.

15. Ribi E, Anacker RL, Barclay WR, Brehmer W, Harris SC, Leif WR, Simmons J. 1971. Efficacy of mycobacterial cell walls as a vaccine against airborne tuberculosis in the Rheesus monkey. *J Infect Dis* 123:527–538.

16. Barclay WR, Busey WM, Dalgard DW, Good RC, Janicki BW, Kasik JE, Ribi E, Ulrich CE, Wolinsky E. 1973. Protection of monkeys against airborne tuberculosis by aerosol vaccination with bacillus Calmette-Guerin. *Am Rev Respir Dis* 107:351–358.

17. Janicki BW, Good RC, Minden P, Affronti LF, Hymes WF. 1973. Immune responses in rhesus monkeys after bacillus Calmette-Guerin vaccination and aerosol challenge with *Mycobacterium tuberculosis*. *Am Rev Respir Dis* 107:359–366.

18. Chaparas SD, Good RC, Janicki BW. 1975. Tuberculin-induced lymphocyte transformation and skin reactivity in monkeys vaccinated or not vaccinated with Bacille Calmette-Guérin, then challenged with virulent *Mycobacterium tuberculosis*. *Am Rev Respir Dis* 112:43–47.

19. Harper GJ, Morton JD. 1953. The respiratory retention of bacterial aerosols: experiments with radioactive spores. *J Hyg (Lond)* 51:372–385.

20. Walsh GP, Tan EV, dela Cruz EC, Abalos RM, Villahermosa LG, Young LJ, Cellona RV, Nazareno JB, Horwitz MA. 1996. The Philippine cynomolgus monkey (*Macaca fasicularis*) provides a new nonhuman primate model of tuberculosis that resembles human disease. *Nat Med* 2:430–436.

21. Gormus BJ, Blanchard JL, Alvarez XH, Didier PJ. 2004. Evidence for a rhesus monkey model of asymptomatic tuberculosis. *J Med Primatol* 33:134–145.

22. Lewinsohn DM, Tydeman IS, Frieder M, Grotzke JE, Lines RA, Ahmed S, Prongay KD, Primack SL, Colgin LM, Lewis AD, Lewinsohn DA. 2006. High resolution radiographic and fine immunologic definition of TB disease progression in the rhesus macaque. *Microbes Infect* 8:2587–2598.

23. Magalhaes I, Sizemore DR, Ahmed RK, Mueller S, Wehlin L, Scanga C, Weichold F, Schirru G, Pau MG, Goudsmit J, Kühlmann-Berenzon S, Spångberg M, Andersson J, Gaines H, Thorstensson R, Skeiky YA, Sadoff J, Maeurer M. 2008. rBCG induces strong antigen-specific T cell responses in rhesus macaques in a prime-boost setting with an adenovirus 35 tuberculosis vaccine vector. *PLoS One* **3**:e3790.

24. Rahman S, Magalhaes I, Rahman J, Ahmed RK, Sizemore DR, Scanga CA, Weichold F, Verreck F, Kondova I, Sadoff J, Thorstensson R, Spångberg M, Svensson M, Andersson J, Maeurer M, Brighenti S. 2012. Prime-boost vaccination with rBCG/rAd35 enhances CD8+ cytolytic T-cell responses in lesions from *Mycobacterium tuberculosis*-infected primates. *Mol Med* **18**:647–658.

25. Verreck FA, Vervenne RA, Kondova I, van Kralingen KW, Remarque EJ, Braskamp G, van der Werff NM, Kersbergen A, Ottenhoff TH, Heidt PJ, Gilbert SC, Gicquel B, Hill AV, Martin C, McShane H, Thomas AW. 2009. MVA.85A boosting of BCG and an attenuated, phoP deficient M. tuberculosis vaccine both show protective efficacy against tuberculosis in rhesus macaques. *PLoS One* **4**:e5264. (Erratum 6:doi:10.1371/annotation/e599dafd-8208-4655-a792-21cb125f7f66).

26. Sharpe SA, McShane H, Dennis MJ, Basaraba RJ, Gleeson F, Hall G, McIntyre A, Gooch K, Clark S, Beveridge NE, Nuth E, White A, Marriott A, Dowall S, Hill AV, Williams A, Marsh PD. 2010. Establishment of an aerosol challenge model of tuberculosis in rhesus macaques and an evaluation of endpoints for vaccine testing. *Clin Vaccine Immunol* **17**:1170–1182.

27. Mehra S, Pahar B, Dutta NK, Conerly CN, Philippi-Falkenstein K, Alvarez X, Kaushal D. 2010. Transcriptional reprogramming in nonhuman primate (rhesus macaque) tuberculosis granulomas. *PLoS One* **5**:e12266.

28. Dutta NK, Mehra S, Didier PJ, Roy CJ, Doyle LA, Alvarez X, Ratterree M, Be NA, Lamichhane G, Jain SK, Lacey MR, Lackner AA, Kaushal D. 2010. Genetic requirements for the survival of tubercle bacilli in primates. *J Infect Dis* **201**:1743–1752.

29. Zhang J, Ye YQ, Wang Y, Mo PZ, Xian QY, Rao Y, Bao R, Dai M, Liu JY, Guo M, Wang X, Huang ZX, Sun LH, Tang ZJ, Ho WZ. 2011. M. *tuberculosis* H37Rv infection of Chinese rhesus macaques. *J Neuroimmune Pharmacol* **6**:362–370.

30. Zhang J, Xian Q, Guo M, Huang Z, Rao Y, Wang Y, Wang X, Bao R, Evans TG, Hokey D, Sizemore D, Ho WZ. 2014. *Mycobacterium tuberculosis* Erdman infection of rhesus macaques of Chinese origin. *Tuberculosis (Edinb)* **94**:634–643.

31. Mehra S, Golden NA, Dutta NK, Midkiff CC, Alvarez X, Doyle LA, Asher M, Russell-Lodrigue K, Monjure C, Roy CJ, Blanchard JL, Didier PJ, Veazey RS, Lackner AA, Kaushal D. 2011. Reactivation of latent tuberculosis in rhesus macaques by coinfection with simian immunodeficiency virus. *J Med Primatol* **40**:233–243.

32. Luciw PA, Oslund KL, Yang XW, Adamson L, Ravindran R, Canfield DR, Tarara R, Hirst L, Christensen M, Lerche NW, Offenstein H, Lewinsohn D, Ventimiglia F, Brignolo L, Wisner ER, Hyde DM. 2011. Stereological

33. Dutta NK, Mehra S, Martinez AN, Alvarez X, Renner NA, Morici LA, Pahar B, Maclean AG, Lackner AA, Kaushal D. 2012. The stress-response factor SigH modulates the interaction between *Mycobacterium tuberculosis* and host phagocytes. *PLoS One* **7**:e28958.

34. Mehra S, Golden NA, Stuckey K, Didier PJ, Doyle LA, Russell-Lodrigue KE, Sugimoto C, Hasegawa A, Sivasubramani SK, Roy CJ, Alvarez X, Kuroda MJ, Blanchard JL, Lackner AA, Kaushal D. 2012. The Mycobacterium tuberculosis stress response factor SigH is required for bacterial burden as well as immunopathology in primate lungs. *J Infect Dis* **205**:1203–1213.

35. Cepeda M, Salas M, Folwarczny J, Leandro AC, Hodara VL, de la Garza MA, Dick EJ Jr, Owston M, Armitige LY, Gauduin MC. 2013. Establishment of a neonatal rhesus macaque model to study *Mycobacterium tuberculosis* infection. *Tuberculosis (Edinb)* **93**(Suppl):S51–S59.

36. Luo Q, Mehra S, Golden NA, Kaushal D, Lacey MR. 2014. Identification of biomarkers for tuberculosis susceptibility via integrated analysis of gene expression and longitudinal clinical data. *Front Genet* **5**:240.

37. Langermans JA, Andersen P, van Soolingen D, Vervenne RA, Frost PA, van der Laan T, van Pinxteren LA, van den Hombergh J, Kroon S, Peekel I, Florquin S, Thomas AW. 2001. Divergent effect of bacillus Calmette-Guérin (BCG) vaccination on *Mycobacterium tuberculosis* infection in highly related macaque species: implications for primate models in tuberculosis vaccine research. *Proc Natl Acad Sci USA* **98**:11497–11502.

38. Ravindran R, Krishnan VV, Dhawan R, Wunderlich ML, Lerche NW, Flynn JL, Luciw PA, Khan IH. 2014. Plasma antibody profiles in non-human primate tuberculosis. *J Med Primatol* **43**:59–71.

39. Phillips BL, Mehra S, Ahsan MH, Selman M, Khader SA, Kaushal D. 2015. LAG3 expression in active *Mycobacterium tuberculosis* infections. *Am J Pathol* **185**: 820–833.

40. Mehra S, Foreman TW, Didier PJ, Ahsan MH, Hudock TA, Kissee R, Golden NA, Gautam US, Johnson AM, Alvarez X, Russell-Lodrigue KE, Doyle LA, Roy CJ, Niu T, Blanchard JL, Khader SA, Lackner AA, Sherman DR, Kaushal D. 2015. The DosR regulon modulates adaptive immunity and is essential for *Mycobacterium tuberculosis* persistence. *Am J Respir Crit Care Med* **191**: 1185–1196.

41. Sibley L, Dennis M, Sarfas C, White A, Clark S, Gleeson F, McIntyre A, Rayner E, Pearson G, Williams A, Marsh P, Sharpe S. 2016. Route of delivery to the airway influences the distribution of pulmonary disease but not the outcome of *Mycobacterium tuberculosis* infection in rhesus macaques. *Tuberculosis (Edinb)* **96**:141–149.

42. Kita Y, Tanaka T, Yoshida S, Ohara N, Kaneda Y, Kuwayama S, Muraki Y, Kanamaru N, Hashimoto S, Takai H, Okada C, Fukunaga Y, Sakaguchi Y, Furukawa I, Yamada K, Inoue Y, Takemoto Y, Naito M, Yamada T, Matsumoto M, McMurray DN, Cruz EC, Tan EV,

Abalos RM, Burgos JA, Gelber R, Skeiky Y, Reed S, Sakatani M, Okada M. 2005. Novel recombinant BCG and DNA-vaccination against tuberculosis in a cynomolgus monkey model. *Vaccine* 23:2132–2135.

43. Okada M, Kita Y, Nakajima T, Kanamaru N, Hashimoto S, Nagasawa T, Kaneda Y, Yoshida S, Nishida Y, Fukamizu R, Tsunai Y, Inoue R, Nakatani H, Namie Y, Yamada J, Takao K, Asai R, Asaki R, Matsumoto M, McMurray DN, Dela Cruz EC, Tan EV, Abalos RM, Burgos JA, Gelber R, Sakatani M. 2007. Evaluation of a novel vaccine (HVJ-liposome/HSP65 DNA+IL-12 DNA) against tuberculosis using the cynomolgus monkey model of TB. *Vaccine* 25:2990–2993.

44. Reed SG, Coler RN, Dalemans W, Tan EV, Dela Cruz EC, Basaraba RJ, Orme IM, Skeiky YA, Alderson MR, Cowgill KD, Prieels JP, Abalos RM, Dubois MC, Cohen J, Mettens P, Lobet Y. 2009. Defined tuberculosis vaccine, Mtb72F/AS02A, evidence of protection in cynomolgus monkeys. *Proc Natl Acad Sci USA* 106:2301–2306 (Erratum 106:7678).

45. Lin PL, Rodgers M, Smith L, Bigbee M, Myers A, Bigbee C, Chiosea I, Capuano SV, Fuhrman C, Klein E, Flynn JL. 2009. Quantitative comparison of active and latent tuberculosis in the cynomolgus macaque model. *Infect Immun* 77:4631–4642.

46. Lin PL, Myers A, Smith L, Bigbee C, Bigbee M, Fuhrman C, Grieser H, Chiosea I, Voitenek NN, Capuano SV, Klein E, Flynn JL. 2010. Tumor necrosis factor neutralization results in disseminated disease in acute and latent *Mycobacterium tuberculosis* infection with normal granuloma structure in a cynomolgus macaque model. *Arthritis Rheum* 62:340–350.

47. Green AM, Mattila JT, Bigbee CL, Bongers KS, Lin PL, Flynn JL. 2010. CD4(+) regulatory T cells in a cynomolgus macaque model of *Mycobacterium tuberculosis* infection. *J Infect Dis* 202:533–541.

48. Diedrich CR, Mattila JT, Klein E, Janssen C, Phuah J, Sturgeon TJ, Montelaro RC, Lin PL, Flynn JL. 2010. Reactivation of latent tuberculosis in cynomolgus macaques infected with SIV is associated with early peripheral T cell depletion and not virus load. *PLoS One* 5:e9611 (Erratum PLoS One 2015).

49. Mattila JT, Diedrich CR, Lin PL, Phuah J, Flynn JL. 2011. Simian immunodeficiency virus-induced changes in T cell cytokine responses in cynomolgus macaques with latent *Mycobacterium tuberculosis* infection are associated with timing of reactivation. *J Immunol* 186:3527–3537.

50. Lin PL, Dietrich J, Tan E, Abalos RM, Burgos J, Bigbee C, Bigbee M, Milk L, Gideon HP, Rodgers M, Cochran C, Guinn KM, Sherman DR, Klein E, Janssen C, Flynn JL, Andersen P. 2012. The multistage vaccine H56 boosts the effects of BCG to protect cynomolgus macaques against active tuberculosis and reactivation of latent *Mycobacterium tuberculosis* infection. *J Clin Invest* 122:303–314.

51. Phuah JY, Mattila JT, Lin PL, Flynn JL. 2012. Activated b cells in the granulomas of nonhuman primates infected with *Mycobacterium tuberculosis*. *Am J Pathol* 181:508–514.

52. Ragheb MN, Ford CB, Chase MR, Lin PL, Flynn JL, Fortune SM. 2013. The mutation rate of mycobacterial repetitive unit loci in strains of *M. tuberculosis* from cynomolgus macaque infection. *BMC Genomics* 14:145.

53. Chen CY, Yao SY, Huang D, Wei HY, Sicard H, Zeng GC, Jomaa H, Larsen MH, Jacobs WR, Wang R, Letvin N, Shen Y, Qiu LY, Shen L, Chen ZW. 2013. Phosphoantigen/IL2 expansion and differentiation of Vγ2Vδ2 T cells increase resistance to tuberculosis in non-human primates. *PLoS Pathog* 9:e1003501.

54. Lin PL, Coleman T, Carney JP, Lopresti BJ, Tomko J, Fillmore D, Dartois V, Scanga C, Frye LJ, Janssen C, Klein E, Barry CE III, Flynn JL. 2013. Radiologic responses in cynomolgous macaques for assessing tuberculosis chemotherapy regimens. *Antimicrob Agents Chemother* 57:4237–4244.

55. Lin PL, Ford CB, Coleman MT, Myers AJ, Gawande R, Ioerger T, Sacchettini J, Fortune SM, Flynn JL. 2014. Sterilization of granulomas is common in active and latent tuberculosis despite within-host variability in bacterial killing. *Nat Med* 20:75–79.

56. Roodgar M, Lackner A, Kaushal D, Sankaran S, Dandekar S, Trask JS, Drake C, Smith DG. 2013. Expression levels of 10 candidate genes in lung tissue of vaccinated and TB-infected cynomolgus macaques. *J Med Primatol* 42:161–164.

57. Dutta NK, McLachlan J, Mehra S, Kaushal D. 2014. Humoral and lung immune responses to *Mycobacterium tuberculosis* infection in a primate model of protection. *Trials Vaccinol* 3:47–51.

58. Marino S, Cilfone NA, Mattila JT, Linderman JJ, Flynn JL, Kirschner DE. 2015. Macrophage polarization drives granuloma outcome during *Mycobacterium tuberculosis* infection. *Infect Immun* 83:324–338.

59. Sharpe S, White A, Gleeson F, McIntyre A, Smyth D, Clark S, Sarfas C, Laddy D, Rayner E, Hall G, Williams A, Dennis M. 2016. Ultra low dose aerosol challenge with *Mycobacterium tuberculosis* leads to divergent outcomes in rhesus and cynomolgus macaques. *Tuberculosis (Edinb)* 96:1–12.

60. Sharpe SA, Eschelbach E, Basaraba RJ, Gleeson F, Hall GA, McIntyre A, Williams A, Kraft SL, Clark S, Gooch K, Hatch G, Orme IM, Marsh PD, Dennis MJ. 2009. Determination of lesion volume by MRI and stereology in a macaque model of tuberculosis. *Tuberculosis (Edinb)* 89:405–416.

61. Vervenne RA, Jones SL, van Soolingen D, van der Laan T, Andersen P, Heidt PJ, Thomas AW, Langermans JA. 2004. TB diagnosis in non-human primates: comparison of two interferon-gamma assays and the skin test for identification of Mycobacterium tuberculosis infection. *Vet Immunol Immunopathol* 100:61–71.

62. Kanaujia GV, Motzel S, Garcia MA, Andersen P, Gennaro ML. 2004. Recognition of ESAT-6 sequences by antibodies in sera of tuberculous nonhuman primates. *Clin Diagn Lab Immunol* 11:222–226.

63. Lyashchenko KP, Greenwald R, Esfandiari J, Greenwald D, Nacy CA, Gibson S, Didier PJ, Washington M, Szczerba P, Motzel S, Handt L, Pollock JM, McNair J, Andersen P, Langermans JA, Verreck F, Ervin S, Ervin F,

McCombs C. 2007. PrimaTB STAT-PAK assay, a novel, rapid lateral-flow test for tuberculosis in nonhuman primates. *Clin Vaccine Immunol* 14:1158–1164.

64. Khan IH, Ravindran R, Yee J, Ziman M, Lewinsohn DM, Gennaro ML, Flynn JL, Goulding CW, DeRiemer K, Lerche NW, Luciw PA. 2008. Profiling antibodies to *Mycobacterium tuberculosis* by multiplex microbead suspension arrays for serodiagnosis of tuberculosis. *Clin Vaccine Immunol* 15:433–438.

65. Rivera-Hernandez T, Carnathan DG, Moyle PM, Toth I, West NP, Young PR, Silvestri G, Walker MJ. 2014. The contribution of non-human primate models to the development of human vaccines. *Discov Med* 18: 313–322.

66. Huang D, Qiu L, Wang R, Lai X, Du G, Seghal P, Shen Y, Shao L, Halliday L, Fortman J, Shen L, Letvin NL, Chen ZW. 2007. Immune gene networks of mycobacterial vaccine-elicited cellular responses and immunity. *J Infect Dis* 195:55–69.

67. Philips JA, Ernst JD. 2012. Tuberculosis pathogenesis and immunity. *Annu Rev Pathol* 7:353–384.

68. Guo M, Ho WZ. 2014. Animal models to study *Mycobacterium tuberculosis* and HIV co-infection. *Dongwuxue Yanjiu* 35:163–169.

69. Shen Y, Shen L, Sehgal P, Zhou D, Simon M, Miller M, Enimi EA, Henckler B, Chalifoux L, Sehgal N, Gastron M, Letvin NL, Chen ZW. 2001. Antiretroviral agents restore *Mycobacterium*-specific T-cell immune responses and facilitate controlling a fatal tuberculosis-like disease in Macaques coinfected with simian immunodeficiency virus and *Mycobacterium bovis* BCG. *J Virol* 75: 8690–8696.

70. Shen Y, Zhou D, Chalifoux L, Shen L, Simon M, Zeng X, Lai X, Li Y, Sehgal P, Letvin NL, Chen ZW. 2002. Induction of an AIDS virus-related tuberculosis-like disease in macaques: a model of simian immunodeficiency virus- *Mycobacterium* coinfection. *Infect Immun* 70: 869–877.

71. Via LE, Weiner DM, Schimel D, Lin PL, Dayao E, Tankersley SL, Cai Y, Coleman MT, Tomko J, Paripati P, Orandle M, Kastenmayer RJ, Tartakovsky M, Rosenthal A, Portevin D, Eum SY, Lahouar S, Gagneux S, Young DB, Flynn JL, Barry CE III. 2013. Differential virulence and disease progression following *Mycobacterium tuberculosis* complex infection of the common marmoset (Callithrix jacchus). *Infect Immun* 81:2909–2919.

72. Lerche NW, Yee JL, Capuano SV, Flynn JL. 2008. New approaches to tuberculosis surveillance in nonhuman primates. *ILAR J* 49:170–178.

73. Foreman TW, Mehra S, Lackner AA, Kaushal D. 2017. Translational research in the nonhuman primate model of tuberculosis. *ILAR J* 1–9.

74. Sharpe SA, Eschelbach E, Basaraba RJ, Gleeson F, Hall GA, McIntyre , Williams A, Kraft SL, Clark S, Gooch K, Hatch G, Orme IM, Marsh PD, Dennis MJ. 2009. Determination of lesion volume by MRI and stereology in a macaque model of tuberculosis. *Tuberculosis* 89:405–416.

75. Sharpe S, White A, Sarfas C, Sibley L, Gleeson F, McIntyre A, Basaraba R, Clark S, Hall G, Rayner E, Williams A, Marsh PD, Dennis M. 2016. Alternative BCG delivery strategies improve protection against *Mycobacterium tuberculosis* in non-human primates: protection associated with mycobacterial antigen-specific CD4 effector memory T-cell populations. *Tuberculosis (Edinb)* 101:174–190.

76. Guo M, Xian QY, Rao Y, Zhang J, Wang Y, Huang ZX, Wang X, Bao R, Zhou L, Liu JB, Tang ZJ, Guo DY, Qin C, Li JL, Ho WZ. 2017. SIV infection facilitates *Mycobacterium tuberculosis* infection of rhesus macaques. *Front Microbiol* 7:2174.

77. Verreck FAW, Tchilian EZ, Vervenne RAW, Sombroek CC, Kondova I, Eissen OA, Sommandas V, van der Werff NM, Verschoor E, Braskamp G, Bakker J, Langermans JAM, Heidt PJ, Ottenhoff THM, van Kralingen KW, Thomas AW, Beverley PCL, Kocken CHM. 2017. Variable BCG efficacy in rhesus populations: pulmonary BCG provides protection where standard intra-dermal vaccination fails. *Tuberculosis (Edinb)* 104:46–57.

78. Billeskov R, Tan EV, Cang M, Abalos RM, Burgos J, Pedersen BV, Christensen D, Agger EM, Andersen P. 2016. Testing the H56 vaccine delivered in four different adjuvants as a BCG-booster in a non-human primate model of tuberculosis. *PLoS One* 11:e0161217.

79. Sharpe SA, White AD, Sibley L, Gleeson F, Hall GA, Basaraba RJ, McIntyre A, Clark SO, Gooch K, Marsh PD, Williams A, Dennis MJ. 2017. An aerosol challenge model of tuberculosis in Mauritian cynomolgus macaques. *PLoS One* 12:e0171906.

80. Mattila JT, Beaino W, Maiello P, Coleman MT, White AG, Scanga CA, Flynn JL, Anderson CJ. 2017. Positron emission tomography imaging of macaques with tuberculosis identifies temporal changes in granuloma glucose metabolism and integrin $\alpha 4\beta 1$-expressing immune cells. *J Immunol.*

Tuberculosis and the Tubercle Bacillus, 2nd ed.
Edited by William R. Jacobs, Jr., Helen McShane, Valerie Mizrahi, and Ian M. Orme
© 2018 American Society for Microbiology, Washington, DC
doi:10.1128/microbiolspec.TBTB2-0017-2016

Experimental Infection Models of Tuberculosis in Domestic Livestock

9

Bryce M. Buddle[1], H. Martin Vordermeier[2], and R. Glyn Hewinson[2]

INTRODUCTION

Tuberculosis (TB) affecting domestic livestock, including cattle, goats, and deer, is predominantly caused by *Mycobacterium bovis*. The disease in cattle, defined as bovine TB, is a major economic animal health problem worldwide, costing U.S. $3 billion annually, with >50 million cattle infected (1). Costs from this disease are related to a reduction in productivity in severely affected animals, testing, culling of affected animals, movement controls, and restriction on trade. Goats and farmed deer are also readily affected by TB, causing economic losses due to trade limitations, culling of affected animals, and depopulation of herds (2, 3). In addition, *M. bovis* affects feral deer, where it may establish a wildlife reservoir, for example, in white-tailed deer in the United States, often resulting in a source of infection to contiguous cattle herds (4). *M. bovis* has a wide host range affecting both domestic and wild animals, but infection of other livestock such as domestic pigs and sheep is relatively rare. *M. bovis* is also infectious to humans, and prior to mandatory pasteurization in many countries, *M. bovis* accounted for about one fourth of TB cases in children (5). Transmission of *M. bovis* to humans has been markedly reduced with the pasteurization of milk and the implementation of bovine TB control programs coupled with abattoir surveillance, although risks remain with the consumption of unpasteurized milk and cohabitation of infected animals with humans.

Experimental infection of cattle, goats, and deer with TB can serve as useful models of the disease in humans because they are outbred, natural hosts of the disease and can be influenced by genetic and environmental factors (6, 7). TB in these animals progresses slowly and is usually confined to the lower or upper respiratory tracts. The disease pathology also has similarities to that observed in humans, with the formation of caseous granulomas and a marked cellular immune response. The genomes of *M. bovis* and *Mycobacterium tuberculosis* are >99.95% identical, with the genome of *M. bovis* being smaller than that of *M. tuberculosis* due to deletion of genetic information (8). Host susceptibility and transmissibility vary between the two species, with a very broad host range for *M. bovis* compared to that for *M. tuberculosis*, and although humans can be infected with *M. bovis*, transmission between humans is rare (9).

The focus of this article is principally on experimental infection of cattle because this model has many features that make it appealing as a model for TB in humans (summarized in Table 1). In addition, studies of experimental infection of TB in goats and deer provide support for the findings from cattle and provide some additional insights into the protection against TB. Aspects from the experimental infection of these three animal species which are particularly relevant to research on human TB include the evaluation of TB vaccines and diagnostic tests as well as the identification of immune correlates of protection and disease.

EXPERIMENTAL INFECTION MODELS

Experimental Infection of Cattle

In the natural disease, tuberculous lesions in cattle are primarily found in the lungs and pulmonary lymph nodes (tracheobronchial and mediastinal) and to a lesser extent in the head and retropharyngeal lymph nodes (10, 11). This distribution of lesions indicates that infection is predominantly from aerosol. However,

[1]AgResearch, Hopkirk Research Institute, Palmerston North, New Zealand; [2]Animal and Plant Health Agency – Weybridge, Addlestone, Surrey, United Kingdom.

Table 1 Use of cattle as a model of TB in humans

Cattle are natural hosts of TB, with infection acquired predominantly via aerosol.
The disease is chronic, taking years to develop and is manifested as caseous, mineralized granulomas with the production of strong cellular immune responses.
A large array of immunological reagents are available to identify possible immune correlates for protection and disease.
The kinetics of the immune responses can be readily followed through the frequent collection of relatively large quantities of blood.
Neonatal vaccination can be undertaken because calves are immunocompetent at birth.
BCG vaccination does not produce complete protection, providing an opportunity to identify vaccines which are better than BCG.
Protection induced by BCG vaccine wanes with time, between 1 and 2 years, providing prospects for revaccination.
Candidate vaccines can be tested in animals subjected to different nutritional or environmental conditions or coinfected with parasitic or viral infections.
Verification of the infection status of the animals can be accurately assessed by slaughter of the animals, which is particularly important for estimating the accuracy of diagnostic tests and reagents as well as the effectiveness of vaccines.
Antigen mining: T cell repertoires between cattle and humans show a high degree of overlap.
Natural transmission and experimental challenge models are available.

oral infection of calves from drinking infected milk can result in mesenteric lymph node lesions. The lesions are typically chronic, caseonecrotic granulomas which are characterized by mantles of lymphocytes, macrophages, and giant cells, often with a mineralized core, with fibrous encapsulation of the granuloma. The lesions contain small numbers of acid-fast bacilli. In contrast to human infections, latency is not considered a common characteristic, and cavitation of lesions is rarely observed. Experimental challenge of cattle with relatively low doses of *M. bovis* (10^2 to 10^3 colony forming units [CFU]) via intratracheal/endobronchial inoculation (12) or by aerosol-generating systems (13, 14) has been shown to mimic the typical lesions observed in the lungs and associated lymph nodes. The severity of the lesions is dose and time dependent (13, 15). These routes of infection have been used for the evaluation of TB vaccines and to assess immunological responses because they allow a presentation of the disease found naturally in the lungs and associated lymph nodes and a more reproducible scoring of pathology. Other routes of infection have included intranasal, with lesions more commonly found in the upper respiratory tract (16), while the intratonsilar route has most commonly produced lesions in the tonsils and retropharnygeal lymph nodes (17).

Protection against *M. bovis* infection is measured by determining the proportion of animals with gross lesions, gross and microscopic lesion scores, and bacterial load in lungs and associated lymph nodes. The infection challenge is more severe than natural exposure to *M. bovis* because the challenge must establish infection in the majority of nonvaccinated cattle to demonstrate statistical differences between vaccinated and nonvaccinated groups, particularly because group sizes must be kept relatively small due to the cost of keeping

animals in high-containment facilities. With this relatively severe challenge system, it is critical to use lesion scores to assess protection rather than the presence of absence of infection, and lesion scores are based on the number and size of the resulting gross lesions (18, 19) as well as a classification of the types of granulomas present in the lesions (20). Radiography has also been used to determine the percentage of lungs containing lesions (21). Mycobacterial counts are usually undertaken by homogenizing samples from pulmonary lymph nodes and expressing counts as per gram of lymph node (18).

A more natural challenge system has been established by housing vaccinated and nonvaccinated cattle with naturally infected cattle (a so-called natural transmission model of infection). This approach to assessing vaccine efficacy was feasible in settings that resulted in high transmission rates such as in Ethiopia and Mexico (22, 23), while it was ineffective in the United Kingdom, where a low rate of transmission was encountered (24). The final assessment of vaccine efficacy must be established in field trials, but these can be expensive when the prevalence of infection is low in herds.

Experimental Infection of Goats

TB infection of goats is caused by *M. bovis* or *Mycobacterium caprae*, and in the natural disease, lesions are predominantly found in the lungs and associated lymph nodes, indicating an aerosol route of infection (25). Goats have some advantages as a model for TB in humans due to easier handling and lower maintenance costs compared to cattle, and the TB lesions are similar to those seen in humans (26). In addition, the availability of diagnostic tests and reagents such as the skin tests and interferon gamma (IFN-γ) assay allows the assessment of immune responses. Recently, it was shown that infection of goats with a low dose of *M. caprae*

(10^3 CFU) via the endobronchial route produced lesions in all infected animals at 14 weeks after infection, showing pathology reflecting the natural disease of caseous necrotic and cavitary lesions in the lungs (27). In contrast, aerosol infection of goats with a similar dose of *M. bovis* produced small pulmonary lesions (28). This difference in pathology may have arisen from differences in routes of infection, because in a subsequent study where groups of goats were challenged transthoracically with either *M. bovis* or *M. caprae*, the total lesion scores and culture results were higher for the *M. bovis*-challenged goats (29). To determine the protective efficacy of vaccines, gross and microscopic lesions have been assessed by qualitative and quantitative analyses, together with mycobacterial culture from lung-associated lymph nodes. The precise determination of the total lung lesion burden related to total lung volume has been achieved using multidetector computed tomography (27).

Experimental Infection of Deer

Tuberculous lesions in wild or farmed deer are predominantly caused by *M. bovis*, but the pathology may be different from that seen in other domestic animals. Commonly, tuberculous lesions are described as liquefied or abscess-like, in contrast to the caseous nature of the lesions seen in cattle and goats (30, 31). In addition to the liquefactive nature of the lesions, they may also be caseous with dystrophic mineralization. The distribution of the tuberculous lesions also differs from those in cattle, with the retropharyngeal lymph nodes being the most common site for lesions in deer, followed by lesions in the lungs and associated lymph nodes. The primary lesion complex in deer appears to be tonsils and retropharyngeal lymph nodes, suggesting an oral or aerosol route of infection. To reproduce the typical pathology seen in naturally infected deer, low doses of *M. bovis* (10^2 CFU) have been instilled into the tonsilar crypts, with lesions developing in the tonsils and retropharyngeal lymph nodes (32, 33).

DEVELOPMENT AND EVALUATION OF TB VACCINES

M. bovis Bacille Calmette-Guérin (BCG) Vaccine

BCG, a live attenuated strain of *M. bovis*, was first reported by Calmette and Guérin in 1911 to induce protection in cattle against experimental challenge with *M. bovis*. A number of trials were undertaken in the first half of the 20th century, and although experimental challenge trials provided encouraging results, more variable results were reported in field trials (reviewed in reference 1). Informative meta-analysis of these trials has been difficult because a number of different BCG strains, doses, and vaccination routes were used, together with different methods to measure protection and varying levels of exposure to *M. bovis*. Over the past 20 years a large number of vaccination/challenge trials have been undertaken in cattle using harmonized models, testing BCG alone, or in comparative studies with other vaccines. Similar BCG strains have been used (initially Pasteur, then BCG Danish SSI) and standardized vaccination/challenge models have been applied. The results have been confirmed in a number of studies and include the following. Doses of 10^4 to 10^6 CFU of BCG administered parenterally induced equivalent protection (12, 34), while higher doses (10^8CFU) were required to induce protection when BCG was administered orally (35). Combinations of administration of BCG by parenteral and mucosal routes have provided mixed results, with a small enhancement of protection observed when BCG was administered subcutaneously and endobronchially on the same day (36), but not with the combination of subcutaneously and orally administered BCG (37). Pasteur and Danish strains of BCG induced similar protection, although the kinetics of the cellular immune response varied with the two strains (38, 39). Neonatal or very young calves were protected at least as well as older calves (40, 41). Protection against experimental challenge was shown to be effective at ≤12 months postvaccination but waned by 24 months postvaccination (42).

Two studies were undertaken to determine the effect of revaccination with BCG. In the first study, calves vaccinated within 8 hours of birth or at 6 weeks of age showed a high level of protection against *M. bovis*, while those vaccinated within 8 hours of birth and revaccinated at 6 weeks of age had a reduced level of protection (40). The revaccinated calves with the lowest level of protection had the strongest antigen-specific IFN-γ and lymphocyte proliferative responses, indicating that revaccination had induced an inappropriate immune response. In neonatal calves, antigen-specific IFN-γ responses remained at elevated levels for longer than those seen in older calves, possibly due to a more active BCG infection, and BCG revaccination when immune responses are at high levels may be contraindicated. In contrast, calves vaccinated with BCG at 2 to 4 weeks of age and revaccinated at 2 years of age, when immunity had waned, showed a significant level of protection when challenged 6 months later, while those receiving only the initial vaccine dose were not protected (43).

Trials in Ethiopia and Mexico which were undertaken in field conditions with exposure of vaccinated and non-vaccinated calves to in-contact, tuberculin-reactor cows both demonstrated a significant level of protection in the vaccinated calves (22, 23). In a large-scale field trial in New Zealand, cattle vaccinated orally with BCG and exposed to tuberculin reactor cattle and a wildlife reservoir of infection had a significant level of protection compared to nonvaccinated cattle, with an estimated vaccine efficacy of 60 to 70% (G. Nugent, personal communication).

A single dose of BCG vaccine administered subcutaneously to goats was shown to significantly induce protection against challenge with *M. caprae* (44, 45). In the first study, significant reductions were observed in pulmonary lymph node pathology and in the bacterial load for the BCG-vaccinated goats (44), and in the second study, the BCG-vaccinated animals had significant reductions in the gross lung and lymph node pathology as well as in the bacterial load compared to the non-vaccinated controls (45).

BCG vaccination studies of deer have been undertaken to assess whether vaccination could be an effective method of protecting farmed deer from TB and to develop a system for vaccinating feral deer to prevent reinfection back into cattle herds. A single dose of BCG administered subcutaneously to 3-month-old deer was shown to protect against disease severity, while re-vaccinating deer at intervals of 8 to 16 weeks induced protection against infection, but revaccination at an interval of 43 weeks did not (46). Parenteral BCG administered to deer at a dose of 10^6 CFU and oral BCG at 10^8 CFU induced a similar degree of protection (47). Evidence has been provided of transmission of BCG by shedding of BCG from parenterally vaccinated deer to in-contact, nonvaccinated deer (48–50). It is not known whether these nonvaccinated deer would be protected against TB. BCG was shown to persist for 3 to 9 months in lymphoid tissues of deer vaccinated parenterally or orally (49).

New-Generation TB Vaccines

In the past 2 decades, there has been a mutually beneficial collaboration between human and animal TB vaccine development, and many of the vaccine strategies being tested in humans have also been tested in cattle and, more recently, in goats. The different types of TB vaccines which have recently been tested in cattle include live attenuated mycobacteria, which could replace BCG, and subunit TB vaccines such as DNA, protein, and virus-vectored vaccines, which could be used to boost immunity induced by BCG (summarized

in Table 2). Two virus-vectored TB vaccines have recently been tested in goats, while the testing of new-generation TB vaccines in deer has yet to be reported.

Published reports evaluating live attenuated mycobacterial vaccines in cattle include modified BCG strains, an *M. bovis* auxotroph, and deletion mutants of *M. tuberculosis* and *M. bovis*. A BCG strain has been developed which overexpressed Ag85B, and cattle vaccinated with this strain had significantly lower histopathological lesion scores in the lungs following challenge with *M. bovis* than those vaccinated with the parent BCG strain (51). Another modification of BCG is the deletion of the *zmp1* gene, based on the concept that the mycobacterial Zmp1 inhibited phagolysosome maturation by preventing inflamasome activation and efficient presentation of mycobacterial antigens by MHC class I and II antigens. Vaccination of cattle with either of two BCG *zmp1* deletion strains resulted in superior T cell memory responses compared to vaccination with a wild-type BCG strain (52). Recent experiments to assess its protective efficacy have demonstrated a trend toward better protection against lesions in the thoracic lymph nodes (B. Khatri, unpublished data). Interestingly, another vaccine developed for humans that has shown promise in small animal models and in safety studies in humans, a recombinant BCG in which the urease genes were deleted and the listeriolysin gene added (BCG Δure::hly) (53, 54), did not protect calves against *M. bovis* infection (G. Dean, B. Villarreal-Ramos, H. M. Vordermeier, unpublished data). However, it is possible that a suboptimal dose of this vaccine was used. Vaccination with a cocktail of four BCG Danish mutants (BCG ΔleuCD, BCG Δfdr8, BCG ΔmmA4, BCG Δpks16) induced significant protection in cattle against *M. bovis* challenge to a level comparable with wild-type BCG Danish (55).

Vaccination with either of two attenuated *M. bovis* strains derived by UV irradiation, with deletions not defined, produced significant protection against challenge with *M. bovis* in calves naturally presensitized to environmental mycobacteria in a study in which BCG vaccine was shown to be ineffective (56). Vaccination with a leucine auxotroph of *M. bovis* was shown to significantly reduce the bacterial burden and histopathology in calves following challenge with virulent *M. bovis* compared to nonvaccinated controls (57). A comparison with BCG was not undertaken in this study. A double deletion mutant of *M. tuberculosis*, a region of difference 1 (RD1) knockout and pantothenate auxotroph, failed to protect calves from an aerosolized *M. bovis* challenge (21), while vaccination with an RD1 deletion mutant of *M. bovis* provided protection

Table 2 Types of new TB vaccines tested in cattle

Type of vaccine	Vaccine	Protection against TB compared to BCG[a]	Reference(s)
Modified BCG	BCG overexpressing Ag85B	+	51
	BCG Δzmp1	+[b]	52; B. Khatri unpublished data
	BCG Δure::listeriolysin	–	53, 54; G. Dean, B. Villarreal-Ramos, and H. M. Vordermeier, unpublished data
	BCG mutants (BCG ΔleuCD, BCG Δfdr8, BCGΔmmA4, BCGΔpks16)	=	55
Attenuated M. tuberculosis strain	M. tuberculosis ΔRD1 ΔpanCD	–	21
Attenuated M. bovis strain	UV-irradiated M. bovis	+	56
	M. bovis ΔleuD	NT	57
	M. bovis ΔRD1	=	58
	M. bovis Δmce2	+	59
DNA vaccine	Mycobacterial DNA	=	60,61
	Mycobacterial DNA + BCG	+	62–64
Adjuvanted protein vaccine	Protein + BCG	+	65, 66
Virus-vectored vaccine	Heterologous prime-boost: BCG + Ad85A	+	67, 68
	Simultaneous systemic BCG and mucosal delivery of Ad85A	+	36

[a]NT, significant protection against TB, but not tested against BCG; +, better than BCG; =, equivalent protection to BCG; –, no protection against TB.
[b]Improved protection against lymph node pathology compared to wild-type BCG.

comparable to BCG (58). For cattle, an attenuated *M. tuberculosis* mutant may be less immunogenic compared to those produced on an *M. bovis* or BCG background strain because cattle are not a natural host for *M. tuberculosis*. An attenuated *M. bovis* strain with a double deletion in the *mce2* gene was shown to induce significant protection against an *M. bovis* challenge and induced significantly lower histopathological scores for the lungs and pulmonary lymph nodes compared to that for BCG (59).

No subunit TB vaccine has been able to induce better protection in cattle than that induced by BCG, although they can produce a synergistic effect when used in combination with BCG. DNA vaccines have induced minimal protection against TB when used alone, although some protection has been observed when mycobacterial DNA was combined with DNA encoding costimulatory molecules CD80 and CD86 (60) or combined with an adjuvant (61). More encouraging results have been reported when DNA vaccines were used in heterologous prime-boost regimens with BCG, and priming or boosting with mycobacterial DNA vaccines induced greater protection than did BCG vaccine alone (62–64). Similarly, TB protein vaccines induced little protection in cattle when used alone, whereas when coadministered at adjacent sites with BCG they induced protection that was better than that observed with BCG alone (65, 66). The major problem encoun-

tered using TB protein vaccines in cattle has been the difficulty of inducing strong cellular immune responses with these vaccines, despite coadministration with a range of adjuvants and immunomodulators.

In contrast, the use of virally vectored vaccines to induce strong cellular immune responses has shown considerable promise when applied in heterologous prime-boost approaches in which the bovine immune response is primed with BCG and then boosted with virally vectored vaccines developed for use as human TB vaccines. Thus, priming with BCG Danish and boosting with a replication-deficient human adenovirus 5 expressing Ag85A (Ad85A) resulted in protection superior to that with BCG alone (67). In a recent study, BCG-vaccinated calves were boosted with either Ad5 expressing Ag85A (Ad5-85A) or Ag85A, Rv0287, Rv0288, and Rv0251 (Ad5-TBF), but only those boosted with Ad5-85A induced a significantly lower histopathological lesion score than that for those vaccinated with BCG alone (68). From an immunogenicity study, the optimal dose and route of immunization of the Ad5-85A used as a boost following a BCG prime was determined to be 2×10^9 infectious units delivered intradermally (69).

It has also been shown that Ad85A boosting of BCG delivered through mucosal (endobronchial) or systemic (intradermal) routes induced comparable peripheral blood responses and that both routes induced bronchoalveolar lavage cells that produced antigen-specific IFN-γ (70). These studies also demonstrated that, regardless of the route of boosting, the kinetics of peripheral blood and bronchoalveolar lavage cell responses differed, with systemic responses being detectable earlier than mucosal responses. Interestingly, when BCG-vaccinated humans were boosted via the aerosol or systemic routes with a modified vaccinia Ankara (MVA) vectored vaccine expressing Ag85A, observations comparable to those described above for cows using Ad85A were reported (71). Namely, specific systemic responses were similar across groups and specific CD4+ T cells were detected in bronchoalveolar lavage cells from both groups, although these mucosal responses were higher in the aerosol-vaccinated than in the intradermally vaccinated group.

Because of the encouraging data suggesting that mucosal delivery of Ad85A boosted T cell responses (70), Ad85A and BCG were also used in a simultaneous vaccination protocol of vaccinating calves at the same time with BCG via the systemic route and with Ad85A via mucosal (endobronchial) application. This vaccination protocol resulted in a trend toward better protective efficacy than vaccination with BCG alone (36).

The testing in goats of a heterologous prime/boost with BCG followed by virus vectored vaccines, Ad5-Ag85A, or Ad5-TBF has provided encouraging results with significant protection against endobronchial *M. caprae* challenge compared to those receiving BCG vaccine alone or the nonvaccinates (44, 45). Confirmation of results using a BCG prime-viral vector boost vaccination strategy to protect against experimental challenge with TB in two domestic livestock species provides additional support for the evaluation of such a vaccination strategy in humans.

IMMUNE CORRELATES OF PROTECTION AND DISEASE

Biomarkers Predicting or Correlating with Vaccine Efficacy

One of the advantages of the bovine model compared to similar studies in humans for identifying host biomarkers that are associated with either vaccine-induced protection or TB-induced disease is that one can perform experimental vaccination and challenge studies of tuberculous infection in a target species using the natural host and its natural pathogen. Thereby, one can immediately relate host responses to relevant clinical endpoints of protection, for example, by assessing the visible pathology or microscopic histopathology estab-

lished following infection. Further, as is the case for humans, the outcome of vaccinating cattle with BCG can be 3-fold: vaccinated animals are either not protected, partially protected (defined as presenting significant reductions in pathology), or present at postmortem without visible or histological signs of disease (e.g., 18, 67, 68). Comparing animals from the same experimental treatment group that were not protected from infection with those that were protected is more informative for biomarker discovery than comparing groups that were vaccinated with different vaccines, as is often done (67).

Applying hypothesis- and data-driven approaches to biomarker discovery has led to the identification of a number of biomarkers in cattle that either correlate with disease status and are generally inversely correlated with vaccine efficacy or predict vaccine efficacy after vaccination but before *M. bovis* challenge (see Table 3 for examples of biomarkers predicting vaccine efficacy). In the next section, we will discuss some of the markers in detail. Parameters that should be considered for a surrogate description of vaccine efficacy against an intracellular pathogen such as *M. bovis* or *M. tuberculosis* that largely depends on T cell-mediated protection include the induction of memory responses, the quality of the T cell responses in relation to the cytokine profiles induced, and response magnitudes, as well as T cell avidity and the breadth of epitopes recognized postvaccination (Table 3).

T cell memory

A promising predictor of vaccine efficacy is based on T cell memory responses measured by the cultured enzyme-linked immunospot (ELISPOT) method (69, 72). These responses were significantly elevated in vaccinated/protected animals compared to matched vaccinated calves that were not protected (58, 67). Furthermore, maintenance of strong cultured ELISPOT responses is associated with the duration of immunity post-BCG vaccination (42). The T cell subset involved in the cultured ELISPOT responses is almost exclusively CD4+, and in particular, is of the CD45RO+ CD62L^high "central memory"-like phenotype (73). In contrast, cells of an effector/effector memory T cell-like phenotype (CD45RO+ CD62L^lo) are the main contributors to *ex vivo* ELISPOT responses that do not necessarily predict vaccine protection. Furthermore, it has been demonstrated that cultured ELISPOT responses can be measured in unvaccinated, infected cattle and ~75% of CD4+ IFN-γ+ cells in long-term cultures expressed a Tcm phenotype (CD45RO+ CD62L^high CCR7+) (74).

Table 3 Potential correlates of protection defined in cattle

Criteria	Example	References
T cell memory	Central memory-like cells (cultured ELISPOT) correlate with protection and duration of immunity	42, 58, 67, 72–74
Quality of T cell responses: cytokine production	IL-17A, IL-22	51, 55, 67, 77
Quality of T cell responses: polyfunctionality	Correlates with vaccine take and disease progression but not predicting protection	68, 81
Magnitude of boost in heterologous-prime boost approaches[a]	Postboost CD4+ T cell frequencies correlate with protection	H. J. Metcalfe, B. Villarreal-Ramos, and H. M. Vordermeier, unpublished data
T cell avidity following heterologous boost approaches[a]	Avidity does not increase postboost = prevention of exhaustion?	H. J. Metcalfe, B. Villarreal-Ramos, and H. M. Vordermeier, unpublished data
Epitope widening following heterologous prime boost[b]	No definitive answer: BCG/MVA85A: epitope spread BCG/Ad85A: no significant epitope spread	85; H. J. Metcalfe, B. Villarreal-Ramos, and H. M. Vordermeier, unpublished data

[a]Based on experiments employing heterologous prime-boost approaches based on BCG prime/recombinant human adenovirus type 5 expressing Ag85A (Ad85A).
[b]Heterologous prime-boost approaches used were based on either BCG boosted with modified vaccinia virus Ankara expressing Ag85A (MVA85A) or BCG with Ad85A.

Quality of the T cell responses

The induction of IFN-γ production after vaccination is not necessarily a predictor of vaccine efficacy. Therefore, T cell subsets producing alternative or additional cytokines have been evaluated. For example, interleukin 17A (IL-17A) expression was found to correlate with protection (67). This finding has been confirmed in recent studies of cattle (51, 55). The role of IL-17A-producing cells in TB has also been highlighted previously in mouse models of human TB. These studies showed that in vaccinated animals the absence of IL-17-producing memory cells resulted in the loss of Th1 responses and protection (75, 76). These results indicated that mixed responses of Th1 and IL-17-producing cells (such as TH17, γδ T cells, or NK cells) seem to cross-regulate themselves and are both important for protective antituberculous responses.

Whole-genome transcriptome analysis of responses of BCG-vaccinated or BCG-primed and adenovirus-vectored vaccine-boosted cattle measured by deep sequencing (RNASeq) has identified IL-22 as a dominant predictor of vaccine success in cattle (77). These results have recently been confirmed by the Waters group as well as by ourselves (55; P. J. Golby, B. Villarreal-Ramos, and H. M. Vordermeier, unpublished data). The role of IL-22 in protective responses is not defined, although one potential effector mechanism could be the production of beta-defensins.

Interestingly, associations between protection and the numbers of such polyfunctional T cells induced post-vaccination have been described mainly in small animal models (e.g., 78–80). However, in cattle polyfunctionality, as defined by the presence of CD4+ T cells pro-

ducing IFN-γ, IL-2, and tumor necrosis factor-α or a combination of at least two of these markers, does not predict vaccine success when measured before challenge but is associated strongly with increased pathology post-*M. bovis* challenge (67, 81).

Magnitude of boosting effect, T cell avidity, and epitope spreading associated with protection induced by heterologous prime-boost schedules of BCG and virally vectored vaccines

These criteria need to be considered when determining whether they can serve as predictive host parameters of vaccine efficacy because they have been implicated in other disease and vaccine systems. In a recent study (H. J. Metcalfe, B. Villarreal-Ramos, and H. M. Vordermeier, unpublished data), we addressed these three parameters using cells from BCG-vaccinated and BCG/adenovirus-vectored vaccine expressing Ag85A (Ad85A) heterologous prime-boost vaccination experiments. Employing an unbiased T cell library approach (82), we found that the increase in the frequencies of Ag85A-specific CD4+ T cells post-Ad85A boost positively correlated with protection. Interestingly, we found no increase in T cell receptor avidity following boosting. Lower, or at least not increased, Ag85A-specific T cell receptor avidity might be advantageous during *M. bovis* infection because these cells may have enhanced functional persistence during recall (83). In situations of antigen persistence (e.g., tumor-associated antigen), it was found that memory CD4+ T cells with low functional avidity are more effective immune cells than those with high functional avidity (84). In this study, we also found little evidence of epitope repertoire widening (i.e., that additional epitopes were recognized after the viral boost). This finding is in contrast to an earlier study (85) in which considerable epitope spread was observed after boosting BCG with recombinant modified vaccinia Ankara expressing Ag95A (modified vaccinia Ankara 85A). However, in that study we did not evaluate protection, and it is therefore not clear whether this epitope repertoire widening was associated with protection.

Biomarkers Correlating with Disease Severity

Host biomarkers can also correlate with host pathology and thus indirectly with vaccine efficacy. The "prototype" read-out parameter of this nature is the *ex vivo* early secretory antigenic target 6 (ESAT-6)-induced production of IFN-γ, which directly correlated with the extent of pathology observed following experimental *M. bovis* infection of cattle. In addition, these responses were lower in BCG-vaccinated calves that presented either without visible pathology or with significantly reduced gross pathology (18).

Another biomarker that falls in the category of a marker of pathology that could be exploited as a diagnostic read-out parameter resulted from studying micro-RNAs. Micro-RNAs are important regulators of gene expression and are known to play a key role in regulating both adaptive and innate immunity. The expression of micro-RNA 155 following *in vitro* stimulation of peripheral blood mononuclear cells with purified protein derivative (PPD) was associated with the degree of pathology observed in *M. bovis*-infected animals (86). The application of systems biology suggested that this micro-RNA regulates the expression of genes that result in stronger immune-pathology. Interestingly, micro-RNA 155 has also been described to be upregulated in human patients with active disease (87).

Markers such as IL-22 and IL-17A were also associated with disease severity (88). This highlights the difficulties of using such biomarkers in field studies of vaccine efficacy because these markers have also been described as promising predictors of vaccine efficacy in experimental cattle studies following vaccination with BCG or with heterologous prime-boost vaccination approaches (see previous section). Additional biomarkers that were upregulated in infected cattle compared to noninfected animals were chemokines such as IP-10 (CXCL10) (88). IP-10 is a diagnostic read-out system that has been described in human studies to complement or substitute IFN-γ-based tests using ELISA assays (reviewed in 89).

To conclude the biomarker section, significant progress has been made to define biomarkers that predict vaccine efficacy or pathology which may serve as accelerators for vaccine development or as additional blood-based test read-outs of infection. However, these markers need to be validated not only in additional experimental vaccination and challenge experiments but also in field trials. This is of particular relevance to markers such as IL-17A and IL-22 that predict both vaccine efficacy and disease progression; the timing of the expression of such markers may be the key to explaining this apparent paradox. This section has also highlighted that there is a significant overlap in the biomarkers defined for human and bovine TB, making the bovine system an attractive model for biomarker discovery and validation for humans in a one health approach. Indeed, the first whole-blood IFN-γ test was developed for the detection of *M. bovis* infection in cattle.

ANTIGEN MINING AND DIVA TESTS

The mainstay of bovine tuberculosis control is the application of tuberculin skin testing and the removal of test-positive animals as part of so-called test and slaughter control policies. However, as is the case for BCG vaccination of humans, BCG vaccination of animals compromises the use of tuberculin-based assays such as skin testing or blood-based IFN-γ release assays due to the antigens shared between BCG and *M. tuberculosis* or *M. bovis* (12, 90–92). Thus, the development of so-called DIVA (differentiating infected from vaccinated animals) tests will be required for countries which intend to use vaccination of cattle alongside conventional test and slaughter control strategies. Development of DIVA tests for human TB is also an integral part of the development of improved human TB vaccines.

The first task of DIVA test development is the identification (mining) of strong and specific antigens recognized by T cells from infected animals but not from those of vaccinated individuals. The elucidation of the genomes for relevant mycobacterial species (including *M. bovis* [93], *M. tuberculosis* [94], *M. bovis* BCG [95], *Mycobacterium avium* subsp. *avium*, and *M. avium* subsp. *paratuberculosis* [96]) and the advent of microarray technology has revolutionized antigen-mining strategies. Before we discuss specific approaches applied to the mining for DIVA antigens, it should be noted that the antigen repertoires recognized by bovine and human T cells following infection with *M. bovis* or *M. tuberculosis* show a remarkable degree of hierarchical overlap (97–102) so that antigens such as ESAT-6 that were identified first in the context of human TB are now also the mainstay of DIVA tests for bovine TB (103–105), and conversely antigens such as Rv3615c, defined first in the bovine system, are also applicable to human TB diagnosis not limited in its use by BCG vaccination (106, 107).

Comparative Genomic Analysis
Comparative genomic analysis has been used to identify *M. bovis* genes that are deleted in BCG (either as individual gene deletions or present in deleted gene regions) or that contain mutations resulting in either truncations or modified amino acid sequences after frame-shifting. Two of the major antigenic targets identified in cattle and humans are the RD1 region encoded antigens ESAT-6 and CFP-10 (103, 104, 108–110). Both ESAT-6 and CFP-10 have the capacity to differentiate *M. tuberculosis* infected from BCG-vaccinated humans or *M. bovis*-infected cattle from BCG-vaccinated animals (91, 92, 104).

Although it demonstrates high specificity in BCG vaccinates, the sensitivity of the ESAT-6/CFP-10 peptide cocktail in identifying infected cattle is below that of tuberculin, thus necessitating the need to identify additional antigens to increase overall test sensitivity. The DIVA potential of other gene products encoded in the RD1 region and two other regions (RD2 and RD14) deleted in BCG (93, 95) has also been assessed (111, 112), but none of the antigens identified in this study complemented ESAT-6 and CFP-10 in increasing overall test sensitivity in cattle. Thus, alternative approaches to comparative genomic analysis were needed to identify potential DIVA antigens to complement ESAT-6/CFP-10 and increase overall test sensitivity.

Comparative Transcriptome Analysis
This approach has been used to explore the link between gene expression level and antigenicity. *M. tuberculosis* and *M. bovis* gene products that were consistently expressed at high levels under a variety of culture conditions (known as the abundant invariome) (106) were prioritized and tested in cattle. These studies identified one antigen, Rv3615c, which was recognized by a significant proportion of infected animals but not in BCG vaccinates (113). Furthermore, Rv3615c responses were detected in a proportion of cattle not detected by ESAT-6/CFP-10; i.e., Rv3615c complemented ESAT-6/CFP-10 to increase overall test sensitivity (113). Later studies conducted in humans confirmed that Rv3615c could also be used as a DIVA diagnostic reagent in humans (107). Although the Rv3615c gene

is present in the genome of BCG, secretion of its gene product is dependent on the esx1 secretion system (107), which is encoded on the RD1 region. Because BCG lacks this region, Rv3615c cannot be secreted by BCG, which explains why it was not immunogenic in vaccinated animals.

Bacterial Cell Biology
In tuberculosis research, it has long been held that secretion of antigenic proteins by mycobacteria induces strong cellular immune responses in the host. To identify potential DIVA reagents, 119 *M. bovis* proteins predicted to be secreted were screened in infected cattle and BCG vaccinates (114, 115). These studies confirmed the immunodominance of members of the ESAT-6 protein family in cattle (114). This immunodominance of members of the ESAT-6 protein family has also been highlighted in human TB in a genome-wide, unbiased evaluation of the human T cell repertoire to latent TB (116). The screen in cattle initially identified Rv3020c as showing DIVA potential (115). However, subsequent evaluation of this protein in a larger cohort of infected animals failed to demonstrate complementation of the ESAT-6/CFP-10 and Rv3615c reagents (P. J. Jones and H. M. Vordermeier, unpublished data).

DIVA Skin Test Development
The above paragraphs discussed antigens in the context of IFN-γ release assay blood testing. However, these antigens were also evaluated for their use in skin testing. Skin test application has a number of advantages compared to blood testing, not least that the costs of skin testing are likely to be significantly lower than those for blood tests. Providing proof of concept for this approach, it has been shown that a combination of ESAT-6, CFP-10, and Rv3615c was effective in detecting *M. bovis*-infected animals while testing negative in uninfected or BCG-vaccinated cattle (117). Recent studies with these three antigens have confirmed their extremely high specificity in unvaccinated or BCG-vaccinated animals (>99.9%) with a sensitivity comparable to the comparative tuberculin test that compares skin test reponses after injection of tuberculin PPD from *M. bovis* and *M. avium* subsp. *avium* (P. J. Jones and H. M. Vordermeier, unpublished data). The costs of these reagents have the potential to be reduced when the proteins are displayed on nanoparticles such as polyester beads produced by bacteria, which enhances their immunogenicity, reducing the concentration of the proteins required to be tested (118). ESAT-6 and CFP-10 are also under development as human skin test reagents (119).

The remarkable overlap between bovine and human antigen repertoires following tuberculous infection has resulted in a large degree of cross-fertilization between the two fields, with the main antigens used for DIVA testing being identical in these two diseases. As far as bovine TB in cattle is concerned, these antigens, and in particular, their application as skin test antigens, need to be validated in larger field trials involving BCG-vaccinated animals. Moreover, it has not escaped our notice that these antigens have the potential to be used as defined skin test antigens in the absence of BCG vaccination, thereby overcoming the major limitations associated with the production and potency testing of human and bovine tuberculin PPDs.

CONCLUSIONS

Experimental models of *M. bovis* infection in domestic livestock are attractive for assessing the efficacy of human TB vaccines because these animals are natural hosts for TB and are influenced by genetic and environmental factors and because the disease in these animals has many pathological features similar to the disease in humans. Both experimental challenge and natural transmission models for *M. bovis* infection in cattle have been developed. Confidence in the effectiveness of TB vaccines can be obtained from testing vaccines in a variety of animal species, and this is particularly important when considering the cost and length of time required for field testing of TB vaccines in humans. Significant progress has been made to define biomarkers in domestic livestock that predict vaccine efficacy or pathology biomarkers to serve as accelerators for vaccine development or as additional blood-based test read-outs of infection. Yet these markers need to be validated not only in additional experimental vaccination and challenge experiments, but also in field trials. There is a significant overlap in markers defined for human and bovine TB, making the bovine system also an attractive model for biomarker discovery and validation for humans in a one health approach. The remarkable overlap between bovine and human antigen repertoires following tuberculous infection has resulted in a large degree of cross-fertilization in the discovery of DIVA antigens. One should also not underestimate the potential of these antigens to be used as defined skin test antigens in the absence of BCG vaccination, thereby overcoming the major limitations associated with the production and potency testing of human and bovine tuberculin PPD.

Overall, the close collaboration and alignment between researchers engaged in human and bovine TB research, and vaccine research in particular, has been highly successful and is benefiting both fields. This one health philosophy should be further cemented by ever closer collaboration and use of the bovine model to address questions specific for human TB.

Acknowledgments. We would like to express our thanks for the generous support obtained from the AgResearch (New Zealand) and the Department for Environment, Food, and Rural Affairs (UK) and to extend our gratitude to all those with whom we have had the pleasure of working over the years and who have contributed to the advances in this field.

Citation. Buddle BM, Vordermeier HM, Hewinson RG. 2016. Experimental infection models of Tuberculosis in domestic livestock. Microbiol Spectrum 4(5):TBTB2-0017-2016.

References

1. **Waters WR, Palmer MV, Buddle BM, Vordermeier HM.** 2012. Bovine tuberculosis vaccine research: historical perspectives and recent advances. *Vaccine* 30:2611–2622.

2. **Daniel R, Evans H, Rolfe S, de la Rua-Domenech R, Crawshaw T, Higgins RJ, Schock A, Clifton-Hadley R.** 2009. Outbreak of tuberculosis caused by *Mycobacterium bovis* in golden Guernsey goats in Great Britain. *Vet Rec* 165:335–342.

3. **More SJ, Cameron AR, Greiner M, Clifton-Hadley RS, Rodeia SC, Bakker D, Salman MD, Sharp JM, De Massis F, Aranaz A, Boniotti MB, Gaffuri A, Have P, Verloo D, Woodford M, Wierup M.** 2009. Defining output-based standards to achieve and maintain tuberculosis freedom in farmed deer, with reference to member states of the European Union. *Prev Vet Med* 90:254–267.

4. **O'Brien DJ, Schmitt SM, Fitzgerald SD, Berry DE, Hickling GJ.** 2006. Managing the wildlife reservoir of *Mycobacterium bovis*: the Michigan, USA, experience. *Vet Microbiol* 112:313–323.

5. **Roswurm JD, Ranney AF.** 1973. Sharpening the attack on bovine tuberculosis. *Am J Public Health* 63:884–886.

6. **Buddle BM, Skinner MA, Wedlock DN, de Lisle GW, Vordermeier HM, Hewinson RG.** 2005. Cattle as a model for development of vaccines against human tuberculosis. *Tuberculosis (Edinb)* 85:19–24.

7. **Waters WR, Palmer MV.** 2015. *Mycobacterium bovis* infection of cattle and white-tailed deer: translational research of relevance to human tuberculosis. *ILAR J* 56:26–43.

8. **Smith NH, Gordon SV, de la Rua-Domenech R, Clifton-Hadley RS, Hewinson RG.** 2006. Bottlenecks and broomsticks: the molecular evolution of *Mycobacterium bovis*. *Nat Rev Microbiol* 4:670–681.

9. **Berg S, Smith NH.** 2014. Why doesn't bovine tuberculosis transmit between humans? *Trends Microbiol* 22:552–553.

10. **McIlroy SG, Neill SD, McCracken RM.** 1986. Pulmonary lesions and *Mycobacterium bovis* excretion from

the respiratory tract of tuberculin reacting cattle. *Vet Rec* 118:718–721.

11. Liebana E, Johnson L, Gough J, Durr P, Jahans K, Clifton-Hadley R, Spencer Y, Hewinson RG, Downs SH. 2008. Pathology of naturally occurring bovine tuberculosis in England and Wales. *Vet J* 176:354–360.

12. Buddle BM, de Lisle GW, Pfeffer A, Aldwell FE. 1995. Immunological responses and protection against *Mycobacterium bovis* in calves vaccinated with a low dose of BCG. *Vaccine* 13:1123–1130.

13. Palmer MV, Waters WR, Whipple DL. 2002. Aerosol delivery of virulent *Mycobacterium bovis* to cattle. *Tuberculosis (Edinb)* 82:275–282.

14. Rodgers JD, Connery NL, McNair J, Welsh MD, Skuce RA, Bryson DG, McMurray DN, Pollock JM. 2007. Experimental exposure of cattle to a precise aerosolised challenge of *Mycobacterium bovis*: a novel model to study bovine tuberculosis. *Tuberculosis (Edinb)* 87:405–414.

15. Buddle BM, Aldwell FE, Pfeffer A, de Lisle GW, Corner LA. 1994. Experimental *Mycobacterium bovis* infection of cattle: effect of dose of M. *bovis* and pregnancy on immune responses and distribution of lesions. *N Z Vet J* 42:167–172.

16. Neill SD, Hanna J, O'Brien JJ, McCracken RM. 1988. Excretion of *Mycobacterium bovis* by experimentally infected cattle. *Vet Rec* 123:340–343.

17. Palmer MV, Whipple DL, Rhyan JC, Bolin CA, Saari DA. 1999. Granuloma development in cattle after intratonsilar inoculation with *Mycobacterium bovis*. *Am J Vet Res* 60:310–315.

18. Vordermeier HM, Chambers MA, Cockle PJ, Whelan AO, Simmons J, Hewinson RG. 2002. Correlation of ESAT-6-specific gamma interferon production with pathology in cattle following *Mycobacterium bovis* BCG vaccination against experimental bovine tuberculosis. *Infect Immun* 70:3026–3032.

19. Wedlock DN, Aldwell FE, Vordermeier HM, Hewinson RG, Buddle BM. 2011. Protection against bovine tuberculosis induced by oral vaccination of cattle with *Mycobacterium bovis* BCG is not enhanced by co-administration of mycobacterial protein vaccines. *Vet Immunol Immunopathol* 144:220–227.

20. Wangoo A, Johnson L, Gough J, Ackbar R, Inglut S, Hicks D, Spencer Y, Hewinson G, Vordermeier M. 2005. Advanced granulomatous lesions in *Mycobacterium bovis*-infected cattle are associated with increased expression of type I procollagen, γδ (WC1+) T cells and CD 68+ cells. *J Comp Pathol* 133:223–234.

21. Waters WR, Palmer MV, Nonnecke BJ, Thacker TC, Scherer CFC, Estes DM, Jacobs WR Jr, Glatman-Freedman A, Larsen MH. 2007. Failure of a Mycobacterium tuberculosis ΔRD1 ΔpanCD double deletion mutant in a neonatal calf aerosol M. *bovis* challenge model: comparisons to responses elicited by M. *bovis* bacille Calmette Guerin. *Vaccine* 25:7832–7840.

22. Ameni G, Vordermeier M, Aseffa A, Young DB, Hewinson RG. 2010. Field evaluation of the efficacy of *Mycobacterium bovis* bacillus Calmette-Guerin against bovine tuberculosis in neonatal calves in Ethiopia. *Clin Vaccine Immunol* 17:1533–1538.

23. Lopez-Valencia G, Renteria-Evangelista T, Williams JJ, Licea-Navarro A, Mora-Valle AL, Medina-Basulto G. 2010. Field evaluation of the protective efficacy of *Mycobacterium bovis* BCG vaccine against bovine tuberculosis. *Res Vet Sci* 88:44–49.

24. Khatri BL, Coad M, Clifford DJ, Hewinson RG, Whelan AO, Vordermeier HM. 2012. A natural-transmission model of bovine tuberculosis provides novel disease insights. *Vet Rec* 171:448

25. Pesciaroli M, Alvarez J, Boniotti MB, Cagiola M, Di Marco V, Marianelli C, Pacciarini M, Pasquali P. 2014. Tuberculosis in domestic animal species. *Res Vet Sci* 97(Suppl):S78–S85.

26. Sanchez J, Tomás L, Ortega N, Buendía AJ, del Rio L, Salinas J, Bezos J, Caro MR, Navarro JA. 2011. Microscopical and immunological features of tuberculoid granulomata and cavitary pulmonary tuberculosis in naturally infected goats. *J Comp Pathol* 145:107–117.

27. Pérez de Val B, López-Soria S, Nofrarías M, Martín M, Vordermeier HM, Villarreal-Ramos B, Romera N, Escobar M, Solanes D, Cardona PJ, Domingo M. 2011. Experimental model of tuberculosis in the domestic goat after endobronchial infection with *Mycobacterium caprae*. *Clin Vaccine Immunol* 18:1872–1881.

28. Gonzalez-Juarrero M, Bosco-Lauth A, Podell B, Soffler C, Brooks E, Izzo A, Sanchez-Campillo J, Bowen R. 2013. Experimental aerosol *Mycobacterium bovis* model of infection in goats. *Tuberculosis (Edinb)* 93:558–564.

29. Bezos J, Casal C, Díez-Delgado I, Romero B, Liandris E, Álvarez J, Sevilla IA, Juan L, Domínguez L, Gortázar C. 2015. Goats challenged with different members of the *Mycobacterium tuberculosis* complex display different clinical pictures. *Vet Immunol Immunopathol* 167:185–189.

30. Beatson NS. 1985. Tuberculosis in red deer, p 147–150. *In* Brown RD (ed), *Biology of Deer Production*. Springer Verlag, New York.

31. Fitzgerald SD, Kaneene JB. 2013. Wildlife reservoirs of bovine tuberculosis worldwide: hosts, pathology, surveillance, and control. *Vet Pathol* 50:488–499.

32. Griffin JFT, Mackintosh CG, Buchan GS. 1995. Animal models of protective immunity in tuberculosis to evaluate candidate vaccines. *Trends Microbiol* 3:418–424.

33. Palmer MV, Waters WR, Whipple DL. 2002. Lesion development in white-tailed deer (*Odocoileus virginianus*) experimentally infected with *Mycobacterium bovis*. *Vet Pathol* 39:334–340

34. Buddle BM, Hewinson RG, Vordermeier HM, Wedlock DN. 2013. Subcutaneous administration of a 10-fold lower dose of a human tuberculosis vaccine, *Mycobacterium bovis* bacille Calmette-Guérin Danish, induced levels of protection against bovine tuberculosis and responses in the tuberculin intradermal test similar to those induced by a standard cattle dose. *Clin Vaccine Immunol* 20:1559–1562.

35. Wedlock DN, Aldwell FE, Vordermeier HM, Hewinson RG, Buddle BM. 2011. Protection against bovine tuberculosis induced by oral vaccination of cattle with *Mycobacterium bovis* BCG is not enhanced

by co-administration of mycobacterial protein vaccines. *Vet Immunol Immunopathol* **144**:220–227.

36. Dean GS, Clifford D, Whelan AO, Tchilian EZ, Beverley PCL, Salguero FJ, Xing Z, Vordermeier HM, Villarreal-Ramos B. 2015. Protection induced by simultaneous subcutaneous and endobronchial vaccination with BCG/BCG and BCG/adenovirus expressing antigen 85A against *Mycobacterium bovis* in cattle. *PLoS One* **10**:e0142270.

37. Buddle BM, Denis M, Aldwell FE, Vordermeier HM, Hewinson RG, Wedlock DN. 2008. Vaccination of cattle with *Mycobacterium bovis* BCG by a combination of systemic and oral routes. *Tuberculosis (Edinb)* **88**:595–600.

38. Wedlock DN, Denis M, Vordermeier HM, Hewinson RG, Buddle BM. 2007. Vaccination of cattle with Danish and Pasteur strains of *Mycobacterium bovis* BCG induce different levels of IFNγ post-vaccination, but induce similar levels of protection against bovine tuberculosis. *Vet Immunol Immunopathol* **118**:50–58.

39. Hope JC, Thom ML, McAulay M, Mead E, Vordermeier HM, Clifford D, Hewinson RG, Villarreal-Ramos B. 2011. Identification of surrogates and correlates of protection in protective immunity against *Mycobacterium bovis* infection induced in neonatal calves by vaccination with *M. bovis* BCG Pasteur and *M. bovis* BCG Danish. *Clin Vaccine Immunol* **18**:373–379.

40. Buddle BM, Wedlock DN, Parlane NA, Corner LA, De Lisle GW, Skinner MA. 2003. Revaccination of neonatal calves with *Mycobacterium bovis* BCG reduces the level of protection against bovine tuberculosis induced by a single vaccination. *Infect Immun* **71**:6411–6419.

41. Hope JC, Thom ML, Villarreal-Ramos B, Vordermeier HM, Hewinson RG, Howard CJ. 2005. Vaccination of neonatal calves with *Mycobacterium bovis* BCG induces protection against intranasal challenge with virulent *M. bovis*. *Clin Exp Immunol* **139**:48–56.

42. Thom ML, McAulay M, Vordermeier HM, Clifford D, Hewinson RG, Villarreal-Ramos B, Hope JC. 2012. Duration of immunity against *Mycobacterium bovis* following neonatal vaccination with bacillus Calmette-Guérin Danish: significant protection against infection at 12, but not 24, months. *Clin Vaccine Immunol* **19**:1254–1260.

43. Parlane NA, Shu D, Subharat S, Wedlock DN, Rehm BH, de Lisle GW, Buddle BM. 2014. Revaccination of cattle with bacille Calmette-Guérin two years after first vaccination when immunity has waned, boosted protection against challenge with *Mycobacterium bovis*. *PLoS One* **9**:e106519.

44. Pérez de Val B, Villarreal-Ramos B, Nofrarías M, López-Soria S, Romera N, Singh M, Abad FX, Xing Z, Vordermeier HM, Domingo M. 2012. Goats primed with *Mycobacterium bovis* BCG and boosted with a recombinant adenovirus expressing Ag85A show enhanced protection against tuberculosis. *Clin Vaccine Immunol* **19**:1339–1347.

45. Pérez de Val B, Vidal E, Villarreal-Ramos B, Gilbert SC, Andaluz A, Moll X, Martín M, Nofrarías M, McShane H, Vordermeier HM, Domingo M. 2013. A

multi-antigenic adenoviral-vectored vaccine improves BCG-induced protection of goats against pulmonary tuberculosis infection and prevents disease progression. *PLoS One* **8**:e81317.

46. Griffin JF, Mackintosh CG, Rodgers CR. 2006. Factors influencing theprotective efficacy of a BCG homologous prime-boost vaccination regime against tuberculosis. *Vaccine* **24**:835–845

47. Nol P, Palmer MV, Waters WR, Aldwell FE, Buddle BM, Triantis JM, Linke LM, Phillips GE, Thacker TC, Rhyan JC, Dunbar MR, Salman MD. 2008. Efficacy of oral and parenteral routes of *Mycobacterium bovis* bacille Calmette-Guerin vaccination against experimental bovine tuberculosis in white-tailed deer (*Odocoileus virginianus*): a feasibility study. *J Wildl Dis* **44**:247–259.

48. Palmer MV, Thacker TC, Waters WR. 2009. Vaccination with *Mycobacterium bovis* BCG strains Danish and Pasteur in white-tailed deer (*Odocoileus virginianus*) experimentally challenged with *Mycobacterium bovis*. *Zoonoses Public Health* **56**:243–251.

49. Palmer MV, Thacker TC, Waters WR, Robbe-Austerman S, Lebepe-Mazur SM, Harris NB. 2010. Persistence of *Mycobacterium bovis* bacillus Calmette-Guérin in white-tailed deer (*Odocoileus virginianus*) after oral or parenteral vaccination. *Zoonoses Public Health* **57**:e206–e212.

50. Nol P, Rhyan JC, Robbe-Austerman S, McCollum MP, Rigg TD, Saklou NT, Salman MD. 2013. The potential for transmission of BCG from orally vaccinated white-tailed deer (*Odocoileus virginianus*) to cattle (*Bos taurus*) through a contaminated environment: experimental findings. *PLoS One* **8**:e60257.

51. Rizzi C, Bianco MV, Blanco FC, Soria M, Gravisaco MJ, Montenegro V, Vagnoni L, Buddle B, Garbaccio S, Delgado F, Leal KS, Cataldi AA, Dellagostin OA, Bigi F. 2012. Vaccination with a BCG strain overexpressing Ag85B protects cattle against *Mycobacterium bovis* challenge. *PLoS One* **7**:e51396.

52. Khatri B, Whelan A, Clifford D, Petrera A, Sander P, Vordermeier HM. 2014. BCG *zmp1* vaccine induces enhanced antigen specific immune responses in cattle. *Vaccine* **32**:779–784

53. Grode L, Ganoza CA, Brohm C, Weiner J III, Eisele B, Kaufmann SH. 2013. Safety and immunogenicity of the recombinant BCG vaccine VPM1002 in a phase 1 open-label clinical trial. *Vaccine* **31**:1340–1348.

54. Grode L, Seiler P, Baumann S, Hess J, Brinkmann V, Nasser Eddine A, Mann P, Goosmann C, Bandermann S, Smith D, Bancroft GJ, Reyrat JM, van Soolingen D, Raupach B, Kaufmann SH. 2005. Increased vaccine efficacy against tuberculosis of recombinant *Mycobacterium bovis* bacille Calmette-Guérin mutants that secrete listeriolysin. *J Clin Invest* **115**:2472–2479.

55. Waters WR, Maggioli MF, Palmer MV, Thacker TC, McGill JL, Vordermeier HM, Berney-Meyer L, Jacobs WR Jr, Larsen MH. 2016. Interleukin-17A as a biomarker for bovine tuberculosis. *Clin Vaccine Immunol* **23**:168–180.

56. Buddle BM, Wards BJ, Aldwell FE, Collins DM, de Lisle GW. 2002. Influence of sensitisation to environ-

mental mycobacteria on subsequent vaccination against bovine tuberculosis. *Vaccine* 20:1126–1133.

57. Khare S, Hondalus MK, Nunes J, Bloom BR, Adams LG. 2007. Mycobacterium bovis ΔleuD auxotroph-induced protective immunity against tissue colonization, burden and distribution in cattle intranasally challenged with *Mycobacterium bovis* Ravenel S. *Vaccine* 25:1743–1755.

58. Waters WR, Palmer MV, Nonnecke BJ, Thacker TC, Scherer CFC, Estes DM, Hewinson RG, Vordermeier HM, Barnes SW, Federe GC, Walker JR, Glynne RJ, Hsu T, Weinrick B, Biermann K, Larsen MH, Jacobs WR Jr. 2009. Efficacy and immunogenicity of *Mycobacterium bovis* ΔRD1 against aerosol M. bovis infection in neonatal calves. *Vaccine* 27:1201–1209.

59. Blanco FC, Bianco MV, Garbaccio S, Meikle V, Gravisaco MJ, Montenegro V, Alfonseca E, Singh M, Barandiaran S, Canal A, Vagnoni L, Buddle BM, Bigi F, Cataldi A. 2013. *Mycobacterium bovis* Δmce2 double deletion mutant protects cattle against challenge with virulent M. bovis. *Tuberculosis (Edinb)* 93:363–372.

60. Maue AC, Waters WR, Palmer MV, Whipple DL, Minion FC, Brown WC, Estes DM. 2004. CD80 and CD86, but not CD154, augment DNA vaccine-induced protection in experimental bovine tuberculosis. *Vaccine* 23:769–779

61. Cai H, Tian X, Hu XD, Li SX, Yu DH, Zhu YX. 2005. Combined DNA vaccines formulated either in DDA or in saline protect cattle from *Mycobacterium bovis* infection. *Vaccine* 23:3887–3895.

62. Skinner MA, Buddle BM, Wedlock DN, Keen D, de Lisle GW, Tascon RE, Ferraz JC, Lowrie DB, Cockle PJ, Vordermeier HM, Hewinson RG. 2003. A DNA prime-*Mycobacterium bovis* BCG boost vaccination strategy for cattle induces protection against bovine tuberculosis. *Infect Immun* 71:4901–4907.

63. Skinner MA, Wedlock DN, de Lisle GW, Cooke MM, Tascon RE, Ferraz JC, Lowrie DB, Vordermeier HM, Hewinson RG, Buddle BM. 2005. The order of prime-boost vaccination of neonatal calves with *Mycobacterium bovis* BCG and a DNA vaccine encoding mycobacterial proteins Hsp65, Hsp70, and Apa is not critical for enhancing protection against bovine tuberculosis. *Infect Immun* 73:4441–4444.

64. Maue AC, Waters WR, Palmer MV, Nonnecke BJ, Minion FC, Brown WC, Norimine J, Foote MR, Scherer CF, Estes DM. 2007. An ESAT-6:CFP10 DNA vaccine administered in conjunction with *Mycobacterium bovis* BCG confers protection to cattle challenged with virulent M. bovis. *Vaccine* 25:4735–4746.

65. Wedlock DN, Denis M, Skinner MA, Koach J, de Lisle GW, Vordermeier HM, Hewinson RG, van Drunen Littel-van den Hurk S, Babiuk LA, Hecker R, Buddle BM. 2005. Vaccination of cattle with a CpG oligodeoxynucleotide-formulated mycobacterial protein vaccine and *Mycobacterium bovis* BCG induces levels of protection against bovine tuberculosis superior to those induced by vaccination with BCG alone. *Infect Immun* 73:3540–3546.

66. Wedlock DN, Denis M, Painter GF, Ainge GD, Vordermeier HM, Hewinson RG, Buddle BM. 2008. Enhanced protec-

tion against bovine tuberculosis after coadministration of *Mycobacterium bovis* BCG with a mycobacterial protein vaccine-adjuvant combination but not after coadministration of adjuvant alone. *Clin Vaccine Immunol* 15:765–772.

67. Vordermeier HM, Villarreal-Ramos B, Cockle PJ, McAulay M, Rhodes SG, Thacker T, Gilbert SC, McShane H, Hill AV, Xing Z, Hewinson RG. 2009. Viral booster vaccines improve *Mycobacterium bovis* BCG-induced protection against bovine tuberculosis. *Infect Immun* 77:3364–3373.

68. Dean G, Whelan A, Clifford D, Salguero FJ, Xing Z, Gilbert S, McShane H, Hewinson RG, Vordermeier M, Villarreal-Ramos B. 2014. Comparison of the immunogenicity and protection against bovine tuberculosis following immunization by BCG-priming and boosting with adenovirus or protein based vaccines. *Vaccine* 32:1304–1310.

69. Dean G, Clifford D, Gilbert S, McShane H, Hewinson RG, Vordermeier HM, Villarreal-Ramos B. 2014. Effect of dose and route of immunisation on the immune response induced in cattle by heterologous Bacille Calmette-Guerin priming and recombinant adenoviral vector boosting. *Vet Immunol Immunopathol* 158:208–213.

70. Whelan A, Court P, Xing Z, Clifford D, Hogarth PJ, Vordermeier M, Villarreal-Ramos B. 2012. Immunogenicity comparison of the intradermal or endobronchial boosting of BCG vaccinates with Ad5-85A. *Vaccine* 30:6294–6300

71. Satti I, Meyer J, Harris SA, Manjaly Thomas ZR, Griffiths K, Antrobus RD, Rowland R, Ramon RL, Smith M, Sheehan S, Bettinson H, McShane H. 2014. Safety and immunogenicity of a candidate tuberculosis vaccine MVA85A delivered by aerosol in BCG-vaccinated healthy adults: a phase 1, double-blind, randomised controlled trial. *Lancet Infect Dis* 14:939–946.

72. Vordermeier HM, Huygen K, Singh M, Hewinson RG, Xing Z. 2006. Immune responses induced in cattle by vaccination with a recombinant adenovirus expressing mycobacterial antigen 85A and *Mycobacterium bovis* BCG. *Infect Immun* 74:1416–1418.

73. Blunt L, Hogarth PJ, Kaveh DA, Webb P, Villarreal-Ramos B, Vordermeier HM. 2015. Phenotypic characterization of bovine memory cells responding to mycobacteria in IFNγ enzyme linked immunospot assays. *Vaccine* 33:7276–7282.

74. Maggioli MF, Palmer MV, Thacker TC, Vordermeier HM, Waters WR. 2015. Characterization of effector and memory T cell subsets in the immune response to bovine tuberculosis in cattle. *PLoS One* 10:e0122571.

75. Khader SA, Bell GK, Pearl JE, Fountain JJ, Rangel-Moreno J, Cilley GE, Shen F, Eaton SM, Gaffen SL, Swain SL, Locksley RM, Haynes L, Randall TD, Cooper AM. 2007. IL-23 and IL-17 in the establishment of protective pulmonary CD4+ T cell responses after vaccination and during *Mycobacterium tuberculosis* challenge. *Nat Immunol* 8:369–377.

76. Khader SA, Cooper AM. 2008. IL-23 and IL-17 in tuberculosis. *Cytokine* 41:79–83.

77. Bhuju S, Aranday-Cortes E, Villarreal-Ramos B, Xing Z, Singh M, Vordermeier HM. 2012. Global gene transcriptome analysis in vaccinated cattle revealed a dominant role of IL-22 for protection against bovine tuberculosis. *PLoS Pathog* 8:e1003077.

78. Aagaard C, Hoang TT, Izzo A, Billeskov R, Troudt J, Arnett K, Keyser A, Elvang T, Andersen P, Dietrich J. 2009. Protection and polyfunctional T cells induced by Ag85B-TB10.4/IC31 against *Mycobacterium tuberculosis* is highly dependent on the antigen dose. *PLoS One* 4:e5930.

79. McShane H. 2009. Vaccine strategies against tuberculosis. *Swiss Med Wkly* 139:156–160.

80. Nambiar JK, Pinto R, Aguilo JI, Takatsu K, Martin C, Britton WJ, Triccas JA. 2012. Protective immunity afforded by attenuated, PhoP-deficient *Mycobacterium tuberculosis* is associated with sustained generation of CD4+ T-cell memory. *Eur J Immunol* 42:385–392.

81. Whelan AO, Villarreal-Ramos B, Vordermeier HM, Hogarth PJ. 2011. Development of an antibody to bovine IL-2 reveals multifunctional CD4 T(EM) cells in cattle naturally infected with bovine tuberculosis. *PLoS One* 6:e29194.

82. Geiger R, Duhen T, Lanzavecchia A, Sallusto F. 2009. Human naive and memory CD4+ T cell repertoires specific for naturally processed antigens analyzed using libraries of amplified T cells. *J Exp Med* 206:1525–1534.

83. Patke DS, Farber DL. 2005. Modulation of memory CD4 T cell function and survival potential by altering the strength of the recall stimulus. *J Immunol* 174:5433–5443.

84. Caserta S, Kleczkowska J, Mondino A, Zamoyska R. 2010. Reduced functional avidity promotes central and effector memory CD4 T cell responses to tumor-associated antigens. *J Immunol* 185:6545–6554.

85. Vordermeier HM, Rhodes SG, Dean G, Goonetilleke N, Huygen K, Hill AV, Hewinson RG, Gilbert SC. 2004. Cellular immune responses induced in cattle by heterologous prime-boost vaccination using recombinant viruses and bacille Calmette-Guérin. *Immunology* 112:461–470.

86. Golby P, Villarreal-Ramos B, Dean G, Jones GJ, Vordermeier M. 2014. MicroRNA expression profiling of PPD-B stimulated PBMC from *M. bovis*-challenged unvaccinated and BCG vaccinated cattle. *Vaccine* 32:5839–5844

87. Huang J, Jiao J, Xu W, Zhao H, Zhang C, Shi Y, Xiao Z. 2015. MiR-155 is up-regulated in patients with active tuberculosis and inhibits apoptosis of monocytes by targeting FOXO3. *Mol Med Rep* 12:7102–7108.

88. Aranday-Cortes E, Hogarth PJ, Kaveh DA, Whelan AO, Villarreal-Ramos B, Lalvani A, Vordermeier HM. 2012. Transcriptional profiling of disease-induced host responses in bovine tuberculosis and the identification of potential diagnostic biomarkers. *PLoS One* 7:e30626.

89. Ruhwald M, Aabye MG, Ravn P. 2012. IP-10 release assays in the diagnosis of tuberculosis infection: current status and future directions. *Expert Rev Mol Diagn* 12:175–187.

90. Berggren SA. 1981. Field experiment with BCG vaccine in Malawi. *Br Vet J* 137:88–96.

91. Buddle BM, Parlane NA, Keen DL, Aldwell FE, Pollock JM, Lightbody K, Andersen P. 1999. Differentiation between *Mycobacterium bovis* BCG-vaccinated and *M. bovis*-infected cattle by using recombinant mycobacterial antigens. *Clin Diagn Lab Immunol* 6:1–5.

92. Vordermeier HM, Cockle PC, Whelan A, Rhodes S, Palmer N, Bakker D, Hewinson RG. 1999. Development of diagnostic reagents to differentiate between *Mycobacterium bovis* BCG vaccination and *M. bovis* infection in cattle. *Clin Diagn Lab Immunol* 6:675–682.

93. Garnier T, Eiglmeier K, Camus JC, Medina N, Mansoor H, Pryor M, Duthoy S, Grondin S, Lacroix C, Monsempe C, Simon S, Harris B, Atkin R, Doggett J, Mayes R, Keating L, Wheeler PR, Parkhill J, Barrell BG, Cole ST, Gordon SV, Hewinson RG. 2003. The complete genome sequence of *Mycobacterium bovis*. *Proc Natl Acad Sci USA* 100:7877–7882.

94. Cole ST, Brosch R, Parkhill J, Garnier T, Churcher C, Harris D, Gordon SV, Eiglmeier K, Gas S, Barry CE III, Tekaia F, Badcock K, Basham D, Brown D, Chillingworth T, Connor R, Davies R, Devlin K, Feltwell T, Gentles S, Hamlin N, Holroyd S, Hornsby T, Jagels K, Krogh A, McLean J, Moule S, Murphy L, Oliver K, Osborne J, Quail MA, Rajandream MA, Rogers J, Rutter S, Seeger K, Skelton J, Squares R, Squares S, Sulston JE, Taylor K, Whitehead S, Barrell BG. 1998. Deciphering the biology of *Mycobacterium tuberculosis* from the complete genome sequence. *Nature* 393:537–544.

95. Brosch R, Gordon SV, Garnier T, Eiglmeier K, Frigui W, Valenti P, Dos Santos S, Duthoy S, Lacroix C, Garcia-Pelayo C, Inwald JK, Golby P, Garcia JN, Hewinson RG, Behr MA, Quail MA, Churcher C, Barrell BG, Parkhill J, Cole ST. 2007. Genome plasticity of BCG and impact on vaccine efficacy. *Proc Natl Acad Sci USA* 104:5596–5601.

96. Li L, Bannantine JP, Zhang Q, Amonsin A, May BJ, Alt D, Banerji N, Kanjilal S, Kapur V. 2005. The complete genome sequence of *Mycobacterium avium* subspecies *paratuberculosis*. *Proc Natl Acad Sci USA* 102:12344–12349.

97. Mustafa AS, Cockle PJ, Shaban F, Hewinson RG, Vordermeier HM. 2002. Immunogenicity of *Mycobacterium tuberculosis* RD1 region gene products in infected cattle. *Clin Exp Immunol* 130:37–42.

98. Wilkinson KA, Stewart GR, Newton SM, Vordermeier HM, Wain JR, Murphy HN, Horner K, Young DB, Wilkinson RJ. 2005. Infection biology of a novel alpha-crystallin of *Mycobacterium tuberculosis*: Acr2. *J Immunol* 174:4237–4243

99. Mustafa AS, Skeiky YA, Al-Attiyah R, Alderson MR, Hewinson RG, Vordermeier HM. 2006. Immunogenicity of *Mycobacterium tuberculosis* antigens in *Mycobacterium bovis* BCG-vaccinated and *M. bovis*-infected cattle. *Infect Immun* 74:4566–4572.

100. Jones GJ, Pirson C, Gideon HP, Wilkinson KA, Sherman DR, Wilkinson RJ, Hewinson RG, Vordermeier HM. 2011. Immune responses to the enduring hypoxic response antigen Rv0188 are preferentially detected in *Mycobacterium bovis* infected cattle with low pathology. *PLoS One* 6:e21371.

101. Gideon HP, Wilkinson KA, Rustad TR, Oni T, Guio H, Sherman DR, Vordermeier HM, Robertson BD, Young DB, Wilkinson RJ. 2012. Bioinformatic and empirical analysis of novel hypoxia-inducible targets of the human antituberculosis T cell response. *J Immunol* **189**:5867–5876.

102. Vordermeier HM, Hewinson RG, Wilkinson RJ, Wilkinson KA, Gideon HP, Young DB, Sampson SL. 2012. Conserved immune recognition hierarchy of mycobacterial PE/PPE proteins during infection in natural hosts. *PLoS One* **7**:e40890.

103. Pollock JM, Andersen P. 1997. The potential of the ESAT-6 antigen secreted by virulent mycobacteria for specific diagnosis of tuberculosis. *J Infect Dis* **175**:1251–1254.

104. Vordermeier HM, Whelan A, Cockle PJ, Farrant L, Palmer N, Hewinson RG. 2001. Use of synthetic peptides derived from the antigens ESAT-6 and CFP-10 for differential diagnosis of bovine tuberculosis in cattle. *Clin Diagn Lab Immunol* **8**:571–578.

105. Buddle BM, Ryan TJ, Pollock JM, Andersen P, de Lisle GW. 2001. Use of ESAT-6 in the interferon-γ test for diagnosis of bovine tuberculosis following skin testing. *Vet Microbiol* **80**:37–46.

106. Sidders B, Withers M, Kendall SL, Bacon J, Waddell SJ, Hinds J, Golby P, Movahedzadeh F, Cox RA, Frita R, Ten Bokum AM, Wernisch L, Stoker NG. 2007. Quantification of global transcription patterns in prokaryotes using spotted microarrays. *Genome Biol* **8**:R265.

107. Millington KA, Fortune SM, Low J, Garces A, Hingley-Wilson SM, Wickremasinghe M, Kon OM, Lalvani A. 2011. Rv3615c is a highly immunodominant RD1 (region of difference 1)-dependent secreted antigen specific for *Mycobacterium tuberculosis* infection. *Proc Natl Acad Sci USA* **108**:5730–5735.

108. Pollock JM, Andersen P. 1997. Predominant recognition of the ESAT-6 protein in the first phase of infection with *Mycobacterium bovis* in cattle. *Infect Immun* **65**:2587–2592.

109. Ravn P, Demissie A, Eguale T, Wondwosson H, Lein D, Amoudy HA, Mustafa AS, Jensen AK, Holm A, Rosenkrands I, Oftung F, Olobo J, von Reyn F, Andersen P. 1999. Human T cell responses to the ESAT-6 antigen from *Mycobacterium tuberculosis*. *J Infect Dis* **179**:637–645.

110. van Pinxteren LA, Ravn P, Agger EM, Pollock J, Andersen P. 2000. Diagnosis of tuberculosis based on the two specific antigens ESAT-6 and CFP10. *Clin Diagn Lab Immunol* **7**:155–160.

111. Cockle PJ, Gordon SV, Lalvani A, Buddle BM, Hewinson RG, Vordermeier HM. 2002. Identification of novel *Mycobacterium tuberculosis* antigens with potential as diagnostic reagents or subunit vaccine candidates by comparative genomics. *Infect Immun* **70**:6996–7003.

112. Cockle PJ, Gordon SV, Hewinson RG, Vordermeier HM. 2006. Field evaluation of a novel differential diagnostic reagent for detection of *Mycobacterium bovis* in cattle. *Clin Vaccine Immunol* **13**:1119–1124.

113. Sidders B, Pirson C, Hogarth PJ, Hewinson RG, Stoker NG, Vordermeier HM, Ewer K. 2008. Screening of highly expressed mycobacterial genes identifies Rv3615c as a useful differential diagnostic antigen for the *Mycobacterium tuberculosis* complex. *Infect Immun* **76**:3932–3939.

114. Jones GJ, Gordon SV, Hewinson RG, Vordermeier HM. 2010. Screening of predicted secreted antigens from *Mycobacterium bovis* reveals the immunodominance of the ESAT-6 protein family. *Infect Immun* **78**:1326–1332.

115. Jones GJ, Hewinson RG, Vordermeier HM. 2010. Screening of predicted secreted antigens from *Mycobacterium bovis* identifies potential novel differential diagnostic reagents. *Clin Vaccine Immunol* **17**:1344–1348.

116. Lindestam Arlehamn CS, Gerasimova A, Mele F, Henderson R, Swann J, Greenbaum JA, Kim Y, Sidney J, James EA, Taplitz R, McKinney DM, Kwok WW, Grey H, Sallusto F, Peters B, Sette A. 2013. Memory T cells in latent *Mycobacterium tuberculosis* infection are directed against three antigenic islands and largely contained in a CXCR3+CCR6+ Th1 subset. *PLoS Pathog* **9**:e1003130.

117. Whelan AO, Clifford D, Upadhyay B, Breadon EL, McNair J, Hewinson GR, Vordermeier MH. 2010. Development of a skin test for bovine tuberculosis for differentiating infected from vaccinated animals. *J Clin Microbiol* **48**:3176–3181.

118. Parlane NA, Chen S, Jones GJ, Vordermeier HM, Wedlock DN, Rehm BHA, Buddle BM. 2015. Display of antigens on polyester inclusions lowers the antigen concentration required for a bovine tuberculosis skin test. *Clin Vaccine Immunol* **23**:19–26.

119. Arend SM, Franken WP, Aggerbeck H, Prins C, van Dissel JT, Thierry-Carstensen B, Tingskov PN, Weldingh K, Andersen P. 2008. Double-blind randomized phase I study comparing rdESAT-6 to tuberculin as skin test reagent in the diagnosis of tuberculosis infection. *Tuberculosis (Edinb)* **88**:249–261.

Tuberculosis and the Tubercle Bacillus, 2nd ed.
Edited by William R. Jacobs, Jr., Helen McShane, Valerie Mizrahi, and Ian M. Orme
© 2018 American Society for Microbiology, Washington, DC
doi:10.1128/microbiolspec.TBTB2-0015-2016

C. VACCINES

Clinical Testing of Tuberculosis Vaccine Candidates

10

Mark Hatherill[1], Dereck Tait[2], and Helen McShane[3]

INDICATIONS FOR VACCINATION AGAINST TUBERCULOSIS

The need for a new tuberculosis (TB) vaccination strategy is clear when we consider the massive burden of TB disease in countries where universal infant bacille Calmette-Guérin (BCG) vaccination is practiced as part of the World Health Organization (WHO) Expanded Program on Immunization (EPI) (1). The lifetime risk for development of TB disease in these high-transmission settings is driven by multiple ongoing *Mycobacterium tuberculosis* exposure-re-exposure episodes, beginning in early childhood, leading to *M. tuberculosis* infection at an early age, and continuing throughout adulthood (Fig. 1). Infants and very young children not only have a higher risk of progression from infection to disease, but have a higher risk of severe disease, including miliary TB and tuberculous meningitis (2). Since BCG vaccine is thought to offer protective efficacy of about 74% against all forms of TB disease in children, BCG vaccination is firmly entrenched in the EPI (3). However, although BCG vaccination is thought to offer modest protection against *M. tuberculosis* infection as defined by interferon-gamma (IFN-γ) release assay (IGRA) conversion, the majority of adults in high-TB-burden countries are *M. tuberculosis*-infected (4). In very high-transmission settings such as South Africa, more than three quarters of adolescents are *M. tuberculosis*-infected by the time they leave high school (5, 6). Given that the rate of infection in some African countries may exceed 10% per annum (7), it is not surprising that

while Africa is responsible for only 28% of the world's new TB cases, 7 of the top 10 countries for TB incidence by population are in Africa, where HIV coinfection, a younger population demographic, and social disadvantage and disruption add susceptibility to TB disease (8). It is against this backdrop that we review the potential indications for TB vaccines, in search of a vaccination strategy that is safe and effective against all forms of TB disease in infants, children, and adults, including *M. tuberculosis*-infected and HIV-infected people.

Prevention of *M. tuberculosis* Infection

It might appear self-evident that the most desirable strategy for TB vaccination, with the greatest potential for public health benefit, would be prevention of infection (POI) (9). Surely, if we could prevent *M. tuberculosis* infection, given that only infected people can develop disease, we could halt the global TB epidemic. The caveat is that 90% of *M. tuberculosis*-infected people control their own infection immunologically and never develop TB disease in their lifetime. It follows that if an effective POI vaccine prevented *M. tuberculosis* infection primarily in those people at lowest risk of progression to disease, a POI vaccination strategy would have little or no impact on the TB epidemic. On the other hand, an effective TB vaccine that prevented infection in the 10% of high-risk people, those who would fail to control their own infection and progress from latency to disease, would have a major impact on the global epidemic (Fig. 2). A POI vaccination strategy

[1]South African Tuberculosis Vaccine Initiative (SATVI) and Institute of Infectious Disease and Molecular Medicine (IDM), University of Cape Town, Cape Town, South Africa 7925; [2]Aeras, Cape Town, South Africa 7925; [3]The Jenner Institute, University of Oxford, Oxford OX3 7DQ, United Kingdom.

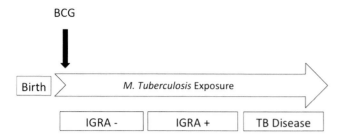

BCG vaccination offers 74% protection against TB in infants and IGRA- children, but little or no protection against pulmonary TB in adults

Figure 1 BCG vaccination, exposure, infection, and TB disease in a high-TB-burden setting.

would be likely to provide maximal benefit to newborns, infants, and adolescents in high-TB-transmission settings, since *M. tuberculosis* exposure and infection occur early in life in high-burden countries (10). Thus, POI vaccination would likely be a long-term strategy, with little immediate impact on TB disease incidence and *M. tuberculosis* transmission in adults. Small proof-of-concept studies of POI vaccines would be relatively easy to conduct in high-transmission settings, since the annual rate of IGRA conversion is several-fold higher than the rate of incident TB disease in the same communities. If proof of concept for a POI vaccine candidate were demonstrated, it would also signal accelerated development of that product into classical phase 2 and 3 prevention of disease (POD) trials.

Is an effective POI vaccine a reasonable prospect, and could we expect such a vaccine to protect against TB disease in vaccinated individuals (11)? There are challenges to developing a POI vaccine, including case definitions and how to evaluate a POI vaccine in preclinical animal models (12). Preclinical data suggest that *M. tuberculosis* infection, defined by tuberculin skin test (TST) conversion, is not a permanent state (13). In a natural infection model, guinea pigs exposed to multidrug-resistant (MDR) TB patients for 18 weeks had a 75% TST conversion rate, but 22% of animals reverted back to a negative TST. Notably, only 2 of 86 TST reverter animals developed TB disease, compared to 47% of animals that exhibited sustained TST conversion. This finding raises the possibility that a TB vaccine that offers protection against sustained TST conversion might reduce the rate of disease in these individuals.

Unfortunately, the data from humans are more difficult to interpret. It has been known for many years that it is not the state of *M. tuberculosis* infection *per se* that is associated with the highest risk of TB disease,

but rather the state of becoming infected. In the classic example, 45% of student nurses entering an Oslo nursing college (1924 to 1936) were TST-positive (14). Among those TST-positive nurses, 3% developed active TB disease and none died. However, among those nurses who were TST-negative, 100% became TST-positive within 3 years, 34% developed active TB disease, and 10 died. Thus, TST conversion was associated with 12-fold increased TB incidence, with considerable mortality, compared to those who were latently *M. tuberculosis*-infected at baseline. This suggests that protection against new *M. tuberculosis* infection is more important than clearing of established or latent infection. Indeed, established latent infection may be protective in high-transmission settings with repeated *M. tuberculosis* exposure. Reports suggest that (BCG-naive) individuals with established latent *M. tuberculosis* infection have a 79% lower risk of developing TB disease after reinfection than uninfected individuals (15).

In recent years, the use of IGRA as an endpoint allows evaluation of the risks associated with *M. tuberculosis* infection in BCG-vaccinated individuals in high TB-burden countries where universal BCG vaccination is practiced. For example, in more than 6,000 South African adolescents (with IGRA-positive prevalence >50%), TB disease incidence was 3-fold higher among IGRA-positive compared to IGRA-negative individuals over 2 years of follow-up (0.22 versus 0.64 per 100 person years) (6). However, with extended follow-up of this cohort, incidence of TB disease in IGRA-negative people who become IGRA-positive was 8-fold that of people who remained IGRA negative and twice that of people who were IGRA-positive at baseline (1.46 versus 0.17 per 100 person years) (16). It would appear from these data that a POI vaccine that offers pro-

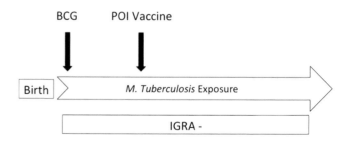

BCG vaccination may offer 20% protection against IGRA+ conversion. An effective POI vaccine strategy would need to offer protection against MTB infection in those persons at highest risk of progression to TB disease

Figure 2 Prevention of *M. tuberculosis* (MTB) infection (POI) vaccine strategy.

tection against an IGRA conversion endpoint would indeed have biological importance, but would it be necessary to prevent any IGRA conversion or only sustained conversion? Data from the guinea pig natural infection model, which suggest that transient TST conversion with subsequent reversion is associated with lower rates of TB disease than sustained TST conversion, are supported by data from humans (13). In a study of almost 4,000 household TB contacts in Philadelphia in the 1920s, 63% became TST-positive, but the 11% who reverted back to TST-negative status had much lower risk of TB disease than sustained TST converters (<1% compared to 23%) (17). Unfortunately, recent human data using the IGRA endpoint are conflicting. TB incidence in South African adolescents who reverted their IGRA status from positive to negative was similar to the rate in individuals with sustained IGRA conversion and was 8-fold higher than those who remained persistently IGRA-negative (7).

Although it might not be clear whether the ideal POI vaccine should prevent all conversion or only sustained IGRA conversion, it is encouraging that data from humans suggest that POI is feasible in principle. Observations from a natural experiment in Greenland during the period from 1991 to 1996, when universal BCG vaccination was temporarily discontinued, showed that IGRA conversion occurred in 23% of BCG-vaccinated people, compared to 57% in BCG-naive people (18). Evidence from several case-control studies now suggests that BCG vaccination provides modest protection in the region of 20% against IGRA conversion (4). However, although it is clear that IGRA conversion and protection against IGRA conversion have biological significance, there are challenges to the use of IGRA as an endpoint, including interpretation of IGRA conversions and reversions that occur near the assay threshold. For example, serial IGRA testing of Canadian health care workers, with expected TST conversion rates of less than 1%, showed unexpectedly high IGRA conversion rates (5%) unrelated to occupational TB exposure risk and associated with a high rate of spontaneous reversion (62%) (19). However, in contrast to reports from low-TB-transmission settings, reports from high-transmission settings suggest good concordance between TST and IGRA conversion and a strong association between IGRA conversion and incident TB disease (7). A clinical trial in South African adolescents is currently evaluating safety, immunogenicity, and prevention of infection by BCG revaccination or by the novel protein/adjuvant vaccine candidate H4: IC31 (AERAS-404) compared to placebo (ClinicalTrials.

gov NCT02075203). The primary endpoint is IGRA conversion, but the trial will also evaluate sustained IGRA conversion and sensitivity to alternative assay threshold values.

Prevention of TB Disease

Regardless of whether a novel TB vaccine could offer protection against *M. tuberculosis* infection, a minimum requirement for a prophylactic TB vaccination strategy is protection against TB disease. Such a POD vaccine should ideally be safe and effective in infants, children, and adults, including HIV-infected and other people at high risk. Historically, TB vaccine development efforts have focused on a POD vaccine targeted at infants, due to the high incidence and the high susceptibility to the most severe forms of disseminated and miliary disease in very young children (20). However, an effective POD vaccine for *M. tuberculosis*-infected and -uninfected adults is likely to have the greatest impact on global TB control in the short term. Modeling suggests that an effective adult POD vaccine is likely to prevent more cases of childhood TB than a POD vaccine targeted at infants, due to interruption of transmission (Fig. 3) (21).

It is likely that the ideal long-term POD strategy would involve some combination of routine infant vaccination with serial mass campaigns among adults. If so, this raises the question of what effect age and prior *M. tuberculosis* infection might have on the efficacy profile of a new TB vaccine or vaccination strategy. We know from a number of systematic reviews that the efficacy of BCG vaccine against TB disease is highest in infants and *M. tuberculosis*-uninfected children (rate ratio 0.26) compared to *M. tuberculosis*-infected and -uninfected adults (rate ratio 0.88) (22). There is thus the theoretical risk that prior *M. tuberculosis* infection, or even sensitization by nontuberculous mycobacteria, might block the effect of new POD vaccines targeted at adults. This risk applies primarily to live mycobacterial vaccines such as BCG, including recombinant BCG and

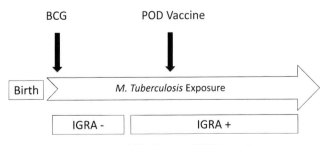

Figure 3 Prevention of TB disease (POD) vaccine strategy.

live attenuated *M. tuberculosis* vaccines (23, 24). Yet there is also the possibility of masking of any additive beneficial effect of subunit or viral-vectored TB vaccines in adults with prior mycobacterial sensitization. These risks are important to consider in light of the fact that 50 to 80% of adults in high-TB-transmission settings are *M. tuberculosis*-infected (5). There are undoubtedly potential advantages to testing POD vaccines in *M. tuberculosis*-infected people, especially since the incidence of TB disease in baseline IGRA-positive individuals is 2- to 3-fold that of IGRA-negative individuals (6). Proof-of-concept efficacy trials that focus only on IGRA-positive people would allow smaller sample sizes and duration of follow-up due to enriched TB case accrual. On the other hand, such trials would be unable to detect a potentially important POI efficacy signal in IGRA-negative people. More importantly, the lack of an efficacy signal among IGRA-positive people in a proof-of-concept trial might halt further clinical development of a candidate vaccine, yet it is very possible that a novel vaccine with efficacy only in *M. tuberculosis*-uninfected people would be discarded prematurely, highlighting the importance of evaluating POD vaccines in both IGRA-positive and IGRA-negative people.

In summary, efforts to target testing of POD vaccines in high-risk study populations, to reduce trial size and cost, risk limiting the generalizability of positive findings and even the possibility of missing an efficacy signal that would have been detected in an unselected study population. The primary risk is that targeted testing of novel TB vaccine candidates in adults, particularly *M. tuberculosis*-infected adults who may be a more challenging study population in whom to demonstrate efficacy, might completely fail to detect a positive efficacy signal in *M. tuberculosis*-uninfected people such as adolescents and children. In this case, the potential for short-term gain, in the form of an effective *M. tuberculosis* transmission-blocking POD vaccine for adults, needs to be balanced against the potential for long-term gain in the form of an effective prophylactic POD vaccine for infants, children, and adolescents.

Prevention of Recurrent TB Disease (Adjunctive Therapeutic Vaccination)

Prevention of TB disease in people with prior *M. tuberculosis* infection may be challenging, in which case, prevention and/or amelioration of TB disease in individuals with previous, recently treated, or active TB disease might be viewed as wholly aspirational. Indeed, the prospect of an effective prevention of recurrence (POR) or truly therapeutic TB vaccine presents a high

bar for any candidate TB vaccine. However, the potential for impact on TB control, particularly advances in therapeutics for drug-sensitive and MDR-TB, warrants discussion of the opportunities and challenges for a POR vaccine.

Cured TB patients, who have completed a course of therapy and have been confirmed *M. tuberculosis* culture-negative, have a higher risk of subsequent TB disease than other people in their community, whether for immunologic, genetic, or epidemiologic reasons. Recurrent disease comprises a combination of true relapse (reactivation disease), usually occurring more proximal to the end of treatment, and reinfection disease, occurring at any time after the end of treatment. Incidence of recurrent TB disease varies between 2 and 8%, depending on the background community TB disease incidence and effectiveness of, and adherence to, the TB treatment regimen, and 70 to 90% of recurrent TB disease occurs within 12 months of treatment completion (25).

An effective POR vaccine would have a modest direct impact on TB control in terms of reducing the burden of retreatment on TB patients and health systems; in countries where MDR-TB is primarily found in retreatment patients, a POR vaccine would be expected to reduce the rate of MDR-TB. However, in many high-TB-burden countries such as South Africa, the majority of MDR-TB is circulating, primary TB disease (8). Perhaps the greatest potential for a POR vaccine is as a therapeutic adjunct. If available, an effective POR vaccine could very quickly make its way into experimental TB treatment-shortening regimens, aimed at reducing the duration and complexity of TB treatment for drug-sensitive TB and MDR-TB (currently 6 and 20 months, respectively). The major limitation on development of new TB drugs, after demonstration of safety, is the rate of recurrent TB disease after treatment completion (26). Any addition to the therapeutic armamentarium that allowed treatment shortening, particularly for MDR-TB, would have a major impact on the financial, logistical, and personal burden of TB treatment.

Testing of potential POR vaccines would allow leverage of the high incidence of recurrent TB disease, relative to community incidence, to show POR efficacy in small, but admittedly complex, trials. A positive signal in any proof-of-concept POR trial would also signal expansion into larger phase 3 trials for the classic prophylactic POD indication, since a POR vaccine that prevented reactivation or reinfection disease might also be expected to prevent progression from latency to active disease. Ideally, any effective POR vaccine would also be tested during the TB treatment phase to evaluate the potential for reduction in rates of treatment failure or for amelioration of disease severity (true therapeutic indications) (Fig. 4).

Is an effective POR vaccine biologically plausible? In the absence of direct evidence from human studies, an effective POR vaccine would seem to set a high bar for novel vaccine candidates. However, the evidence from non-human primate (NHP) studies that subunit TB vaccines are capable of limiting TB disease severity, and prevent reactivation from latency, suggests that an effective POR vaccine is feasible (27, 28). The evidence from humans that *Mycobacterium vaccae*, in a meta-analysis of 54 studies, offers therapeutic benefit to TB patients by reducing time to sputum smear conversion and chest radiographic resolution also supports the notion that TB vaccination may alter the course of therapy and disease (29). The first step in the evaluation of potential POR and therapeutic TB vaccines is demonstration of safety and immunogenicity in TB patients upon completion of treatment, and two such clinical trials of subunit TB vaccine candidates are ongoing in this study population (ClinicalTrials.gov NCT02465216; NCT02375698).

TB VACCINE CANDIDATES IN CLINICAL TRIALS

The development and availability of new TB vaccines is an essential part of the WHO End TB Strategy. WHO has noted that without new effective TB vaccines the targets of reducing TB deaths by 95% and new cases of TB by 90%, between 2015 and 2035 will not be met (30). Thirteen TB vaccine candidates are currently in clinical development, and besides Vaccae, which is in phase 3 in China, the others are all either in phase 1 or phase 2 clinical development (Fig. 5).

The critical need for new TB vaccines is driven by the need for greater efficacy to prevent TB disease and transmission of *M. tuberculosis* to uninfected individuals. TB vaccines could be used for prophylaxis

and/or immunotherapy. The majority of TB vaccine candidates are being developed for TB prophylaxis indications.

Pathways for TB vaccine development currently follow one of three strategies:

- **Prime:** To replace BCG with a safer and more effective vaccine
- **Prime-boost:** TB vaccine administered to recently or remotely BCG-vaccinated individuals or administered as a booster after administration of a non-BCG TB vaccine
- **Immunotherapy:** A TB vaccine administered to patients with TB to influence the outcome of treatment of active TB disease by reducing either the duration of treatment and/or the incidence of posttreatment recurrence

Clinical trials are an essential component of vaccine development, and the different stages and outcomes are well defined. Phase 1 clinical trials, which include first-time-in-humans studies in which new candidate vaccines are evaluated for the first time, are often conducted in small numbers of healthy volunteers. The primary outcome in phase 1 studies is usually safety. Additional phase 1 and/or phase 2a studies further evaluate safety in larger numbers and potentially within the target population. For TB vaccines, this can include studies in adolescents, infants, and *M. tuberculosis*-and/or HIV-infected subjects. A secondary outcome in these phase 1/2a studies is immunogenicity, using predefined markers of a vaccine-induced host immune response. For pathogens for which defined and validated immunological correlates of protection exist, for example, *Neisseria meningitides* or *Streptococcus pneumoniae*, such safety and immunogenicity studies can provide the essential data required for vaccine licensure (31). However, for TB vaccines, such correlates have yet to be defined. This means that a new TB vaccine can and will only be licensed after the demonstration of efficacy in an appropriately powered phase 3 efficacy trial. Proof-of-concept efficacy might be demonstrable in a smaller phase 2b trial, but it is unlikely that such a single trial would ever be sufficient for licensure. Such efficacy trials require large sample sizes, even in high-incidence populations, take many years to complete, and are extremely costly. In TB vaccine development, immunological readouts in phase 1/2a trials focus primarily on markers of cell-mediated immunity such as Th1 immunity, which are known to be essential for protection (32). There is now increased interest in other aspects of vaccine-induced innate and adaptive immunity, because it is unlikely that

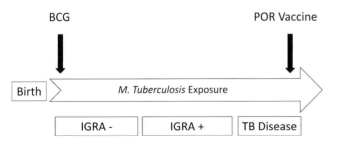

Figure 4 Prevention of recurrence (POR) and therapeutic TB vaccine strategies.

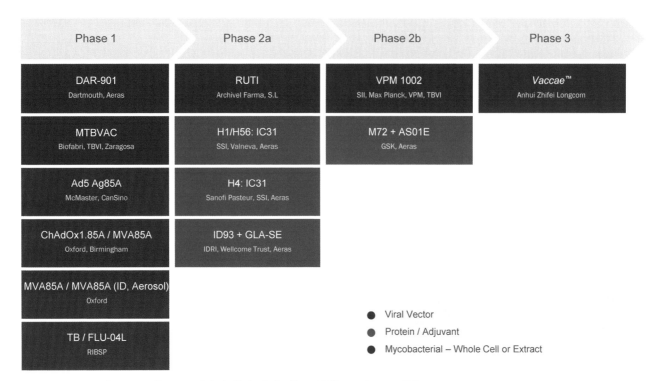

Figure 5   Current global clinical pipeline of TB vaccine candidates.

cell-mediated immunity alone is sufficient for protection (33).

TB vaccine candidates currently in clinical development fall into the following broad classes:

- Recombinant mycobacterial vaccines (MTBVAC, VPM1002)
- Adjuvanted subunit booster vaccines (H1:IC31, H56:IC31, H4:IC31, ID93+GLA-SE, M72/AS01E)
- Viral-vectored vaccines (MVA85A, Crucell Ad35, Ad5Ag85A, TB/Flu-04L)
- Inactivated whole-cell and fragmented TB vaccines (DAR-901, RUTI, Vaccae)

In the following section we will review those candidates currently in clinical development.

Protein-Adjuvant TB Vaccines

H1:IC31 and H1:CAF01

Hybrid I (H1) (Statens Serum Institut, Denmark) is a recombinant fusion protein of antigen 85B (Ag85B) and early secretory antigenic target 6 (ESAT-6) adjuvanted with IC31, a combination of an immunopotentiating antibacterial peptide (KLKL[5]KLK) and a synthetic oligodeoxynucleotide Toll-like 9 receptor agonist (34). Phase 1 studies have been conducted in non-BCG-vaccinated individuals, remotely BCG-vaccinated-individuals, and IGRA-positive individuals (34, 35).

H1-IC31 was demonstrated to be safe and well tolerated. It was immunogenic in all populations studied, and antigen-specific responses were evident for 2.5 years of follow-up. H1 has also been formulated with a two-component liposomal adjuvant system (CAF01) and administered in one phase 1 study to non-BCG-vaccinated adults, where it was demonstrated to be well tolerated and immunogenic with antigen-specific cell-mediated immune responses evident for 3 years (36).

H56:IC31

H56:IC31 (Statens Serum Institut, Denmark) is a fusion protein consisting of Ag85B, ESAT-6, and Rv2660c formulated with the adjuvant IC31, antigens that are characteristic of early infection and latency (37). High levels of protection by H56:IC31 have been demonstrated in murine models both pre- and postexposure compared with BCG alone or adjuvant control mice (37). H56:IC31 administered as a boost to BCG has been demonstrated to delay and reduce clinical disease in cynomolgus monkeys challenged with *M. tuberculosis* and also to prevent reactivation of latent infection compared with BCG alone (28). A phase 1 open-label, dose ranging, safety and immunogenicity study has been completed in IGRA-positive and -negative individuals who received three vaccinations with H56:IC31 or placebo 2 months apart. A dominant CD4+ T cell response that persisted for up to 3 months after the last vaccination was demonstrated, and immune responses were greater in IGRA-positive individuals than in IGRA-negative individuals (38). A double-blind, dose-finding H56:IC31 study in HIV-negative adults with and without latent TB infection is ongoing to investigate doses of 5 g, 15 g, and 150 g formulated with 500 nmol IC31 (ClinicalTrials.gov NCT01865487). Safety and immunogenicity is being investigated in a study enrolling individuals who have recently completed a course of treatment for pulmonary TB (ClinicalTrials.gov NCT02375698).

H4:IC31

H4:IC31 (Sanofi Pasteur), is a recombinant fusion protein of Ag85B and TB10.4 coformulated with the adjuvant IC31. In preclinical animal studies the vaccine was well tolerated, induced strong immune responses, and significantly reduced pulmonary bacterial loads in a mouse challenge model compared to unvaccinated mice and mice in which the vaccine antigens were administered individually. In these studies the level of protection from the vaccine was similar to that observed in BCG-vaccinated mice (39). In studies in guinea pigs, boosting BCG with H4:IC31 significantly reduced bacterial loads in the lung and spleen compared to BCG alone (40). A number of safety, immunogenicity, and dose-ranging (antigen and adjuvant) phase 1 studies have been completed in BCG-naive and BCG-vaccinated healthy adults. H4:IC31 was well tolerated with mild to moderate injection site reactions and systemic adverse events. In one study in which a TST was performed to determine *M. tuberculosis* infection status, mild to severe hypersensitivity reactions were observed at the TST injection site following vaccination, even in individuals who were TST-negative. In another study, in which BCG was administered 42 days before H4:IC31 vaccination, no similar severe acute hypersensitivity reactions were noted at the BCG injection site. H4:IC31 elicited antigen-specific polyfunctional CD4 T cell responses, with the highest levels of response noted in the 15-g H4 and 500-nmol IC31 dose regimen, and this combination, administered on two occasions 2 months apart, has been selected for further study (41). An ongoing safety and immunogenicity study to investigate escalating doses of H4:IC31 is being conducted in BCG-primed infants 64 to 196 days of age (ClinicalTrials.gov NCT01861730). A randomized, partially blinded placebo-controlled study to investigate the safety, immunogenicity, and prevention of *M. tuberculosis* infection is ongoing in 990 IGRA-negative adolescents between 12 and 17 years of age randomized to receive H4:IC31; BCG, or placebo

(ClinicalTrials.gov NCT02075203). A phase 1b clinical trial to evaluate the safety and immunogenicity of BCG revaccination, H4:IC31, and H56:IC31 in healthy, IGRA-negative adolescent participants is ongoing (ClinicalTrials.gov NCT02378207). The major goal of this latter study is to generate immunological data on a wide range of immune responses to increase the likelihood of detecting responses correlating with risk or protection in ongoing and planned prevention of infection phase 2 studies.

ID93+GLA-SE

ID93+GLA-SE (Infectious Diseases Research Institute) is a recombinant fusion protein containing four *M. tuberculosis* antigens (Rv2608, Rv3619, Rv3620, and Rv1813) administered with GLA-SE, a glucopyranosyl lipid adjuvant-stable squalene-based oil-in-water emulsion which acts like a Toll-like receptor 4. In a prime-boost guinea pig model, higher ID93+GLA-SE protective efficacy was demonstrated in animals challenged with *M. tuberculosis* which had received BCG followed by ID93+GLA-SE compared to those which had not been vaccinated or those which received only BCG (42). Mice immunized with the ID93+GLA-SE vaccine displayed antigen-specific Th1-type immune responses and upon challenge with *M. tuberculosis* showed significantly lower bacterial burdens in lungs and/or spleens compared with mice injected with saline, antigen alone, or adjuvant alone (42). A phase 1, randomized, double-blind, dose-escalation evaluation of two dose levels of the ID93 antigen administered intramuscularly either alone or in combination with two dose levels of the GLA-SE adjuvant has been completed in 60 HIV-negative, healthy, BCG-naive, and IGRA-negative adults (ClinicalTrials.gov NCT01599897). A phase 1b, randomized, double-blind, placebo-controlled, dose-escalation evaluation of two dose levels of the ID93 antigen administered intramuscularly in combination with two dose levels of the GLA-SE adjuvant is ongoing in 66 HIV-negative, healthy, IGRA-negative or IGRA-positive adults (ClinicalTrials.gov NCT01927159). A phase 2a study to evaluate the safety and immunogenicity of different doses of ID93 and GLA-SE administered to adults with pulmonary TB who have successfully completed TB treatment is ongoing and is being conducted in preparation for a future phase 2b prevention of TB recurrence trial in the same population (ClinicalTrials.gov NCT02465216).

M72/AS01E

M72 (GlaxoSmithKline) is a fusion protein consisting of two *M. tuberculosis* antigens, *MTB*32A and *MTB*39A, and the adjuvant AS01E. AS01E is a liposome-based adjuvant containing MPL, a purified nontoxic endo-toxin derivative which has strong immunostimulatory effects on both cellular and humoral immune responses (43), and QS21, a natural saponin molecule which stimulates TH1-type cell-mediated immunity and cyto-toxic T lymphocyte activity (44). Strong interferon-gamma and antibody responses to both antigens were demonstrated in a mouse challenge model, as was pro-tection following challenge with *M. tuberculosis* com-pared to saline- or adjuvant-injected mice (45). Guinea pigs immunized with M72 had prolonged survival (>1 year) after aerosol challenge with *M. tuberculosis* compared to those that received saline or adjuvant alone, and survival was similar to those that received BCG (45). Coadministration of BCG and rM72F to guinea pigs resulted in significantly prolonged survival times compared to those that received BCG only (46). Cynomolgus monkeys vaccinated with M72-AS02A following vaccination with BCG had strong immu-nogenic responses and a nonsignificant trend toward greater protection from disease compared to those who received BCG alone (47). A number of phase 1 studies with different ASO formulations have been conducted to select the adjuvant (ASO1$_E$) for progression into further studies (48). The safety and immunogenicity of M72/AS01E has been studied in IGRA-negative and IGRA-positive adults, healthy HIV-positive adults on antiretroviral treatment, and healthy adolescents. The vaccine has demonstrated a clinically acceptable safety profile in these populations and induces poly-functional CD4+ T cells (49–53). A study of this vac-cine in adults successfully treated for pulmonary TB or receiving treatment for pulmonary TB was terminated due to a safety signal found at a planned interim safety review (ClinicalTrials.gov NCT01424501). A double-blind, randomized, placebo-controlled, phase 2b effi-cacy study in up to 3,506 IGRA-positive, HIV-negative adults with prevention of pulmonary TB disease as the primary endpoint is ongoing (ClinicalTrials.gov NCT01755598). A substudy is being conducted in parallel to the phase 2b study during which biological samples will be collected for future investigations of biological correlates, markers, or prognostic factors for TB disease (ClinicalTrials.gov NCT02097095).

Viral-Vectored Vaccines
MVA85A
MVA85A (Oxford University) is a subunit viral-vectored vaccine in which a recombinant strain of modified vaccinia virus Ankara is used as a vector for the *M. tuberculosis* antigen 85A. Preclinical studies in

BCG-vaccinated mice, guinea pigs, NHPs, and cattle have demonstrated significant improvement in efficacy in some but not all studies. In mice, boosting of BCG with MVA85A induced significantly higher levels of protection, reduction in bacterial load postchallenge with *M. tuberculosis*, than BCG alone (54). Boosting of BCG with MVA85A in guinea pigs prolonged survival significantly longer than saline controls but not longer than BCG alone, and boosting BCG with MVA85A and a second recombinant viral vector, FP85A, led to a sig-nificant improvement in efficacy compared with BCG alone (55, 56). Intratracheal challenge with *M. tuber-culosis* in NHPs following BCG prime and MVA85A boost was better than BCG alone on all outcome mea-sures in the study (CFU counts, pathology scores, chest X-ray score, and weight loss) (57), but when a simi-lar experiment was conducted using high-dose aerosol challenge there was no difference compared to BCG alone (58). Cattle vaccinated with a BCG prime and MVA85A boost had lower lesion scores and CFU counts than those vaccinated with BCG alone (59).

Safety and immunogenicity has been demonstrated in a number of phase 1 studies which have explored different doses, dose regimens, and routes of admin-istration (intradermal, intramuscular, and aerosol). The populations studied include BCG-naive (60), BCG-vaccinated (60–64), and IGRA-positive adults (65), children, and infants (66–68); HIV-infected adults (69, 70); and HIV and *M. tuberculosis* coinfected indi-viduals (71). In these studies MVA85A has been dem-onstrated to be capable of inducing IFN-γ-producing polyfunctional CD4+ T cells, IFN-γ-producing CD8+ T cells, and expansion of long-lasting memory cell pop-ulations. A phase 2b safety, immunogenicity, and effi-cacy (TB disease and *M. tuberculosis* infection) trial has been completed in South Africa in 2,797 HIV-uninfected, BCG-vaccinated infants aged between 4 and 6 months (20). MVA85A was safe and well tolerated but did not confer additional protection against *M. tuberculosis* in-fection or TB disease compared to BCG alone. It is un-certain what the reason for the lack of efficacy was, but it could, among other reasons, be due to the modest immunological responses demonstrated in infants com-pared to those observed in earlier United Kingdom adult studies or prior BCG vaccination which may have masked an MVA85A effect, or the effect of MVA85A on severe disease was masked in a study which predom-inantly detected mild forms of TB (20). A randomized, placebo-controlled phase 2 safety, immunogenicity, and efficacy (TB disease and *M. tuberculosis* infection) study of MVA85A has been completed in healthy adults infected with HIV-1 (72). This study was designed to enroll 1,400 participants, but following the results of the phase 2 infant study, the sample size was revised to 650 participants, with safety as the primary objective. MVA85A was shown to be well tolerated and immunogenic with immunogenic profiles similar to those observed in previous studies. There was no evidence of efficacy against *M. tuberculosis* infection or disease compared to placebo, but the study was not powered for the endpoint after revision of the sample size.

Continued development of MVA85A includes study of an aerosolized MVA85A formulation in BCG-vaccinated individuals to evaluate whether aerosol administration improves immune responses and avoids antivector immunity (ClinicalTrials.gov NCT01954563) (73). Potent immune responses were observed in the first two participants, and subsequently the MVA85A dose was reduced by an order of magnitude for subsequent volunteers. Aerosolized MVA85A was well tolerated and produced more potent CD4+ T cell responses in blood and lung than those induced by intradermal MVA85A vaccination. Novel prime-boost studies are being conducted in combination with other vaccine candidates. A phase 1 safety and immunogenicity study conducted in adults who received one or two doses of Crucell Ad35 boosted by MVA85A demonstrated that MVA85A boosted both CD4+ and CD8+ T cell responses. As MVA85A primarily stimulates CD4+ T cell responses and Crucell Ad35 stimulates predominantly CD8+ T cell responses, these data suggest that there is some immunological synergy with the combination regimen (74). MVA85A is also currently being evaluated in a phase 1 study in BCG-vaccinated adults as a boost to ChAdOx1.85A, a simian adenovirus-expressing antigen 85A (NCT01829490).

Crucell Ad35

Crucell Ad35 is a replication-deficient adenovirus type 35 vector containing the *M. tuberculosis* antigens 85A, 85B, and TB10.4. The vector was selected due to a low frequency of neutralizing antibodies. The protective ability of the vaccine against intranasal *M. tuberculosis* challenge was studied in two strains of mice following intramuscular and intranasal administration of the vaccine. In both strains the intranasal route provided significant protection (reduced CFUs in lung and spleen and reduced histological lung tissue score) against *M. tuberculosis* compared to BCG. However, following intramuscular injection significant protection was observed only in one strain (75). Aerosol vaccination of NHPs with Crucell Ad35 elicited robust pulmonary cellular immune responses, but there was no evidence of protection against aerosol challenge with high-dose

M. tuberculosis (76). A number of phase 1 safety and immunogenicity studies of healthy adults which have included BCG-naive, BCG-vaccinated, IGRA-negative, and IGRA-positive populations investigating a variety of doses and dosing regimens have been completed, and the vaccine was demonstrated to be well tolerated and immunogenic with robust polyfunctional CD4+ T cell and CD8+ T cell responses (74, 77, 78). The vaccine was well tolerated and immunogenic in a phase 2 study in HIV-positive participants with CD4 counts of >350/ml^3, did not appear to influence CD4 counts or HIV load over the course of the study, and induced predominantly polyfunctional CD4+ and CD8+ T cell responses to vaccine (79). A phase 1 randomized, double-blind, placebo-controlled, dose-escalation study was conducted in BCG-vaccinated infants aged 6 to 9 months and was well tolerated and induced a specific T cell response (80).

A planned phase 2b randomized, placebo-controlled, dose-finding, safety and immunogenicity, and efficacy study in healthy infants aged 16 to 26 weeks was amended to exclude efficacy from the objectives due to lower than expected immune responses to the vaccine. The vaccine was well tolerated with one reported serious adverse event of tachypnea which was considered to be related to study vaccine. Lower-magnitude CD4+ and CD8+ polyfunctional T cell responses were observed at all dose levels compared to responses seen in adults; the addition of a third dose to the two-dose regimen at the highest dose level did not increase the magnitude of the responses (80).

Ad5Ag85A

Ad5Ag85A (McMaster) is composed of a replication-deficient serotype 5 adenoviral vector expressing the *M. tuberculosis* antigen 85A. Intranasal administration but not intramuscular delivery of the vaccine demonstrated increased protection against *M. tuberculosis* aerosol challenge compared to subcutaneously administered BCG, and enhanced protection was evident when the vaccine was given as a boost to BCG in both mice and guinea pigs (81–83). The vaccine was well tolerated and immunogenic in a phase 1 safety and immunogenicity study in BCG-naive and BCG-vaccinated healthy adults. Polyfunctional CD4+ and CD8+ T cells were boosted more potently in BCG-vaccinated individuals (84). Concerns have been raised about using Ad5 as a vaccine vector due to the high prevalence of preexisting serotype 5 adenovirus-neutralizing antibodies, but in this small study there was little evidence that preexisting immunity dampened the vaccine immune response (84).

TB/Flu-04L

TB/Flu-04L (Research Institute of Influenza, Saint Petersburg, Russia) is a live attenuated influenza A virus vector containing the *M. tuberculosis* antigens ESAT-6 and Ag85A. Preclinical studies, including NHPs, have demonstrated the vaccine to be safe and immunogenic and to provide greater protective efficacy than BCG in mice and guinea pigs following intranasal administration (85). A phase 1 randomized, double-blind, placebo-controlled study has been conducted on 36 previously BCG-vaccinated, IGRA-negative, healthy volunteers who received two intranasal doses of TB/Flu-04L 21 days apart (ClinicalTrials.gov NCT02501421). In this study TB/Flu-04L had an acceptable safety profile not appreciably different from placebo and with no vaccine-related serious adverse events. Influenza virus-specific RNA, but no infectious virus, was detected in nasal swabs on day 2 in 5/18 (13.9%) TB/Flu-04L volunteers and in no volunteers on day 3 or day 5 post-vaccination, suggesting that shedding of this attenuated virus is unlikely to occur. Immunogenicity was evaluated by assaying nasal cytokines in nasal secretions obtained prior to vaccination and 24 and 48 hours post-vaccination, and by intracellular cytokine staining in whole blood. Vaccination induced local innate immune responses and CD4+ and CD8+ IFN-γ responses to both antigens. There was a detectable increase in antibody to influenza A virus postvaccination (85). A phase 2a clinical trial is planned in IGRA-positive individuals.

Inactivated Whole-Cell and Fragmented TB Vaccines

DAR-901

DAR-901 (Dartmouth University) is a heat-inactivated vaccine derived from an environmental nontuberculous mycobacterium, *Mycobacterium obuense*. SRL-172, a vaccine closely related to DAR-901, differing only in a change in the method of production, has been extensively studied. Randomized, double-blind, controlled immunotherapeutic studies have produced variable results. Positive outcomes with faster bacteriological and radiological improvement have been reported in two studies (86, 87), while there was no difference in outcome compared to placebo in another study (88). SRL-72 demonstrated a vaccine efficacy of 39% against definite TB, defined as culture-positive disease, compared to placebo in a 2013 participant phase 3 efficacy trial (89). DAR-901 is now being developed as a prophylactic vaccine. A placebo-controlled phase 1 study is ongoing to compare the safety and immunogenicity of DAR-901 to BCG (ClinicalTrials.gov NCT02063555).

Vaccae

An inactivated whole-cell strain of *M. vaccae*, dubbed Vaccae, has been studied for many years as a potential immunotherapeutic agent for the treatment of TB. A meta-analysis of 54 studies in which *M. vaccae* was administered with or without a placebo control concluded that sputum conversion, at month 2 of treatment but not at the end of treatment, and X-ray appearance were improved when *M. vaccae* was administered to patients who had not previously been treated for TB (29). A 10,000-participant phase 3 randomized, placebo-controlled, double-blind study, sponsored by Anhui Zhifei Longcom Biologic Pharmacy Co., Ltd., is ongoing in China in IGRA-positive individuals aged 16 to 65 using a six-dose regimen with doses administered 2 weeks apart to determine efficacy in preventing TB disease (ClinicalTrials.gov NCT01979900).

RUTI

RUTI (Archivel Farma SL) is a therapeutic TB vaccine candidate based on fragmented and detoxified cellular fragments of *M. tuberculosis* contained within liposomes. Protective efficacy has been demonstrated in guinea pig and mouse models of TB in conjunction with short-course chemotherapy (90). A double-blind, placebo-controlled, randomized safety and immunogenicity study of four increasing doses (5, 25, 100, and 200 g) of RUTI has been completed in 24 healthy, non-BCG-vaccinated, IGRA-negative volunteers. Two doses of vaccine 28 days apart were administered to each volunteer. The vaccine was well tolerated with local, generally mild, adverse events reported more frequently in participants receiving RUTI compared to placebo, and these reactions were observed to be dose related (91). A phase 2 study has been conducted in 48 HIV-negative and 47 HIV-positive IGRA- and TST-positive participants who were given two doses of vaccine or placebo starting after 1 month of isoniazid to compare the safety and immunogenicity of three doses of vaccine (5, 25, and 50 g) and placebo. The immunogenicity profile suggested that future studies should be conducted using only a single administration of one of the higher doses. RUTI was generally well tolerated, although local reactogenicity was marked, and drainage of abscesses was required in four participants (92).

Recombinant Mycobacterial Vaccines

MTBVAC

MTBVAC (University of Zaragoza and Biofabri) is the first live attenuated *M. tuberculosis* vaccine to enter clinical trials. It is a recombinant *M. tuberculosis* strain that lacks the genes *phoP*, which codes for a transcription factor key for the regulation of *M. tuberculosis* virulence, and *fadD26*, which is essential for the synthesis of the complex lipid phthiocerol dimycocerosate, a major mycobacterial virulence factor (93). Genomic comparison of BCG with *M. tuberculosis* clinical isolates shows that several major antigens and human T cell epitopes are missing from BCG. MTBVAC contains all the genes present in BCG vaccine together with the genes deleted from *Mycobacterium bovis* and therefore presents a wider collection of mycobacterial antigens to the host immune system than BCG (93). MTBVAC demonstrated a safety profile comparable to BCG in mice and significantly greater protective efficacy, as measured by reduction in CFUs in both lung and spleen, compared to BCG in mice vaccinated with MTBVAC or BCG prior to intranasal challenge with virulent *M. tuberculosis* (93). The vaccine candidate is being developed as a BCG replacement. A phase 1 dose escalation study in IGRA-negative adults comparing three doses of MTBVAC (5×10^3 CFU, 5×10^4 CFU, 5×10^5 CFU) to BCG (5×10^5 CFU) demonstrated that MTBVAC had comparable safety and was at least as immunogenic as BCG (24).

VPM 1002

VPM 1002 (Vakzine Projekt Management GmbH) is a recombinant BCG mutant that expresses listeriolysin O, a virulence factor from *Listeria monocytogenes*, which mediates the perforation of the phagosome membrane, allowing the egress of recombinant BCG antigens to the cytosol and thereby facilitating CD8+ T cell priming (94). The vaccine is being developed as a BCG replacement. VPM 1002 protected mice against *M. tuberculosis* aerosol challenge significantly better than BCG (95). Administration of the vaccine to SCID mice, at doses higher than the target human dose, demonstrated that the safety profile of VPM 1002 was indistinguishable from BCG and normal saline (94). As the target population is BCG replacement in neonates, a preclinical study in newborn rabbits was conducted and demonstrated that VPM 1002 did not disseminate for up to 90 days after vaccination (94). Two phase 1 studies have been completed, and VPM 1002 was well tolerated and immunogenic in vaccinated participants (23, 94). A phase 2 study of HIV-unexposed, BCG-naive newborn infants has been completed and demonstrated that VPM 1002 is at least as safe as BCG (94). A phase 2 double-blind, randomized, controlled study to evaluate the safety and immunogenicity of VPM 1002 compared with BCG is currently ongoing in up

to 416 HIV-exposed and HIV-unexposed, BCG-naive newborn infants (ClinicalTrials.gov NCT02391415).

THE ROLE OF EXPERIMENTAL MEDICINE IN TB VACCINE DEVELOPMENT

In the absence of defined and validated immunological correlates of protection, and coupled with the fact that the predictive value of the preclinical TB animal models for human efficacy is uncertain, TB vaccine development is a risky and expensive business. The failure of MVA85A, one of the most advanced TB vaccine candidates in clinical development, to confer protection in either BCG-vaccinated infants or in HIV-infected adults, has highlighted how difficult vaccine development and vaccine selection is (19, 20). While the presence of the current TB vaccine pipeline described above, with several candidate vaccines currently being tested in early-stage studies, is a welcome improvement on the situation in 2001, when there were no candidate TB vaccines in clinical development, it will never be possible to evaluate all these candidates in expensive and time-consuming human efficacy trials. There is an urgent need for better models, and better clinical models, with which we can rationally select which vaccines should progress to efficacy testing. Experimental Medicine describes a paradigm whereby novel concepts are tested in humans within a clinical trial. Experimental Medicine can be defined as "investigation undertaken in humans, relating where appropriate to model systems, to identify mechanisms of pathophysiology or disease, or to demonstrate proof-of-concept evidence of the validity and importance of new discoveries or treatments" (96). Such studies are usually small scale and often first time in humans. However, Experimental Medicine studies need not be limited to small-scale phase 1 studies and can include, for example, proof-of-concept efficacy studies. These studies can also be combined with, or lead to, further clinical trials within a more conventional product development setting. The primary role of Experimental Medicine studies is to further scientific understanding, in contrast to product development, where the primary aim is the development of the product being tested.

There are several ways in which an Experimental Medicine approach may help reduce the risk of early-stage clinical development. Such an approach allows proof-of-concept testing in the target species, humans. This is important given the myriad ways in which animal, particularly murine, and human immunity differ. Experimental Medicine allows hypotheses concerning vaccine development to be tested which will inform whether products that induce similar immunologic responses are worthy of further development. One can test whether potentially protective immune mechanisms observed in animal models can similarly be induced in humans. Such an approach allows the identification and refinement of criteria by which vaccine selection is conducted, either for very specific products or for a more global class of candidates. This ability would potentially help reduce the risk of clinical development by shifting the risk curve to the left, i.e., to earlier-stage clinical trials. Given that the disproportionate burden of cost for TB vaccine development is in efficacy testing, such an approach would potentially allow decision making at an earlier stage of investment. Furthermore, an Experimental Medicine approach would allow mechanistic insights and understanding and may generate critical human samples for the development of assays needed to further vaccine development. An important additional component of this paradigm is that it facilitates the identification of best-in-class candidates by head-to-head comparative testing.

The Difference between Experimental Medicine and Product Development

To a certain extent, the distinction between Experimental Medicine and Product Development is artificial. Any particular clinical study or trial could potentially address an Experimental Medicine question and also fulfill a product development focus. Experimental Medicine may use product candidates or nonproduct candidates as well as licensed products (e.g., BCG), depending on the question being addressed and the availability of material manufactured under good manufacturing practices (GMPs). In such trials, a candidate vaccine being tested may or may not be in current clinical development, because there may be reasons why a particular candidate, which belongs to a particular class of vaccine or induces a particular immunological profile, may need to be tested for proof of concept, even if that particular candidate is not in clinical development at the time. A candidate vaccine could move between the two categories of Experimental Medicine and Product Development depending on the results of such trials. Products for which further development is not indicated can still be useful to test hypotheses or be used as probes in Experimental Medicine studies to add to the body of knowledge about that class of product. Given the number of candidate vaccines that have been manufactured under GMP conditions and evaluated in clinical trials since 2002, it is important to utilize and exploit available material where possible to minimize new manufacturing costs.

Potential Users of an Experimental Medicine Strategy

There are multiple potential users of an Experimental Medicine strategy. These include TB vaccine researchers, TB vaccine developers, and funders and sponsors of TB vaccine research. Given the potential scientific benefits of an Experimental Medicine approach to TB vaccine development, it may be necessary to create incentives, because not all vaccine developers may be interested in their vaccine and GMP material being utilized in an Experimental Medicine study. Additional funding should be provided to facilitate this if there are Experimental Medicine questions that can be addressed in an "added-value" way within an ongoing or planned clinical trial. If a candidate vaccine is being used, then it is important to be clear which aspect of the trial may or may not inform the development of the candidate actually being used. It should also be clear that Experimental Medicine questions concerning TB vaccine development, such as dose, route of delivery, and the nature of immune responses, may be answered by using vaccines from other fields and not just candidate TB vaccines.

Potential Outcomes in Experimental Medicine Studies

There are many potential outcomes in TB vaccine Experimental Medicine studies. Proof-of-concept safety studies might be conducted for novel classes of vaccine; novel routes of immunization, e.g., aerosol; high-risk target populations, e.g., latent *M. tuberculosis* infection; HIV; and head-to-head safety comparisons with different candidate vaccines. As part of these safety studies, or as separate studies, immunogenicity and biomarker studies might be conducted with novel classes of vaccine, e.g., CD1-restricted and other nonconventional *M. tuberculosis* antigens; novel routes of immunization, e.g., aerosol, new combinations of vaccines, and prime boost strategies; and comparison with parallel NHP immunogenicity and challenge experiments. *In vitro* mycobacterial growth inhibition assays and other relevant candidate functional assays can be evaluated in an Experimental Medicine context, with blood, cells, and serum from vaccinated subjects. Furthermore, leukophoresis studies can be conducted to generate large volumes of material for very detailed immunogenicity studies. Smaller-scale, intensive (detailed) longitudinal analyses can also be conducted to capture early and late immune responses, because durability of immunity, and therefore protection, is a critical component of a TB vaccine. As above with safety, an important component of proof-of-concept immunogenicity studies is the potential to conduct head-to-head immunogenicity comparisons with different candidate vaccines. Given the large and increasing number of candidates in phase 1/2a testing, such an approach will increasingly be necessary to allow the selection of the candidate most likely to be efficacious in efficacy testing.

Experimental Medicine studies do not always have to be small. Proof-of-concept efficacy studies might be conducted, for example, on prevention of TB disease in selected high-incidence study populations or evaluation of potential surrogate endpoints, such as IGRA conversion or transcriptomic signatures of risk for TB disease. Such proof-of-concept efficacy trials also create the potential to conduct immune correlate studies to identify immune correlates, and even if such trials do not demonstrate efficacy, correlate samples can still be utilized for correlate of risk analyses.

Controlled Human Challenge Models

Human challenge models are an example of Experimental Medicine studies and have played an essential role in vaccine development for malaria, influenza, typhoid, etc. (97–99). The development of a human mycobacterial challenge model would greatly facilitate TB vaccine development by allowing the demonstration of proof-of-concept efficacy in a small challenge study before progressing to large field efficacy trials. Such a model could not use virulent *M. tuberculosis*, for obvious ethical reasons, but could potentially use attenuated strains of *M. tuberculosis* which had been rendered safe for human use. One pragmatic approach to such a model has been to utilize BCG, an attenuated but replicating strain of *M. bovis* which is licensed for human use. Two human Experimental Medicine studies have demonstrated that prior BCG vaccination can confer some protection against subsequent BCG challenge in a population which BCG is known to protect (100, 101). These data provide important biological validation that such a model may be useful in the evaluation of candidate TB vaccines. To date, the development of a BCG challenge model has utilized an intradermal route of challenge, which is the licensed route of delivery of BCG. However, the natural route of exposure to *M. tuberculosis* is by aerosol, and further studies to evaluate the safety and tolerability of an aerosol BCG challenge are planned.

There are other limitations of BCG as a challenge organism within a human mycobacterial challenge model. A BCG challenge would not be appropriate to evaluate the potential efficacy of any vaccine containing the region of difference-1 antigens not present in BCG, e.g., the hybrid I fusion protein ESAT6 and Ag85B (34). The development of attenuated strains

of *M. tuberculosis*, which would be safe for human challenge, are currently being developed. Furthermore, the labeling of such strains may increase the utility and predictive power of a challenge model by allowing repeated, noninvasive measurements of mycobacterial load. Once developed, a mycobacterial challenge model would ultimately need validating against field efficacy trials. While it would never be possible to validate against human virulent *M. tuberculosis* challenge, this validation against virulent mycobacterial challenge is possible in preclinical animal models. Studies of mice and cattle have demonstrated that BCG vaccination confers similar levels of protection against BCG challenge compared with known levels of efficacy against virulent *M. tuberculosis*/*M. bovis* challenge (102, 103).

One further use of a human challenge model would be in the identification of potential immune correlates of protection, which can again be validated, both in preclinical animal challenge studies and ultimately in field efficacy studies.

Examples of Experimental Medicine

Some examples of Experimental Medicine studies include the use of aerosol BCG or recombinant BCG vaccine candidates to define key lung immunologic measures; the use of DNA or RNA to understand the immunogenicity of subdominant or poorly recognized epitopes; the use of aerosol MVA85A, adenovirus, BCG, or other vectors to understand the risk of using vectors or antigens delivered into the lung in *M. tuberculosis* infected subjects; the use of one adenovirus (+/− MVA prime-boost regimen) to optimize vaccine kinetics, dose, and route; and the formulation of a specific adjuvant combined with different antigens to better understand the function of adjuvant and prioritize antigens. Intensive immunogenicity studies can be conducted with a particular class of vaccine (for example, days 0, 1, 2, 3, 5, 7, 14) to define the best timing for drawing RNA and other samples in larger trials, and leukopheresis studies with BCG and/or a new class of vaccine can be conducted to generate 200 peripheral blood mononuclear cell samples per time point for intensive study of new immunologic reagents, assays, or techniques.

The Role of Preclinical Studies in Experimental Medicine Studies

There are many reasons why conducting parallel preclinical studies alongside human Experimental Medicine studies adds value to both studies. Such an approach allows the use of appropriate animal models to maximize the relevance of information to human vaccine development. One example is bridging between clinical immunogenicity and preclinical immunogenicity, which facilitates meaningful interpretation of the relevance of preclinical efficacy to human efficacy. Such parallel studies can also be used to identify candidate biomarkers of protection which can then be evaluated in clinical studies (product development and Experimental Medicine). To exploit the maximum potential from this approach, preclinical and clinical studies need to be performed with parallel study designs to maximize the ability to bridge between species. It is particularly important for studies of NHPs to feed back into and optimally inform further clinical testing and development. It is also important to recognize that data arising from human Experimental Medicine studies can also inform preclinical studies.

The Added Value of Experimental Medicine for Funders and for the Scientific Community

Given the many scientific uncertainties and unknowns within the field of TB vaccine development, an Experimental Medicine approach offers an opportunity to potentially shift the development risk curve to the left, i.e., to facilitate vaccine selection at an earlier stage of investment and development. This approach would facilitate the refining of stage gating criteria for vaccine selection, which, together with portfolio management, will increasingly be a necessary approach for the global TB vaccine community. This will allow the determination, in a proof-of-concept setting, of whether candidate immune responses can be induced; will allow studies to optimize dose, route, and regimen; will allow assay evaluation versus clinical parameters; and will allow the identification of candidate biomarkers to facilitate vaccine development. Ultimately, an Experimental Medicine approach to TB vaccine development has the potential to increase the chances of success in efficacy trials. To retain the momentum gained in the field over the last decade, it is essential that this potential be evaluated. A coordinated and harmonized approach is critical to ensuring the maximum generation of knowledge from all clinical trials, which has the potential to benefit the field and expedite the ultimate development of an effective TB vaccine regimen.

Citation. Hatherill M, Tait D, McShane H. 2016. Clinical testing of tuberculosis vaccine candidates. Microbiol Spectrum 4(5):TBTB2-0015-2016.

References

1. Zwerling A, Behr MA, Verma A, Brewer TF, Menzies D, Pai M. 2011. The BCG World Atlas: a database of global BCG vaccination policies and practices. *PLoS Med* 8: e1001012.

2. Marais BJ, Gie RP, Schaaf HS, Hesseling AC, Obihara CC, Starke JJ, Enarson DA, Donald PR, Beyers N. 2004. The natural history of childhood intra-thoracic tuberculosis: a critical review of literature from the pre-chemotherapy era. *Int J Tuberc Lung Dis* 8:392–402.

3. Colditz GA, Berkey CS, Mosteller F, Brewer TF, Wilson ME, Burdick E, Fineberg HV. 1995. The efficacy of bacillus Calmette-Guérin vaccination of newborns and infants in the prevention of tuberculosis: meta-analyses of the published literature. *Pediatrics* 96:29–35.

4. Roy A, Eisenhut M, Harris RJ, Rodrigues LC, Sridhar S, Habermann S, Snell L, Mangtani P, Adetifa I, Lalvani A, Abubakar I. 2014. Effect of BCG vaccination against *Mycobacterium tuberculosis* infection in children: systematic review and meta-analysis. *BMJ* 349:g4643.

5. Mahomed H, Hughes EJ, Hawkridge T, Minnies D, Simon E, Little F, Hanekom WA, Geiter L, Hussey GD. 2006. Comparison of mantoux skin test with three generations of a whole blood IFN-gamma assay for tuberculosis infection. *Int J Tuberc Lung Dis* 10:310–316.

6. Mahomed H, Hawkridge T, Verver S, Abrahams D, Geiter L, Hatherill M, Ehrlich R, Hanekom WA, Hussey GD. 2011. The tuberculin skin test versus QuantiFERON TB Gold in predicting tuberculosis disease in an adolescent cohort study in South Africa. *PLoS One* 6:e17984. (Erratum, 6:6)

7. Andrews JR, Hatherill M, Mahomed H, Hanekom WA, Campo M, Hawn TR, Wood R, Scriba TJ. 2015. The dynamics of QuantiFERON-TB gold in-tube conversion and reversion in a cohort of South African adolescents. *Am J Respir Crit Care Med* 191:584–591.

8. WHO. 2015. *Global Tuberculosis Control Report.* http://www.who.int/tb/publications/global_report/en/.

9. Ellis RD, Hatherill M, Tait D, Snowden M, Churchyard G, Hanekom W, Evans T, Ginsberg AM. 2015. Innovative clinical trial designs to rationalize TB vaccine development. *Tuberculosis (Edinb)* 95:352–357.

10. Mahomed H, Hawkridge T, Verver S, Geiter L, Hatherill M, Abrahams DA, Ehrlich R, Hanekom WA, Hussey GD, Team SAS, SATVI Adolescent Study Team. 2011. Predictive factors for latent tuberculosis infection among adolescents in a high-burden area in South Africa. *Int J Tuberc Lung Dis* 15:331–336.

11. Hawn TR, Day TA, Scriba TJ, Hatherill M, Hanekom WA, Evans TG, Churchyard GJ, Kublin JG, Bekker LG, Self SG. 2014. Tuberculosis vaccines and prevention of infection. *Microbiol Mol Biol Rev* 78:650–671.

12. Orme IM. 2014. Vaccines to prevent tuberculosis infection rather than disease: physiological and immunological aspects. *Tuberculosis (Edinb)* S1472-9792(14)20550-6.

13. Dharmadhikari AS, Basaraba RJ, Van Der Walt ML, Weyer K, Mphahlele M, Venter K, Jensen PA, First MW, Parsons S, McMurray DN, Orme IM, Nardell EA. 2011. Natural infection of guinea pigs exposed to patients with highly drug-resistant tuberculosis. *Tuberculosis (Edinb)* 91:329–338.

14. Bjartveit K. 2003. Olaf Scheel and Johannes Heimbeck: their contribution to understanding the pathogenesis and prevention of tuberculosis. *Int J Tuberc Lung Dis* 7: 306–311.

15. Andrews JR, Noubary F, Walensky RP, Cerda R, Losina E, Horsburgh CR. 2012. Risk of progression to active tuberculosis following reinfection with *Mycobacterium tuberculosis*. *Clin Infect Dis* **54**:784–791.

16. Machingaidze S, Verver S, Mulenga H, Abrahams DA, Hatherill M, Hanekom W, Hussey GD, Mahomed H. 2012. Predictive value of recent QuantiFERON conversion for tuberculosis disease in adolescents. *Am J Respir Crit Care Med* **186**:1051–1056.

17. Dahlstrom A. 1940. The instabiity of the tuberculin reaction. *Am Rev Tuberc* **42**:471–487.

18. Michelsen SW, Soborg B, Koch A, Carstensen L, Hoff ST, Agger EM, Lillebaek T, Sorensen HC, Wohlfahrt J, Melbye M. 2014. The effectiveness of BCG vaccination in preventing *Mycobacterium tuberculosis* infection and disease in Greenland. *Thorax* **69**:851–856.

19. Zwerling A, Benedetti A, Cojocariu M, McIntosh F, Pietrangelo F, Behr MA, Schwartzman K, Menzies D, Pai M. 2013. Repeat IGRA testing in Canadian health workers: conversions or unexplained variability? *PLoS One* **8**:e54748.

20. Tameris MD, Hatherill M, Landry BS, Scriba TJ, Snowden MA, Lockhart S, Shea JE, McClain JB, Hussey GD, Hanekom WA, Mahomed H, McShane H, MVA85A 020 Trial Study Team. 2013. Safety and efficacy of MVA85A, a new tuberculosis vaccine, in infants previously vaccinated with BCG: a randomised, placebo-controlled phase 2b trial. *Lancet* **381**:1021–1028.

21. Knight GM, Griffiths UK, Sumner T, Laurence YV, Gheorghe A, Vassall A, Glaziou P, White RG. 2014. Impact and cost-effectiveness of new tuberculosis vaccines in low- and middle-income countries. *Proc Natl Acad Sci USA* **111**:15520–15525.

22. Mangtani P, Abubakar I, Ariti C, Beynon R, Pimpin L, Fine PE, Rodrigues LC, Smith PG, Lipman M, Whiting PF, Sterne JA. 2014. Protection by BCG vaccine against tuberculosis: a systematic review of randomized controlled trials. *Clin Infect Dis* **58**:470–480.

23. Grode L, Ganoza CA, Brohm C, Weiner J III, Eisele B, Kaufmann SH. 2013. Safety and immunogenicity of the recombinant BCG vaccine VPM1002 in a phase 1 open-label randomized clinical trial. *Vaccine* **31**:1340–1348.

24. Spertini F, Audran R, Chakour R, Karoui O, Steiner-Monard V, Thierry AC, Mayor CE, Rettby N, Jaton K, Vallotton L, Lazor-Blanchet C, Doce J, Puentes E, Marinova D, Aguilo N, Martin C. 2015. Safety of human immunisation with a live-attenuated *Mycobacterium tuberculosis* vaccine: a randomised, double-blind, controlled phase I trial. *Lancet Respir Med* **3**:953–962.

25. Nunn AJ, Phillips PP, Mitchison DA. 2010. Timing of relapse in short-course chemotherapy trials for tuberculosis. *Int J Tuberc Lung Dis* **14**:241–242.

26. Gillespie SH, Crook AM, McHugh TD, Mendel CM, Meredith SK, Murray SR, Pappas F, Phillips PP, Nunn AJ, REMoxTB Consortium. 2014. Four-month moxifloxacin-based regimens for drug-sensitive tuberculosis. *N Engl J Med* **371**:1577–1587.

27. Coler RN, Bertholet S, Pine SO, Orr MT, Reese V, Windish HP, Davis C, Kahn M, Baldwin SL, Reed SG. 2013. Therapeutic immunization against *Mycobacterium tuberculosis* is an effective adjunct to antibiotic treatment. *J Infect Dis* **207**:1242–1252 10.1093/infdis/jis425.

28. Lin PL, Dietrich J, Tan E, Abalos RM, Burgos J, Bigbee C, Bigbee M, Milk L, Gideon HP, Rodgers M, Cochran C, Guinn KM, Sherman DR, Klein E, Janssen C, Flynn JL, Andersen P. 2012. The multistage vaccine H56 boosts the effects of BCG to protect cynomolgus macaques against active tuberculosis and reactivation of latent *Mycobacterium tuberculosis* infection. *J Clin Invest* **122**:303–314.

29. Yang XY, Chen QF, Li YP, Wu SM. 2011. *Mycobacterium vaccae* as adjuvant therapy to anti-tuberculosis chemotherapy in never-treated tuberculosis patients: a meta-analysis. *PLoS One* **6**:e23826.

30. WHO. 2015. *The end TB strategy*. http://www.who.int/tb/post2015_TBstrategy.pdf.

31. Plotkin SA. 2008. Vaccines: correlates of vaccine-induced immunity. *Clin Infect Dis* **47**:401–409.

32. Ottenhoff TH, Kumararatne D, Casanova JL. 1998. Novel human immunodeficiencies reveal the essential role of type-I cytokines in immunity to intracellular bacteria. *Immunol Today* **19**:491–494.

33. Kagina BM, Abel B, Scriba TJ, Hughes EJ, Keyser A, Soares A, Gamieldien H, Sidibana M, Hatherill M, Gelderbloem S, Mahomed H, Hawkridge A, Hussey G, Kaplan G, Hanekom WA, other members of the South African Tuberculosis Vaccine Initiative. 2010. Specific T cell frequency and cytokine expression profile do not correlate with protection against tuberculosis after bacillus Calmette-Guérin vaccination of newborns. *Am J Respir Crit Care Med* **182**:1073–1079.

34. van Dissel JT, Arend SM, Prins C, Bang P, Tingskov PN, Lingnau K, Nouta J, Klein MR, Rosenkrands I, Ottenhoff TH, Kromann I, Doherty TM, Andersen P. 2010. Ag85B-ESAT-6 adjuvanted with IC31 promotes strong and long-lived *Mycobacterium tuberculosis* specific T cell responses in naïve human volunteers. *Vaccine* **28**:3571–3581.

35. Ottenhoff TH, Doherty TM, van Dissel JT, Bang P, Lingnau K, Kromann I, Andersen P. 2010. First in humans: a new molecularly defined vaccine shows excellent safety and strong induction of long-lived *Mycobacterium tuberculosis*-specific Th1-cell like responses. *Hum Vaccin* **6**:1007–1015.

36. van Dissel JT, Joosten SA, Hoff ST, Soonawala D, Prins C, Hokey DA, O'Dee DM, Graves A, Thierry-Carstensen B, Andreasen LV, Ruhwald M, de Visser AW, Agger EM, Ottenhoff TH, Kromann I, Andersen P. 2014. A novel liposomal adjuvant system, CAF01, promotes long-lived *Mycobacterium tuberculosis*-specific T-cell responses in human. *Vaccine* **32**:7098–7107.

37. Aagaard C, Hoang T, Dietrich J, Cardona PJ, Izzo A, Dolganov G, Schoolnik GK, Cassidy JP, Billeskov R, Andersen P. 2011. A multistage tuberculosis vaccine that confers efficient protection before and after exposure. *Nat Med* **17**:189–194.

38. Luabeya AK, Kagina BM, Tameris MD, Geldenhuys H, Hoff ST, Shi Z, Kromann I, Hatherill M, Mahomed H, Hanekom WA, Andersen P, Scriba TJ, Schoeman E, Krohn C, Day CL, Africa H, Makhethe L, Smit E,

Brown Y, Suliman S, Hughes EJ, Bang P, Snowden MA, McClain B, Hussey GD, H56-032 Trial Study Group. 2015. First-in-human trial of the post-exposure tuberculosis vaccine H56:IC31 in *Mycobacterium tuberculosis* infected and non-infected healthy adults. *Vaccine* 33: 4130–4140.

39. Dietrich J, Aagaard C, Leah R, Olsen AW, Stryhn A, Doherty TM, Andersen P. 2005. Exchanging ESAT6 with TB10.4 in an Ag85B fusion molecule-based tuberculosis subunit vaccine: efficient protection and ESAT6-based sensitive monitoring of vaccine efficacy. *J Immunol* 174: 6332–6339.

40. Billeskov R, Elvang TT, Andersen PL, Dietrich J. 2012. The HyVac4 subunit vaccine efficiently boosts BCG-primed anti-mycobacterial protective immunity. *PLoS One* 7:e39909.

41. Shi Z, Ginsberg A, Hockey D, Ishmukhamedov S, Kromann I, Hoff S, Andersen P, de Bruyn G. 2015. H4: IC31 as a booster vaccine to BCG: results of four phase 1 trials. Poster presentation, TB Vaccines 4th Global Forum; Shanghai, China.

42. Bertholet S, Ireton GC, Ordway DJ, Windish HP, Pine SO, Kahn M, Phan T, Orme IM, Vedvick TS, Baldwin SL, Coler RN, Reed SG. 2010. A defined tuberculosis vaccine candidate boosts BCG and protects against multidrug-resistant *Mycobacterium tuberculosis*. *Sci Transl Med* 2:53ra74.

43. Garçon N, Chomez P, Van Mechelen M. 2007. Glaxo SmithKline Adjuvant Systems in vaccines: concepts, achievements and perspectives. *Expert Rev Vaccines* 6: 723–739.

44. Campbell JB, Peerbaye YA. 1992. Saponin. *Res Immunol* 143:526–530; discussion 577–528.

45. Skeiky YA, Alderson MR, Ovendale PJ, Guderian JA, Brandt L, Dillon DC, Campos-Neto A, Lobet Y, Dalemans W, Orme IM, Reed SG. 2004. Differential immune responses and protective efficacy induced by components of a tuberculosis polyprotein vaccine, Mtb72F, delivered as naked DNA or recombinant protein. *J Immunol* 172: 7618–7628.

46. Brandt L, Skeiky YA, Alderson MR, Lobet Y, Dalemans W, Turner OC, Basaraba RJ, Izzo AA, Lasco TM, Chapman PL, Reed SG, Orme IM. 2004. The protective effect of the *Mycobacterium bovis* BCG vaccine is increased by coadministration with the *Mycobacterium tuberculosis* 72-kilodalton fusion polyprotein Mtb72F in *M. tuberculosis*-infected guinea pigs. *Infect Immun* 72:6622–6632.

47. Reed SG, Coler RN, Dalemans W, Tan EV, DeLa Cruz EC, Basaraba RJ, Orme IM, Skeiky YA, Alderson MR, Cowgill KD, Prieels JP, Abalos RM, Dubois MC, Cohen J, Mettens P, Lobet Y. 2009. Defined tuberculosis vaccine, Mtb72F/AS02A, evidence of protection in cynomolgus monkeys. *Proc Natl Acad Sci USA* 106: 2301–2306.

48. Leroux-Roels I, Forgus S, De Boever F, Clement F, Demoitié MA, Mettens P, Moris P, Ledent E, Leroux-Roels G, Ofori-Anyinam O, M72 Study Group. 2013. Improved CD4+ T cell responses to *Mycobacterium tuberculosis* in PPD-negative adults by M72/AS01 as

compared to the M72/AS02 and Mtb72F/AS02 tuberculosis candidate vaccine formulations: a randomized trial. *Vaccine* 31:2196–2206.

49. Spertini F, Audran R, Lurati F, Ofori-Anyinam O, Zysset F, Vandepapelière P, Moris P, Demoitié MA, Mettens P, Vinals C, Vastiau I, Jongert E, Cohen J, Ballou WR. 2013. The candidate tuberculosis vaccine Mtb72F/AS02 in PPD positive adults: a randomized controlled phase I/II study. *Tuberculosis (Edinb)* 93:179–188.

50. Montoya J, Solon JA, Cunanan SR, Acosta L, Bollaerts A, Moris P, Janssens M, Jongert E, Demoitié MA, Mettens P, Gatchalian S, Vinals C, Cohen J, Ofori-Anyinam O. 2013. A randomized, controlled dose-finding phase II study of the M72/AS01 candidate tuberculosis vaccine in healthy PPD-positive adults. *J Clin Immunol* 33:1360–1375.

51. Day CL, Tameris M, Mansoor N, van Rooyen M, de Kock M, Geldenhuys H, Erasmus M, Makhethe L, Hughes EJ, Gelderbloem S, Bollaerts A, Bourguignon P, Cohen J, Demoitié MA, Mettens P, Moris P, Sadoff JC, Hawkridge A, Hussey GD, Mahomed H, Ofori-Anyinam O, Hanekom WA. 2013. Induction and regulation of T-cell immunity by the novel tuberculosis vaccine M72/AS01 in South African adults. *Am J Respir Crit Care Med* 188:492–502.

52. Penn-Nicholson A, Geldenhuys H, Burny W, van der Most R, Day CL, Jongert E, Moris P, Hatherill M, Ofori-Anyinam O, Hanekom W, Bollaerts A, Demoitie MA, Kany Luabeya AK, De Ruymaeker E, Tameris M, Lapierre D, Scriba TJ, Vaccine Study Team. 2015. Safety and immunogenicity of candidate vaccine M72/AS01E in adolescents in a TB endemic setting. *Vaccine* 33:4025–4034.

53. Thacher EG, Cavassini M, Audran R, Thierry AC, Bollaerts A, Cohen J, Demoitié MA, Ejigu D, Mettens P, Moris P, Ofori-Anyinam O, Spertini F. 2014. Safety and immunogenicity of the M72/AS01 candidate tuberculosis vaccine in HIV-infected adults on combination antiretroviral therapy: a phase I/II, randomized trial. *AIDS* 28:1769–1781.

54. Goonetilleke NP, McShane H, Hannan CM, Anderson RJ, Brookes RH, Hill AV. 2003. Enhanced immunogenicity and protective efficacy against *Mycobacterium tuberculosis* of bacille Calmette-Guérin vaccine using mucosal administration and boosting with a recombinant modified vaccinia virus Ankara. *J Immunol* 171:1602–1609.

55. Williams A, Hatch GJ, Clark SO, Gooch KE, Hatch KA, Hall GA, Huygen K, Ottenhoff TH, Franken KL, Andersen P, Doherty TM, Kaufmann SH, Grode L, Seiler P, Martin C, Gicquel B, Cole ST, Brodin P, Pym AS, Dalemans W, Cohen J, Lobet Y, Goonetilleke N, McShane H, Hill A, Parish T, Smith D, Stoker NG, Lowrie DB, Källenius G, Svenson S, Pawlowski A, Blake K, Marsh PD. 2005. Evaluation of vaccines in the EU TB Vaccine Cluster using a guinea pig aerosol infection model of tuberculosis. *Tuberculosis (Edinb)* 85: 29–38.

56. Williams A, Goonetilleke NP, McShane H, Clark SO, Hatch G, Gilbert SC, Hill AV. 2005. Boosting with poxviruses enhances *Mycobacterium bovis* BCG effi-

cacy against tuberculosis in guinea pigs. *Infect Immun* 73:3814–3816.

57. Verreck FA, Vervenne RA, Kondova I, van Kralingen KW, Remarque EJ, Braskamp G, van der Werff NM, Kersbergen A, Ottenhoff TH, Heidt PJ, Gilbert SC, Gicquel B, Hill AV, Martin C, McShane H, Thomas AW. 2009. MVA.85A boosting of BCG and an attenuated, phoP deficient *M. tuberculosis* vaccine both show protective efficacy against tuberculosis in rhesus macaques. *PLoS One* 4:e5264. (Erratum, 6:2.)

58. White AD, Sibley L, Dennis MJ, Gooch K, Betts G, Edwards N, Reyes-Sandoval A, Carroll MW, Williams A, Marsh PD, McShane H, Sharpe SA. 2013. Evaluation of the safety and immunogenicity of a candidate tuberculosis vaccine, MVA85A, delivered by aerosol to the lungs of macaques. *Clin Vaccine Immunol* 20: 663–672.

59. Vordermeier HM, Villarreal-Ramos B, Cockle PJ, McAulay M, Rhodes SG, Thacker T, Gilbert SC, McShane H, Hill AV, Xing Z, Hewinson RG. 2009. Viral booster vaccines improve *Mycobacterium bovis* BCG-induced protection against bovine tuberculosis. *Infect Immun* 77:3364–3373.

60. McShane H, Pathan AA, Sander CR, Keating SM, Gilbert SC, Huygen K, Fletcher HA, Hill AV. 2004. Recombinant modified vaccinia virus Ankara expressing antigen 85A boosts BCG-primed and naturally acquired antimycobacterial immunity in humans. *Nat Med* 10: 1240–1244.

61. Hawkridge T, Scriba TJ, Gelderbloem S, Smit E, Tameris M, Moyo S, Lang T, Veldsman A, Hatherill M, Merwe L, Fletcher HA, Mahomed H, Hill AV, Hanekom WA, Hussey GD, McShane H. 2008. Safety and immunogenicity of a new tuberculosis vaccine, MVA85A, in healthy adults in South Africa. *J Infect Dis* 198:544–552.

62. Pathan AA, Minassian AM, Sander CR, Rowland R, Porter DW, Poulton ID, Hill AV, Fletcher HA, McShane H. 2012. Effect of vaccine dose on the safety and immunogenicity of a candidate TB vaccine, MVA85A, in BCG vaccinated UK adults. *Vaccine* 30:5616–5624.

63. Rowland R, Pathan AA, Satti I, Poulton ID, Matsumiya MM, Whittaker M, Minassian AM, O'Hara GA, Hamill M, Scott JT, Harris SA, Poyntz HC, Bateman C, Meyer J, Williams N, Gilbert SC, Lawrie AM, Hill AV, McShane H. 2013. Safety and immunogenicity of an FP9-vectored candidate tuberculosis vaccine (FP85A), alone and with candidate vaccine MVA85A in BCG-vaccinated healthy adults: a phase I clinical trial. *Hum Vaccin Immunother* 9:50–62.

64. Meyer J, Harris SA, Satti I, Poulton ID, Poyntz HC, Tanner R, Rowland R, Griffiths KL, Fletcher HA, McShane H. 2013. Comparing the safety and immunogenicity of a candidate TB vaccine MVA85A administered by intramuscular and intradermal delivery. *Vaccine* 31:1026–1033.

65. Sander CR, Pathan AA, Beveridge NE, Poulton I, Minassian A, Alder N, Van Wijgerden J, Hill AV, Gleeson FV, Davies RJ, Pasvol G, McShane H. 2009. Safety and immunogenicity of a new tuberculosis vac-

cine, MVA85A, in *Mycobacterium tuberculosis*-infected individuals. *Am J Respir Crit Care Med* 179:724–733.

66. Ota MO, Odutola AA, Owiafe PK, Donkor S, Owolabi OA, Brittain NJ, Williams N, Rowland-Jones S, Hill AV, Adegbola RA, McShane H. 2011. Immunogenicity of the tuberculosis vaccine MVA85A is reduced by coadministration with EPI vaccines in a randomized controlled trial in Gambian infants. *Sci Transl Med* 3:88ra56

67. Scriba TJ, Tameris M, Mansoor N, Smit E, van der Merwe L, Isaacs F, Keyser A, Moyo S, Brittain N, Lawrie A, Gelderbloem S, Veldsman A, Hatherill M, Hawkridge A, Hill AV, Hussey GD, Mahomed H, McShane H, Hanekom WA. 2010. Modified vaccinia Ankara-expressing Ag85A, a novel tuberculosis vaccine, is safe in adolescents and children, and induces polyfunctional CD4+ T cells. *Eur J Immunol* 40:279–290.

68. Scriba TJ, Tameris M, Mansoor N, Smit E, van der Merwe L, Mauff K, Hughes EJ, Moyo S, Brittain N, Lawrie A, Mulenga H, de Kock M, Gelderbloem S, Veldsman A, Hatherill M, Geldenhuys H, Hill AV, Hussey GD, Mahomed H, Hanekom WA, McShane H. 2011. Dose-finding study of the novel tuberculosis vaccine, MVA85A, in healthy BCG-vaccinated infants. *J Infect Dis* 203:1832–1843.

69. Minassian AM, Rowland R, Beveridge NE, Poulton ID, Satti I, Harris S, Poyntz H, Hamill M, Griffiths K, Sander CR, Ambrozak DR, Price DA, Hill BJ, Casazza JP, Douek DC, Koup RA, Roederer M, Winston A, Ross J, Sherrard J, Rooney G, Williams N, Lawrie AM, Fletcher HA, Pathan AA, McShane H. 2011. A phase I study evaluating the safety and immunogenicity of MVA85A, a candidate TB vaccine, in HIV-infected adults. *BMJ Open* 1:e000223.

70. Dieye TN, Ndiaye BP, Dieng AB, Fall M, Brittain N, Vermaak S, Camara M, Diop-Ndiaye H, Ngom-Gueye NF, Diaw PA, Toure-Kane C, Sow PS, Mboup S, McShane H. 2013. Two doses of candidate TB vaccine MVA85A in antiretroviral therapy (ART) naïve subjects gives comparable immunogenicity to one dose in ART+ subjects. *PLoS One* 8:e67177.

71. Scriba TJ, Tameris M, Smit E, van der Merwe L, Hughes EJ, Kadira B, Mauff K, Moyo S, Brittain N, Lawrie A, Mulenga H, de Kock M, Makhethe L, Janse van Rensburg E, Gelderbloem S, Veldsman A, Hatherill M, Geldenhuys H, Hill AV, Hawkridge A, Hussey GD, Hanekom WA, McShane H, Mahomed H. 2012. A phase IIa trial of the new tuberculosis vaccine, MVA85A, in HIV- and/or *Mycobacterium tuberculosis*-infected adults. *Am J Respir Crit Care Med* 185:769–778.

72. Ndiaye BP, Thienemann F, Ota M, Landry BS, Camara M, Dièye S, Dieye TN, Esmail H, Goliath R, Huygen K, January V, Ndiaye I, Oni T, Raine M, Romano M, Satti I, Sutton S, Thiam A, Wilkinson KA, Mboup S, Wilkinson RJ, McShane H, MVA85A 030 Trial Investigators. 2015. Safety, immunogenicity, and efficacy of the candidate tuberculosis vaccine MVA85A in healthy adults infected with HIV-1: a randomised, placebo-controlled, phase 2 trial. *Lancet Respir Med* 3:190–200.

73. Satti I, Meyer J, Harris SA, Manjaly Thomas ZR, Griffiths K, Antrobus RD, Rowland R, Ramon RL, Smith M, Sheehan S, Bettinson H, McShane H. 2014. Safety and immunogenicity of a candidate tuberculosis vaccine MVA85A delivered by aerosol in BCG-vaccinated healthy adults: a phase 1, double-blind, randomised controlled trial. *Lancet Infect Dis* 14:939–946.

74. Sheehan S, Harris SA, Satti I, Hokey DA, Dheenadhayalan V, Stockdale L, Manjaly Thomas ZR, Minhinnick A, Wilkie M, Vermaak S, Meyer J, O'Shea MK, Pau MG, Versteege I, Douoguih M, Hendriks J, Sadoff J, Landry B, Moss P, McShane H. 2015. A phase I, open-label trial, evaluating the safety and immunogenicity of candidate tuberculosis vaccines AERAS-402 and MVA85A, administered by prime-boost regime in BCG-vaccinated healthy adults. *PLoS One* 10:e0141687.

75. Radosevic K, Wieland CW, Rodriguez A, Weverling GJ, Mintardjo R, Gillissen G, Vogels R, Skeiky YA, Hone DM, Sadoff JC, van der Poll T, Havenga M, Goudsmit J. 2007. Protective immune responses to a recombinant adenovirus type 35 tuberculosis vaccine in two mouse strains: CD4 and CD8 T-cell epitope mapping and role of gamma interferon. *Infect Immun* 75:4105–4115.

76. Darrah PA, Bolton DL, Lackner AA, Kaushal D, Aye PP, Mehra S, Blanchard JL, Didier PJ, Roy CJ, Rao SS, Hokey DA, Scanga CA, Sizemore DR, Sadoff JC, Roederer M, Seder RA. 2014. Aerosol vaccination with AERAS-402 elicits robust cellular immune responses in the lungs of rhesus macaques but fails to protect against high-dose *Mycobacterium tuberculosis* challenge. *J Immunol* 193:1799–1811.

77. Hoft DF, Blazevic A, Stanley J, Landry B, Sizemore D, Kpamegan E, Gearhart J, Scott A, Kik S, Pau MG, Goudsmit J, McClain JB, Sadoff J. 2012. A recombinant adenovirus expressing immunodominant TB antigens can significantly enhance BCG-induced human immunity. *Vaccine* 30:2098–2108.

78. Abel B, Tameris M, Mansoor N, Gelderbloem S, Hughes J, Abrahams D, Makhethe L, Erasmus M, de Kock M, van der Merwe L, Hawkridge A, Veldsman A, Hatherill M, Schirru G, Pau MG, Hendriks J, Weverling GJ, Goudsmit J, Sizemore D, McClain JB, Goetz M, Gearhart J, Mahomed H, Hussey GD, Sadoff JC, Hanekom WA. 2010. The novel tuberculosis vaccine, AERAS-402, induces robust and polyfunctional CD4+ and CD8+ T cells in adults. *Am J Respir Crit Care Med* 181:1407–1417.

79. Churchyard GJ, Snowden MA, Hokey D, Dheenadhayalan V, McClain JB, Douoguih M, Pau MG, Sadoff J, Landry B. 2015. The safety and immunogenicity of an adenovirus type 35-vectored TB vaccine in HIV-infected, BCG-vaccinated adults with CD4(+) T cell counts >350 cells/mm(3). *Vaccine* 33:1890–1896.

80. Tameris M, Hokey DA, Nduba V, Sacarlal J, Laher F, Kiringa G, Gondo K, Lazarus EM, Gray GE, Nachman S, Mahomed H, Downing K, Abel B, Scriba TJ, McClain JB, Pau MG, Hendriks J, Dheenadhayalan V, Ishmukhamedov S, Luabeya AK, Geldenhuys H, Shepherd B, Blatner G, Cardenas V, Walker R, Hanekom WA, Sadoff J, Douoguih M, Barker L, Hatherill M. 2015. A double-blind, randomised, placebo-controlled, dose-finding trial of the novel tuberculosis vaccine AERAS-402, an adenovirus-vectored fusion protein, in healthy, BCG-vaccinated infants. *Vaccine* 33:2944–2954.

81. Santosuosso M, McCormick S, Zhang X, Zganiacz A, Xing Z. 2006. Intranasal boosting with an adenovirus-vectored vaccine markedly enhances protection by parenteral *Mycobacterium bovis* BCG immunization against pulmonary tuberculosis. *Infect Immun* 74:4634–4643.

82. Wang J, Thorson L, Stokes RW, Santosuosso M, Huygen K, Zganiacz A, Hitt M, Xing Z. 2004. Single mucosal, but not parenteral, immunization with recombinant adenoviral-based vaccine provides potent protection from pulmonary tuberculosis. *J Immunol* 173:6357–6365.

83. Xing Z, McFarland CT, Sallenave JM, Izzo A, Wang J, McMurray DN. 2009. Intranasal mucosal boosting with an adenovirus-vectored vaccine markedly enhances the protection of BCG-primed guinea pigs against pulmonary tuberculosis. *PLoS One* 4:e5856.

84. Smaill F, Jeyanathan M, Smieja M, Medina MF, Thanthrige-Don N, Zganiacz A, Yin C, Heriazon A, Damjanovic D, Puri L, Hamid J, Xie F, Foley R, Bramson J, Gauldie J, Xing Z. 2013. A human type 5 adenovirus-based tuberculosis vaccine induces robust T cell responses in humans despite preexisting anti-adenovirus immunity. *Sci Transl Med* 5:205ra134.

85. Stukova M, Khairullin B, Bekembaeva G, Erofeeva M, Shurygina AP, Pisareva M, Buzitskaya J, Grudinin M, Kassenov M, Sandybaev N, Nurpeisova A, Sarsenbaeva G, Bogdanov N, Volgin E, Isagulov T, Kudryavstev I, Egorov A, Abildaev T, Kiselev OSA. 2015. Randomized double-blind placebo-controlled phase 1 trial of intranasal TB/FLU-04L tuberculosis vaccine in BCG vaccinated healthy adults aged 18-50 years. Poster presentation. TB Vaccines 4th Global Forum; Shanghai, China.

86. Dlugovitzky D, Fiorenza G, Farroni M, Bogue C, Stanford C, Stanford J. 2006. Immunological consequences of three doses of heat-killed *Mycobacterium vaccae* in the immunotherapy of tuberculosis. *Respir Med* 100:1079–1087.

87. Johnson JL, Kamya RM, Okwera A, Loughlin AM, Nyole S, Hom DL, Wallis RS, Hirsch CS, Wolski K, Foulds J, Mugerwa RD, Ellner JJ, The Uganda-Case Western Reserve University Research Collaboration. 2000. Randomized controlled trial of *Mycobacterium vaccae* immunotherapy in non-human immunodeficiency virus-infected Ugandan adults with newly diagnosed pulmonary tuberculosis. *J Infect Dis* 181:1304–1312.

88. Mwinga A, Nunn A, Ngwira B, Chintu C, Warndorff D, Fine P, Darbyshire J, Zumla A, LUSKAR Collaboration. 2002. *Mycobacterium vaccae* (SRL172) immunotherapy as an adjunct to standard antituberculosis treatment in HIV-infected adults with pulmonary tuberculosis: a randomised placebo-controlled trial. *Lancet* 360:1050–1055.

89. von Reyn CF, Mtei L, Arbeit RD, Waddell R, Cole B, Mackenzie T, Matee M, Bakari M, Tvaroha S, Adams LV, Horsburgh CR, Pallangyo K, DarDar Study Group. 2010. Prevention of tuberculosis in BACILLE Calmette-Guérin-primed, HIV-infected adults boosted with an inactivated whole-cell mycobacterial vaccine. *AIDS* 24:675–685.

90. Cardona PJ. 2006. RUTI: a new chance to shorten the treatment of latent tuberculosis infection. *Tuberculosis (Edinb)* 86:273–289.

91. Vilaplana C, Montané E, Pinto S, Barriocanal AM, Domenech G, Torres F, Cardona PJ, Costa J. 2010. Double-blind, randomized, placebo-controlled phase I clinical trial of the therapeutical antituberculous vaccine RUTI. *Vaccine* 28:1106–1116.

92. Nell AS, D'lom E, Bouic P, Sabaté M, Bosser R, Picas J, Amat M, Churchyard G, Cardona PJ. 2014. Safety, tolerability, and immunogenicity of the novel antituberculous vaccine RUTI: randomized, placebo-controlled phase II clinical trial in patients with latent tuberculosis infection. *PLoS One* 9:e89612.

93. Arbues A, Aguilo JI, Gonzalo-Asensio J, Marinova D, Uranga S, Puentes E, Fernandez C, Parra A, Cardona PJ, Vilaplana C, Ausina V, Williams A, Clark S, Malaga W, Guilhot C, Gicquel B, Martin C. 2013. Construction, characterization and preclinical evaluation of MTBVAC, the first live-attenuated *M. tuberculosis*-based vaccine to enter clinical trials. *Vaccine* 31:4867–4873.

94. Kaufmann SH, Cotton MF, Eisele B, Gengenbacher M, Grode L, Hesseling AC, Walzl G. 2014. The BCG replacement vaccine VPM1002: from drawing board to clinical trial. *Expert Rev Vaccines* 13:619–630.

95. Velmurugan K, Grode L, Chang R, Fitzpatrick M, Laddy D, Hokey D, Derrick S, Morris S, McCown D, Kidd R, Gengenbacher M, Eisele B, Kaufmann SH, Fulkerson J, Brennan MJ. 2013. Nonclinical development of BCG replacement vaccine candidates. *Vaccines (Basel)* 1:120–138.

96. Medical Research Council. 2016. *Experimental medicine.* http://www.mrc.ac.uk/research/initiatives/experimental-medicine/.

97. Spring M, Polhemus M, Ockenhouse C. 2014. Controlled human malaria infection. *J Infect Dis* 209 (Suppl 2):S40–S45.

98. Oxford JS. 2013. Towards a universal influenza vaccine: volunteer virus challenge studies in quarantine to speed the development and subsequent licensing. *Br J Clin Pharmacol* 76:210–216.

99. Tacket CO, Forrest B, Morona R, Attridge SR, LaBrooy J, Tall BD, Reymann M, Rowley D, Levine MM. 1990. Safety, immunogenicity, and efficacy against cholera challenge in humans of a typhoid-cholera hybrid vaccine derived from *Salmonella typhi* Ty21a. *Infect Immun* 58:1620–1627.

100. Minassian AM, Satti I, Poulton ID, Meyer J, Hill AV, McShane H. 2012. A human challenge model for *Mycobacterium tuberculosis* using *Mycobacterium bovis* bacille Calmette-Guerin. *J Infect Dis* 205:1035–1042.

101. Harris SA, Meyer J, Satti I, Marsay L, Poulton ID, Tanner R, Minassian AM, Fletcher HA, McShane H. 2014. Evaluation of a human BCG challenge model to assess antimycobacterial immunity induced by BCG and a candidate tuberculosis vaccine, MVA85A, alone and in combination. *J Infect Dis* 209:1259–1268.

102. Minassian AM, Ronan EO, Poyntz H, Hill AV, McShane H. 2011. Preclinical development of an *in vivo* BCG challenge model for testing candidate TB vaccine efficacy. *PLoS One* 6:e19840.

103. Villarreal-Ramos B, Berg S, Chamberlain L, McShane H, Hewinson RG, Clifford D, Vordermeier M. 2014. Development of a BCG challenge model for the testing of vaccine candidates against tuberculosis in cattle. *Vaccine* 32:5645–5649.

Tuberculosis and the Tubercle Bacillus, 2nd ed.
Edited by William R. Jacobs, Jr., Helen McShane, Valerie Mizrahi, and Ian M. Orme
© 2018 American Society for Microbiology, Washington, DC
doi:10.1128/microbiolspec.TBTB2-0016-2016

D. HUMAN IMMUNOLOGY

Human Immunology of Tuberculosis

11

Thomas J. Scriba[1], Anna K. Coussens[2], and Helen A. Fletcher[3]

Immunity to *Mycobacterium tuberculosis* is an inter-play between the innate and adaptive immune response, both cellular and humoral. This interplay is not static but changes over time as we grow, age, and respond to our environment. Animal models enable examination of individual components of the immune response at distinct time points during the course of infection. This has enabled identification and understanding of key immune mechanisms for *M. tuberculosis* control. However, rational development of interventions, such as more effective vaccines and other host-directed therapies, has to take into consideration the enormous heterogeneity of the interactions between *M. tuberculosis* with human innate and adaptive immune responses, which are profoundly influenced by genetic variation, environment, and comorbidities.

Recent technological advances now being applied to the field of tuberculosis (TB) have pushed the boundaries of our understanding of the host-pathogen interactions. These include the use of highly sensitive imaging such as positron emission tomography/computed tomography (PET/CT; [18]fluorodeoxyglucose positron emission and computerized axial tomographic scanning) to identify subclinical TB lesions in asymptomatic individuals to study early stages of human infection; the explosion of high-throughput "omics" technologies for unbiased transcriptomic, genomic, proteomic, and metabolomic investigation of blood and tissues isolated from the site of disease; and the ability to isolate human *M. tuberculosis*-specific T cell populations by the use of *M. tuberculosis* peptide-specific tetramers and flow cytometry. Moreover, rigorous design of clinical studies, improved and standardized clinical definitions, and

extensive collection of clinical data and appropriate specimens for immunological studies have significantly advanced our understanding of human immunology. Together, these advances have led to a revolution in how we understand the different stages of *M. tuberculosis* infection and the interplay of innate and adaptive immunity in humans (Fig. 1).

ACQUISITION OF *M. TUBERCULOSIS* INFECTION

The host-pathogen interaction between *M. tuberculosis* and humans has been honed by thousands of years of coevolution (1). The estimation that a third of the global population is sensitized to *M. tuberculosis* (2) bears testament to the supreme success with which the bacterium infects, survives, and spreads within its human host. Billions of humans have experienced acquisition of *M. tuberculosis* infection. Despite this, our knowledge of the immunological events that occur during exposure and acute infection in humans is very limited. This is primarily due to the lack of diagnostic tests that directly identify *M. tuberculosis* in those with infection and to our limited ability to study early disease processes at the site of disease, such that the majority of human studies investigate immune responses *ex vivo* in peripheral blood or after *in vitro* infection of primary cells or cell lines.

Primary Response to *M. tuberculosis* Infection

Meticulous clinical observation of TB contacts, combined with serial tuberculin skin testing (TST) to detect

[1]South African Tuberculosis Vaccine Initiative, Division of Immunology, Department of Pathology and Institute of Infectious Disease and Molecular Medicine, University of Cape Town, South Africa; [2]Clinical Infectious Diseases Research Initiative, Division of Medical Microbiology, Department of Pathology and Institute of Infectious Disease and Molecular Medicine, University of Cape Town, South Africa; [3]Immunology and Infection Department, London School of Hygiene and Tropical Medicine, London, United Kingdom.

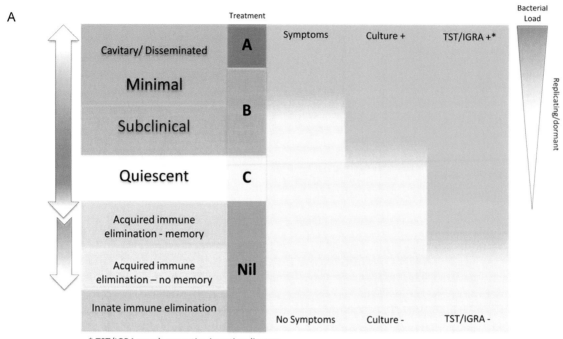

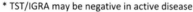

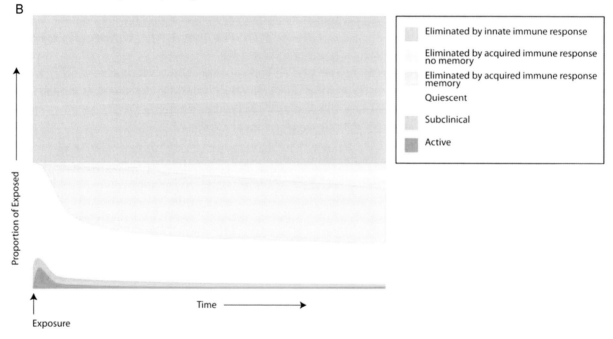

Figure 1 (**A**) Hypothesized stages of response to *M. tuberculosis* infection, beginning with elimination mediated by innate immune cells without induction of a long-lasting memory response; further stages of elimination may be mediated via acquired immune mechanisms. If antigen-specific effector memory persists, this can be measured via IFN-γ release assays (IGRA) or tuberculin skin test (TST) and may provide protection from infection for a variable period of time. If the acquired immunity does not eliminate the bacteria, then infection will persist over a range of bacterial states. Increasing bacterial load is hypothesized to correlate with progression to active TB. (**B**) For all exposed individuals, the risk of developing TB is highest immediately following exposure and changes over time. The longitudinal risk of developing TB, predicted in the exposed individual, is presented (adapted from references 204 and 205).

the onset of hypersensitivty to *M. tuberculosis* antigens, allowed Arvid Wallgren to document the symptomology of incident *M. tuberculosis* infection in 1948 (3). He reported that most people who converted from a negative to a positive TST presented with erythema nodosum and/or fever, while many also had elevated erythrocyte sedimentation rates (3). This suggests that acute infection is associated with a systemic innate inflammatory response that precedes the induction of a detectable adaptive immune response. Erythema nodosum is still a symptomatic trigger that may lead to investigation and diagnosis of human infection with *M. tuberculosis* (4–6) or *Mycobacterium bovis* (7).

The inflammatory processes that underlie erythema nodosum, febrile illness, and erythrocyte sedimentation are thought to be causally linked to the delayed hypersensitivity reaction that underlies priming of the *M. tuberculosis*-specific T cell response. However, at least in people without prior sensitization to mycobacteria, it is likely that innate immune responses to the infecting pathogen precede these T cell-driven reactions. It is thought that the first event that occurs upon inhalation of *M. tuberculosis*-containing microdroplets is that the bacilli are taken up by alveolar macrophages (AMs). A number of important barriers and antimicrobial hurdles must be negotiated by aerosolized *M. tuberculosis* particles to reach the alveoli, most of which are poorly understood in humans and are often neglected. However, it is likely that the pathogen is particularly susceptible to mechanical and immunological attack during its journey through the upper airways. A better understanding of these events, and of the cellular and humoral components that frequent the mucosal surfaces, could lead to interventions that prevent infection at the port of entry. In fact, a sizable proportion of people who are heavily exposed to *M. tuberculosis* do not develop any evidence for immune sensitization (8, 9), suggesting that prevention of infection is possible (10).

Alveolar macrophages

AMs are regarded as the sentinels of *M. tuberculosis* infection. Their role in initial *M. tuberculosis* phagocytosis is unquestionable, according to animal models of infection. Defining their role in the human response to *M. tuberculosis* infection has been more problematic, and our knowledge can only be inferred from studies of cells collected by invasive bronchoalveolar lavage (BAL), investigation of tissue sections from autopsies, or lung resections (generally only indicated due to severe disease pathology). As a consequence, our picture of macrophage responses to *in vitro M. tuberculosis* infection is confounded by their removal from their tissue matrix and surrounding immunological milieu, including activated cytokines and other interacting cell populations. Although reductionist, the latter has provided enormous insight into differences between human AMs and peripheral monocytes.

A number of studies of BAL-isolated AMs from healthy donors have compared responses to *in vitro* infection with virulent (H37Rv) or avirulent (H37Ra) laboratory strains of *M. tuberculosis* (11–14). In comparison to mouse studies indicating that tumor necrosis factor (TNF) provides a protective response against *M. tuberculosis* infection and that it is vital for granuloma formation, these studies showed that virulent *M. tuberculosis* induces higher levels of TNF secretion from AMs than avirulent *M. tuberculosis*, that TNF levels correlated with increased *M. tuberculosis* growth, that TNF induces apoptotic cell death in culture, that cytoxicity can be inhibited by anti-TNF treatment, and that exogenous application of TNF increases both the intracellular bacterial load and the number of infected AMs (13, 14). It is further hypothesized that increased apoptosis may spread the infection to neighboring AMs via efferocytosis, and extensive apoptosis has been demonstrated within caseating granulomas of lung tissue samples from TB patients (12).

Phagocytosis by AMs is mediated primarily by complement receptor 4 (CR4), whereas blood monocytes utilize CR1, CR3, and CR4. As such, uptake of *M. tuberculosis* can be enhanced by increasing concentrations of serum and decreased by heat inactivation of serum (15). AMs are also more efficient than monocytes at limiting intracellular growth of *M. tuberculosis*, and they produce high levels of TNF (15). Interestingly, phagocytosis alone is not responsible for TNF production, as uninfected AMs within the same culture also produce TNF. However, this does not occur if uninfected AMs are separated from infected AMs via a 0.4-μm transwell, indicating that cell-cell interaction or a soluble factor larger than 0.4 μm is required for TNF production in uninfected AMs (13).

AMs are highly heterogeneous in *M. tuberculosis* phagocytic potential, despite homogeneity in phagocytosis of latex beads, such that up to only 20% of AMs in culture become infected with *M. tuberculosis*, even with excessive infection (multiplicity of infection of 10:1 for 18 h) (13). This may be mediated by variable surface expression levels of CR, while differential cytokine response can be linked to expression of pattern recognition receptor (PRR) expression. Nucleotide-binding oligomerization domain-containing protein 2 (NOD2), Toll-like receptor 2 (TLR2), and TLR4 expression on AMs is highly correlated and variable between each AM (16). The expression of PPR also changes on AMs from TB patients following treatment, indicating that the phenotype of AM changes during infection (16). The differential expression of these PPRs may be important for primary restriction of *M. tuberculosis* replication because NOD2 activation in AMs by muramyldipeptide (MDP) induces expression of interleukin-1β (IL-1β), IL-6, and TNF; the antimicrobial peptide cathelicidin (LL-37); and the autophagy enzyme IRGM, and it restricts intracellular growth of *M. tuberculosis* (17). Interestingly, LL-37 is not detected in AMs in tuberculous granulomas, suggesting that LL-37 participates only during early infection or that defects in LL-37 production can lead to *M. tuberculosis* growth and progression to disease (18).

When comparing BAL from TB patients versus healthy controls, TB AMs express higher concentrations of IL-1β, IL-6, and TNF, and this correlates with higher protein levels in BAL fluid and with IL-6 and TNF in serum (19). AMs from TB patients also show higher levels of chemokines CXCL10 (IP-10), CXCL8 (IL-8), and nuclear factor-kappa B (NF-κB) repressing factor (NRF), and these levels correlate with higher bacillary loads in the AMs. Interestingly, peripheral blood mononuclear cells (PBMCs) from patients with high bacillary load also have high expression of CXCL10 and CXCL8, while NRF levels are higher in AMs than in PBMCs (20).

The hyperreactivity of AMs in TB patients may be either due to an innate defect leading to susceptibility to TB or because *M. tuberculosis* infection changes the phenotype of AMs. The observation that the AM phenotype changes during therapy (16) supports the finding that the infection is modifying AM function. Recent evidence of a shift in the metabolic state of AMs following infection also supports this hypothesis. Macrophages can be classified as classical (M1) or alternatively activated (M2), with pro- and anti-inflammatory properties, respectively. M1s derive ATP via aerobic glycolysis and M2s via oxidative phosphorylation. *M. tuberculosis* infection of healthy donor AMs induces a shift from oxidative phosphorylation to aerobic glycolysis, leading to increased IL-1β and prostaglandin synthase PTGS2 and decreased IL-10, while blocking this shift to aerobic glycolysis leads to increased intracellular *M. tuberculosis* survival (21), suggesting that AM polarization to M1 activates antimicrobial activity.

Neutrophils

Peripheral neutrophilia is a hallmark of TB disease in humans and a predictor of poor outcome and mor-

bidity (22, 23). The lack of neutrophil involvement in murine TB and the difficulties associated with studying neutrophils *in vitro* have led to limited investigation of their role in human TB. A resurgence of interest in neutrophils occurred after the first whole-blood microarray study of TB patients compared with healthy controls, which showed profound neutrophil involvement in the gene expression signature that differentiated between TB patients and controls (24). While it seems clear that neutrophils promote pathology during disease development, an understanding of their role in initial infection is more difficult to acquire. Recent TB contacts show increased peripheral blood neutrophil counts compared to healthy controls, and risk of *M. tuberculosis* infection has been shown to be inversely associated with neutrophil count (25). Neutrophil depletion from whole blood also decreases *M. tuberculosis* killing, which is primarily mediated through phagocytosis and the respiratory burst. In addition, neutrophils can kill through the release of antimicrobial peptides including human neutrophil peptides (HNPs) 1–3, LL-37, and lipocalin 2 (25). Neutrophils can also capture mycobacteria in neutrophil extracellular traps (NETs) composed of DNA coated with antimicrobial peptides (26). Interestingly, individuals of African ancestry have lower circulating neutrophil numbers and lower serum levels of HNP1–3 and lipocalin 2 compared to Caucasian individuals (25, 27). CXCL8, one of the chemokines most highly expressed by *M. tuberculosis*-infected AMs, with neutrophil recruiting activity, has recently been shown to bind *M. tuberculosis* directly and enhance phagocytosis and killing by neutrophils (28). These data suggest that neutrophils may have an early protective effect against *M. tuberculosis* infection.

Innate T cells

Interest in lung-resident and germline-encoded lymphocyte populations has recently been growing, with the rationale that these cells may act rapidly upon *M. tuberculosis* infection. These cells naturally reside at mucosal sites in the airways and are thus ideally located to respond to invading pathogens (reviewed in reference 29). This is an important advantage over conventional T cell responses that require priming in primary lymphoid tissue and subsequent differentiation into effector cells before trafficking to the site of infection. Tissue-resident T cells, such as mucosal-associated invariant T (MAIT) cells, also possess immediate effector functions, including cytokine expression and cytotoxicity, which further enable immediate antimicrobial activity. It is currently not known whether airway-resident lymphocytes play a key role in resistance to infection with *M. tuberculosis* in humans.

Most individuals who are exposed to *M. tuberculosis* do appear to acquire an established infection and develop readily detectable CD4 T cell responses to protein components of *M. tuberculosis*. This immune response, which typically persists for years and even decades, forms the basis for the diagnosis of human infection with *M. tuberculosis*, using TST or interferon gamma (IFN-γ) release assays (IGRAs). The utility of these diagnostic methods has been extensively reviewed (30).

The Granuloma

The structure of the granuloma is formed primarily through the coalescence of recruited macrophages around *M. tuberculosis*-infected macrophages, of which some differentiate into epithelioid cells and some can fuse to become multinucleated giant cells. In the typical granuloma structure these macrophages are interspersed with recruited neutrophils and are surrounded by a lymphocyte cuff, including T cells and B cells. A recent review of the historical literature has shown that granulomata are highly diverse, displaying a wide spectrum of structures and sizes and cell composition, and that this diversity can be observed even within a single host (Fig. 2; reviewed in references 31 and 32). It is thought that the granuloma functions to contain the spread of *M. tuberculosis*, although it can also act as a physical barrier, preventing the penetration of TB drugs and protecting the organism from the adaptive immune response. The phenotype of macrophages within the granuloma can affect the likelihood that the granuloma will contain *M. tuberculosis*, break down and transmit *M. tuberculosis*, and initiate an inflammatory response (33).

Adaptive Responses and the Spectrum of *M. tuberculosis* Infection

B cells

The dominance of T cell responses and the concealment of *M. tuberculosis* within the infected macrophage suggest that antibodies would play a minor role in possible prevention of infection with *M. tuberculosis* during exposure. However, it has recently been recognized that B cells and antibodies have a variety of mechanisms for the modulation of the immune response to intracellular bacteria that are likely to be important in the control of *M. tuberculosis* (reviewed in references 34–37) (Fig. 3). B cells are a major cellular component of the lung granuloma, where they can

process and present antigen to T cells, secrete antibodies, and modulate inflammation through the production of IL-10 (reviewed in reference 37). Although likely to be important, few clinical studies have examined the B cell response in *M. tuberculosis* infection. Plasmablasts and memory B cells are elevated in *M. tuberculosis*-infected compared to uninfected controls (38), and *in vitro* human B cells have been shown to ingest mycobacteria, produce IgM, and upregulate the expression of the costimulatory molecules CD80 and CD86 and the chemokine CXCL10 (39, 40). Further studies of the role of B cells in *M. tuberculosis* infection are required.

T cells

A lot of emphasis has been placed on the *M. tuberculosis* antigens targeted by T cell responses. Early literature has focused on T cell responses that recognize a relatively small set of immunodominant antigens, including early secretory antigenic target-6 (ESAT-6), 10-kDa culture filtrate protein antigen (CFP-10), TB10.4, and antigen 85A (Ag85A) and Ag85B (41–45). These were the first to be incorporated as antigens into subunit vaccines (46, 47). However, a recent unbiased, genome-wide analysis of CD4 T cell responses to *M. tuberculosis* antigens in adults with latent *M. tuberculosis* infection (LTBI) revealed that the human CD4 T cell response targets a very broad array of more than 80 antigens (48). These responses were predominantly restricted to CD4 T cells and highly enriched for a CXCR3+CCR6+ subset that exhibits Th1-response characteristics (48). Nearly half of the epitopes identified in this study were derived from proteins that had not previously been identified as T cell antigens. This study and subsequent others demonstrate that the human immune response to *M. tuberculosis* is very heterogeneous and as yet poorly defined (48–50). An intriguing question is whether T cell recognition of distinct *M. tuberculosis* antigens is associated with TB disease risk.

Functional and phenotypic characteristics of *M. tuberculosis*-specific T cell responses have received particular attention in recent times, and interesting associations with the presentation of *M. tuberculosis* infection have been described. While the *M. tuberculosis*-specific T cell response in healthy people is dominated by CD4 T cells (48), a number of studies have revealed an increased contribution by CD8 T cells in patients with TB disease (51–53). The mechanism for this finding is currently not clear, but this pattern appears robust and has been proposed as a diagnostic approach for TB disease (53).

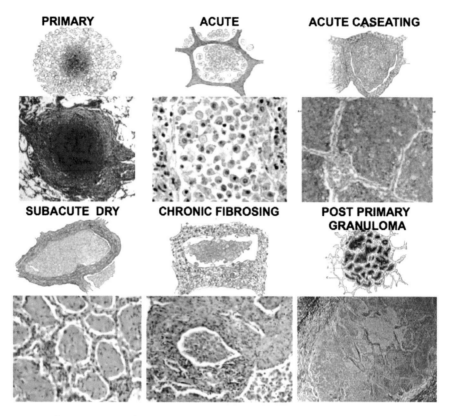

Figure 2 The spectrum of pulmonary TB lesions that can be found in the same host and that represent different stages of disease. Primary TB is characterized by the hallmark circular granuloma with caseating necrosis which forms within the center, surrounded by a lymphocytic cuff. Conversely, post-primary TB is typically represented by a diverse range of pathologies. Acute post-primary lesions are composed of paucibacillary lobular pneumonia; these may either resolve (subacute dry), fibrose (chronic fibrosing) or necrose (acute caseating). Caseating granulomas in post-primary TB are distinct from the granulomas of primary TB in that they form around and in response to caseous necrosis of pneumonic lesions (post-primary granuloma) rather than necrosis occurring in the center of preformed lesions as occurs in primary TB. Cavities are formed from the dissolution of these caseating pneumonic lesions. Six stages are represented by a 19th century drawing and a 21st century photomicrograph of sections stained with hematoxylin and eosin or trichrome, imaged at 40 to 400×. (Reproduced from references 31, 220, and 221).

A prominent theme has been the pattern of Th1 cytokine coexpression, shown to be associated with the degree of T cell differentiation in viral infections (54). Comparative studies of patients with TB disease and latently infected people have reported elevated frequencies of *M. tuberculosis*-specific CD4 T cells expressing only TNF or TNF+IFN-γ+ CD4 T cells in TB patients, while those with latent infection have higher frequencies of polyfunctional TNF+IFN-γ+IL-2+ *M. tuberculosis*-specific CD4+ T cell responses (51, 55, 56). Furthermore, successful TB treatment appears to reverse this functional pattern, because CD4 T cells coexpress IFN-γ, TNF, and IL-2 to a greater degree after cure (51, 56). However, other studies have reported the opposite: active TB disease was accompanied by greater frequen-

cies of polyfunctional TNF+IFN-γ+IL-2+ CD4 T cells than was LTBI (57–59). An immune correlates study in bacillus Calmette-Guérin (BCG)-vaccinated infants aimed to determine whether frequencies or cytokine coexpression patterns of mycobacteria-specific Th1-cytokine-expressing CD4 or CD8 cells, measured at 10 weeks of age, were associated with subsequent risk of TB disease (60). The study reported no association between frequencies or cytokine expression patterns in BCG-specific CD4 and CD8 T cells (61). However, more recently, BCG-specific IFN-γ-secreting T cells measured by enzyme-linked immunosorbent spot assay (ELIspot) were found to be associated with reduced risk of developing TB disease in a South African infant cohort from the same population (62).

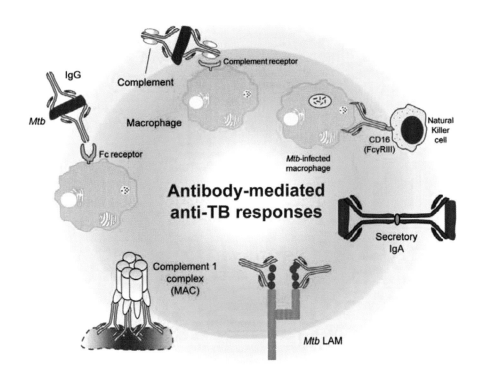

Figure 3 Role of antibodies in anti-*M. tuberculosis* (*Mtb*) infection. Antibodies may directly bind to mycobacteria, triggering complement deposition and lysis of *M. tuberculosis*, or complement may mediate opsonophagocytosis of the organism. Alternatively, *M. tuberculosis*-bound antibody may enhance macrophage uptake through Fc receptor binding or activate NK cell activity through Fc receptor engagement. It is also possible for immune complexes to form between mycobacterial antigen and antibody. Abbreviations: FcγRIII, Fc gamma receptor III; IgA, immunoglobulin A; IgG, immunoglobulin G; LAM, lipoarabinomannan; MAC, membrane-attack complex. (From reference 37 with permission.)

Such functional differences in T cell cytokine expression may simply reflect differential levels of T cell exposure to *M. tuberculosis* antigens, indicating *in vivo* bacterial load (51). This hypothesis is supported by phenotypic analyses of *M. tuberculosis*-specific T cells, which suggest that higher bacterial load in active disease is associated with greater T cell activation.

Activation of antigen-specific CD4 T cells, measured by HLA-DR, CD38, or Ki67 expression, was significantly higher in patients with active TB compared to controls with LTBI (63). These activation markers seemed to track antigen load well, as expression levels gradually decreased during treatment of active disease, suggesting that T cell expression of these activation markers can be useful as treatment response markers (63). A recent study investigated T cell activation as a biomarker of risk of TB (see section on progression to TB disease).

B cells and antibody responses

Many studies have assessed the ability of antibodies to accurately diagnose active TB, and these studies will be discussed below. In some studies the ability of antibodies to differentiate *M. tuberculosis*-infected subjects (defined as either TST+ or IGRA+) and uninfected controls has also been assessed (Table 1). It is estimated that a third of the world's population is latently infected with *M. tuberculosis*, although this varies greatly from region to region (2) and latency is likely to represent a spectrum from transient exposure to subclinical TB disease (64). Analysis of antibodies in those with *M. tuberculosis* infection, approximately 90% of whom are able to contain infection, versus uninfected controls enables the identification of antibody responses that may be important in the control of *M. tuberculosis* infection. *M. tuberculosis* infection induces mycobacteria-specific antibodies against a broad range of antigens, with no single antigen or group of antigens emerging as a preferential target for an antibody response (Table 1). Mycobacterial antigen-specific IgG, IgA, and IgM have all been reported in *M. tuberculosis* infection (Table 1). Perley et al. report approximately equal ratios of IgG and IgM in response to live cell surface, whole cell lysate, lipoarabinomannan (LAM), and cell wall and secreted mycobacterial proteins in *M. tuberculosis*-infected and uninfected controls (65). There are few studies in HIV-infected populations and little evidence for elevation of mycobacterial antibodies in HIV-infected, *M. tuberculosis*-infected versus HIV-1-infected, *M. tuberculosis*-uninfected populations (66, 67). All studies agree that antibody levels in *M. tuberculosis* infection are highly variable, with a high degree of overlap between infected individuals and uninfected controls. The greatest separation between *M. tuberculosis*-infected and uninfected control populations was reported by Baumann et al. (68), who found discrimination between *M. tuberculosis*-infected (defined as IGRA+ or TST+) and uninfected controls with 80% sensitivity and 93% specificity using AlaDH (Rv2780)-specific IgA, and 84.2% sensitivity and 93% specificity using NARL (Rv0844c)-specific IgA. In a separate study, they reported 74% sensitivity and 83% specificity using a combination of IgA and IgG specific for LAM and PE35 (Rv3872) (68). Perley et al. found better discrimination when measuring antibodies directed against the live cell surface of mycobacteria when compared to cell wall, LAM, or secreted proteins from *M. tuberculosis* (65).

T cell responses to *M. tuberculosis*-specific antigens, including ESAT-6 and CFP-10, are used as the basis for IGRAs to discriminate between *M. tuberculosis*-infected and uninfected individuals (30). However, antibody responses against *M. tuberculosis*-specific antigens are generally poor at discriminating between infected and uninfected individuals, although Hoff et al. found that they performed better in low-burden settings (69–72). It is important to note the potential bias because *M. tuberculosis* infection is defined by a cellular immune response measured by either TST reaction or IGRA response to an *M. tuberculosis*-specific antigen. There is currently no method that does not depend upon detection of a cell-mediated immune response for the detection of *M. tuberculosis* infection. While antibody responses are higher in those with a positive TST or IGRA, several studies have described high levels of *M. tuberculosis* antibodies in individuals with TST anergy, suggesting that antibodies can be elevated following *M. tuberculosis* exposure in the absence of a cell-mediated immune response (73, 74).

BCG vaccination and antibodies

A detectable increase in mycobacterial specific antibody is not always observed following BCG immunization (75), most likely due to pre-existing high-titer antibody induced by exposure to environmental mycobacteria (76, 77). BCG, however, has been found to induce modest levels of mycobacterial antigen-specific antibodies in several studies (78–81). Higher levels of Ag85A IgG antibodies in 4- to 6-month-old South African infants vaccinated with BCG at birth were found to be associated with reduced risk of developing TB disease over the next 3 years of life (62). BCG-induced antibodies may contribute toward a protective immune response through mechanisms including the opsonization of mycobacterial cells for uptake by phagocytes (82).

Mechanisms of antibody action

Kumar et al. found that treatment with sera from *M. tuberculosis*-infected, healthy subjects enhanced uptake and intracellular killing of mycobacteria by donor myeloid-derived macrophages (MDM). Interestingly, not all mycobacterial antigens opsonized mycobacteria, and two antigens with approximate molecular weights of 48 and 80 kDa (possibly *M. tuberculosis* 48 and *M. tuberculosis* 81) were absent from opsonizing antibody extracts (83). Opsonized mycobacteria were killed more rapidly with enhanced IFN-γ and IL-6 production, enhanced phagosome acidification, and increased inducible nitric oxide synthase and nitric oxide production (83). The enhanced uptake of serum-coated mycobacteria by neutrophils and monocyte/macrophages was found to be IgG dependent in a separate study (82).

Antibody-inducing vaccines

There are no TB vaccine candidates currently in clinical development that are designed for the specific enhancement of a B cell or antibody response, although whole-cell mycobacterial vaccines such as VPM1002 (recombinant BCG) (84) and VAC (attenuated *M. tuberculosis*) (85) will induce a broad-spectrum response including antibodies. It is possible to enhance antibody responses to subunit TB vaccines through the use of specific adjuvants (86). Alum is widely used for the induction of antibodies, although it also skews toward a Th2 type immune response and does not protect against *M. tuberculosis* (86). There are, however, adjuvants such as MF59 which induce both a Th1 type cellular response and antibody and have been shown to enhance protection in mice challenged with *M. tuberculosis* (86).

Table 1 Antibodies in *M. tuberculosis* infection

Author	Study design	HIV-1 pos/neg	Class of antibody	Antigen	Detected difference[a] (% sensitivity; % specificity)
Chen J et al., 2010 (70)	LTBI versus controls (China)	Neg	IgG	Rv1985c	62; 97
Baumann R et al., 2015 (68)	LTBI versus controls (South Africa)	Neg	IgA	NARL (Rv0844c)	84.2; 93
			IgA	MPT83 (Rv2873)	63.2; 93
			IgA	19 kDa (Rv3763)	78.9; 93
			IgA,	AlaDH (Rv2780)	89.5; 93
			IgG	AlaDH (Rv2780)	26.3; 93
					NS
			IgA	PstS3 (Rv0928)	57.9
Baumann R et al., 2014 (222)	LTBI versus controls (South Africa)	Neg	IgM, IgA	MPT32 (Rv1860)	49; 100 IgA
			IgA, IgG	PE35 (Rv3872)	PE35 + LAM
			IgA, IgG	LAM	74; 83 IgA and IgG combined
			IgA, IgG	Tpx (Rv1932)	NS
			IgA, IgG	16 kDa (Rv2031c)	NS
			IgA	HSP20 (Rv251c)	NS
Hur Y et al., 2015 (71)	LTBI versus controls, TST+ and IGRA+ (South Korea)	Neg	IgG	38 kDa (Rv0934)	NS
			IgG	16 kDa (Rv2031c)	NS
			IgG	ESAT-6 (Rv3875)	NS
			IgG	CFP-10 (Rv3874)	NS
			IgG	LAM	NS
Niki M et al., 2015 (72)	LTBI versus controls, IGRA+ (Tokyo)	Neg	IgG/IgA	HrpA (Rv0251c/hsp)	IgG, $P < 0.01$
			IgG/IgA	MDP1 (Rv2986c)	IgA, $P < 0.05$[b]
			IgG/IgA	ESAT-6 (Rv3875)	NS
			IgG/IgA	CFP-10 (Rv3874)	NS
			IgG/IgA	Ag85A (Rv3804c)	NS
			IgG/IgA	16 kDa (Rv2031c)	NS
			IgG/IgA	HBHA (Rv0475)	NS
Hoff S et al., 2007 (69)	Control versus LTBI (Denmark, Brazil, Ethiopia, Tanzania)	Neg	IgG	ESAT-6-CFP10 fusion	$P < 0.01$
			IgG	Denmark	$P = 0.043$
			IgG	Brazil, Ethiopia	$P = 0.038$
Siev M et al., 2014 (67)	Control versus TST+ (U.S.)	Pos	IgG	MPT51 (Rv3803c)	NS
			IgG	echA1 (Rv0222)	NS
			IgG	MS (Rv1837c)	NS
			IgG	38 kDa (Rv0934)	NS
Yu X et al., 2012 (66)	Control versus TST+ (U.S.)	Pos	IgG	Arabinomannan	NS
			IgM	Arabinomannan	NS
			IgA	Arabinomannan	NS
		Neg	IgG	Arabinomannan	$P = 0.02$[b]
			IgM	Arabinomannan	NS
			IgA	Arabinomannan	NS
Perley CC et al., 2014 (65)	Control versus IGRA+ (U.S.)	Neg	IgG	Live cell surface	$P < 0.001$
			IgG	Whole cell lysate	$P < 0.01$
			IgG	IgG avidity, live cell surface	$P < 0.05$[b]
			IgG	IgG avidity, whole cell lysate	NS
			IgG	LAM	NS
			IgG	Cell wall	NS
			IgG	Secreted proteins	NS
			IgG	IgG avidity, LAM	$P < 0.05$
			IgG	IgG avidity, cell wall	NS
			IgG	IgG avidity, secreted proteins	$P < 0.001$

[a]NS, not significant.
[b]Decreased in LTBI.

PROGRESSION FROM *M. TUBERCULOSIS* INFECTION TO TB DISEASE

Although most individuals who become infected with *M. tuberculosis* remain asymptomatic, in some the immune response fails to contain the infection and clinical symptoms develop, including fevers, night sweats, weight loss, and chronic coughing, among many others. Definitive diagnosis of TB disease is based on detection of acid-fast bacilli, most often in sputum from the patient. The risk of progression to disease is greatest immediately following infection (87, 88); however, *M. tuberculosis* can persist for years in asymptomatic individuals. Long-term persistence of viable bacilli was reported in 1927, when *M. tuberculosis* was cultured from apparently healthy tissues of individuals with no pathological evidence of TB who died from other causes (89). Progression to active disease is possible even decades after exposure (88) and is typically triggered by immune compromise. This was elegantly demonstrated by reactivation of LTBI in rheumatoid arthritis patients who received anti-TNF blocking antibodies or other immunotherapies (90, 91). Many factors, including the magnitude of the infectious dose, the bacterial strain, time since exposure, and a multitude of other risk factors have been associated with risk of TB. Innate and adaptive immune mechanisms are clearly very important for successful control of *M. tuberculosis*, since impairment of immunity through steroids, chemotherapy, biologics, and HIV coinfection predisposes to TB disease (reviewed in reference 92).

Immune Mediators of TB Risk

TB susceptibility is driven by immune dysfunction, whether during acute or chronic latent stages of *M. tuberculosis* infection. The control of infection requires a precise balance between immune-mediated eradication of *M. tuberculosis* and limitation of inflammation to prevent immunopathology. As such, it is thought that any immune dysfunction which tips the balance in either direction can lead to disease progression. Among the greatest risk factors for TB are HIV-1 infection, malnutrition, diabetes mellitus, smoking, vitamin D deficiency, drug/alcohol abuse, male gender, age, and anti-TNF therapy (93–97). These risk factors are not mutually exclusive and can exacerbate each other (98–102). However, the phenotype of immunodeficiency induced by each is different, and therefore the interrelationship between comorbidities and disease susceptibility is complex. Studies of the underlying causes of each of these risk factors and their effects on TB risk can provide important insights into the mechanisms of protective immunity against *M. tuberculosis* in humans.

HIV

The resurgence of TB in sub-Saharan Africa is linked to the onset of the HIV-1 pandemic (103). Coinfection with HIV-1 is thought to increase susceptibility to TB via a number of mechanisms, primarily through dysfunctional and decreased numbers of CD4 T cells and impaired activation of T cell responses by phagocytes (100, 104–106). However, increased risk of TB typically occurs in HIV-infected individuals prior to significant T cell depletion (107), suggesting that HIV may alter cellular responses to *M. tuberculosis* infection. HIV-1 and *M. tuberculosis* coinfection of PBMCs or macrophages has been shown to synergistically increase replication of both pathogens *in vitro* (108, 109). *M. tuberculosis* infection induces HIV-1 replication via a number of mechanisms, including upregulating the transcription factors, NF-κB (108), nuclear factor of activated T cells-5 (NFAT5), positive transcription elongation factor (P-TEFb), and loss of an inhibitory C/EBPβ (110–112). Induction of chemokines during *M. tuberculosis* infection also increases cellular recruitment of CCR5-positive monocytes and CD4 T cells into the site of infection, increasing the pool of cells that can be infected by HIV-1 (113). Conversely, the effect of HIV-1 on the macrophage response is variable and subtle, modifying cytokine and chemokine production required for T cell recruitment and activation (109, 114). In a large multicenter study in India, Lagrange et al. found higher levels and greater sensitivity for antibody-based TB diagnostic tests among HIV-positive compared to HIV-negative TB patients (115). In HIV-positive TB, secretion of BCG-specific IgG antibodies from peripheral plasmablasts was higher than in HIV-negative TB, and it increased further as CD4 T cell counts declined (116). The higher levels of antibody in HIV-positive TB likely reflect increased systemic mycobacterial load. The interaction of HIV with *M. tuberculosis* susceptibility is discussed in detail in reference 117.

Diabetes mellitus

The link between type 2 diabetes mellitus (T2DM) and increased TB risk has long been recognized (118), but the immunological mechanisms are poorly understood. Up to 22% of TB cases are attributed to T2DM in countries where both conditions are endemic (119). Recent systematic reviews have shown that individuals with T2DM have a 3-fold greater risk of TB and increased risk of mortality, delayed sputum conversion, treatment failure, and relapse, as well as developing drug resistance due to T2DM, interfering with rifampin metabolism (120–124). TB patients with T2DM are also more likely to have cavitary TB (124), while HIV-1 decreases this risk (125). Therefore, while HIV-1 increases TB risk up to 50-fold (126), the increasing prevalence of T2DM could have a relatively greater impact on TB control in the future (127).

Two mechanisms underlying the T2DM-associated risk for TB have been hypothesized: (i) dysregulated glucose metabolism results in hyperglycemia and insulin resistance, enhancing *M. tuberculosis* replication, and (ii) increased inflammation by adipose-resident monocytes activated by free fatty acids and lipid intermediates, associated with insulin resistance, promotes a generalized proinflammatory environment that favors progression to TB disease (118, 128). In support of the second hypothesis, it has recently been shown that TB patients with T2DM have increased circulating Th1 (IFN-γ, TNF, IL-2), Th17 (IL-17A), and other proinflammatory (IL-1β, IL-6, IL-18) cytokines, hyperreactive T-helper cells, and reduced frequencies of regulatory T cells (Tregs) (129–131). How T2DM-associated inflammation impacts TB susceptibility, TB immunopathology, and *M. tuberculosis* killing is unknown, but longitudinal studies investigating HbA1c levels in TB patients during TB treatment have shown that glucose intolerance decreases following successful TB treatment (132, 133). This suggests that in some cases T2DM may result from infection-induced impaired glucose metabolism, rather than prior T2DM increasing TB risk. Irrespective of the sequence of attainment, screening and treatment for glucose intolerance during TB are likely to improve treatment outcome.

Vitamin D

Vitamin D deficiency is common in active TB patients (102, 134), is exacerbated in TB patients with HIV-1, and is more prevalent in people with LTBI who progress to active TB (135). Furthermore, individuals who carry a vitamin D receptor (VDR) polymorphism at the Taq1 locus (rs731236) or the vitamin D binding protein Gc2 haplotype (T420K amino acid change) and are vitamin D deficient are more susceptible to TB (134, 136). The effects of vitamin D on the immune system are pleiotropic (137). Consequently, the exact mechanisms by which vitamin D may help prevent TB remain a subject of contention. Moreover, the unique antimicrobial effect of vitamin D metabolites, mediated by expression of cathelicidin antimicrobial peptide (*CAMP*), is unique to humans (and other primates), who have evolved three vitamin D response elements in the *CAMP* promoter. These promoter elements are missing from rodents and cattle (138), species commonly studied as models of human TB.

Vitamin D has two modes of action. One is fast-activating via membrane VDR, increasing reactive oxygen species (139), nitric oxide (140), and phagolysosome fusion during mycobacterial infection (141). The other occurs via binding to the nuclear VDR, forming a transcription factor complex which targets more than 900 promoters (142). VDR activation induces expression of cathelicidin (proteolytically cleaved into LL-37), which has direct antimycobacterial effects and also induces autophagy (25, 101, 143). Vitamin D treatment also reduces matrix metalloproteinase (MMP) activity, which is linked to lung matrix degradation and chemokine processing (144, 145). Conversely, vitamin D drives the adaptive response toward an anti-inflammatory state, increasing IL-10 production and regulatory T cell differentiation and inhibiting proinflammatory cytokines (99, 146, 147). While a decrease in proinflammatory responses during initial infection is counterintuitive to a protective response, the anti-inflammatory effects of vitamin D are likely to enhance resolution of pathologic inflammation during TB treatment (148). The same may occur during initial infection, limiting excessive inflammation while enhancing antimycobacterial activity.

The antimicrobial effects of vitamin D metabolites have also been shown to be crucial for the protective activity of IFN-γ. We and others have shown that stimulating human monocytes and MDM with IFN-γ in vitamin D-sufficient media prior to infection increased *CAMP* expression and autophagolysosomal fusion and reduced intracellular *M. tuberculosis* growth (149, 150). Conversely, pre- and postinfection treatment of MDM with IFN-γ had no effect on vitamin D-mediated *M. tuberculosis* growth restriction when vitamin D metabolites were added postinfection (149). This suggests that maintaining vitamin D sufficiency prior to infection will enhance macrophage and T cell-mediated innate cell responses during *M. tuberculosis* infection.

Malnutrition

Malnutrition has historically been associated with peaks in TB incidence, but the direct effect of malnutrition on TB risk is ill-defined (151). Body mass index (BMI) and TB incidence have been demonstrated to have an inverse relationship, with a 13.8% reduction in TB per unit increase in BMI (152). Malnutrition can encompass both macronutrient and micronutrient deficiencies; however, the underlying interaction of each with host immunity to increase TB risk is poorly understood. Studies have shown that TB patients from various populations have deficiencies of vitamins A, C, D, and E, zinc, and iron

(153). Vitamin D, being the most studied, has been described above. Recent evidence suggests that vitamin C has direct anti-*M. tuberculosis* activity, dependent on high ferrous ion levels and reactive oxygen species production (154). Vitamin A (retinol) deficiency is also associated with TB and may synergize with vitamin D, as the retinol X receptor RXR forms a heterodimer with the VDR to form a transcription factor complex, and cotreatment with vitamin D_3 plus retinoic acid inhibits *M. tuberculosis* entry and survival within macrophages, possibly through rescue of phagosome maturation arrest (155). Vitamin A, via its active metabolite all-trans retinoic acid, has recently been shown to induce myeloid cells to express *NPC2*, which helps the cell effectively remove cholesterol from the lysosomes so *M. tuberculosis* bacteria cannot access it. This increases lysosome acidification and *M. tuberculosis* killing (156). Moreover, vitamin A adjunct therapy during intensive-phase TB treatment enhances sputum smear conversion (157).

Inflammation and Progression to TB

TB disease is a chronic inflammatory condition, and the pathology of the disease is a consequence of the host immune response to the mycobacterium, rather than direct destruction of tissue by *M. tuberculosis* itself. The balance of sufficient inflammation for containment of infection and immune pathology as a result of excessive inflammation is critical to our understanding of human TB disease. In 1891 Robert Koch reported results of a study in which he repeatedly injected TB patients with tuberculin (158). This treatment did not cure TB but, rather, induced inflammation, swollen lymph nodes, and tissue necrosis and in some patients resulted in death (158). In addition to the magnitude of the inflammatory response, the timing and location of the response are also likely to be key for the balance between control of infection and progression to active disease (reviewed in reference 33). While animal models have revealed the importance of individual cell types such as neutrophils, classically and alternatively activated macrophages, and specific cytokines such as IL-10 and TNF (159) in a balanced inflammatory response, it has been harder to understand these processes in human populations. Genetics can influence the inflammatory response, but the strongest driver of variability in the human inflammatory response appears to be our environment. In an immune phenotyping study, differences in immune cell populations were largely associated with environmental and not genetic factors, with cytomegalovirus identified as the major microbial driver of immune variation (160).

Type I interferons in TB

The type I interferon response is classically a response to viral infection, and yet human biomarker studies have identified IFN-α/β proinflammatory immune signatures as key components of active TB disease (24, 161–164). This response is likely driven by mycobacterial load because it associates with disease pathology and declines in response to TB treatment (164, 165). *In vitro* experiments show that type I interferons reduce the expression of IFN-γ and the ability of macrophages to respond to IFN-γ and control intracellular growth of *M. tuberculosis* (166). IL-1 can limit excessive type 1 interferon activity in mice, suggesting that this pathway could provide a target for host-directed therapy in TB (167).

Monocytes in TB disease

Monocytes are the primary target of mycobacterial growth among PBMCs infected *in vitro*, and in peripheral blood, monocyte numbers expand during active TB disease (168). In the 1930s it was recognized that the ratio of monocytes to lymphocytes in peripheral blood may be important for the resistance or susceptibility to TB disease. During healing of lesions, an increase of lymphocytes around the granuloma has also been detected, and this correlated with an increase in lymphocyte:monocytes in the periphery (169).

Monocytes can be phenotypically and functionally distinct and can differentiate into M1 or M2 macrophages with pro- and anti-inflammatory properties, respectively, although this bipolar nomenculature is becoming more contentious with the increasing emergence of more polarization states which are relative to the activation agent (170). CD16+ "inflammatory" monocytes have recently been shown to modulate immunity to mycobacteria through the production of IL-10 (171). Monocytes can also modulate immunity through amino acid catabolism, in particular tryptophan and arginine, through the induction of indoleamine 2,3-dioxygenase and arginase (reviewed in reference 172). T cells are sensitive to amino acid levels in the microenvironment, and depletion of arginine and tryptophan can result in T cell anergy. Increased ratios of monocytes in peripheral blood are associated with increased type I interferon-related transcript signatures and a reduction in ability to inhibit mycobacterial growth (173). The frequency of monocytes relative to lymphocytes has also been associated with risk of progression to TB disease (174–177). Typically, M1 macrophages are associated with killing of mycobacteria, whereas M2 macrophages are associated with tissue repair and bacterial persistence (178, 179). Therefore, in addition to monocyte quantity, the polarization state of monocytes is likely important for maintenance of balance in the inflammatory response in TB disease.

Tissue Remodeling

The ability of *M. tuberculosis* to induce degradation of pulmonary extracellular matrix (ECM) contributes to its success as a pathogen. Induction of lung cavitation allows bacilli to replicate in an immunologically privileged site, promoting persistence and transmission, while penetration of the alveolar basement membrane allows extrapulmonary dissemination of infection. MMPs, a family of zinc- and calcium-dependent endopeptidases, are capable of degrading all components of the pulmonary ECM. Moreover, MMPs also regulate the innate immune response by controlling cytokine and chemokine processing, apoptosis, and antimicrobial peptide activation (for review, see reference 180). These potent enzymes are expressed by a wide variety of cells, including lymphocytes, resting monocytes, and activated macrophages. MMP-1 (interstitial collagenase) and MMP-9 (92-kDa gelatinase B) are the major secreted MMPs of human monocytes and alveolar macrophages under basal conditions (181). *M. tuberculosis* induces expression of *MMP-1, MMP-7,* and *MMP-10* in infected human macrophages (144, 182), and increased expression of *MMP-1, MMP-7,* and *MMP-9* has also been demonstrated in cells isolated from the lungs of TB patients. MMP-1 and MMP-7 have been shown to colocalize to macrophages around the central area of necrosis in tuberculous granulomata (182, 183). *M. tuberculosis*-induced MMP-1, MMP-7, and MMP-9 secretion by mononuclear phagocytes has been shown to be prostaglandin E2 (PGE2) dependent (182, 184, 185), and IL-4 and IL-10 can inhibit monocyte secretion of MMP-1, MMP-7, and MMP-9 (184, 186, 187). Together this suggests that inhibiting MMP production though reduced PGE2 signaling may limit cavitation and potentially resolve pulmonary pathology during treatment.

T Cell Responses during TB

A recent analysis of immune correlates in infants who participated in the recent Phase IIb efficacy trial of MVA85A (188) suggests that elevated CD4 T cell activation is associated with risk of TB. Infants who developed TB disease during follow-up in the trial had significantly higher levels of total CD4 T cells expressing HLA-DR at study baseline than infants who remained healthy (62). Importantly, this association was replicated in an independent cohort, *M. tuberculosis*-infected adolescents, in whom elevated CD4 T cell

activation was also found to correlate with risk of TB (62).

Positive TST or IGRA tests can spontaneously revert to negative (reviewed in reference 10). Reversion has been reported in many studies throughout the last century at rates of 10 to 50% (189–194). The mechanisms of reversion are not understood, and immune suppression, egress of *M. tuberculosis*-specific T cells from the peripheral blood to sites of infection, or decreases in bacillary load are possible underlying causes. However, TST or IGRA reversion may also be indicative of clearance of *M. tuberculosis* infection. The most comprehensive study of TST reversion was performed in the 1920s in household contacts of TB cases (193). Among household contacts with at least two TSTs, 11.1% reverted from positive to negative. These TST reverters had a very low risk of active TB over the subsequent 5 years (0.72%). By contrast, 23.3% of the entire cohort developed disease. The largest study of Quantiferon Gold In-Tube (QFT) reversion was performed in South African adolescents, in whom annual reversion rates of 5.1% were reported (189). Although the number of TB cases was too low for robust stratification of disease risk in this study, incident TB was 8-fold higher among QFT reverters than among individuals with consistently negative QFT results (1.47 versus 0.18 cases/100 person-years) (189). Additional studies are necessary to establish the clinical significance of TST and IGRA reversion.

B Cells and TB Antibody Responses

Although antibodies are induced against a broad range of protein and nonprotein antigens in active TB disease, they are not useful for diagnosis due to a lack of sensitivity and specificity. There is evidence for reduced antibody avidity in active TB disease and for perturbation in Fc receptor expression, suggesting that phagocytosis and antibody-mediated cellular cytotoxicity could be dysregulated. Transcriptomic signatures for B cells are also depressed in TB, suggesting downregulation or exhaustion of the B cell response. B cells and antibodies are involved in the immune response to TB, and the interaction of antibodies with phagocytic cells through Fc receptor engagement is emerging as a key area for research.

The quantity of antibody produced during *M. tuberculosis* infection is related to bacterial load, and higher antibody responses are observed in those at risk of disease and are correlated with mycobacterial load during disease (195). This suggests that antibodies are important in the control of active TB disease and has also led to the development of antibody-based assays for TB diagnosis. Antibody-based diagnostic assays are cheap to produce and amenable to development as point-of-care tests which can be used in remote settings because they do not require specialist equipment. Much effort has been invested in developing an antibody-based assay for TB diagnosis, with limited success (196). In a systematic review and meta-analysis of the literature, which included 67 studies amounting to 5,147 participants, the sensitivity was 0 to 100% and specificity was 31 to 100% (196). It was concluded that antibody assays produce inconsistent and inaccurate results, and these data were used to inform a World Health Organization policy statement against the use of serological tests (http://whqlibdoc.who.int/publications/2011/978924150 2054_eng.pdf).

However, poor performance of antibodies as a diagnostic test does not translate to lack of importance in immune control of TB disease. This section discusses evidence from human studies of a role for antibodies in the control of TB disease.

Antibody quality

The primary purpose of antibody measurement in human studies has been the diagnosis of TB disease, and most studies focus on the quantity of antibody detected and not antibody quality. Antibody avidity is variable in TB patients (197) and shortly following TB treatment there is an increase in antibody quantity and a decrease in avidity, suggesting exhaustion of the B cell response (198). Perley et al. found a decrease in avidity of antibody specific for the live cell surface of mycobacteria in TB patients, suggesting conversion of antibodies to low-avidity IgG or B cell exhaustion (65). Antibody avidity was also higher in those previously immunized with BCG, which raises the possibility of using vaccination to improve antibody avidity as a potential mechanism for protection against TB.

Antibody function

Given the extensive literature on antibody quantity in TB, there are few studies assessing antibody function using clinical samples. It is known that complement binds efficiently to the surface of mycobacteria and that the classical, lectin, and alternative complement pathways are activated (15, 199). Preincubation with human serum containing mycobacterial specific IgG and IgM further enhances complement binding to mycobacteria (200). The ability of human sera to enhance uptake of mycobacteria into the macrophage is retained after heat treatment to inactivate complement, suggesting that uptake of mycobacteria also occurs via en-

gagement of Fc gamma receptors on the phagocyte cell surface (83). Fc gamma receptor expression has consistently been identified in active TB disease biomarker studies with decreased expression in TB disease, indicating that downregulation of Fc gamma receptor may play a role in pathogenesis of TB disease (161, 162, 201, 202).

BIOMARKERS IN HUMAN TB

A major limitation of IGRA tests and TST is their inability to differentiate between LTBI and active TB disease (reviewed in reference 203). These tests cannot predict risk for progression to TB disease (30). Moreover, whole-blood transcriptomic signatures comparing TB, LTBI, and healthy controls support the recent change in dogma that LTBI represents a spectrum of disease states (Fig. 1), rather than a single clinical stage (204, 205). An important finding from whole-blood transcriptional profiling is that the gene expression signatures of some individuals clinically classified as LTBI cluster with the signature of active TB patients. These data suggest that these asymptomatic individuals may have subclinical TB disease (24, 206).

A biomarker that accurately identifies those at high risk for progression would allow targeted preventive antimicrobial therapy to prevent TB disease. This would be especially useful in settings of TB endemicity, where treating all latently infected people for 6 to 9 months is not feasible. Many investigators are therefore engaged in projects aimed at identifying correlates of risk of TB. The first study to report an association between gene expression in peripheral blood cells and risk of TB disease compared 15 HIV-infected drug users who ultimately progressed to active TB with 16 who remained disease free. Expression of two transcripts, IL-13 and AIRE, was found to correlate with risk of TB (207).

Transcriptomic Profiling

The unprecedented increase in our understanding of the human immune response to *M. tuberculosis* in the past decade is largely attributed to studies using whole-genome transcriptional profiling during various stages of pathogenesis and treatment (reviewed in reference 208). In general, these studies have characterized gene expression in whole blood. While these studies have been able to identify biomarkers with impressive diagnostic sensitivity for active TB, it is not possible to infer correlates of protection against disease from such cross-sectional study designs. To learn about mechanisms that underlie protective responses or progression from infection to disease, longitudinal studies in which individuals transition from LTBI to active TB are necessary. Three recent studies with such longitudinal designs have been completed. The first two were in BCG-vaccinated infants, and the results are discussed in the T cell and antibody sections above. The third was a large cohort study of 6,363 adolescents, half of whom were *M. tuberculosis* infected, who were followed up for 2 years. Incident TB disease was diagnosed during follow-up in 47 adolescents (209). A prominent IFN response signature distinguished asymptomatic, HIV-uninfected persons who progressed to TB disease from those who remained asymptomatic. An additional fourth study adopted an alternate study design using PET/CT imaging of HIV-infected individuals with *M. tuberculosis* infection to identify those with sublinical TB and those at risk of TB (210). In those with underlying HIV infection, IFN response signatures did not readily discriminate between persons with subclinical TB and controls, most likely because HIV infection leads to increased expression of interferon transcripts in peripheral blood (H. Esmail, personal communication). This suggests that discriminating interferon signatures for TB risk may perform with reduced accuracy as predictive biomarkers of disease risk in HIV-infected individuals. However, additional signatures implicating myeloid inflammation and complement components were also identified as correlates of TB risk in both studies. It is clear that more such studies are required to delve deeper into the processes that underlie the transitions between the stages of *M. tuberculosis* infection in HIV-infected and uninfected individuals.

Treatment Response

A large number of studies across various populations have investigated serum biomarkers of TB and their response during therapy. In addition to the classical acute-phase markers C-reactive protein (CRP), serum amyloid A (SAA), and albumin, other highly regulated proteins in TB which change during TB therapy include CXCL9, CXCL10, S100A9, MMP1, MMP9, D-dimer, PGE-2, HGF, VEGF, and sIL-2R (148, 211, 212). Serum markers that can predict fast versus slow response to therapy have also been identified in multiple studies. However, performance of these biomarkers varies depending on the cohort and the cut-off used to define fast response. Some of the most consistent markers include CRP, SAA, sTNF-R1, sIL-2R, and neutrophil-associated proteins, including granzyme B and MMP1 (27, 213–216). Ethnic genetic variation has been identified as a key variable affecting the performance of

biomarkers of TB response (149), a finding that should be considered if protein biomarkers are to be used in TB diagnosis and the monitoring of therapy.

The measurement of antibody levels during TB drug treatment has been inconsistent, with some studies reporting a decline in antibody over time of treatment and others finding that antibody levels rise or do not change (217, 218). As described above, biomarker studies have identified changes in Fc gamma receptor expression in active TB disease (164, 219).

Transcriptomic signatures associated with B cells and humoral immunity have also been identified in biomarker studies focused on the response to TB treatment (164). Gene signatures associated with B cells are initially depressed and rise through therapy. This suggests that B cells are depleted or less functional during active disease, which is consistent with the observation of reduced antibody avidity in active TB (65).

CONCLUSION

Remarkable advances in our understanding of the immune response have been made since the advent of molecular biology and modern immunology. Among the themes are the incredible heterogeneity in infection states, disease presentation, and the complexity of the host response to *M. tuberculosis*. However, the exact immune mechanisms that underlie protective immunity against *M. tuberculosis* in humans remain unknown. Continued concerted research efforts and application of modern technologies are likely to enhance our understanding of the immunopathogenesis of TB in humans and facilitate rational development of highly effective interventions.

Citation. Scriba TJ, Coussens AK, Fletcher HA. 2017. Human immunology of tuberculosis. Microbiol Spectrum 5(1):TBTB2-0016-2016.

References

1. **Gagneux S.** 2012. Host-pathogen coevolution in human tuberculosis. *Philos Trans R Soc Lond B Biol Sci* **367:** 850–859.
2. **Dye C, Scheele S, Dolin P, Pathania V, Raviglione MC.** 1999. Consensus statement. Global burden of tuberculosis: estimated incidence, prevalence, and mortality by country. WHO Global Surveillance and Monitoring Project. *JAMA* **282:**677–686.
3. **Wallgren A.** 1948. The time-table of tuberculosis. *Tubercle* **29:**245–251.
4. **Chen S, Chen J, Chen L, Zhang Q, Luo X, Zhang W.** 2013. *Mycobacterium tuberculosis* infection is associated with the development of erythema nodosum and nodular vasculitis. *PLoS One* **8:**e62653.

5. Mert A, Kumbasar H, Ozaras R, Erten S, Tasli L, Tabak F, Ozturk R. 2007. Erythema nodosum: an evaluation of 100 cases. *Clin Exp Rheumatol* 25:563–570.

6. Nicol MP, Kampmann B, Lawrence P, Wood K, Pienaar S, Pienaar D, Eley B, Levin M, Beatty D, Anderson ST. 2007. Enhanced anti-mycobacterial immunity in children with erythema nodosum and a positive tuberculin skin test. *J Invest Dermatol* 127:2152–2157.

7. Méchaï F, Soler C, Aoun O, Fabre M, Mérens A, Imbert P, Rapp C. 2011. Primary *Mycobacterium bovis* infection revealed by erythema nodosum. *Int J Tuberc Lung Dis* 15:1131–1132.

8. Mahan CS, Zalwango S, Thiel BA, Malone LL, Chervenak KA, Baseke J, Dobbs D, Stein CM, Mayanja H, Joloba M, Whalen CC, Boom WH. 2012. Innate and adaptive immune responses during acute *M. tuberculosis* infection in adult household contacts in Kampala, Uganda. *Am J Trop Med Hyg* 86:690–697.

9. Stein CM, Zalwango S, Malone LL, Won S, Mayanja-Kizza H, Mugerwa RD, Leontiev DV, Thompson CL, Cartier KC, Elston RC, Iyengar SK, Boom WH, Whalen CC, Mugerwa RD, Routy JP, Leontiev DV, Sekaly RP, Thompson CL, Cartier KC, Elston RC, Iyengar SK, Boom WH, Whalen CC. 2008. Genome scan of *M. tuberculosis* infection and disease in Ugandans. *PLoS One* 3:e4094.

10. Hawn TR, Day TA, Scriba TJ, Hatherill M, Hanekom WA, Evans TG, Churchyard GJ, Kublin JG, Bekker L-G, Self SG. 2014. Tuberculosis vaccines and prevention of infection. *Microbiol Mol Biol Rev* 78:650–671.

11. Hirsch CS, Ellner JJ, Russell DG, Rich EA. 1994. Complement receptor-mediated uptake and tumor necrosis factor-alpha-mediated growth inhibition of *Mycobacterium tuberculosis* by human alveolar macrophages. *J Immunol* 152:743–753.

12. Keane J, Balcewicz-Sablinska MK, Remold HG, Chupp GL, Meek BB, Fenton MJ, Kornfeld H. 1997. Infection by *Mycobacterium tuberculosis* promotes human alveolar macrophage apoptosis. *Infect Immun* 65:298–304.

13. Engele M, Stössel E, Castiglione K, Schwerdtner N, Wagner M, Bölcskei P, Röllinghoff M, Stenger S. 2002. Induction of TNF in human alveolar macrophages as a potential evasion mechanism of virulent *Mycobacterium tuberculosis*. *J Immunol* 168:1328–1337.

14. Silver RF, Walrath J, Lee H, Jacobson BA, Horton H, Bowman MR, Nocka K, Sypek JP. 2009. Human alveolar macrophage gene responses to *Mycobacterium tuberculosis* strains H37Ra and H37Rv. *Am J Respir Cell Mol Biol* 40:491–504.

15. Hirsch CS, Ellner JJ, Russell DG, Rich EA. 1994. Complement receptor-mediated uptake and tumor necrosis factor-alpha-mediated growth inhibition of *Mycobacterium tuberculosis* by human alveolar macrophages. *J Immunol* 152:743–753.

16. Lala S, Dheda K, Chang JS, Huggett JF, Kim LU, Johnson MA, Rook GA, Keshav S, Zumla A. 2007. The pathogen recognition sensor, NOD2, is variably expressed in patients with pulmonary tuberculosis. *BMC Infect Dis* 7:96.

17. Juárez E, Carranza C, Hernández-Sánchez F, León-Contreras JC, Hernández-Pando R, Escobedo D, Torres M, Sada E. 2012. NOD2 enhances the innate response of alveolar macrophages to *Mycobacterium tuberculosis* in humans. *Eur J Immunol* 42:880–889.

18. Rivas-Santiago B, Hernandez-Pando R, Carranza C, Juarez E, Contreras JL, Aguilar-Leon D, Torres M, Sada E. 2008. Expression of cathelicidin LL-37 during *Mycobacterium tuberculosis* infection in human alveolar macrophages, monocytes, neutrophils, and epithelial cells. *Infect Immun* 76:935–941.

19. Tsao TC, Hong J, Huang C, Yang P, Liao SK, Chang KS. 1999. Increased TNF-alpha, IL-1 beta and IL-6 levels in the bronchoalveolar lavage fluid with the up-regulation of their mRNA in macrophages lavaged from patients with active pulmonary tuberculosis. *Tuber Lung Dis* 79:279–285.

20. Huang KH, Wang CH, Lee KY, Lin SM, Lin CH, Kuo HP. 2013. NF-κB repressing factor inhibits chemokine synthesis by peripheral blood mononuclear cells and alveolar macrophages in active pulmonary tuberculosis. *PLoS One* 8:e77789.

21. Gleeson LE, Sheedy FJ, Palsson-McDermott EM, Triglia D, O'Leary SM, O'Sullivan MP, O'Neill LA, Keane J. 2016. Cutting Edge: *Mycobacterium tuberculosis* induces aerobic glycolysis in human alveolar macrophages that is required for control of intracellular bacillary replication. *J Immunol* 196:2444–2449.

22. Barnes PF, Leedom JM, Chan LS, Wong SF, Shah J, Vachon LA, Overturf GD, Modlin RL. 1988. Predictors of short-term prognosis in patients with pulmonary tuberculosis. *J Infect Dis* 158:366–371.

23. Lowe DM, Bandara AK, Packe GE, Barker RD, Wilkinson RJ, Griffiths CJ, Martineau AR. 2013. Neutrophilia independently predicts death in tuberculosis. *Eur Respir J* 42:1752–1757.

24. Berry MP, Graham CM, McNab FW, Xu Z, Bloch SA, Oni T, Wilkinson KA, Banchereau R, Skinner J, Wilkinson RJ, Quinn C, Blankenship D, Dhawan R, Cush JJ, Mejias A, Ramilo O, Kon OM, Pascual V, Banchereau J, Chaussabel D, O'Garra A. 2010. An interferon-inducible neutrophil-driven blood transcriptional signature in human tuberculosis. *Nature* 466: 973–977.

25. Martineau AR, Newton SM, Wilkinson KA, Kampmann B, Hall BM, Nawroly N, Packe GE, Davidson RN, Griffiths CJ, Wilkinson RJ. 2007. Neutrophil-mediated innate immune resistance to mycobacteria. *J Clin Invest* 117:1988–1994.

26. Ramos-Kichik V, Mondragón-Flores R, Mondragón-Castelán M, Gonzalez-Pozos S, Muñiz-Hernandez S, Rojas-Espinosa O, Chacón-Salinas R, Estrada-Parra S, Estrada-García I. 2009. Neutrophil extracellular traps are induced by *Mycobacterium tuberculosis*. *Tuberculosis (Edinb)* 89:29–37.

27. Coussens AK, Wilkinson RJ, Nikolayevskyy V, Elkington PT, Hanifa Y, Islam K, Timms PM, Bothamley GH, Claxton AP, Packe GE, Darmalingam M, Davidson RN, Milburn HJ, Baker LV, Barker RD, Drobniewski FA, Mein CA, Bhaw-Rosun L, Nuamah RA, Griffiths CJ, Martineau AR. 2013. Ethnic variation in inflammatory profile in tuberculosis. *PLoS Pathog* 9:e1003468.

28. Krupa A, Fol M, Dziadek BR, Kepka E, Wojciechowska D, Brzostek A, Torzewska A, Dziadek J, Baughman RP, Griffith D, Kurdowska AK. 2015. Binding of CXCL8/IL-8 to *Mycobacterium tuberculosis* modulates the innate immune response. *Mediators Inflamm* 2015:124762.

29. Park H, Li Z, Yang XO, Chang SH, Nurieva R, Wang YH, Wang Y, Hood L, Zhu Z, Tian Q, Dong C. 2005. A distinct lineage of CD4 T cells regulates tissue inflammation by producing interleukin 17. *Nat Immunol* 6:1133–1141.

30. Pai M, Denkinger CM, Kik SV, Rangaka MX, Zwerling A, Oxlade O, Metcalfe JZ, Cattamanchi A, Dowdy DW, Dheda K, Banaei N. 2014. Gamma interferon release assays for detection of *Mycobacterium tuberculosis* infection. *Clin Microbiol Rev* 27:3–20.

31. Hunter RL. 2016. Tuberculosis as a three-act play: a new paradigm for the pathogenesis of pulmonary tuberculosis. *Tuberculosis (Edinb)* 97:8–17.

32. Hunter RL. 2011. Pathology of post primary tuberculosis of the lung: an illustrated critical review. *Tuberculosis (Edinb)* 91:497–509.

33. Dorhoi A, Kaufmann SH. 2014. Perspectives on host adaptation in response to *Mycobacterium tuberculosis*: modulation of inflammation. *Semin Immunol* 26:533–542.

34. Chan J, Mehta S, Bharrhan S, Chen Y, Achkar JM, Casadevall A, Flynn J. 2014. The role of B cells and humoral immunity in *Mycobacterium tuberculosis* infection. *Semin Immunol* 26:588–600.

35. Achkar JM, Chan J, Casadevall A. 2015. B cells and antibodies in the defense against *Mycobacterium tuberculosis* infection. *Immunol Rev* 264:167–181.

36. du Plessis WJ, Walzl G, Loxton AG. 2016. B cells as multi-functional players during *Mycobacterium tuberculosis* infection and disease. *Tuberculosis (Edinb)* 97: 118–125. https://www.ncbi.nlm.nih.gov/pubmed/26611659

37. Rao M, Valentini D, Poiret T, Dodoo E, Parida S, Zumla A, Brighenti S, Maeurer M. 2015. B in TB: B cells as mediators of clinically relevant immune responses in tuberculosis. *Clin Infect Dis* 61(Suppl 3):S225–S234.

38. Sebina I, Biraro IA, Dockrell HM, Elliott AM, Cose S. 2014. Circulating B-lymphocytes as potential biomarkers of tuberculosis infection activity. *PLoS One* 9:e106796.

39. Hoff ST, Salman AM, Ruhwald M, Ravn P, Brock I, Elsheikh N, Andersen P, Agger EM. 2015. Human B cells produce chemokine CXCL10 in the presence of *Mycobacterium tuberculosis* specific T cells. *Tuberculosis (Edinb)* 95:40–47.

40. Zhu Q, Zhang M, Shi M, Liu Y, Zhao Q, Wang W, Zhang G, Yang L, Zhi J, Zhang L, Hu G, Chen P, Yang Y, Dai W, Liu T, He Y, Feng G, Zhao G. 2016. Human B cells have an active phagocytic capability and undergo immune activation upon phagocytosis of *Mycobacterium tuberculosis*. *Immunobiology* 221:558–567.

41. Covert BA, Spencer JS, Orme IM, Belisle JT. 2001. The application of proteomics in defining the T cell antigens of *Mycobacterium tuberculosis*. *Proteomics* 1:574–586.

42. Boesen H, Jensen BN, Wilcke T, Andersen P. 1995. Human T-cell responses to secreted antigen fractions of *Mycobacterium tuberculosis*. *Infect Immun* 63:1491–1497.

43. Wilkinson KA, Wilkinson RJ, Pathan A, Ewer K, Prakash M, Klenerman P, Maskell N, Davies R, Pasvol G, Lalvani A. 2005. Ex vivo characterization of early secretory antigenic target 6-specific T cells at sites of active disease in pleural tuberculosis. *Clin Infect Dis* 40:184–187.

44. Lalvani A, Nagvenkar P, Udwadia Z, Pathan AA, Wilkinson KA, Shastri JS, Ewer K, Hill AV, Mehta A, Rodrigues C. 2001. Enumeration of T cells specific for RD1-encoded antigens suggests a high prevalence of latent *Mycobacterium tuberculosis* infection in healthy urban Indians. *J Infect Dis* 183:469–477.

45. Pathan AA, Wilkinson KA, Klenerman P, McShane H, Davidson RN, Pasvol G, Hill AV, Lalvani A. 2001. Direct ex vivo analysis of antigen-specific IFN-gamma-secreting CD4 T cells in *Mycobacterium tuberculosis*-infected individuals: associations with clinical disease state and effect of treatment. *J Immunol* 167:5217–5225.

46. McShane H, Pathan AA, Sander CR, Keating SM, Gilbert SC, Huygen K, Fletcher HA, Hill AV. 2004. Recombinant modified vaccinia virus Ankara expressing antigen 85A boosts BCG-primed and naturally acquired antimycobacterial immunity in humans. *Nat Med* 10:1240–1244.

47. Abel B, Tameris M, Mansoor N, Gelderbloem S, Hughes J, Abrahams D, Makhethe L, Erasmus M, de Kock M, van der Merwe L, Hawkridge A, Veldsman A, Hatherill M, Schirru G, Pau MG, Hendriks J, Weverling GJ, Goudsmit J, Sizemore D, McClain JB, Goetz M, Gearhart J, Mahomed H, Hussey GD, Sadoff JC, Hanekom WA. 2010. The novel tuberculosis vaccine, AERAS-402, induces robust and polyfunctional CD4+ and CD8+ T cells in adults. *Am J Respir Crit Care Med* 181:1407–1417.

48. Lindestam Arlehamn CS, Gerasimova A, Mele F, Henderson R, Swann J, Greenbaum JA, Kim Y, Sidney J, James EA, Taplitz R, McKinney DM, Kwok WW, Grey H, Sallusto F, Peters B, Sette A. 2013. Memory T cells in latent *Mycobacterium tuberculosis* infection are directed against three antigenic islands and largely contained in a CXCR3+CCR6+ Th1 subset. *PLoS Pathog* 9:e1003130.

49. Carpenter C, Sidney J, Kolla R, Nayak K, Tomiyama H, Tomiyama C, Padilla OA, Rozot V, Ahamed SF, Ponte C, Rolla V, Antas PR, Chandele A, Kenneth J, Laxmi S, Makgotlho E, Vanini V, Ippolito G, Kazanova AS, Panteleev AV, Hanekom W, Mayanja-Kizza H, Lewinsohn D, Saito M, McElrath MJ, Boom WH, Goletti D, Gilman R, Lyadova IV, Scriba TJ, Kallas EG, Murali-Krishna K, Sette A, Lindestam Arlehamn CS. 2015. A side-by-side comparison of T cell reactivity to fifty-nine *Mycobacterium tuberculosis* antigens in diverse populations from five continents. *Tuberculosis (Edinb)* 95:713–721.

50. Lindestam Arlehamn CS, Paul S, Mele F, Huang C, Greenbaum JA, Vita R, Sidney J, Peters B, Sallusto F, Sette A. 2015. Immunological consequences of intragenus conservation of *Mycobacterium tuberculosis* T-cell epitopes. *Proc Natl Acad Sci USA* 112:E147–E155.

51. Day CL, Abrahams DA, Lerumo L, Janse van Rensburg E, Stone L, O'rie T, Pienaar B, de Kock M, Kaplan G, Mahomed H, Dheda K, Hanekom WA. 2011. Functional capacity of *Mycobacterium tuberculosis*-specific T cell responses in humans is associated with mycobacterial load. *J Immunol* 187:2222–2232.

52. Rozot V, Vigano S, Mazza-Stalder J, Idrizi E, Day CL, Perreau M, Lazor-Blanchet C, Petruccioli E, Hanekom W, Goletti D, Bart PA, Nicod L, Pantaleo G, Harari A. 2013. *Mycobacterium tuberculosis*-specific CD8+ T cells are functionally and phenotypically different between latent infection and active disease. *Eur J Immunol* 43: 1568–1577.

53. Rozot V, Patrizia A, Vigano S, Mazza-Stalder J, Idrizi E, Day CL, Perreau M, Lazor-Blanchet C, Ohmiti K, Goletti D, Bart P-A, Hanekom W, Scriba TJ, Nicod L, Pantaleo G, Harari A. 2015. Combined use of *Mycobacterium tuberculosis*-specific CD4 and CD8 T-cell responses is a powerful diagnostic tool of active tuberculosis. *Clin Infect Dis* 60:432–437.

54. Seder RA, Darrah PA, Roederer M. 2008. T-cell quality in memory and protection: implications for vaccine design. *Nat Rev Immunol* 8:247–258.

55. Harari A, Rozot V, Bellutti Enders F, Perreau M, Stalder JM, Nicod LP, Cavassini M, Calandra T, Blanchet CL, Jaton K, Faouzi M, Day CL, Hanekom WA, Bart PA, Pantaleo G. 2011. Dominant TNF-α+ *Mycobacterium tuberculosis*-specific CD4+ T cell responses discriminate between latent infection and active disease. *Nat Med* 17:372–376.

56. Riou C, Gray CM, Lugongolo M, Gwala T, Kiravu A, Deniso P, Stewart-Isherwood L, Omar SV, Grobusch MP, Coetzee G, Conradie F, Ismail N, Kaplan G, Fallows D. 2014. A subset of circulating blood mycobacteria-specific CD4 T cells can predict the time to *Mycobacterium tuberculosis* sputum culture conversion. *PLoS One* 9:e102178.

57. Sutherland JS, Adetifa IM, Hill PC, Adegbola RA, Ota MO. 2009. Pattern and diversity of cytokine production differentiates between *Mycobacterium tuberculosis* infection and disease. *Eur J Immunol* 39:723–729.

58. Caccamo N, Guggino G, Joosten SA, Gelsomino G, Di Carlo P, Titone L, Galati D, Bocchino M, Matarese A, Salerno A, Sanduzzi A, Franken WPJ, Ottenhoff THM, Dieli F. 2010. Multifunctional CD4(+) T cells correlate with active *Mycobacterium tuberculosis* infection. *Eur J Immunol* 40:2211–2220.

59. Mueller H, Detjen AK, Schuck SD, Gutschmidt A, Wahn U, Magdorf K, Kaufmann SH, Jacobsen M. 2008. *Mycobacterium tuberculosis*-specific CD4+, IFNgamma+, and TNFalpha+ multifunctional memory T cells coexpress GM-CSF. *Cytokine* 43:143–148.

60. Kagina BM, Abel B, Bowmaker M, Scriba TJ, Gelderbloem S, Smit E, Erasmus M, Nene N, Walzl G, Black G, Hussey GD, Hesseling AC, Hanekom WA. 2009. Delaying BCG vaccination from birth to 10 weeks of age may result in an enhanced memory CD4 T cell response. *Vaccine* 27:5488–5495.

61. Kagina BM, Abel B, Scriba TJ, Hughes EJ, Keyser A, Soares A, Gamieldien H, Sidibana M, Hatheril M, Gelderbloem S, Mahomed H, Hawkridge A, Hussey G, Kaplan G, Hanekom WA. 2010. Specific T cell frequency and cytokine expression profile do not correlate with protection against tuberculosis, following BCG vaccination of newborns. *Am J Respir Crit Care Med* 182:1073–1079.

62. Fletcher HA, Snowden MA, Landry B, Rida W, Satti I, Harris SA, Matsumiya M, Tanner R, O'Shea MK, Dheenadhayalan V, Bogardus L, Stockdale L, Marsay L, Chomka A, Harrington-Kandt R, Manjaly-Thomas Z-R, Naranbhai V, Stylianou E, Darboe F, Penn-Nicholson A, Nemes E, Hatheril M, Hussey G, Mahomed H, Tameris M, McClain JB, Evans TG, Hanekom WA, Scriba TJ, McShane H. 2016. T-cell activation is an immune correlate of risk in BCG vaccinated infants. *Nat Commun* 7:11290.

63. Adekambi T, Ibegbu CC, Cagle S, Kalokhe AS, Wang YF, Hu Y, Day CL, Ray SM, Rengarajan J. 2015. Biomarkers on patient T cells diagnose active tuberculosis and monitor treatment response. *J Clin Invest* 125: 1827–1838.

64. Esmail H, Barry CE III, Young DB, Wilkinson RJ. 2014. The ongoing challenge of latent tuberculosis. *Philos Trans R Soc Lond B Biol Sci* 369:20130437.

65. Perley CC, Frahm M, Click EM, Dobos KM, Ferrari G, Stout JE, Frothingham R. 2014. The human antibody response to the surface of *Mycobacterium tuberculosis*. *PLoS One* 9:e98938.

66. Yu X, Prados-Rosales R, Jenny-Avital ER, Sosa K, Casadevall A, Achkar JM. 2012. Comparative evaluation of profiles of antibodies to mycobacterial capsular polysaccharides in tuberculosis patients and controls stratified by HIV status. *Clin Vaccine Immunol* 19:198–208.

67. Siev M, Wilson D, Kainth S, Kasprowicz VO, Feintuch CM, Jenny-Avital ER, Achkar JM. 2014. Antibodies against mycobacterial proteins as biomarkers for HIV-associated smear-negative tuberculosis. *Clin Vaccine Immunol* 21:791–798.

68. Baumann R, Kaempfer S, Chegou NN, Oehlmann W, Spallek R, Loxton AG, van Helden PD, Black GF, Singh M, Walzl G. 2015. A subgroup of latently *Mycobacterium tuberculosis* infected individuals is characterized by consistently elevated IgA responses to several mycobacterial antigens. *Mediators Inflamm* 2015:364758.

69. Hoff ST, Abebe M, Ravn P, Range N, Malenganisho W, Rodriques DS, Kallas EG, Søborg C, Mark Doherty T, Andersen P, Weldingh K. 2007. Evaluation of *Mycobacterium tuberculosis*-specific antibody responses in populations with different levels of exposure from Tanzania, Ethiopia, Brazil, and Denmark. *Clin Infect Dis* 45:575–582.

70. Chen J, Wang S, Zhang Y, Su X, Wu J, Shao L, Wang F, Zhang S, Weng X, Wang H, Zhang W. 2010. Rv1985c, a promising novel antigen for diagnosis of tuberculosis infection from BCG-vaccinated controls. *BMC Infect Dis* 10:273.

71. Hur YG, Kim A, Kang YA, Kim AS, Kim DY, Kim Y, Kim Y, Lee H, Cho SN. 2015. Evaluation of antigen-specific immunoglobulin g responses in pulmonary

tuberculosis patients and contacts. *J Clin Microbiol* 53: 904–909.

72. Niki M, Suzukawa M, Akashi S, Nagai H, Ohta K, Inoue M, Niki M, Kaneko Y, Morimoto K, Kurashima A, Kitada S, Matsumoto S, Suzuki K, Hoshino Y. 2015. Evaluation of humoral immunity to *Mycobacterium tuberculosis*-specific antigens for correlation with clinical status and effective vaccine development. *J Immunol Res* 2015:527395.

73. Bothamley GH, Beck JS, Potts RC, Grange JM, Kardjito T, Ivanyi J. 1992. Specificity of antibodies and tuberculin response after occupational exposure to tuberculosis. *J Infect Dis* 166:182–186.

74. Sousa AO, Salem JI, Lee FK, Verçosa MC, Cruaud P, Bloom BR, Lagrange PH, David HL. 1997. An epidemic of tuberculosis with a high rate of tuberculin anergy among a population previously unexposed to tuberculosis, the Yanomami Indians of the Brazilian Amazon. *Proc Natl Acad Sci USA* 94:13227–13232.

75. Das S, Cheng SH, Lowrie DB, Walker KB, Mitchison DA, Vallishayee RS, Narayanan PR. 1992. The pattern of mycobacterial antigen recognition in sera from Mantoux-negative individuals is essentially unaffected by bacille Calmette-Guérin (BCG) vaccination in either south India or London. *Clin Exp Immunol* 89:402–406.

76. Pilkington C, Costello AM, Rook GA, Stanford JL. 1993. Development of IgG responses to mycobacterial antigens. *Arch Dis Child* 69:644–649.

77. Stainsby KJ, Lowes JR, Allan RN, Ibbotson JP. 1993. Antibodies to *Mycobacterium paratuberculosis* and nine species of environmental mycobacteria in Crohn's disease and control subjects. *Gut* 34:371–374.

78. Lagercrantz R, Enell H. 1953. Tuberculin-sensitivity and antibodies (agglutinins) after BCG-vaccination. *Acta Paediatr* 42:316–322.

79. Turneer M, Van Vooren JP, Nyabenda J, Legros F, Lecomte A, Thiriaux J, Serruys E, Yernault JC. 1988. The humoral immune response after BCG vaccination in humans: consequences for the serodiagnosis of tuberculosis. *Eur Respir J* 1:589–593.

80. Beyazova U, Rota S, Cevheroğlu C, Karsligil T. 1995. Humoral immune response in infants after BCG vaccination. *Tuber Lung Dis* 76:248–253.

81. Hoft DF, Kemp EB, Marinaro M, Cruz O, Kiyono H, McGhee JR, Belisle JT, Milligan TW, Miller JP, Belshe RB. 1999. A double-blind, placebo-controlled study of *Mycobacterium*-specific human immune responses induced by intradermal bacille Calmette-Guérin vaccination. *J Lab Clin Med* 134:244–252.

82. de Vallière S, Abate G, Blazevic A, Heuertz RM, Hoft DF. 2005. Enhancement of innate and cell-mediated immunity by antimycobacterial antibodies. *Infect Immun* 73:6711–6720.

83. Kumar SK, Singh P, Sinha S. 2015. Naturally produced opsonizing antibodies restrict the survival of *Mycobacterium tuberculosis* in human macrophages by augmenting phagosome maturation. *Open Biol* 5:150171.

84. Grode L, Seiler P, Baumann S, Hess J, Brinkmann V, Nasser Eddine A, Mann P, Goosmann C, Bandermann S, Smith D, Bancroft GJ, Reyrat J-M, van Soolingen D,

Raupach B, Kaufmann SHE. 2005. Increased vaccine efficacy against tuberculosis of recombinant *Mycobacterium bovis* bacille Calmette-Guérin mutants that secrete listeriolysin. *J Clin Invest* 115:2472–2479.

85. Spertini F, Audran R, Chakour R, Karoui O, Steiner-Monard V, Thierry A-C, Mayor CE, Rettby N, Jaton K, Vallotton L, Lazor-Blanchet C, Doce J, Puentes E, Marinova D, Aguilo N, Martin C. 2015. Safety of human immunisation with a live-attenuated *Mycobacterium tuberculosis* vaccine: a randomised, double-blind, controlled phase I trial. *Lancet Respir Med* 3:953–962.

86. Knudsen NP, Olsen A, Buonsanti C, Follmann F, Zhang Y, Coler RN, Fox CB, Meinke A, D'Oro U, Casini D, Bonci A, Billeskov R, De Gregorio E, Rappuoli R, Harandi AM, Andersen P, Agger EM. 2016. Different human vaccine adjuvants promote distinct antigen-independent immunological signatures tailored to different pathogens. *Sci Rep* 6:19570.

87. Ferebee SH. 1970. Controlled chemoprophylaxis trials in tuberculosis. A general review. *Bibl Tuberc* 26:28–106.

88. Wiker HG, Mustafa T, Bjune GA, Harboe M. 2010. Evidence for waning of latency in a cohort study of tuberculosis. *BMC Infect Dis* 10:37.

89. Opie EL, Aronson JD. 1927. Tubercle bacilli in latent tuberculous lesions and in lung tissue without tuberculous lesions. *Arch Pathol Lab Med* 4:1.

90. Keane J, Gershon S, Wise RP, Mirabile-Levens E, Kasznica J, Schwieterman WD, Siegel JN, Braun MM. 2001. Tuberculosis associated with infliximab, a tumor necrosis factor alpha-neutralizing agent. *N Engl J Med* 345:1098–1104.

91. Singh JA, Wells GA, Christensen R, Tanjong Ghogomu E, Maxwell L, Macdonald JK, Filippini G, Skoetz N, Francis D, Lopes LC, Guyatt GH, Schmitt J, La Mantia L, Weberschock T, Roos JF, Siebert H, Hershan S, Lunn MP, Tugwell P, Buchbinder R. 2011. Adverse effects of biologics: a network meta-analysis and Cochrane overview. *Cochrane Database Syst Rev* (2):CD008794.

92. Ernst JD. 2012. The immunological life cycle of tuberculosis. *Nat Rev Immunol* 12:581–591.

93. Corbett EL, Watt CJ, Walker N, Maher D, Williams BG, Raviglione MC, Dye C. 2003. The growing burden of tuberculosis: global trends and interactions with the HIV epidemic. *Arch Intern Med* 163:1009–1021.

94. Cegielski JP, McMurray DN. 2004. The relationship between malnutrition and tuberculosis: evidence from studies in humans and experimental animals. *Int J Tuberc Lung Dis* 8:286–298.

95. Nnoaham KE, Clarke A. 2008. Low serum vitamin D levels and tuberculosis: a systematic review and meta-analysis. *Int J Epidemiol* 37:113–119.

96. Oeltmann JE, Kammerer JS, Pevzner ES, Moonan PK. 2009. Tuberculosis and substance abuse in the United States, 1997–2006. *Arch Intern Med* 169:189–197.

97. Ferrara G, Murray M, Winthrop K, Centis R, Sotgiu G, Migliori GB, Maeurer M, Zumla A. 2012. Risk factors associated with pulmonary tuberculosis: smoking, diabetes and anti-TNFα drugs. *Curr Opin Pulm Med* 18:233–240.

98. Haug CJ, Aukrust P, Haug E, Mørkrid L, Müller F, Frøland SS. 1998. Severe deficiency of 1,25-dihydroxyvitamin D3 in human immunodeficiency virus infection: association with immunological hyperactivity and only minor changes in calcium homeostasis. *J Clin Endocrinol Metab* **83:**3832–3838.

99. Martineau AR, Wilkinson KA, Newton SM, Floto RA, Norman AW, Skolimowska K, Davidson RN, Sørensen OE, Kampmann B, Griffiths CJ, Wilkinson RJ. 2007. IFN-gamma- and TNF-independent vitamin D-inducible human suppression of mycobacteria: the role of cathelicidin LL-37. *J Immunol* **178:**7190–7198.

100. Kalsdorf B, Scriba TJ, Wood K, Day CL, Dheda K, Dawson R, Hanekom WA, Lange C, Wilkinson RJ. 2009. HIV-1 infection impairs the bronchoalveolar T-cell response to mycobacteria. *Am J Respir Crit Care Med* **180:**1262–1270.

101. Campbell GR, Spector SA. 2011. Hormonally active vitamin D3 (1alpha,25-dihydroxycholecalciferol) triggers autophagy in human macrophages that inhibits HIV-1 infection. *J Biol Chem* **286:**18890–18902.

102. Martineau AR, Nhamoyebonde S, Oni T, Rangaka MX, Marais S, Bangani N, Tsekela R, Bashe L, de Azevedo V, Caldwell J, Venton TR, Timms PM, Wilkinson KA, Wilkinson RJ. 2011. Reciprocal seasonal variation in vitamin D status and tuberculosis notifications in Cape Town, South Africa. *Proc Natl Acad Sci USA* **108:**19013–19017.

103. Chaisson RE, Martinson NA. 2008. Tuberculosis in Africa—combating an HIV-driven crisis. *N Engl J Med* **358:**1089–1092.

104. Coleman CM, Wu L. 2009. HIV interactions with monocytes and dendritic cells: viral latency and reservoirs. *Retrovirology* **6:**51.

105. Tsang J, Chain BM, Miller RF, Webb BL, Barclay W, Towers GJ, Katz DR, Noursadeghi M. 2009. HIV-1 infection of macrophages is dependent on evasion of innate immune cellular activation. *AIDS* **23:**2255–2263.

106. Diedrich CR, Flynn JL. 2011. HIV-1/mycobacterium tuberculosis coinfection immunology: how does HIV-1 exacerbate tuberculosis? *Infect Immun* **79:**1407–1417.

107. Sonnenberg P, Glynn JR, Fielding K, Murray J, Godfrey-Faussett P, Shearer S. 2005. How soon after infection with HIV does the risk of tuberculosis start to increase? A retrospective cohort study in South African gold miners. *J Infect Dis* **191:**150–158.

108. Ranjbar S, Boshoff HI, Mulder A, Siddiqi N, Rubin EJ, Goldfeld AE. 2009. HIV-1 replication is differentially regulated by distinct clinical strains of *Mycobacterium tuberculosis*. *PLoS One* **4:**e6116.

109. Pathak S, Wentzel-Larsen T, Asjö B. 2010. Effects of in vitro HIV-1 infection on mycobacterial growth in peripheral blood monocyte-derived macrophages. *Infect Immun* **78:**4022–4032.

110. Ranjbar S, Jasenosky LD, Chow N, Goldfeld AE. 2012. Regulation of *Mycobacterium tuberculosis*-dependent HIV-1 transcription reveals a new role for NFAT5 in the toll-like receptor pathway. *PLoS Pathog* **8:**e1002620.

111. Toossi Z, Wu M, Hirsch CS, Mayanja-Kizza H, Baseke J, Aung H, Canaday DH, Fujinaga K. 2012. Activation of P-TEFb at sites of dual HIV/TB infection, and inhibition of MTB-induced HIV transcriptional activation by the inhibitor of CDK9, indirubin-3′-monoxime. *AIDS Res Hum Retroviruses* **28:**182–187.

112. Hoshino Y, Nakata K, Hoshino S, Honda Y, Tse DB, Shioda T, Rom WN, Weiden M. 2002. Maximal HIV-1 replication in alveolar macrophages during tuberculosis requires both lymphocyte contact and cytokines. *J Exp Med* **195:**495–505.

113. Toossi Z, Mayanja-Kizza H, Baseke J, Peters P, Wu M, Abraha A, Aung H, Okwera A, Hirsch C, Arts E. 2005. Inhibition of human immunodeficiency virus-1 (HIV-1) by beta-chemokine analogues in mononuclear cells from HIV-1-infected patients with active tuberculosis. *Clin Exp Immunol* **142:**327–332.

114. Maddocks S, Scandurra GM, Nourse C, Bye C, Williams RB, Slobedman B, Cunningham AL, Britton WJ. 2009. Gene expression in HIV-1/*Mycobacterium tuberculosis* co-infected macrophages is dominated by *M. tuberculosis*. *Tuberculosis (Edinb)* **89:**285–293.

115. Lagrange PH, Thangaraj SK, Dayal R, Deshpande A, Ganguly NK, Girardi E, Joshi B, Katoch K, Katoch VM, Kumar M, Lakshmi V, Leportier M, Longuet C, Malladi SV, Mukerjee D, Nair D, Raja A, Raman B, Rodrigues C, Sharma P, Singh A, Singh S, Sodha A, Kabeer BS, Vernet G, Goletti D. 2014. A toolbox for tuberculosis (TB) diagnosis: an Indian multi-centric study (2006-2008); evaluation of serological assays based on PGL-Tb1 and ESAT-6/CFP10 antigens for TB diagnosis. *PLoS One* **9:**e96367.

116. Ashenafi S, Aderaye G, Zewdie M, Raqib R, Bekele A, Magalhaes I, Lema B, Habtamu M, Rekha RS, Aseffa G, Maeurer M, Aseffa A, Svensson M, Andersson J, Brighenti S. 2013. BCG-specific IgG-secreting peripheral plasmablasts as a potential biomarker of active tuberculosis in HIV negative and HIV positive patients. *Thorax* **68:**269–276.

117. du Bruyn E, Wilkinson RJ. 2016. The immune interaction between HIV-1 infection and *Mycobacterium tuberculosis*. *Microbiol Spectrum* **4**(5):TBTB2-0012-2016.

118. Dooley KE, Chaisson RE. 2009. Tuberculosis and diabetes mellitus: convergence of two epidemics. *Lancet Infect Dis* **9:**737–746.

119. Stevenson CR, Forouhi NG, Roglic G, Williams BG, Lauer JA, Dye C, Unwin N. 2007. Diabetes and tuberculosis: the impact of the diabetes epidemic on tuberculosis incidence. *BMC Public Health* **7:**234.

120. Restrepo BI. 2007. Convergence of the tuberculosis and diabetes epidemics: renewal of old acquaintances. *Clin Infect Dis* **45:**436–438.

121. Jeon CY, Murray MB. 2008. Diabetes mellitus increases the risk of active tuberculosis: a systematic review of 13 observational studies. *PLoS Med* **5:**e152.

122. Baker MA, Harries AD, Jeon CY, Hart JE, Kapur A, Lönnroth K, Ottmani SE, Goonesekera SD, Murray MB. 2011. The impact of diabetes on tuberculosis treatment outcomes: a systematic review. *BMC Med* **9:**81.

123. Wang JY, Lee MC, Shu CC, Lee CH, Lee LN, Chao KM, Chang FY. 2015. Optimal duration of anti-TB treatment

in patients with diabetes: nine or six months? *Chest* 147:520–528.

124. Gil-Santana L, Almeida-Junior JL, Oliveira CA, Hickson LS, Daltro C, Castro S, Kornfeld H, Netto EM, Andrade BB. 2016. Diabetes is associated with worse clinical presentation in tuberculosis patients from Brazil: a retrospective cohort study. *PLoS One* 11:e0146876.

125. Restrepo BI, Fisher-Hoch SP, Crespo JG, Whitney E, Perez A, Smith B, McCormick JB, Nuevo Santander Tuberculosis Trackers. 2007. Type 2 diabetes and tuberculosis in a dynamic bi-national border population. *Epidemiol Infect* 135:483–491.

126. Corbett EL, Watt CJ, Walker N, Maher D, Williams BG, Raviglione MC, Dye C. 2003. The growing burden of tuberculosis: global trends and interactions with the HIV epidemic. *Arch Intern Med* 163:1009–1021.

127. Restrepo BI, Schlesinger LS. 2013. Host-pathogen interactions in tuberculosis patients with type 2 diabetes mellitus. *Tuberculosis (Edinb)* 93(Suppl):S10–S14.

128. Shoelson SE, Lee J, Goldfine AB. 2006. Inflammation and insulin resistance. *J Clin Invest* 116:1793–1801.

129. Restrepo BI, Fisher-Hoch SP, Pino PA, Salinas A, Rahbar MH, Mora F, Cortes-Penfield N, McCormick JB. 2008. Tuberculosis in poorly controlled type 2 diabetes: altered cytokine expression in peripheral white blood cells. *Clin Infect Dis* 47:634–641.

130. Jagannathan-Bogdan M, McDonnell ME, Shin H, Rehman Q, Hasturk H, Apovian CM, Nikolajczyk BS. 2011. Elevated proinflammatory cytokine production by a skewed T cell compartment requires monocytes and promotes inflammation in type 2 diabetes. *J Immunol* 186:1162–1172.

131. Kumar NP, Sridhar R, Banurekha VV, Jawahar MS, Fay MP, Nutman TB, Babu S. 2013. Type 2 diabetes mellitus coincident with pulmonary tuberculosis is associated with heightened systemic type 1, type 17, and other proinflammatory cytokines. *Ann Am Thorac Soc* 10:441–449.

132. Jawad F, Shera AS, Memon R, Ansari G. 1995. Glucose intolerance in pulmonary tuberculosis. *J Pak Med Assoc* 45:237–238.

133. Tabarsi P, Baghaei P, Marjani M, Vollmer WM, Masjedi M-R, Harries AD. 2014. Changes in glycosylated haemoglobin and treatment outcomes in patients with tuberculosis in Iran: a cohort study. *J Diabetes Metab Disord* 13:123.

134. Wilkinson RJ, Llewelyn M, Toossi Z, Patel P, Pasvol G, Lalvani A, Wright D, Latif M, Davidson RN. 2000. Influence of vitamin D deficiency and vitamin D receptor polymorphisms on tuberculosis among Gujarati Asians in west London: a case-control study. *Lancet* 355:618–621.

135. Talat N, Perry S, Parsonnet J, Dawood G, Hussain R. 2010. Vitamin D deficiency and tuberculosis progression. *Emerg Infect Dis* 16:853–855.

136. Martineau AR, Leandro AC, Anderson ST, Newton SM, Wilkinson KA, Nicol MP, Pienaar SM, Skolimowska KH, Rocha MA, Rolla VC, Levin M, Davidson RN, Bremner SA, Griffiths CJ, Eley BS, Bonecini-Almeida MG, Wilkinson RJ. 2010. Association between Gc

genotype and susceptibility to TB is dependent on vitamin D status. *Eur Respir J* 35:1106–1112.

137. Coussens AK. 2011. Immunomodulatory actions of vitamin D metabolites and their potential relevance to human lung disease. *Curr Rep Med Rev* 7:444–453.

138. Gombart AF, Borregaard N, Koeffler HP. 2005. Human cathelicidin antimicrobial peptide (CAMP) gene is a direct target of the vitamin D receptor and is strongly up-regulated in myeloid cells by 1,25-dihydroxyvitamin D3. *FASEB J* 19:1067–1077.

139. Sly LM, Lopez M, Nauseef WM, Reiner NE. 2001. 1alpha,25-Dihydroxyvitamin D3-induced monocyte antimycobacterial activity is regulated by phosphatidylinositol 3-kinase and mediated by the NADPH-dependent phagocyte oxidase. *J Biol Chem* 276: 35482–35493.

140. Rockett KA, Brookes R, Udalova I, Vidal V, Hill AV, Kwiatkowski D. 1998. 1,25-Dihydroxyvitamin D3 induces nitric oxide synthase and suppresses growth of *Mycobacterium tuberculosis* in a human macrophage-like cell line. *Infect Immun* 66:5314–5321.

141. Fratti RA, Backer JM, Gruenberg J, Corvera S, Deretic V. 2001. Role of phosphatidylinositol 3-kinase and Rab5 effectors in phagosomal biogenesis and mycobacterial phagosome maturation arrest. *J Cell Biol* 154: 631–644.

142. Wang TT, Tavera-Mendoza LE, Laperriere D, Libby E, MacLeod NB, Nagai Y, Bourdeau V, Konstorum A, Lallemant B, Zhang R, Mader S, White JH. 2005. Large-scale in silico and microarray-based identification of direct 1,25-dihydroxyvitamin D3 target genes. *Mol Endocrinol* 19:2685–2695.

143. Liu PT, Stenger S, Tang DH, Modlin RL. 2007. Cutting edge: vitamin D-mediated human antimicrobial activity against *Mycobacterium tuberculosis* is dependent on the induction of cathelicidin. *J Immunol* 179:2060–2063.

144. Coussens A, Timms PM, Boucher BJ, Venton TR, Ashcroft AT, Skolimowska KH, Newton SM, Wilkinson KA, Davidson RN, Griffiths CJ, Wilkinson RJ, Martineau AR. 2009. 1alpha,25-dihydroxyvitamin D3 inhibits matrix metalloproteinases induced by *Mycobacterium tuberculosis* infection. *Immunology* 127:539–548.

145. Elkington P, Shiomi T, Breen R, Nuttall RK, Ugarte-Gil CA, Walker NF, Saraiva L, Pedersen B, Mauri F, Lipman M, Edwards DR, Robertson BD, D'Armiento J, Friedland JS. 2011. MMP-1 drives immunopathology in human tuberculosis and transgenic mice. *J Clin Invest* 121:1827–1833.

146. Boonstra A, Barrat FJ, Crain C, Heath VL, Savelkoul HF, O'Garra A. 2001. 1alpha,25-Dihydroxyvitamin d3 has a direct effect on naive CD4(+) T cells to enhance the development of Th2 cells. *J Immunol* 167:4974–4980.

147. Xystrakis E, Kusumakar S, Boswell S, Peek E, Urry Z, Richards DF, Adikibi T, Pridgeon C, Dallman M, Loke TK, Robinson DS, Barrat FJ, O'Garra A, Lavender P, Lee TH, Corrigan C, Hawrylowicz CM. 2006. Reversing the defective induction of IL-10-secreting regulatory T cells in glucocorticoid-resistant asthma patients. *J Clin Invest* 116:146–155.

148. Coussens AK, Wilkinson RJ, Hanifa Y, Nikolayevskyy V, Elkington PT, Islam K, Timms PM, Venton TR, Bothamley GH, Packe GE, Darmalingam M, Davidson RN, Milburn HJ, Baker LV, Barker RD, Mein CA, Bhaw-Rosun L, Nuamah R, Young DB, Drobniewski FA, Griffiths CJ, Martineau AR. 2012. Vitamin D accelerates resolution of inflammatory responses during tuberculosis treatment. *Proc Natl Acad Sci USA* **109**: 15449–15454.

149. Coussens AK, Martineau AR, Wilkinson RJ. 2014. Anti-inflammatory and antimicrobial actions of vitamin D in combating TB/HIV. *Scientifica (Cairo)* **2014**: 903680.

150. Fabri M, Stenger S, Shin DM, Yuk JM, Liu PT, Realegeno S, Lee HM, Krutzik SR, Schenk M, Sieling PA, Teles R, Montoya D, Iyer SS, Bruns H, Lewinsohn DM, Hollis BW, Hewison M, Adams JS, Steinmeyer A, Zügel U, Cheng G, Jo EK, Bloom BR, Modlin RL. 2011. Vitamin D is required for IFN-gamma-mediated antimicrobial activity of human macrophages. *Sci Transl Med* **3**:104ra102.

151. Schaible UE, Kaufmann SH. 2007. Malnutrition and infection: complex mechanisms and global impacts. *PLoS Med* **4**:e115.

152. Lönnroth K, Williams BG, Cegielski P, Dye C. 2010. A consistent log-linear relationship between tuberculosis incidence and body mass index. *Int J Epidemiol* **39**: 149–155.

153. Papathakis P, Piwoz E. 2008. *Nutrition and Tuberculosis: A Review of the Literature and Considerations for TB Control Programs.* USAID / Africa's Health in 2010 Project. http://digitalcommons.calpoly.edu/cgi/viewcontent.cgi?article=1009&context=fsn_fac

154. Vilchèze C, Hartman T, Weinrick B, Jacobs WRJ Jr. 2013. *Mycobacterium tuberculosis* is extraordinarily sensitive to killing by a vitamin C-induced Fenton reaction. *Nat Commun* **4**:1881.

155. Anand PK, Kaul D, Sharma M. 2008. Synergistic action of vitamin D and retinoic acid restricts invasion of macrophages by pathogenic mycobacteria. *J Microbiol Immunol Infect* **41**:17–25.

156. Wheelwright M, Kim EW, Inkeles MS, De Leon A, Pellegrini M, Krutzik SR, Liu PT. 2014. All-trans retinoic acid-triggered antimicrobial activity against *Mycobacterium tuberculosis* is dependent on NPC2. *J Immunol* **192**:2280–2290.

157. Karyadi E, West CE, Schultink W, Nelwan RH, Gross R, Amin Z, Dolmans WM, Schlebusch H, van der Meer JW. 2002. A double-blind, placebo-controlled study of vitamin A and zinc supplementation in persons with tuberculosis in Indonesia: effects on clinical response and nutritional status. *Am J Clin Nutr* **75**:720–727.

158. Koch R. 1891. A further communication on a remedy for tuberculosis. *BMJ* **1**:125–127.

159. Roca FJ, Ramakrishnan L. 2013. TNF dually mediates resistance and susceptibility to mycobacteria via mitochondrial reactive oxygen species. *Cell* **153**:521–534.

160. Brodin P, Jojic V, Gao T, Bhattacharya S, Angel CJ, Furman D, Shen-Orr S, Dekker CL, Swan GE, Butte AJ, Maecker HT, Davis MM. 2015. Variation in the human immune system is largely driven by non-heritable influences. *Cell* **160**:37–47.

161. Maertzdorf J, Ota M, Repsilber D, Mollenkopf HJ, Weiner J, Hill PC, Kaufmann SH. 2011. Functional correlations of pathogenesis-driven gene expression signatures in tuberculosis. *PLoS One* **6**:e26938.

162. Maertzdorf J, Repsilber D, Parida SK, Stanley K, Roberts T, Black G, Walzl G, Kaufmann SH. 2011. Human gene expression profiles of susceptibility and resistance in tuberculosis. *Genes Immun* **12**:15–22.

163. Ottenhoff TH, Dass RH, Yang N, Zhang MM, Wong HE, Sahiratmadja E, Khor CC, Alisjahbana B, van Crevel R, Marzuki S, Seielstad M, van de Vosse E, Hibberd ML. 2012. Genome-wide expression profiling identifies type 1 interferon response pathways in active tuberculosis. *PLoS One* **7**:e45839.

164. Cliff JM, Lee JS, Constantinou N, Cho JE, Clark TG, Ronacher K, King EC, Lukey PT, Duncan K, Van Helden PD, Walzl G, Dockrell HM. 2013. Distinct phases of blood gene expression pattern through tuberculosis treatment reflect modulation of the humoral immune response. *J Infect Dis* **207**:18–29.

165. Bloom CI, Graham CM, Berry MP, Rozakeas F, Redford PS, Wang Y, Xu Z, Wilkinson KA, Wilkinson RJ, Kendrick Y, Devouassoux G, Ferry T, Miyara M, Bouvry D, Valeyre D, Gorochov G, Blankenship D, Saadatian M, Vanhems P, Beynon H, Vancheeswaran R, Wickremasinghe M, Chaussabel D, Banchereau J, Pascual V, Ho LP, Lipman M, O'Garra A. 2013. Transcriptional blood signatures distinguish pulmonary tuberculosis, pulmonary sarcoidosis, pneumonias and lung cancers. *PLoS One* **8**:e70630.

166. de Paus RA, van Wengen A, Schmidt I, Visser M, Verdegaal EM, van Dissel JT, van de Vosse E. 2013. Inhibition of the type I immune responses of human monocytes by IFN-α and IFN-β. *Cytokine* **61**:645–655.

167. Mayer-Barber KD, Andrade BB, Oland SD, Amaral EP, Barber DL, Gonzales J, Derrick SC, Shi R, Kumar NP, Wei W, Yuan X, Zhang G, Cai Y, Babu S, Catalfamo M, Salazar AM, Via LE, Barry CE III, Sher A. 2014. Host-directed therapy of tuberculosis based on interleukin-1 and type I interferon crosstalk. *Nature* **511**:99–103.

168. Rogers PM. 1928. A study of the blood monocytes in children with tuberculosis. *N Engl J Med* **198**:740–749.

169. Doan CA, Sabin FR. 1930. Studies on tuberculosis. IV. The relation of the tubercle and the monocyte:lymphocyte ratio to resistance and susceptibility in tuberculosis. *J Exp Med* **52**(Suppl 3):113–152.

170. Murray PJ, Allen JE, Biswas SK, Fisher EA, Gilroy DW, Goerdt S, Gordon S, Hamilton JA, Ivashkiv LB, Lawrence T, Locati M, Mantovani A, Martinez FO, Mege J-L, Mosser DM, Natoli G, Saeij JP, Schultze JL, Shirey KA, Sica A, Suttles J, Udalova I, van Ginderachter JA, Vogel SN, Wynn TA. 2014. Macrophage activation and polarization: nomenclature and experimental guidelines. *Immunity* **41**:14–20.

171. Lastrucci C, Bénard A, Balboa L, Pingris K, Souriant S, Poincloux R, Al Saati T, Rasolofo V, González-Montaner P, Inwentarz S, Moraña EJ, Kondova I,

Verreck FA, Sasiain MC, Neyrolles O, Maridonneau-Parini I, Lugo-Villarino G, Cougoule C. 2015. Tuberculosis is associated with expansion of a motile, permissive and immunomodulatory CD16(+) monocyte population via the IL-10/STAT3 axis. *Cell Res* **25:** 1333–1351.

172. Dorhoi A, Kaufmann SH. 2014. Perspectives on host adaptation in response to *Mycobacterium tuberculosis*: modulation of inflammation. *Semin Immunol* **26:**533–542.

173. Naranbhai V, Fletcher HA, Tanner R, O'Shea MK, McShane H, Fairfax BP, Knight JC, Hill AV. 2015. Distinct transcriptional and anti-mycobacterial profiles of peripheral blood monocytes dependent on the ratio of monocytes: lymphocytes. *EBioMedicine* **2:**1619–1626.

174. Naranbhai V, Hill AV, Abdool Karim SS, Naidoo K, Abdool Karim Q, Warimwe GM, McShane H, Fletcher H. 2014. Ratio of monocytes to lymphocytes in peripheral blood identifies adults at risk of incident tuberculosis among HIV-infected adults initiating antiretroviral therapy. *J Infect Dis* **209:**500–509.

175. Naranbhai V, Moodley D, Chipato T, Stranix-Chibanda L, Nakabaiito C, Kamateeka M, Musoke P, Manji K, George K, Emel LM, Richardson P, Andrew P, Fowler M, Fletcher H, McShane H, Coovadia HM, Hill AV, HPTN 046 Protocol Team. 2014. The association between the ratio of monocytes: lymphocytes and risk of tuberculosis among HIV-infected postpartum women. *J Acquir Immune Defic Syndr* **67:** 573–575.

176. Naranbhai V, Kim S, Fletcher H, Cotton MF, Violari A, Mitchell C, Nachman S, McSherry G, McShane H, Hill AV, Madhi SA. 2014. The association between the ratio of monocytes:lymphocytes at age 3 months and risk of tuberculosis (TB) in the first two years of life. *BMC Med* **12:**120.

177. Rakotosamimanana N, Richard V, Raharimanga V, Gicquel B, Doherty TM, Zumla A, Rasolofo Razanamparany V. 2015. Biomarkers for risk of developing active tuberculosis in contacts of TB patients: a prospective cohort study. *Eur Respir J* **46:**1095–1103.

178. Schaale K, Brandenburg J, Kispert A, Leitges M, Ehlers S, Reiling N. 2013. Wnt6 is expressed in granulomatous lesions of *Mycobacterium tuberculosis*-infected mice and is involved in macrophage differentiation and proliferation. *J Immunol* **191:**5182–5195.

179. Labonte AC, Tosello-Trampont AC, Hahn YS. 2014. The role of macrophage polarization in infectious and inflammatory diseases. *Mol Cells* **37:**275–285.

180. Parks WC, Wilson CL, López-Boado YS. 2004. Matrix metalloproteinases as modulators of inflammation and innate immunity. *Nat Rev Immunol* **4:**617–629.

181. Welgus HG, Campbell EJ, Cury JD, Eisen AZ, Senior RM, Wilhelm SM, Goldberg GI. 1990. Neutral metalloproteinases produced by human mononuclear phagocytes. Enzyme profile, regulation, and expression during cellular development. *J Clin Invest* **86:**1496–1502.

182. Elkington PT, Nuttall RK, Boyle JJ, O'Kane CM, Horncastle DE, Edwards DR, Friedland JS. 2005. *Mycobacterium tuberculosis*, but not vaccine BCG, specifi-

cally upregulates matrix metalloproteinase-1. *Am J Respir Crit Care Med* **172:**1596–1604.

183. Chang JC, Wysocki A, Tchou-Wong KM, Moskowitz N, Zhang Y, Rom WN. 1996. Effect of *Mycobacterium tuberculosis* and its components on macrophages and the release of matrix metalloproteinases. *Thorax* **51:** 306–311.

184. Busiek DF, Baragi V, Nehring LC, Parks WC, Welgus HG. 1995. Matrilysin expression by human mononuclear phagocytes and its regulation by cytokines and hormones. *J Immunol* **154:**6484–6491.

185. Zhang Y, McCluskey K, Fujii K, Wahl LM. 1998. Differential regulation of monocyte matrix metalloproteinase and TIMP-1 production by TNF-alpha, granulocyte-macrophage CSF, and IL-1 beta through prostaglandin-dependent and -independent mechanisms. *J Immunol* **161:**3071–3076.

186. Lacraz S, Nicod L, Galve-de Rochemonteix B, Baumberger C, Dayer JM, Welgus HG. 1992. Suppression of metalloproteinase biosynthesis in human alveolar macrophages by interleukin-4. *J Clin Invest* **90:**382–388.

187. Lacraz S, Nicod LP, Chicheportiche R, Welgus HG, Dayer JM. 1995. IL-10 inhibits metalloproteinase and stimulates TIMP-1 production in human mononuclear phagocytes. *J Clin Invest* **96:**2304–2310.

188. Tameris MD, Hatherill M, Landry BS, Scriba TJ, Snowden MA, Lockhart S, Shea JE, McClain JB, Hussey GD, Hanekom WA, Mahomed H, McShane H, MVA85A 020 Trial Study Team. 2013. Safety and efficacy of MVA85A, a new tuberculosis vaccine, in infants previously vaccinated with BCG: a randomised, placebo-controlled phase 2b trial. *Lancet* **381:**1021–1028.

189. Andrews JR, Hatherill M, Mahomed H, Hanekom WA, Campo M, Hawn TR, Wood R, Scriba TJ. 2015. The dynamics of QuantiFERON-TB gold in-tube conversion and reversion in a cohort of South African adolescents. *Am J Respir Crit Care Med* **191:**584–591.

190. Vynnycky E, Fine PE. 1999. Interpreting the decline in tuberculosis: the role of secular trends in effective contact. *Int J Epidemiol* **28:**327–334.

191. Vynnycky E, Fine PE. 2000. Lifetime risks, incubation period, and serial interval of tuberculosis. *Am J Epidemiol* **152:**247–263.

192. Fine PE, Bruce J, Ponnighaus JM, Nkhosa P, Harawa A, Vynnycky E. 1999. Tuberculin sensitivity: conversions and reversions in a rural African population. *Int J Tuberc Lung Dis* **3:**962–975.

193. Dahlstrom AW. 1940. The instability of the tuberculin reaction. *Am Rev Tuberc* **42:**471.

194. Gordin FM, Perez-Stable EJ, Reid M, Schecter G, Cosgriff L, Flaherty D, Hopewell PC. 1991. Stability of positive tuberculin tests: are boosted reactions valid? *Am Rev Respir Dis* **144:**560–563.

195. Kunnath-Velayudhan S, Davidow AL, Wang HY, Molina DM, Huynh VT, Salamon H, Pine R, Michel G, Perkins MD, Xiaowu L, Felgner PL, Flynn JL, Catanzaro A, Gennaro ML. 2012. Proteome-scale antibody responses and outcome of *Mycobacterium tuberculosis* infection in nonhuman primates and in tuberculosis patients. *J Infect Dis* **206:**697–705.

196. Steingart KR, Flores LL, Dendukuri N, Schiller I, Laal S, Ramsay A, Hopewell PC, Pai M. 2011. Commercial serological tests for the diagnosis of active pulmonary and extrapulmonary tuberculosis: an updated systematic review and meta-analysis. *PLoS Med* 8:e1001062.

197. Maes RF. 1991. Evaluation of the avidity of IgG anti-mycobacterial antibodies in tuberculous patients serum by an A-60 immunoassay. *Eur J Epidemiol* 7: 188–190.

198. Arias-Bouda LM, Kuijper S, Van der Werf A, Nguyen LN, Jansen HM, Kolk AH. 2003. Changes in avidity and level of immunoglobulin G antibodies to *Mycobacterium tuberculosis* in sera of patients undergoing treatment for pulmonary tuberculosis. *Clin Diagn Lab Immunol* 10:702–709.

199. Carroll MV, Lack N, Sim E, Krarup A, Sim RB. 2009. Multiple routes of complement activation by Mycobacterium bovis BCG. *Mol Immunol* 46:3367–3378.

200. Carroll MV, Lack N, Sim E, Krarup A, Sim RB. 2009. Multiple routes of complement activation by *Mycobacterium bovis* BCG. *Mol Immunol* 46:3367–3378.

201. Jacobsen M, Repsilber D, Gutschmidt A, Neher A, Feldmann K, Mollenkopf HJ, Ziegler A, Kaufmann SH. 2007. Candidate biomarkers for discrimination between infection and disease caused by *Mycobacterium tuberculosis*. *J Mol Med Berl* 85:613–621.

202. Laux da Costa L, Delcroix M, Dalla Costa ER, Prestes IV, Milano M, Francis SS, Unis G, Silva DR, Riley LW, Rossetti ML. 2015. A real-time PCR signature to discriminate between tuberculosis and other pulmonary diseases. *Tuberculosis (Edinb)* 95:421–425.

203. Pai M. 2010. Spectrum of latent tuberculosis – existing tests cannot resolve the underlying phenotypes. *Nat Rev Microbiol* 8:242.

204. Young DB, Gideon HP, Wilkinson RJ. 2009. Eliminating latent tuberculosis. *Trends Microbiol* 17:183–188.

205. Esmail H, Barry CE III, Wilkinson RJ. 2012. Understanding latent tuberculosis: the key to improved diagnostic and novel treatment strategies. *Drug Discov Today* 17:514–521.

206. Kaforou M, Wright VJ, Oni T, French N, Anderson ST, Bangani N, Banwell CM, Brent AJ, Crampin AC, Dockrell HM, Eley B, Heyderman RS, Hibberd ML, Kern F, Langford PR, Ling L, Mendelson M, Ottenhoff TH, Zgambo F, Wilkinson RJ, Coin LJ, Levin M. 2013. Detection of tuberculosis in HIV-infected and -uninfected African adults using whole blood RNA expression signatures: a case-control study. *PLoS Med* 10:e1001538.

207. Sloot R, Schim van der Loeff MF, van Zwet EW, Haks MC, Keizer ST, Scholing M, Ottenhoff THM, Borgdorff MW, Joosten SA. 2014. Biomarkers can identify pulmonary tuberculosis in HIV-infected drug users months prior to clinical diagnosis. *EBioMedicine* 2:172–179.

208. Deffur A, Wilkinson RJ, Coussens AK. 2015. Tricks to translating TB transcriptomics. *Ann Transl Med* 3 (Suppl 1):S43.

209. Zak DE, Penn-Nicholson A, Scriba TJ, Thompson E, Suliman S, Amon LM, Mahomed H, Erasmus M, Whatney W, Hussey GD, Abrahams D, Kafaar F, Hawkridge T, Verver S, Hughes EJ, Ota M, Sutherland J, Howe R, Dockrell HM, Boom WH, Thiel B, Ottenhoff THM, Mayanja-Kizza H, Crampin AC, Downing K, Hatherill M, Valvo J, Shankar S, Parida SK, Kaufmann SHE, Walzl G, Aderem A, Hanekom WA, ACS and GC6-74 cohort study groups. 2016. A blood RNA signature for tuberculosis disease risk: a prospective cohort study. *Lancet* 387:2312–2322.

210. Esmail H, Lai RP, Lesosky M, Wilkinson KA, Graham CM, Coussens AK, Oni T, Warwick JM, Said-Hartley Q, Koegelenberg CF, Walzl G, Flynn JL, Young DB, Barry CE III, O'Garra A, Wilkinson RJ. 2016. Characterization of progressive HIV-associated tuberculosis using 2-deoxy-2-[(18)F]fluoro-D-glucose positron emission and computed tomography. *Nat Med* 22:1090–1093.

211. De Groote MA, Nahid P, Jarlsberg L, Johnson JL, Weiner M, Muzanyi G, Janjic N, Sterling DG, Ochsner UA. 2013. Elucidating novel serum biomarkers associated with pulmonary tuberculosis treatment. *PLoS One* 8: e61002.

212. Wergeland I, Pullar N, Assmus J, Ueland T, Tonby K, Feruglio S, Kvale D, Damås JK, Aukrust P, Mollnes TE, Dyrhol-Riise AM. 2015. IP-10 differentiates between active and latent tuberculosis irrespective of HIV status and declines during therapy. *J Infect* 70: 381–391.

213. Agranoff D, Fernandez-Reyes D, Papadopoulos MC, Rojas SA, Herbster M, Loosemore A, Tarelli E, Sheldon J, Schwenk A, Pollok R, Rayner CF, Krishna S. 2006. Identification of diagnostic markers for tuberculosis by proteomic fingerprinting of serum. *Lancet* 368:1012–1021.

214. Brahmbhatt S, Black GF, Carroll NM, Beyers N, Salker F, Kidd M, Lukey PT, Duncan K, van Helden P, Walzl G. 2006. Immune markers measured before treatment predict outcome of intensive phase tuberculosis therapy. *Clin Exp Immunol* 146:243–252.

215. Djoba Siawaya JF, Bapela NB, Ronacher K, Beyers N, van Helden P, Walzl G. 2008. Differential expression of interleukin-4 (IL-4) and IL-4 delta 2 mRNA, but not transforming growth factor beta (TGF-beta), TGF-beta RII, Foxp3, gamma interferon, T-bet, or GATA-3 mRNA, in patients with fast and slow responses to antituberculosis treatment. *Clin Vaccine Immunol* 15: 1165–1170.

216. Djoba Siawaya JF, Bapela NB, Ronacher K, Veenstra H, Kidd M, Gie R, Beyers N, van Helden P, Walzl G. 2008. Immune parameters as markers of tuberculosis extent of disease and early prediction of anti-tuberculosis chemotherapy response. *J Infect* 56:340–347.

217. Baumann R, Kaempfer S, Chegou NN, Nene NF, Veenstra H, Spallek R, Bolliger CT, Lukey PT, van Helden PD, Singh M, Walzl G. 2013. Serodiagnostic markers for the prediction of the outcome of intensive phase tuberculosis therapy. *Tuberculosis (Edinb)* 93: 239–245.

218. Feng X, Yang X, Xiu B, Qie S, Dai Z, Chen K, Zhao P, Zhang L, Nicholson RA, Wang G, Song X, Zhang H.

2014. IgG, IgM and IgA antibodies against the novel polyprotein in active tuberculosis. *BMC Infect Dis* **14:**336.

219. **Cliff JM, Kaufmann SH, McShane H, van Helden P, O'Garra A.** 2015. The human immune response to tuberculosis and its treatment: a view from the blood. *Immunol Rev* **264:**88–102.

220. **Cornil V, Ranvier L.** 1880. *A Manual of Pathological Histology. Part III.* Henry G. Lea, Philadelphia, PA.

221. **Hamilton DJ.** 1883. *On the Pathology of Bronchitis, Catarrhal Pneumonia, Tubercle, and Allied Lesions of the Human Lung.* Macmillan and Co., London, United Kingdom.

222. **Baumann R, Kaempfer S, Chegou NN, Oehlmann W, Loxton AG, Kaufmann SH, van Helden PD, Black GF, Singh M, Walzl G.** 2014. Serologic diagnosis of tuberculosis by combining Ig classes against selected mycobacterial targets. *J Infect* **69:**581–589.

Tuberculosis and the Tubercle Bacillus, 2nd ed.
Edited by William R. Jacobs, Jr., Helen McShane, Valerie Mizrahi, and Ian M. Orme
© 2018 American Society for Microbiology, Washington, DC
doi:10.1128/microbiolspec.TBTB2-0012-2016

The Immune Interaction between HIV-1 Infection and *Mycobacterium tuberculosis*

12

Elsa du Bruyn[1] and Robert John Wilkinson[1,2]

INTRODUCTION

HIV-1-infected people are approximately 26 times more likely to develop tuberculosis (TB) than HIV-1-uninfected people (1). This increased risk of developing TB is apparent early after HIV-1 seroconversion: a large study of South African miners found that TB incidence doubled within the first year of HIV-1 infection (2). Of the 9.6 million reported TB cases in 2014, 1.2 million were coinfected with HIV-1, with 74% of reported HIV-1-infected TB cases being from Africa (1). The HIV-1 burden in sub-Saharan Africa is particularly high, where 25.8 million people were living with HIV in 2014 and only 41% had access to antiretroviral therapy (ART) (3). The relatively low ART access may arise in part from a lack of eligibility as determined by local guidelines. It is hoped that more people living with HIV might access ART as a result of the 2015 World Health Organization (WHO) recommendation that ART be initiated for everyone living with HIV at any CD4 cell count (4). ART reduces TB risk among HIV-1-infected people by 54 to 90% and halves the TB recurrence rate (5). Despite this risk reduction, HIV-1-infected people established on ART in high TB burden settings remain at higher risk than HIV-1-uninfected people, even in higher CD4 strata (6).

The higher risk of incident TB reflects both increased risk of reactivation of latent TB (7, 8) and increased risk of progression to active TB following recent infection or reinfection by *Mycobacterium tuberculosis* in HIV-1-infected individuals (9). In high-incidence regions such as South Africa (10), Malawi (11), and India (12) TB recurrence after successful treatment in HIV-1-coinfected people may often be attributable to reinfection, not relapse. Epidemiological studies have shown that TB risk increases in HIV-1-infected people as the CD4 count declines (13) and in advanced clinical stages of disease (WHO stages 3/4) (Fig. 1) (14, 15). Although unsuppressed HIV-1 viral load during ART treatment has been associated with increased TB risk in a large retrospective study (16), others have not shown it to be an independent risk factor (14, 17).

In addition to ART, another intervention that decreases the risk of TB in HIV-1 infected patients is isoniazid preventive therapy (IPT), which reduces TB risk by 32% in ART-naive people (18) and 37% in patients on ART (19). The influence of tuberculin skin test/interferon gamma release assay (IGRA) status on the preventive effects of IPT is controversial because some studies have reported risk reduction to be greatest in tuberculin skin test /IGRA-positive people (20). However, these tests lose diagnostic sensitivity in latent TB infection (LTBI) with advanced immunosuppression (21), and a recent large randomized placebo-control trial in South Africa showed benefit in the tuberculin skin test/IGRA-negative group (19). It is therefore reasonable to consider IPT in all HIV-1-infected people, especially in TB-endemic areas.

HIV-1-MEDIATED IMMUNOSUPPRESSION

HIV virus descends from the *Lentivirus* genus of the *Retroviridae* family, which has—through multiple zoonotic transmissions from non-human primates to

[1]Clinical Infectious Diseases Research Initiative, Institute of Infectious Diseases and Molecular Medicine, University of Cape Town, Observatory 7925, Republic of South Africa; [2]Department of Medicine, Imperial College London, London W2 1PG and The Francis Crick Institute Mill Hill Laboratory, London NW7 1AA, United Kingdom.

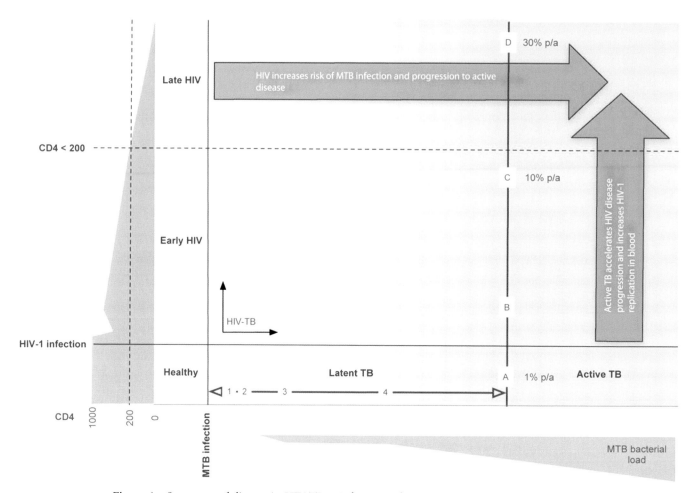

Figure 1 Spectrum of disease in HIV-TB coinfection. The *x* axis represents stages of tuberculosis, from infection through to active disease, while the *y* axis represents stages of HIV-1 infection. *M. tuberculosis* bacterial burden and CD4 count are shown in blue along the respective axes. The spectrum of latent TB is represented as follows: (**1**) infection eliminated without priming antigen-specific T cells; (**2**) infection eliminated in association with T-cell priming; (**3**) infection contained with some bacteria persisting in a nonreplicating form; (**4**) bacterial replication maintained at the subclinical level by the immune system. Clinical disease (pulmonary and extrapulmonary tuberculosis) occurs in a subset of individuals who are latently infected or who develop primary tuberculosis directly following infection or reinfection. The annual risk is represented as follows: (**A**) HIV-1-uninfected: about 10% lifetime risk or about 1% per annum (p/a); (**B**) shortly after HIV-1 infection and prior to substantial CD4 T-cell depletion, the risk of active tuberculosis increases; (**C**) during the early stages of HIV-1 infection, this risk rises to approximately 10% p/a; (**D**) in late-stage HIV-1 infection, the risk of active tuberculosis increases to 30% p/a. The effects of HIV-1 on tuberculosis and of tuberculosis on HIV-1 disease are shown by the red arrows. Reproduced from *Pathogens and Disease* (286) with permission of the publisher.

humans—given rise to several lineages that constitute the greater HIV pandemic. There are two types of HIV: HIV-1 and HIV-2. The former is associated with greater TB risk, greater TB disease severity, and greater TB mortality risk. However, HIV-2 does impart greater TB risk, severity, and mortality when compared to uninfected patients (22). HIV-2 contributes comparatively little to the global HIV burden, with the total number

of HIV-2 infections being few and largely limited to West Africa, due to its poor transmission capabilities (23). HIV-2 is generally less virulent than HIV-1 and has a much longer disease-free survival period but responds poorly to standard ART used in HIV-1 (23–25). The important HIV-1 pandemic is predominantly driven by the group M lineage—a group with great genetic diversity comprising nine subtypes and multiple circulating recombinant forms. This genetic diversity and the ability of HIV-1 to subvert acquired immune responses through sequence mutations and recombination makes HIV-1 vaccine development a complex task (26).

The most characteristic feature of HIV-1-induced immunosuppression is CD4 T lymphocyte depletion. The initial cellular targets of HIV-1 infection are the mucosal CD4 T lymphocytes, resident macrophages, and dendritic cells (DCs) (27). Cellular uptake of HIV-1 is mediated by the CD4 receptor in conjunction with several coreceptors: in the setting of acute infection, most notably the CC-chemokine receptor 5 (CCR5) (28). This accounts for the rapid depletion of the memory subset of CD4 T cells expressing CCR5, with the effector memory phenotype being particularly vulnerable due to CCR5 upregulation during intermediate stages of differentiation (29). Effector memory CD4 T cells are found in high numbers in the gastrointestinal tract lamina propria and other mucosal sites, including the lung mucosa, with their depletion initially compensated for by migration and maturation of their precursors that are predominantly CCR5⁻. Although transmitted HIV-1 strains do not commonly use the CXC chemokine receptor 4 (CXCR4) during early infection, a proportion of strains acquire the ability to do so through mutation as the disease progresses (30). CXCR4 tropism is associated with more rapid progression to AIDS and significant CD4 T cell depletion (28). This is thought to be due to the fact that the viral population not only infects $CCR5^+CXCR4^+$ and $CCR5^+CXCR4^-$ expressing memory CD4 lymphocytes, but additionally targets the $CCR5^-CXCR4^+$-expressing naive CD4 lymphocyte subset recruited to compensate for effector memory CD4 T cell loss (31). This results in a highly immunodeficient state where both effector memory CD4 T cells and their precursors are severely depleted.

Although great emphasis is placed on the depletion of CD4 T cell numbers as a measure of disease progression, it is also recognized that the initial depletion seen in acute infection occurs in the setting of generalized immune activation and dysregulation that persists for the duration of infection (32, 33). Peripheral blood CD4 counts may not adequately reflect the degree of CD4 T cell depletion at mucosal sites, with 60% of all mucosal memory CD4 T cells being infected at the peak of HIV-1 viremia (34). Although in most cases of acute HIV-1 infection the initial dramatic increase in CD8 T lymphocytes and HIV-1-specific responses causes a decline in viral load and a modest increase in CD4 T lymphocyte counts, this is not sustained (33). In chronic infection there is a continued slow depletion of CD4 T lymphocytes driven by immune activation, apoptosis

of both infected and uninfected cells, and generalized immune dysfunction with ongoing viral replication (32).

HIV-TB COINFECTION: ABERRATION IN INNATE IMMUNITY

Macrophages in Coinfection

The importance of macrophage apoptosis

The principal phagocytes involved in the uptake of *M. tuberculosis* in the lung parenchyma are the alveolar macrophages (AMs) and myeloid DCs. HIV-1 infects only 1 to 10% of AMs *in vivo* (35), with limited cytopathic effect. However, these infected AMs become HIV-1 reservoirs that are deficient in key aspects of macrophage immunity such as receptor-mediated phagocytosis (36, 37), antigen presentation (38), and intracellular pathogen elimination (39, 40), all of which have a deleterious effect on the innate immune response to *M. tuberculosis*. Additionally, CCR5-tropic HIV-1 infection of macrophage colony-stimulating factor-differentiated monocyte-derived macrophages (MDMs) induces an inhibitory effect on nuclear factor kappa-light-chain-enhancer of activated B cells (NF-κB) signaling downstream of Toll-like receptor (TLR) 2 and TLR4 (41), with the two latter being involved in *M. tuberculosis* recognition (42).

M. tuberculosis in turn establishes its persistent infective niche in AMs through arrest of phagosomal acidification and maturation (43, 44). Apoptosis, defined as programmed cell death, is mediated by the activation of the proteolytic caspase cascade that leads to cleavage of cellular proteins, with degraded cellular cytoplasmic content eventually being confined to membrane-bound apoptotic bodies that can be recognized and cleared by phagocytes via efferocytosis (45). This is an important host defense mechanism that promotes antigen recognition, phagosome maturation, and *M. tuberculosis* clearance in AMs. Virulent *M. tuberculosis* manipulates apoptotic pathways and instead promotes cellular necrosis, thus avoiding immune-mediated clearance by the host (46).

In HIV-TB coinfection it has been shown that HIV-1-infected macrophages undergo even less apoptosis in response to *M. tuberculosis* than do HIV-1-uninfected macrophages. This is partly mediated by impaired tumor necrosis factor alpha (TNFα) release and reduced TNFα bioavailability in HIV-1-infected macrophages in response to *M. tuberculosis* (39). The latter may be a consequence of binding of TNFα by the soluble TNFα receptors (sTNFαR), because both sTNFαR1 and sTNFαR2 are increased in concentration in cell-free bronchoalveolar lavage (BAL) fluid of healthy HIV-1-infected people compared with controls (39). Virulent (H37Rv) *M. tuberculosis* induces the release of higher concentrations of sTNFαR2 from infected macrophages than avirulent *M. tuberculosis* does, resulting in a decrease in macrophage apoptosis. This is thought to be in part mediated by interleukin 10 (IL-10), because virulent *M. tuberculosis* infection of macrophages results in greater production of IL-10 than avirulent (H37Ra) *M. tuberculosis* does, which in turn promotes sTNFαR2 release. Addition of exogenous recombinant IL-10 to H37Ra *M. tuberculosis*-infected macrophage cultures decreased apoptosis in a dose-dependent manner (47). HIV-1 infection *per se* influences the extrinsic apoptosis pathway through the release of HIV-1 *nef* protein, which attenuates macrophage apoptosis by inhibition of apoptosis signal regulating kinase 1 (ASK1), a key serine/threonine kinase upstream of the TNFα apoptotic pathway (48). Additionally, HIV-1 *nef* and the *M. tuberculosis* antigen Rv3416 have been reported to synergistically contribute to antiapoptotic signaling through TLR2-induced altered calcium homeostasis and downmodulation of reactive oxygen species in macrophages (49).

Both HIV-1 *nef* and *tat* trigger IL-10 release in monocytes (50, 51), which is supported by the finding of higher IL-10 levels in BAL fluid from asymptomatic HIV-1-infected people compared with uninfected controls (52). IL-10 has also been found to directly decrease TNFα mRNA in AMs treated with irradiated H37Rv *M. tuberculosis*, with a proposed mechanism being IL-10-induced B-cell lymphoma 3-encoded protein (BCL-3) release, BCL-3 being a known inhibitor of NF-κB nuclear activity (52). It has been shown that exogenous 1,25-dihydroxycholecalciferol treatment of HIV-1-infected U1 macrophages before infection with *M. tuberculosis* restores deficient TNFα secretion through repair of IκB/NFκB signaling and upregulation of CD14, a known coreceptor of TLR4 (53). Vitamin D has additionally been shown to be a critical factor in the TLR8-mediated autophagy pathway leading to suppression of HIV-1 replication in macrophages (54, 55). In contrast, alveolar macrophages isolated from HIV-1-infected people showed robust TNFα secretion in response to *M. tuberculosis*, and the authors attributed this difference to the fact that alveolar macrophages exhibit 10-fold lower expression of the HIV-1 genome than U1 macrophages (35, 53). Although others also found slightly elevated TNFα levels in human MDMs cocultured with *M. tuberculosis* in response to 1,25-dihydroxycholecalciferol treatment, this elevation was not statistically significant (56). Martineau et al., however, found decreased gene transcription and levels of

TNFα and other proinflammatory cytokines (interferon gamma [IFN-γ] and IL-12p40) in peripheral blood mononuclear cells (PBMCs) and macrophages cocultured with *M. tuberculosis* and 1,25-dihydroxycholecalciferol compared to controls (57). These findings implicate a possible role for vitamin D in influencing the cytokine milieu and apoptosis in coinfected macrophages.

Another pathway possibly contributing to decreased TNFα production by HIV-1-infected macrophages is the mitogen-activated protein (MAP) kinase phosphatase-1 pathway. HIV-1 infection induces increased MAP kinase phosphatase-1 activity (58), resulting in reduced extracellular signal-regulated kinase 1/2 phosphorylation, with both extracellular signal-regulated kinase 1/2 and p38 MAP kinases being shown to be important in mediating TNFα release by *M. tuberculosis*-infected AM (59).

Some controversy exists surrounding the role of IL-10 in the setting of HIV-TB coinfection. In contrast to the finding that BAL fluid from asymptomatic HIV-1 mono-infected people contained increased IL-10 levels compared with uninfected controls, it was recently reported that BAL fluid from HIV-TB coinfected people contained lower concentrations of IL-10 and higher concentrations of proinflammatory cytokines, most notably IL-1β, than people with nonmycobacterial lung infections (60). In contrast to the site of disease, plasma levels of IL-10 have been found to be elevated in HIV-TB coinfected people, with significantly lower IL-10 plasma levels being found in those with HIV-1 only and those with HIV-1 and LTBI, respectively (61). There is evidence that may to some extent account for the effect seen at the site of disease with the finding of attenuated IL-10 production by macrophages through HIV-1-mediated inhibition of p38 phosphorylation of MAP kinase. Extracellular signal-regulated kinase 1/2 inhibition was shown to play an auxiliary role in this setting. It was additionally demonstrated that recombinant IL-10 could inhibit HIV-1-replication *in vitro* and, conversely, that HIV-1's role in attenuation of IL-10 production was maintained, irrespective of the rate of viral replication and adjunctive administration of protease inhibitors (60). In the setting of HIV-TB coinfection, gene polymorphisms associated with increased IL-10 production have been implicated in contributing to the predisposition of HIV-1-infected people to develop TB (62). This suggests that in established *M. tuberculosis* infection the macrophage cytokine production may be skewed to promote a proinflammatory environment and thus favor HIV-1 replication, while a microenvironment rich in IL-10 as seen in HIV-1-mono-infection may promote the establishment of *M. tuberculosis* infection by compounding existing *M. tuberculosis* virulence factors aimed at escaping apoptotic cell death in macrophages.

Determinants of mycobacterial growth and HIV-1 viral replication in macrophages

Phagocytosis of *M. tuberculosis* by macrophages induces a state of cellular activation mediated by the production of a host of proinflammatory cytokines. It has been shown that gene expression of coinfected primary human macrophages is influenced to a much greater degree by *M. tuberculosis* than by HIV-1 (63), with HIV-1 exerting very little effect on the immune activation status and transcriptional profile of coinfected macrophages (64). Important in this respect is evidence that different *M. tuberculosis* strains may differ in their ability to induce HIV-1 replication (65).

MDMs coinfected with HIV-1 and *M. tuberculosis* have been shown to exhibit enhanced growth of *M. tuberculosis* (66), increased HIV-1 replication, and decreased macrophage viability (67), although this has not been consistently shown (44, 68). In a coinfection model using the promonocytic U1 cell line, irradiated H37Rv *M. tuberculosis* increased HIV-1 p24 levels in a dose-dependent manner, and the 6-kDa early secretory antigenic target (ESAT-6) also induced HIV-1 viral replication up to 100-fold at noncytotoxic concentrations in cell culture (69). Hoshino et al. found a 2-fold increase in CXCR4 mRNA in the BAL fluid of people with TB compared with healthy controls. Alveolar macrophages isolated from the BAL fluid of people with TB showed relatively higher levels of CXCR4 expression than CCR5 expression (70). *In vitro* experiments using MDMs revealed enhanced CXCR4-tropic HIV-1 cDNA production in *M. tuberculosis*-infected MDMs compared to uninfected MDMs, with similar enhancement in CCR5-tropic HIV-1 cDNA not being demonstrated. Findings of high BAL fluid levels of the CCR5 ligands macrophage inflammatory protein-1β (MIP-1β) and CCL5 (RANTES) in people with TB was thought to account for decreased CCR5-tropic HIV-1 virus entry because it is known that these inhibit CCR5-tropic, but not CXCR4-tropic HIV-1 cellular entry (71, 72). The authors suggest that enhanced proliferation of CXCR4-tropic HIV-1 strains in the lung is a possible mechanism whereby *M. tuberculosis* may contribute to accelerated disease progression to AIDS (70). However, this observation may be specific to alveolar macrophages because predominantly CCR5-tropic HIV-1 has been demonstrated in pleural fluid of people with TB (73, 74), and PBMCs, monocytes, and CD4 T lymphocytes isolated from whole blood show upregulation of CCR5 (75) and CXCR4 (76–78).

It has been consistently shown that a proinflammatory microenvironment for the most part favors both pathogens, a prime example being where exogenous TNFα enhanced *M. tuberculosis* growth in HIV-1-infected MDMs *in vitro*, whereas it had no effect in HIV-1-uninfected MDMs (79). This emphasizes the precarious balance of the cytokine milieu in HIV-TB coinfection. Although TNFα is required to trigger the extrinsic apoptotic pathway to facilitate clearance of *M. tuberculosis*, it also seems to contribute to a proinflammatory microenvironment where both HIV-1-replication (80) and *M. tuberculosis* growth (79) are enhanced. This may impact HIV-1 transmission to T lymphocytes: enhanced HIV-1 transmission between H37Rv-*M. tuberculosis* infected MDMs and T lymphocytes has been demonstrated *in vitro* (81).

Neutrophils in Coinfection

An interferon-inducible neutrophil-driven blood transcriptional signature characterizes active TB (82), and elevated peripheral blood neutrophil count independently associates with active pulmonary TB and *M. tuberculosis* burden in sputum of HIV-1-infected people and is an independent predictor of mortality in those with TB (83, 84). However, little work has been done on the role of neutrophils in HIV-TB coinfection. Neutrophils can restrict *M. tuberculosis* growth in whole blood, with human neutrophil peptides 1–3 being shown to kill mycobacteria in culture (85). This is of particular significance because it is known that HIV-1-infected people are at greater risk of mycobacteremia and disseminated TB (86, 87). Neutrophils in whole blood of ART-naive HIV-1-infected people could not restrict *M. tuberculosis* growth as effectively as neutrophils from uninfected control patients (85). The reduced capability of neutrophils to control *M. tuberculosis* growth in whole blood correlated with HIV-1 viral load and was associated with decreased neutrophil survival compared with that of uninfected controls. The ability of neutrophils to restrict *M. tuberculosis* growth was restored after 6 months of ART (88). This is in keeping with findings by others that HIV-1 induces increased rates of neutrophil apoptosis (89), especially at lower CD4 counts (90), with reversal of this phenomenon occurring with ART (91).

These findings are interesting considering that *M. tuberculosis* induces neutrophil apoptosis (92–94) and that *M. tuberculosis*-induced apoptosis of neutrophils is required to facilitate *M. tuberculosis*-induced DC maturation (95, 96). *M. tuberculosis*-induced neutrophil apoptosis induces DC maturation via direct neutrophil-DC cross talk with DC-specific intracellular adhesion molecule-3-grabbing nonintegrin (DC-SIGN) and Mac-1 receptor binding, while conversely, nonspecific neutrophil apoptosis inhibits DC maturation (96). Nonspecific neutrophil apoptosis results in reduced expression of HLA class II, costimulatory molecules (CD86, CD83) and in a lack of Th1 polarizing cytokine (IL-12, IFN-γ) production by immature DCs in response to *M. tuberculosis*. The consequence of this is a decreased *in vitro* lymphoproliferative response to *M. tuberculosis* and possibly immune tolerance (95, 97, 98). Taken together, these findings may be indicative of a potential contributory mechanism whereby coinfection delays and inhibits the development of a strong adaptive immune response to *M. tuberculosis*.

DCs in Coinfection

DC, especially plasmacytoid DC, numbers decrease markedly in acute HIV-1 infection, with plasmacytoid DC numbers not being adequately restored upon ART, in contrast to the myeloid DC subset (99, 100). Only 1 to 3% of DCs become productively infected with HIV-1 (101). However, their ability to transmit the HIV-1 virus to other cells, most importantly to T lymphocytes, is notable. The capability of DCs to transmit HIV-1 infection without viral fusion events occurring is well documented, so much so that they have been described as "Trojan horses" containing intact viral particles in intracellular vesicles (102–104). DCs have the ability to efficiently transmit HIV-1 to T lymphocytes through a process called *trans*-infection, where the HIV-1 envelope glycoprotein gp120 binds to DC-SIGN but the DC itself does not become productively infected (104–106), although DC-SIGN-independent pathways have subsequently also been identified (107, 108).

Several compounds with affinity for DC-SIGN including dextrans and gp120 antagonists have been shown to decrease HIV *gag* RNA levels in B-THP-1/DC-SIGN cell cultures (109). DC-SIGN has also been investigated in the setting of *M. tuberculosis* infection because it has high affinity for the mycobacterial mannose-capped cell wall component lipoarabinomannan (ManLAM) found in both *M. tuberculosis* and *Mycobacterium bovis* bacillus Calmette-Guérin (BCG) (110). Binding of mycobacterial ManLAM to DC-SIGN has been shown to inhibit DC maturation, increase DC IL-10 production, and decrease DC IL-12 production in response to lipopolysaccharides (110, 111), which may hamper the initiation of the adaptive immune response to *M. tuberculosis*. However, subsequent studies of transgenic mice with human DC-SIGN suggest that DC-SIGN may be important to limit tissue pathology in the setting of chronic infection and that DC-SIGN

ligands other than ManLAM may play a greater role in *M. tuberculosis*-mediated immune evasion (112, 113; reviewed in 114). Further work is needed to evaluate if DC-SIGN presents a potentially important intersection in the copathogenesis of *M. tuberculosis* and HIV-1.

Natural Killer (NK) Cells in Coinfection

NK cells are innate immune cells that mediate non-major histocompatibility complex-restricted cytotoxic killing of target cells through the release of cytoplasmic granules containing granulysin, perforin, granzymes and several death receptors that mediate apoptosis (reviewed in 115). NK cells from HIV-1-infected people have significantly lower surface expression of the NK-activating receptors NKp46, NKp30, and NKp44 that are involved in target cell lysis (116), with significantly diminished cytolytic function being apparent in HIV-1 infection (117).

A specific subpopulation (CD7$^+$CD56$^-$CD16$^+$) of NK cells lacking CD57, a marker of terminal differentiation in NK cells (118), were found to be significantly expanded in HIV-1-infected individuals (119) compared to HIV-1-uninfected controls. This subpopulation expressed CD95$^+$, a cell death receptor, with high frequency, suggesting that this subset may undergo apoptosis before being able to undergo terminal differentiation. Both the CD7$^+$CD56$^-$ NK cell subset and the CD7$^+$CD56$^+$ showed similar expression of the killer-cell immunoglobulin-like receptors (KIRs) in people with and without HIV-1, but the density of the cytotoxicity receptors NKp30 and NKp46 were found to be decreased in the CD7$^+$CD56$^-$ NK cell subset in HIV-1-infected individuals. Furthermore, CD7$^+$CD56$^-$CD16$^+$ NK cells exhibited reduced expression of granzyme B and perforin with increased expression of CD107a, a degranulation marker. NK cells have been shown to be able to engage with multiple target cells during their lifespan, with each encounter resulting in a decrease in their perforin and granzyme B content (120). Thus, this phenotype (CD7$^+$CD56$^-$CD16$^+$) is reminiscent of a target-cell-experienced subpopulation. Both CD56$^+$ and CD56$^-$ NK cells in HIV-1-infected people exhibited minimal IFN-γ response to NK-cell-stimulating cytokines (IL-12 and IL-18) (119). NK cell IFN-γ secretion and cytotoxicity are inhibited by HIV-1 *tat* and the gp120 envelope protein of HIV-1 (121–124). Granulysin production by NK cells in response to IL-15 stimulation is reduced in PBMC from HIV-1-infected people, while it is relatively preserved in response to BCG (125). NK cells have been shown to contribute to the control of *M. tuberculosis* infection in monocytes and macrophage cultures *in vitro* through cytolysis and of induction of apoptosis of infected cells and thereby of inhibition of *M. tuberculosis* growth (126–129). Although the murine model failed to demonstrate a reciprocal increase in *M. tuberculosis* load upon NK cell depletion with a lytic antibody (130), NK cell-derived IFN-γ was required for *M. tuberculosis* control in the absence of T cells in a model using T cell-deficient RAG⁻/⁻ mice (131), suggesting a role for NK cells in the context of immunodeficiency.

Glutathione is a nonprotein thiol with an antioxidant effect that has been found at decreased concentrations in macrophages, NK cells, and T lymphocytes from HIV-1-infected people and in the PBMC and red blood cells of those with pulmonary TB (132). In the case of HIV-1, it is thought that the reduction is mediated by high levels of free radicals and decreased catalytic subunits of glutamine-cysteine ligase production coupled with decreased gene transcription for glutathione (133, 134), while the reason for low glutathione levels in TB is less clear but is thought to be attributable to increased synthesis of reactive oxygen intermediates in TB (132). Glutathione has been found to control intracellular *M. tuberculosis* growth in human MDMs, where manipulation of redox metabolism in *M. tuberculosis* has been suggested as the bacteriostatic mechanism involved, although it is unknown what significance its structural similarity to that of penicillin precursors imparts (135, 136). N-acetyl cysteine plays a role in intracellular glutathione maintenance. Coculture of H37Rv-infected monocytes with NK cells, N-acetyl cysteine, IL-12, and IL-2 leads to *M. tuberculosis* growth stasis through enhanced expression of NK cytotoxic ligands (CD40L and FasL) and NK cytotoxic receptors NK-44 and NKP30 (137). A guinea pig model of tuberculosis illustrated that treatment with N-acetyl cysteine resulted in increased glutathione levels and increased total serum antioxidant capacity as measured by an assay detecting capacity to reduce radical cation production. This was also associated with decreased spleen mycobacterial burden and a decrease in both spleen and lung lesion burden and necrosis (138). These findings provide insight into the role of NK cells in the control of *M. tuberculosis* in HIV-TB coinfected people and reveal the potential utility of antioxidants such as glutathione in enhancing this capacity.

COINFECTION AT THE SITE OF DISEASE

HIV-1 Replication at the Site of Disease

There is evidence that *M. tuberculosis* increases HIV-1 replication, especially at the site of disease. The en-

hancement of HIV-1 replication by *M. tuberculosis* can occur through multiple mechanisms. BAL fluid from *M. tuberculosis*-infected lung zones displayed increased HIV-1 p24 levels compared with uninfected lung zones in coinfected patients (139). This was shown to be mediated by the 16-kDa CCAAT/enhancer-binding protein β (C/EPβ), a transcriptional repressor of the HIV-1 long terminal repeat (LTR) expressed in alveolar macrophages (140). The HIV-1 LTR functions as a control center for HIV-1 gene expression, and its induction of HIV-1 replication can be regulated by numerous host- and pathogen-derived factors, with three binding sites for C/EPβ having been identified in the negative regulatory element of the HIV LTR (141, 142). The 16-kDa, in contrast to the 37-kDa stimulatory, isoform of C/EPβ functions as a negative transcription factor and abrogates HIV-1 replication and LTR promoter function (143). Honda et al. demonstrated that *M. tuberculosis* infection inhibits the 16-kDa C/EPβ *in vivo* and thus proposed that this mechanism derepresses the HIV-1 LTR with subsequent increased HIV-1 replication.

Contact of activated lymphocytes with alveolar macrophages was shown to result in a loss of inhibitory C/EPβ and activation of the NF-κB pathway (144). The mechanism behind contact-mediated inhibition of C/EPβ was shown to occur via cross-linking of the macrophage costimulatory receptors CD40 and CD80/86 and intracellular adhesion molecule-1 with their respective ligands on polymorphonuclear neutrophils (145). Similarly, HIV-1 viral load has been shown to be up to 4 times that of plasma in coinfected patients with TB pleurisy (146). This has been shown to be mediated by the positive transcription elongation factor, composed of cyclin T1 and cyclin-dependent kinase 9, in concert with HIV-1 *tat* protein activating HIV-1 transcription in pleural mononuclear cells (147). HIV-1 replication can be directly enhanced by the recognition of mycobacterial pathogen-associated molecular patterns by their respective pattern recognition receptors, thus triggering cellular signaling pathways involved in the activation of the HIV-1 LTR promoting viral replication. There are increasing numbers of *M. tuberculosis* lipoproteins, cell wall components, and other pathogen-derived molecules that stimulate HIV-1 replication *in vitro*, e.g., phosphatidylinositol mannoside 6 from the mycobacterial cell wall (148) and the mycobacterial proline-proline-glutamic acid protein Rv1168c (149). Similarly, the pattern recognition receptors that have been most frequently associated with recognition of *M. tuberculosis* pathogen-associated molecular patterns include TLR2, -4, and -9; nucleotide-binding oligomerization domain 2; Dectin-1; and DC-SIGN, with associated signaling pathways including NF-κB, nuclear factor of activated T cells 5, MAP kinase, the positive transcription elongation factor, and C/EβP (150–152). In addition, HIV-1 replication is enhanced by the predominantly proinflammatory cellular immune response to *M. tuberculosis* infection, leading to the binding of cytokines such as IL-1α, IL-1β, IL-6, IL-8, TNF, IFN-γ, monocyte chemoattractant protein-1, and transforming growth factor-β to their respective receptors and in so doing activating transcription of the HIV-1 LTR (Tables 1 and 2) (150, 153).

HIV-1 viral replication specifically in T lymphocytes also occurs by a number of mechanisms, with overlap with those observed in phagocytes. HIV-1 replication in T lymphocytes is initiated by *M. tuberculosis*-driven activation of the T cell receptor (TCR), which activates the nuclear factor of activated T cells-c, leading to enhanced HIV-1 viral replication (154). As in phagocytes, activation of the NF-κB pathway is also likely to be an important enhancer of HIV-1 transcription. In T lymphocytes NF-κB is activated following TCR stimulation along with costimulatory signaling through CD2 and CD28 (155).

Table 1 *M. tuberculosis*-derived PAMPs and cytokines mediating enhanced HIV-1 replication[a]: PAMP-mediated activation of HIV-LTR

PAMP	Pattern recognition receptor	Adaptor proteins/upstream kinases	Downstream kinases	Transcription factors
M. tuberculosis cell wall components, e.g., LAM, PIM, lipomannan, trehalose dimycolate, LpqH (19-kDa lipoprotein)	TLR2 (heterodimerizes with TLR1 and TLR6)	TIRAP, MyD88→ IRAK1, IRAK2, IRAK4→ TRAF6→ TAB2, TAB3, TAK1		
Heat-sensitive *M. tuberculosis* components, 38-kDa glycoprotein, HSP70	TLR4	MyD88-dependent pathway (as above for TLR2)		
		MyD88-independent pathway: endosomal translocation of TLR4 and signaling through either TRAM, TRIF→ TRAF6→ TAB2, TAB3, TAK1 or TRAM, TRIF→ TRADD, Pellino-1, RIP1→ TAB2, TAB3, TAK1	MAPKs: JNK, p38 and NEMO, IKKα, IKKβ	AP-1, ATF, ATF-2/c-jun and NF-κB, IκB C/EBPβ, C/EPBδ
Unmethylated CpG motifs from bacterial genome	TLR9 (through endosomal translocation)	MyD88→ IRAK4→ TRAF6→ TAB2, TAB3, TAK1		
Muramyl dipeptide (MDP)	NOD2	RIP2→ TRAF6→ TAB2, TAB3, TAK1		
		CARD9	MAPKs: JNK, p38	AP-1, ATF, ATF-2/c-jun
manLAM, PIMs, e.g., PIM₆, arabinomannan, lipomannan, LpqH	DC-SIGN	Ras Src Pak	Raf-1	NF-κB
Unknown *M. tuberculosis* ligand	Dectin-1	Ras	Raf-1	NF-κB
		Syk→ CARD9, Bcl-10, MALT1	NEMO, IKKα, IKKβ	

[a]Adapted from reference 150 with permission from the publisher. Abbreviations: AP-1, activator protein 1; ATF, activating transcription factor; BCL10, B-cell CLL/lymphoma 10; CARD9, caspase recruitment domain family member 9; C/EBP, CCAAT/enhancer binding protein; DC-SIGN, dendritic cell-specific intracellular adhesion molecule-3-grabbing nonintegrin; HSP70, the 70-kDa heat shock proteins; IFN-γ, interferon gamma; IKK, IκB kinase; IL, interleukin; IRAK, interleukin 1 receptor-associated kinase; LAM, lipoarabinomannan; LTR, long terminal repeat; MALT1, mucosa-associated lymphoid tissue lymphoma translocation protein 1; ManLAM, mannosylated LAMs; MAPK, mitogen-activated protein kinase; MLK, mixed lineage kinase; MyD88, myeloid differentiation factor 88; NEMO, NF-κB essential modulator; NOD2, nucleotide-binding oligomerization domain; PAMP, pathogen-associated molecular pattern; PIM, phosphatidylinositol mannoside; RIP, receptor-interacting protein; TAB, transforming growth factor β-activated kinase (TAK) 1-binding protein; TAF, TATA (thymine-adenine-thymine-adenine)-binding protein-associated factors; TIRAP, Toll-interleukin 1 receptor (TIR) domain containing adaptor protein; TLR, Toll-like receptor; TNF, tumor necrosis factor; TRADD, TNFR1-associated DEATH domain protein; TRAF, TNF receptor-associated factor; TRAM, TRIF-related adaptor molecule; TRIF, TIR-domain-containing adapter-inducing interferon-β.

Table 2 *M. tuberculosis*-derived cytokines mediating enhanced HIV-1 replication: cytokines produced in *M. tuberculosis* response activating HIV-1 LTR[a]

Cytokine	Receptor	Adaptor proteins/upstream kinases	Downstream kinases	Transcription factors
TNF	TNFR-1	TRADD, RIP1, TRAF2, TRAF5→ TAB2, TAB3, TAK1		
	TNFR-2	TRAF2, TRAF5→ TAB2, TAB3, TAK1	MAPKs: JNK, p38 NEMO, IKKα, IKKβ	AP-1, ATF, ATF-2/c-jun NF-κB, IκB
IL-1α, IL-1β	IL-1R, IL-1RAcP	MyD88→ IRAK4, IRAK2, IRAK1, Pellino-1, TRAF6→ TAB2, TAB3, TAK1		
Transforming growth factor β	TβRI, TβRII	TRAF6→ TAB2, TAB3, TAK1		
Monocyte chemoattractant protein-1	CC-chemokine receptor 2	Gα/Gβγ, phospholipase C	Protein kinase C phospholipase→ MAPKs: JNK, p38	
IFN-γ	IFN-γRα, IFN-γRβ	Unknown→ MLK3	Unknown	C/EBPβ
		MyD88→ MLK3	MAPKs: JNK, p38	AP-1, ATF, ATF-2/c-jun
		Unknown→ MEKK1→ MEK1/2	ERK1/2	C/EBPβ
IL-6	IL-6Rα, gp130	Ras→ unknown	ERK1/2→ unknown	C/EBPβ

[a]Adapted from reference 150 with permission from the publisher. Abbreviations: AP-1, activator protein 1; ATF, activating transcription factor; C/EBP, CCAAT/enhancer binding protein; ERK1/2, extracellular signal-regulated kinase 1/2; HSP70, the 70-kDa heat shock proteins; IFN-γ, interferon gamma; IKK, IκB kinase; IL, interleukin; IL-1RAcP, IL-1 receptor accessory protein; LAM, lipoarabinomannan; LTR, long terminal repeat; MAPK, mitogen-activated protein kinase; MEK1/2, MAPK/Erk kinase MAPK/Erk kinase; MEKK1, mitogen-activated protein kinase kinase kinase 1; MLK, mixed lineage kinase; NEMO, NF-κB essential modulator; PAMP, pathogen-associated molecular pattern; PIM, phosphatidylinositol mannoside; RIP, receptor-interacting protein; TAB, transforming growth factor β-activated kinase (TAK) binding protein; TAF, TATA (thymine-adenine-thymine-adenine)-binding protein-associated factors; TIRAP, Toll-interleukin 1 receptor (TIR) domain containing adaptor protein; TLR, Toll-like receptor; TNF, tumor necrosis factor; TRAF, TNF receptor-associated factor; TRAM, TRIF-related adaptor molecule; TRIF, TIR-domain-containing adapter-inducing interferon-β.

It is likely that ongoing HIV-1 viral replication mediates its most detrimental effects in the host through its induction of constant immune activation, which is associated with disease progression and mortality (156, 157).

HIV-1 Heterogeneity at the Site of Disease

The full implications of enhanced viral replication at the site of *M. tuberculosis* disease are not fully understood, but the error-prone transcriptional process of HIV-1 replication has prompted investigation into a possible influence on HIV-1 heterogeneity in the host. In cases of active pulmonary TB the degree of viral heterogeneity was greater in *M. tuberculosis*-infected lung segments than in uninfected lung segments (158). Furthermore, Collins et al. (159) found that pulmonary TB in HIV-1-infected people gave rise to 2- to 3-fold greater mutation frequency when compared to CD4 matched HIV-1 mono-infected people, findings reproduced by a similar study (160). TB pleurisy exhibited modest influence on HIV-1 quasispecies heterogeneity when the pleural compartment was compared with blood. However, this became more pronounced once compensated for migration events between the blood

and pleura (73). Spinal TB granulomas of HIV-1-coinfected people have a higher viral load than plasma (161, 162). Divergent HIV-1 evolution of predominantly CCR5-tropic virus was demonstrated in the spinal granulomas, with both *M. tuberculosis* and virus particles being observed in granuloma macrophages (162). This builds on the hypothesis put forward by Lawn et al. that trafficking of HIV-1-infected cells contributes to granuloma disruption, thus creating a micro-environment conducive to both HIV-1 replication and *M. tuberculosis* growth (163). Further investigation is required to elucidate the repercussions of increased HIV-1 heterogeneity at the site of *M. tuberculosis* infection, whether it persists after antituberculosis treatment (ATT) as previously suggested (164), whether these disease sites are adequately penetrated by ART, and if divergent HIV-1 quasispecies upon migration contribute to increased systemic HIV-1 viral fitness and accelerated progression to AIDS (165).

IMMUNE ACTIVATION IN COINFECTION

It is well-recognized that *M. tuberculosis* infection contributes to immune activation observed in HIV-TB-coinfected people, with this effect persisting beyond clinical cure of TB and contributing to accelerated progression to AIDS, higher risk of concomitant opportunistic infection, and death (166, 167). Indeed, cellular activation status in HIV-TB coinfection has been found to be a key correlate of the rate of HIV-1 replication, with immature macrophages (CD36[+]) and activated CD4 T cells (CD26[+]) being major cellular contributors to viral burden at treatment commencement and early time points postinitiation of ATT. Thereafter, it was shown that CD3+ T lymphocytes become the predominant source of HIV-1 viral replication, with elevated levels of viral replication still being apparent up to 6 months after completion of successful ATT (168). Active TB in HIV-1-coinfected people has been shown to induce both higher levels of soluble markers of monocyte activation (soluble CD14, IL-6, IL-8, etc.) and T cell surface activation markers (CD38 and HLA-DR) when compared to HIV-1 mono-infected people. Interestingly, coinfected participants with latent TB also had increased levels of T cell, but not monocyte, activation (169). This once again underscores the potential of IPT, although it has not been determined if IPT in conjunction with ART can reduce T cell activation status and thus slow HIV-1 disease progression in patients with latent TB.

DISSEMINATION AND MYCOBACTEREMIA IN COINFECTION

As previously noted in the section "Neutrophils in Coinfection," disseminated TB and mycobacteremia occur with greater frequency in HIV-1-infected people and are associated with high mortality (86, 87). Recent findings from the murine model have potential implications for understanding how M. tuberculosis disseminates from the granuloma. Antigen transfer and T cell priming by M. tuberculosis-infected migratory DCs in infected tissue has been shown to be inefficient, whereas lymph-node-resident DCs activate T cells with much greater efficiency (170, 171). M. tuberculosis-infected inflammatory DCs express less CCR7 and have impaired migration capabilities compared with uninfected inflammatory DCs. Upon encountering M. tuberculosis-specific T cells in the infected tissue, the migration of infected DCs is halted and, depending on the distance traveled from the granuloma, either the existing inflammatory focus expands or a new focus of infection is established. Consequently, reduced priming of T cells in the lymph node occurs with impairment in M. tuberculosis-specific T cell expansion. Arrested DC migration due to capture by M. tuberculosis-specific

T cells in the tissue surrounding the site of infection with resultant expansion of existing granulomas or establishment of a new satellite granulomas was shown to be dependent on the availability of M. tuberculosis-specific T cells (171). Given the decline of M. tuberculosis-specific T cells in HIV-1 infection, it is therefore unsurprising that systemic dissemination of M. tuberculosis is observed with greater frequency than in uninfected people (86). It has been suggested that blood-borne M. tuberculosis alters its transcription toward greater virulence, with ESAT-6 transcript levels being higher in the blood of HIV-1-infected people than in that of HIV-1-uninfected people (69). ESAT-6 has been associated with alveolar cytolysis, dissemination of M. tuberculosis from the lungs (172), and release of matrix metalloproteinase-9 (MMP-9) with consequent enhancement of M. tuberculosis growth and macrophage recruitment in the Mycobacterium marinum zebrafish model (173). This assumes greater significance when considering that the HIV-1-infected donors in the aforementioned study of the blood gene transcriptome (69) were prescribed ART at the time of blood sampling.

It was recently shown that antagonism of vascular endothelial growth factor can reduce granuloma angiogenesis (174, 175) and thereby reduce M. tuberculosis burden and dissemination in the zebrafish model of TB (175). Furthermore, improved small molecule delivery to the granuloma through normalization of granuloma vasculature was demonstrated in rabbits, suggesting the possibility for improved ART and ATT delivery to the granuloma (174). These findings merit further investigation because it is tempting to speculate that they may find particular applicability in the setting of drug-resistant TB, where adequate drug penetration to the site of infection is crucial and where HIV-1 coinfection still significantly enhances mortality when compared to uninfected people (176).

ACQUIRED IMMUNITY

CD4 T Cells in Coinfection

Numeric depletion of CD4 T lymphocytes

HIV-1 infection is characterized not only by a quantitative decline in CD4 lymphocytes, but also by generalized impairment of T cell helper function that is already apparent at early clinical stages of HIV-1 infection, before a substantial decline in the peripheral CD4 count (177, 178). It is important to note that HIV-1 mediates general numeric depletion of T lymphocytes through multiple mechanisms including decreased production and maturation as well as increased destruction through direct cellular infection by the virus and so-called bystander cell death in the absence of direct infection. In the first instance T lymphocyte production may be altered by HIV-1 infection of the bone marrow with attendant suppression of lymphopoiesis, with these effects persisting in some people despite ART (179). In addition, it has been shown that HIV-1 infection impairs the rate of naive lymphocyte maturation in the thymus. This may lead to failure to compensate for CD4 lymphocyte losses, increases in short-lived T lymphocytes, and decreases in the amount of long-lived T lymphocytes with potential as progenitors in circulation; importantly, this may be restored by ART (180, 181). It has additionally been shown that HIV-1 disrupts the paracortical T cell zone in lymphoid tissue through enhanced collagen deposition, with the amount of collagen being found to be inversely proportional to both the lymphoid tissue and peripheral CD4 count (182). The degree of T cell zone fibrosis due to collagen deposition also impacts the extent of reconstitution of the peripheral CD4 T cell pool after ART initiation (183) and may continue to do so despite ART because, indeed, the coadministration of the antifibrotic pirfenidone with ART was shown to increase the magnitude of CD4 T cell populations in the peripheral blood and lymphoid tissues of SIV-infected rhesus macaques when compared to ART alone (184). Lastly, it has been shown that HIV-1 can induce pyroptotic cell death in HIV-1-uninfected lymphocytes through sensing of incomplete HIV-1 reverse transcripts via interferon-γ-inducible protein 16 and subsequent activation of caspase-1 in lymphoid tissues (185, 186).

Depletion in CD4 T cell numbers and impaired function is also apparent in the lung, where CD4 T cells are depleted in BAL from HIV-1-infected healthy people compared to uninfected people, with significantly impaired *M. tuberculosis*-specific T cell responses also being observed in T cells from HIV-1-infected people when compared with those who are not HIV-1 infected (187, 188). Similarly, CD4 lymphocytes were depleted in BAL from HIV-1-infected people with active pulmonary tuberculosis (PTB) compared to HIV-1-uninfected people with TB (189, 190): these findings were supported in the cynomolgus macaque model of SIV-TB coinfection, where significant CD4 depletion was found in granulomas of coinfected macaques versus TB-mono-infected macaques (191). Numeric depletion of CD4 T cells in human spinal granulomas compared to peripheral blood of HIV-TB-coinfected patients has also been observed (161). Peripheral CD4 count has been shown to correlate with TB risk, with CD4 counts

of ≥300 cells/mm³ associated with a one-third smaller risk of active TB during a 3- to 6-month follow-up compared to those with CD4 counts ≤100 cells/mm³ in HIV-1-infected people on ART (16). The peripheral CD4 counts of HIV-1-infected individuals show an inverse correlation with bacterial burden as determined by acid fast bacilli staining in TB lymphadenitis. Higher acid fast bacilli grades are associated with more extensive necrosis and disrupted granuloma architecture in lymph nodes (192, 193). Although peripheral CD4 counts provide an estimate of the degree of immunodeficiency in HIV-1-infected people, it is important to realize that this measure may incompletely reflect the degree of CD4 depletion at the site of *M. tuberculosis* disease, which may be far greater than that of the periphery in the setting of coinfection (187).

One mechanism through which *M. tuberculosis*-specific CD4 T cells form a target for HIV-1 infection is through their relatively high CCR5 expression on the cellular surface, which is thought to be mediated by TCR activation and IL-12 production resulting from the Th1 response to *M. tuberculosis* infection (194, 195). CCR5 upregulation is not specific to *M. tuberculosis* infection and has similarly been found in response to cytomegalovirus (CMV) infection, although CMV-specific T cells appear relatively resistant to depletion by HIV-1 (196). Geldmacher et al. demonstrated that this difference could be contributed to by differences in CCR5-ligand and cytokine production between these two cellular subsets. The majority of CMV-specific T cells were potent producers of MIP-1α and poor producers of IL-2 (197). In an earlier study the less frequent subpopulation of CMV-specific T cells not expressing either of the CCR5 ligands MIP-1α or MIP-1β were found to express 10 times the amount of HIV-1 *gag* DNA when compared to T cells that do express these ligands (196). This is attributable to the known inhibitory effect of the CCR5 ligands on CCR5-tropic HIV-1 viral entry (71, 72). *M. tuberculosis*-specific T cells were found to be less mature than the effector memory CMV-specific T cells and, by contrast, produced comparatively little MIP-1α and more IL-2. MIP-1α is a known ligand of the CCR5 receptor, and IL-2-mediated stimulation of cells expressing the IL-2 receptor CD25 promotes HIV-1 reverse transcription (198–200). The combination of low MIP-1α production and high IL-2 production of *M. tuberculosis*-specific T cells was shown to contribute to the high levels of HIV-1 *gag* DNA found in these cells and their rapid depletion *in vivo* (197).

There are, however, some discrepancies in the literature on the selective depletion of *M. tuberculosis*-

specific T cells. One study involving healthy HIV-1-infected, ART-naive people reported that the proportion of CD4 T cells producing IFN-γ in response to ESAT-6/CFP-10 as measured by enzyme-linked immunospot (ELISpot) assay increased with a decline in peripheral CD4 count, whereas responses to tuberculin-purified protein derivative (PPD) stimulation decreased (201). However, another study also measuring IFN-γ responses to ESAT-6/CFP-10 by ELISpot in healthy HIV-1 infected (median CD4 of 300 cells/mm^3) and uninfected people found that the HIV-1-infected group had a lower percentage of responders than the uninfected group (47% versus 19%) with a 9-fold reduction in M. tuberculosis-specific cells observed in the HIV-1-infected group. The PPD-stimulated ELISpot response was similarly decreased in the HIV-1-infected group, and there was no correlation found between either the ESAT-6/CFP-10 responses or the PPD responses and peripheral CD4 count in the HIV-1-infected people (197). A third study reported that IFN-γ responses to ESAT-6/CFP-10 and PPD as measured by ELISpot decreased with CD4 count in HIV-1-infected people without active PTB, with only PPD

responses correlating significantly with CD4 count in all HIV-1-infected people both with and without active PTB. In the same study a whole-blood assay mirrored the decreased IFN-γ responses to PPD in the HIV-1-infected versus HIV-1-uninfected group (both without active PTB), with ESAT-6/CFP-10 responses once again being decreased in the former group, but not significantly so (202).

Functional impairment of CD4 T cells in HIV-1 infection

Even in people on ART where CD4 T cells are numerically reconstituted, there is still a significantly increased risk of tuberculosis. This is hypothesized either to be due to persistent impairment of the quality of CD4 T cell responses to M. tuberculosis or to be because certain subsets of CD4 T cells do not recover quantitatively, regardless of ART. As previously mentioned, functional impairment of M. tuberculosis-specific CD4 lymphocytes in HIV-1 infection plays a key role in coinfection with TB (Table 3). HIV-1 not only impacts the pathogen-specific cytokine production of T lymphocytes, but also affects antigen presentation. HIV-1

Table 3 T lymphocyte dysfunction in the setting of HIV-TB coinfection and the effect of ART

Functional impairment of T cells in HIV-TB coinfection with and without ART	Pre-ART	With ART
Factors mediating global T cell dysfunction	Endocytic relocation of MHC I/II, CD80, and CD86 → impaired antigen-specific T cell activation	Unknown
	↓IL-2 production	Proportion of IL-2 producing M. tuberculosis-specific CD4 T cells is inversely proportional to HIV-1 viral load, thus possibly improved
	↓IL-2Rα expression	
	Decreased T cell proliferation and differentiation	
	↑PD1 expression → ↓TCR activation and signaling	PD1 expression correlated with HIV-1 viral load, thus possibly reduced
M. tuberculosis-specific T cell dysfunction	↓M. tuberculosis-specific CD4 T cell responses to PPD stimulation	Improved, but not fully restored
	PPD responses correlate with CD4 count	
	↓M. tuberculosis-specific CD4 T cell responses to ESAT-6/CFP-10 stimulation	Unchanged or improved, but not fully restored
	↓BAL M. tuberculosis-specific CD4 T cell responses to PPD, ESAT-6/CFP-10 and BCG	Improved
	↓ Proportion and frequency of IFN-γ⁺ TNF⁺ M. tuberculosis-specific CD4 T cells	Similar frequency to HIV-1-uninfected after 4 years on ART
		Improved, but not restored proportion irrespective of ART duration
	↓ Frequency of IFN-γ⁺ TNF⁺ IL-2⁺M. tuberculosis-specific CD4 T cells	Unchanged or improved
	↓Degranulation and proliferation of CD8 T cells in response to M. tuberculosis	Unknown

^{a}Abbreviations: ART, antiretroviral therapy; MHC, major histocompatibility complex; ESAT-6, 6-kDa early secretory antigenic target; TCR, T cell receptor; PPD, purified protein derivative; BAL, bronchoalveolar lavage; BCG, bacillus Calmette-Guérin; IFN-γ, interferon gamma; TNF, tumor necrosis factor; IL, interleukin.

nef can mediate endocytic relocation of both major histocompatibility complex proteins I and II from the cell surface, along with the costimulatory molecules CD80 and CD86 (203, 204) with resultant impaired naive T cell activation by monocytoid cells. Furthermore, the HIV-1 envelope glycoprotein gp120, as well as the HIV-1 *tat* protein, mediates decreased IL-2 production and decreased surface IL-2 receptor (IL-2R) alpha-chain expression in T cells (205, 206), impairing the IL-2 response required for lymphocyte differentiation and proliferation in the response to infection. The frequency of programmed cell death protein 1 expression has been found to be increased on T cells producing IFN-γ in response to PPD stimulation in HIV-TB-coinfected people compared with IFN-γ-producing T cells from those with TB alone, LTBI and HIV-1 infection, or LTBI alone (207). Programmed cell death protein 1 is a negative regulator of TCR signaling and activation (208), and its expression on T lymphocytes has been associated with failure of immune reconstitution after ART-mediated suppression of HIV-1 viral replication (209, 210).

Influence of ART on T cell responses to *M. tuberculosis* in coinfection

While highly beneficial, ART does not fully restore the TB-specific immune response, despite long-term HIV-1 viral suppression and recovery of CD4 count (13). There is heterogeneity in the capacity of HIV-1-infected people to reconstitute various CD4 T cell subsets, and baseline CD4 counts below 350 cells/mm^3 at ART initiation are particularly associated with an inability to reconstitute the naive:memory CD4 T cell ratio to that of HIV-1-uninfected levels (211). The differentiation state of antigen-specific CD4 T cells before ART initiation may also play a role as shown by a study of *M. tuberculosis*- and CMV-specific memory CD4 T cells and their reconstitution after a year of ART. The predominant late differentiated phenotype (CD45RO$^+$, CD27$^-$) prior to ART initiation showed less capacity to reconstitute than that of predominantly early differentiated phenotype (CD45RO$^+$, CD27$^+$) (212). The memory CD4 T cell subset is the first to be reconstituted on ART (213, 214), with the naive subset taking somewhat longer to be reconstituted, and it may not fully reconstitute in all people despite long-term ART-mediated viral suppression (213, 215). Wilkinson et al. examined CD4 T cell reconstitution during the first 48 weeks of ART and showed that terminally differentiated effector CD4 T cells (CD4$^+$CD27$^-$CCR7$^-$) increase in total number but decrease as a proportion of the total CD4 T cell pool (213). The ability of reconsti-

tuted cell populations to respond to antigen stimulation is also improved, with an increase in responses to PPD (216, 217) and both unchanged (218) and increased (213, 219) responses to *M. tuberculosis*-specific ESAT-6/CFP-10 being reported with increasing duration of ART-mediated viral suppression. However, IFN-γ secreting capacity in response to both PPD and ESAT-6/CFP-10 is not fully restored to that of HIV-1-uninfected people (213, 220, 221).

As mentioned previously, a similar phenomenon also applies to BAL CD4 T cell responses to ESAT-6/CFP-10, BCG, and PPD stimulation, which were significantly decreased despite ART (187, 222). In a cross-sectional study by Jambo et al. only the participant group on ART for longer than 4 years showed frequency of IFN-γ and TNF double positive CD4 T cells in BAL comparable to that of the HIV-1-uninfected group, and the proportion of this subset to the overall CD4 population remained diminished. Indeed, both blood and BAL CD4 T cells of the all-HIV-1-infected groups, irrespective of ART duration, showed diminished proportions of double positive CD4 T cells (222). Furthermore, polyfunctional T cells producing IFN-γ, TNF, and IL-2 in response to *M. tuberculosis* antigen stimulation were found to be significantly decreased in BAL from HIV-1-infected people when compared to HIV-1-uninfected people (187). These findings were mirrored by a prospective study that also showed expansion of the polyfunctional *M. tuberculosis*-specific T cell subset in HIV-1-infected people between the pre-ART time point and 1 year after ART initiation (219), although a similar study showed no significant change in this subset pre- and post-ART (212). Considering the finding that IL-2 production in *M. tuberculosis*-specific CD4 T cells showed an inverse correlation with HIV-1 viral load (223), the authors of the latter study suggested that this discrepancy may be explained by differences in cohort immune status with a generally more advanced disease state and relatively higher viral loads being the case in the former. The presumption is thus that with a greater magnitude of ART-induced decreases in viral load, the early differentiated *M. tuberculosis*-specific T cells would show greater recovery of polyfunctionality.

Cytotoxic Lymphocytes in Coinfection

CD8 T cells form an important component of the immune response to intracellular pathogens, especially viruses but also *M. tuberculosis* (224, 225). CD8 T cells mediate their effect via major histocompatibility complex class I recognition of infected cells, are cytolytic via secretion of granzymes and perforins, and can also induce apoptosis by activating cell death receptors on target cells (226). In a study comparing HIV-1-infected and -uninfected LTBI participants it was shown that CD8 T cells from coinfected people exhibited decreased expression of the degranulation marker CD107a and impaired proliferative capacity in response to ESAT-6/CFP-10 (227). The murine model of *M. tuberculosis* has suggested that CD8 lymphocyte depletion does not affect survival but does play a role in bacterial control in the latent phase of infection (228, 229). Similarly, a role for *M. tuberculosis*-specific CD8 T cells has been suggested in the setting of human LTBI. Reactivated LTBI in people treated with anti-TNF immunotherapy is associated with decreased frequency of circulating *M. tuberculosis*-specific CD8 T cells of the effector memory phenotype (230). HIV-1-infected people with LTBI have been shown to have a greater proportion of effector memory phenotype *M. tuberculosis*-specific CD8 T cells compared with people with active PTB and HIV-1 infection (231). However, a subsequent study reported increased effector memory (CD45RA⁻CCR7⁻) and terminal effector (CD45RA⁺CCR7⁻) CD8 T cell proportions in both *M. tuberculosis*-specific IFN-γ⁺ CD8 T cell and CD107a/b⁺ CD8 T cell subsets sorted from HIV-TB-coinfected people compared to healthy controls (232).

Although the effector memory CD8 T cell subset was expanded in HIV-TB-coinfected people, the mean fluorescence intensity of CD45RA was significantly decreased in comparison to healthy controls. This may indicate dysfunctional TCR signaling in this subset of CD8 T cells because CD45 has been shown to be a mediator of TCR activation and gene transcription (233, 234). Additionally, both latent and active TB cases with HIV-1 had higher ratios of terminal effector: naive CD8 T cells than healthy controls. ART seemed to some extent to restore the bulk percentage of naive CD8 T cells in people with HIV-TB coinfection who were on ART, where significantly increased percentages of naive (CD45RA⁺CCR7⁺) CD8 T cells and significantly decreased percentages of effector memory CD8 T cells are observed. Furthermore, HIV-TB-coinfected and HIV-1-infected people had higher expression of programmed cell death protein 1, a marker of CD8 T cell dysfunction in chronic viral infection (235), on CD8 T cells than healthy controls, and this was found to be especially marked in the CD27⁺ CD8 T cell population (232). Although the CD27 receptor has been shown to be involved in providing costimulatory signaling affecting T cell and B cell proliferation, it can also mediate apoptosis (236). Further work is needed to fully elucidate the role of *M. tuberculosis*-specific CD8 T cells in the setting of HIV-TB coinfection.

HIV-TUBERCULOSIS-ASSOCIATED IMMUNE RECONSTITUTION INFLAMMATORY SYNDROME (IRIS)

Introduction

Although ART effectively restores the HIV-1-infected immune system, it can ironically also give rise to clinical worsening of previously unrecognized, or pre-existing, inflammatory or infective conditions known as IRIS. Two types of TB-IRIS have been identified: paradoxical and unmasking. The former occurs when tuberculosis is diagnosed prior to ART initiation and clinical improvement or stabilization of the TB infection is noticeable in response to ATT. However, upon initiation of ART new, recurrent, or worsening features of TB appear. Unmasking TB-IRIS occurs when previously undiagnosed and untreated TB is "unmasked" by ART initiation (237). TB-IRIS occurs in approximately 18% of HIV-TB coinfected people upon ART initiation, necessitates hospital admission in 25%, and is associated with mortality in 2% of patients. TB meningitis patients are at increased risk of TB-IRIS, and this is one of the most severe forms of TB-IRIS, resulting in higher rates of mortality than other forms of TB-IRIS (238–240). Risk factors for paradoxical IRIS include low pre-ART CD4, with rapid reconstitution following ART initiation (241, 242), high pre-ART viral load (243), extrapulmonary TB (244, 245), and a short time interval between starting ATT and ART initiation (244, 246). Although early ART initiation (between 2 and 4 weeks on ATT) is associated with an increased rate of TB-IRIS and TB-IRIS-associated mortality, significantly decreased all-cause mortality is observed compared to deferred ART initiation (247). Thus, it is rarely recommended that TB-IRIS is managed by withdrawal, or prevented by delay, of ART.

Innate Immunity and TB-IRIS

Although initial TB-IRIS research focused on the adaptive immune response, the central role of the innate immune system in the pathogenesis of TB-IRIS is increasingly recognized. Transcriptomic profiling of whole blood from HIV-TB coinfected people has clearly highlighted the importance of the innate immune system in TB-IRIS, with a transcriptomic signature predominated by innate immune components such as TLR and triggering receptor expressed on myeloid cells 1 (TREM-1)-induced inflammasome signaling being apparent at 2 weeks (the usual median time of onset of IRIS) post-ART initiation (248).

The well-recognized dysfunction of macrophages in the setting of HIV-TB coinfection has led to investigation of the role of monocytes and macrophages in TB-IRIS. TB-IRIS is associated with increased plasma markers of monocyte activation, namely, sCD14, sCD163, and soluble tissue factor, with the latter two found to be elevated before ART initiation in those who develop TB-IRIS, whereas sCD14 was found to be elevated at the time of TB-IRIS. Different monocyte subsets were also prevalent at different time points in people who develop TB-IRIS; most notably, $CD14^{++}CD16^{-}$ monocyte frequency was found to be an independent predictor of TB-IRIS that closely associated with proinflammatory cytokine production (249).

Monocytes and DCs exhibit increased TLR2 expression pre-ART in TB-IRIS patients when compared to healthy controls. This increased TLR2 expression was associated with lipomannan-induced TNF-α and IL-12p40 responses (250). *M. tuberculosis*-mediated signaling via TLR2, TLR4, and the NF-κB pathway has been established in the pathogenesis of TB-IRIS, where proinflammatory cytokine release could be abrogated by peptide blockade of the MyD88 adapter in PBMC from TB-IRIS patients (Fig. 2) (248).

NK cells may play a role in the setting of unmasking TB-IRIS, because it has been shown that they exhibit increased activation status compared to NK cells from chronic HIV-1-infected people and HIV-TB coinfected people without IRIS (251). In paradoxical TB-IRIS, NK cells were shown to have increased degranulation capacity prior to ART initiation, whereas this normalized with increased duration of ART and at occurrence of IRIS (252). Furthermore, the transcripts from the perforin 1 and granzyme B genes were found to be elevated in PBMC from people with TB-IRIS compared to non-IRIS individuals, with this being confirmed at the protein level. Additionally, granzyme B levels showed a decline over a 2-week period in people with TB-IRIS treated with prednisone, a corticosteroid known to mediate clinical improvement in TB-IRIS, compared to placebo. It was also demonstrated that iNKT cell proportions were increased at the time of TB-IRIS, suggesting that this cell population may contribute to the increased levels of these cytotoxic mediators (253). Neutrophils may contribute to increased levels of cytotoxic mediators, with elevated neutrophil levels, IL-17 concentration, and neutrophil mediator S100A8/A9 being elevated in the cerebrospinal fluid of patients who developed TB meningitis-IRIS compared to controls who did not (238, 254).

Hypercytokinemia in TB-IRIS

Compared to non-IRIS controls, TB-IRIS is characterized by hypercytokinemia, as demonstrated by the increased

presence of a range of pro- and anti-inflammatory cytokines including IL-1, IL-5, IL-6, IL-10, IL-13, IL-17A, IFN-γ, granulocyte-macrophage colony-stimulating factor, and TNF from PBMC sampled from TB-IRIS patients at presentation and stimulated with heat-killed *M. tuberculosis* compared to non-IRIS controls (255). Plasma concentrations of a number of proinflammatory cytokines including IL-6 and TNF were found to significantly increase over 4 weeks following ART initiation in patients who developed TB-IRIS compared to controls (256). Hypercytokinemia in TB-IRIS may compound the hyperinflammatory state that characterizes vitamin D3 deficiency, because higher plasma IL-8 and IL-18 concentrations were found at baseline, with significantly increased IL-8 still being apparent at 2 weeks post-ART initiation in people with TB-IRIS and vitamin D3 deficiency. Deficiency in vitamin D3 itself was not found to be a risk factor for TB-IRIS (257).

A randomized placebo-controlled trial of prednisone treatment for TB-IRIS demonstrated decreased IL-6, IL-10, IL-12p40, TNF-α, IFN-γ, and IFN-γ-induced protein-10 in the serum of the treatment group at weeks 2 and 4 (258). Similarly, a number of chemokines have been shown to be differentially expressed in TB-IRIS versus non-IRIS patients: most notably, CCL2 and CXCL10 (257, 259–261). In plasma of people with TB-IRIS it was found that CCL2 concentrations were lower and CXCL10 and IL-18 concentrations were elevated relative to controls (259). CXCL10 or IFN-γ-induced protein 10 (IP-10) expression is mediated by *M. tuberculosis*-induced type I interferon and is important in the context of TB in mediating chemotaxis of activated T cells expressing its ligand, CXCR3, to the site of infection (262, 263). Aberrant interferon signaling appears to be an important mechanism in TB-IRIS because both type I and II interferon gene transcripts were shown to be differentially expressed at as early as 0.5 weeks in people who develop TB-IRIS (248). Although the role of type I interferon in *M. tuberculosis* seems to be principally that of immunomodulation, with increased IL-10 and decreased IL-1α, IL-1β, and IL-12 being observed (264, 265), the opposite was shown in TB-IRIS, with increased IL-1α, IL-1β, and IL-12p40 concentrations in PBMC and plasma being observed (248, 266). Indeed, as hypothesized by Lai et al. (248), it is probable that high *M. tuberculosis* load in TB-IRIS coupled with disregulation of innate immune signaling and hypercytokinemia are important factors in the pathogenesis of TB-IRIS, with differential chemokine expression such as CXCL10 and CCR5 perhaps compounding the heightened state of inflamma-

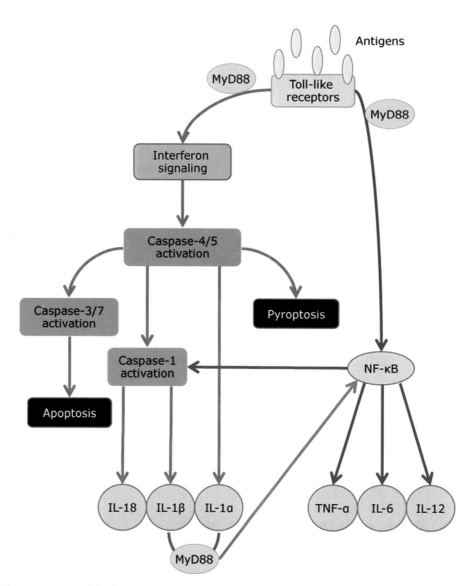

Figure 2 A model of innate receptor signaling in mediating TB-IRIS pathogenesis as proposed by Lai et al. Microarray profiling revealed that TLR signaling and inflammasome activation are critical in mediating TB-IRIS pathogenesis. The proposed model begins with *M. tuberculosis* antigen recognition by surface-expressing TLRs, which triggers the downstream signaling cascade with adaptor molecules such as MyD88 and IRAK4 to activate IRF7, thereby triggering the production of type I IFN. Paracrine signaling of type I IFN to IFNAR recruits and phosphorylates STAT1/2 dimers, leading to further recruitment of IRF9 and the formation of ISGF3, thereby inducing pro-caspase-11 (caspase-4/5 in human) and AIM-2 inflammasome (caspase-1). Caspase-11 cleaves IL-1α into its mature form and can lead to pyroptosis. The noncanonical inflammasome (caspase-11) can also activate the canonical inflammasome (caspase-1), which cleaves IL-1β and IL-18 into their mature form. Alternatively, TLR signaling via MyD88 can also activate NF-κB via the TAK1/IKK complex. Activation of NF-κB triggers the production of an array of cytokines, including TNF-α, IL-6, and IL-12. In addition, NF-κB also activates NLRP1/3 inflammasomes and subsequently leads to the production of IL-1β and IL-18. Reproduced from *Seminars in Immunopathology* (287) with permission of the publisher.

tion at the site of disease by enhanced homing of highly activated T lymphocytes.

Matrix metalloproteinases (MMPs) are a group of enzymes that are responsible for degradation of extracellular matrix proteins. MMP-1 gene transcription is upregulated in response to TB, and concentrations in sputum and BAL have been shown to be increased compared with controls (267, 268). HIV-1 coinfection has been associated with lower concentrations of MMP-1, -2, -8, and -9 in induced sputum of TB patients (269), but in PBMC of patients with TB-IRIS there was increased gene transcription and protein levels of MMP-1, -3, -7, and -10 compared to controls (270). In TB meningitis-IRIS it was shown that cerebrospinal fluid MMP-9 concentrations were elevated pre-ART initiation, with further increases observed after ART was started (254).

Acquired Immunity and TB-IRIS

CD4 T cells in TB-IRIS

Initial work in the TB-IRIS field focused on the role of expansion of the *M. tuberculosis*-specific Th1 response. Bourgarit et al. reported an increased frequency of PPD-responsive IFN-γ-producing T cells measured by ELISpot in people with TB-IRIS and compared with CMV-specific T cells as controls. Additionally, Th1-associated cytokines and chemokines (IFN-γ, IL-2, IL-12, CXCL10, and monokine induced by IFN-gamma) were shown to be increased at the time of TB-IRIS (271). However, it was subsequently shown in a study following up HIV-TB-coinfected people over 8 weeks following ART initiation that significant expansion of *M. tuberculosis*-specific IFN-γ-producing T cells was not unique to TB-IRIS and occurred in both IRIS and non-IRIS cases (272). Furthermore, the proposed association between elevated Th1 cytokines in TB-IRIS as opposed to non-IRIS cases was not consistently demonstrated, and IGRA measurement of IFN-γ responses also did not show any differences between these two groups at early time points (273, 274). It has been shown that TB-IRIS is associated with a state of heightened T cell activation, with CD45RO+HLA-DR+ CD4 T cells being observed at significantly greater frequency pre-ART in TB-IRIS cases than in non-IRIS cases (266). This is in keeping with other reports of higher T cell activation states in IRIS (275), and thus a role for regulatory T cells (Treg) was postulated for TB-IRIS. However, no difference in the frequency of FoxP3 positive cells was found in TB-IRIS when compared with non-IRIS controls (272, 275), illustrating that regulation of this subset in IRIS may be pathogen-specific because a

relative Treg expansion was demonstrated in people who developed IRIS with underlying CMV and *M. avium* infection (276, 277).

In support of the aforementioned findings, there was no difference found in TB-IRIS and non-IRIS CD25+CD127lo CD4+ Tregs at ART initiation in the study by Haridas et al. (266); however, this subset showed rapid decline with increasing ART duration, amounting to a significantly decreased proportion at week 34 post-ATT in TB-IRIS compared to non-IRIS cases. It was also demonstrated that there was no pre-ART difference in central memory and effector memory subsets of people who developed TB-IRIS compared with non-IRIS controls, but the effector memory subset showed significant increases while the central memory subset significantly declined over 34 weeks of ATT in people who developed TB-IRIS. CD95 expression on effector memory CD4 T cells was similar in TB-IRIS and non-IRIS cases but also increased to significantly higher frequency by week 34 in TB-IRIS cases. OX40 expressing CD4 T cells was significantly increased at ART initiation and showed significant decline with duration on ART, where no difference in frequency between the two groups was observed at 34 weeks. This may be significant because OX40 expression on activated T cells has been shown to enhance HIV-LTR-dependent viral replication through HIV protein gp34 binding of OX40, with subsequent NF-κB activation occurring (278). Thus, the expanded OX40+ CD4 T cell population could contribute to increased HIV-1 viral load that predisposes to IRIS (243), as well as the observed hypercytokinemia through activation of NF-κB signaling.

Cytotoxic T cells in TB-IRIS

TCRγδ T cells form a small subset of T cells that are enriched at epithelial borders, recognize bacteria and parasites through their TCR, and can exert their effector function by cytokines with or without cytotoxic granule (e.g., perforin, granzyme B) production (279). Although a model of γδ knockout mice demonstrated that they may be dispensable for the control of *M. avium* (280), TCRγδ T cells have capability to efficiently kill *M. tuberculosis*-infected macrophages *in vitro* (281). Deficiency of the Vγ9Vδ2+ T cell subset has been associated with the occurrence of active pulmonary tuberculosis (282), and TCRγδ T cells have been shown to be dysfunctional in the setting of HIV-TB coinfection (283). In paradoxical TB-IRIS the KIR−Vδ2+ TCRγδ T cells were shown to be significantly elevated pre-ART and at various time points thereafter compared with non-IRIS controls. The TCRγδ T cells expressing

KIR, a receptor predominantly mediating inhibition of cytotoxic responses, were of lower frequency pre-ART and at subsequent time points in TB-IRIS (284).

Although one study has reported pre-ART CD8 T cell percentage as an independent predictor of TB-IRIS, with expansion of the naive and $CD38^+HLA-DR^+$ CD8 T cell subsets being found (285), this has not been consistently demonstrated (253, 266). Two other studies found no difference in CD8 T cell number or frequency between TB-IRIS and non-IRIS groups pre-ART. However, Haridas et al. (266) found that compared with the TB-IRIS group, the non-IRIS group showed significant decline in the frequency of activated ($HLA-DR^+$) CD8 T cells in response to ART. Significantly higher proportions of the TB-IRIS group expressed CD95 on effector memory CD8 T cells at ART initiation, although overall effector memory phenotype was similar between both groups. At ART-initiation there were reduced proportions of central memory/ early effector memory or "transitional" phenotype in the TB-IRIS group, with no detectable difference between any of these at 34 weeks in TB-IRIS and non-IRIS groups (266).

CONCLUDING REMARKS

The HIV-TB syndemic represents the two greatest contributors to global infectious disease mortality. Although advances have been made in understanding how each pathogen compounds the immunopathology associated with the other, a great deal remains incompletely understood. It is yet to be defined what constitutes a protective or a pathogenic immune response to TB, and this may be particularly challenging in HIV-TB coinfection, where widespread aberration in innate and adaptive immunity adds complexity. There is currently no effective vaccine for either HIV or TB, and the development of a TB vaccine that is safe and immunogenic in both HIV-1-infected and -uninfected people is crucial. The lack of accurate TB diagnostics and robust biomarkers to diagnose and monitor both LTBI and active TB in HIV-1 coinfection also represents an unmet need. Animal models are useful to study HIV-TB coinfection, and although the murine model of T cell depletion does not fully recapitulate HIV-1-induced immunopathology, the non-human primate model of SIV is a useful tool to confirm or refute the hypotheses generated. ART-mediated immune reconstitution is clearly beneficial, and investigating the nature of residual immune dysfunction after ART initiation may be informative in defining factors that still contribute to increased TB risk in this population. Biomarkers that can assist in early identification and monitoring of TB-IRIS are needed, particularly as the use of corticosteroids has already illustrated the potential benefit of immunomodulation in this condition.

Acknowledgments. RJW is supported by the Wellcome Trust (104803, 084323), National Institutes for Health (NIH 1U01AI115940-01), Medical Research Council (UK) (U1175.02.002.00014), Medical Research Council of South Africa (Strategic Health Innovations Partnership), European Commission (FP7 HEALTH-F3-2012-305578), and National Research Foundation of South Africa (96841).

Citation. du Bruyn E, Wilkinson RJ. 2016. The immune interaction between HIV-1 infection and *Mycobacterium tuberculosis*. Microbiol Spectrum 4(6):TBTB2-0012-2016.

References

1. **WHO.** 2015. *Global tuberculosis report 2015.* WHO, Geneva, Switzerland. http://www.who.int/tb/publications/global_report/en/.
2. **Sonnenberg P, Glynn JR, Fielding K, Murray J, Godfrey-Faussett P, Shearer S.** 2005. How soon after infection with HIV does the risk of tuberculosis start to increase? A retrospective cohort study in South African gold miners. *J Infect Dis* **191:**150–158.
3. **UNAIDS.** *UNAIDS fact sheet 2015: the Joint United Nations Programme on HIV/AIDS 2015.* http://www.unaids.org/sites/default/files/media_asset/20150901_FactSheet_2015_en.pdf.
4. **WHO.** 2015. *Guideline on When to Start Antiretroviral Therapy and on Pre-Exposure Prophylaxis for HIV.* World Health Organization, Geneva, Switzerland.
5. **Lawn SD, Harries AD, Williams BG, Chaisson RE, Losina E, De Cock KM, Wood R.** 2011. Antiretroviral therapy and the control of HIV-associated tuberculosis. Will ART do it? *Int J Tuberc Lung Dis* **15:**571–581.
6. **Gupta A, Wood R, Kaplan R, Bekker LG, Lawn SD.** 2012. Tuberculosis incidence rates during 8 years of follow-up of an antiretroviral treatment cohort in South Africa: comparison with rates in the community. *PLoS One* **7:**e34156.
7. **Selwyn PA, Hartel D, Lewis VA, Schoenbaum EE, Vermund SH, Klein RS, Walker AT, Friedland GH.** 1989. A prospective study of the risk of tuberculosis among intravenous drug users with human immunodeficiency virus infection. *N Engl J Med* **320:**545–550.
8. **Girardi E, Raviglione MC, Antonucci G, Godfrey-Faussett P, Ippolito G.** 2000. Impact of the HIV epidemic on the spread of other diseases: the case of tuberculosis. *AIDS* **14**(Suppl 3):S47–S56.
9. **Houben RM, Crampin AC, Ndhlovu R, Sonnenberg P, Godfrey-Faussett P, Haas WH, Engelmann G, Lombard CJ, Wilkinson D, Bruchfeld J, Lockman S, Tappero J, Glynn JR.** 2011. Human immunodeficiency virus associated tuberculosis more often due to recent infection than reactivation of latent infection. *Int J Tuberc Lung Dis* **15:**24–31.
10. **Charalambous S, Grant AD, Moloi V, Warren R, Day JH, van Helden P, Hayes RJ, Fielding KL, De Cock**

KM, Chaisson RE, Churchyard GJ. 2008. Contribution of reinfection to recurrent tuberculosis in South African gold miners. *Int J Tuberc Lung Dis* 12:942–948.

11. Crampin AC, Mwaungulu JN, Mwaungulu FD, Mwafulirwa DT, Munthali K, Floyd S, Fine PE, Glynn JR. 2010. Recurrent TB: relapse orreinfection? The effect of HIV in a general population cohort in Malawi. *AIDS* 24:417–426.

12. Narayanan S, Swaminathan S, Supply P, Shanmugam S, Narendran G, Hari L, Ramachandran R, Locht C, Jawahar MS, Narayanan PR. 2010. Impact of HIV infection on the recurrence of tuberculosis in South India. *J Infect Dis* 201:691–703.

13. Lawn SD, Myer L, Edwards D, Bekker LG, Wood R. 2009. Short-term and long-term risk of tuberculosis associated with CD4 cell recovery during antiretroviral therapy in South Africa. *AIDS* 23:1717–1725.

14. Lawn SD, Badri M, Wood R. 2005. Tuberculosis among HIV-infected patients receiving HAART: long term incidence and risk factors in a South African cohort. *AIDS* 19:2109–2116.

15. Wood R, Maartens G, Lombard CJ. 2000. Risk factors for developing tuberculosis in HIV-1-infected adults from communities with a low or very high incidence of tuberculosis. *J Acquir Immune Defic Syndr* 23:75–80.

16. Chang CA, Meloni ST, Eisen G, Chaplin B, Akande P, Okonkwo P, Rawizza HE, Tchetgen Tchetgen E, Kanki PJ. 2015. Tuberculosis incidence and risk factors among human immunodeficiency virus (HIV)-infected adults receiving antiretroviral therapy in a large HIV program in Nigeria. *Open Forum Infect Dis* 2:ofv154.

17. Martín-Echevarría E, Serrano-Villar S, Sainz T, Moreno A, Casado JL, Dronda F, Elías MJ, Navas E, Zapata MR, Moreno S. 2014. Development of tuberculosis in human immunodeficiency virus infected patients receiving antiretroviral therapy. *Int J Tuberc Lung Dis* 18:1080–1084.

18. Akolo C, Adetifa I, Shepperd S, Volmink J. 2010. Treatment of latent tuberculosis infection in HIV infected persons. *Cochrane Database Syst Rev* (1):CD000171.

19. Rangaka MX, Wilkinson RJ, Boulle A, Glynn JR, Fielding K, van Cutsem G, Wilkinson KA, Goliath R, Mathee S, Goemaere E, Maartens G. 2014. Isoniazid plus antiretroviral therapy to prevent tuberculosis: a randomised double-blind, placebo-controlled trial. *Lancet* 384:682–690.

20. Briggs MA, Emerson C, Modi S, Taylor NK, Date A. 2015. Use of isoniazid preventive therapy for tuberculosis prophylaxis among people living with HIV/AIDS: a review of the literature. *J Acquir Immune Defic Syndr* 68(Suppl 3):S297–S305.

21. Lagrange PH, Herrmann JL. 2008. Diagnosing latent tuberculosis infection in the HIV era. *Open Respir Med J* 2:52–59.

22. Wejse C, Patsche CB, Kühle A, Bamba FJ, Mendes MS, Lemvik G, Gomes VF, Rudolf F. 2015. Impact of HIV-1, HIV-2, and HIV-1+2 dual infection on the outcome of tuberculosis. *Int J Infect Dis* 32:128–134.

23. Marlink R, Kanki P, Thior I, Travers K, Eisen G, Siby T, Traore I, Hsieh C, Dia M, Gueye E, et. 1994. Reduced rate of disease development after HIV-2 infection as compared to HIV-1. *Science* 265:1587–1590.

24. Campbell-Yesufu OT, Gandhi RT. 2011. Update on human immunodeficiency virus (HIV)-2 infection. *Clin Infect Dis* 52:780–787.

25. Ekouevi DK, Tchounga BK, Coffie PA, Tegbe J, Anderson AM, Gottlieb GS, Vitoria M, Dabis F, Eholie SP. 2014. Antiretroviral therapy response among HIV-2 infected patients: a systematic review. *BMC Infect Dis* 14:461.

26. Girard MP, Osmanov S, Assossou OM, Kieny MP. 2011. Human immunodeficiency virus (HIV) immuno-pathogenesis and vaccine development: a review. *Vaccine* 29:6191–6218.

27. Dezzutti CS, Hladik F. 2013. Use of human mucosal tissue to study HIV-1 pathogenesis and evaluate HIV-1 prevention modalities. *Curr HIV/AIDS Rep* 10:12–20.

28. Cicala C, Arthos J, Fauci AS. 2011. HIV-1 envelope, integrins and co-receptor use in mucosal transmission of HIV. *J Transl Med* 9(Suppl 1):S2.

29. Monteiro P, Gosselin A, Wacleche VS, El-Far M, Said EA, Kared H, Grandvaux N, Boulassel MR, Routy JP, Ancuta P. 2011. Memory CCR6+CD4+ T cells are preferential targets for productive HIV type 1 infection regardless of their expression of integrin β7. *J Immunol* 186:4618–4630.

30. Ruibal-Ares BH, Belmonte L, Baré PC, Parodi CM, Massud I, de Bracco MM. 2004. HIV-1 infection and chemokine receptor modulation. *Curr HIV Res* 2:39–50.

31. Hazenberg MD, Otto SA, Hamann D, Roos MT, Schuitemaker H, de Boer RJ, Miedema F. 2003. Depletion of naive CD4 T cells by CXCR4-using HIV-1 variants occurs mainly through increased T-cell death and activation. *AIDS* 17:1419–1424.

32. Okoye AA, Picker LJ. 2013. CD4(+) T-cell depletion in HIV infection: mechanisms of immunological failure. *Immunol Rev* 254:54–64.

33. Krebs SJ, Ananworanich J. 2015. Immune activation during acute HIV infection and the impact of early antiretroviral therapy. *Curr Opin HIV AIDS* 11:163–172.

34. Brenchley JM, Price DA, Douek DC. 2006. HIV disease: fallout from a mucosal catastrophe? *Nat Immunol* 7:235–239.

35. Koziel H, Kim S, Reardon C, Li X, Garland R, Pinkston P, Kornfeld H. 1999. Enhanced *in vivo* human immunodeficiency virus-1 replication in the lungs of human immunodeficiency virus-infected persons with *Pneumocystis carinii* pneumonia. *Am J Respir Crit Care Med* 160:2048–2055.

36. Jambo KC, Banda DH, Kankwatira AM, Sukumar N, Allain TJ, Heyderman RS, Russell DG, Mwandumba HC. 2014. Small alveolar macrophages are infected preferentially by HIV and exhibit impaired phagocytic function. *Mucosal Immunol* 7:1116–1126.

37. Azzam R, Kedzierska K, Leeansyah E, Chan H, Doischer D, Gorry PR, Cunningham AL, Crowe SM, Jaworowski A. 2006. Impaired complement-mediated phagocytosis by HIV type-1-infected human monocyte-derived macrophages involves a cAMP-dependent mechanism. *AIDS Res Hum Retroviruses* 22:619–629.

38. Leeansyah E, Wines BD, Crowe SM, Jaworowski A. 2007. The mechanism underlying defective Fcgamma receptor-mediated phagocytosis by HIV-1-infected human monocyte-derived macrophages. *J Immunol* 178: 1096–1104.

39. Patel NR, Zhu J, Tachado SD, Zhang J, Wan Z, Saukkonen J, Koziel H. 2007. HIV impairs TNF-alpha mediated macrophage apoptotic response to *Mycobacterium tuberculosis*. *J Immunol* 179:6973–6980.

40. Biggs BA, Hewish M, Kent S, Hayes K, Crowe SM. 1995. HIV-1 infection of human macrophages impairs phagocytosis and killing of *Toxoplasma gondii*. *J Immunol* 154:6132–6139.

41. Noursadeghi M, Tsang J, Miller RF, Straschewski S, Kellam P, Chain BM, Katz DR. 2009. Genome-wide innate immune responses in HIV-1-infected macrophages are preserved despite attenuation of the NF-kappa B activation pathway. *J Immunol* 182:319–328.

42. Harding CV, Boom WH. 2010. Regulation of antigen presentation by *Mycobacterium tuberculosis*: a role for Toll-like receptors. *Nat Rev Microbiol* 8:296–307.

43. Podinovskaia M, Lee W, Caldwell S, Russell DG. 2013. Infection of macrophages with *Mycobacterium tuberculosis* induces global modifications to phagosomal function. *Cell Microbiol* 15:843–859.

44. Mwandumba HC, Russell DG, Nyirenda MH, Anderson J, White SA, Molyneux ME, Squire SB. 2004. *Mycobacterium tuberculosis* resides in nonacidified vacuoles in endocytically competent alveolar macrophages from patients with tuberculosis and HIV infection. *J Immunol* 172:4592–4598.

45. Parandhaman DK, Narayanan S. 2014. Cell death paradigms in the pathogenesis of *Mycobacterium tuberculosis* infection. *Front Cell Infect Microbiol* 4:31.

46. Behar SM, Martin CJ, Booty MG, Nishimura T, Zhao X, Gan HX, Divangahi M, Remold HG. 2011. Apoptosis is an innate defense function of macrophages against *Mycobacterium tuberculosis*. *Mucosal Immunol* 4: 279–287.

47. Balcewicz-Sablinska MK, Keane J, Kornfeld H, Remold HG. 1998. Pathogenic *Mycobacterium tuberculosis* evades apoptosis of host macrophages by release of TNF-R2, resulting in inactivation of TNF-alpha. *J Immunol* 161:2636–2641.

48. Geleziunas R, Xu W, Takeda K, Ichijo H, Greene WC. 2001. HIV-1 Nef inhibits ASK1-dependent death signalling providing a potential mechanism for protecting the infected host cell. *Nature* 410:834–838.

49. Mehto S, Antony C, Khan N, Arya R, Selvakumar A, Tiwari BK, Vashishta M, Singh Y, Jameel S, Natarajan K. 2015. *Mycobacterium tuberculosis* and human immunodeficiency virus type 1 cooperatively modulate macrophage apoptosis via toll like receptor 2 and calcium homeostasis. *PLoS One* 10:e0131767.

50. Brigino E, Haraguchi S, Koutsonikolis A, Cianciolo GJ, Owens U, Good RA, Day NK. 1997. Interleukin 10 is induced by recombinant HIV-1 Nef protein involving the calcium/calmodulin-dependent phosphodiesterase signal transduction pathway. *Proc Natl Acad Sci USA* 94:3178–3182.

51. Bennasser Y, Bahraoui E. 2002. HIV-1 Tat protein induces interleukin-10 in human peripheral blood monocytes: involvement of protein kinase C-betaII and -delta. *FASEB J* 16:546–554.

52. Patel NR, Swan K, Li X, Tachado SD, Koziel H. 2009. Impaired *M. tuberculosis*-mediated apoptosis in alveolar macrophages from HIV+ persons: potential role of IL-10 and BCL-3. *J Leukoc Biol* 86:53–60.

53. Anandaiah A, Sinha S, Bole M, Sharma SK, Kumar N, Luthra K, Li X, Zhou X, Nelson B, Han X, Tachado SD, Patel NR, Koziel H. 2013. Vitamin D rescues impaired *Mycobacterium tuberculosis*-mediated tumor necrosis factor release in macrophages of HIV-seropositive individuals through an enhanced Toll-like receptor signaling pathway *in vitro*. *Infect Immun* 81:2–10.

54. Campbell GR, Spector SA. 2012. Vitamin D inhibits human immunodeficiency virus type 1 and *Mycobacterium tuberculosis* infection in macrophages through the induction of autophagy. *PLoS Pathog* 8:e1002689.

55. Campbell GR, Spector SA. 2012. Toll-like receptor 8 ligands activate a vitamin D mediated autophagic response that inhibits human immunodeficiency virus type 1. *PLoS Pathog* 8:e1003017.

56. Eklund D, Persson HL, Larsson M, Welin A, Idh J, Paues J, Fransson SG, Stendahl O, Schön T, Lerm M. 2013. Vitamin D enhances IL-1β secretion and restricts growth of *Mycobacterium tuberculosis* in macrophages from TB patients. *Int J Mycobacteriol* 2:18–25.

57. Martineau AR, Wilkinson KA, Newton SM, Floto RA, Norman AW, Skolimowska K, Davidson RN, Sørensen OE, Kampmann B, Griffiths CJ, Wilkinson RJ. 2007. IFN-gamma- and TNF-independent vitamin D-inducible human suppression of mycobacteria: the role of cathelicidin LL-37. *J Immunol* 178:7190–7198.

58. Tachado SD, Zhang J, Zhu J, Patel N, Koziel H. 2005. HIV impairs TNF-alpha release in response to Toll-like receptor 4 stimulation in human macrophages *in vitro*. *Am J Respir Cell Mol Biol* 33:610–621.

59. Song CH, Lee JS, Lee SH, Lim K, Kim HJ, Park JK, Paik TH, Jo EK. 2003. Role of mitogen-activated protein kinase pathways in the production of tumor necrosis factor-alpha, interleukin-10, and monocyte chemotactic protein-1 by *Mycobacterium tuberculosis* H37Rv-infected human monocytes. *J Clin Immunol* 23:194–201.

60. Tomlinson GS, Bell LC, Walker NF, Tsang J, Brown JS, Breen R, Lipman M, Katz DR, Miller RF, Chain BM, Elkington PT, Noursadeghi M. 2014. HIV-1 infection of macrophages dysregulates innate immune responses to *Mycobacterium tuberculosis* by inhibition of interleukin-10. *J Infect Dis* 209:1055–1065.

61. Chetty S, Porichis F, Govender P, Zupkosky J, Ghebremichael M, Pillay M, Walker BD, Ndung'u T, Kaufmann DE, Kasprowicz VO. 2014. Tuberculosis distorts the inhibitory impact of interleukin-10 in HIV infection. *AIDS* 28:2671–2676.

62. Ramaseri Sunder S, Hanumanth SR, Nagaraju RT, Venkata SKN, Suryadevara NC, Pydi SS, Gaddam S, Jonnalagada S, Valluri VL. 2012. IL-10 high producing genotype predisposes HIV infected individuals to TB infection. *Hum Immunol* 73:605–611.

63. Maddocks S, Scandurra GM, Nourse C, Bye C, Williams RB, Slobedman B, Cunningham AL, Britton WJ. 2009. Gene expression in HIV-1/*Mycobacterium tuberculosis* co-infected macrophages is dominated by *M. tuberculosis*. *Tuberculosis (Edinb)* 89:285–293.

64. Tsang J, Chain BM, Miller RF, Webb BL, Barclay W, Towers GJ, Katz DR, Noursadeghi M. 2009. HIV-1 infection of macrophages is dependent on evasion of innate immune cellular activation. *AIDS* 23:2255–2263.

65. Ranjbar S, Boshoff HI, Mulder A, Siddiqi N, Rubin EJ, Goldfeld AE. 2009. HIV-1 replication is differentially regulated by distinct clinical strains of *Mycobacterium tuberculosis*. *PLoS One* 4:e6116.

66. Toossi Z, Wu M, Liu S, Hirsch CS, Walrath J, van Ham M, Silver RF. 2014. Role of protease inhibitor 9 in survival and replication of *Mycobacterium tuberculosis* in mononuclear phagocytes from HIV-1-infected patients. *AIDS* 28:679–687.

67. Pathak S, Wentzel-Larsen T, Asjö B. 2010. Effects of *in vitro* HIV-1 infection on mycobacterial growth in peripheral blood monocyte-derived macrophages. *Infect Immun* 78:4022–4032.

68. Meylan PR, Munis JR, Richman DD, Kornbluth RS. 1992. Concurrent human immunodeficiency virus and mycobacterial infection of macrophages *in vitro* does not reveal any reciprocal effect. *J Infect Dis* 165:80–86.

69. Ryndak MB, Singh KK, Peng Z, Zolla-Pazner S, Li H, Meng L, Laal S. 2014. Transcriptional profiling of *Mycobacterium tuberculosis* replicating *ex vivo* in blood from HIV- and HIV+ subjects. *PLoS One* 9:e94939.

70. Hoshino Y, Tse DB, Rochford G, Prabhakar S, Hoshino S, Chitkara N, Kuwabara K, Ching E, Raju B, Gold JA, Borkowsky W, Rom WN, Pine R, Weiden M. 2004. *Mycobacterium tuberculosis*-induced CXCR4 and chemokine expression leads to preferential X4 HIV-1 replication in human macrophages. *J Immunol* 172:6251–6258.

71. Deng H, Liu R, Ellmeier W, Choe S, Unutmaz D, Burkhart M, Di Marzio P, Marmon S, Sutton RE, Hill CM, Davis CB, Peiper SC, Schall TJ, Littman DR, Landau NR. 1996. Identification of a major co-receptor for primary isolates of HIV-1. *Nature* 381:661–666.

72. Dragic T, Litwin V, Allaway GP, Martin SR, Huang Y, Nagashima KA, Cayanan C, Maddon PJ, Koup RA, Moore JP, Paxton WA. 1996. HIV-1 entry into CD4+ cells is mediated by the chemokine receptor CC-CKR-5. *Nature* 381:667–673.

73. Collins KR, Quiñones-Mateu ME, Wu M, Luzze H, Johnson JL, Hirsch C, Toossi Z, Arts EJ. 2002. Human immunodeficiency virus type 1 (HIV-1) quasispecies at the sites of *Mycobacterium tuberculosis* infection contribute to systemic HIV-1 heterogeneity. *J Virol* 76:1697–1706.

74. Toossi Z, Johnson JL, Kanost RA, Wu M, Luzze H, Peters P, Okwera A, Joloba M, Mugyenyi P, Mugerwa RD, Aung H, Ellner JJ, Hirsch CS. 2001. Increased replication of HIV-1 at sites of *Mycobacterium tuberculosis* infection: potential mechanisms of viral activation. *J Acquir Immune Defic Syndr* 28:1–8.

75. Mayanja-Kizza H, Wajja A, Wu M, Peters P, Nalugwa G, Mubiru F, Aung H, Vanham G, Hirsch C, Whalen C, Ellner J, Toossi Z. 2001. Activation of beta-chemokines and CCR5 in persons infected with human immunodeficiency virus type 1 and tuberculosis. *J Infect Dis* 183:1801–1804.

76. Juffermans NP, Paxton WA, Dekkers PE, Verbon A, de Jonge E, Speelman P, van Deventer SJ, van der Poll T. 2000. Up-regulation of HIV coreceptors CXCR4 and CCR5 on CD4(+) T cells during human endotoxemia and after stimulation with (myco)bacterial antigens: the role of cytokines. *Blood* 96:2649–2654.

77. Rosas-Taraco AG, Arce-Mendoza AY, Caballero-Olín G, Salinas-Carmona MC. 2006. *Mycobacterium tuberculosis* upregulates coreceptors CCR5 and CXCR4 while HIV modulates CD14 favoring concurrent infection. *AIDS Res Hum Retroviruses* 22:45–51.

78. Wolday D, Tegbaru B, Kassu A, Messele T, Coutinho R, van Baarle D, Miedema F. 2005. Expression of chemokine receptors CCR5 and CXCR4 on CD4+ T cells and plasma chemokine levels during treatment of active tuberculosis in HIV-1-coinfected patients. *J Acquir Immune Defic Syndr* 39:265–271.

79. Imperiali FG, Zaninoni A, La Maestra L, Tarsia P, Blasi F, Barcellini W. 2001. Increased *Mycobacterium tuberculosis* growth in HIV-1-infected human macrophages: role of tumour necrosis factor-alpha. *Clin Exp Immunol* 123:435–442.

80. Lederman MM, Georges DL, Kusner DJ, Mudido P, Giam CZ, Toossi Z. 1994. *Mycobacterium tuberculosis* and its purified protein derivative activate expression of the human immunodeficiency virus. *J Acquir Immune Defic Syndr* 7:727–733.

81. Mancino G, Placido R, Bach S, Mariani F, Montesano C, Ercoli L, Zembala M, Colizzi V. 1997. Infection of human monocytes with *Mycobacterium tuberculosis* enhances human immunodeficiency virus type 1 replication and transmission to T cells. *J Infect Dis* 175:1531–1535.

82. Berry MP, Graham CM, McNab FW, Xu Z, Bloch SA, Oni T, Wilkinson KA, Banchereau R, Skinner J, Wilkinson RJ, Quinn C, Blankenship D, Dhawan R, Cush JJ, Mejias A, Ramilo O, Kon OM, Pascual V, Banchereau J, Chaussabel D, O'Garra A. 2010. An interferon-inducible neutrophil-driven blood transcriptional signature in human tuberculosis. *Nature* 466:973–977.

83. Kerkhoff AD, Wood R, Lowe DM, Vogt M, Lawn SD. 2013. Blood neutrophil counts in HIV-infected patients with pulmonary tuberculosis: association with sputum mycobacterial load. *PLoS One* 8:e67956.

84. Lowe DM, Bandara AK, Packe GE, Barker RD, Wilkinson RJ, Griffiths CJ, Martineau AR. 2013. Neutrophilia independently predicts death in tuberculosis. *Eur Respir J* 42:1752–1757.

85. Martineau AR, Newton SM, Wilkinson KA, Kampmann B, Hall BM, Nawroly N, Packe GE, Davidson RN, Griffiths CJ, Wilkinson RJ. 2007. Neutrophil-mediated innate immune resistance to mycobacteria. *J Clin Invest* 117:1988–1994.

86. Crump JA, Ramadhani HO, Morrissey AB, Saganda W, Mwako MS, Yang LY, Chow SC, Njau BN, Mushi GS, Maro VP, Reller LB, Bartlett JA. 2012. Bacteremic

disseminated tuberculosis in sub-Saharan Africa: a prospective cohort study. *Clin Infect Dis* **55**:242–250.

87. Bouza E, Díaz-López MD, Moreno S, Bernaldo de Quirós JC, Vicente T, Berenguer J. 1993. *Mycobacterium tuberculosis* bacteremia in patients with and without human immunodeficiency virus infection. *Arch Intern Med* **153**:496–500.

88. Lowe DM, Bangani N, Goliath R, Kampmann B, Wilkinson KA, Wilkinson RJ, Martineau AR. 2015. Effect of antiretroviral therapy on HIV-mediated impairment of the neutrophil antimycobacterial response. *Ann Am Thorac Soc* **12**:1627–1637.

89. Baldelli F, Preziosi R, Francisci D, Tascini C, Bistoni F, Nicoletti I. 2000. Programmed granulocyte neutrophil death in patients at different stages of HIV infection. *AIDS* **14**:1067–1069.

90. Pitrak DL, Tsai HC, Mullane KM, Sutton SH, Stevens P. 1996. Accelerated neutrophil apoptosis in the acquired immunodeficiency syndrome. *J Clin Invest* **98**:2714–2719.

91. Mastroianni CM, Mengoni F, Lichtner M, D'Agostino C, d'Ettorre G, Forcina G, Marzi M, Russo G, Massetti AP, Vullo V. 2000. *Ex vivo* and *in vitro* effect of human immunodeficiency virus protease inhibitors on neutrophil apoptosis. *J Infect Dis* **182**:1536–1539.

92. Perskvist N, Long M, Stendahl O, Zheng L. 2002. *Mycobacterium tuberculosis* promotes apoptosis in human neutrophils by activating caspase-3 and altering expression of Bax/Bcl-xL via an oxygen-dependent pathway. *J Immunol* **168**:6358–6365.

93. Alemán M, García A, Saab MA, De La Barrera SS, Finiasz M, Abbate E, Sasiain MC. 2002. *Mycobacterium tuberculosis*-induced activation accelerates apoptosis in peripheral blood neutrophils from patients with active tuberculosis. *Am J Respir Cell Mol Biol* **27**:583–592.

94. Persson A, Blomgran-Julinder R, Eklund D, Lundström C, Stendahl O. 2009. Induction of apoptosis in human neutrophils by *Mycobacterium tuberculosis* is dependent on mature bacterial lipoproteins. *Microb Pathog* **47**:143–150.

95. Alemán M, de la Barrera S, Schierloh P, Yokobori N, Baldini M, Musella R, Abbate E, Sasiain M. 2007. Spontaneous or *Mycobacterium tuberculosis*-induced apoptotic neutrophils exert opposite effects on the dendritic cell-mediated immune response. *Eur J Immunol* **37**:1524–1537.

96. Hedlund S, Persson A, Vujic A, Che KF, Stendahl O, Larsson M. 2010. Dendritic cell activation by sensing *Mycobacterium tuberculosis*-induced apoptotic neutrophils via DC-SIGN. *Hum Immunol* **71**:535–540.

97. Heath WR, Carbone FR. 2001. Cross-presentation, dendritic cells, tolerance and immunity. *Annu Rev Immunol* **19**:47–64.

98. Jonuleit H, Schmitt E, Schuler G, Knop J, Enk AH. 2000. Induction of interleukin 10-producing, nonproliferating CD4(+) T cells with regulatory properties by repetitive stimulation with allogeneic immature human dendritic cells. *J Exp Med* **192**:1213–1222.

99. Pacanowski J, Kahi S, Baillet M, Lebon P, Deveau C, Goujard C, Meyer L, Oksenhendler E, Sinet M,

Hosmalin A. 2001. Reduced blood CD123+ (lymphoid) and CD11c+ (myeloid) dendritic cell numbers in primary HIV-1 infection. *Blood* **98**:3016–3021.

100. Chehimi J, Campbell DE, Azzoni L, Bacheller D, Papasavvas E, Jerandi G, Mounzer K, Kostman J, Trinchieri G, Montaner LJ. 2002. Persistent decreases in blood plasmacytoid dendritic cell number and function despite effective highly active antiretroviral therapy and increased blood myeloid dendritic cells in HIV-infected individuals. *J Immunol* **168**:4796–4801.

101. Smed-Sörensen A, Loré K, Vasudevan J, Louder MK, Andersson J, Mascola JR, Spetz AL, Koup RA. 2005. Differential susceptibility to human immunodeficiency virus type 1 infection of myeloid and plasmacytoid dendritic cells. *J Virol* **79**:8861–8869.

102. Turville SG, Santos JJ, Frank I, Cameron PU, Wilkinson J, Miranda-Saksena M, Dable J, Stössel H, Romani N, Piatak M Jr, Lifson JD, Pope M, Cunningham AL. 2004. Immunodeficiency virus uptake, turnover, and 2-phase transfer in human dendritic cells. *Blood* **103**:2170–2179.

103. Izquierdo-Useros N, Naranjo-Gómez M, Erkizia I, Puertas MC, Borràs FE, Blanco J, Martinez-Picado J. 2010. HIV and mature dendritic cells: Trojan exosomes riding the Trojan horse? *PLoS Pathog* **6**:e1000740.

104. Nobile C, Petit C, Moris A, Skrabal K, Abastado JP, Mammano F, Schwartz O. 2005. Covert human immunodeficiency virus replication in dendritic cells and in DC-SIGN-expressing cells promotes long-term transmission to lymphocytes. *J Virol* **79**:5386–5399.

105. Geijtenbeek TB, Kwon DS, Torensma R, van Vliet SJ, van Duijnhoven GC, Middel J, Cornelissen IL, Nottet HS, KewalRamani VN, Littman DR, Figdor CG, van Kooyk Y. 2000. DC-SIGN, a dendritic cell-specific HIV-1-binding protein that enhances trans-infection of T cells. *Cell* **100**:587–597.

106. Gurney KB, Elliott J, Nassanian H, Song C, Soilleux E, McGowan I, Anton PA, Lee B. 2005. Binding and transfer of human immunodeficiency virus by DC-SIGN+ cells in human rectal mucosa. *J Virol* **79**:5762–5773.

107. Wu L, Bashirova AA, Martin TD, Villamide L, Mehlhop E, Chertov AO, Unutmaz D, Pope M, Carrington M, KewalRamani VN. 2002. Rhesus macaque dendritic cells efficiently transmit primate lentiviruses independently of DC-SIGN. *Proc Natl Acad Sci USA* **99**:1568–1573.

108. Gummuluru S, Rogel M, Stamatatos L, Emerman M. 2003. Binding of human immunodeficiency virus type 1 to immature dendritic cells can occur independently of DC-SIGN and mannose binding C-type lectin receptors via a cholesterol-dependent pathway. *J Virol* **77**:12865–12874.

109. Pustylnikov S, Dave RS, Khan ZK, Porkolab V, Rashad AA, Hutchinson M, Fieschi F, Chaiken I, Jain P. 2016. Short communication: inhibition of DC-SIGN-mediated HIV-1 infection by complementary actions of dendritic cell receptor antagonists and env-targeting virus inactivators. *AIDS Res Hum Retroviruses* **32**:93–100.

110. Geijtenbeek TB, Van Vliet SJ, Koppel EA, Sanchez-Hernandez M, Vandenbroucke-Grauls CM, Appelmelk

B, Van Kooyk Y. 2003. Mycobacteria target DC-SIGN to suppress dendritic cell function. *J Exp Med* 197: 7–17.

111. Nigou J, Zelle-Rieser C, Gilleron M, Thurnher M, Puzo G. 2001. Mannosylated lipoarabinomannans inhibit IL-12 production by human dendritic cells: evidence for a negative signal delivered through the mannose receptor. *J Immunol* 166:7477–7485.

112. Driessen NN, Ummels R, Maaskant JJ, Gurcha SS, Besra GS, Ainge GD, Larsen DS, Painter GF, Vandenbroucke-Grauls CM, Geurtsen J, Appelmelk BJ. 2009. Role of phosphatidylinositol mannosides in the interaction between mycobacteria and DC-SIGN. *Infect Immun* 77: 4538–4547.

113. Schaefer M, Reiling N, Fessler C, Stephani J, Taniuchi I, Hatam F, Yildirim AO, Fehrenbach H, Walter K, Ruland J, Wagner H, Ehlers S, Sparwasser T. 2008. Decreased pathology and prolonged survival of human DC-SIGN transgenic mice during mycobacterial infection. *J Immunol* 180:6836–6845.

114. Ehlers S. 2010. DC-SIGN and mannosylated surface structures of *Mycobacterium tuberculosis*: a deceptive liaison. *Eur J Cell Biol* 89:95–101.

115. Vivier E, Tomasello E, Baratin M, Walzer T, Ugolini S. 2008. Functions of natural killer cells. *Nat Immunol* 9: 503–510.

116. De Maria A, Fogli M, Costa P, Murdaca G, Puppo F, Mavilio D, Moretta A, Moretta L. 2003. The impaired NK cell cytolytic function in viremic HIV-1 infection is associated with a reduced surface expression of natural cytotoxicity receptors (NKp46, NKp30 and NKp44). *Eur J Immunol* 33:2410–2418.

117. Fogli M, Costa P, Murdaca G, Setti M, Mingari MC, Moretta L, Moretta A, De Maria A. 2004. Significant NK cell activation associated with decreased cytolytic function in peripheral blood of HIV-1-infected patients. *Eur J Immunol* 34:2313–2321.

118. Lopez-Vergès S, Milush JM, Pandey S, York VA, Arakawa-Hoyt J, Pircher H, Norris PJ, Nixon DF, Lanier LL. 2010. CD57 defines a functionally distinct population of mature NK cells in the human CD56dimCD16+ NK-cell subset. *Blood* 116:3865–3874.

119. Milush JM, López-Vergès S, York VA, Deeks SG, Martin JN, Hecht FM, Lanier LL, Nixon DF. 2013. CD56negCD16+ NK cells are activated mature NK cells with impaired effector function during HIV-1 infection. *Retrovirology* 10:158.

120. Bhat R, Watzl C. 2007. Serial killing of tumor cells by human natural killer cells: enhancement by therapeutic antibodies. *PLoS One* 2:e326.

121. Zocchi MR, Rubartelli A, Morgavi P, Poggi A. 1998. HIV-1 Tat inhibits human natural killer cell function by blocking L-type calcium channels. *J Immunol* 161: 2938–2943.

122. Poggi A, Carosio R, Spaggiari GM, Fortis C, Tambussi G, Dell'Antonio G, Dal Cin E, Rubartelli A, Zocchi MR. 2002. NK cell activation by dendritic cells is dependent on LFA-1-mediated induction of calcium-calmodulin kinase II: inhibition by HIV-1 Tat C-terminal domain. *J Immunol* 168:95–101.

123. Poggi A, Zocchi MR. 2006. HIV-1 Tat triggers TGF-beta production and NK cell apoptosis that is prevented by pertussis toxin B. *Clin Dev Immunol* 13:369–372.

124. Kottilil S, Shin K, Jackson JO, Reitano KN, O'Shea MA, Yang J, Hallahan CW, Lempicki R, Arthos J, Fauci AS. 2006. Innate immune dysfunction in HIV infection: effect of HIV envelope-NK cell interactions. *J Immunol* 176:1107–1114.

125. Hogg A, Huante M, Ongaya A, Williams J, Ferguson M, Cloyd M, Amukoye E, Endsley J. 2011. Activation of NK cell granulysin by mycobacteria and IL-15 is differentially affected by HIV. *Tuberculosis (Edinb)* 91(Suppl 1):S75–S81.

126. Vankayalapati R, Klucar P, Wizel B, Weis SE, Samten B, Safi H, Shams H, Barnes PF. 2004. NK cells regulate CD8+ T cell effector function in response to an intracellular pathogen. *J Immunol* 172:130–137.

127. Denis M. 1994. Interleukin-12 (IL-12) augments cytolytic activity of natural killer cells toward *Mycobacterium tuberculosis*-infected human monocytes. *Cell Immunol* 156:529–536.

128. Brill KJ, Li Q, Larkin R, Canaday DH, Kaplan DR, Boom WH, Silver RF. 2001. Human natural killer cells mediate killing of intracellular *Mycobacterium tuberculosis* H37Rv via granule-independent mechanisms. *Infect Immun* 69:1755–1765.

129. Yoneda T, Ellner JJ. 1998. CD4(+) T cell and natural killer cell-dependent killing of *Mycobacterium tuberculosis* by human monocytes. *Am J Respir Crit Care Med* 158:395–403.

130. Junqueira-Kipnis AP, Kipnis A, Jamieson A, Juarrero MG, Diefenbach A, Raulet DH, Turner J, Orme IM. 2003. NK cells respond to pulmonary infection with *Mycobacterium tuberculosis*, but play a minimal role in protection. *J Immunol* 171:6039–6045.

131. Feng CG, Kaviratne M, Rothfuchs AG, Cheever A, Hieny S, Young HA, Wynn TA, Sher A. 2006. NK cell-derived IFN-gamma differentially regulates innate resistance and neutrophil response in T cell-deficient hosts infected with *Mycobacterium tuberculosis*. *J Immunol* 177:7086–7093.

132. Venketaraman V, Millman A, Salman M, Swaminathan S, Goetz M, Lardizabal A, David Hom, Connell ND. 2008. Glutathione levels and immune responses in tuberculosis patients. *Microb Pathog* 44:255–261.

133. Morris D, Guerra C, Donohue C, Oh H, Khurasany M, Venketaraman V. 2012. Unveiling the mechanisms for decreased glutathione in individuals with HIV infection. *Clin Dev Immunol* 2012:734125.

134. Morris D, Guerra C, Khurasany M, Guilford F, Saviola B, Huang Y, Venketaraman V. 2013. Glutathione supplementation improves macrophage functions in HIV. *J Interferon Cytokine Res* 33:270–279.

135. Dayaram YK, Talaue MT, Connell ND, Venketaraman V. 2006. Characterization of a glutathione metabolic mutant of *Mycobacterium tuberculosis* and its resistance to glutathione and nitrosoglutathione. *J Bacteriol* 188:1364–1372.

136. Spallholz JE. 1987. Glutathione: is it an evolutionary vestige of the penicillins? *Med Hypotheses* 23:253–257.

137. Guerra C, Johal K, Morris D, Moreno S, Alvarado O, Gray D, Tanzil M, Pearce D, Venketaraman V. 2012. Control of *Mycobacterium tuberculosis* growth by activated natural killer cells. *Clin Exp Immunol* 168:142–152.

138. Palanisamy GS, Kirk NM, Ackart DF, Shanley CA, Orme IM, Basaraba RJ. 2011. Evidence for oxidative stress and defective antioxidant response in guinea pigs with tuberculosis. *PLoS One* 6:e26254.

139. Zhang Y, Nakata K, Weiden M, Rom WN. 1995. *Mycobacterium tuberculosis* enhances human immunodeficiency virus-1 replication by transcriptional activation at the long terminal repeat. *J Clin Invest* 95:2324–2331.

140. Honda Y, Rogers L, Nakata K, Zhao BY, Pine R, Nakai Y, Kurosu K, Rom WN, Weiden M. 1998. Type I interferon induces inhibitory 16-kD CCAAT/ enhancer binding protein (C/EBP)beta, repressing the HIV-1 long terminal repeat in macrophages: pulmonary tuberculosis alters C/EBP expression, enhancing HIV-1 replication. *J Exp Med* 188:1255–1265.

141. Wu Y. 2004. HIV-1 gene expression: lessons from provirus and non-integrated DNA. *Retrovirology* 1:13

142. Tesmer VM, Rajadhyaksha A, Babin J, Bina M. 1993. NF-IL6-mediated transcriptional activation of the long terminal repeat of the human immunodeficiency virus type 1. *Proc Natl Acad Sci USA* 90:7298–7302.

143. Ossipow V, Descombes P, Schibler U. 1993. CCAAT/ enhancer-binding protein mRNA is translated into multiple proteins with different transcription activation potentials. *Proc Natl Acad Sci USA* 90:8219–8223.

144. Hoshino Y, Nakata K, Hoshino S, Honda Y, Tse DB, Shioda T, Rom WN, Weiden M. 2002. Maximal HIV-1 replication in alveolar macrophages during tuberculosis requires both lymphocyte contact and cytokines. *J Exp Med* 195:495–505.

145. Hoshino Y, Hoshino S, Gold JA, Raju B, Prabhakar S, Pine R, Rom WN, Nakata K, Weiden M. 2007. Mechanisms of polymorphonuclear neutrophil-mediated induction of HIV-1 replication in macrophages during pulmonary tuberculosis. *J Infect Dis* 195:1303–1310.

146. Lawn SD, Pisell TL, Hirsch CS, Wu M, Butera ST, Toossi Z. 2001. Anatomically compartmentalized human immunodeficiency virus replication in HLA-DR+ cells and CD14+ macrophages at the site of pleural tuberculosis coinfection. *J Infect Dis* 184:1127–1133.

147. Toossi Z, Wu M, Hirsch CS, Mayanja-Kizza H, Baseke J, Aung H, Canaday DH, Fujinaga K. 2012. Activation of P-TEFb at sites of dual HIV/TB infection, and inhibition of *MTB*-induced HIV transcriptional activation by the inhibitor of CDK9, Indirubin-3′-monoxime. *AIDS Res Hum Retroviruses* 28:182–187.

148. Rodriguez ME, Loyd CM, Ding X, Karim AF, McDonald DJ, Canaday DH, Rojas RE. 2013. Mycobacterial phosphatidylinositol mannoside 6 (PIM6) up-regulates TCR-triggered HIV-1 replication in CD4+ T cells. *PLoS One* 8:e80938.

149. Bhat KH, Chaitanya CK, Parveen N, Varman R, Ghosh S, Mukhopadhyay S. 2012. Proline-proline-glutamic acid (PPE) protein Rv1168c of *Mycobacterium tubercu-*

150. *losis* augments transcription from HIV-1 long terminal repeat promoter. *J Biol Chem* 287:16930–16946.

150. Falvo JV, Ranjbar S, Jasenosky LD, Goldfeld AE. 2011. Arc of a vicious circle: pathways activated by *Mycobacterium tuberculosis* that target the HIV-1 long terminal repeat. *Am J Respir Cell Mol Biol* 45:1116–1124.

151. Toor JS, Singh S, Sharma A, Arora SK. 2014. *Mycobacterium tuberculosis* modulates the gene interactions to activate the HIV replication and faster disease progression in a co-infected host. *PLoS One* 9:e106815.

152. Ranjbar S, Jasenosky LD, Chow N, Goldfeld AE. 2012. Regulation of *Mycobacterium tuberculosis*-dependent HIV-1 transcription reveals a new role for NFAT5 in the toll-like receptor pathway. *PLoS Pathog* 8:e1002620.

153. Mamik MK, Ghorpade A. 2014. Chemokine CXCL8 promotes HIV-1 replication in human monocyte-derived macrophages and primary microglia via nuclear factor-κB pathway. *PLoS One* 9:e92145.

154. Robichaud GA, Barbeau B, Fortin JF, Rothstein DM, Tremblay MJ. 2002. Nuclear factor of activated T cells is a driving force for preferential productive HIV-1 infection of CD45RO-expressing CD4+ T cells. *J Biol Chem* 277:23733–23741.

155. Costello R, Lipcey C, Algarté M, Cerdan C, Baeuerle PA, Olive D, Imbert J. 1993. Activation of primary human T-lymphocytes through CD2 plus CD28 adhesion molecules induces long-term nuclear expression of NF-kappa B. *Cell Growth Differ* 4:329–339.

156. Deeks SG, Kitchen CM, Liu L, Guo H, Gascon R, Narváez AB, Hunt P, Martin JN, Kahn JO, Levy J, McGrath MS, Hecht FM. 2004. Immune activation set point during early HIV infection predicts subsequent CD4+ T-cell changes independent of viral load. *Blood* 104:942–947.

157. Giorgi JV, Hultin LE, McKeating JA, Johnson TD, Owens B, Jacobson LP, Shih R, Lewis J, Wiley DJ, Phair JP, Wolinsky SM, Detels R. 1999. Shorter survival in advanced human immunodeficiency virus type 1 infection is more closely associated with T lymphocyte activation than with plasma virus burden or virus chemokine coreceptor usage. *J Infect Dis* 179:859–870.

158. Nakata K, Rom WN, Honda Y, Condos R, Kanegasaki S, Cao Y, Weiden M. 1997. *Mycobacterium tuberculosis* enhances human immunodeficiency virus-1 replication in the lung. *Am J Respir Crit Care Med* 155:996–1003.

159. Collins KR, Mayanja-Kizza H, Sullivan BA, Quiñones-Mateu ME, Toossi Z, Arts EJ. 2000. Greater diversity of HIV-1 quasispecies in HIV-infected individuals with active tuberculosis. *J Acquir Immune Defic Syndr* 24:408–417.

160. Biru T, Lennemann T, Stürmer M, Stephan C, Nisius G, Cinatl J, Staszewski S, Gürtler LG. 2010. Human immunodeficiency virus type-1 group M quasispecies evolution: diversity and divergence in patients co-infected with active tuberculosis. *Med Microbiol Immunol (Berl)* 199:323–332.

161. Danaviah S, Sacks JA, Kumar KP, Taylor LM, Fallows DA, Naicker T, Ndung'u T, Govender S, Kaplan G. 2013. Immunohistological characterization of spinal

TB granulomas from HIV-negative and -positive patients. *Tuberculosis (Edinb)* 93:432–441.

162. Danaviah S, de Oliveira T, Gordon M, Govender S, Chelule P, Pillay S, Naicker T, Cassol S, Ndung'u T. 2015. Analysis of dominant HIV quasispecies suggests independent viral evolution within spinal granulomas coinfected with *Mycobacterium tuberculosis* and HIV-1 subtype C. *AIDS Res Hum Retroviruses* 32:262–270.

163. Lawn SD, Butera ST, Shinnick TM. 2002. Tuberculosis unleashed: the impact of human immunodeficiency virus infection on the host granulomatous response to *Mycobacterium tuberculosis*. *Microbes Infect* 4:635–646.

164. Kizza HM, Rodriguez B, Quinones-Mateu M, Mirza M, Aung H, Yen-Lieberman B, Starkey C, Horter L, Peters P, Baseke J, Johnson JL, Toossi Z. 2005. Persistent replication of human immunodeficiency virus type 1 despite treatment of pulmonary tuberculosis in dually infected subjects. *Clin Diagn Lab Immunol* 12:1298–1304.

165. Collins KR, Quiñones-Mateu ME, Toossi Z, Arts EJ. 2002. Impact of tuberculosis on HIV-1 replication, diversity, and disease progression. *AIDS Rev* 4:165–176.

166. Badri M, Ehrlich R, Wood R, Pulerwitz T, Maartens G. 2001. Association between tuberculosis and HIV disease progression in a high tuberculosis prevalence area. *Int J Tuberc Lung Dis* 5:225–232.

167. Whalen C, Horsburgh CR, Hom D, Lahart C, Simberkoff M, Ellner J. 1995. Accelerated course of human immunodeficiency virus infection after tuberculosis. *Am J Respir Crit Care Med* 151:129–135.

168. Toossi Z, Mayanja-Kizza H, Lawn SD, Hirsch CS, Lupo LD, Butera ST. 2007. Dynamic variation in the cellular origin of HIV type 1 during treatment of tuberculosis in dually infected subjects. *AIDS Res Hum Retroviruses* 23:93–100.

169. Sullivan ZA, Wong EB, Ndung'u T, Kasprowicz VO, Bishai WR. 2015. Latent and active tuberculosis infection increase immune activation in individuals co-infected with HIV. *EBioMedicine* 2:334–340.

170. Srivastava S, Ernst JD. 2014. Cell-to-cell transfer of *M. tuberculosis* antigens optimizes CD4 T cell priming. *Cell Host Microbe* 15:741–752.

171. Harding JS, Rayasam A, Schreiber HA, Fabry Z, Sandor M. 2015. *Mycobacterium*-infected dendritic cells disseminate granulomatous inflammation. *Sci Rep* 5:15248.

172. Krishnan N, Robertson BD, Thwaites G. 2010. The mechanisms and consequences of the extra-pulmonary dissemination of *Mycobacterium tuberculosis*. *Tuberculosis (Edinb)* 90:361–366.

173. Volkman HE, Pozos TC, Zheng J, Davis JM, Rawls JF, Ramakrishnan L. 2010. Tuberculous granuloma induction via interaction of a bacterial secreted protein with host epithelium. *Science* 327:466–469.

174. Datta M, Via LE, Kamoun WS, Liu C, Chen W, Seano G, Weiner DM, Schimel D, England K, Martin JD, Gao X, Xu L, Barry CE III, Jain RK. 2015. Anti-vascular endothelial growth factor treatment normalizes tuberculosis granuloma vasculature and improves small molecule delivery. *Proc Natl Acad Sci USA* 112:1827–1832.

175. Oehlers SH, Cronan MR, Scott NR, Thomas MI, Okuda KS, Walton EM, Beerman RW, Crosier PS, Tobin DM. 2015. Interception of host angiogenic signalling limits mycobacterial growth. *Nature* 517:612–615.

176. Isaakidis P, Casas EC, Das M, Tseretopoulou X, Ntzani EE, Ford N. 2015. Treatment outcomes for HIV and MDR-TB co-infected adults and children: systematic review and meta-analysis. *Int J Tuberc Lung Dis* 19:969–978.

177. Munier ML, Kelleher AD. 2007. Acutely dysregulated, chronically disabled by the enemy within: t-cell responses to HIV-1 infection. *Immunol Cell Biol* 85:6–15.

178. Clerici M, Stocks NI, Zajac RA, Boswell RN, Lucey DR, Via CS, Shearer GM. 1989. Detection of three distinct patterns of T helper cell dysfunction in asymptomatic, human immunodeficiency virus-seropositive patients. Independence of CD4+ cell numbers and clinical staging. *J Clin Invest* 84:1892–1899.

179. Isgrò A, Leti W, De Santis W, Marziali M, Esposito A, Fimiani C, Luzi G, Pinti M, Cossarizza A, Aiuti F, Mezzaroma I. 2008. Altered clonogenic capability and stromal cell function characterize bone marrow of HIV-infected subjects with low CD4+ T cell counts despite viral suppression during HAART. *Clin Infect Dis* 46:1902–1910.

180. Hellerstein M, Hanley MB, Cesar D, Siler S, Papageorgopoulos C, Wieder E, Schmidt D, Hoh R, Neese R, Macallan D, Deeks S, McCune JM. 1999. Directly measured kinetics of circulating T lymphocytes in normal and HIV-1-infected humans. *Nat Med* 5:83–89.

181. Hellerstein MK, Hoh RA, Hanley MB, Cesar D, Lee D, Neese RA, McCune JM. 2003. Subpopulations of long-lived and short-lived T cells in advanced HIV-1 infection. *J Clin Invest* 112:956–966.

182. Schacker TW, Nguyen PL, Beilman GJ, Wolinsky S, Larson M, Reilly C, Haase AT. 2002. Collagen deposition in HIV-1 infected lymphatic tissues and T cell homeostasis. *J Clin Invest* 110:1133–1139.

183. Schacker TW, Reilly C, Beilman GJ, Taylor J, Skarda D, Krason D, Larson M, Haase AT. 2005. Amount of lymphatic tissue fibrosis in HIV infection predicts magnitude of HAART-associated change in peripheral CD4 cell count. *AIDS* 19:2169–2171.

184. Estes JD, Reilly C, Trubey CM, Fletcher CV, Cory TJ, Piatak M Jr, Russ S, Anderson J, Reimann TG, Star R, Smith A, Tracy RP, Berglund A, Schmidt T, Coalter V, Chertova E, Smedley J, Haase AT, Lifson JD, Schacker TW. 2015. Antifibrotic therapy in simian immunodeficiency virus infection preserves CD4+ T-cell populations and improves immune reconstitution with antiretroviral therapy. *J Infect Dis* 211:–754.

185. Doitsh G, Cavrois M, Lassen KG, Zepeda O, Yang Z, Santiago ML, Hebbeler AM, Greene WC. 2010. Abortive HIV infection mediates CD4 T cell depletion and inflammation in human lymphoid tissue. *Cell* 143:789–801. (Erratum, 156:1112–1113).

186. Monroe KM, Yang Z, Johnson JR, Geng X, Doitsh G, Krogan NJ, Greene WC. 2014. IFI16 DNA sensor is required for death of lymphoid CD4 T cells abortively infected with HIV. *Science* 343:428–432.

187. Kalsdorf B, Scriba TJ, Wood K, Day CL, Dheda K, Dawson R, Hanekom WA, Lange C, Wilkinson RJ. 2009. HIV-1 infection impairs the bronchoalveolar T-cell response to mycobacteria. *Am J Respir Crit Care Med* **180**:1262–1270.

188. Jambo KC, Sepako E, Fullerton DG, Mzinza D, Glennie S, Wright AK, Heyderman RS, Gordon SB. 2011. Bronchoalveolar CD4+ T cell responses to respiratory antigens are impaired in HIV-infected adults. *Thorax* **66**: 375–382.

189. Law KF, Jagirdar J, Weiden MD, Bodkin M, Rom WN. 1996. Tuberculosis in HIV-positive patients: cellular response and immune activation in the lung. *Am J Respir Crit Care Med* **153**:1377–1384.

190. Breen RA, Janossy G, Barry SM, Cropley I, Johnson MA, Lipman MC. 2006. Detection of mycobacterial antigen responses in lung but not blood in HIV-tuberculosis co-infected subjects. *AIDS* **20**:1330–1332.

191. Diedrich CR, Mattila JT, Klein E, Janssen C, Phuah J, Sturgeon TJ, Montelaro RC, Lin PL, Flynn JL. 2010. Reactivation of latent tuberculosis in cynomolgus macaques infected with SIV is associated with early peripheral T cell depletion and not virus load. *PLoS One* **5**:e9611.

192. Mondal K, Mandal R. 2015. Cytopathological and microbiological profile of tuberculous lymphadenitis in HIV-infected patients with special emphasis on its corroboration with CD4+ T-cell counts. *Acta Cytol* **59**: 156–162.

193. Rao JS, Kumari SJ, Kini U. 2015. Correlation of CD4 counts with the FNAC patterns of tubercular lymphadenitis in patients with HIV: a cross sectional pilot study. *Diagn Cytopathol* **43**:16–20.

194. Geldmacher C, Schuetz A, Ngwenyama N, Casazza JP, Sanga E, Saathoff E, Boehme C, Geis S, Maboko L, Singh M, Minja F, Meyerhans A, Koup RA, Hoelscher M. 2008. Early depletion of *Mycobacterium tuberculosis*-specific T helper 1 cell responses after HIV-1 infection. *J Infect Dis* **198**:1590–1598.

195. Yang YF, Tomura M, Iwasaki M, Mukai T, Gao P, Ono S, Zou JP, Shearer GM, Fujiwara H, Hamaoka T. 2001. IL-12 as well as IL-2 upregulates CCR5 expression on T cell receptor-triggered human CD4+ and CD8+ T cells. *J Clin Immunol* **21**:116–125.

196. Casazza JP, Brenchley JM, Hill BJ, Ayana R, Ambrozak D, Roederer M, Douek DC, Betts MR, Koup RA. 2009. Autocrine production of beta-chemokines protects CMV-specific CD4 T cells from HIV infection. *PLoS Pathog* **5**:e1000646.

197. Geldmacher C, Ngwenyama N, Schuetz A, Petrovas C, Reither K, Heeregrave EJ, Casazza JP, Ambrozak DR, Louder M, Ampofo W, Pollakis G, Hill B, Sanga E, Saathoff E, Maboko L, Roederer M, Paxton WA, Hoelscher M, Koup RA. 2010. Preferential infection and depletion of *Mycobacterium tuberculosis*-specific CD4 T cells after HIV-1 infection. *J Exp Med* **207**: 2869–2881.

198. Ramilo O, Bell KD, Uhr JW, Vitetta ES. 1993. Role of CD25+ and CD25-T cells in acute HIV infection in vitro. *J Immunol* **150**:5202–5208.

199. Arlen PA, Brooks DG, Gao LY, Vatakis D, Brown HJ, Zack JA. 2006. Rapid expression of human immunodeficiency virus following activation of latently infected cells. *J Virol* **80**:1599–1603.

200. Goletti D, Weissman D, Jackson RW, Graham NM, Vlahov D, Klein RS, Munsiff SS, Ortona L, Cauda R, Fauci AS. 1996. Effect of *Mycobacterium tuberculosis* on HIV replication. Role of immune activation. *J Immunol* **157**:1271–1278.

201. Hammond AS, McConkey SJ, Hill PC, Crozier S, Klein MR, Adegbola RA, Rowland-Jones S, Brookes RH, Whittle H, Jaye A. 2008. Mycobacterial T cell responses in HIV-infected patients with advanced immunosuppression. *J Infect Dis* **197**:295–299.

202. Rangaka MX, Diwakar L, Seldon R, van Cutsem G, Meintjes GA, Morroni C, Mouton P, Shey MS, Maartens G, Wilkinson KA, Wilkinson RJ. 2007. Clinical, immunological, and epidemiological importance of antituberculosis T cell responses in HIV-infected Africans. *Clin Infect Dis* **44**:1639–1646.

203. Chaudhry A, Das SR, Hussain A, Mayor S, George A, Bal V, Jameel S, Rath S. 2005. The Nef protein of HIV-1 induces loss of cell surface costimulatory molecules CD80 and CD86 in APCs. *J Immunol* **175**:4566–4574.

204. Chaudhry A, Verghese DA, Das SR, Jameel S, George A, Bal V, Mayor S, Rath S. 2009. HIV-1 Nef promotes endocytosis of cell surface MHC class II molecules via a constitutive pathway. *J Immunol* **183**:2415–2424.

205. Oyaizu N, Chirmule N, Kalyanaraman VS, Hall WW, Pahwa R, Shuster M, Pahwa S. 1990. Human immunodeficiency virus type 1 envelope glycoprotein gp120 produces immune defects in CD4+ T lymphocytes by inhibiting interleukin 2 mRNA. *Proc Natl Acad Sci USA* **87**:2379–2383.

206. Puri RK, Leland P, Aggarwal BB. 1995. Constitutive expression of human immunodeficiency virus type 1 tat gene inhibits interleukin 2 and interleukin 2 receptor expression in a human CD4+ T lymphoid (H9) cell line. *AIDS Res Hum Retroviruses* **11**:31–40.

207. Pollock KM, Montamat-Sicotte DJ, Grass L, Cooke GS, Kapembwa MS, Kon OM, Sampson RD, Taylor GP, Lalvani A. 2016. PD-1 expression and cytokine secretion profiles of *Mycobacterium tuberculosis*-specific CD4+ T-cell subsets: potential correlates of containment in HIV-TB co-infection. *PLoS One* **11**:e0146905.

208. Fife BT, Pauken KE. 2011. The role of the PD-1 pathway in autoimmunity and peripheral tolerance. *Ann N Y Acad Sci* **1217**:45–59.

209. Nakanjako D, Ssewanyana I, Mayanja-Kizza H, Kiragga A, Colebunders R, Manabe YC, Nabatanzi R, Kamya MR, Cao H. 2011. High T-cell immune activation and immune exhaustion among individuals with suboptimal CD4 recovery after 4 years of antiretroviral therapy in an African cohort. *BMC Infect Dis* **11**:43.

210. Grabmeier-Pfistershammer K, Steinberger P, Rieger A, Leitner J, Kohrgruber N. 2011. Identification of PD-1 as a unique marker for failing immune reconstitution in HIV-1-infected patients on treatment. *J Acquir Immune Defic Syndr* **56**:118–124.

211. Robbins GK, Spritzler JG, Chan ES, Asmuth DM, Gandhi RT, Rodriguez BA, Skowron G, Skolnik PR, Shafer RW, Pollard RB, AIDS Clinical Trials Group 384 Team. 2009. Incomplete reconstitution of T cell subsets on combination antiretroviral therapy in the AIDS Clinical Trials Group protocol 384. *Clin Infect Dis* 48:350–361.

212. Riou C, Tanko RF, Soares AP, Masson L, Werner L, Garrett NJ, Samsunder N, Abdool Karim Q, Abdool Karim SS, Burgers WA. 2015. Restoration of CD4+ responses to copathogens in HIV-infected individuals on antiretroviral therapy is dependent on T cell memory phenotype. *J Immunol* 195:2273–2281.

213. Wilkinson KA, Seldon R, Meintjes G, Rangaka MX, Hanekom WA, Maartens G, Wilkinson RJ. 2009. Dissection of regenerating T-cell responses against tuberculosis in HIV-infected adults sensitized by *Mycobacterium tuberculosis*. *Am J Respir Crit Care Med* 180:674–683.

214. Evans TG, Bonnez W, Soucier HR, Fitzgerald T, Gibbons DC, Reichman RC. 1998. Highly active antiretroviral therapy results in a decrease in CD8+ T cell activation and preferential reconstitution of the peripheral CD4+ T cell population with memory rather than naive cells. *Antiviral Res* 39:163–173.

215. Rönsholt FF, Ullum H, Katzenstein TL, Gerstoft J, Ostrowski SR. 2012. T-cell subset distribution in HIV-1-infected patients after 12 years of treatment-induced viremic suppression. *J Acquir Immune Defic Syndr* 61:270–278.

216. Wendland T, Furrer H, Vernazza PL, Frutig K, Christen A, Matter L, Malinverni R, Pichler WJ. 1999. HAART in HIV-infected patients: restoration of antigen-specific CD4 T-cell responses *in vitro* is correlated with CD4 memory T-cell reconstitution, whereas improvement in delayed type hypersensitivity is related to a decrease in viraemia. *AIDS* 13:1857–1862.

217. Li TS, Tubiana R, Katlama C, Calvez V, Ait Mohand H, Autran B. 1998. Long-lasting recovery in CD4 T-cell function and viral-load reduction after highly active antiretroviral therapy in advanced HIV-1 disease. *Lancet* 351:1682–1686.

218. Hsu DC, Kerr SJ, Thongpaeng P, Iamsirnsin T, Pett SL, Zaunders JJ, Avihingsanon A, Ubolyam S, Ananworanich J, Kelleher AD, Cooper DA. 2014. Incomplete restoration of *Mycobacterium tuberculosis*-specific-CD4 T cell responses despite antiretroviral therapy. *J Infect* 68:344–354.

219. Sutherland JS, Young JM, Peterson KL, Sanneh B, Whittle HC, Rowland-Jones SL, Adegbola RA, Jaye A, Ota MO. 2010. Polyfunctional CD4(+) and CD8(+) T cell responses to tuberculosis antigens in HIV-1-infected patients before and after anti-retroviral treatment. *J Immunol* 184:6537–6544.

220. Sutherland R, Yang H, Scriba TJ, Ondondo B, Robinson N, Conlon C, Suttill A, McShane H, Fidler S, McMichael A, Dorrell L. 2006. Impaired IFN-gamma-secreting capacity in mycobacterial antigen-specific CD4 T cells during chronic HIV-1 infection despite long-term HAART. *AIDS* 20:821–829.

221. Mendonça M, Tanji MM, Silva LC, Silveira GG, Oliveira SC, Duarte AJ, Benard G. 2007. Deficient *in vitro* anti-mycobacterial immunity despite successful long-term highly active antiretroviral therapy in HIV-infected patients with past history of tuberculosis infection or disease. *Clin Immunol* 125:60–66.

222. Jambo KC, Banda DH, Afran L, Kankwatira AM, Malamba RD, Allain TJ, Gordon SB, Heyderman RS, Russell DG, Mwandumba HC. 2014. Asymptomatic HIV-infected individuals on antiretroviral therapy exhibit impaired lung CD4(+) T-cell responses to mycobacteria. *Am J Respir Crit Care Med* 190:938–947.

223. Day CL, Mkhwanazi N, Reddy S, Mncube Z, van der Stok M, Klenerman P, Walker BD. 2008. Detection of polyfunctional *Mycobacterium tuberculosis*-specific T cells and association with viral load in HIV-1-infected persons. *J Infect Dis* 197:990–999.

224. Canaday DH, Wilkinson RJ, Li Q, Harding CV, Silver RF, Boom WH. 2001. CD4(+) and CD8(+) T cells kill intracellular *Mycobacterium tuberculosis* by a perforin and Fas/Fas ligand-independent mechanism. *J Immunol* 167:2734–2742.

225. Woodworth JS, Wu Y, Behar SM. 2008. *Mycobacterium tuberculosis*-specific CD8+ T cells require perforin to kill target cells and provide protection *in vivo*. *J Immunol* 181:8595–8603.

226. Gulzar N, Copeland KF. 2004. CD8+ T-cells: function and response to HIV infection. *Curr HIV Res* 2:23–37.

227. Kalokhe AS, Adekambi T, Ibegbu CC, Ray SM, Day CL, Rengarajan J. 2015. Impaired degranulation and proliferative capacity of *Mycobacterium tuberculosis*-specific CD8+ T cells in HIV-infected individuals with latent tuberculosis. *J Infect Dis* 211:635–640.

228. van Pinxteren LA, Cassidy JP, Smedegaard BH, Agger EM, Andersen P. 2000. Control of latent *Mycobacterium tuberculosis* infection is dependent on CD8 T cells. *Eur J Immunol* 30:3689–3698.

229. Mogues T, Goodrich ME, Ryan L, LaCourse R, North RJ. 2001. The relative importance of T cell subsets in immunity and immunopathology of airborne *Mycobacterium tuberculosis* infection in mice. *J Exp Med* 193:271–280.

230. Bruns H, Meinken C, Schauenberg P, Härter G, Kern P, Modlin RL, Antoni C, Stenger S. 2009. Anti-TNF immunotherapy reduces CD8+ T cell-mediated antimicrobial activity against *Mycobacterium tuberculosis* in humans. *J Clin Invest* 119:1167–1177.

231. Chiacchio T, Petruccioli E, Vanini V, Cuzzi G, Pinnetti C, Sampaolesi A, Antinori A, Girardi E, Goletti D. 2014. Polyfunctional T-cells and effector memory phenotype are associated with active TB in HIV-infected patients. *J Infect* 69:533–545.

232. Suarez GV, Angerami MT, Vecchione MB, Laufer N, Turk G, Ruiz MJ, Mesch V, Fabre B, Maidana P, Ameri D, Cahn P, Sued O, Salomón H, Bottasso OA, Quiroga MF. 2015. HIV-TB coinfection impairs CD8(+) T-cell differentiation and function while dehydroepiandrosterone improves cytotoxic antitubercular immune responses. *Eur J Immunol* 45:2529–2541.

233. Wu L, Fu J, Shen SH. 2002. SKAP55 coupled with CD45 positively regulates T-cell receptor-mediated gene transcription. *Mol Cell Biol* 22:2673–2686.

234. Wang Y, Johnson P. 2005. Expression of CD45 lacking the catalytic protein tyrosine phosphatase domain modulates Lck phosphorylation and T cell activation. *J Biol Chem* 280:14318–14324.

235. Barber DL, Wherry EJ, Masopust D, Zhu B, Allison JP, Sharpe AH, Freeman GJ, Ahmed R. 2006. Restoring function in exhausted CD8 T cells during chronic viral infection. *Nature* 439:682–687.

236. Prasad KV, Ao Z, Yoon Y, Wu MX, Rizk M, Jacquot S, Schlossman SF. 1997. CD27, a member of the tumor necrosis factor receptor family, induces apoptosis and binds to Siva, a proapoptotic protein. *Proc Natl Acad Sci USA* 94:6346–6351.

237. Meintjes G, Lawn SD, Scano F, Maartens G, French MA, Worodria W, Elliott JH, Murdoch D, Wilkinson RJ, Seyler C, John L, van der Loeff MS, Reiss P, Lynen L, Janoff EN, Gilks C, Colebunders R, International Network for the Study of HIV-associated IRIS. 2008. Tuberculosis-associated immune reconstitution inflammatory syndrome: case definitions for use in resource-limited settings. *Lancet Infect Dis* 8:516–523.

238. Marais S, Meintjes G, Pepper DJ, Dodd LE, Schutz C, Ismail Z, Wilkinson KA, Wilkinson RJ. 2013. Frequency, severity, and prediction of tuberculous meningitis immune reconstitution inflammatory syndrome. *Clin Infect Dis* 56:450–460.

239. Asselman V, Thienemann F, Pepper DJ, Boulle A, Wilkinson RJ, Meintjes G, Marais S. 2010. Central nervous system disorders after starting antiretroviral therapy in South Africa. *AIDS* 24:2871–2876.

240. Pepper DJ, Marais S, Maartens G, Rebe K, Morroni C, Rangaka MX, Oni T, Wilkinson RJ, Meintjes G. 2009. Neurologic manifestations of paradoxical tuberculosis-associated immune reconstitution inflammatory syndrome: a case series. *Clin Infect Dis* 48:e96–e107.

241. Lawn SD, Myer L, Bekker LG, Wood R. 2007. Tuberculosis-associated immune reconstitution disease: incidence, risk factors and impact in an antiretroviral treatment service in South Africa. *AIDS* 21:335–341.

242. Ratnam I, Chiu C, Kandala NB, Easterbrook PJ. 2006. Incidence and risk factors for immune reconstitution inflammatory syndrome in an ethnically diverse HIV type 1-infected cohort. *Clin Infect Dis* 42:418–427.

243. Namale PE, Abdullahi LH, Fine S, Kamkuemah M, Wilkinson RJ, Meintjes G. 2015. Paradoxical TB-IRIS in HIV-infected adults: a systematic review and meta-analysis. *Future Microbiol* 10:1077–1099.

244. Burman W, Weis S, Vernon A, Khan A, Benator D, Jones B, Silva C, King B, LaHart C, Mangura B, Weiner M, El-Sadr W. 2007. Frequency, severity and duration of immune reconstitution events in HIV-related tuberculosis. *Int J Tuberc Lung Dis* 11:1282–1289.

245. Manosuthi W, Kiertiburanakul S, Phoorisri T, Sungkanuparph S. 2006. Immune reconstitution inflammatory syndrome of tuberculosis among HIV-infected patients receiving antituberculous and antiretroviral therapy. *J Infect* 53:357–363.

246. Naidoo K, Yende-Zuma N, Padayatchi N, Naidoo K, Jithoo N, Nair G, Bamber S, Gengiah S, El-Sadr WM, Friedland G, Abdool Karim S. 2012. The immune reconstitution inflammatory syndrome after antiretroviral therapy initiation in patients with tuberculosis: findings from the SAPiT trial. *Ann Intern Med* 157:313–324.

247. Abay SM, Deribe K, Reda AA, Biadgilign S, Datiko D, Assefa T, Todd M, Deribew A. 2015. The effect of early initiation of antiretroviral therapy in TB/HIV-coinfected patients: a systematic review and meta-analysis. *J Int Assoc Provid AIDS Care* 14:560–570.

248. Lai RP, Meintjes G, Wilkinson KA, Graham CM, Marais S, Van der Plas H, Deffur A, Schutz C, Bloom C, Munagala I, Anguiano E, Goliath R, Maartens G, Banchereau J, Chaussabel D, O'Garra A, Wilkinson RJ. 2015. HIV-tuberculosis-associated immune reconstitution inflammatory syndrome is characterized by Toll-like receptor and inflammasome signalling. *Nat Commun* 6:8451.

249. Andrade BB, Singh A, Narendran G, Schechter ME, Nayak K, Subramanian S, Anbalagan S, Jensen SM, Porter BO, Antonelli LR, Wilkinson KA, Wilkinson RJ, Meintjes G, van der Plas H, Follmann D, Barber DL, Swaminathan S, Sher A, Sereti I. 2014. Mycobacterial antigen driven activation of CD14++CD16- monocytes is a predictor of tuberculosis-associated immune reconstitution inflammatory syndrome. *PLoS Pathog* 10:e1004433.

250. Tan DB, Lim A, Yong YK, Ponnampalavanar S, Omar S, Kamarulzaman A, French MA, Price P. 2011. TLR2-induced cytokine responses may characterize HIV-infected patients experiencing mycobacterial immune restoration disease. *AIDS* 25:1455–1460.

251. Conradie F, Foulkes AS, Ive P, Yin X, Roussos K, Glencross DK, Lawrie D, Stevens W, Montaner LJ, Sanne I, Azzoni L. 2011. Natural killer cell activation distinguishes *Mycobacterium tuberculosis*-mediated immune reconstitution syndrome from chronic HIV and HIV/MTB coinfection. *J Acquir Immune Defic Syndr* 58:309–318.

252. Pean P, Nerrienet E, Madec Y, Borand L, Laureillard D, Fernandez M, Marcy O, Sarin C, Phon K, Taylor S, Pancino G, Barré-Sinoussi F, Scott-Algara D, Cambodian Early versus Late Introduction of Antiretroviral Drugs (CAMELIA) Study Team. 2012. Natural killer cell degranulation capacity predicts early onset of the immune reconstitution inflammatory syndrome (IRIS) in HIV-infected patients with tuberculosis. *Blood* 119:3315–3320.

253. Wilkinson KA, Walker NF, Meintjes G, Deffur A, Nicol MP, Skolimowska KH, Matthews K, Tadokera R, Seldon R, Maartens G, Rangaka MX, Besra GS, Wilkinson RJ. 2015. Cytotoxic mediators in paradoxical HIV-tuberculosis immune reconstitution inflammatory syndrome. *J Immunol* 194:1748–1754.

254. Marais S, Wilkinson KA, Lesosky M, Coussens AK, Deffur A, Pepper DJ, Schutz C, Ismail Z, Meintjes G, Wilkinson RJ. 2014. Neutrophil-associated central nervous system inflammation in tuberculous meningitis immune reconstitution inflammatory syndrome. *Clin Infect Dis* 59:1638–1647.

255. Tadokera R, Meintjes G, Skolimowska KH, Wilkinson KA, Matthews K, Seldon R, Chegou NN, Maartens G, Rangaka MX, Rebe K, Walzl G, Wilkinson RJ. 2011. Hypercytokinaemia accompanies HIV-tuberculosis immune reconstitution inflammatory syndrome. *Eur Respir J* 37:1248–1259.

256. Ravimohan S, Tamuhla N, Steenhoff AP, Letlhogile R, Nfanyana K, Bellamy SL, MacGregor RR, Gross R, Weissman D, Bisson GP. 2015. Immunological profiling of tuberculosis-associated immune reconstitution inflammatory syndrome and non-immune reconstitution inflammatory syndrome death in HIV-infected adults with pulmonary tuberculosis starting antiretroviral therapy: a prospective observational cohort study. *Lancet Infect Dis* 15:429–438.

257. Conesa-Botella A, Meintjes G, Coussens AK, van der Plas H, Goliath R, Schutz C, Moreno-Reyes R, Mehta M, Martineau AR, Wilkinson RJ, Colebunders R, Wilkinson KA. 2012. Corticosteroid therapy, vitamin D status, and inflammatory cytokine profile in the HIV-tuberculosis immune reconstitution inflammatory syndrome. *Clin Infect Dis* 55:1004–1011.

258. Meintjes G, Skolimowska KH, Wilkinson KA, Matthews K, Tadokera R, Conesa-Botella A, Seldon R, Rangaka MX, Rebe K, Pepper DJ, Morroni C, Colebunders R, Maartens G, Wilkinson RJ. 2012. Corticosteroid-modulated immune activation in the tuberculosis immune reconstitution inflammatory syndrome. *Am J Respir Crit Care Med* 186:369–377.

259. Oliver BG, Elliott JH, Price P, Phillips M, Saphonn V, Vun MC, Kaldor JM, Cooper DA, French MA. 2010. Mediators of innate and adaptive immune responses differentially affect immune restoration disease associated with *Mycobacterium tuberculosis* in HIV patients beginning antiretroviral therapy. *J Infect Dis* 202:1728–1737.

260. Oliver BG, Elliott JH, Price P, Phillips M, Cooper DA, French MA. 2012. Tuberculosis after commencing antiretroviral therapy for HIV infection is associated with elevated CXCL9 and CXCL10 responses to *Mycobacterium tuberculosis* antigens. *J Acquir Immune Defic Syndr* 61:287–292.

261. Tan HY, Yong YK, Andrade BB, Shankar EM, Ponnampalavanar S, Omar SF, Narendran G, Kamarulzaman A, Swaminathan S, Sereti I, Crowe SM, French MA. 2015. Plasma interleukin-18 levels are a biomarker of innate immune responses that predict and characterize tuberculosis-associated immune reconstitution inflammatory syndrome. *AIDS* 29:421–431.

262. Lande R, Giacomini E, Grassi T, Remoli ME, Iona E, Miettinen M, Julkunen I, Coccia EM. 2003. IFN-alpha beta released by *Mycobacterium tuberculosis*-infected human dendritic cells induces the expression of CXCL10: selective recruitment of NK and activated T cells. *J Immunol* 170:1174–1182.

263. Moser B, Loetscher P. 2001. Lymphocyte traffic control by chemokines. *Nat Immunol* 2:123–128.

264. Mayer-Barber KD, Andrade BB, Barber DL, Hieny S, Feng CG, Caspar P, Oland S, Gordon S, Sher A. 2011. Innate and adaptive interferons suppress IL-1α and IL-1β production by distinct pulmonary myeloid subsets during *Mycobacterium tuberculosis* infection. *Immunity* 35:1023–1034.

265. McNab FW, Ewbank J, Howes A, Moreira-Teixeira L, Martirosyan A, Ghilardi N, Saraiva M, O'Garra A. 2014. Type I IFN induces IL-10 production in an IL-27-independent manner and blocks responsiveness to IFN-γ for production of IL-12 and bacterial killing in *Mycobacterium tuberculosis*-infected macrophages. *J Immunol* 193:3600–3612.

266. Haridas V, Pean P, Jasenosky LD, Madec Y, Laureillard D, Sok T, Sath S, Borand L, Marcy O, Chan S, Tsitsikov E, Delfraissy JF, Blanc FX, Goldfeld AE, CAPRI-T (ANRS 12164) Study Team. 2015. TB-IRIS, T-cell activation, and remodeling of the T-cell compartment in highly immunosuppressed HIV-infected patients with TB. *AIDS* 29:263–273.

267. Elkington P, Shiomi T, Breen R, Nuttall RK, Ugarte-Gil CA, Walker NF, Saraiva L, Pedersen B, Mauri F, Lipman M, Edwards DR, Robertson BD, D'Armiento J, Friedland JS. 2011. MMP-1 drives immunopathology in human tuberculosis and transgenic mice. *J Clin Invest* 121:1827–1833.

268. Elkington PT, Nuttall RK, Boyle JJ, O'Kane CM, Horncastle DE, Edwards DR, Friedland JS. 2005. *Mycobacterium tuberculosis*, but not vaccine BCG, specifically upregulates matrix metalloproteinase-1. *Am J Respir Crit Care Med* 172:1596–1604.

269. Walker NF, Clark SO, Oni T, Andreu N, Tezera L, Singh S, Saraiva L, Pedersen B, Kelly DL, Tree JA, D'Armiento JM, Meintjes G, Mauri FA, Williams A, Wilkinson RJ, Friedland JS, Elkington PT. 2012. Doxycycline and HIV infection suppress tuberculosis-induced matrix metalloproteinases. *Am J Respir Crit Care Med* 185:989–997.

270. Tadokera R, Meintjes GA, Wilkinson KA, Skolimowska KH, Walker N, Friedland JS, Maartens G, Elkington PT, Wilkinson RJ. 2014. Matrix metalloproteinases and tissue damage in HIV-tuberculosis immune reconstitution inflammatory syndrome. *Eur J Immunol* 44:127–136.

271. Bourgarit A, Carcelain G, Martinez V, Lascoux C, Delcey V, Gicquel B, Vicaut E, Lagrange PH, Sereni D, Autran B. 2006. Explosion of tuberculin-specific Th1-responses induces immune restoration syndrome in tuberculosis and HIV co-infected patients. *AIDS* 20:F1–F7.

272. Meintjes G, Wilkinson KA, Rangaka MX, Skolimowska K, van Veen K, Abrahams M, Seldon R, Pepper DJ, Rebe K, Mouton P, van Cutsem G, Nicol MP, Maartens G, Wilkinson RJ. 2008. Type 1 helper T cells and FoxP3-positive T cells in HIV-tuberculosis-associated immune reconstitution inflammatory syndrome. *Am J Respir Crit Care Med* 178:1083–1089.

273. Tieu HV, Ananworanich J, Avihingsanon A, Apateerapong W, Sirivichayakul S, Siangphoe U, Klongugkara S, Boonchokchai B, Hammer SM, Manosuthi W. 2009. Immunologic markers as predictors of tuberculosis-associated immune reconstitution inflammatory syndrome in HIV and tuberculosis coinfected persons in Thailand. *AIDS Res Hum Retroviruses* 25:1083–1089.

274. Elliott JH, Vohith K, Saramony S, Savuth C, Dara C, Sarim C, Huffam S, Oelrichs R, Sophea P, Saphonn V, Kaldor J, Cooper DA, Chhi Vun M, French MA. 2009. Immunopathogenesis and diagnosis of tuberculosis and tuberculosis-associated immune reconstitution inflammatory syndrome during early antiretroviral therapy. *J Infect Dis* **200**:1736–1745.

275. Antonelli LR, Mahnke Y, Hodge JN, Porter BO, Barber DL, DerSimonian R, Greenwald JH, Roby G, Mican J, Sher A, Roederer M, Sereti I. 2010. Elevated frequencies of highly activated CD4+ T cells in HIV+ patients developing immune reconstitution inflammatory syndrome. *Blood* **116**:3818–3827.

276. Seddiki N, Sasson SC, Santner-Nanan B, Munier M, van Bockel D, Ip S, Marriott D, Pett S, Nanan R, Cooper DA, Zaunders JJ, Kelleher AD. 2009. Proliferation of weakly suppressive regulatory CD4+ T cells is associated with over-active CD4+ T-cell responses in HIV-positive patients with mycobacterial immune restoration disease. *Eur J Immunol* **39**:391–403.

277. Tan DB, Yong YK, Tan HY, Kamarulzaman A, Tan LH, Lim A, James I, French M, Price P. 2008. Immunological profiles of immune restoration disease presenting as mycobacterial lymphadenitis and cryptococcal meningitis. *HIV Med* **9**:307–316.

278. Takahashi Y, Tanaka Y, Yamashita A, Koyanagi Y, Nakamura M, Yamamoto N. 2001. OX40 stimulation by gp34/OX40 ligand enhances productive human immunodeficiency virus type 1 infection. *J Virol* **75**: 6748–6757.

279. Kabelitz D, Wesch D. 2003. Features and functions of gamma delta T lymphocytes: focus on chemokines and their receptors. *Crit Rev Immunol* **23**:339–370.

280. Saunders BM, Frank AA, Cooper AM, Orme IM. 1998. Role of gamma delta T cells in immunopathology of pulmonary *Mycobacterium avium* infection in mice. *Infect Immun* **66**:5508–5514.

281. Dieli F, Troye-Blomberg M, Ivanyi J, Fournié JJ, Bonneville M, Peyrat MA, Sireci G, Salerno A. 2000. Vgamma9/Vdelta2 T lymphocytes reduce the viability of intracellular *Mycobacterium tuberculosis*. *Eur J Immunol* **30**:1512–1519.

282. Gioia C, Agrati C, Casetti R, Cairo C, Borsellino G, Battistini L, Mancino G, Goletti D, Colizzi V, Pucillo LP, Poccia F. 2002. Lack of CD27-CD45RA-V gamma 9V delta 2+ T cell effectors in immunocompromised hosts and during active pulmonary tuberculosis. *J Immunol* **168**:1484–1489.

283. Rojas RE, Chervenak KA, Thomas J, Morrow J, Nshuti L, Zalwango S, Mugerwa RD, Thiel BA, Whalen CC, Boom WH. 2005. Vdelta2+ gammadelta T cell function in *Mycobacterium tuberculosis*- and HIV-1-positive patients in the United States and Uganda: application of a whole-blood assay. *J Infect Dis* **192**:1806–1814.

284. Bourgarit A, Carcelain G, Samri A, Parizot C, Lafaurie M, Abgrall S, Delcey V, Vicaut E, Sereni D, Autran B, PARADOX Study Group. 2009. Tuberculosis-associated immune restoration syndrome in HIV-1-infected patients involves tuberculin-specific CD4 Th1 cells and KIR-negative gammadelta T cells. *J Immunol* **183**:3915–3923.

285. Espinosa E, Ormsby CE, Vega-Barrientos RS, Ruiz-Cruz M, Moreno-Coutiño G, Peña-Jiménez A, Peralta-Prado AB, Cantoral-Díaz M, Romero-Rodríguez DP, Reyes-Terán G. 2010. Risk factors for immune reconstitution inflammatory syndrome under combination antiretroviral therapy can be aetiology-specific. *Int J STD AIDS* **21**:573–579.

286. Deffur A, Mulder NJ, Wilkinson RJ. 2013. Co-infection with *Mycobacterium tuberculosis* and human immunodeficiency virus: an overview and motivation for systems approaches. *Pathog Dis* **69**:101–113.

287. Lai RP, Meintjes G, Wilkinson RJ. 2015. HIV-1 tuberculosis-associated immune reconstitution inflammatory syndrome. *Semin Immunopathol* **38**:185–198.

Drug Discovery and Development: State of the Art and Future Directions

II

Tuberculosis and the Tubercle Bacillus, 2nd ed.
Edited by William R. Jacobs, Jr., Helen McShane, Valerie Mizrahi, and Ian M. Orme
© 2018 American Society for Microbiology, Washington, DC
doi:10.1128/microbiolspec.TBTB2-0034-2017

Preclinical Efficacy Testing of New Drug Candidates

13

Eric L. Nuermberger

INTRODUCTION

Since the early 1950s, combination chemotherapy has remained the strongest line of defense against the ancient scourge of tuberculosis (TB). Between the years 2000 and 2015 alone, it was estimated that TB treatment averted 39 million deaths among people without HIV infection and, together with antiretroviral therapy, another 9.6 million deaths among people with HIV infection (1). Despite these successes, TB continues to exert a terrible toll on humanity. In 2015, TB was estimated to be the cause of 10.4 million new cases and 1.4 million deaths, making *Mycobacterium tuberculosis* the leading microbial cause of death in the world (1). The failure to achieve greater control of TB over the past half century is partly attributable to several important limitations of current chemotherapy regimens, including the prolonged treatment durations necessary to prevent relapse after treatment completion and the inability to effectively suppress resistance emergence when treatment is applied on a global scale. These deficiencies are especially notable for current second-line and salvage regimens used to treat drug-resistant TB (2–4), which are also complicated by excessive toxicity, poor tolerability, high cost, and the inconvenience of injections, multiple daily doses, and large pill burdens. As a result, shortening or otherwise simplifying regimens to treat TB without sacrificing efficacy is a major goal of TB drug development research (5).

Successful treatment of active TB requires the use of drug combinations to efficiently eradicate the diverse population of bacteria present in the infected host, including actively replicating bacilli, smaller subpopulations of persistent bacilli that are phenotypically tolerant to the bactericidal action of drugs, as well as small subpopulations of spontaneous drug-resistant mutants (6–9). Shortening the duration of TB treatment requires more rapid elimination of drug-tolerant persisters, while preventing the development of drug resistance requires more effective killing of spontaneous drug-resistant mutants by the remaining drugs in the regimen to which the mutants remain susceptible. Although promising results from recent phase 2 trials suggest that optimizing the dosing of existing rifamycin drugs may significantly shorten the duration of therapy for drug-susceptible TB (10, 11), a clear need exists for new drugs with treatment-shortening effects driven by novel mechanisms of action, especially against rifampin-resistant forms of TB. Such new drugs may also be expected to shorten the duration of treatment for latent TB infection, which would remove a major impediment to greater implementation of treatment strategies aimed at preventing development of active disease.

Fortunately, after a drought of over 40 years in which no new class of drugs was approved for use against TB, renewed discovery efforts and repurposing of existing antibacterial agents have produced a global portfolio of new drug candidates for TB. The portfolio of agents that are currently under evaluation in clinical trials is summarized in Table 1. It includes agents from six novel classes that are not approved or in development for other indications, including the newly approved drugs bedaquiline and delamanid. Other previously approved TB drugs are being re-examined to determine whether more effective dosing strategies will improve their contribution to TB treatment. Promising compounds also continue to emerge at earlier stages of discovery and preclinical development. A curated description of this preclinical portfolio is available at http://www.newtbdrugs.org/pipeline/discovery.

Center for Tuberculosis Research, Department of Medicine, Johns Hopkins University School of Medicine, and Department of International Health, Johns Hopkins Bloomberg School of Public Health, Baltimore, MD 21231-1002.

Table 1 New drugs in clinical development for the treatment of active TB, including ongoing clinical trials and the preclinical evidence base that supports each trial[a]

Drug (abbreviation)	Class	Mechanism(s) of action	Target	Trial objective (clinicaltrials.gov identifier)	Preclinical evidence base (references)
Existing TB drugs in dose optimization studies					
Isoniazid (INH)	Nicotinamide analog	Inhibition of mycolic acid synthesis	2-*trans*-Enoyl-acyl carrier protein reductase (InhA)	Dose-ranging EBA vs. INH-resistant mutants (NCT01936831)	19, 150, 151
				EBA of high-dose INH vs. INH-resistant mutants (NCT02236078)	
Rifampin (RIF)	Rifamycin	Inhibition of RNA synthesis	DNA-dependent RNA polymerase (RpoB)	Dose-ranging activity of RIF in the intensive phase (NCT00760149, NCT01408914, NCT02153528)	110, 152, 153
				Dose-ranging activity of RIF in a 4-month regimen (NCT02581527)	
Rifapentine (RPT)	Rifamycin	Inhibition of RNA synthesis	DNA-dependent RNA polymerase (RpoB)	Efficacy of 4-month regimens based on high-dose RPT (NCT02410772)	153–155
Repurposing of anti-infectives for TB treatment					
Moxifloxacin (MXF)	Fluoroquinolone	Inhibition of DNA synthesis	DNA gyrase (GyrA)	Efficacy of 4-month regimens based on high-dose RPT with or without MXF (NCT02410772)	155, 156
				Efficacy of MXF in place of EMB in retreatment of TB (NCT02114684)	73, 74, 157, 158
				Efficacy of regimens containing BDQ, PA-824, and PZA ± MXF (NCT02193776)	77, 78
				Efficacy of 4- and 6-month regimens containing PA-824, MXF, and PZA (NCT02342886)	75, 77, 109
				EBA of MXF vs. ofloxacin-resistant mutants (NCT02236078)	159–161
				Efficacy of MDR-TB regimens containing BDQ, PA-824, LZD ± MXF, or CFZ (NCT02589782)	E. Nuermberger, unpublished; 70*, 76
Levofloxacin (LVFX)	Fluoroquinolone	Inhibition of DNA synthesis	DNA gyrase (GyrA)	Dose-ranging activity of LVFX in MDR-TB (NCT01918397)	161–163
				Efficacy of MDR-TB regimen containing DLM, LZD, LVFX, and PZA (NCT02619994)	76
				Efficacy of a 4.5-month regimen containing 1st-line drugs + LVFX (NCT02901288)	157
Clofazimine (CFZ)	Riminophenazine	Redox cycling, production of reactive oxygen species	N/A	Efficacy of a short-course CFZ-containing regimen for MDR-TB (NCT02409290)	164
				Efficacy of MDR-TB regimens containing BDQ, PA-824, LZD ± MXF, or CFZ (NCT02589782)	Nuermberger, unpublished; 70, 76
Linezolid (LZD)	Oxazolidinone	Inhibition of protein synthesis	Ribosomal initiation complex	Dose-ranging EBA of LZD (NCT02279875)	29, 33, 40, 165
				Efficacy of a short-course regimen of BDQ, PA-824, and LZD for MDR/XDR-TB (NCT02333799)	76

				Clinical trial status	Reference(s)
				Efficacy of MDR-TB regimen containing DLM, LZD, LVFX, and PZA (NCT02619994)	76*
				Efficacy of MDR-TB regimens containing BDQ, PA-824, LZD ± MXF, or CFZ (NCT02589782)	Nuermberger, unpublished; 70*, 76
New chemical entities in clinical development for TB					
Bedaquiline (BDQ)	Diarylquinoline	Inhibition of ATP synthesis	F1F0 proton ATP synthase (AtpE)	Efficacy of a short-course regimen of BDQ, PA-824, and LZD for MDR/XDR-TB (NCT02333799)	76
				Efficacy of regimens containing BDQ, PA-824, and PZA ± MXF (NCT02193776)	77, 78
				Efficacy of MDR-TB regimens containing BDQ, PA-824, LZD ± MXF, or CFZ (NCT02589782)	Nuermberger, unpublished; 70*, 76
Delamanid (DLM)	Nitroimidazo-oxazole	Inhibition of mycolic acid synthesis, production of reactive nitrogen species	Unknown	Efficacy of a short-course CFZ-containing regimen for MDR-TB (NCT02409290)	
				Efficacy of MDR-TB regimen containing DLM, LVFX, and PZA (NCT02619994)	76*
Pretomanid (PA-824)	Nitroimidazo-oxazine	Inhibition of mycolic acid synthesis, production of reactive nitrogen species	Unknown	Efficacy of a short-course regimen of BDQ, PA-824, and LZD for MDR/XDR-TB (NCT02333799)	76
				Efficacy of regimens containing BDQ, PA-824, and PZA ± MXF (NCT02193776)	77, 78
				Efficacy of MDR-TB regimens containing BDQ, PA-824, LZD ± MXF, or CFZ (NCT02589782)	Nuermberger, unpublished; 70*, 76
SQ109	Diethylamine	Dissipation of proton motive force, inhibition of menaquinone synthesis	Mycobacterial membrane protein-large 3 (MmpL3), MenA, MenG	Completed phase 1 No active trials**	
Sutezolid (SZD)	Oxazolidinone	Inhibition of protein synthesis	Ribosomal initiation complex	Completed phase 1 No active trials**	
PBTZ169	Benzothiazinone	Inhibition of arabinogalactan synthesis	Decaprenylphosphoryl-b-D-ribose 2'-epimerase (DprE1)	Phase 1	
OPC-167832	3,4-Carbostyril derivative	Inhibition of arabinogalactan synthesis	Decaprenylphosphoryl-b-D-ribose 2'-epimerase (DprE1)	Phase 1	
Q203	Imidazopyridine amide	Inhibition of electron transport chain	Cytochrome bc_1 complex (QcrB)	Phase 1	

a*, regimen(s) tested in pre-clinical study and clinical trial may differ by at least one drug in the same class. **, no active trials registered on clinicaltrials.gov (last confirmed on May 18, 2017). EBA, early bactericidal activity; PZA, pyrazinamide.

The overarching objective of these efforts is to develop novel drug regimens containing one or more new agents capable of shortening or otherwise simplifying the treatment of drug-susceptible as well as drug-resistant forms of active and latent TB infection.

As for most infectious disease indications, drug and regimen developers focused on TB rely on preclinical models to provide evidence of efficacy suitable for selecting and advancing new drugs and drug regimens and for informing clinical trial designs. Indeed, given the many challenges inherent in the clinical development pathway for new TB therapies, including limited financial resources for phase 3 trials and lack of reliable biomarkers predictive of long-term efficacy in such trials (12), TB drug development efforts may rely more on preclinical models than many other infectious indications. This dependency and the recent availability of new investigational and repurposed drugs have brought increased scrutiny to preclinical efficacy testing and its clinical translation (12–14). Currently, there is no consensus on what preclinical tools and studies might constitute a "critical path" for development of new TB drugs or regimens (15). On the contrary, substantial gaps in knowledge exist regarding the predictive accuracy of commonly used preclinical models and the most efficient and effective manner in which to utilize the outputs of these models to optimally inform key decisions, including the design and interpretation of clinical trials (16). This review will describe existing dynamic *in vitro* and *in vivo* models of TB chemotherapy and their utility in preclinical evaluations of promising new drugs and combination regimens, with an effort to highlight recent developments.

GOALS OF PRECLINICAL EFFICACY STUDIES

Simply stated, the primary goal of preclinical efficacy studies is to evaluate the potential of a new candidate drug or drug regimen to shorten or otherwise improve the treatment of drug-susceptible and/or drug-resistant TB. Initial studies focus on comparing the efficacy of new compounds to existing TB drugs and identifying drug exposures expected to produce optimal anti-TB effects while minimizing the risk of toxicity and selective amplification of drug-resistant mutants. More advanced studies seek to identify the best strategies for combining a new drug candidate with other new and existing drugs to produce superior new regimens. Once potentially superior regimens are identified, further studies may seek to refine the optimal dose and dose schedule for each drug and estimate the duration of

treatment needed to produce outcomes equivalent or superior to existing comparator regimens.

The more specific objectives of preclinical efficacy studies are to characterize the drug's (or regimen's) activity against actively and nonactively multiplying *M. tuberculosis*, its potential to selectively amplify resistant bacterial subpopulations, and the pharmacokinetic and pharmacodynamic (PK/PD) relationships that govern these activities. Knowledge of the drug's ability to reach *M. tuberculosis* and exert its effect in various sublesional locations and microenvironments characteristic of TB lesions (e.g., necrotic [caseous] foci and cavities) is expected to further inform dose and regimen selection (17).

While dose optimization is nothing new to TB drug development efforts, the importance of quantitative PK/PD-based dose selection is increasingly recognized (18). Indeed, there are compelling arguments for further dose optimization of three of the four first-line TB drugs (i.e., isoniazid, rifampin, and pyrazinamide) (11, 19–21) and the two most important second-line drug classes (i.e., fluoroquinolones and aminoglycosides) (22–24), all of which have been used to treat TB patients for at least 3 decades and, in most cases, longer. The most important example is the rifamycin class, where continued use of suboptimal doses and dramatic interpatient variability in PK and drug exposure, despite receiving the same dose, likely interact to drive the current length of TB therapy and the emergence of multidrug-resistant (MDR) TB (10, 25–27). As with other anti-infectives, both the magnitude of drug concentrations achievable at the site of the infection as well as the shape of the concentration-time curve are important determinants of activity for some anti-TB drugs (21, 28–33). PK/PD relationships established in simpler, more tractable *in vitro* models are likely to be relevant for more complex *in vivo* disease models (18), although it will be necessary to account for factors that modify the concentrations of biologically active drug that are achievable at the site of infection *in vivo* (e.g., plasma protein binding, intracellular penetration, diffusion through caseum or blood-brain barrier) and the influence of microenvironmental conditions or the host immune response (13, 17, 34, 35).

No single preclinical *in vitro* or animal model recapitulates all aspects of human TB within a cost-effective and ethically acceptable framework (16). Therefore, it is unlikely that a critical path for development of novel drugs and drug regimens can rely on a single model to provide data sufficient to inform all key development decisions (15). Instead, sound knowledge of the utility of a variety of models and methods will be necessary to employ all available tools in the most integrative and complementary fashion to guide drug and regimen selection and optimization. In the ideal critical path, the predictive accuracy of each model and its fitness for each designated purpose would be well established through a set of validating experiments and quantitative analyses (15).

PRECLINICAL EFFICACY MODELS

In Vitro Models
In general, there are two categories of in vitro models used to study the activity of anti-TB drugs: static models in which drug concentrations remain fixed over time and dynamic models in which drug concentrations change over time.

Static drug concentration models
Static models evaluate the bacterial response to drug concentrations that are fixed over time. Response measures include colony-forming unit (CFU) counts or surrogates such as optical density or other markers of bacterial growth or viability in liquid culture systems (36). The most common output from static models is the minimum inhibitory concentration (MIC). The greatest value of MIC may be its relative simplicity as a quantitative measure of potency for ranking compounds and for indexing microbial susceptibility to drug exposure in PK/PD analyses. However, by definition, it measures only growth inhibitory effects and cannot be used under conditions in which there is little or no growth. Bactericidal effects, as measured by the minimum bactericidal concentration and quantitative time-kill curves, are more informative but more costly and time-consuming to measure. Classically, MIC and minimum bactericidal concentration measurements are obtained against actively multiplying bacteria in optimal growth conditions. However, given the important role of persistent bacterial subpopulations in the treatment of TB, a wide variety of alternative models have been developed to test static drug concentrations against bacteria under stressful conditions that alter bacterial growth and metabolism in a manner that may reproduce mechanisms that drive bacterial persistence in vivo (8, 36). To date, there is limited evidence based on which to favor one particular persister model over another, and a detailed discussion of this topic is outside the scope of this review.

Because the shape of the concentration-time curve can have a profound effect on drug activity (37), PK/PD parameters associated with optimal efficacy in static concentration models may be significantly different from those derived from models that expose bacteria to changing drug concentrations over time.

Dynamic drug concentration models, including the hollow fiber system model of tuberculosis
Hollow fiber systems (HFSs) and related dynamic in vitro models are useful to study the bacterial response to fluctuating drug concentrations over time. They have been employed to derive information on PK/PD relationships for antibacterial agents and used in regulatory filings for decades, but HFS-TB models emerged only in the past 15 years (23, 38). HFS units (Fig. 1) consist of a bioreactor cartridge, the interior of which is traversed by multiple hollow fiber capillary tubes to create two compartments: an extracapillary compartment for culturing M. tuberculosis and an intracapillary compartment through which drug-containing media is supplied to the cartridge. The semipermeable nature of the hollow fibers allows small molecules (e.g., drugs, nutrients, bacterial metabolites) to diffuse between the two compartments but prevents the movement of bacteria into the intracapillary compartment. The intracapillary compartment of each cartridge is linked to a vascular system of tubing through which the flow of media is controlled by an adjustable perfusion pump. Drugs are introduced into the system using a programmable drug delivery pump and cleared by dilution in a central compartment at a rate controlled by additional pumps linked to input (fresh media) and output (waste media) reservoirs.

In many respects, the HFS-TB model is an ideal tool for developing a quantitative understanding of PK/PD relationships to inform drug and regimen development. As in static concentration models, bacteria in HFS units can be cultivated under a variety of environmental conditions by manipulating aspects of the media (e.g., pH, nutritional content) or the external environment (e.g., HFS enclosed in an anaerobic chamber) (21, 39). Even the intracellular niche of M. tuberculosis can be studied by cultivating infected macrophage-like cells (e.g., THP-1 or J774 cells) in the extracapillary space (40). Tight control of the culture conditions enables the study of PK/PD relationships against specific phenotypic subpopulations of bacteria that may be similar to in vivo subpopulations and relevant to clinical outcomes. Various culture conditions have been studied, including log-phase growth in nutrient-rich media, slower growth under acidic conditions (e.g., pH 5.8), nonreplicating persistence under low oxygen tension (e.g., ≤10 parts per billion), and intracellular infection

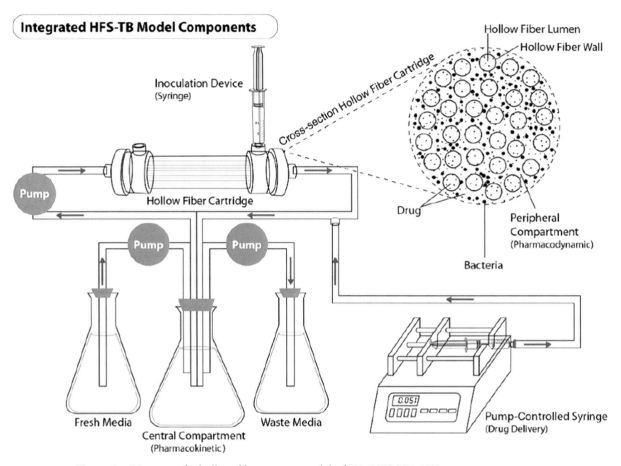

Figure 1   Diagram of a hollow fiber system model of TB (HFS-TB) (49).

(41). Another advantage of the HFS-TB over animal models is that its compartments can be serially sampled to measure viable bacterial counts, bacterial metabolites, and drug concentrations over time. This facilitates time-to-event and repeated event analyses that increase statistical power and enable construction of more dynamic and robust systems pharmacology models (41).

Perhaps the greatest advantage of the HFS-TB over static drug concentration models (and most animal models) is the precise control of the drug concentration-time profiles to which the bacteria are exposed. Concentration-time profiles may be designed to mimic *in vivo* (human or animal) PK profiles or to produce concentration-time profiles that are unattainable in animal models but have clinical or experimental value. For example, the activity of carbapenems and related β-lactams correlates best with the proportion of the dosing interval for which drug concentrations exceed the MIC (37). Because they are cleared much faster in mice than in humans, it is difficult to attain clinically relevant exposures in mice for many drugs in this class

(42). In contrast, producing human-like exposures is quite straightforward in the HFS (29).

With appropriate attention to sterile technique to prevent contamination of the HFS, treatment durations of 28 to 56 days are feasible, and treatment durations as long as 6 months have been studied. Experimental designs have included dose-ranging and dose fractionation studies of single agents and comparisons of drug combinations, including drug sequencing studies (41). Data output, typically in the form of CFU counts, has been used to identify PK/PD parameters correlated with antibacterial effect and to derive target drug exposures associated with optimal microbial kill (e.g., as defined by the exposure associated with 80% or 90% of the maximal effect [EC_{80} or EC_{90}, respectively]) and suppression of drug-resistant mutants (41, 43). Output from HFS-TB models also has been used to perform computer-aided clinical trial simulations based on Monte Carlo analyses (19, 23, 43, 44). In some studies, key PK/PD parameters and target exposures derived from HFS-TB experiments were used together with population PK data and wild-type MIC distributions to predict the probability of different clinical antibiotic doses achieving optimal drug exposures and rates of sterilizing effect in sputum in patient populations and to predict the proportion of patients that would develop acquired drug resistance despite receiving combination therapy as a result of population-level PK variability (26, 43). Finally, although more prospective study is required, HFS-TB data have been used to derive PK/PD-based breakpoints for drug susceptibility testing that could distinguish clinical scenarios in which treatment response is likely or unlikely (45, 46). In a formal statistical analysis, kill rates in sputum of patients, PK/PD parameters, and targets associated with optimal effect and even probability and time to emergence of drug resistance were found to be similar between patients and results of analyses based on HFS-TB outputs (43, 44).

The demonstrated predictive accuracy of the HFS-TB model should give confidence to drug developers and regulatory agencies that they are a valuable tool for PK/PD profiling to support regulatory activities (47, 48). Indeed, the European Medicines Agency's Committee for Medicinal Products for Human Use recently rendered a positive qualification opinion that the HFS-TB model may be used in anti-TB drug development programs as an additional and complementary tool to existing methodologies (including animal models) to inform dose and regimen selection, including combinations of two or more drugs, to maximize bactericidal effects and minimize emergence of drug resistance (Table 2) (49). Specifically, the group endorsed the HFS-TB as a model fit to provide preliminary proof of concept for developing a specific drug or combination to treat TB, to select the PK/PD target for optimal effect, and to provide data to support PK/PD analyses leading to initial dose selection for preclinical and clinical studies. As a tractable dynamic *in vitro* PK/PD

model, the HFS-TB model is expected to reduce the complexity and size of dose-finding studies in animal models and clinical trials and thereby shorten the duration of TB drug development programs. The HFS-TB model is also expected to assist in confirming dose regimens for later clinical trials taking into account any accumulated human PK data and available information on exposure-response relationships.

Despite its advantages, the HFS-TB model cannot replace preclinical animal efficacy studies or clinical trials (16, 47). Moreover, because most studies included in the predictive accuracy analysis of the model were performed after the clinical trials that the HFS-TB output was compared to, it is important to prospectively collect and analyze data on the performance of the model (16, 47). Finally, the use of the HFS-TB model has thus far been limited to a small number of laboratories. It will be important to study the reproducibility of the method and any operational issues related to model performance as it is taken up by other investigators.

Animal Infection Models of Active TB Suitable for Efficacy Testing

While drug exposure-response relationships derived in the HFS-TB or other dynamic *in vitro* models are expected to translate to *in vivo* models and to the clinic, *in vivo* drug efficacy occurs in the complex milieu of the infected host, where a variety of factors may be encountered that modify the relationship between plasma drug exposures and drug effect at the site of infection. These factors include various host defense mechanisms, protein binding, drug diffusion through caseum, unique environmental determinants of drug effect, and more diverse bacterial heterogeneity under conditions that cannot be fully reproduced *in vitro*. Moreover, tuberculous lesions are three-dimensional structures that introduce temporal and spatial gradients of these modifying

---

Table 2 Qualification opinion of the European Medicines Agency's Committee for Medicinal Products for Human Use regarding the HFS-TB (48)

The HFS-TB is qualified to be used in anti-TB drug development programs as an additional and complementary tool to existing methodology to inform selection of dose and treatment regimen, to maximize bactericidal effects and minimize emergence of resistance. More specifically, the HFS-TB may be useful as follows:

- To provide preliminary proof of concept for developing a specific drug or combination to treat tuberculosis
- To select the pharmacodynamic target (e.g., T/MIC, AUC/MIC)
- To provide data to support PK/PD analyses leading to initial dose selection for nonclinical and clinical studies, with the aim of limiting the number of regimens that are to be tested *in vivo*; it is anticipated that HFS-TB may be used to limit doses tested both in single-drug and combination regimen studies *in vivo*
- To assist in confirming dose regimens for later clinical trials, taking into account the accumulated human PK data in healthy volunteers and then patients as well as available information on exposure-response relationships

factors that influence drug distribution and effect. Used appropriately, *in vivo* models enable study of the antibacterial effects of dynamic drug concentration-time profiles to derive PK/PD relationships or to confirm those derived in *in vitro* models. Many animal models also enable simultaneous study of multiple subpopulations, perhaps in clinically relevant proportions, to better understand the sterilizing potential of drug regimens and thus their potential to shorten TB treatment. Mice are by far the most commonly used preclinical efficacy model. However, because they do not form caseating lung lesions, the most commonly used mouse strains do not mimic the three-dimensional structure and heterogeneity of TB lesions. As a result, emerging mouse models and larger non-mouse species may have a key role to play in TB drug development.

The major premise behind the use of non-mouse species is that tuberculous lesions in species such as guinea pigs, rabbits, and non-human primates more closely represent the pathological hallmarks of human TB (e.g., caseation necrosis, and in rabbits and non-human primates, cavitation). If such lesions or the microenvironmental conditions found therein are important determinants of drug effect, by altering drug distribution, the mechanism or kinetics of drug action, or the susceptibility of the pathogen to the drug effect, then the presence or absence of such pathology could have an important influence on drug efficacy and the PK/PD relationships that govern it. Within the architecture of active caseous lung lesions, whether they are organized caseous granulomas, more disorganized areas of caseous pneumonia, or cavities, most bacilli are found extracellularly in the caseum, and only a minority reside intracellularly in neutrophils, epithelioid macrophages, and foamy macrophages in the cellular borders of the caseous lesions and in other cellular lesions (50–54). Detailed descriptions of caseating graulomas in some models have noted relatively small numbers of extracellular bacilli in caseum (55). However, such lesions are frequently sterilized by host immune mechanisms and resolve without treatment (56) and should not be confused with more poorly contained caseous lesions (e.g., caseous pneumonia and cavities) where host immune mechanisms are less effective and extracellular bacillary populations are disproportionately large (54, 56, 57). The latter progressive caseating lesions better reflect those that determine treatment outcomes in patients presenting with active TB.

Bacilli in different types of tuberculous lesions and in different compartments of caseous lesions experience different microenvironmental conditions that may affect a drug's concentration-response relationship. Bac-

terial responses to stress conditions such as hypoxia, low pH, and oxidant stress have long been known to cause phenotypic tolerance and persistence in the face of drug exposure, affecting some drugs more than others. On the other hand, certain drugs require specific microenvironmental conditions for optimal effect. For example, pyrazinamide's anti-TB effect is inversely proportional to pH (58). Metronidazole requires very low oxygen tension for bioactivation and activity against *M. tuberculosis* (59). These drugs may exhibit very different effects in different models and in different lesion compartments despite achieving similar concentrations at the site (35, 53, 60–63). Finally, although some drugs (e.g., small polar molecules such as pyrazinamide and isoniazid) distribute quite evenly through the various lesion types and sublesional compartments, other drugs partition differently into cells or into acellular caseum, creating the potential for markedly different drug exposures for bacilli in different lesion compartments (17, 34, 64, 65). Drugs exhibiting high lipophilicity as measured by logP and high protein binding tend to accumulate inside cells and to diffuse poorly through caseum. Examples include bedaquiline and clofazimine (34, 65). When compared to plasma concentrations, these drugs may achieve much higher concentrations where bacilli reside in macrophages but lower concentrations against extracellular bacilli in caseous lesions. Other interesting drug distribution profiles have recently been revealed. For example, unlike pyrazinamide and isoniazid, which diffuse rapidly in and out of caseous regions, rifampin diffuses relatively slowly into caseum but accumulates there with repeated dosing (65). The heterogeneous nature of human TB lesions and the various influences on drug concentration and concentration-response relationships illustrate the importance of understanding how a given drug candidate may be affected so that it can be taken into account in drug and regimen development.

Animal species used as preclinical efficacy models

Mice

Mice are the most commonly used species in TB drug development owing to their ease of handling and relatively low procurement and housing costs (36, 66). Particularly in the early phases of drug development, their ubiquity, tractability, cost, and small compound requirements make mice the most practical model. Nevertheless, the absence of caseating lung lesions and cavities is a potential limitation of commonly used mouse strains.

Instead of developing caseating lung lesions, commonly used mouse strains (e.g., Swiss, BALB/c, C57BL/6) contain the infection in nonnecrotic cellular granulomas composed predominantly of lymphocytes, epithelioid macrophages, and foamy macrophages. Here, virtually all tubercle bacilli reside in macrophages and may not be exposed to all of the microenvironmental conditions found in caseous lesions that are closed to the airways (e.g., hypoxia) (60, 63, 67). Thus, at least for some drugs that partition very differently in various lesion compartments, commonly used mouse strains may best represent the intracellular compartment and not other lesion compartments found in caseous disease models. The utility of these mouse strains for evaluating new drugs and drug regimens may therefore depend on several factors. Of perhaps the greatest importance is whether a drug requires conditions found only in caseous lesions to be active. This is an unusual scenario but is exemplified by metronidazole, which requires very low oxygen tension for activation and has demonstrable anti-TB activity in closed caseous foci of rabbits and macaques but not in mice (53, 60, 62, 63, 68). A second factor is the extent to which a drug partitions differently into cells and caseum. Drugs that diffuse evenly into these compartments are likely to be well represented in mice. On the other hand, the activity of drugs that show markedly greater partitioning into cells compared to caseum, such as clofazimine and bedaquiline (34, 65), could be overestimated in mice that do not develop caseous lesions (69, 70). However, it is important to emphasize that the treatment-shortening potential of such drugs demonstrated in mice may yet be relevant to human TB, provided that the intracellular bacterial populations modeled in mice are similar to intracellular bacilli found in human TB lesions and that these populations, even if they are minority subpopulations, persist there and play a role in determining the duration of treatment needed to cure human TB.

Despite their limitations, mice have been instrumental in drug and regimen development for TB. The greater use of mouse models relative to any other species means that there is a larger evidence base on which to judge their utility. To date, no other animal model has demonstrated the same or superior predictive value for drug regimens in clinical use (16). Despite developing rather homogeneous intracellular infections, commonly used mouse strains such as Swiss and BALB/c mice have a good track record in predicting the clinical utility of new TB drugs and regimens. For example, rifampin and pyrazinamide are the only drugs with a clinically validated ability to shorten the duration of TB treatment to 12 months or less. These treatment-

shortening effects were first demonstrated in mice (71). More recently, a large phase 3 trial (72) sought to shorten the treatment duration from 6 months to 4 months by replacing isoniazid or ethambutol with the late-generation fluoroquinolone moxifloxacin, based in part on results from murine models (73, 74). Despite shortening the time to sputum culture conversion, the 4-month moxifloxacin-containing regimens were not as effective as the 6-month control regimen (72). Although this result prompted criticism of mouse models as well as surrogate markers used in phase 2 clinical trials leading up to the phase 3 trial, an objective appraisal of the available mouse model and clinical data suggests that a treatment-shortening effect of less than 2 months is entirely consistent with both the murine and clinical data (14). More novel regimens with new and repurposed drugs (e.g., bedaquiline, pretomanid, linezolid) have also demonstrated treatment-shortening potential in mice (75–78). Although early clinical data are promising (79–81), confirmation of their treatment-shortening effects in patients and comparisons to results in mouse models will require phase 3 trials using relapse as an endpoint.

Experimental infection of mice
Experimental infection of mice is generally via the respiratory tract (e.g., aerosol or intratracheal inoculation) or intravenous injection. In either case, virulent *M. tuberculosis* multiplies exponentially in the lungs and spleen of naive mice for the first 2 to 3 weeks postinfection. Thereafter, in immunocompetent mice, the adaptive immune response reduces the net bacterial multiplication rate (82). In the absence of treatment, the outcome of the infection depends on the virulence of the *M. tuberculosis* strain, the size of the infectious dose, and the susceptibility of the mouse strain. High-dose infection (e.g., implantation of approximately 5×10^3 or more CFU in the lungs by any route) with a virulent *M. tuberculosis* strain typically results in overwhelming infection and death within 4 to 6 weeks postinfection in any mouse strain. Lower infectious doses produce the same fate in immunodeficient mice (e.g., athymic nude mice or gamma-interferon knockout mice) (36). In contrast, similar low-dose infections (e.g., 10 to 500 CFU implanted in the lungs) in immunocompetent strains such as BALB/c and C57BL/6 mice result in containment of infection by the adaptive immune response, a plateau in lung CFU counts beginning at approximately 4 weeks postinfection, and long-term survival of the animal with chronic infection (36, 66). Among inbred mouse strains, there are clear differences in susceptibility to infection (83) that may translate

into differences in disease susceptibility and treatment outcomes. However, there are unlikely to be distinct differences in drug efficacy between commonly used immunocompetent mouse strains, especially with respect to ranking drug regimens (36).

Common experimental designs

The natural history of infection in mice enables three basic experimental designs for initial drug efficacy studies (Fig. 2). The first is an acute infection model in which treatment is initiated within the first week (often the first 1 to 3 days) postinfection, and drug effects against logarithmically multiplying bacteria are measured over 1 to 4 weeks of treatment. Use of "real-time" efficacy measures such as mouse survival, body weight, prevention of macroscopic lung lesions and splenomegaly, and *in vivo* or *ex vivo* biomarkers of bacterial viability other than culture-based outcomes (e.g., CFU counts) may permit relatively high throughput but may not reliably discriminate bactericidal and bacteriostatic effects (36). Whether non-culture-based or culture-based readouts are used, it is clear that assessments using acute infection models favor compounds with rapid onset of antibacterial effects and bactericidal mechanisms of action and may misrepresent the sterilizing activity of compounds or doses having a slower onset of action or activity predominantly against slowly replicating or nonreplicating bacilli (84). One has to look no farther than the performance of isoniazid versus rifampin and pyrazinamide for an example. In acute infection models, isoniazid, which has celebrated early bactericidal activity and limited sterilizing activity in TB patients (6, 7), markedly outperforms rifampin and pyrazinamide, the two first-line drugs with

bona fide treatment-shortening effects (84, 85). Therefore, such acute infection models are most useful for rapid screening for *in vivo* anti-TB activity and perhaps some measure of a drug's ability to kill mutants resistant to companion agents in the absence of a suitable host response.

A chronic infection model, in which treatment is initiated at least 3 weeks, and often 4 to 6 weeks, after low-dose infection, is more effective for demonstrating the superior sterilizing efficacy of compounds such as rifampin and pyrazinamide that are most active against the slowly replicating or nonreplicating bacilli that predominate during the plateau in lung CFU counts brought about by the adaptive immune response (84). Thus, although it takes longer to set up compared to an acute infection model, a chronic infection model is more likely to differentiate between compounds or doses of the same compound on the basis of their potential sterilizing activity. However, since there is no net multiplication in untreated animals (82, 86), the chronic model is unable to distinguish bacteriostatic effects from no effect.

Both the acute and chronic models defined above have the disadvantage of significantly lower bacterial burdens at the initiation of treatment relative to the bacterial burden in patients with cavitary lesions, where estimates suggest 10^7 to 10^9 cultivable bacteria reside in the cavity wall alone (87). Larger bacterial populations are more diverse, have higher numbers of spontaneous drug-resistant mutants, and require longer treatment durations to attain cure with combination chemotherapy. Thus, a subacute infection model, in which treatment begins 2 weeks after high-dose infection (e.g., 10^4 CFU inoculated via aerosol or 5×10^6 CFU inoculated intravenously), may be preferable for evaluating multidrug regimens for their effects on actively and nonactively replicating bacilli and drug-resistant subpopulations, and for estimation of the treatment duration necessary for cure (88). Whether the route of infection is via the aerosol or intravenous route, the bacterial burden at the initiation of treatment is close to 10^8 CFU in the lungs in this subacute model, and the modern short-course regimen of 2 months of rifampin, isoniazid, pyrazinamide and ethambutol followed by rifampin and isoniazid requires approximately 6 months of treatment to prevent relapse in the great majority of mice, as it does in TB patients (66, 88).

C3HeB/FeJ mice

C3HeB/FeJ mice have garnered significant interest recently because, unlike commonly used mouse strains, they develop caseating lesions after *M. tuberculosis* in-

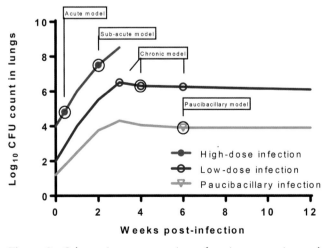

Figure 2   Schematic representation of various experimental models.

fection under the proper experimental conditions (52, 53, 89). Development of the caseating lesions is primarily determined by a natural deficiency in the *Ipr1* (for intracellular pathogen resistance 1) gene in the *sst1* (for supersusceptibility to TB 1) locus, which promotes necrosis, rather than apoptosis, of infected macrophages (89–91). The closest human homolog of Ipr1 is SP110b, an interferon-inducible protein that normally downregulates proinflammatory cytokines, including tumor necrosis factor-alpha (TNF-α), and limits excessive tissue damage and development of necrotic lung lesions (92). The increased susceptibility of C3HeB/FeJ mice appears limited to virulent intracellular pathogens (93). However, they do not appear to have difficulty containing infections with nontuberculous mycobacteria, *Mycobacterium bovis* bacille Calmette-Guérin (BCG), and even less virulent isolates of *M. tuberculosis* (52, 89, 94). Although the role of *SP110* in human susceptibility to TB is debated, evidence is mounting that variations in this locus do contribute (92).

Considerable heterogeneity in lung pathology may be observed in C3HeB/FeJ mice, even among those infected in the same experiment (52, 53). After infecting mice via aerosol with 50 to 75 CFU of virulent *M. tuberculosis*, Irwin et al. (52) performed detailed histopathological analyses at various time points over the course of infection. They described three distinct types of lung lesions: fulminant necrotizing alveolitis, well-organized caseating granulomas, and cellular granulomas typical of those predominating in other commonly used mouse strains. Although they may develop features of caseous necrosis, mice exhibiting the fulminant granulocytic alveolitis typically succumb to infection within 5 to 6 weeks of infection and are therefore of limited utility for drug efficacy studies. In contrast, the well-organized caseating granulomas developing in one-third to two-thirds of mice display central caseation, fibrous encapsulation, and hypoxia characteristic of larger species, including humans (52, 67). Some large caseating granulomas or foci of caseous pneumonia contain more than 10^9 bacilli and eventually cavitate, although this tends to be a late event (53, 60, 95). Cavities in association with a more stable clinical condition can be promoted specifically by allowing caseous granulomas to form, then treating with a noncurative course of combination chemotherapy (e.g., 8 weeks for the first-line regimen) before allowing the disease to recur (95). Mice with cavities in this scenario can be identified by serial computed tomography (CT) and may live for months once cavities are found (95), thereby enabling drug distribution studies and efficacy testing against this lesion type.

Given the potential impact of caseous lesions on the PK/PD of TB drugs, there is substantial optimism that the histopathological changes observed in C3HeB/FeJ mice will enable better representation of human drug efficacy in mice. The potential value of C3HeB/FeJ mice may be indicated by the differential response to some anti-TB drugs in this strain compared to commonly used mouse strains, as indicated by recent experiences with pyrazinamide and clofazimine. As in humans and larger species (64, 65), pyrazinamide distributes evenly through various caseous lesion compartments, including acellular caseum, in C3HeB/FeJ mice (34, 35). However, unlike in BALB/c mice and in C3HeB/FeJ mice harboring only cellular granulomas, where it exerts a significant bactericidal effect, pyrazinamide has only limited effect against the numerous extracellular bacilli in the caseum of large caseous granulomas in C3HeB/FeJ mice (35). This discrepant activity was ultimately shown to be due to the elevated pH of the caseum, which prevented pyrazinamide from exerting a bactericidal effect (34, 35). Nevertheless, pyrazinamide does exert a sterilizing effect even in C3HeB/FeJ mice with large caseous lesions (96), an effect that is presumably restricted to bacteria engulfed by activated macrophages, where the pH falls to a level sufficient for pyrazinamide effect. This result suggests that the bacterial persisters targeted by the treatment-shortening effects of pyrazinamide in the first-line regimen reside intracellularly.

Unlike pyrazinamide, clofazimine partitions very differently into cellular compartments compared to acellular caseum, a trait evident in C3HeB/FeJ mice as well as rabbits and humans (65). This provides at least one explanation for the poor initial activity of clofazimine observed in C3HeB/FeJ mice relative to BALB/c mice, but the hypoxic conditions observed in caseous granulomas of the former are another potential explanation (69). Whether clofazimine, like pyrazinamide, exerts bactericidal activity against intracellular bacilli and contributes sterilizing activity to regimens in C3HeB/FeJ mice remains to be seen. Likewise, several novel regimens now in clinical development based on results in BALB/c mice have been evaluated in C3HeB/FeJ mice (67, 76). The clinical outcomes observed relative to the standard of care should allow further evaluation of the potential utility of the latter strain.

Rats

Although commonly utilized in the pharmaceutical industry for PK and toxicology studies, rats were long considered too resistant to *M. tuberculosis* infection to be a suitable model for TB drug development. However, aerosol and intratracheal infections of outbred Wistar rats produce pathological features similar to those observed in commonly used mouse strains other than C3HeB/FeJ (97, 98). Advantages of working with this species include the ability to study efficacious drug exposures in a commonly used toxicity model, greater feasibility to control drug exposures through long-term vascular catheters or implantable infusion pumps, and sometimes lower compound clearance compared to mice (99). For example, a low-dose aerosol infection model was employed at AstraZeneca to test a series of DprE1 inhibitors alone in part because the compounds were cleared too rapidly in mice to attain optimal drug exposures (100). The cotton rat (*Sigmodon hispidus*) can develop caseating lung lesions more characteristic of human TB. However, the presence of conflicting reports (101, 102) suggests that such lesions are dependent on experimental conditions that will require further optimization.

Guinea pigs

Once the favored *in vivo* model for TB drug development due to their marked susceptibility to *M. tuberculosis* infection, guinea pigs are now used infrequently for this purpose. However, they remain an alternative or complementary model to mice given the occurrence of caseating primary lung lesions. The histopathology of *M. tuberculosis* infection is well characterized. Moreover, elegant staining studies during chemotherapy have mapped the location of the most numerous persistently acid-fast bacilli to the necrotic core of such lesions, where the organisms reside extracellularly (51, 103), suggesting that this is an important persister population. Smaller numbers of extracellular bacilli are found in the acellular rim of these necrotic lesions. Still smaller numbers of intracellular bacilli are found in the cellular rim of necrotic primary lesions and in the secondary disseminated lesions that do not typically undergo necrosis (51).

Guinea pigs are typically used in chronic infection schemes to allow time for caseous lesions to develop. Infection is most often via the aerosol route, although parenteral routes are possible. Recent experiments have recapitulated the combined treatment-shortening effects of rifampin and pyrazinamide compared to streptomycin and isoniazid (104–106). Remarkably, however, cure without relapse of disease is obtained with shorter durations of treatment in guinea pigs compared to BALB/c mice, despite similar bacterial population sizes and drug exposures in the two models, suggesting that infections in BALB/c mice harbor more persistent

bacteria (104, 107). Another interesting observation of guinea pigs is the apparent difficulty in selecting isoniazid-resistant mutants harboring mutations in the mycobacterial catalase-peroxidase *katG* (105). This suggests greater fitness costs associated with these mutations in guinea pigs, compared to mice and possibly cavitary disease in humans, perhaps a result of enhanced oxidative stress experienced by *M. tuberculosis* in guinea pigs.

Several novel drugs and drug regimens now in clinical trials have been compared to standard therapies in guinea pigs, and results seem generally consistent with those in BALB/c mice (61, 103, 105, 106, 108–111), although the guinea pig may have better demonstrated the rifapentine doses needed to achieve efficacy superior to that of rifampin in phase 2 trials (10, 109, 112). Although this may be attributable to the caseous lesions occurring in guinea pigs and not in mice, further study is required. Compared to rifampin, rifapentine accumulates to a greater extent inside cells and diffuses and accumulates less readily in caseum compared to rifampin (65, 113). Thus, for a given plasma drug exposure, rifapentine may exhibit superior activity relative to rifampin against intracellular bacilli in the lesions of BALB/c mice and the cellular regions of caseous lesions but inferior activity in the caseous regions (13, 113, 114). Pharmacometric analyses of ongoing phase 3 trials of high-dose rifamycin-containing regimens and more advanced modeling of drug distribution and compartmentalization of drug effect may shed further light on the predictive accuracy and most complementary applications of guinea pig and mouse models for preclinical drug development.

Despite their potential advantages relative to non-C3HeB/FeJ mouse strains, guinea pigs only infrequently develop cavitary lesions and have other disadvantages that limit their use. They are both more expensive to maintain and more fragile than mice, being especially susceptible to the adverse effects of broad-spectrum antimicrobials on the normal intestinal flora. Surprisingly, guinea pigs also clear a number of drugs, including first-line TB drugs as well as moxifloxacin and pretomanid, faster than mice do (107, 109). Combined with their larger size, higher clearance in guinea pigs leads to large compound requirements that discourage their use in early drug development. Nevertheless, guinea pigs may be useful as a relatively economical model for confirming or revising results obtained in mice, especially when microenvironmental conditions such as hypoxia (51, 63) or other aspects of larger caseous lesions are expected to influence drug distribution or drug action.

Rabbits

Rabbits are highly susceptible to virulent *M. bovis* strains (115), whereas infection with common laboratory strains of *M. tuberculosis*, such as H37Rv and Erdman, does not result in progressive infection (116). In contrast, aerosol infection of outbred New Zealand white rabbits with the HN878 strain of the *M. tuberculosis* Beijing subfamily was recently shown to cause progressive infection with caseating lung lesions by 8 weeks and cavitary lung disease by 16 weeks postinfection (117). Cavitary disease also can be produced with a wider range of *M. tuberculosis* strains using sensitization with heat-killed bacilli followed by bronchoscopic instillation of viable cultures (118). The creation of lung cavities is the major potential advantage of rabbit models for preclinical drug efficacy testing because cavitary disease is associated with slower response to TB treatment, relapse, and emergence of drug resistance and because cavities are not a feature of non-C3HeB/FeJ mouse or guinea pig models. Although cavity formation may not occur uniformly in all animals at the same time, CT imaging is useful for predicting when and where cavities will occur (119, 120). CT also allows for serial quantification of lesion/cavity volume and cavity surface area as biomarkers of treatment response (120).

The larger size of rabbits and their caseous lung lesions makes them well suited for studying the impact of specific lesion types on drug distribution and efficacy. Recent lesion-specific drug distribution and PK studies demonstrating similarities between results in rabbits and humans are promising in this regard (64, 65, 113, 121–123). To date, however, studies of drug efficacy in rabbits are very limited. One tantalizing finding is that large, closed caseous lesions in rabbits are likely to harbor more extensive zones where *M. tuberculosis* encounters severe hypoxia, as demonstrated by the anti-TB activity of metronidazole in rabbits but not in mice (53, 60, 63, 68). Unfortunately, evidence confirming that metronidazole is useful in human TB remains elusive (*vide infra*) (124). Combination therapy has been studied more rarely in rabbits, although a recent study characterized the response to therapy with first-line TB drugs, including evaluation of positron emission tomography (PET)-CT as a potential surrogate marker for antimicrobial effects (125).

Disadvantages of rabbits include the high acquisition and housing costs, the limited number of reagents for characterizing immunological responses, and greater pathogen containment concerns. Too expensive to be a "workhorse" model for preclinical efficacy studies, rabbits will likely remain most useful in drug development for informing PK/PD models incorporating lesion-specific drug distribution, exploring hypotheses related to the effects of microenvironmental conditions on drug efficacy, and perhaps bridging efficacy studies using surrogate markers that can be used in clinical trials such as PET-CT.

Non-human primates

Non-human primates, primarily macaques, were used as preclinical TB drug efficacy models as early as the 1950s and have recently garnered renewed interest. Unlike other animal models considered here, they may represent the full spectrum of pathology and outcomes of *M. tuberculosis* infection in humans.

Infection of cynomolgus macaques via intrabronchial instillation of approximately 25 CFU of *M. tuberculosis* produces active TB or subclinical/latent infection in roughly equal proportions over the ensuing 6 to 8 months (126, 127). Serial PET-CT imaging beginning as early as 3 weeks postinfection appears useful for identifying animals destined to develop active versus latent disease (128). A higher proportion of animals with active disease can be obtained more rapidly (e.g., within 10 weeks) with instillation of approximately 10^3 CFU (129). Active disease is evidenced by symptoms (e.g., cough, weight loss), elevated erythrocyte sedimentation rate, abnormal chest radiograph, and positive cultures from gastric aspirate and bronchoalveolar lavage specimens (126, 127). Potential endpoints for drug efficacy studies include serial measures of viable bacterial counts from gastric aspirates or bronchoalveolar lavages, serial PET-CT imaging endpoints, and terminal measures such as organ CFU scores and gross pathology scores (62, 128). To date, however, these endpoints have not been proven to be useful in discriminating between active regimens with differing potencies. The responses to monotherapy with the oxazolidinones linezolid and AZD5847 were superior to no treatment but indistinguishable from each other after 1 to 2 months of treatment in macaques using various scores based on bacterial burden and PET-CT imaging (130). However, linezolid has demonstrably greater bactericidal activity in human sputum over the first 2 weeks of treatment (131) than AZD5847 (132), despite achieving higher AZD5847 plasma exposures in patients than in macaques (130, 132). Metronidazole was also evaluated in macaques with active disease, where it did not appear to increase the activity of a rifampin-isoniazid combination (62). In one small clinical trial with MDR-TB, addition of metronidazole to a background regimen of second-line drugs was associated with higher rates of sputum smear conversion and culture conversion in liquid, but not solid, media at 1 month, but these differences did not persist after the second month (124). Clearly, further study is needed to determine the predictive accuracy of endpoints measured in macaques for clinical outcomes.

Many challenges are associated with the use of macaques for preclinical drug efficacy models, including limited availability, great expense, requirements for special husbandry and enrichment, and ethical concerns. With respect to drug development, the challenge to the field is to demonstrate whether the potential advantages of working with these primates are unique to this model or whether similar information can be gained from more economical and more ethically acceptable models.

Common marmosets (*Callithrix jacchus*) are New World primates that, at 250 to 500 grams as adults, are much smaller than macaques (and even rabbits) yet develop similar caseous lesions, including cavities, in response to *M. tuberculosis* infection (133). In addition to being much more economical, marmosets have the advantage of frequent twinning, which provides opportunities for ideal experimental controls (133). Despite these promising features, there are currently few published data affirming the utility of the marmoset in drug efficacy studies. The first description of experimental *M. tuberculosis* infection in marmosets was published only recently (133). Since then, a study compared the efficacy of the modern, four-drug short-course regimen to that of a more primitive streptomycin-isoniazid combination over 6 weeks of treatment (134). Intriguingly, the former regimen showed greater effect in cavitary lesions, significantly reducing the proportion of animals with cultivable bacilli and the total number of bacilli in cavities. No significant difference was noted in noncavitary lesions or other body sites, except that the streptomycin-isoniazid combination was more active in the spleen. These results suggest that the marmosets are a more economically viable alternative to macaques for identifying the impact of drug distribution and microenvironmental conditions on drug effect at the site of action in caseous lesions. As with C3HeB/FeJ mice, additional studies are warranted to demonstrate the relative value of marmosets as alternative or complementary models to more commonly used mouse strains.

MODELING THE CHEMOTHERAPY OF LATENT TB INFECTION

Treatment of latent TB infection (LTBI) is critical to improving TB control and essential to TB elimination with available tools (135). Thus, it is a key component

of the WHO End TB Strategy. LTBI is defined by evidence of *M. tuberculosis* infection in the absence of clinical symptoms. Only approximately 5 to 10% of immunocompetent individuals with LTBI will ultimately develop active TB, with half of the risk occurring within the first 2 years after infection. The principal objective of drug development for treatment of LTBI is to develop shorter or otherwise simpler regimens to promote adherence and treatment completion. This is especially true for treatment of LTBI among people exposed to MDR and extensively drug-resistant (XDR) TB cases, for which existing rifamycin- and isoniazid-based LTBI regimens are expected to be less effective and second-line drug regimens are longer and less well tolerated.

Although the pathogenesis of LTBI and reactivation remains incompletely understood, there is growing appreciation that LTBI represents a spectrum of conditions resulting from different outcomes of the host-pathogen interaction (136). These conditions range from cleared infection (and thus no risk of reactivation) with residual immunological memory, to controlled or dormant infection with viable bacilli (with intermediate risk of progression), to percolating or incipient disease (with the highest risk of progression to active disease). With respect to evaluating experimental models of LTBI chemotherapy, an important question is whether it is necessary to model the entire spectrum of viable infectious states including dormant, possibly noncultivable, bacilli or whether most people with LTBI who will subsequently reactivate (especially in the timeframe studied in clinical trials) harbor chronic, low-level infection with cultivable bacilli that can be modeled successfully in a variety of species.

Mice are not generally considered to develop LTBI because they are incapable, on their own, of preventing progression to disease after experimental infection. However, mice have still proven useful as models of LTBI treatment and contributed directly to the development of treatment-shortening LTBI regimens used in the clinic. Grosset et al. developed a mouse model of LTBI chemotherapy in which mice are immunized with *M. bovis* BCG 4 to 6 weeks before infection with virulent *M. tuberculosis* (137). The enhanced immune response promoted by BCG immunization limits multiplication of *M. tuberculosis*, leading to a lower-burden infection with stable CFU counts over time. Unlike the more commonly used Cornell model, in which the paucibacillary state is created by treatment of mice with high doses of first-line TB drugs, the paucibacillary state of the BCG immunization model is created by the host immune response and is therefore more likely to represent the phenotypic state of bacteria in people with LTBI (138).

The BCG immunization model garnered attention after being used to demonstrate that treatment with 2 months of rifampin plus pyrazinamide (2RZ) had sterilizing activity superior to 6 months of isoniazid (139). This finding gave rise to clinical trials (140, 141) that subsequently established the efficacy of this short-course LTBI regimen that enjoyed clinical usage until being abandoned due to toxicity concerns (142). Once-weekly administration of isoniazid and rifapentine for 3 months (3HP$_{1/7}$) was later studied and shown to be at least as effective as daily administration of isoniazid for 6 months (143), a finding that was also confirmed in a large clinical trial (144).

Use of a more immunogenic recombinant BCG strain overexpressing antigen 85B and a very low aerosol challenge dose with M. tuberculosis produces a stable paucibacillary state ($\leq 10^4$ CFU) contained within compact cellular granulomas that may be even more representative of LTBI (145). This refined paucibacillary model has been validated by comparing the efficacy of five clinically recommended LTBI regimens (145, 146). The ranking of the regimens in order of increasing activity and the decreasing duration needed to cure the infection in this model are consistent with the decreasing treatment durations recommended when these regimens are used in humans (i.e., 6 to 9 months of daily isoniazid, 4 months of daily rifampin, 3 months of daily rifampin-isoniazid, 3 months of once-weekly isoniazid-rifapentine, and 2 months of daily rifampin-pyrazinamide (Table 3). Moreover, the duration of treatment necessary to prevent relapse in approximately 50% or more of mice appears to give a good general estimate of the effective treatment duration in clinical use. No other LTBI chemotherapy model, including the Cornell model, is validated in this way. Recent studies

identified other effective regimens containing new drugs in development that may be capable of treating LTBI caused by both drug-susceptible and MDR/XDR M. tuberculosis (146–148).

As species relatively resistant to M. tuberculosis infection, rabbits and non-human primates may also prove to be useful models of LTBI treatment. However, there is limited relevant experience with chemotherapy to date. Infection of rabbits with many commonly used M. tuberculosis strains results in apparent clearance of the infection (116). Infection of New Zealand white rabbits with the CDC1551 strain under conditions similar to those that cause progressive caseating disease and cavitation after HN878 strain infection also resulted in an apparently abortive infection in which the bacterial burden peaked around 4 weeks and subsequently declined, leaving few or no cultivable bacilli and only rare organized granulomas by 16 to 20 weeks postinfection (149). However, viable bacteria persisted and reactivated to cause disease upon treatment with corticosteroids (149). In contrast to the murine model, which arguably best represents the percolating or incipient disease portion of the LTBI spectrum, this rabbit model may better represent the more dormant range of the spectrum. To the author's knowledge, this rabbit model has not yet been used to study the chemotherapy of LTBI. Given the different states of infection in the murine and rabbit models, a fascinating experiment would be to compare the efficacy of isoniazid versus one or more rifamycin-containing regimens to determine how results compare to the outcomes of clinical trials. In addition to validating the model, such a comparison might shed light on the persistent question of how isoniazid, which is not believed to be active against dormant bacilli, is as effective as it is in preventing reactivation of LTBI. Beyond the absence of data indicating its predictive value, the key

Table 3 Ranking of regimens to treat latent TB infection in the paucibacillary mouse model and correspondence with clinical guidelines[a]

Regimen	Clinically recommended duration for treatment of latent TB infection (166–168)	% of mice with positive M. tuberculosis cultures 3 months after completing the indicated treatment duration (146, 148)			
		2 months	3 months	4 months	6 months
INH	9 months	100		100	100
RIF	3–4 months	100	87	**30–46**	
RIF+INH	3 months	93	54		
RPT+INH (1/7)[b]	3 months	87	47		
RIF+PZA[c]	2 months	**60**		0	

[a]For comparison purposes, treatment durations producing treatment success in ~50% of mice are in bold font. Abbreviations: INH, isoniazid; PZA, pyrazinamide; RIF, rifampin; RPT, rifapentine.
[b](1/7) indicates once weekly treatment; all other regimens are daily (5 to 7 days per week).
[c]The RIF+PZA regimen is no longer clinically recommended due to excessive hepatotoxicity (142).

challenge facing the rabbit LTBI model is the exponentially higher cost required to run the model.

As the most pathologically similar animal models of *M. tuberculosis* infection, non-human primates also could be considered the most relevant LTBI models. Roughly half of cynomolgus macaques infected with approximately 25 CFU of *M. tuberculosis* Erdman develop lung lesions representing the full LTBI spectrum within 6 to 8 months of infection. The presentations range from sterilized infection and dormant infection with no cultivable bacilli (and predominantly fibrocalcific or sclerotic granulomas), to quasi-stable, low-burden infections with 10^1 to 10^4 detectable CFU per lesion, to percolating disease with a higher bacterial load (126, 127). Spontaneous reactivation of the more dormant end of the spectrum was rare. In contrast, some percolators manifested pathologic features of active disease. Lower-dose infection may be useful to enrich for more latently infected animals, with or without as many percolators. Compared to no treatment, treatment of latently infected macaques with isoniazid for 6 months (n = 5 animals) or rifampin-isoniazid for 2 months (n = 7) prevented progression of disease after challenge with an inhibitor of TNF-α, as measured by gross pathology, bacterial burden, and dissemination scores (62).

In an interesting departure from negative results in the murine Cornell model (68), metronidazole appeared to reduce the bacterial burden after TNF-α inhibitor challenge in the same experiment (62). This result indicates the potential value of the macaque model in presenting conditions not found in mice. Unfortunately, due to toxicity concerns, it is unlikely that the efficacy of metronidazole will ever be evaluated against human LTBI to further validate the model. More recently, once-weekly isoniazid-rifapentine for 3 months appeared efficacious in a similar model using rhesus macaques, although only five animals were studied (169). As discussed for rabbits, further study of isoniazid versus various rifamycin-containing regimens in dormant versus percolating infections would again help to understand the reactivation potential of these two states and the relative merits of focusing experimental LTBI chemotherapy work on one state or the other. Study of responses to LTBI treatment also may be especially valuable for biomarker discovery to facilitate early phase 2 clinical trials evaluating new LTBI treatments since phase 3 trials require thousands of patients and many years to complete. It would also be of interest to determine whether a paucibacillary infection in marmosets could be produced by BCG immunization followed by low-dose challenge.

Citation. Nuermberger EL. 2017. Preclinical efficacy testing of new drug candidates. *Microbiol Spectrum* 5(3):TBTB2-0034-2017.

References

1. **World Health Organization.** 2016. Global tuberculosis report 2016. http://www.who.int/tb/publications/global_report/en/.

2. **Cegielski JP, Dalton T, Yagui M, Wattanaamornkiet W, Volchenkov GV, Via LE, Van Der Walt M, Tupasi T, Smith SE, Odendaal R, Leimane V, Kvasnovsky C, Kuznetsova T, Kurbatova E, Kummik T, Kuksa L, Kliiman K, Kiryanova EV, Kim H, Kim CK, Kazennyy BY, Jou R, Huang WL, Ershova J, Erokhin VV, Diem L, Contreras C, Cho SN, Chernousova LN, Chen MP, Caoili JC, Bayona J, Akksilp S, Global Preserving Effective TB Treatment Study (PETTS) Investigators.** 2014. Extensive drug resistance acquired during treatment of multidrug-resistant tuberculosis. *Clin Infect Dis* 59:1049–1063.

3. **Cegielski JP, Kurbatova E, van der Walt M, Brand J, Ershova J, Tupasi T, Caoili JC, Dalton T, Contreras C, Yagui M, Bayona J, Kvasnovsky C, Leimane V, Kuksa L, Chen MP, Via LE, Hwang SH, Wolfgang M, Volchenkov GV, Somova T, Smith SE, Akksilp S, Wattanaamornkiet W, Kim HJ, Kim CK, Kazennyy BY, Khorosheva T, Kliiman K, Viiklepp P, Jou R, Huang AS, Vasilyeva IA, Demikhova OV, Global PETTS Investigators.** 2016. Multidrug-resistant tuberculosis treatment outcomes in relation to treatment and initial versus acquired second-line drug resistance. *Clin Infect Dis* 62:418–430.

4. **Diacon AH, Pym A, Grobusch MP, de los Rios JM, Gotuzzo E, Vasilyeva I, Leimane V, Andries K, Bakare N, De Marez T, Haxaire-Theeuwes M, Lounis N, Meyvisch P, De Paepe E, van Heeswijk RP, Dannemann B, TMC207-C208 Study Group.** 2014. Multidrug-resistant tuberculosis and culture conversion with bedaquiline. *N Engl J Med* 371:723–732.

5. **Lienhardt C, Lönnroth K, Menzies D, Balasegaram M, Chakaya J, Cobelens F, Cohn J, Denkinger CM, Evans TG, Källenius G, Kaplan G, Kumar AM, Matthiessen L, Mgone CS, Mizrahi V, Mukadi YD, Nguyen VN, Nordström A, Sizemore CF, Spigelman M, Squire SB, Swaminathan S, Van Helden PD, Zumla A, Weyer K, Weil D, Raviglione M.** 2016. Translational research for tuberculosis elimination: priorities, challenges, and actions. *PLoS Med* 13:e1001965.

6. **Grosset J.** 1980. Bacteriologic basis of short-course chemotherapy for tuberculosis. *Clin Chest Med* 1:231–241.

7. **Mitchison DA.** 2000. Role of individual drugs in the chemotherapy of tuberculosis. *Int J Tuberc Lung Dis* 4:796–806.

8. **Warner DF, Mizrahi V.** 2006. Tuberculosis chemotherapy: the influence of bacillary stress and damage response pathways on drug efficacy. *Clin Microbiol Rev* 19:558–570.

9. **Torrey HL, Keren I, Via LE, Lee JS, Lewis K.** 2016. High persister mutants in *Mycobacterium tuberculosis*. *PLoS One* 11:e0155127.

10. Dorman SE, Savic RM, Goldberg S, Stout JE, Schluger N, Muzanyi G, Johnson JL, Nahid P, Hecker EJ, Heilig CM, Bozeman L, Feng PJ, Moro RN, MacKenzie W, Dooley KE, Nuermberger EL, Vernon A, Weiner M, Tuberculosis Trials Consortium. 2015. Daily rifapentine for treatment of pulmonary tuberculosis. A randomized, dose-ranging trial. *Am J Respir Crit Care Med* **191**:333–343.

11. Boeree MJ, Heinrich N, Aarnoutse R, Diacon AH, Dawson R, Rehal S, Kibiki GS, Churchyard G, Sanne I, Ntinginya NE, Minja LT, Hunt RD, Charalambous S, Hanekom M, Semvua HH, Mpagama SG, Manyama C, Mtafya B, Reither K, Wallis RS, Venter A, Narunsky K, Mekota A, Henne S, Colbers A, van Balen GP, Gillespie SH, Phillips PP, Hoelscher M, PanACEA consortium. 2017. High-dose rifampicin, moxifloxacin, and SQ109 for treating tuberculosis: a multi-arm, multi-stage randomised controlled trial. *Lancet Infect Dis* **17**:39–49.

12. Warner DF, Mizrahi V. 2014. Shortening treatment for tuberculosis: to basics. *N Engl J Med* **371**:1642–1643.

13. Bartelink IH, Zhang N, Keizer RJ, Strydom N, Converse PJ, Dooley KE, Nuermberger EL, Savic RM. A new paradigm for translational modeling to predict long-term tuberculosis treatment response. *Clin Transl Sci.* In press.

14. Lanoix JP, Chaisson RE, Nuermberger EL. 2016. Shortening tuberculosis treatment with fluoroquinolones: lost in translation? *Clin Infect Dis* **62**:484–490.

15. Nuermberger E, Sizemore C, Romero K, Hanna D. 2016. Toward an evidence-based nonclinical road map for evaluating the efficacy of new tuberculosis (TB) drug regimens: Proceedings of a Critical Path to TB Drug Regimens-National Institute of Allergy and Infectious Diseases *In Vivo* Pharmacology Workshop for TB Drug Development. *Antimicrob Agents Chemother* **60**:1177–1182.

16. Gumbo T, Lenaerts AJ, Hanna D, Romero K, Nuermberger E. 2015. Nonclinical models for antituberculosis drug development: a landscape analysis. *J Infect Dis* **211** (Suppl 3):S83–S95.

17. Dartois V. 2014. The path of anti-tuberculosis drugs: from blood to lesions to mycobacterial cells. *Nat Rev Microbiol* **12**:159–167.

18. Gumbo T, Angulo-Barturen I, Ferrer-Bazaga S. 2015. Pharmacokinetic-pharmacodynamic and dose-response relationships of antituberculosis drugs: recommendations and standards for industry and academia. *J Infect Dis* **211**(Suppl 3):S96–S106.

19. Gumbo T, Louie A, Liu W, Brown D, Ambrose PG, Bhavnani SM, Drusano GL. 2007. Isoniazid bactericidal activity and resistance emergence: integrating pharmacodynamics and pharmacogenomics to predict efficacy in different ethnic populations. *Antimicrob Agents Chemother* **51**:2329–2336.

20. Dooley KE, Mitnick CD, DeGroote MA, Obuku E, Belitsky V, Hamilton CD, Makhene M, Shah S, Brust JC, Durakovic N, Nuermberger E, Efficacy Subgroup, RESIST-TB. 2012. Old drugs, new purpose: retooling existing drugs for optimized treatment of resistant tuberculosis. *Clin Infect Dis* **55**:572–581.

21. Gumbo T, Siyambalapitiyage Dona CSW, Meek C, Leff R. 2009. Pharmacokinetics-pharmacodynamics of pyrazinamide in a novel *in vitro* model of tuberculosis for sterilizing effect: a paradigm for faster assessment of new antituberculosis drugs. *Antimicrob Agents Chemother* **53**:3197–3204.

22. Yew WW, Nuermberger E. 2013. High-dose fluoroquinolones in short-course regimens for treatment of MDR-TB: the way forward? *Int J Tuberc Lung Dis* **17**: 853–854.

23. Gumbo T, Louie A, Deziel MR, Parsons LM, Salfinger M, Drusano GL. 2004. Selection of a moxifloxacin dose that suppresses drug resistance in *Mycobacterium tuberculosis*, by use of an i pharmacodynamic infection model and mathematical modeling. *J Infect Dis* **190**: 1642–1651.

24. Srivastava S, Modongo C, Siyambalapitiyage Dona CW, Pasipanodya JG, Deshpande D, Gumbo T. 2016. Amikacin optimal exposure targets in the hollow-fiber system model of tuberculosis. *Antimicrob Agents Chemother* **60**:5922–5927.

25. Peloquin C. 2003. What is the 'right' dose of rifampin? *Int J Tuberc Lung Dis* **7**:3–5.

26. Pasipanodya JG, Srivastava S, Gumbo T. 2012. Meta-analysis of clinical studies supports the pharmacokinetic variability hypothesis for acquired drug resistance and failure of antituberculosis therapy. *Clin Infect Dis* **55**: 169–177.

27. Srivastava S, Pasipanodya JG, Meek C, Leff R, Gumbo T. 2011. Multidrug-resistant tuberculosis not due to noncompliance but to between-patient pharmacokinetic variability. *J Infect Dis* **204**:1951–1959.

28. Gumbo T, Louie A, Liu W, Ambrose PG, Bhavnani SM, Brown D, Drusano GL. 2007. Isoniazid's bactericidal activity ceases because of the emergence of resistance, not depletion of *Mycobacterium tuberculosis* in the log phase of growth. *J Infect Dis* **195**:194–201.

29. Srivastava S, Deshpande D, Pasipanodya J, Nuermberger E, Swaminathan S, Gumbo T. 2016. Optimal clinical doses of faropenem, linezolid, and moxifloxacin in children with disseminated tuberculosis: Goldilocks. *Clin Infect Dis* **63**(Suppl 3):S102–S109.

30. Ahmad Z, Peloquin CA, Singh RP, Derendorf H, Tyagi S, Ginsberg A, Grosset JH, Nuermberger EL. 2011. PA-824 exhibits time-dependent activity in a murine model of tuberculosis. *Antimicrob Agents Chemother* **55**:239–245.

31. Jayaram R, Gaonkar S, Kaur P, Suresh BL, Mahesh BN, Jayashree R, Nandi V, Bharat S, Shandil RK, Kantharaj E, Balasubramanian V. 2003. Pharmacokinetics-pharmacodynamics of rifampin in an aerosol infection model of tuberculosis. *Antimicrob Agents Chemother* **47**:2118–2124.

32. Jayaram R, Shandil RK, Gaonkar S, Kaur P, Suresh BL, Mahesh BN, Jayashree R, Nandi V, Bharath S, Kantharaj E, Balasubramanian V. 2004. Isoniazid pharmacokinetics-pharmacodynamics in an aerosol infection model of tuberculosis. *Antimicrob Agents Chemother* **48**:2951–2957.

33. Brown AN, Drusano GL, Adams JR, Rodriquez JL, Jambunathan K, Baluya DL, Brown DL, Kwara A,

Mirsalis JC, Hafner R, Louie A. 2015. Preclinical evaluations to identify optimal linezolid regimens for tuberculosis therapy. *MBio* 6:e01741-15.

34. Irwin SM, Prideaux B, Lyon ER, Zimmerman MD, Brooks EJ, Schrupp CA, Chen C, Reichlen MJ, Asay BC, Voskuil MI, Nuermberger EL, Andries K, Lyons MA, Dartois V, Lenaerts AJ. 2016. Bedaquiline and pyrazinamide treatment responses are affected by pulmonary lesion heterogeneity in *Mycobacterium tuberculosis* infected C3HeB/FeJ mice. *ACS Infect Dis* 2: 251–267.

35. Lanoix JP, Ioerger T, Ormond A, Kaya F, Sacchettini J, Dartois V, Nuermberger E. 2015. Selective inactivity of pyrazinamide against tuberculosis in C3HeB/FeJ mice is best explained by neutral pH of caseum. *Antimicrob Agents Chemother* 60:735–743.

36. Franzblau SG, DeGroote MA, Cho SH, Andries K, Nuermberger E, Orme IM, Mdluli K, Angulo-Barturen I, Dick T, Dartois V, Lenaerts AJ. 2012. Comprehensive analysis of methods used for the evaluation of compounds against *Mycobacterium tuberculosis*. *Tuberculosis (Edinb)* 92:453–488.

37. Craig WA. 1998. Pharmacokinetic/pharmacodynamic parameters: rationale for antibacterial dosing of mice and men. *Clin Infect Dis* 26:1–10, quiz 11–12.

38. Ginsburg AS, Lee J, Woolwine SC, Grosset JH, Hamzeh FM, Bishai WR. 2005. Modeling *in vivo* pharmacokinetics and pharmacodynamics of moxifloxacin therapy for *Mycobacterium tuberculosis* infection by using a novel cartridge system. *Antimicrob Agents Chemother* 49:853–856.

39. Drusano GL, Sgambati N, Eichas A, Brown DL, Kulawy R, Louie A. 2010. The combination of rifampin plus moxifloxacin is synergistic for suppression of resistance but antagonistic for cell kill of *Mycobacterium tuberculosis* as determined in a hollow-fiber infection model. *MBio* 1:e00139-10.

40. Deshpande D, Srivastava S, Pasipanodya JG, Bush SJ, Nuermberger E, Swaminathan S, Gumbo T. 2016. Linezolid for infants and toddlers with disseminated tuberculosis: first steps. *Clin Infect Dis* 63(Suppl 3):S80–S87.

41. Pasipanodya JG, Nuermberger E, Romero K, Hanna D, Gumbo T. 2015. Systematic analysis of hollow fiber model of tuberculosis experiments. *Clin Infect Dis* 61 (Suppl 1):S10–S17.

42. Rullas J, Dhar N, McKinney JD, García-Pérez A, Lelievre J, Diacon AH, Hugonnet JE, Arthur M, Angulo-Barturen I, Barros-Aguirre D, Ballell L. 2015. Combinations of β-lactam antibiotics currently in clinical trials are efficacious in a DHP-I-deficient mouse model of tuberculosis infection. *Antimicrob Agents Chemother* 59:4997–4999.

43. Gumbo T, Pasipanodya JG, Nuermberger E, Romero K, Hanna D. 2015. Correlations between the hollow fiber model of tuberculosis and therapeutic events in tuberculosis patients: learn and confirm. *Clin Infect Dis* 61 (Suppl 1):S18–S24.

44. Gumbo T, Pasipanodya JG, Romero K, Hanna D, Nuermberger E. 2015. Forecasting accuracy of the

hollow fiber model of tuberculosis for clinical therapeutic outcomes. *Clin Infect Dis* 61(Suppl 1):S25–S31.

45. Gumbo T. 2010. New susceptibility breakpoints for first-line antituberculosis drugs based on antimicrobial pharmacokinetic/pharmacodynamic science and population pharmacokinetic variability. *Antimicrob Agents Chemother* 54:1484–1491.

46. Gumbo T, Chigutsa E, Pasipanodya J, Visser M, van Helden PD, Sirgel FA, McIlleron H. 2014. The pyrazinamide susceptibility breakpoint above which combination therapy fails. *J Antimicrob Chemother* 69:2420–2425.

47. Chilukuri D, McMaster O, Bergman K, Colangelo P, Snow K, Toerner JG. 2015. The hollow fiber system model in the nonclinical evaluation of antituberculosis drug regimens. *Clin Infect Dis* 61(Suppl 1):S32–S33.

48. Cavaleri M, Manolis E. 2015. Hollow fiber system model for tuberculosis: the European Medicines Agency experience. *Clin Infect Dis* 61(Suppl 1):S1–S4.

49. European Medicines Agency. 2015. *Final qualification opinion.* http://www.ema.europa.eu/docs/en_GB/document_library/Regulatory_and_procedural_guideline/2015/02/WC500181899.pdf.

50. Canetti G. 1955. *The Tubercle Bacillus in the Pulmonary Lesion of Man.* Springer, New York, NY.

51. Hoff DR, Ryan GJ, Driver ER, Ssemakulu CC, De Groote MA, Basaraba RJ, Lenaerts AJ. 2011. Location of intra- and extracellular *M. tuberculosis* populations in lungs of mice and guinea pigs during disease progression and after drug treatment. *PLoS One* 6:e17550.

52. Irwin SM, Driver E, Lyon E, Schrupp C, Ryan G, Gonzalez-Juarrero M, Basaraba RJ, Nuermberger EL, Lenaerts AJ. 2015. Presence of multiple lesion types with vastly different microenvironments in C3HeB/FeJ mice following aerosol infection with *Mycobacterium tuberculosis*. *Dis Model Mech* 8:591–602.

53. Lanoix JP, Lenaerts AJ, Nuermberger EL. 2015. Heterogeneous disease progression and treatment response in a C3HeB/FeJ mouse model of tuberculosis. *Dis Model Mech* 8:603–610.

54. Hunter RL. 2011. Pathology of post primary tuberculosis of the lung: an illustrated critical review. *Tuberculosis (Edinb)* 91:497–509.

55. Mattila JT, Ojo OO, Kepka-Lenhart D, Marino S, Kim JH, Eum SY, Via LE, Barry CE III, Klein E, Kirschner DE, Morris SM Jr, Lin PL, Flynn JL. 2013. Microenvironments in tuberculous granulomas are delineated by distinct populations of macrophage subsets and expression of nitric oxide synthase and arginase isoforms. *J Immunol* 191:773–784.

56. Lin PL, Ford CB, Coleman MT, Myers AJ, Gawande R, Ioerger T, Sacchettini J, Fortune SM, Flynn JL. 2014. Sterilization of granulomas is common in active and latent tuberculosis despite within-host variability in bacterial killing. *Nat Med* 20:75–79.

57. Kaplan G, Post FA, Moreira AL, Wainwright H, Kreiswirth BN, Tanverdi M, Mathema B, Ramaswamy SV, Walther G, Steyn LM, Barry CE III, Bekker LG. 2003. *Mycobacterium tuberculosis* growth at the cavity surface: a microenvironment with failed immunity. *Infect Immun* 71:7099–7108.

58. Zhang Y, Permar S, Sun Z. 2002. Conditions that may affect the results of susceptibility testing of *Mycobacterium tuberculosis* to pyrazinamide. *J Med Microbiol* **51:**42–49.

59. Wayne LG, Sramek HA. 1994. Metronidazole is bactericidal to dormant cells of *Mycobacterium tuberculosis*. *Antimicrob Agents Chemother* **38:**2054–2058.

60. Driver ER, Ryan GJ, Hoff DR, Irwin SM, Basaraba RJ, Kramnik I, Lenaerts AJ. 2012. Evaluation of a mouse model of necrotic granuloma formation using C3HeB/FeJ mice for testing of drugs against *Mycobacterium tuberculosis*. *Antimicrob Agents Chemother* **56:**3181–3195.

61. Hoff DR, Caraway ML, Brooks EJ, Driver ER, Ryan GJ, Peloquin CA, Orme IM, Basaraba RJ, Lenaerts AJ. 2008. Metronidazole lacks antibacterial activity in guinea pigs infected with *Mycobacterium tuberculosis*. *Antimicrob Agents Chemother* **52:**4137–4140.

62. Lin PL, Dartois V, Johnston PJ, Janssen C, Via L, Goodwin MB, Klein E, Barry CE III, Flynn JL. 2012. Metronidazole prevents reactivation of latent *Mycobacterium tuberculosis* infection in macaques. *Proc Natl Acad Sci USA* **109:**14188–14193.

63. Via LE, Lin PL, Ray SM, Carrillo J, Allen SS, Eum SY, Taylor K, Klein E, Manjunatha U, Gonzales J, Lee EG, Park SK, Raleigh JA, Cho SN, McMurray DN, Flynn JL, Barry CE III. 2008. Tuberculous granulomas are hypoxic in guinea pigs, rabbits, and nonhuman primates. *Infect Immun* **76:**2333–2340.

64. Kjellsson MC, Via LE, Goh A, Weiner D, Low KM, Kern S, Pillai G, Barry CE III, Dartois V. 2012. Pharmacokinetic evaluation of the penetration of antituberculosis agents in rabbit pulmonary lesions. *Antimicrob Agents Chemother* **56:**446–457.

65. Prideaux B, Via LE, Zimmerman MD, Eum S, Sarathy J, O'Brien P, Chen C, Kaya F, Weiner DM, Chen PY, Song T, Lee M, Shim TS, Cho JS, Kim W, Cho SN, Olivier KN, Barry CE III, Dartois V. 2015. The association between sterilizing activity and drug distribution into tuberculosis lesions. *Nat Med* **21:**1223–1227.

66. Nuermberger E. 2008. Using animal models to develop new treatments for tuberculosis. *Semin Respir Crit Care Med* **29:**542–551.

67. Harper J, Skerry C, Davis SL, Tasneen R, Weir M, Kramnik I, Bishai WR, Pomper MG, Nuermberger EL, Jain SK. 2012. Mouse model of necrotic tuberculosis granulomas develops hypoxic lesions. *J Infect Dis* **205:**595–602.

68. Dhillon J, Allen BW, Hu YM, Coates AR, Mitchison DA. 1998. Metronidazole has no antibacterial effect in Cornell model murine tuberculosis. *Int J Tuberc Lung Dis* **2:**736–742.

69. Irwin SM, Gruppo V, Brooks E, Gilliland J, Scherman M, Reichlen MJ, Leistikow R, Kramnik I, Nuermberger EL, Voskuil MI, Lenaerts AJ. 2014. Limited activity of clofazimine as a single drug in a mouse model of tuberculosis exhibiting caseous necrotic granulomas. *Antimicrob Agents Chemother* **58:**4026–4034.

70. Williams K, Minkowski A, Amoabeng O, Peloquin CA, Taylor D, Andries K, Wallis RS, Mdluli KE, Nuermberger EL. 2012. Sterilizing activities of novel combinations lacking first- and second-line drugs in a murine model of tuberculosis. *Antimicrob Agents Chemother* **56:**3114–3120.

71. Grosset J. 1978. The sterilizing value of rifampicin and pyrazinamide in experimental short-course chemotherapy. *Bull Int Union Tuberc* **53:**5–12.

72. Gillespie SH, Crook AM, McHugh TD, Mendel CM, Meredith SK, Murray SR, Pappas F, Phillips PP, Nunn AJ, REMoxTB Consortium. 2014. Four-month moxifloxacin-based regimens for drug-sensitive tuberculosis. *N Engl J Med* **371:**1577–1587.

73. Nuermberger EL, Yoshimatsu T, Tyagi S, O'Brien RJ, Vernon AN, Chaisson RE, Bishai WR, Grosset JH. 2004. Moxifloxacin-containing regimen greatly reduces time to culture conversion in murine tuberculosis. *Am J Respir Crit Care Med* **169:**421–426.

74. Nuermberger EL, Yoshimatsu T, Tyagi S, Williams K, Rosenthal I, O'Brien RJ, Vernon AA, Chaisson RE, Bishai WR, Grosset JH. 2004. Moxifloxacin-containing regimens of reduced duration produce a stable cure in murine tuberculosis. *Am J Respir Crit Care Med* **170:**1131–1134.

75. Nuermberger E, Tyagi S, Tasneen R, Williams KN, Almeida D, Rosenthal I, Grosset JH. 2008. Powerful bactericidal and sterilizing activity of a regimen containing PA-824, moxifloxacin, and pyrazinamide in a murine model of tuberculosis. *Antimicrob Agents Chemother* **52:**1522–1524.

76. Tasneen R, Betoudji F, Tyagi S, Li SY, Williams K, Converse PJ, Dartois V, Yang T, Mendel CM, Mdluli KE, Nuermberger EL. 2015. Contribution of oxazolidinones to the efficacy of novel regimens containing bedaquiline and pretomanid in a mouse model of tuberculosis. *Antimicrob Agents Chemother* **60:**270–277.

77. Tasneen R, Li SY, Peloquin CA, Taylor D, Williams KN, Andries K, Mdluli KE, Nuermberger EL. 2011. Sterilizing activity of novel TMC207- and PA-824-containing regimens in a murine model of tuberculosis. *Antimicrob Agents Chemother* **55:**5485–5492.

78. Tasneen R, Williams K, Amoabeng O, Minkowski A, Mdluli KE, Upton AM, Nuermberger EL. 2015. Contribution of the nitroimidazoles PA-824 and TBA-354 to the activity of novel regimens in murine models of tuberculosis. *Antimicrob Agents Chemother* **59:**129–135.

79. Dawson R, Diacon AH, Everitt D, van Niekerk C, Donald PR, Burger DA, Schall R, Spigelman M, Conradie A, Eisenach K, Venter A, Ive P, Page-Shipp L, Variava E, Reither K, Ntinginya NE, Pym A, von Groote-Bidlingmaier F, Mendel CM. 2015. Efficiency and safety of the combination of moxifloxacin, pretomanid (PA-824), and pyrazinamide during the first 8 weeks of antituberculosis treatment: a phase 2b, open-label, partly randomised trial in patients with drug-susceptible or drug-resistant pulmonary tuberculosis. *Lancet* **385:**1738–1747.

80. Diacon AH, Dawson R, von Groote-Bidlingmaier F, Symons G, Venter A, Donald PR, van Niekerk C, Everitt D, Hutchings J, Burger DA, Schall R, Mendel CM. 2015. Bactericidal activity of pyrazinamide and

clofazimine alone and in combinations with pretomanid and bedaquiline. *Am J Respir Crit Care Med* **191**: 943–953.

81. Diacon AH, Dawson R, von Groote-Bidlingmaier F, Symons G, Venter A, Donald PR, van Niekerk C, Everitt D, Winter H, Becker P, Mendel CM, Spigelman MK. 2012. 14-day bactericidal activity of PA-824, bedaquiline, pyrazinamide, and moxifloxacin combinations: a randomised trial. *Lancet* **380**:986–993.

82. Gill WP, Harik NS, Whiddon MR, Liao RP, Mittler JE, Sherman DR. 2009. A replication clock for *Mycobacterium tuberculosis*. *Nat Med* **15**:211–214.

83. Medina E, North RJ. 1998. Resistance ranking of some common inbred mouse strains to *Mycobacterium tuberculosis* and relationship to major histocompatibility complex haplotype and Nramp1 genotype. *Immunology* **93**:270–274.

84. Nuermberger EL. 2011. The role of the mouse model in the evaluation of new antituberculosis drugs, p 145–152. *In* Donald PR, van Helden PD (ed), *Antituberculosis Chemotherapy*, vol 40. Karger, Basel, Switzerland.

85. Rullas J, García JI, Beltrán M, Cardona PJ, Cáceres N, García-Bustos JF, Angulo-Barturen I. 2010. Fast standardized therapeutic-efficacy assay for drug discovery against tuberculosis. *Antimicrob Agents Chemother* **54**: 2262–2264.

86. Muñoz-Elías EJ, Timm J, Botha T, Chan WT, Gomez JE, McKinney JD. 2005. Replication dynamics of *Mycobacterium tuberculosis* in chronically infected mice. *Infect Immun* **73**:546–551.

87. Canetti G. 1965. Present aspects of bacterial resistance in tuberculosis. *Am Rev Respir Dis* **92**:687–703.

88. Grosset J, Ji B. 1998. Experimental chemotherapy of mycobacterial diseases, p 51–97. *In* Gangadharam PRJ, Jenkins PA (ed), *Mycobacteria*, vol II. Chapman & Hall, New York, NY.

89. Pan H, Yan BS, Rojas M, Shebzukhov YV, Zhou H, Kobzik L, Higgins DE, Daly MJ, Bloom BR, Kramnik I. 2005. Ipr1 gene mediates innate immunity to tuberculosis. *Nature* **434**:767–772.

90. Kramnik I, Dietrich WF, Demant P, Bloom BR. 2000. Genetic control of resistance to experimental infection with virulent *Mycobacterium tuberculosis*. *Proc Natl Acad Sci USA* **97**:8560–8565.

91. Pichugin AV, Yan BS, Sloutsky A, Kobzik L, Kramnik I. 2009. Dominant role of the sst1 locus in pathogenesis of necrotizing lung granulomas during chronic tuberculosis infection and reactivation in genetically resistant hosts. *Am J Pathol* **174**:2190–2201.

92. Leu JS, Chen ML, Chang SY, Yu SL, Lin CW, Wang H, Chen WC, Chang CH, Wang JY, Lee LN, Yu CJ, Kramnik I, Yan BS. 2017. SP110b controls host immunity and susceptibility to tuberculosis. *Am J Respir Crit Care Med* **195**:369–382.

93. He X, Berland R, Mekasha S, Christensen TG, Alroy J, Kramnik I, Ingalls RR. 2013. The sst1 resistance locus regulates evasion of type I interferon signaling by *Chlamydia pneumoniae* as a disease tolerance mechanism. *PLoS Pathog* **9**:e1003569.

94. Obregón-Henao A, Arnett KA, Henao-Tamayo M, Massoudi L, Creissen E, Andries K, Lenaerts AJ, Ordway DJ. 2015. Susceptibility of *Mycobacterium abscessus* to antimycobacterial drugs in preclinical models. *Antimicrob Agents Chemother* **59**:6904–6912.

95. Ordonez AA, Tasneen R, Pokkali S, Xu Z, Converse PJ, Klunk MH, Mollura DJ, Nuermberger EL, Jain SK. 2016. Mouse model of pulmonary cavitary tuberculosis and expression of matrix metalloproteinase-9. *Dis Model Mech* **9**:779–788.

96. Lanoix JP, Betoudji F, Nuermberger E. 2015. Sterilizing activity of pyrazinamide in combination with first-line drugs in a C3HeB/FeJ mouse model of tuberculosis. *Antimicrob Agents Chemother* **60**:1091–1096.

97. Gaonkar S, Bharath S, Kumar N, Balasubramanian V, Shandil RK. 2010. Aerosol infection model of tuberculosis in wistar rats. *Int J Microbiol* **2010**:426035

98. Singhal A, Aliouat M, Hervé M, Mathys V, Kiass M, Creusy C, Delaire B, Tsenova L, Fleurisse L, Bertout J, Camacho L, Foo D, Tay HC, Siew JY, Boukhouchi W, Romano M, Mathema B, Dartois V, Kaplan G, Bifani P. 2011. Experimental tuberculosis in the Wistar rat: a model for protective immunity and control of infection. *PLoS One* **6**:e18632.

99. Kumar N, Vishwas KG, Kumar M, Reddy J, Parab M, Manikanth CL, Pavithra BS, Shandil RK. 2014. Pharmacokinetics and dose response of anti-TB drugs in rat infection model of tuberculosis. *Tuberculosis (Edinb)* **94**:282–286.

100. Chatterji M, Shandil R, Manjunatha MR, Solapure S, Ramachandran V, Kumar N, Saralaya R, Panduga V, Reddy J, Prabhakar KR, Sharma S, Sadler C, Cooper CB, Mdluli K, Iyer PS, Narayanan S, Shirude PS. 2014. 1,4-azaindole, a potential drug candidate for treatment of tuberculosis. *Antimicrob Agents Chemother* **58**: 5325–5331.

101. Elwood RL, Wilson S, Blanco JC, Yim K, Pletneva L, Nikonenko B, Samala R, Joshi S, Hemming VG, Trucksis M. 2007. The American cotton rat: a novel model for pulmonary tuberculosis. *Tuberculosis (Edinb)* **87**:145–154.

102. McFarland CT, Ly L, Jeevan A, Yamamoto T, Weeks B, Izzo A, McMurray D. 2010. BCG vaccination in the cotton rat (*Sigmodon hispidus*) infected by the pulmonary route with virulent *Mycobacterium tuberculosis*. *Tuberculosis (Edinb)* **90**:262–267.

103. Lenaerts AJ, Hoff D, Aly S, Ehlers S, Andries K, Cantarero L, Orme IM, Basaraba RJ. 2007. Location of persisting mycobacteria in a guinea pig model of tuberculosis revealed by r207910. *Antimicrob Agents Chemother* **51**:3338–3345.

104. Ahmad Z, Fraig MM, Pinn ML, Tyagi S, Nuermberger EL, Grosset JH, Karakousis PC. 2011. Effectiveness of tuberculosis chemotherapy correlates with resistance to *Mycobacterium tuberculosis* infection in animal models. *J Antimicrob Chemother* **66**:1560–1566.

105. Ahmad Z, Klinkenberg LG, Pinn ML, Fraig MM, Peloquin CA, Bishai WR, Nuermberger EL, Grosset JH, Karakousis PC. 2009. Biphasic kill curve of isoniazid reveals the presence of drug-tolerant, not drug-resistant,

Mycobacterium tuberculosis in the guinea pig. *J Infect Dis* 200:1136–1143.

106. Ahmad Z, Pinn ML, Nuermberger EL, Peloquin CA, Grosset JH, Karakousis PC. 2010. The potent bactericidal activity of streptomycin in the guinea pig model of tuberculosis ceases due to the presence of persisters. *J Antimicrob Chemother* 65:2172–2175.

107. Ahmad Z, Nuermberger EL, Tasneen R, Pinn ML, Williams KN, Peloquin CA, Grosset JH, Karakousis PC. 2010. Comparison of the 'Denver regimen' against acute tuberculosis in the mouse and guinea pig. *J Antimicrob Chemother* 65:729–734.

108. Ahmad Z, Fraig MM, Bisson GP, Nuermberger EL, Grosset JH, Karakousis PC. 2011. Dose-dependent activity of pyrazinamide in animal models of intracellular and extracellular tuberculosis infections. *Antimicrob Agents Chemother* 55:1527–1532.

109. Dutta NK, Alsultan A, Gniadek TJ, Belchis DA, Pinn ML, Mdluli KE, Nuermberger EL, Peloquin CA, Karakousis PC. 2013. Potent rifamycin-sparing regimen cures guinea pig tuberculosis as rapidly as the standard regimen. *Antimicrob Agents Chemother* 57:3910–3916.

110. Dutta NK, Illei PB, Peloquin CA, Pinn ML, Mdluli KE, Nuermberger EL, Grosset JH, Karakousis PC. 2012. Rifapentine is not more active than rifampin against chronic tuberculosis in guinea pigs. *Antimicrob Agents Chemother* 56:3726–3731.

111. Shang S, Shanley CA, Caraway ML, Orme EA, Henao-Tamayo M, Hascall-Dove L, Ackart D, Lenaerts AJ, Basaraba RJ, Orme IM, Ordway DJ. 2011. Activities of TMC207, rifampin, and pyrazinamide against *Mycobacterium tuberculosis* infection in guinea pigs. *Antimicrob Agents Chemother* 55:124–131.

112. Dorman SE, Goldberg S, Stout JE, Muzanyi G, Johnson JL, Weiner M, Bozeman L, Heilig CM, Feng PJ, Moro R, Narita M, Nahid P, Ray S, Bates E, Haile B, Nuermberger EL, Vernon A, Schluger NW, Tuberculosis Trials Consortium. 2012. Substitution of rifapentine for rifampin during intensive phase treatment of pulmonary tuberculosis: study 29 of the tuberculosis trials consortium. *J Infect Dis* 206:1030–1040.

113. Rifat DPB, Urbanowski M, Luna B, Marzinke M, Dartois V, Savic R, Bishai W, Dooley K. 2015. Penetration of rifampin and rifapentine into diseased lung in the rabbit cavity pulmonary disease model of TB, abstr 8th International Workshop on Clinical Pharmacology of Tuberculosis Drugs, San Diego, CA.

114. Savic RM, Weiner M, Mac Kenzie WR, Engle M, Whitworth WC, Johnson JL, Nsubuga P, Nahid P, Nguyen NV, Peloquin CA, Dooley KE, Dorman SE, Tuberculosis Trials Consortium of the Centers for Disease Control and Prevention. 2017. Defining the optimal dose of rifapentine for pulmonary tuberculosis: exposure-response relations from two phase 2 clinical trials. *Clin Pharmacol Ther*.

115. Converse PJ, Dannenberg AM Jr, Estep JE, Sugisaki K, Abe Y, Schofield BH, Pitt ML. 1996. Cavitary tuberculosis produced in rabbits by aerosolized virulent tubercle bacilli. *Infect Immun* 64:4776–4787.

116. Manabe YC, Dannenberg AM Jr, Tyagi SK, Hatem CL, Yoder M, Woolwine SC, Zook BC, Pitt ML, Bishai WR. 2003. Different strains of *Mycobacterium tuberculosis* cause various spectrums of disease in the rabbit model of tuberculosis. *Infect Immun* 71:6004–6011.

117. Subbian S, Tsenova L, Yang G, O'Brien P, Parsons S, Peixoto B, Taylor L, Fallows D, Kaplan G. 2011. Chronic pulmonary cavitary tuberculosis in rabbits: a failed host immune response. *Open Biol* 1:110016.

118. Nedeltchev GG, Raghunand TR, Jassal MS, Lun S, Cheng QJ, Bishai WR. 2009. Extrapulmonary dissemination of *Mycobacterium bovis* but not *Mycobacterium tuberculosis* in a bronchoscopic rabbit model of cavitary tuberculosis. *Infect Immun* 77:598–603.

119. Luna B, Kubler A, Larsson C, Foster B, Bagci U, Mollura DJ, Jain SK, Bishai WR. 2015. *In vivo* prediction of tuberculosis-associated cavity formation in rabbits. *J Infect Dis* 211:481–485.

120. Xu Z, Bagci U, Kubler A, Luna B, Jain S, Bishai WR, Mollura DJ. 2013. Computer-aided detection and quantification of cavitary tuberculosis from CT scans. *Med Phys* 40:113701.

121. Prideaux B, ElNaggar MS, Zimmerman M, Wiseman JM, Li X, Dartois V. 2015. Mass spectrometry imaging of levofloxacin distribution in TB-infected pulmonary lesions by MALDI-MSI and continuous liquid microjunction surface sampling. *Int J Mass Spectrom* 377:699–708.

122. Via LE, Savic R, Weiner DM, Zimmerman MD, Prideaux B, Irwin SM, Lyon E, O'Brien P, Gopal P, Eum S, Lee M, Lanoix JP, Dutta NK, Shim T, Cho JS, Kim W, Karakousis PC, Lenaerts A, Nuermberger E, Barry CE III, Dartois V. 2015. Host-mediated bioactivation of pyrazinamide: implications for efficacy, resistance, and therapeutic alternatives. *ACS Infect Dis* 1:203–214.

123. Prideaux B, Dartois V, Staab D, Weiner DM, Goh A, Via LE, Barry CE III, Stoeckli M. 2011. High-sensitivity MALDI-MRM-MS imaging of moxifloxacin distribution in tuberculosis-infected rabbit lungs and granulomatous lesions. *Anal Chem* 83:2112–2118.

124. Carroll MW, Jeon D, Mountz JM, Lee JD, Jeong YJ, Zia N, Lee M, Lee J, Via LE, Lee S, Eum SY, Lee SJ, Goldfeder LC, Cai Y, Jin B, Kim Y, Oh T, Chen RY, Dodd LE, Gu W, Dartois V, Park SK, Kim CT, Barry CE III, Cho SN. 2013. Efficacy and safety of metronidazole for pulmonary multidrug-resistant tuberculosis. *Antimicrob Agents Chemother* 57:3903–3909.

125. Via LE, Schimel D, Weiner DM, Dartois V, Dayao E, Cai Y, Yoon YS, Dreher MR, Kastenmayer RJ, Laymon CM, Carny JE, Flynn JL, Herscovitch P, Barry CE III. 2012. Infection dynamics and response to chemotherapy in a rabbit model of tuberculosis using [18F] 2-fluoro-deoxy-D-glucose positron emission tomography and computed tomography. *Antimicrob Agents Chemother* 56:4391–4402.

126. Capuano SV III, Croix DA, Pawar S, Zinovik A, Myers A, Lin PL, Bissel S, Fuhrman C, Klein E, Flynn JL. 2003. Experimental *Mycobacterium tuberculosis* infection of cynomolgus macaques closely resembles the

various manifestations of human *M. tuberculosis* infection. *Infect Immun* 71:5831–5844.

127. Lin PL, Rodgers M, Smith L, Bigbee M, Myers A, Bigbee C, Chiosea I, Capuano SV, Fuhrman C, Klein E, Flynn JL. 2009. Quantitative comparison of active and latent tuberculosis in the cynomolgus macaque model. *Infect Immun* 77:4631–4642.

128. Lin PL, Coleman T, Carney JP, Lopresti BJ, Tomko J, Fillmore D, Dartois V, Scanga C, Frye LJ, Janssen C, Klein E, Barry CE III, Flynn JL. 2013. Radiologic responses in cynomolgus macaques for assessing tuberculosis chemotherapy regimens. *Antimicrob Agents Chemother* 57:4237–4244.

129. Walsh GP, Tan EV, dela Cruz EC, Abalos RM, Villahermosa LG, Young LJ, Cellona RV, Narareno JB, Horwitz MA. 1996. The Philippine cynomolgus monkey (*Macaca fasicularis*) provides a new nonhuman primate model of tuberculosis that resembles human disease. *Nat Med* 2:430–436.

130. Coleman MT, Chen RY, Lee M, Lin PL, Dodd LE, Maiello P, Via LE, Kim Y, Marriner G, Dartois V, Scanga C, Janssen C, Wang J, Klein E, Cho SN, Barry CE III, Flynn JL. 2014. PET/CT imaging reveals a therapeutic response to oxazolidinones in macaques and humans with tuberculosis. *Sci Transl Med* 6:265ra167.

131. Dietze R, Hadad DJ, McGee B, Molino LP, Maciel EL, Peloquin CA, Johnson DF, Debanne SM, Eisenach K, Boom WH, Palaci M, Johnson JL. 2008. Early and extended early bactericidal activity of linezolid in pulmonary tuberculosis. *Am J Respir Crit Care Med* 178:1180–1185.

132. Furin JJ, Du Bois J, van Brakel E, Chheng P, Venter A, Peloquin CA, Alsultan A, Thiel BA, Debanne SM, Boom WH, Diacon AH, Johnson JL. 2016. Early bactericidal activity of AZD5847 in patients with pulmonary tuberculosis. *Antimicrob Agents Chemother* 60:6591–6599.

133. Via LE, Weiner DM, Schimel D, Lin PL, Dayao E, Tankersley SL, Cai Y, Coleman MT, Tomko J, Paripati P, Orandle M, Kastenmayer RJ, Tartakovsky M, Rosenthal A, Portevin D, Eum SY, Lahouar S, Gagneux S, Young DB, Flynn JL, Barry CE III. 2013. Differential virulence and disease progression following *Mycobacterium tuberculosis* complex infection of the common marmoset (*Callithrix jacchus*). *Infect Immun* 81:2909–2919.

134. Via LE, England K, Weiner DM, Schimel D, Zimmerman MD, Dayao E, Chen RY, Dodd LE, Richardson M, Robbins KK, Cai Y, Hammoud D, Herscovitch P, Dartois V, Flynn JL, Barry CE III. 2015. A sterilizing tuberculosis treatment regimen is associated with faster clearance of bacteria in cavitary lesions in marmosets. *Antimicrob Agents Chemother* 59:4181–4189.

135. Dye C, Glaziou P, Floyd K, Raviglione M. 2013. Prospects for tuberculosis elimination. *Annu Rev Public Health* 34:271–286.

136. Barry CE III, Boshoff HI, Dartois V, Dick T, Ehrt S, Flynn J, Schnappinger D, Wilkinson RJ, Young D. 2009. The spectrum of latent tuberculosis: rethinking the biology and intervention strategies. *Nat Rev Microbiol* 7:845–855.

137. Lecoeur HF, Lagrange PH, Truffot-Pernot C, Gheorghiu M, Grosset J. 1989. Relapses after stopping chemotherapy for experimental tuberculosis in genetically resistant and susceptible strains of mice. *Clin Exp Immunol* 76:458–462.

138. Nuermberger EL, Yoshimatsu T, Tyagi S, Bishai WR, Grosset JH. 2004. Paucibacillary tuberculosis in mice after prior aerosol immunization with *Mycobacterium bovis* BCG. *Infect Immun* 72:1065–1071.

139. Lecoeur HF, Truffot-Pernot C, Grosset JH. 1989. Experimental short-course preventive therapy of tuberculosis with rifampin and pyrazinamide. *Am Rev Respir Dis* 140:1189–1193.

140. Gordin F, Chaisson RE, Matts JP, Miller C, de Lourdes Garcia M, Hafner R, Valdespino JL, Coberly J, Schechter M, Klukowicz AJ, Barry MA, O'Brien RJ. 2000. Rifampin and pyrazinamide vs isoniazid for prevention of tuberculosis in HIV-infected persons: an international randomized trial. *JAMA* 283:1445–1450.

141. Halsey NA, Coberly JS, Desormeaux J, Losikoff P, Atkinson J, Moulton LH, Contave M, Johnson M, Davis H, Geiter L, Johnson E, Huebner R, Boulos R, Chaisson RE. 1998. Randomised trial of isoniazid versus rifampicin and pyrazinamide for prevention of tuberculosis in HIV-1 infection. *Lancet* 351:786–792.

142. Centers for Disease Control and Prevention (CDC), American Thoracic Society. 2003. Update: adverse event data and revised American Thoracic Society/CDC recommendations against the use of rifampin and pyrazinamide for treatment of latent tuberculosis infection–United States, 2003. *MMWR Morb Mortal Wkly Rep* 52:735–739.

143. Nuermberger E, Tyagi S, Williams KN, Rosenthal I, Bishai WR, Grosset JH. 2005. Rifapentine, moxifloxacin, or DNA vaccine improves treatment of latent tuberculosis in a mouse model. *Am J Respir Crit Care Med* 172:1452–1456.

144. Sterling TR, Scott NA, Miro JM, Calvet G, La Rosa A, Infante R, Chen MP, Benator DA, Gordin F, Benson CA, Chaisson RE, Villarino ME, Tuberculosis Trials Consortium, the AIDS Clinical Trials Group for the PREVENT TB Trial (TBTC Study 26ACTG 5259). 2016. Three months of weekly rifapentine and isoniazid for treatment of *Mycobacterium tuberculosis* infection in HIV-coinfected persons. *AIDS* 30:1607–1615.

145. Zhang T, Zhang M, Rosenthal IM, Grosset JH, Nuermberger EL. 2009. Short-course therapy with daily rifapentine in a murine model of latent tuberculosis infection. *Am J Respir Crit Care Med* 180:1151–1157.

146. Zhang T, Li SY, Williams KN, Andries K, Nuermberger EL. 2011. Short-course chemotherapy with TMC207 and rifapentine in a murine model of latent tuberculosis infection. *Am J Respir Crit Care Med* 184:732–737.

147. Lanoix JP, Betoudji F, Nuermberger E. 2014. Novel regimens identified in mice for treatment of latent tuberculosis infection in contacts of patients with multidrug-resistant tuberculosis. *Antimicrob Agents Chemother* 58:2316–2321.

148. Dutta NK, Illei PB, Jain SK, Karakousis PC. 2014. Characterization of a novel necrotic granuloma model

of latent tuberculosis infection and reactivation in mice. *Am J Pathol* **184:**2045–2055.

149. Subbian S, Tsenova L, O'Brien P, Yang G, Kushner NL, Parsons S, Peixoto B, Fallows D, Kaplan G. 2012. Spontaneous latency in a rabbit model of pulmonary tuberculosis. *Am J Pathol* **181:**1711–1724.

150. Cynamon MH, Zhang Y, Harpster T, Cheng S, DeStefano MS. 1999. High-dose isoniazid therapy for isoniazid-resistant murine *Mycobacterium tuberculosis* infection. *Antimicrob Agents Chemother* **43:**2922–2924.

151. Almeida D, Nuermberger E, Tasneen R, Rosenthal I, Tyagi S, Williams K, Peloquin C, Grosset J. 2009. Paradoxical effect of isoniazid on the activity of rifampin-pyrazinamide combination in a mouse model of tuberculosis. *Antimicrob Agents Chemother* **53:**4178–4184.

152. de Steenwinkel JE, Aarnoutse RE, de Knegt GJ, ten Kate MT, Teulen M, Verbrugh HA, Boeree MJ, van Soolingen D, Bakker-Woudenberg IA. 2013. Optimization of the rifampin dosage to improve the therapeutic efficacy in tuberculosis treatment using a murine model. *Am J Respir Crit Care Med* **187:**1127–1134.

153. Rosenthal IM, Tasneen R, Peloquin CA, Zhang M, Almeida D, Mdluli KE, Karakousis PC, Grosset JH, Nuermberger EL. 2012. Dose-ranging comparison of rifampin and rifapentine in two pathologically distinct murine models of tuberculosis. *Antimicrob Agents Chemother* **56:**4331–4340.

154. Lenaerts AM, Chase SE, Chmielewski AJ, Cynamon MH. 1999. Evaluation of rifapentine in long-term treatment regimens for tuberculosis in mice. *Antimicrob Agents Chemother* **43:**2356–2360.

155. Rosenthal IM, Zhang M, Williams KN, Peloquin CA, Tyagi S, Vernon AA, Bishai WR, Chaisson RE, Grosset JH, Nuermberger EL. 2007. Daily dosing of rifapentine cures tuberculosis in three months or less in the murine model. *PLoS Med* **4:**e344.

156. Rosenthal IM, Zhang M, Almeida D, Grosset JH, Nuermberger EL. 2008. Isoniazid or moxifloxacin in rifapentine-based regimens for experimental tuberculosis? *Am J Respir Crit Care Med* **178:**989–993.

157. Li SY, Irwin SM, Converse PJ, Mdluli KE, Lenaerts AJ, Nuermberger EL. 2015. Evaluation of moxifloxacin-containing regimens in pathologically distinct murine tuberculosis models. *Antimicrob Agents Chemother* **59:**4026–4030.

158. De Groote MA, Gilliland JC, Wells CL, Brooks EJ, Woolhiser LK, Gruppo V, Peloquin CA, Orme IM, Lenaerts AJ. 2011. Comparative studies evaluating mouse models used for efficacy testing of experimental drugs against *Mycobacterium tuberculosis*. *Antimicrob Agents Chemother* **55:**1237–1247.

159. Fillion A, Aubry A, Brossier F, Chauffour A, Jarlier V, Veziris N. 2013. Impact of fluoroquinolone resistance on bactericidal and sterilizing activity of a moxifloxacin-containing regimen in murine tuberculosis. *Antimicrob Agents Chemother* **57:**4496–4500.

160. Poissy J, Aubry A, Fernandez C, Lott MC, Chauffour A, Jarlier V, Farinotti R, Veziris N. 2010. Should moxifloxacin be used for the treatment of extensively drug-resistant tuberculosis? An answer from a murine model. *Antimicrob Agents Chemother* **54:**4765–4771.

161. Veziris N, Truffot-Pernot C, Aubry A, Jarlier V, Lounis N. 2003. Fluoroquinolone-containing third-line regimen against *Mycobacterium tuberculosis in vivo*. *Antimicrob Agents Chemother* **47:**3117–3122.

162. Ahmad Z, Tyagi S, Minkowski A, Peloquin CA, Grosset JH, Nuermberger EL. 2013. Contribution of moxifloxacin or levofloxacin in second-line regimens with or without continuation of pyrazinamide in murine tuberculosis. *Am J Respir Crit Care Med* **188:**97–102.

163. Ji B, Lounis N, Truffot-Pernot C, Grosset J. 1995. *In vitro* and *in vivo* activities of levofloxacin against *Mycobacterium tuberculosis*. *Antimicrob Agents Chemother* **39:**1341–1344.

164. Grosset JH, Tyagi S, Almeida DV, Converse PJ, Li SY, Ammerman NC, Bishai WR, Enarson D, Trébucq A. 2013. Assessment of clofazimine activity in a second-line regimen for tuberculosis in mice. *Am J Respir Crit Care Med* **188:**608–612.

165. Williams KN, Stover CK, Zhu T, Tasneen R, Tyagi S, Grosset JH, Nuermberger E. 2009. Promising antituberculosis activity of the oxazolidinone PNU-100480 relative to that of linezolid in a murine model. *Antimicrob Agents Chemother* **53:**1314–1319.

166. American Thoracic Society, Centers for Disease Control. 2000. Targeted tuberculin testing and treatment of latent tuberculosis infection. *MMWR Recommend Rep* **49(RR-6):**1–51.

167. Centers for Disease Control and Prevention (CDC). 2011. Recommendations for use of an isoniazid-rifapentine regimen with direct observation to treat latent *Mycobacterium tuberculosis* infection. *MMWR Morb Mortal Wkly Rep* **60:**1650–1653.

168. World Health Organization. 2015. *Guidelines on the Management of Latent Tuberculosis Infection*. World Health Organization, Geneva, Switzerland.

169. Blumberg H. 2016. Rifpentine plus isoniazid eradicates *Mycobacterium tuberculosis* among rhesus macaques with latent TB infection. Abstr 9th International Workshop on Clinical Pharmacology of Tuberculosis Drugs, Liverpool, UK, 24 October 2016.

Tuberculosis and the Tubercle Bacillus, 2nd ed.
Edited by William R. Jacobs, Jr., Helen McShane, Valerie Mizrahi, and Ian M. Orme
© 2018 American Society for Microbiology, Washington, DC
doi:10.1128/microbiolspec.TBTB2-0014-2016

Oxidative Phosphorylation as a Target Space for Tuberculosis: Success, Caution, and Future Directions

14

Gregory M. Cook,[1,2] Kiel Hards,[1] Elyse Dunn,[1] Adam Heikal,[1,2]
Yoshio Nakatani,[1,2] Chris Greening,[3,4] Dean C. Crick,[5]
Fabio L. Fontes,[5] Kevin Pethe,[6] Erik Hasenoehrl,[7] and Michael Berney[7]

OVERVIEW OF RESPIRATION AND OXIDATIVE PHOSPHORYLATION IN *MYCOBACTERIUM TUBERCULOSIS*

The genus *Mycobacterium* comprises a group of obligately aerobic bacteria that have adapted to inhabit a wide range of intracellular and extracellular environments. Fundamental to this adaptation is the ability to respire and generate energy from variable sources and to sustain metabolism in the absence of growth. The pioneering work of Brodie and colleagues on *Mycobacterium phlei* established much of the primary information on the electron transport chain and oxidative phosphorylation system in mycobacteria (reviewed in 1). Mycobacteria can only generate sufficient energy for growth by coupling the oxidation of electron donors derived from organic carbon catabolism (e.g., NADH, succinate, malate) to the reduction of O_2 as a terminal electron acceptor. Mycobacterial genome sequencing revealed that branched pathways exist in mycobacterial species for electron transfer from many low-potential reductants, via quinol, to oxygen (Fig. 1).

During aerobic growth, electrons are transferred to oxygen via two terminal respiratory oxidases: an aa_3-type cytochrome *c* oxidase (encoded by *ctaBCDE*) belonging to the heme-copper respiratory oxidase family and cytochrome *bd*-type menaquinol oxidase (*cydABCD*) (Fig. 1). Despite the acknowledged importance of oxy-gen in the physiology and pathobiology of *M. tuberculosis*, the molecular mechanisms governing the regulation of terminal oxidase expression remain largely unknown. In the absence of oxygen, mycobacterial growth is inhibited, even if alternative electron acceptors are present (e.g., nitrate, fumarate). Despite growth being inhibited, mycobacteria are able to metabolize exogenous and endogenous energy sources under low oxygen for maintenance functions. The electron acceptors and mechanisms to recycle reducing equivalents under these conditions are poorly understood. ATP synthesis is obligatorily coupled to the electron transport chain and the F_1F_0-ATP synthase, irrespective of the oxygen concentration or the proton motive force (PMF), but the reasons for this remain unexplained. The aim of this review is to discuss the progress in understanding the role of energetic targets in mycobacterial physiology and pathogenesis and the opportunities for drug discovery.

TARGETING THE PMF IN *M. TUBERCULOSIS*

All bacteria require a PMF to grow and remain viable under replicating and nonreplicating conditions. During respiration, energy is conserved by the generation of a PMF across a proton-impermeable membrane. The PMF (electrochemical potential) consists of two

[1]University of Otago, Department of Microbiology and Immunology, Otago School of Medical Sciences, Dunedin, New Zealand; [2]Maurice Wilkins Center for Molecular Biodiscovery, The University of Auckland, Auckland 1042, New Zealand; [3]The Commonwealth Scientific and Industrial Research Organization, Land and Water Flagship, Acton ACT, Australia; [4]Monash University, School of Biological Sciences, Clayton VIC, Australia; [5]Colorado State University, Department of Microbiology, Immunology, and Pathology, Fort Collins, CO 80523; [6]Lee Kong Chian School of Medicine, Nanyang Technological University, Singapore; [7]Albert Einstein School of Medicine, Department of Microbiology and Immunology, Bronx, NY 10461.

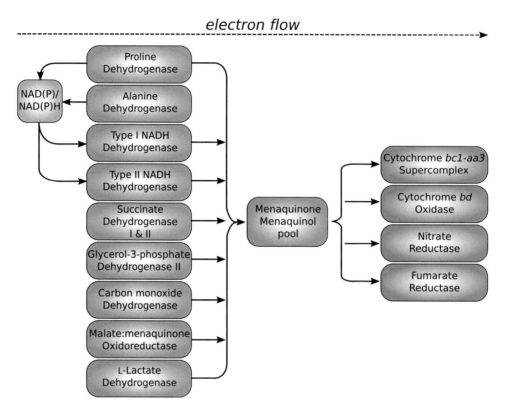

Figure 1 Generalized schematic overview of relevant electron transfer components of *M. tuberculosis*. Complexes indicated in blue oxidize various substrates to reduce quinones. The resulting (mena)quinol molecules (orange) can be oxidized to result in reduction of various terminal electron acceptors, mediated by the complexes shown in purple.

gradients: an electrical potential ($\Delta\psi$), due to the charge separation across the membrane (positive$_{outside}$/negative$_{inside}$), and a chemical transmembrane gradient of protons (ΔpH, acidic$_{outside}$/alkaline$_{inside}$) (Fig. 2). At neutral pH, the PMF is predominantly in the form of a $\Delta\psi$, but as the external pH drops, the ΔpH increases and the $\Delta\psi$ decreases to maintain a constant PMF. Dissipation of the PMF leads to a rapid loss of cell viability and cell death.

A variety of mechanisms are used to generate the PMF in mycobacteria (Fig. 2). Mycobacteria generally grow at neutral pH and under these conditions generate a PMF of approximately −180 mV (2). Under hypoxia, *M. tuberculosis* generates a total PMF of −113 mV (−73 mV of $\Delta\psi$ and −41 mV of ZΔpH) (3). In obligately aerobic bacteria like *M. tuberculosis*, the generation of a PMF is mediated primarily by the proton-pumping components of the electron transport chain (Fig. 2, mechanism 3). As oxygen becomes limiting for growth, many bacterial pathogens switch to alternative electron acceptors (e.g., nitrate, fumarate), and proton release is coupled to a terminal reductase (e.g., nitrate reductase) via a PMF redox loop mecha-

nism (4) (Fig. 2, mechanism 2). *M. tuberculosis* harbors both nitrate reductase and fumarate reductase, but few direct experimental data have accumulated to suggest that they contribute to PMF generation under hypoxia. The membrane-bound F_1F_0-ATP synthase can usually operate as a reversible ATP-driven proton pump to generate the PMF (5). However, in *M. tuberculosis* the enzyme shows extreme latency in the hydrolysis reaction (6). End-product (e.g., lactate) efflux can generate a PMF (7) (Fig. 2, mechanism 1), and it has been proposed that fumarate may be used as a mechanism to generate succinate as an excreted end product for maintenance of the membrane potential, under hypoxia, in *M. tuberculosis* (8).

A number of compounds target the PMF in bacteria (Fig. 3A), including agents that inhibit the major proton pumps (e.g., rotenone) and those that facilitate proton transport through the cytoplasmic membrane (protonophores, e.g., CCCP). The majority of protonophores are nonspecific and functional in both prokaryotic and eukaryotic cell membranes. Individual components of the PMF can be collapsed using specific inhibitors. For example, the membrane potential can be collapsed by

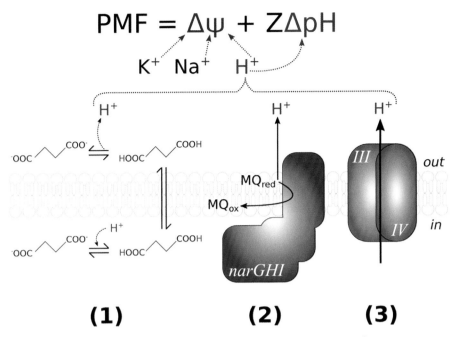

$$PMF = \Delta\psi + Z\Delta pH$$

Figure 2   Mechanisms by which a proton motive (membrane potential [$\Delta\psi$] + transmembrane pH gradient [$Z\Delta pH$]) force can be generated in mycobacteria. (**1**) Cotransport of protons driven by solute (succinate) symport into the periplasm. (**2**) Redox-loop separation of charge; (mena)quinol oxidation results in proton release into the periplasm by virtue of (mena)quinol site proximity to the periplasm, while electrons are transferred to reduce a terminal electron acceptor (e.g., nitrate, fumarate) in the cytoplasm that results in neutralization of charge. (**3**) Proton translocation mediated by primary proton-pumping complexes (bc_1-aa_3 supercomplex).

compounds that catalyze electrogenic cation transport across the cell membrane (e.g., valinomycin) (Fig. 3a). Valinomycin is a dodecaepsipeptide that forms a macrocyclic molecule allowing for rapid K^+ movement down its electrochemical gradient. The chemical transmembrane gradient of protons (ΔpH) can be collapsed by nigericin through its K^+/H^+ antiporter (electroneutral) activity (Fig. 3a). Growth of mycobacteria is sensitive to compounds that dissipate the membrane potential (e.g., protonophores and valinomycin), and these compounds are bactericidal toward growing and nongrowing (aerobic or hypoxic) cells, further highlighting the importance of the membrane potential in mycobacterial viability (2, 3). Rao et al. (3) have reported that thioridazine, a compound purported to target NDH-2, results in dissipation of the $\Delta\psi$ and significant cell death. They suggested that NADH is an important electron donor for the generation of the $\Delta\psi$ under hypoxic conditions. Inhibitors of succinate dehydrogenase (SDH) (e.g., 3-propionate) are also able to dissipate the $\Delta\psi$ under hypoxia, suggesting that SDH is an important generator of the $\Delta\psi$ under hypoxia (9).

As the external pH of the growth medium changes and becomes mildly acidic, mycobacteria are able to generate a considerable transmembrane pH gradient ($Z\Delta pH$) and maintain a constant PMF (2). While proton translocation via the respiratory chain generates the PMF, during respiration with oxygen as the terminal electron acceptor, it is not clear how the PMF is established in the absence of oxygen under microaerobic growth conditions. Anaerobic bacteria are able to generate a significant PMF (-100 mV) using their membrane-bound F_1F_0-ATP synthase in the ATP hydrolysis direction (5). The ATPase activity (proton-pumping) of the enzyme is fueled by ATP produced by substrate-level phosphorylation. This mechanism does not appear to operate in mycobacterial cells where the F_1F_0-ATP synthase has been reported to have latent ATPase activity when measured in inverted membrane vesicles (6, 10). Whether the enzyme is also latent in actively growing cells is not known, and therefore the potential does exist for this enzyme to function as a primary proton pump in the absence of oxygen and a functional respiratory chain to generate the PMF. The mechanisms controlling this extreme latency in the ATP hydrolysis direction are an area that could unlock new avenues for drug development and requires further investigation at a molecular and structural level.

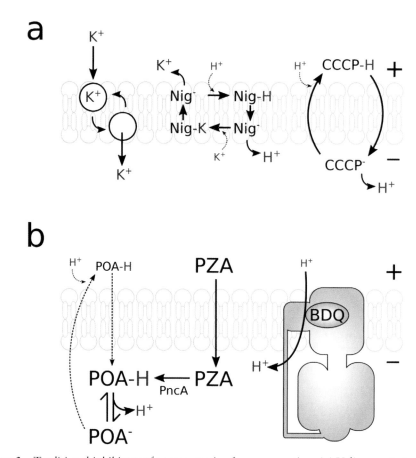

Figure 3 Traditional inhibitors of proton motive force generation. (**a**) Valinomycin is an ionophore, selective for potassium ions, which equilibrates the potassium gradient—dissipating the $\Delta\psi$ (electrogenic). Nigericin is a hydrophobic weak carboxylic acid which can traverse the membrane as its either protonated acid or neutral salt. It dissipates chemical gradients (i.e., ΔpH) but maintains the charge (one positive charge exchanged for one positive charge—electroneutral) (3). Carbonyl cyanide m-chlorophenyl hydrazine (CCCP) is an electrogenic protonophore. CCCP$^-$ is driven to the periplasm by the $\Delta\psi$, while CCCPH is driven to the cytoplasm by the ΔpH. It can equilibrate both $\Delta\psi$ and ΔpH. (**b**) Model for uncoupling by either pyrazinamide (PZA) or BDQ. (Left side) PZA diffuses into the cell and is converted to pyrazinoic acid (POA) by PncA (pyrazinamidase). Anionic POA could effectively inhibit growth through anion accumulation in the neutral pH of the cytoplasm and/or efflux from the cells to become protonated in the acidic extracellular environment (POA-H). POA-H would then diffuse back into the cell driven by the ΔpH gradient and dissociate in the cytoplasm (neutral pH), leading to intracellular acidification and cell death. (Right side) In a typical mycobacterial cell, the majority of ATP synthesis is respiratory, driven by the PMF. The binding of BDQ to the c-ring most likely perturbs the a-c subunit interface, causing an uncontrolled proton leak uncoupled from ATP synthesis and resulting in a futile proton cycle. Compensation by the exchange of other cations (i.e., K$^+$) would allow the process to remain electroneutral.

The clinically approved antimycobacterial bedaquiline (Sirturo, TMC207) is a potent nanomolar inhibitor of the mycobacterial F_1F_0-ATP synthase that binds to the enzyme's oligomeric c-ring to inhibit ATP synthesis (11–16). We have recently reported that bedaquiline activates respiration and is a potent uncoupler of respiration-driven ATP synthesis in mycobacteria (17). However, unlike classical uncouplers/protonophores, bedaquiline does not translocate protons *per se* but perturbs respiration by binding to F_0 (oligomeric c-ring) of the ATP synthase, likely disrupting the subunit a-c subunit interface in F_0, thereby uncoupling proton flow from ATP synthesis by the F_1F_0-ATP synthase (Fig. 3b). This uncoupling is electroneutral, consistent with no observed change in the membrane potential. Feng et al. (18) further demonstrated the potential of targeting the

PMF of *M. tuberculosis* and reported that a number of tuberculosis (TB) drugs (e.g., clofazimine, bedaquiline [BDQ], SQ109) are active uncouplers of the PMF in addition to binding to enzyme targets, highlighting the multitargeting nature of these molecules.

M. tuberculosis encounters acidic microenvironments in the host and must maintain its intracellular pH homeostasis to survive. Compounds that dissipate the transmembrane pH gradient lead to a rapid loss in cell viability at acidic pH and the lethal intracellular pH for mycobacterial species in the pH range of 5.5 to 6 (2). To address pH homeostasis as a drug target, Nathan and colleagues developed a whole-cell screen to identify compounds that dissipate the ΔpH gradient in *M. tuberculosis* (19). This study identified a number of candidate molecules, including PZA, that disrupted intracellular pH homeostasis and caused cell killing (loss of viability), highlighting this as a potential pathway for drug development (19) (Fig. 3b).

TARGETING PRIMARY DEHYDROGENASES IN *M. TUBERCULOSIS*: THE UNTAPPED SOURCE OF METABOLIC DRUG DISCOVERY

M. tuberculosis encodes several primary dehydrogenases that serve as direct reductants for electron transport (Fig. 1). Many of these have attractive properties for drug development, such as essentiality or lack of presence in the human genome. Unfortunately, the unifying feature of these enzymes is a paucity of information regarding their physiological and biochemical roles. Increasing our understanding of these processes will likely reveal mechanisms to perturb the viability within, and reactivation from, dormant mycobacteria.

NADH:Menaquinone Oxidoreductases

M. tuberculosis possesses two classes of NADH: menaquinone oxidoreductase to couple the oxidation of NADH from central metabolism to energize the electron transport chain (20) (Fig. 1). Like mitochondria, *M. tuberculosis* harbors a proton-pumping type I NADH dehydrogenase complex (NDH-1, complex I) that transfers electrons to menaquinone, conserving energy by translocating protons across the membrane to generate a PMF (Fig. 1 and Fig. 2). In *M. tuberculosis*, the *nuo* operon is not essential for either growth or persistence in an *in vitro* Wayne model (3). Moreover, the *nuo* operon has been lost from the genome of the intracellular parasite *Mycobacterium leprae* except for a single remaining *nuoN* pseudogene (21). These data suggest that NDH-1 does not represent a compelling target for drug development. However, *M. tuberculosis* mutants

lacking the NDH-1 subunit *nuoG* had reduced virulence in mice (22). There is evidence that *nuoG* and potentially other subunits of NDH-1 are antiapoptosis factors and are indeed potential candidates for vaccine development.

The second class of NADH:menaquinone oxidoreductase is the non-proton translocating type II NADH dehydrogenase (NDH-2) that does not conserve energy (Fig. 1). NDH-2 is a small monotopic membrane protein (50 to 60 kDa) that catalyzes electron transfer from NADH via FAD (noncovalently bound redox prosthetic group) to quinone. *M. tuberculosis* harbors two copies of NDH-2 (*ndh* Rv1854c and *ndhA* Rv0392c) (20), which are well conserved among slow-growing mycobacterial species. In *M. tuberculosis*, Ndh (1,392 bp) and NdhA (1,413 bp) share 65% identity, and the FAD- and NADH-binding motifs are highly conserved. The Ndh and NdhA proteins of *M. tuberculosis* have been shown to be functional NADH dehydrogenases that transfer electrons to the quinone pool via a two-site ping-pong reaction mechanism (23, 24). Several studies have suggested that *ndh* is essential for growth of *M. tuberculosis* (20, 25, 26), but the reasons for this essentiality remain unknown.

Unlike NDH-1, NDH-2 has not been reported in mammalian mitochondria, leading to the proposal that NDH-2 may represent a potential drug target for TB. Several antimycobacterial compounds have been reported to target NDH-2 (3, 20, 23, 27–30) (Fig. 4). For example, drugs of the phenothiazine family (e.g., thioridazine, trifluoperazine, chlorpromazine) have potent activity *in vitro* against drug-susceptible and drug-resistant *M. tuberculosis* strains (31, 32) and show activity in a mouse model of pulmonary TB (20). However, the levels of phenothiazines required for antitubercular activity (>0.5 mg/liter of plasma) appear to be clinically unachievable in patients (33); the development of phenothiazines as antitubercular drugs is currently limited by the wide range of potentially serious off-target effects displayed during use, including cognitive effects in the central nervous system at concentrations lower than their antimycobacterial activity (34). In contrast to the phenothiazines, quinolinyl pyrimidines inhibit NDH-2 from *M. tuberculosis* in the nanomolar range and show no toxicity to the eukaryotic organism *Saccharomyces cerevisiae*, and no membrane disruption activity in a red blood cell hemolysis assay (30). The high potency and preliminary lack of toxicity against higher-order species are promising. Scopafungin, gramicidin S, and polymyxin B have been identified as inhibitors of *Mycobacterium smegmatis* NDH-2, and further work with *M. tuberculosis*

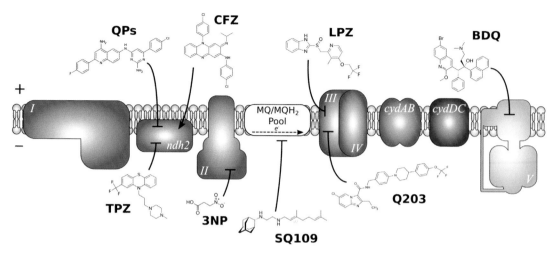

Figure 4   Inhibitors of the electron transport chain and F_1F_0-ATP synthase of *M. tuberculosis*. Selected inhibitors of these complexes are indicated with flathead arrows and do not reflect the binding site of the inhibitors. Abbreviations: QPs, quinolinyl pyrimidines; TPZ, trifluoperazine; CFZ, clofazimine; 3-NP, 3-nitropropionate; SQ109, *N*-adamantan-2-yl-*N*´-((*E*)-3,7-dimethyl-octa-2,6-dienyl)-ethane-1,2-diamine; LPZ, lansoprazole; Q203, imidazopyridine amide; BDQ, bedaquiline.

is needed to determine their efficacy against the pathogen (35, 36).

Mode of action studies are required to understand how NDH-2 inhibitors work at a molecular and structural level and why inhibition of NDH-2 activity leads to cell death. Yano et al. (37) have shown that clofazimine (CFZ), a long-standing clinical drug for leprosy, is a redox-active (phenazine derivative) prodrug activated by NDH-2. The authors proposed a model in which the drug inhibits the growth of mycobacteria by a redox cycling pathway involving the enzymatic reduction of CFZ by NDH-2 followed by nonenzymatic reoxidation of CFZ by O_2, leading to the production of toxic reactive oxygen species (37). Hartkoorn et al. (38) reported that CFZ-resistant mutants of *M. tuberculosis* map to the transcriptional regulator *Rv0678*, leading to the upregulation of the multisubstrate efflux pump, MmpL5. The authors showed that CFZ-resistant mutants are cross-resistant to bedaquiline, suggesting a common mechanism of resistance (38). In slow- and fast-growing mycobacterial species, reduction in NDH-2 activity has been linked to isoniazid and ethambutol resistance (39). Taken together, these studies suggest that the development of NDH-2 inhibitors will need to determine what effect these compounds have on current drug therapy regimens, particularly in regard to the development of cross-resistance.

Structure-aided drug design against NDH-2 is now possible with the first high-resolution bacterial structures published (40, 41). The bacterial NDH-2 structure reveals a homodimeric organization and localization to the cytoplasmic membrane by the membrane-anchoring domain highlighted with two amphipathic C-terminal helices (40, 41). Unique binding sites for quinone and NADH sites were also proposed, allowing concomitant oxidation of NADH from the cytoplasm with reduction of quinone from the membrane, with the ability of both substrates to access the FAD cofactor sequentially (40). This implies that NDH-2 harbors two potential drug target sites, and both warrant investigation. Most common structure-based drug design approaches rely on the protein-ligand complex structure model (42). The ligand-complex structures have been solved for both yeast (43) and bacterial NDH-2 (Y. Nakatani, unpublished data), allowing for the rational design of small inhibitor molecules targeting the NADH-binding site, and with further quinone-ligand structures, the quinone-binding site.

Succinate:Quinone Oxidoreductase: A Chink in the Carbon-Metabolic Armor

Succinate dehydrogenase (SDH), or complex II (Fig. 1), enzymes are well known for their role in the citric acid cycle. They couple the oxidation of succinate to the reduction of quinone via both FAD and heme cofactors (44), thereby playing important roles in both carbon metabolism and PMF generation. *M. tuberculosis* encodes two SDH enzymes (*sdh1*, *Rv0249c-Rv0247c*; *sdh2*, *Rv3316-Rv3319*), as well as a separate fumarate reductase with possible bidirectional behavior. It is unprecedented in the current literature for an organism to encode three functionally redundant enzymes for this reaction, which complicates both physiological analysis and drug design. Furthermore, while a vast amount of literature exists regarding the SDHs of *Escherichia coli* and mitochondria, the SDHs encoded by mycobacteria have distinct phylogeny, prosthetic groups, and predicted biochemistry (9, 45). Despite these challenges, using SDHs as drug targets remains promising, because succinate is a major focal point in both the central carbon metabolism and respiratory chain of *M. tuberculosis*. The bacilli must find a way to drive the endergonic oxidation of succinate (E_m = +113 mV versus E_m = −74 for menaquinone): a reaction required for generating a membrane potential under hypoxia (9) and maintaining the balance of menaquinone:menaquinol (46). Under hypoxia, succinate can be electronically secreted or stored until a suitable electron acceptor is accessed (47). The versatility of succinate therefore suggests that disrupting its oxidation may result in clinically advantageous outcomes: inhibitors may have primary lethality, force a premature exit from nonreplicating persistence, or compromise bacilli reactivation, depending on which aspect of succinate metabolism is affected by modulating SDH activity.

Drug development targeting SDH enzymes will need to consider how to achieve selectivity for the multiple *M. tuberculosis* enzymes without off-target effects on human counterparts. Fortunately, several key differences between these homologues exist within the hydrophobic, menaquinone-binding portion of the complex. Enzymes are classified as types A to E according to their heme content and number of transmembrane subunits (45, 48). Sdh2 is a type A enzyme (two subunits, two hemes) (49), while Sdh1 was proposed to be similar to the *Bacillus*-like type B enzymes (one subunit, two hemes) (9). The mammalian SDH and *M. tuberculosis* fumarate reductase are of different types (types C and D, respectively), and thus are different in terms of electron transfer and menaquinone reduction. It follows that compounds targeting the hydrophobic subunits of SDH are ideally suited for achieving selective inhibition.

There have been no reported screens for inhibitors of mycobacterial SDH activity. A commonly used inhibitor of SDH is 3-nitropropionate, targeting the A subunit (50, 51), which has been reported to inhibit mycobacterial SDHs (9, 47). However, inhibitors developed against the dicarboxylate-binding site are likely to also inhibit mitochondrial SDH due to high A subunit similarity, and hence this is likely to be a poor direction for lead candidate identification. Despite this, routine inhibitors such as the A subunit-targeting carboxin and

quinone-mimic HQNO have been found to display selectivity between organisms (52), so this enzyme may yet serve as a lesson about the development of drugs against targets also present in mitochondrial genomes.

Alternative Dehydrogenases: Oxidative Phosphorylation Intrinsically Linked to Growth Reactivation

While mycobacteria are primarily heterotrophs, there is strong evidence that they can support chemolithotrophic growth on certain gases. *M. tuberculosis* is capable of supporting carboxydotrophic growth by utilizing carbon monoxide dehydrogenases (53) (CODH structural subunits, *Rv0375c-Rv0373c*) (Fig. 1). These enzymes oxidize CO to CO_2 concomitant with the reduction of various types of acceptors, ferredoxins, or cytochromes, for example (54, 55). The mycobacterial enzymes have additionally been proposed to oxidize NO (56). Aerobic CODHs are three-subunit enzymes that can be distinguished from their anaerobic counterparts by their molybdenum active sites (57, 58). They are typically induced under autotrophic conditions (59), although catabolite repression has been implicated in mycobacterial CODH regulation (60). Genetic essentiality has not been rigorously confirmed, although several transposon mutagenesis studies have putatively identified that the large subunit of CODH is essential (26, 61). The physiological electron acceptor of CODH has not been identified in mycobacteria, and doing so would likely reveal a more robust site for drug design, as opposed to targeting the gas-binding catalytic site.

While CO is abundant during host infection (62) and is likely an important energy source for the bacillus, the possibility of deleterious effects during CODH inhibition must be considered. CO and NO are inducers of the mycobacterial DosR response (63–65), both being apparent substrates of the mycobacterial CODH (56). As suggested previously (66), the metabolism of CO by CODH could serve as a reactivation signal by depleting the inducer. The potential metabolism of NO by CODH only further serves this hypothesis. It is therefore possible that inhibiting CODH will force a greater proportion of bacilli into a nonreplicating persistent state, by allowing accumulation of DosR inducers. Instead, CODH is a very promising target for activators, as opposed to inhibitors, because it could force these drug-resistant persisters to reactivate growth. This would allow the repurposing of classical antitubercular compounds in effective short-term regimens. Currently, only molecules with broad-spectrum inhibitory activity, such as cyanide and derivative isonitriles, have been reported (67), and no activators have been reported at the time of writing.

Another potential respiratory electron donor in mycobacteria is $F_{420}H_2$. A low-potential two-electron carrier, F_{420} plays a unique and central role in the redox metabolism of mycobacteria but is absent from human cells and gut microbiota (68). F_{420} is reduced during central carbon catabolism of *M. tuberculosis* by an F_{420}-dependent glucose 6-phosphate dehydrogenase (69). Multiple $F_{420}H_2$-dependent reductases in turn couple the reoxidation of $F_{420}H_2$ to the reduction of diverse endogenous and exogenous heterocyclic organic compounds (68, 70, 71), among them quinones. It has been demonstrated that three such reductases of the split β-barrel family in *M. tuberculosis*, Rv3547, Rv1558, and Rv3178, can reduce quinone compounds through hydride transfer (72). It has been proposed that this activity maintains the quinone pool in a reduced state during oxidative stress (72); while rapid activity has been observed with nonphysiological quinones (72), it has yet to be confirmed if $F_{420}H_2$ oxidation can reduce menaquinone and generate PMF in whole cells. Irrespectively, mutants unable to synthesize or reduce F_{420} are hypersusceptible to oxidative stress, antibiotic treatment, and hypoxia (72–74); hence, inhibitors of the F_{420} system (including F_{420} analogues) might selectively kill persistent mycobacteria and would act synergistically with first-line antimycobacterials. However, there may be even more promise in exploiting the mycobacterial FDORs to activate prodrugs. The 5-nitroimidazoles delamanid and pretomanid are reductively activated by Rv3547, resulting in production of reactive nitrogen species and *des*-nitro products that are proposed to kill *M. tuberculosis* through a combination of respiratory poisoning and inhibition of mycolic acid synthesis (71, 75–77). Delamanid is the second new drug in 40 years (following bedaquiline) to be clinically approved for TB treatment (78). Acquired resistance to delamanid in extensively drug-resistant TB has been reported to be mediated by mutations in *fbiA* (F_{420} biosynthesis protein) and *fgd1* (F_{420}-dependent glucose-6-phosphate dehydrogenase) (79).

The enzymes discussed above demonstrate the potential array of treatment options that could be achieved with sufficient ingenuity. Valuable outcomes, such as direct lethality and modulation of growth state, can be hypothesized, and the potential to overcome undesirable target properties is readily apparent. NDH-2 has been extensively studied, and large high-throughput screens for inhibitors performed with some success (20, 30, 80). Other primary dehydrogenases have received little attention. *M. tuberculosis* encodes far more primary dehydrogenases that are not covered here due to paucity of understanding in the context of mycobac-

terial oxidative phosphorylation. Most notably, there is a need to understand the role of the tricarboxylic acid cycle-linked malate:quinone oxidoreductase (*Rv2852c*) in the redox and ion homeostasis of *M. tuberculosis* (81, 82). Two quinone-linked glycerol-3-phosphate dehydrogenases (Rv3302c and Rv2249c) need to be dissected from a further two NAD(P)H-linked counterparts (Rv0564c and Rv2982c). In addition, the physiological conditions that would promote the activity of two L-lactate dehydrogenases (Rv0694 and Rv1872) need to be assessed, and it is not yet determined if quinone reduction by proline dehydrogenase occurs purely as a consequence of its previously demonstrated methylglyoxal-detoxification activity (83).

MENAQUINONE BIOSYNTHESIS: PROMISING DRUG TARGETS

Lipoquinones serve as the membrane-bound electron shuttles between primary dehydrogenases and terminal reductases in respiratory chains. Whereas ubiquinone serves as the predominant quinone in mitochondria and many Gram-negative bacteria, menaquinones are the predominant lipoquinones of mycobacteria and many other Gram-positive bacteria (84). It has recently been reported that polyketide-derived quinones are alternate lipoquinones that are expressed and function as electron carriers in mycobacterial biofilms (85). The biosynthesis of menaquinone requires two separate pathways (Fig. 5). 1,4-Dihydroxy-2-naphthoate is synthesized from chorismate. The naphthoate ring is then prenylated with a polyisoprenyldiphosphate, derived from isopentenyl diphosphate and dimethylallyl diphosphate, to form demethylmenaquinone, and subsequently, the C2 position of the ring structure is methylated. In mycobacteria the β-isoprene unit of the prenyl group is reduced to form menaquinone-9 (II-H_2) after the formation of menaquinone (86). Menaquinone synthesis has been relatively extensively studied in *E. coli* (due in part to the availability of the *men* mutants, which can easily be generated in this organism, because it can utilize ubiquinone as an electron carrier in aerobic conditions). In *E. coli* the synthesis of menaquinone is accomplished by 10 enzymes (MenA-MenI and UbiE; see Fig. 5). These enzymes are encoded by two clusters of genes: the *men* cluster, consisting of *menB, C, D, E, F, H*, and a separate cluster containing *menA* and *ubiE*. It was originally thought that MenB catalyzed the conversion of 2-succinylbenzoyl-CoA to 1,4-dihydroxy-2-naphthoate; however, recent evidence indicates that MenB forms 1,4-dihydroxy-2-naphthoyl-CoA, which MenI then hydrolyzes to 1,4-dihydroxy-2-naphthoate (87).

Menaquinone synthesis in Gram-positive bacteria in general has largely been underrepresented in the literature; however, the general pathway in *M. tuberculosis* appears to be similar to that of *E. coli*. In *M. tuberculosis* the *menA-E* genes appear to be found in a single cluster along with the two genes annotated as possible methyl transferases involved in lipoquinone synthesis (*Rv0558* and *Rv0560c*). One or both of these genes presumably encode the protein(s) (MenG, which has an analogous function to UbiE in *E. coli*) that methylate demethylmenaquinone. The gene encoding the protein with the most similarity to MenF in *E. coli* is *Rv3215*, annotated as *entC* (isochorismate synthase), and the gene encoding the protein most similar to MenI is *Rv1847*. In addition, *M. tuberculosis* harbors *Rv0561c*, which is clustered with *menA-E* and encodes MenJ, the enzyme that reduces the β-isoprene of menaquinone (86). Interestingly, *M. tuberculosis* does not have a gene that is easily identifiable as encoding a protein with similar function to MenH. *Rv0045c*, *Rv1938*, and *Rv2715* are all potential candidates, although none encode a protein with a high degree of similarity to MenH from *E. coli*. The isoprenoid tail of the menaquinone must be generated by an isoprenyl diphosphate synthase as described above, and together with 1,4-dihydroxy-2-napthoic acid these are the substrates for MenA (*Rv0534c*). However, the specific synthase generating this isoprenyl diphosphate has yet to be identified.

Surprisingly, not all of the enzymes involved in the mycobacterial menaquinone biosynthetic pathway appear to be viable drug targets, or even essential. Initial studies (25) predicted that the mycobacterial *menC*, *menD*, *menE*, and *menF* genes were essential for bacterial survival. Subsequently, these predictions were supported by high-resolution phenotypic profiling experiments (26), which added *menF* and *menA* to the list of predicted essential genes. MenA (demethylmenaquinone synthase, Rv0534c [88, 89]), MenB (1,4-dihydroxy-2-naphthoyl-CoA synthase, Rv0548c [20–22]), and MenE (*o*-succinylbenzoyl-CoA synthase, Rv0542c [90–92]) from mycobacteria are being studied as potential drug targets, having been genetically or pharmacologically demonstrated to be essential. This is exemplified by the development of aurachin RE analogues, which inhibit MenA and result in growth inhibition of drug-resistant *M. tuberculosis* (89). It seems probable that MenC, D, and F are potential drug targets in addition to MenA, B, and E. MenG has yet to be definitively identified in mycobacteria. As noted above, two genes are annotated as possible methyl transferases involved in lipoquinone synthesis (*Rv0558* and *Rv0560c*). Both of these genes reside in the Men

cluster in *M. tuberculosis*; however, only *Rv0558* is predicted to be essential (25, 26, 93). Thus, further study is indicated.

MenI has only recently been identified as the enzyme that hydrolyzes 1,4-dihydroxy-2-naphthoyl-CoA to 1,4-dihydroxy-2-naphthoate in *E. coli* (87). An orthologous gene has not been positively identified in mycobacteria, although *Rv1847* appears to be the highest probability match. This gene is predicted to be nonessential for mycobacterial survival (25, 26, 93). This is perhaps unremarkable because deletion of MenI in *E. coli* does not eliminate menaquinone synthesis; it only reduces the levels of menaquinone in the bacteria by 67% (87), suggesting that other nonspecific thioesterase activities can compensate. Similarly *Rv0045c*, *Rv1938*, and *Rv2715* encode potential, but low probability, candidates for 2-succinyl-6-hydroxy-2,4-cyclohexadiene-1-carboxylate synthase (MenH) in *M. tuberculosis*, none of which are predicted to be essential. It should be noted that 2-succinyl-5-enolpyruvyl-6-hydroxy-3-cyclohexadiene-1-carboxylate can undergo spontaneous elimination to form 2-succinyl-6-hydroxy-2,4-cyclohexadiene-1-carboxylate (94). Thus, mycobacterial MenI and MenH do not appear to be likely drug targets. MenJ is unique among the *men* genes in that it is nonessential for growth in culture (25, 26, 86) but is essential for bacterial survival in mouse macrophages (86, 95). Thus, menaquinone with partially saturated isoprenyl moieties appears to be a novel virulence factor, and MenJ is a contextually essential enzyme and a potential drug target (86). Sulfated menaquinone synthesis does not appear to present an important drug target. The function of this unique lipid is, as yet, unknown; however, it has been reported that the synthesis of sulfated menaquinone reduces the virulence of the organism in mouse infection models (96).

TARGETING OXYGEN REDUCTION IN MYCOBACTERIA

All mycobacteria sequenced to date harbor genes for a cytochrome *c* pathway consisting of a cytochrome *bc*₁ (related to the mitochondrial complex III) and an *aa*₃-type cytochrome *c* oxidase (complex IV) (Fig. 1). The cytochrome *bc*₁ transfers electrons from menaquinol to the cytochrome *c* oxidase, a process linked to proton translocation across the membrane. Since the cytochrome *c* oxidase is also capable of pumping protons, this pathway is the most energetically favorable respiratory branch in mycobacteria. In contrast to mitochondria, actinobacteria do not possess genes for soluble cytochrome *c* or any other *c*-type cytochrome (97, 98).

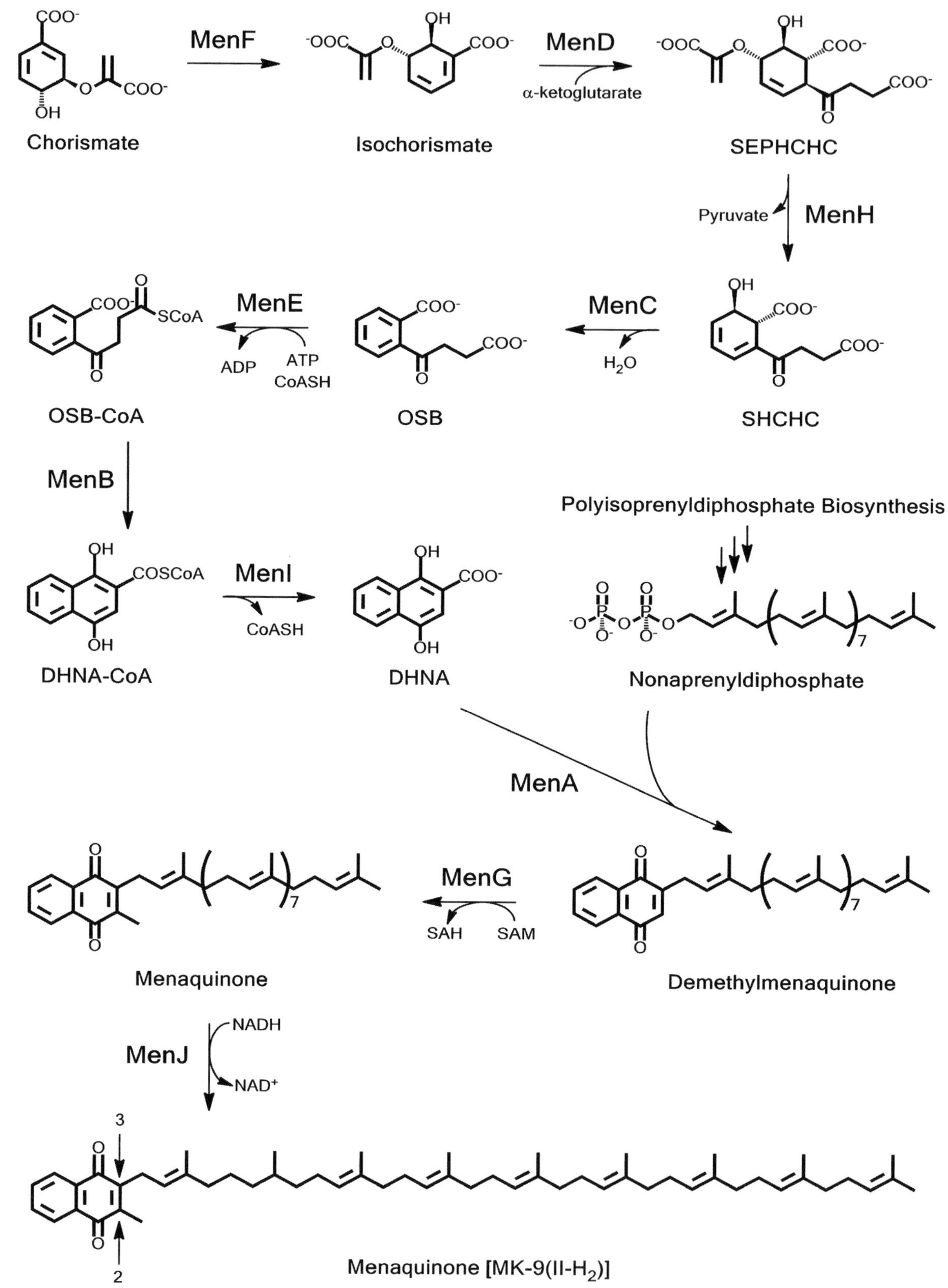

Chorismate
MenF
Isochorismate
MenD
α-ketoglutarate
SEPHCHC
Pyruvate
MenH
SHCHC
MenC
H_2O
OSB
MenE
ADP
ATP
CoASH
OSB-CoA
MenB
DHNA-CoA
MenI
CoASH
DHNA
Polyisoprenyldiphosphate Biosynthesis
Nonaprenyldiphosphate
MenA
Demethylmenaquinone
MenG
SAH
SAM
Menaquinone
MenJ
NADH
NAD+
Menaquinone [MK-9(II-H_2)]

Instead, the complexes III and IV form a supercomplex that facilitates the direct transfer of electrons from menaquinol to oxygen (98–100). The bc_1 complex (encoded by the *qcrCAB* operon) is composed of the cytochrome *b* (*qcrB*), which contains two *b*-type heme groups, a 2Fe-2S iron-sulfur cluster located on the Riske protein QcrA, and a di-heme *c*-type cytochrome c_1 (*qcrC*), as initially described in *Corynebacterium glutamicum* (101).

The aa_3-type cytochrome *c* oxidase is encoded by the *ctaB*, *ctaC*, *ctaD*, and *ctaE* genes. The genes *ctaD* and *ctaC* are in close proximity to the *qcrCAB* operon, whereas *ctaB* and *ctaE* are located elsewhere in the genome. The cytochrome *c* oxidase contains three redox centers: CuA (located on CtaC, subunit II) and the heme *a* (located on CtaD, subunit I) are the primary electron acceptors from the bc_1 complex, whereas the a_3-CuB unit (located on CtaD) is the oxygen-reducing element. The cytochrome *c* oxidase is annotated as essential (25), whereas attempts to delete *qcrCAB* in *M. tuberculosis* were unsuccessful (102), suggesting that the cytochrome *c* pathway is required for the survival of slow-growing mycobacteria. *qcrCAB* could be deleted in *M. smegmatis* but led to a profound growth impairment *in vitro* (102). Recently, the thioredoxin CcsX was shown to be required for heme insertion into membrane-bound heme-containing proteins (103). Deletion of *ccsX* in *M. tuberculosis* had a marked growth defect due to a deficient heme insertion in membrane-proteins, including QcrC. Nevertheless, the mutant strain could still multiply (103), suggesting that the perturbation, or inactivation, of the cytochrome *c* branch may be viable under certain circumstances. Interestingly, the cytochrome *bd* oxidase was upregulated in the *ccsX* mutant strain, suggesting that the cytochrome *bd* oxidase can act as a robust alternate terminal oxidase when the integrity of the cytochrome *c* branch is compromised (103).

Several inhibitors of the cytochrome bc_1 are known. The archetype is stigmatellin, a natural antibiotic that inhibits most cytochrome bc_1 by impeding the interaction of the quinol with the QcrB subunit. The recent discovery of small molecules targeting QcrB has triggered interest in the respiratory cytochrome *c* pathway (104–107). A number of groups have identified a series of imidazopyridine amide (IPA) compounds that interfere with energy metabolism (104–106, 108). The most advanced derivatives of the IPA series are active in the low nanomolar range *in vitro* (106, 108, 109). The series is surprisingly highly selective to mycobacteria since it does not inhibit the growth of any other bacteria or microorganism classes that were tested (104, 106). Whole-genome sequencing of spontaneous-resistant mutants to the IPA drugs revealed that a single amino acid substitution at position 313 in QcrB confers high resistance to Q203 (104, 106). Subsequently, additional mutations were identified in a strain deficient for the expression of the cytochrome *bd* oxidase (105). Since all the mutations conferring resistance are in close proximity to the Qp menaquinone-binding site, it is likely that the IPA compounds inhibit respiration by interfering with the binding of menaquinol at the Qp site of QcrB. Even though target engagement remains to be demonstrated, the observation that the IPA series triggers a rapid ATP depletion (105, 106) suggests that the cytochrome bc_1 is the direct target. The drug candidate Q203 recently progressed to clinical development phase I under a U.S. FDA investigational new drug application, marking the first step to validate the vulnerability of the cytochrome *c* pathway in human TB.

Several other compound series targeting QcrB have been reported (105, 107), arguing for a high level of vulnerability of this respiratory branch under conditions used for compound screening. Of particular interest, the approved drug lansoprazole is a prodrug targeting QcrB in mycobacteria (107). Despite the high vulnerability of the cytochrome bc_1, it is puzzling to note that all the inhibitors discovered to date bind to a narrow region of the QcrB subunit that is predicted to interact with menaquinol. A better understanding of the biology of the cytochrome *c* branch may allow for the identification of lead molecules that bind to alternate positions. Although exciting drug development advances have been made, much work remains to be done to under-

Figure 5 Proposed menaquinone biosynthesis pathway in mycobacteria based on the known pathway in *E. coli*. In this scheme the product of MenA is depicted as the quinone rather than the quinol. This is consistent with the majority of the menaquinone literature (167), which indicates that the oxidation from quinol to quinone is spontaneous but differs from ubiquinone synthesis. The arrows indicate C2 and C3 of menaquinone-9(II-H$_2$). Abbreviations: DHNA, 1,4-dihydroxy-2-naphthoate; DHNA-CoA, 1,4-dihydroxy-2-naphthoyl-CoA; OSB, *o*-succinylbenzoate; OSB-CoA, *o*-succinylbenzoyl-CoA; SEPHCHC, 2-succinyl-5-enolpyruvyl-6-hydroxy-3-cyclohexadiene-1-carboxylate; SHCHC, 2-succinyl-6-hydroxy-2,4-cyclohexadiene-1-carboxylate.

stand the biology of cytochrome bc_1 and under which conditions the cytochrome c branch is essential for survival. As such, it was observed that the high expression of the cytochrome bd-type oxidase in laboratory strains of M. tuberculosis can partly alleviate the potency of cytochrome bc_1 inhibitors (105). Although this was not the case for clinical isolates that seem to regulate cytochrome bd expression more tightly (105), it is imperative to clarify the synthetic genetic interaction between the two terminal oxidases to exploit the full potential of QcrB inhibitors for the treatment of TB. Furthermore, the conditions under which alternate terminal acceptors can compensate for the inhibition of the bc_1 complex must also be delineated to develop a rational drug combination targeting oxidative phosphorylation. It is interesting to note that ongoing reductive evolution in M. leprae and Mycobacterium ulcerans resulted in the deletion of the cytochrome bd oxidase, nitrate reductase, and fumarate reductase (21, 110), leaving the cytochrome c oxidase branch as the only functional terminal electron acceptor. Therefore, drugs targeting cytochrome bc_1 hold great promise for the treatment of leprosy and Buruli ulcer infections.

Cytochrome bd-Type Oxidase and CydDC

M. tuberculosis and other mycobacterial species harbor genes for the cytochrome bd-type menaquinol oxidase (cydAB) (111) (Fig. 1). Cytochrome bd oxidase (CbdO) could be viewed as one of the most scientifically neglected and least understood respiratory enzymes in the electron transport chain of M. tuberculosis. The rather modest interest in this M. tuberculosis enzyme might stem from its dispensability for optimal growth and survival in mouse models (25, 61). In the absence of structural or biochemical data for CbdO of M. tuberculosis, it is assumed that this enzyme functions similarly to its well-characterized E. coli homologue as a high-affinity terminal oxidase that accepts electrons from menaquinol to reduce oxygen under hypoxic conditions (112–114). This enzyme activity contributes to the maintenance of a PMF and facilitates the scavenging of oxygen necessary to colonize oxygen-poor niches or to protect oxygen-labile enzymes (112, 114–116). From an energetic point of view, cytochrome bd oxidase is less efficient than cytochrome c oxidases because it does not pump protons but instead generates a PMF by transmembrane charge separation at an H^+/e ratio of 1 (113). This would appear useful for cells under conditions where the role of CbdO is not primarily to create a PMF, but to serve as an electron sink, for example, during reductive, oxidative, or nitrosative stress defenses (117) or during disulfide-bond formation (114).

Downstream of the cydAB gene locus of M. tuberculosis, another operon, cydDC, encodes a putative ABC-transporter. In E. coli this transporter was shown to transport glutathione and cysteine to the periplasm, where these molecules contribute to redox homeostasis and disulfide bond formation (114). Similar to CbdO, CydDC of M. tuberculosis is largely uncharacterized, and its physiological role is unclear. Mouse infection studies with transposon mutant libraries indicate that mutants with insertions in CydDC are at a disadvantage compared to the wild-type cells (118). However, mouse challenge with single cydC mutants shows no growth attenuation and only a subtle decrease in bacillary loads in lungs during latent infection (119), although a subsequent study was unable to reproduce this phenotype (120). It is important to note that mice do not form hypoxic granulomas, which could explain why neither cydAB nor cydDC mutants are attenuated in this animal model.

Cytochrome bd oxidase and the CydDC transporter appear to protect mycobacteria from chemotherapeutic challenge. For example, disruption of cydC in M. tuberculosis caused increased bacterial clearance in mouse model infections treated with isoniazid when compared to wild-type infections (120). An even more striking observation has been the role of CbdO, specifically in protection of M. tuberculosis from respiratory chain inhibitors. Berney et al. demonstrated that cydA deletion greatly enhances the early bactericidal activity (eBA), killing in the first 7 days, in M. tuberculosis treated with the F_1F_0-ATP synthase inhibitor bedaquiline (121). In another study, cydA inactivation in M. tuberculosis H37Rv enhanced the MIC of cytochrome c oxidoreductase inhibitors by more than 4 orders of magnitude (105). Consistent with these data, deletion of cydA in M. smegmatis greatly decreased the MIC of bedaquiline (17) and led to complete sterilization after clofazimine treatment for 72 hours, while effects on the wild-type and the cytochrome bc_1 mutant were only bacteriostatic (122). However, the mechanism of action of this phenotypic resistance and the more pronounced role in protection from respiratory chain inhibitors is unclear.

CdbO and CydDC enzymes also appear important in adaptation to adverse conditions and persistence. Kana et al. showed that inactivation of cydA in M. smegmatis inhibits cell growth under hypoxic conditions (111). It is intriguing to note that inactivation of the cytochrome c maturation pathway in M. tuberculosis led to upregulation of CbdO concomitant with increased resistance to hydrogen peroxide (103). Accordingly, cydA deletion in M. smegmatis (122) and

M. tuberculosis (M. Berney, unpublished results) increases susceptibility to peroxide. Taken together with the observed protection from antibiotics, this can lead one to assume that cytochrome *bd* oxidase and potentially CydDC are important in pathogenicity and adaptation to adverse conditions. Interestingly, *cydAB* and *cydDC* are upregulated as part of hypoxia-induced dormancy (123) and may facilitate *M. tuberculosis* transition to nonreplicating persistence (124). Bacilli in this state are tolerant to antibiotics (125, 126), and it is possible that the phenotypic resistance to drugs is due in part to a CbdO-facilitated transition to persistence.

Neither cytochrome *bd* oxidase nor the CydDC transporter appears to be essential for the survival or normal growth of *M. tuberculosis* under standard conditions. However, their unique roles discussed above and the lack of mammalian homologues warrant their investigation as potential drug targets. When *M. tuberculosis* is treated with bedaquiline, the dormancy regulon and ATP-generating pathways, including *cydAB* and *cydDC* genes, are activated and induce metabolic remodeling that delays bactericidal activity (127). As noted, inactivation of CbdO inhibits this phenotypic resistance and promotes *de novo* early bactericidal activity of BDQ (121). It is possible that similar mechanisms of resistance are employed in response to a broad range of chemotherapeutics (128). Furthermore, CbdO is likely the predominant terminal oxidase under low oxygen tensions (111, 119, 129) such as those found in hypoxic granulomas (130) and may facilitate the survival of latent or persistent bacilli (131, 132). Therefore, it is conceivable that inhibitors of CbdO or CydDC would enhance the eBA of existing chemotherapeutics and target nonreplicating bacilli populations, which could effectively reduce the currently lengthy therapy timelines (133).

The only cytochrome *bd* oxidase-selective inhibitors currently identified are aurachin D and its analogues (134). Aurachin D is a quinolone-type drug that prevents menaquinol reduction (134) by competitive inhibition at the quinol-binding domain of CbdO (135). Its selective inhibition of CbdO has been validated in *M. smegmatis* by measuring oxygen consumption of membrane vesicles (122). Its efficacy as a chemotherapeutic and toxicity to mammals have not been studied. To our knowledge, no inhibitors of the CydDC transporter have been identified. This general lack of development is likely because inhibitors of these enzymes are not a promising source of stand-alone drugs for treatment of *M. tuberculosis* under aerobic conditions. However, the attributes of CbdO and CydDC discussed here suggest that they may be valuable drug targets to enhance the efficacy and reduce the treatment timelines of current chemotherapy regimens.

Alternative Reductases: Critical for Redox Homeostasis during Hypoxia

There is strong evidence that *M. tuberculosis* uses the alternative electron sinks nitrate, nitrite, and fumarate to maintain redox balance during hypoxia. *M. tuberculosis* exploits host defenses to generate the respiratory electron acceptor nitrate. The organism converts the nitric oxide (NO) produced by host inducible NO synthase (iNOS) in the human macrophage to nitrate by secreting the nitric oxide dioxygenase HbN (136, 137). It in turn imports the nitrate produced with a specific transporter (NarK2), reduces nitrate to nitrite with a membrane-bound respiratory nitrate reductase (NarGHJI), and detoxifies the nitrite to ammonium with a cytosolic NADH-dependent nitrite reductase (NirBD) (138, 139). While nitrate reductase and nitrite reductase are constitutively expressed, the nitrate transporter is under tight transcriptional control by the NO- and hypoxia-induced DosS/DosT-DosR system (119, 140, 141), and hence the rate of nitrate reduction increases in hypoxic cells concurrent with reduction of the respiratory chain (139). While the physiological role of this pathway is incompletely understood, it appears to enhance the flexibility of mycobacteria in response to reductive stress: nitrate supplementation enhances the survival of *M. tuberculosis* cultures following sudden anaerobiosis or phenothiazine treatment (142, 143). The nitrite produced can be exported from the cell or alternatively reduced to ammonium; the nitrite reductase that mediates this process is essential for survival of *M. tuberculosis* both in the Wayne model and in human macrophages, likely due to its combined roles in nitrite detoxification and nitrogen assimilation (138, 144, 145). Given the multifaceted roles of nitrate and nitrite reduction in this pathogen, there may be potential in developing small-molecule inhibitors of nitrate reductase and nitrite reductase. Host-directed therapies aimed at reducing NO production also show promise (146), though they could also be counterproductive given that NO also has innate cytotoxic effects: administration of the iNOS2 inhibitor N^6-(1-iminoethyl)-L-lysine accelerated progress of *M. tuberculosis* infection in a murine model (147).

There is also a weight of evidence that *M. tuberculosis* depends on fumarate reduction to adapt to hypoxia. Two groups have independently demonstrated that *M. tuberculosis* operates a reverse tricarboxylic acid cycle during hypoxia, resulting in fumarate production and succinate excretion (8, 47). Given that succinate is a multifunctional molecule, this remodeling may serve several purposes: (i) respiratory electron transport to fumarate generates PMF by a redox-loop mechanism, (ii) fermentative succinate excretion to the extracellular milieu dissipates excess reductant, and (iii) succinate may be used for anaplerosis or respiration according to cellular needs (8, 47). In contrast to its saprophytic relatives, *M. tuberculosis* has acquired a canonical fumarate reductase that likely mediates the majority of these activities. There is evidence that the two afore-mentioned annotated succinate dehydrogenases in its genome (Sdh1, Sdh2) can operate in a reversed direc-tion to compensate for loss of this enzyme (8, 9, 46, 47). Consistent with such roles, both the canonical fu-marate reductase and Sdh2 are strongly upregulated and highly active under hypoxia (8, 9, 46, 148). Given this functional redundancy, genes encoding these en-zymes can be individually but not collectively deleted (8, 9, 47), and hence it may be difficult to develop effective inhibitors against the fumarate reduction path-way. However, an exciting precedent has been set by the discovery of nanomolar affinity natural products (e.g., nafured, verticipyrone) that inhibit eukaryotic parasites by targeting mitochondrial fumarate reduc-tases (149). The finding that succinate may be excreted as a fermentative end-product in mycobacteria is also worthy of special attention (8). Other recent work has suggested that, while mycobacteria strictly require res-piration for growth, they may resort to fermentation if all respiratory electron acceptors are exhausted (150). It is important to gain a further understanding of the electron sinks that *M. tuberculosis* uses to maintain re-dox balance in order to evaluate current and discover new drug targets in mycobacterial energetics.

ATP SYNTHESIS BY THE F_1F_0 ATP SYNTHASE: A CLINICALLY VALIDATED TARGET

In *M. tuberculosis* and other mycobacterial species, ATP is synthesized via substrate-level phosphorylation and oxidative phosphorylation using the membrane-bound F_1F_0-ATP synthases (encoded by the *atpBEFHAGDC* op-eron, Rv1304-1311). The F_1F_0-ATP synthase catalyzes ATP synthesis by utilizing the electrochemical gradient of protons to generate ATP from ADP and inorganic phosphate (P_i) and operates under conditions of a high PMF and low intracellular ATP. The enzyme is also capable of working as an ATPase under conditions of high intracellular ATP and an overall low PMF (151). As an ATPase, the enzyme hydrolyzes ATP while pump-ing protons from the cytoplasm to the outside of the cell. The ATP synthase of mycobacteria has been studied in detail at a biochemical level in *M. phlei* and shown to exhibit latent ATPase activity (10). ATPase activity could be activated by trypsin treatment and magnesium ions, but the mechanism of activation was not elucidated. Recent experiments with inverted membrane vesicles of *Mycobacterium bovis* BCG and *M. smegmatis* demonstrate latent ATPase activity that could be activated by methanol and the PMF, sug-gesting regulation by the epsilon subunit and ADP in-hibition (6). The reason for the extreme latency in ATP hydrolysis of the mycobacterial ATP synthase is un-known but may represent an adaptation to function at low PMF and under hypoxia. Hypoxic nonreplicating cells of *M. tuberculosis* generate a PMF on the order of −100 mV, and the ATP synthase inhibitor TMC207 is bactericidal toward these cells, demonstrating that the ATP synthase still continues to function at relatively low PMF (3).

The F_1F_0-ATP synthase in *M. tuberculosis* and *M. smegmatis* has been shown to be essential for opti-mal growth (25, 152). In other bacteria, the F_1F_0-ATP synthase is dispensable for growth on fermentable car-bon sources (153, 154), where increased glycolytic flux can compensate for the loss of oxidative phosphoryl-ation. This strategy does not appear to be exploited by *M. smegmatis*: the F_1F_0-ATP synthase is essential for growth even on fermentable substrates, suggesting that ATP production from substrate-level phosphorylation alone, despite increased glycolytic flux, may be insuffi-cient to sustain growth of these bacteria (152). This may be due to an extraordinarily high value for the amount of ATP required to synthesize a mycobacterial cell, a possibility that requires further investigation (155). Alternatively, in conjunction with a high ATP demand for growth, the ATP synthase may be an oblig-atory requirement for the oxidation of NADH by pro-viding a sink for translocated protons during NADH oxidation coupled to oxygen reduction (152). Such strict coupling would imply that mycobacteria do not support uncoupled respiration; either they lack a con-duit for proton re-entry in the absence of the F_1F_0-ATP synthase or they are unable to adjust the proton perme-ability of the cytoplasmic membrane to allow a futile cycle of protons to operate. In this context, the cyto-plasmic membrane of *M. smegmatis* has been shown to be extremely impermeable to protons (156). In *M. tu-berculosis*, the *atp* operon is downregulated during growth in macrophages (157), in the mouse lung, and in cells exposed to NO or hypoxia (119). The *atp* operon of *M. bovis* BCG and *M. smegmatis* is down-regulated in response to slow growth rate (158, 159).

When slow-growing cells of *M. smegmatis* (70 h doubling time) with low levels of *atp* operon expression are exposed to hypoxia (0.6% oxygen saturation), the *atp* operon is upregulated 3-fold, suggesting an important role for this enzyme during adaptation to hypoxia (158).

Several new antitubercular compounds have been reported that target oxidative phosphorylation in mycobacteria (11, 20, 88). The most promising compounds clinically, the diarylquinolines, have been shown to target the F_1F_0-ATP synthase and inhibit ATP synthesis (11–13). The FDA approved the use of a diarylquinoline (i.e., first-in-class compound BDQ) for treatment of multidrug-resistant TB in 2012, which was the first drug licensed in 40 years for TB disease. BDQ was developed in an attempt to improve outcomes in multidrug-resistant TB patients due to the suboptimal effectiveness and toxicity of currently available drugs and regimens. BDQ has fast-acting bactericidal *in vivo* activity in different animal models and in TB patients against several mycobacterial species, both susceptible and resistant to all first-line and many second-line drugs (160, 161). However, resistance to BDQ has already been reported (127), and phase 2 clinical trials showed a higher mortality rate in subjects assigned to the bedaquiline cohort compared to the placebo group (162). Additionally, BDQ accumulates in tissues and has a prolonged half-life, taking 8 weeks to reach peak exposure and displaying a terminal half-life of 4 to 5 months.

Genome sequencing of both *M. tuberculosis* and *M. smegmatis* mutants that are resistant to diarylquinolines (i.e., TMC207) revealed that the target of these compounds is the oligomeric c-ring (encoded by *atpE*) of the enzyme (11, 14, 15). The high-resolution X-ray structure of the oligomeric c-ring of *M. phlei* has been solved complexed with BDQ. The structure reveals that BDQ interacts with the oligomeric c-ring via numerous interactions (hydrophobic, hydrophilic, and electrostatic) completely covering the c-ring's proton-binding sites, thus explaining the high-affinity (nM) binding of BDQ to the *M. phlei* c-ring and the measured low MIC values of BDQ toward *M. tuberculosis* (11). The binding of BDQ to the c-ring prevents the rotor ring from acting as a proton shuttle and stalls ATP synthase operation (16). The structures explain how diarylquinolines specifically inhibit the mycobacterial ATP synthase and thus will enable structure-based drug design for next-generation ATP synthase inhibitors against *M. tuberculosis* (16, 163, 164).

When mycobacterial cells (growing or nongrowing) are treated with BDQ, time-dependent (not dose-dependent) killing is observed (11, 127). The mechanism of killing is not clear but does not involve the dissipation of the membrane potential, which is lethal to all living cells. A dose-dependent decrease in intracellular ATP has been observed when *M. tuberculosis* cells are treated with TMC207 (12, 13), but these data do not explain cell death because mycobacterial cells can be depleted of ATP and yet remain viable (165). We have shown that BDQ kills nonreplicating mycobacterial cells by a unique mechanism that involves uncoupling of the electron transport chain (through ATP synthase), leading to a futile cycling of protons that causes cell death (17). A striking observation during this work was the activation of respiration by BDQ, suggesting a protonophoric-like activity. As discussed above, this was due to binding the c subunit of the F_0 subunit.

A NEED TO UNDERSTAND ENERGETIC PLASTICITY AND ANTIMICROBIAL RESISTANCE/SUSCEPTIBILITY

The energetic targets discussed in this chapter play essential roles in mycobacterial metabolism and respiration under different host conditions. There is a need for continued fundamental research to clarify the molecular interactions and compensatory expression between various energetic targets to develop a rational drug combination targeting oxidative phosphorylation. The discovery of bedaquiline demonstrates that energetic targets provide a pathway to discover fast-acting drugs that eradicate replicating and nonreplicating cells. The mode of bedaquiline action further highlights the multitargeting nature of these molecules. The promise of respiration and oxidative phosphorylation as a new target space is highlighted by the discovery that bacterial respiration is essential for the killing of *E. coli* by ampicillin, gentamicin, and norfloxacin (166). In *E. coli*, cytochrome *bo* and cytochrome *bd* mutants are resistant to the killing effects of ampicillin, gentamicin, and norfloxacin (166). In contrast to *E. coli*, cytochrome *bd* mutants of *M. tuberculosis* (121) and *M. smegmatis* (17, 122) become hypersusceptible to bedaquiline, clofazimine, and hydrogen peroxide (17, 121, 122). These data suggest that the inhibitors of cytochrome *bd* would indeed be synergistic with bedaquiline and clofazimine, making this a priority target for inhibitor discovery.

When *M. tuberculosis* is grown in aerobic batch culture, the rate of oxygen consumption is precisely regulated as a function of percentage air saturation (46). Under these conditions, cells are able to direct electron flow to both terminal respiratory oxidases (cytochrome *bd* and *aa_3*-type cytochrome c oxidase), allowing the cell to rapidly adjust to changes in the PMF and direct electrons to the appropriate oxidase (proton pumping or non-proton pumping) in response to physiological demand (17, 122). The mechanisms that control the rate of oxygen consumption by *M. tuberculosis* are not known. Succinate dehydrogenase and NADH dehydrogenase mutants of *M. tuberculosis* are perturbed in oxygen management, leading to higher rates of oxygen consumption during normal growth and a survival defect in stationary phase (46). These data suggest that the identification of molecules that activate respiration in *M. tuberculosis* may be effective in killing nonreplicating cells and synergizing with current TB drugs. The scope that exists for modulating TB metabolism sets the scene for several exciting innovations and discoveries, a promising contrast to other targets that may soon reach the point of saturation.

Acknowledgments. Research in the authors' laboratory is funded by Health Research Council, Lottery Health, Marsden Fund, Royal Society New Zealand, and the Maurice Wilkins Centre. D.C.C. acknowledges the support of NIH/NIAID grant AI049151. M.B. was supported by NIH grant R21AI119573.

Citation. Cook GM, Hards K, Dunn E, Heikal A, Nakatani Y, Greening C, Crick DC, Fontes FL, Pethe K, Hasenoehrl E, Berney M. 2017. Oxidative phosphorylation as a target space for tuberculosis: success, caution, and future directions. Microbiol Spectrum 5(3):TBTB2-0014-2016.

References

1. Brodie AF, Gutnik DL (ed). 1972. *Electron Transport and Oxidative Phosphorylation in Microbial Systems.* Marcel Dekker Inc., New York, NY.

2. Rao M, Streur TL, Aldwell FE, Cook GM. 2001. Intracellular pH regulation by *Mycobacterium smegmatis* and *Mycobacterium bovis* BCG. *Microbiology* 147:1017–1024.

3. Rao SP, Alonso S, Rand L, Dick T, Pethe K. 2008. The protonmotive force is required for maintaining ATP homeostasis and viability of hypoxic, nonreplicating *Mycobacterium tuberculosis. Proc Natl Acad Sci USA* 105:11945–11950.

4. Jormakka M, Byrne B, Iwata S. 2003. Protonmotive force generation by a redox loop mechanism. *FEBS Lett* 545:25–30.

5. Dimroth P, Cook GM. 2004. Bacterial Na+ - or H+ -coupled ATP synthases operating at low electrochemical potential. *Adv Microb Physiol* 49:175–218.

6. Haagsma AC, Driessen NN, Hahn MM, Lill H, Bald D. 2010. ATP synthase in slow- and fast-growing mycobacteria is active in ATP synthesis and blocked in ATP hydrolysis direction. *FEMS Microbiol Lett* 313:68–74.

7. Otto R, Sonnenberg AS, Veldkamp H, Konings WN. 1980. Generation of an electrochemical proton gradient in *Streptococcus cremoris* by lactate efflux. *Proc Natl Acad Sci USA* 77:5502–5506.

8. Watanabe S, Zimmermann M, Goodwin MB, Sauer U, Barry CE III, Boshoff HI. 2011. Fumarate reductase activity maintains an energized membrane in anaerobic *Mycobacterium tuberculosis. PLoS Pathog* 7:e1002287.

9. Pecsi I, Hards K, Ekanayaka N, Berney M, Hartman T, Jacobs WR Jr, Cook GM. 2014. Essentiality of succinate dehydrogenase in *Mycobacterium smegmatis* and its role in the generation of the membrane potential under hypoxia. *MBio* 5:e01093-14.

10. Higashi T, Kalra VK, Lee SH, Bogin E, Brodie AF. 1975. Energy-transducing membrane-bound coupling factor-ATPase from *Mycobacterium phlei.* I. Purification, homogeneity, and properties. *J Biol Chem* 250: 6541–6548.

11. Andries K, Verhasselt P, Guillemont J, Göhlmann HW, Neefs JM, Winkler H, Van Gestel J, Timmerman P, Zhu M, Lee E, Williams P, de Chaffoy D, Huitric E, Hoffner S, Cambau E, Truffot-Pernot C, Lounis N, Jarlier V. 2005. A diarylquinoline drug active on the ATP synthase of *Mycobacterium tuberculosis. Science* 307: 223–227.

12. Koul A, Dendouga N, Vergauwen K, Molenberghs B, Vranckx L, Willebrords R, Ristic Z, Lill H, Dorange I, Guillemont J, Bald D, Andries K. 2007. Diarylquinolines target subunit c of mycobacterial ATP synthase. *Nat Chem Biol* 3:323–324.

13. Koul A, Vranckx L, Dendouga N, Balemans W, Van den Wyngaert I, Vergauwen K, Göhlmann HW, Willebrords R, Poncelet A, Guillemont J, Bald D, Andries K. 2008. Diarylquinolines are bactericidal for dormant mycobacteria as a result of disturbed ATP homeostasis. *J Biol Chem* 283:25273–25280.

14. Huitric E, Verhasselt P, Andries K, Hoffner SE. 2007. *In vitro* antimycobacterial spectrum of a diarylquinoline ATP synthase inhibitor. *Antimicrob Agents Chemother* 51:4202–4204.

15. Huitric E, Verhasselt P, Koul A, Andries K, Hoffner S, Andersson DI. 2010. Rates and mechanisms of resistance development in *Mycobacterium tuberculosis* to a novel diarylquinoline ATP synthase inhibitor. *Antimicrob Agents Chemother* 54:1022–1028.

16. Preiss L, Langer JD, Yildiz Ö, Eckhardt-Strelau L, Guillemont JE, Koul A, Meier T. 2015. Structure of the mycobacterial ATP synthase Fo rotor ring in complex with the anti-TB drug bedaquiline. *Sci Adv* 1:e1500106

17. Hards K, Robson JR, Berney M, Shaw L, Bald D, Koul A, Andries K, Cook GM. 2015. Bactericidal mode of action of bedaquiline. *J Antimicrob Chemother* 70: 2028–2037.

18. Feng X, Zhu W, Schurig-Briccio LA, Lindert S, Shoen C, Hitchings R, Li J, Wang Y, Baig N, Zhou T, Kim BK, Crick DC, Cynamon M, McCammon JA, Gennis RB, Oldfield E. 2015. Antiinfectives targeting enzymes and the proton motive force. *Proc Natl Acad Sci USA* 112:E7073–E7082.

19. Darby CM, Ingólfsson HI, Jiang X, Shen C, Sun M, Zhao N, Burns K, Liu G, Ehrt S, Warren JD, Andersen OS, Brickner SJ, Nathan C. 2013. Whole cell screen for inhibitors of pH homeostasis in *Mycobacterium tuberculosis. PLoS One* 8:e68942.

20. Weinstein EA, Yano T, Li LS, Avarbock D, Avarbock A, Helm D, McColm AA, Duncan K, Lonsdale JT, Rubin H. 2005. Inhibitors of type II NADH:menaquinone oxidoreductase represent a class of antitubercular drugs. *Proc Natl Acad Sci USA* 102:4548–4553.

21. Cole ST, Eiglmeier K, Parkhill J, James KD, Thomson NR, Wheeler PR, Honoré N, Garnier T, Churcher C, Harris D, Mungall K, Basham D, Brown D, Chillingworth T, Connor R, Davies RM, Devlin K, Duthoy S, Feltwell T, Fraser A, Hamlin N, Holroyd S, Hornsby T, Jagels K, Lacroix C, Maclean J, Moule S, Murphy L, Oliver K, Quail MA, Rajandream MA, Rutherford KM, Rutter S, Seeger K, Simon S, Simmonds M, Skelton J, Squares R, Squares S, Stevens K, Taylor K, Whitehead S, Woodward JR, Barrell BG. 2001. Massive gene decay in the leprosy bacillus. *Nature* 409:1007–1011.

22. Velmurugan K, Chen B, Miller JL, Azogue S, Gurses S, Hsu T, Glickman M, Jacobs WR Jr, Porcelli SA, Briken V. 2007. *Mycobacterium tuberculosis* nuoG is a virulence gene that inhibits apoptosis of infected host cells. *PLoS Pathog* 3:e110

23. Yano T, Li LS, Weinstein E, Teh JS, Rubin H. 2006. Steady-state kinetics and inhibitory action of antitubercular phenothiazines on mycobacterium tuberculosis type-II NADH-menaquinone oxidoreductase (NDH-2). *J Biol Chem* 281:11456–11463.

24. Yano T, Rahimian M, Aneja KK, Schechter NM, Rubin H, Scott CP. 2014. *Mycobacterium tuberculosis* type II NADH-menaquinone oxidoreductase catalyzes electron transfer through a two-site ping-pong mechanism and has two quinone-binding sites. *Biochemistry* 53:1179–1190.

25. Sassetti CM, Boyd DH, Rubin EJ. 2003. Genes required for mycobacterial growth defined by high density mutagenesis. *Mol Microbiol* 48:77–84.

26. Griffin JE, Gawronski JD, Dejesus MA, Ioerger TR, Akerley BJ, Sassetti CM. 2011. High-resolution phenotypic profiling defines genes essential for mycobacterial growth and cholesterol catabolism. *PLoS Pathog* 7:e1002251.

27. Warman AJ, Rito TS, Fisher NE, Moss DM, Berry NG, O'Neill PM, Ward SA, Biagini GA. 2013. Antitubercular pharmacodynamics of phenothiazines. *J Antimicrob Chemother* 68:869–880.

28. Teh JS, Yano T, Rubin H. 2007. Type II NADH:menaquinone oxidoreductase of *Mycobacterium tuberculosis*. *Infect Disord Drug Targets* 7:169–181.

29. Dunn EA, Roxburgh M, Larsen L, Smith RA, McLellan AD, Heikal A, Murphy MP, Cook GM. 2014. Incorporation of triphenylphosphonium functionality improves the inhibitory properties of phenothiazine derivatives in *Mycobacterium tuberculosis*. *Bioorg Med Chem* 22:5320–5328.

30. Shirude PS, Paul B, Roy Choudhury N, Kedari C, Bandodkar B, Ugarkar BG. 2012. Quinolinyl pyrimidines: potent inhibitors of NDH-2 as a novel class of anti-TB agents. *ACS Med Chem Lett* 3:736–740.

31. Ordway D, Viveiros M, Leandro C, Bettencourt R, Almeida J, Martins M, Kristiansen JE, Molnar J, Amaral L. 2003. Clinical concentrations of thioridazine kill intracellular multidrug-resistant *Mycobacterium tuberculosis*. *Antimicrob Agents Chemother* 47:917–922.

32. Amaral L, Kristiansen JE, Abebe LS, Millett W. 1996. Inhibition of the respiration of multi-drug resistant clinical isolates of *Mycobacterium tuberculosis* by thioridazine: potential use for initial therapy of freshly diagnosed tuberculosis. *J Antimicrob Chemother* 38:1049–1053.

33. Bettencourt MV, Bosne-David S, Amaral L. 2000. Comparative *in vitro* activity of phenothiazines against multidrug-resistant *Mycobacterium tuberculosis*. *Int J Antimicrob Agents* 16:69–71.

34. Madrid PB, Polgar WE, Toll L, Tanga MJ. 2007. Synthesis and antitubercular activity of phenothiazines with reduced binding to dopamine and serotonin receptors. *Bioorg Med Chem Lett* 17:3014–3017.

35. Mogi T, Matsushita K, Murase Y, Kawahara K, Miyoshi H, Ui H, Shiomi K, Omura S, Kita K. 2009. Identification of new inhibitors for alternative NADH dehydrogenase (NDH-II). *FEMS Microbiol Lett* 291:157–161.

36. Mogi T, Murase Y, Mori M, Shiomi K, Omura S, Paranagama MP, Kita K. 2009. Polymyxin B identified as an inhibitor of alternative NADH dehydrogenase and malate: quinone oxidoreductase from the Gram-positive bacterium *Mycobacterium smegmatis*. *J Biochem* 146:491–499.

37. Yano T, Kassovska-Bratinova S, Teh JS, Winkler J, Sullivan K, Isaacs A, Schechter NM, Rubin H. 2011. Reduction of clofazimine by mycobacterial type 2 NADH:quinone oxidoreductase: a pathway for the generation of bactericidal levels of reactive oxygen species. *J Biol Chem* 286:10276–10287.

38. Hartkoorn RC, Uplekar S, Cole ST. 2014. Cross-resistance between clofazimine and bedaquiline through upregulation of MmpL5 in *Mycobacterium tuberculosis*. *Antimicrob Agents Chemother* 58:2979–2981.

39. Vilchèze C, Weisbrod TR, Chen B, Kremer L, Hazbón MH, Wang F, Alland D, Sacchettini JC, Jacobs WR Jr. 2005. Altered NADH/NAD+ ratio mediates coresistance to isoniazid and ethionamide in mycobacteria. *Antimicrob Agents Chemother* 49:708–720.

40. Heikal A, Nakatani Y, Dunn E, Weimar MR, Day CL, Baker EN, Lott JS, Sazanov LA, Cook GM. 2014. Structure of the bacterial type II NADH dehydrogenase: a monotopic membrane protein with an essential role in energy generation. *Mol Microbiol* 91:950–964.

41. Sena FV, Batista AP, Catarino T, Brito JA, Archer M, Viertler M, Madl T, Cabrita EJ, Pereira MM. 2015. Type-II NADH:quinone oxidoreductase from *Staphylococcus aureus* has two distinct binding sites and is rate limited by quinone reduction. *Mol Microbiol* 98:272–288.

42. Anderson AC. 2003. The process of structure-based drug design. *Chem Biol* 10:787–797.

43. Feng Y, Li W, Li J, Wang J, Ge J, Xu D, Liu Y, Wu K, Zeng Q, Wu JW, Tian C, Zhou B, Yang M. 2012. Structural insight into the type-II mitochondrial NADH dehydrogenases. *Nature* 491:478–482.

44. Maklashina E, Cecchini G, Dikanov SA. 2013. Defining a direction: electron transfer and catalysis in *Escherichia coli* complex II enzymes. *Biochim Biophys Acta* **1827**: 668–678.

45. Lancaster CR. 2013. The di-heme family of respiratory complex II enzymes. *Biochim Biophys Acta* **1827**: 679–687.

46. Hartman T, Weinrick B, Vilchèze C, Berney M, Tufariello J, Cook GM, Jacobs WR Jr. 2014. Succinate dehydrogenase is the regulator of respiration in *Mycobacterium tuberculosis*. *PLoS Pathog* **10**:e1004510.

47. Eoh H, Rhee KY. 2013. Multifunctional essentiality of succinate metabolism in adaptation to hypoxia in *Mycobacterium tuberculosis*. *Proc Natl Acad Sci USA* **110**:6554–6559.

48. Hägerhäll C. 1997. Succinate: quinone oxidoreductases. Variations on a conserved theme. *Biochim Biophys Acta* **1320**:107–141.

49. Lemos RS, Fernandes AS, Pereira MM, Gomes CM, Teixeira M. 2002. Quinol:fumarate oxidoreductases and succinate:quinone oxidoreductases: phylogenetic relationships, metal centres and membrane attachment. *Biochim Biophys Acta* **1553**:158–170.

50. Huang LS, Sun G, Cobessi D, Wang AC, Shen JT, Tung EY, Anderson VE, Berry EA. 2006. 3-nitropropionic acid is a suicide inhibitor of mitochondrial respiration that, upon oxidation by complex II, forms a covalent adduct with a catalytic base arginine in the active site of the enzyme. *J Biol Chem* **281**:5965–5972.

51. Alston TA, Mela L, Bright HJ. 1977. 3-Nitropropionate, the toxic substance of *Indigofera*, is a suicide inactivator of succinate dehydrogenase. *Proc Natl Acad Sci USA* **74**:3767–3771.

52. Cecchini G, Schröder I, Gunsalus RP, Maklashina E. 2002. Succinate dehydrogenase and fumarate reductase from *Escherichia coli*. *Biochim Biophys Acta* **1553**: 140–157.

53. Park SW, Hwang EH, Park H, Kim JA, Heo J, Lee KH, Song T, Kim E, Ro YT, Kim SW, Kim YM. 2003. Growth of mycobacteria on carbon monoxide and methanol. *J Bacteriol* **185**:142–147.

54. Kim YM, Hegeman GD. 1983. Oxidation of carbon monoxide by bacteria. *Int Rev Cytol* **81**:1–32.

55. Ragsdale SW. 2004. Life with carbon monoxide. *Crit Rev Biochem Mol Biol* **39**:165–195.

56. Park SW, Song T, Kim SY, Kim E, Oh JI, Eom CY, Kim YM. 2007. Carbon monoxide dehydrogenase in mycobacteria possesses a nitric oxide dehydrogenase activity. *Biochem Biophys Res Commun* **362**:449–453.

57. Dobbek H, Svetlitchnyi V, Gremer L, Huber R, Meyer O. 2001. Crystal structure of a carbon monoxide dehydrogenase reveals a [Ni-4Fe-5S] cluster. *Science* **293**: 1281–1285.

58. Dobbek H, Svetlitchnyi V, Liss J, Meyer O. 2004. Carbon monoxide induced decomposition of the active site [Ni-4Fe-5S] cluster of CO dehydrogenase. *J Am Chem Soc* **126**:5382–5387.

59. Santiago B, Schübel U, Egelseer C, Meyer O. 1999. Sequence analysis, characterization and CO-specific

transcription of the *cox* gene cluster on the megaplasmid pHCG3 of *Oligotropha carboxidovorans*. *Gene* **236**:115–124.

60. Oh JI, Park SJ, Shin SJ, Ko IJ, Han SJ, Park SW, Song T, Kim YM. 2010. Identification of trans- and cis-control elements involved in regulation of the carbon monoxide dehydrogenase genes in *Mycobacterium* sp. strain JC1 DSM 3803. *J Bacteriol* **192**:3925–3933.

61. Zhang YJ, Ioerger TR, Huttenhower C, Long JE, Sassetti CM, Sacchettini JC, Rubin EJ. 2012. Global assessment of genomic regions required for growth in *Mycobacterium tuberculosis*. *PLoS Pathog* **8**:e1002946 (Erratum, **9**:10.1371/annotation/4669e9e7-fd12-4a01-be2a-617b956ec0bb.)

62. Shiloh MU, Manzanillo P, Cox JS. 2008. *Mycobacterium tuberculosis* senses host-derived carbon monoxide during macrophage infection. *Cell Host Microbe* **3**: 323–330.

63. Sousa EH, Tuckerman JR, Gonzalez G, Gilles-Gonzalez MA. 2007. DosT and DevS are oxygen-switched kinases in *Mycobacterium tuberculosis*. *Protein Sci* **16**:1708–1719.

64. Kumar A, Deshane JS, Crossman DK, Bolisetty S, Yan BS, Kramnik I, Agarwal A, Steyn AJ. 2008. Heme oxygenase-1-derived carbon monoxide induces the *Mycobacterium tuberculosis* dormancy regulon. *J Biol Chem* **283**:18032–18039.

65. Kumar A, Toledo JC, Patel RP, Lancaster JR Jr, Steyn AJ. 2007. *Mycobacterium tuberculosis* DosS is a redox sensor and DosT is a hypoxia sensor. *Proc Natl Acad Sci USA* **104**:11568–11573.

66. Shi T, Xie J. 2011. Molybdenum enzymes and molybdenum cofactor in mycobacteria. *J Cell Biochem* **112**: 2721–2728.

67. Dobbek H, Gremer L, Kiefersauer R, Huber R, Meyer O. 2002. Catalysis at a dinuclear [CuSMo(==O)OH] cluster in a CO dehydrogenase resolved at 1.1-A resolution. *Proc Natl Acad Sci USA* **99**:15971–15976.

68. Ahmed FH, Carr PD, Lee BM, Afriat-Jurnou L, Mohamed AE, Hong NS, Flanagan J, Taylor MC, Greening C, Jackson CJ. 2015. Sequence-structure-function classification of a catalytically diverse oxidoreductase superfamily in mycobacteria. *J Mol Biol* **427**: 3554–3571.

69. Purwantini E, Gillis TP, Daniels L. 1997. Presence of F420-dependent glucose-6-phosphate dehydrogenase in *Mycobacterium* and *Nocardia* species, but absence from *Streptomyces* and *Corynebacterium* species and methanogenic Archaea. *FEMS Microbiol Lett* **146**:129–134.

70. Taylor MC, Jackson CJ, Tattersall DB, French N, Peat TS, Newman J, Briggs LJ, Lapalikar GV, Campbell PM, Scott C, Russell RJ, Oakeshott JG. 2010. Identification and characterization of two families of F420 H2-dependent reductases from mycobacteria that catalyse aflatoxin degradation. *Mol Microbiol* **78**:561–575.

71. Cellitti SE, Shaffer J, Jones DH, Mukherjee T, Gurumurthy M, Bursulaya B, Boshoff HI, Choi I, Nayyar A, Lee YS, Cherian J, Niyomrattanakit P, Dick T, Manjunatha UH, Barry CE III, Spraggon G, Geierstanger BH. 2012. Struc-

ture of Ddn, the deazaflavin-dependent nitroreductase from *Mycobacterium tuberculosis* involved in bioreductive activation of PA-824. *Structure* 20:101–112.

72. Gurumurthy M, Rao M, Mukherjee T, Rao SP, Boshoff HI, Dick T, Barry CE III, Manjunatha UH. 2013. A novel F(420) -dependent anti-oxidant mechanism protects *Mycobacterium tuberculosis* against oxidative stress and bactericidal agents. *Mol Microbiol* 87:744–755.

73. Purwantini E, Mukhopadhyay B. 2009. Conversion of NO2 to NO by reduced coenzyme F420 protects mycobacteria from nitrosative damage. *Proc Natl Acad Sci USA* 106:6333–6338.

74. Hasan MR, Rahman M, Jaques S, Purwantini E, Daniels L. 2010. Glucose 6-phosphate accumulation in mycobacteria: implications for a novel F420-dependent anti-oxidant defense system. *J Biol Chem* 285:19135–19144.

75. Stover CK, Warrener P, VanDevanter DR, Sherman DR, Arain TM, Langhorne MH, Anderson SW, Towell JA, Yuan Y, McMurray DN, Kreiswirth BN, Barry CE, Baker WR. 2000. A small-molecule nitroimidazopyran drug candidate for the treatment of tuberculosis. *Nature* 405:962–966.

76. Singh R, Manjunatha U, Boshoff HI, Ha YH, Niyomrattanakit P, Ledwidge R, Dowd CS, Lee IY, Kim P, Zhang L, Kang S, Keller TH, Jiricek J, Barry CE III. 2008. PA-824 kills nonreplicating *Mycobacterium tuberculosis* by intracellular NO release. *Science* 322:1392–1395.

77. Gurumurthy M, Mukherjee T, Dowd CS, Singh R, Niyomrattanakit P, Tay JA, Nayyar A, Lee YS, Cherian J, Boshoff HI, Dick T, Barry CE III, Manjunatha UH. 2012. Substrate specificity of the deazaflavin-dependent nitroreductase from *Mycobacterium tuberculosis* responsible for the bioreductive activation of bicyclic nitroimidazoles. *FEBS J* 279:113–125.

78. Lewis JM, Sloan DJ. 2015. The role of delamanid in the treatment of drug-resistant tuberculosis. *Ther Clin Risk Manag* 11:779–791.

79. Bloemberg GV, Keller PM, Stucki D, Trauner A, Borrell S, Latshang T, Coscolla M, Rothe T, Hömke R, Ritter C, Feldmann J, Schulthess B, Gagneux S, Böttger EC. 2015. Acquired resistance to bedaquiline and delamanid in therapy for tuberculosis. *N Engl J Med* 373:1986–1988.

80. Mak PA, Rao SP, Ping Tan M, Lin X, Chyba J, Tay J, Ng SH, Tan BH, Cherian J, Duraiswamy J, Bifani P, Lim V, Lee BH, Ling Ma N, Beer D, Thayalan P, Kuhen K, Chatterjee A, Supek F, Glynne R, Zheng J, Boshoff HI, Barry CE III, Dick T, Pethe K, Camacho LR. 2012. A high-throughput screen to identify inhibitors of ATP homeostasis in non-replicating *Mycobacterium tuberculosis*. *ACS Chem Biol* 7:1190–1197.

81. Molenaar D, van der Rest ME, Drysch A, Yücel R. 2000. Functions of the membrane-associated and cytoplasmic malate dehydrogenases in the citric acid cycle of *Corynebacterium glutamicum*. *J Bacteriol* 182:6884–6891.

82. van der Rest ME, Frank C, Molenaar D. 2000. Functions of the membrane-associated and cytoplasmic malate dehydrogenases in the citric acid cycle of *Escherichia coli*. *J Bacteriol* 182:6892–6899.

83. Berney M, Weimar MR, Heikal A, Cook GM. 2012. Regulation of proline metabolism in mycobacteria and its role in carbon metabolism under hypoxia. *Mol Microbiol* 84:664–681.

84. Collins MD, Jones D. 1981. Distribution of isoprenoid quinone structural types in bacteria and their taxonomic implication. *Microbiol Rev* 45:316–354.

85. Anand A, Verma P, Singh AK, Kaushik S, Pandey R, Shi C, Kaur H, Chawla M, Elechalawar CK, Kumar D, Yang Y, Bhavesh NS, Banerjee R, Dash D, Singh A, Natarajan VT, Ojha AK, Aldrich CC, Gokhale RS. 2015. Polyketide quinones are alternate intermediate electron carriers during mycobacterial respiration in oxygen-deficient niches. *Mol Cell* 60:637–650.

86. Upadhyay A, Fontes FL, Gonzalez-Juarrero M, McNeil MR, Crans DC, Jackson M, Crick DC. 2015. Partial saturation of menaquinone in *Mycobacterium tuberculosis*: function and essentiality of a novel reductase. MenJ. *ACS Cent Sci* 1:292–302.

87. Chen M, Ma X, Chen X, Jiang M, Song H, Guo Z. 2013. Identification of a hotdog fold thioesterase involved in the biosynthesis of menaquinone in *Escherichia coli*. *J Bacteriol* 195:2768–2775.

88. Dhiman RK, Mahapatra S, Slayden RA, Boyne ME, Lenaerts A, Hinshaw JC, Angala SK, Chatterjee D, Biswas K, Narayanasamy P, Kurosu M, Crick DC. 2009. Menaquinone synthesis is critical for maintaining mycobacterial viability during exponential growth and recovery from non-replicating persistence. *Mol Microbiol* 72:85–97.

89. Debnath J, Siricilla S, Wan B, Crick DC, Lenaerts AJ, Franzblau SG, Kurosu M. 2012. Discovery of selective menaquinone biosynthesis inhibitors against *Mycobacterium tuberculosis*. *J Med Chem* 55:3739–3755.

90. Lu X, Zhou R, Sharma I, Li X, Kumar G, Swaminathan S, Tonge PJ, Tan DS. 2012. Stable analogues of OSB-AMP: potent inhibitors of MenE, the o-succinylbenzoate-CoA synthetase from bacterial menaquinone biosynthesis. *ChemBioChem* 13:129–136.

91. Lu X, Zhang H, Tonge PJ, Tan DS. 2008. Mechanism-based inhibitors of MenE, an acyl-CoA synthetase involved in bacterial menaquinone biosynthesis. *Bioorg Med Chem Lett* 18:5963–5966.

92. Truglio JJ, Theis K, Feng Y, Gajda R, Machutta C, Tonge PJ, Kisker C. 2003. Crystal structure of *Mycobacterium tuberculosis* MenB, a key enzyme in vitamin K2 biosynthesis. *J Biol Chem* 278:42352–42360.

93. Sassetti CM, Rubin EJ. 2003. Genetic requirements for mycobacterial survival during infection. *Proc Natl Acad Sci USA* 100:12989–12994.

94. Jiang M, Cao Y, Guo ZF, Chen M, Chen X, Guo Z. 2007. Menaquinone biosynthesis in *Escherichia coli*: identification of 2-succinyl-5-enolpyruvyl-6-hydroxy-3-cyclohexene-1-carboxylate as a novel intermediate and re-evaluation of MenD activity. *Biochemistry* 46:10979–10989.

95. Rengarajan J, Bloom BR, Rubin EJ. 2005. Genome-wide requirements for *Mycobacterium tuberculosis* adaptation and survival in macrophages. *Proc Natl Acad Sci USA* 102:8327–8332.

96. Mougous JD, Senaratne RH, Petzold CJ, Jain M, Lee DH, Schelle MW, Leavell MD, Cox JS, Leary JA, Riley LW, Bertozzi CR. 2006. A sulfated metabolite produced by stf3 negatively regulates the virulence of *Mycobacterium tuberculosis*. *Proc Natl Acad Sci USA* **103**:4258–4263.

97. Bott M, Niebisch A. 2003. The respiratory chain of *Corynebacterium glutamicum*. *J Biotechnol* **104**:129–153.

98. Niebisch A, Bott M. 2003. Purification of a cytochrome bc-aa3 supercomplex with quinol oxidase activity from *Corynebacterium glutamicum*. Identification of a fourth subunity of cytochrome *aa*3 oxidase and mutational analysis of diheme cytochrome c1. *J Biol Chem* **278**:4339–4346.

99. Kim MS, Jang J, Ab Rahman NB, Pethe K, Berry EA, Huang LS. 2015. Isolation and characterization of a hybrid respiratory supercomplex consisting of *Mycobacterium tuberculosis* cytochrome *bcc* and *Mycobacterium smegmatis* cytochrome *aa*3. *J Biol Chem* **290**:14350–14360.

100. Megehee JA, Hosler JP, Lundrigan MD. 2006. Evidence for a cytochrome *bcc-aa*3 interaction in the respiratory chain of *Mycobacterium smegmatis*. *Microbiology* **152**:823–829.

101. Niebisch A, Bott M. 2001. Molecular analysis of the cytochrome bc_1-aa_3 branch of the *Corynebacterium glutamicum* respiratory chain containing an unusual diheme cytochrome c_1. *Arch Microbiol* **175**:282–294.

102. Matsoso LG, Kana BD, Crellin PK, Lea-Smith DJ, Pelosi A, Powell D, Dawes SS, Rubin H, Coppel RL, Mizrahi V. 2005. Function of the cytochrome bc_1-aa_3 branch of the respiratory network in mycobacteria and network adaptation occurring in response to its disruption. *J Bacteriol* **187**:6300–6308.

103. Small JL, Park SW, Kana BD, Ioerger TR, Sacchettini JC, Ehrt S. 2013. Perturbation of cytochrome *c* maturation reveals adaptability of the respiratory chain in *Mycobacterium tuberculosis*. *MBio* **4**:e00475-13.

104. Abrahams KA, Cox JA, Spivey VL, Loman NJ, Pallen MJ, Constantinidou C, Fernández R, Alemparte C, Remuiñán MJ, Barros D, Ballell L, Besra GS. 2012. Identification of novel imidazo[1,2-a]pyridine inhibitors targeting *M. tuberculosis* QcrB. *PLoS One* **7**:e52951.

105. Arora K, Ochoa-Montaño B, Tsang PS, Blundell TL, Dawes SS, Mizrahi V, Bayliss T, Mackenzie CJ, Cleghorn LA, Ray PC, Wyatt PG, Uh E, Lee J, Barry CE III, Boshoff HI. 2014. Respiratory flexibility in response to inhibition of cytochrome *c* oxidase in *Mycobacterium tuberculosis*. *Antimicrob Agents Chemother* **58**:6962–6965.

106. Pethe K, et al. 2013. Discovery of Q203, a potent clinical candidate for the treatment of tuberculosis. *Nat Med* **19**:1157–1160.

107. Rybniker J, Vocat A, Sala C, Busso P, Pojer F, Benjak A, Cole ST. 2015. Lansoprazole is an antituberculous prodrug targeting cytochrome bc_1. *Nat Commun* **6**:7659.

108. Moraski GC, Markley LD, Cramer J, Hipskind PA, Boshoff H, Bailey M, Alling T, Ollinger J, Parish T, Miller MJ. 2013. Advancement of imidazo[1,2-a]pyridines with improved pharmacokinetics and nM activity vs. *Mycobacterium tuberculosis*. *ACS Med Chem Lett* **4**:675–679.

109. Kang S, Kim RY, Seo MJ, Lee S, Kim YM, Seo M, Seo JJ, Ko Y, Choi I, Jang J, Nam J, Park S, Kang H, Kim HJ, Kim J, Ahn S, Pethe K, Nam K, No Z, Kim J. 2014. Lead optimization of a novel series of imidazo[1,2-a]pyridine amides leading to a clinical candidate (Q203) as a multi- and extensively-drug resistant antituberculosis agent. *J Med Chem* **57**:5293–5305.

110. Demangel C, Stinear TP, Cole ST. 2009. Buruli ulcer: reductive evolution enhances pathogenicity of *Mycobacterium ulcerans*. *Nat Rev Microbiol* **7**:50–60.

111. Kana BD, Weinstein EA, Avarbock D, Dawes SS, Rubin H, Mizrahi V. 2001. Characterization of the cydAB-encoded cytochrome *bd* oxidase from *Mycobacterium smegmatis*. *J Bacteriol* **183**:7076–7086.

112. Poole RK, Cook GM. 2000. Redundancy of aerobic respiratory chains in bacteria? Routes, reasons and regulation. *Adv Microb Physiol* **43**:165–224.

113. Borisov VB, Murali R, Verkhovskaya ML, Bloch DA, Han H, Gennis RB, Verkhovsky MI. 2011. Aerobic respiratory chain of *Escherichia coli* is not allowed to work in fully uncoupled mode. *Proc Natl Acad Sci USA* **108**:17320–17324.

114. Holyoake LV, Poole RK, Shepherd M. 2015. The CydDC family of transporters and their roles in oxidase assembly and homeostasis. *Adv Microb Physiol* **66**:1–53.

115. Borisov VB, Gennis RB, Hemp J, Verkhovsky MI. 2011. The cytochrome *bd* respiratory oxygen reductases. *Biochim Biophys Acta* **1807**:1398–1413.

116. Cook GM, Greening C, Hards K, Berney M. 2014. Energetics of pathogenic bacteria and opportunities for drug development. *Adv Microb Physiol* **65**:1–62.

117. Giuffre A, Borisov VB, Arese M, Sarti P, Forte E. 2014. Cytochrome *bd* oxidase and bacterial tolerance to oxidative and nitrosative stress. *Biochim Biophys Acta* **1837**:1178–1187.

118. Zhang YJ, Reddy MC, Ioerger TR, Rothchild AC, Dartois V, Schuster BM, Trauner A, Wallis D, Galaviz S, Huttenhower C, Sacchettini JC, Behar SM, Rubin EJ. 2013. Tryptophan biosynthesis protects mycobacteria from CD4 T-cell-mediated killing. *Cell* **155**:1296–1308.

119. Shi L, Sohaskey CD, Kana BD, Dawes S, North RJ, Mizrahi V, Gennaro ML. 2005. Changes in energy metabolism of *Mycobacterium tuberculosis* in mouse lung and under *in vitro* conditions affecting aerobic respiration. *Proc Natl Acad Sci USA* **102**:15629–15634.

120. Dhar N, McKinney JD. 2010. *Mycobacterium tuberculosis* persistence mutants identified by screening in isoniazid-treated mice. *Proc Natl Acad Sci USA* **107**:12275–12280.

121. Berney M, Hartman TE, Jacobs WR Jr. 2014. A *Mycobacterium tuberculosis* cytochrome *bd* oxidase mutant is hypersensitive to bedaquiline. *MBio* **5**:e01275-14.

122. Lu P, Heineke MH, Koul A, Andries K, Cook GM, Lill H, van Spanning R, Bald D. 2015. The cytochrome *bd*-type quinol oxidase is important for survival of *Mycobacterium smegmatis* under peroxide and antibiotic-induced stress. *Sci Rep* **5**:10333.

123. Voskuil MI, Visconti KC, Schoolnik GK. 2004. *Mycobacterium tuberculosis* gene expression during adaptation to stationary phase and low-oxygen dormancy. *Tuberculosis (Edinb)* **84**:218–227.

124. Wayne LG, Sohaskey CD. 2001. Nonreplicating persistence of *Mycobacterium tuberculosis*. *Annu Rev Microbiol* **55**:139–163.

125. Keren I, Kaldalu N, Spoering A, Wang Y, Lewis K. 2004. Persister cells and tolerance to antimicrobials. *FEMS Microbiol Lett* **230**:13–18.

126. Wayne LG, Hayes LG. 1996. An *in vitro* model for sequential study of shiftdown of *Mycobacterium tuberculosis* through two stages of nonreplicating persistence. *Infect Immun* **64**:2062–2069.

127. Koul A, Vranckx L, Dhar N, Göhlmann HW, Özdemir E, Neefs JM, Schulz M, Lu P, Mørtz E, McKinney JD, Andries K, Bald D. 2014. Delayed bactericidal response of *Mycobacterium tuberculosis* to bedaquiline involves remodelling of bacterial metabolism. *Nat Commun* **5**:3369.

128. Boshoff HI, Myers TG, Copp BR, McNeil MR, Wilson MA, Barry CE III. 2004. The transcriptional responses of *Mycobacterium tuberculosis* to inhibitors of metabolism: novel insights into drug mechanisms of action. *J Biol Chem* **279**:40174–40184.

129. Aung HL, Berney M, Cook GM. 2014. Hypoxia-activated cytochrome *bd* expression in *Mycobacterium smegmatis* is cyclic AMP receptor protein dependent. *J Bacteriol* **196**:3091–3097.

130. Barry CE III, Boshoff HI, Dartois V, Dick T, Ehrt S, Flynn J, Schnappinger D, Wilkinson RJ, Young D. 2009. The spectrum of latent tuberculosis: rethinking the biology and intervention strategies. *Nat Rev Microbiol* **7**:845–855.

131. Boshoff HI, Barry CE III. 2005. Tuberculosis: metabolism and respiration in the absence of growth. *Nat Rev Microbiol* **3**:70–80.

132. Gomez JE, McKinney JD. 2004. M. tuberculosis persistence, latency, and drug tolerance. *Tuberculosis (Edinb)* **84**:29–44.

133. Dick T. 2001. Dormant tubercle bacilli: the key to more effective TB chemotherapy? *J Antimicrob Chemother* **47**:117–118.

134. Meunier B, Madgwick SA, Reil E, Oettmeier W, Rich PR. 1995. New inhibitors of the quinol oxidation sites of bacterial cytochromes *bo* and *bd*. *Biochemistry* **34**:1076–1083.

135. Jünemann S, Wrigglesworth JM, Rich PR. 1997. Effects of decyl-aurachin D and reversed electron transfer in cytochrome *bd*. *Biochemistry* **36**:9323–9331.

136. Jung JY, Madan-Lala R, Georgieva M, Rengarajan J, Sohaskey CD, Bange FC, Robinson CM. 2013. The intracellular environment of human macrophages that produce nitric oxide promotes growth of mycobacteria. *Infect Immun* **81**:3198–3209.

137. Arya S, Sethi D, Singh S, Hade MD, Singh V, Raju P, Chodisetti SB, Verma D, Varshney GC, Agrewala JN, Dikshit KL. 2013. Truncated hemoglobin, HbN, is post-translationally modified in *Mycobacterium tuberculosis* and modulates host-pathogen interactions during intracellular infection. *J Biol Chem* **288**:29987–29999.

138. Malm S, Tiffert Y, Micklinghoff J, Schultze S, Joost I, Weber I, Horst S, Ackermann B, Schmidt M, Wohlleben W, Ehlers S, Geffers R, Reuther J, Bange FC. 2009. The roles of the nitrate reductase NarGHJI, the nitrite reductase NirBD and the response regulator GlnR in nitrate assimilation of *Mycobacterium tuberculosis*. *Microbiology* **155**:1332–1339.

139. Sohaskey CD, Wayne LG. 2003. Role of narK2X and narGHJI in hypoxic upregulation of nitrate reduction by *Mycobacterium tuberculosis*. *J Bacteriol* **185**:7247–7256.

140. Voskuil MI, Schnappinger D, Visconti KC, Harrell MI, Dolganov GM, Sherman DR, Schoolnik GK. 2003. Inhibition of respiration by nitric oxide induces a *Mycobacterium tuberculosis* dormancy program. *J Exp Med* **198**:705–713.

141. Sohaskey CD. 2005. Regulation of nitrate reductase activity in *Mycobacterium tuberculosis* by oxygen and nitric oxide. *Microbiology* **151**:3803–3810.

142. Tan MP, Sequeira P, Lin WW, Phong WY, Cliff P, Ng SH, Lee BH, Camacho L, Schnappinger D, Ehrt S, Dick T, Pethe K, Alonso S. 2010. Nitrate respiration protects hypoxic *Mycobacterium tuberculosis* against acid- and reactive nitrogen species stresses. *PLoS One* **5**:e13356.

143. Sohaskey CD. 2008. Nitrate enhances the survival of *Mycobacterium tuberculosis* during inhibition of respiration. *J Bacteriol* **190**:2981–2986.

144. Cunningham-Bussel A, Bange FC, Nathan CF. 2013. Nitrite impacts the survival of *Mycobacterium tuberculosis* in response to isoniazid and hydrogen peroxide. *Microbiologyopen* **2**:901–911

145. Akhtar S, Khan A, Sohaskey CD, Jagannath C, Sarkar D. 2013. Nitrite reductase NirBD is induced and plays an important role during *in vitro* dormancy of *Mycobacterium tuberculosis*. *J Bacteriol* **195**:4592–4599.

146. Holden JK, Li H, Jing Q, Kang S, Richo J, Silverman RB, Poulos TL. 2013. Structural and biological studies on bacterial nitric oxide synthase inhibitors. *Proc Natl Acad Sci USA* **110**:18127–18131.

147. MacMicking JD, North RJ, LaCourse R, Mudgett JS, Shah SK, Nathan CF. 1997. Identification of nitric oxide synthase as a protective locus against tuberculosis. *Proc Natl Acad Sci USA* **94**:5243–5248.

148. Rustad TR, Harrell MI, Liao R, Sherman DR. 2008. The enduring hypoxic response of *Mycobacterium tuberculosis*. *PLoS One* **3**:e1502.

149. Sakai C, Tomitsuka E, Esumi H, Harada S, Kita K. 2012. Mitochondrial fumarate reductase as a target of chemotherapy: from parasites to cancer cells. *Biochim Biophys Acta* **1820**:643–651.

150. Berney M, Greening C, Conrad R, Jacobs WR Jr, Cook GM. 2014. An obligately aerobic soil bacterium activates fermentative hydrogen production to survive reductive stress during hypoxia. *Proc Natl Acad Sci USA* **111**:11479–11484.

151. von Ballmoos C, Cook GM, Dimroth P. 2008. Unique rotary ATP synthase and its biological diversity. *Annu Rev Biophys* **37**:43–64.

152. Tran SL, Cook GM. 2005. The F_1F_o-ATP synthase of *Mycobacterium smegmatis* is essential for growth. *J Bacteriol* **187**:5023–5028.

153. Friedl P, Hoppe J, Gunsalus RP, Michelsen O, von Meyenburg K, Schairer HU. 1983. Membrane integration and function of the three F_0 subunits of the ATP synthase of *Escherichia coli* K12. *EMBO J* **2**:99–103.

154. Santana M, Ionescu MS, Vertes A, Longin R, Kunst F, Danchin A, Glaser P. 1994. *Bacillus subtilis* F_0F_1 ATPase: DNA sequence of the *atp* operon and characterization of *atp* mutants. *J Bacteriol* **176**:6802–6811.

155. Cox RA, Cook GM. 2007. Growth regulation in the mycobacterial cell. *Curr Mol Med* **7**:231–245.

156. Tran SL, Rao M, Simmers C, Gebhard S, Olsson K, Cook GM. 2005. Mutants of *Mycobacterium smegmatis* unable to grow at acidic pH in the presence of the protonophore carbonyl cyanide m-chlorophenylhydrazone. *Microbiology* **151**:665–672.

157. Schnappinger D, Ehrt S, Voskuil MI, Liu Y, Mangan JA, Monahan IM, Dolganov G, Efron B, Butcher PD, Nathan C, Schoolnik GK. 2003. Transcriptional adaptation of *Mycobacterium tuberculosis* within macrophages: insights into the phagosomal environment. *J Exp Med* **198**:693–704.

158. Berney M, Cook GM. 2010. Unique flexibility in energy metabolism allows mycobacteria to combat starvation and hypoxia. *PLoS One* **5**:e8614.

159. Beste DJ, Laing E, Bonde B, Avignone-Rossa C, Bushell ME, McFadden JJ. 2007. Transcriptomic analysis identifies growth rate modulation as a component of the adaptation of mycobacteria to survival inside the macrophage. *J Bacteriol* **189**:3969–3976.

160. Diacon AH, Donald PR, Pym A, Grobusch M, Patientia RF, Mahanyele R, Bantubani N, Narasimooloo R, De Marez T, van Heeswijk R, Lounis N, Meyvisch P, Andries K, McNeeley DF. 2012. Randomized pilot trial of eight weeks of bedaquiline (TMC207) treatment for multidrug-resistant tuberculosis: long-term outcome, tolerability, and effect on emergence of drug resistance. *Antimicrob Agents Chemother* **56**:3271–3276.

161. Diacon AH, Pym A, Grobusch M, Patientia R, Rustomjee R, Page-Shipp L, Pistorius C, Krause R, Bogoshi M, Churchyard G, Venter A, Allen J, Palomino JC, De Marez T, van Heeswijk RP, Lounis N, Meyvisch P, Verbeeck J, Parys W, de Beule K, Andries K, McNeeley DF. 2009. The diarylquinoline TMC207 for multidrug-resistant tuberculosis. *N Engl J Med* **360**:2397–2405.

162. Diacon AH, Pym A, Grobusch MP, de los Rios JM, Gotuzzo E, Vasilyeva I, Leimane V, Andries K, Bakare N, De Marez T, Haxaire-Theeuwes M, Lounis N, Meyvisch P, De Paepe E, van Heeswijk RP, Dannemann B, TMC207-C208 Study Group. 2014. Multidrug-resistant tuberculosis and culture conversion with bedaquiline. *N Engl J Med* **371**:723–732.

163. Haagsma AC, Podasca I, Koul A, Andries K, Guillemont J, Lill H, Bald D. 2011. Probing the interaction of the diarylquinoline TMC207 with its target mycobacterial ATP synthase. *PLoS One* **6**:e23575.

164. Lu P, Lill H, Bald D. 2014. ATP synthase in mycobacteria: special features and implications for a function as drug target. *Biochim Biophys Acta* **1837**:1208–1218.

165. Frampton R, Aggio RB, Villas-Bôas SG, Arcus VL, Cook GM. 2012. Toxin-antitoxin systems of *Mycobacterium smegmatis* are essential for cell survival. *J Biol Chem* **287**:5340–5356.

166. Lobritz MA, Belenky P, Porter CB, Gutierrez A, Yang JH, Schwarz EG, Dwyer DJ, Khalil AS, Collins JJ. 2015. Antibiotic efficacy is linked to bacterial cellular respiration. *Proc Natl Acad Sci USA* **112**:8173–8180.

167. Meganathan R. 2001. Biosynthesis of menaquinone (vitamin K2) and ubiquinone (coenzyme Q): a perspective on enzymatic mechanisms. *Vitam Horm* **61**:173–218.

Tuberculosis and the Tubercle Bacillus, 2nd ed.
Edited by William R. Jacobs, Jr., Helen McShane, Valerie Mizrahi, and Ian M. Orme
© 2018 American Society for Microbiology, Washington, DC
doi:10.1128/microbiolspec.TBTB2-0031-2016

Targeting Phenotypically Tolerant
Mycobacterium tuberculosis

15

Ben Gold and Carl Nathan

INTRODUCTION

Two parallel revolutions were born in the golden era of antibiotics (~1940 to 1960). One was a revolution in medicine as physicians went to war with microbes. The second was a revolution in biology as microbiologists and geneticists used anti-infectives as tools to reveal how microbes function on a molecular level. Scientists converged on a surprisingly short list of essential biological processes that appeared to make up an Achilles' heel shared by diverse bacterial pathogens: the biosynthesis of nucleic acids (DNA and RNA), protein, cell walls (peptidoglycan and lipids), and folate. Only later were the far wider dimensions of potential target space appreciated (1). The discovery of targets led to the development of methods to improve existing antibiotics and find new ones.

The success of chemical biology at advancing antibiotic development was spectacular but short-lived. New antibiotics quickly encountered genetically encoded drug resistance (2). The selective pressure imposed by antibiotics presented bacteria with a seemingly impossible task of becoming drug resistant by modifying the antibiotic's target, modifying the antibiotic's structure, effluxing the antibiotic, or altering their cell wall's permeability to the drug without a major fitness cost. Yet bacteria solve this problem routinely in laboratories, the environment, animal models of disease, and patients. Resistant mutants distribute drug resistance by vertical transmission (passing chromosomal DNA to their progeny) and horizontal transmission (via phages and plasmids). Antibiotic research concentrated on understanding the basis of genetically encoded drug resistance, and medical chemistry campaigns focused on bypassing it.

However, genetic drug resistance was not the only hurdle. Pioneering observations published by Hobby, Meyer, and Chaffee in 1942 (3) and by Bigger in 1944 (4) cast an ominous cloud over the remnants of optimism that antibiotics could eradicate diseases of bacterial origin. Hobby and her colleagues observed that about 1 streptococcus of 10^6 in a replicating culture survived exposure to penicillin, while in a culture whose replication was halted by cold, nearly all the cocci survived (3). Bigger made the same observation with staphylococcus and additionally noted that the cocci became tolerant to penicillin when their replication was halted by acidification or hypotonicity of the medium (4). Microbiologists had long assumed that logarithmically growing bacterial cultures were uniform. Use of penicillin as a tool allowed Hobby, Meyer, Chafee, and Bigger to discover that the assumption of bacterial homogeneity was incorrect. Moreover, they demonstrated that bacteria could resist killing by antibiotics through a nonheritable mechanism. The penicillin-resistant cells were as sensitive to penicillin as the population from which they came when they were expanded in fresh medium and exposed to penicillin a second time. Bigger used the term "persisters" for bacteria that survived antibiotics without heritable resistance. The property allowing persisters to survive was later termed "phenotypic drug resistance" or "phenotypic tolerance." These historic studies have important implications for anti-infective discovery paradigms today (3, 4).

Two decades later, Hobby and Lenert extended the observation of phenotypic tolerance to a different organism, *Mycobacterium tuberculosis*, and additional drugs, isoniazid and para-aminosalicylate (5). Isoniazid targets the synthesis of mycolic acids, para-

Department of Microbiology and Immunology, Weill Cornell Medical College, New York, NY 10065.

aminosalicylate targets the synthesis of folate, and penicillin targets the synthesis of peptidoglycan. Thus, the phenomenon of phenotypic tolerance was independent of the chemical class of antibiotics and of the pathways they inhibit.

The problem of persisters is central to the chemotherapy of tuberculosis. It is believed to be a major reason why the current WHO-approved treatment regimen for drug-sensitive tuberculosis takes 6 months to achieve cure in ~95% of participants in formal studies; the cure rate is about 86% in routine practice. Drug-resistant tuberculosis generally requires treatment for over 2 years, and cure is often not achieved (6). In the "Cornell model," mice with drug-sensitive tuberculosis that are treated with isoniazid and pyrazinamide for 2 months harbor no detectable CFU of *M. tuberculosis* when their organ homogenates are spread on bacteriologic agar. However, about one-third of the remaining members of the same cohort of mice relapse spontaneously some months later, and nearly all of them relapse if immunosuppressed with corticosteroids, anti-interferon-γ (IFN-γ), anti-tumor necrosis factor, or inhibitors of inducible nitric oxide synthase (7–9). The *M. tuberculosis* recovered at relapse is as sensitive to isoniazid and pyrazinamide as the population used for inoculation. These observations indicate the presence of drug-tolerant persister populations after antibiotic treatment, even if they are temporarily undetectable by

standard microbiologic methods. Likewise, sputa from about 80% of treatment-naive tuberculosis patients contained *M. tuberculosis* that was not quantifiable by CFU analysis (10, 11).

Experience with metronidazole illustrates the challenge of translating the foregoing knowledge into a faster and more effective treatment of tuberculosis. In some animal models, *M. tuberculosis* encounters hypoxia in necrotic granulomas (Table 1). *In vitro*, hypoxia causes mycobacteria to cease replicating and become phenotypically tolerant to most drugs. In contrast, the antibacterial and antiparasitic drug metronidazole kills hypoxic mycobacteria *in vitro*. Thus, metronidazole seemed well suited to kill nonreplicating *M. tuberculosis*. However, metronidazole's activity in animal models of tuberculosis correlated imperfectly with hypoxia in granulomas (Table 1) (12–19). Metronidazole improved the proportion of patients whose sputum became smear- or culture-negative at 1 month of treatment but did not impact treatment outcome at 6 months, other than contributing to peripheral neuropathy (14). In retrospect, the ability of metronidazole to kill hypoxic *M. tuberculosis in vitro* was studied in the absence of an alternative electron acceptor, putting the organism at a greater disadvantage than it is likely to face *in vivo*. *M. tuberculosis* is not restricted to using oxygen as an electron acceptor; it can also use nitrate or fumarate (20–22). Nitrate is a physiologic constitu-

Table 1 Evaluating the relationship between hypoxia and metronidazole activity *in vitro* and *in vivo*

Model	Method to measure or demonstrate hypoxia	Evidence of hypoxia?	Caseating granulomas?	Activity of metronidazole	References
Wayne *in vitro* model of dormancy	<0.06% O_2, methylene blue decolorization	Yes	No	Active	19, 95
Mouse: C57Bl/6	Pimonidazole (immunohistochemistry), EF5/ELK3-51 antibody	No	No	Inactive	13, 17, 294, 295
Mouse: BALB/c	Copper(II)-diacetyl-bis(N^4-methyl-thiosemicarbazone), pimonidazole (immunohistochemistry)	No	No	Inactive	17, 64, 296, 297
Mouse: C3HeB/FeJ "Kramnik model"	Copper(II)-diacetyl-bis(N^4-methyl-thiosemicarbazone), pimonidazole (immunohistochemistry), gene expression of hypoxia-associated genes in *M. tuberculosis*	Yes	Yes	Inactive	64, 296, 297
Guinea pig	Pimonidazole (immunohistochemistry)	Yes	Yes	Inactive	15, 17
Rabbit	Pimonidazole (immunohistochemistry), fiber-optic O_2 probe	Yes	Yes	Active	17
Non-human primates	Pimonidazole (immunohistochemistry)	Yes	Yes	Active	16, 17
Human	EF5/ELK3-51 antibody, HIF-1α (hypoxia inducible factor) (immunohistochemistry), [^{18}F]-fluoromisonidazole (positron emission tomography imaging)	Yes	Yes	Clinically ineffective	14, 245, 294, 298

ent of human body fluids. Inclusion of nitrate markedly diminished the *in vitro* efficacy of pyrazinamide (23).

The experience with metronidazole suggests that it may not be enough to find antibiotics with the exceptional property of killing bacteria that are phenotypically tolerant to most other antibiotics; it matters how the bacteria are rendered phenotypically tolerant. If phenotypic tolerance is achieved by using conditions that prevent the bacteria from replicating, it matters how they are prevented from replicating. The more the conditions resemble those in the host, the more likely that drugs that work under those conditions may also work in the host.

The foregoing statements are a hypothesis whose testing is just beginning. After Bigger's report (4), it took another 40 years until Coates proposed large-scale screening to target nonreplicating *M. tuberculosis* (24). His proposal came at a time when many pharmaceutical companies were scaling back or abandoning anti-infective discovery. Other firms stuck to the industry's standard practice of seeking broad-spectrum agents that could cure infections prevalent in economically advantaged regions. Only after 1999 did a new funding landscape emerge that supported academic-industrial partnerships for drug discovery for infectious diseases that are prevalent chiefly in economically disadvantaged regions (1, 25–27). Only about 10 years ago did pharmaceutical companies and their academic partners begin large-scale screens for drugs targeting phenotypically tolerant mycobacteria (28, 29).

This chapter describes and categorizes approximately 100 compounds that have been reported to kill mycobacteria rendered nonreplicating in one or another *in vitro* model. We also offer comments about the biology of drug tolerance, strategies for screening compounds against phenotypically tolerant mycobacteria, progressing the "actives" through secondary assays, and pitfalls in data interpretation.

SUMMARY OF KEY OBSERVATIONS

- At least two types of phenotypic tolerance are important to distinguish because different strategies will probably be needed to overcome them (25, 27). Class I phenotypic tolerance is manifest by a small proportion of bacteria in a replicating population. Existing evidence, while incomplete, suggests that different individual bacteria in the population can be phenotypically tolerant to different antibiotics by different mechanisms. To the degree that this is the case, phenotypic tolerance can be overcome by

treating the overall population with a combination of drugs. Class II phenotypic tolerance is manifest by almost all the cells in a population whose number is not changing during the period of observation. Almost every cell must be phenotypically tolerant to all the antibiotics to which the population as a whole is tolerant. Overcoming class II phenotypic tolerance will likely require new kinds of drugs that are highly active on nonreplicating bacteria.

- While nonreplication imposed by diverse stresses is closely associated with phenotypic tolerance, mycobacteria that become nonreplicating under different conditions may be phenotypically diverse.
- While nonreplication is a state associated with phenotypic tolerance, nonreplication is not a mechanistic explanation for phenotypic tolerance. Nonreplication is not equivalent to dormancy and does not connote a lack of dependence on biosynthetic pathways.
- Nonreplicating mycobacteria are reportedly killed by a large number of chemically diverse compounds. However, only a few of these compounds have been tested and found to be active against mycobacteria rendered nonreplicating in multiple ways.
- Only a few of the compounds reported to kill nonreplicating mycobacteria have been tested under conditions designed to exclude false-positive results that can arise from drug carryover from the nonreplicating phase of the assay to the replicating phase, such as by enumerating viable bacilli on a solid bacteriologic medium containing activated charcoal (30–33).
- Some approved drugs for tuberculosis, such as rifampin and moxifloxacin, are genuinely active *in vitro* against nonreplicating *M. tuberculosis*, but at far higher concentrations and with far less reduction in bacterial numbers than under replicating conditions. For others, such as bedaquiline, the apparent activity against nonreplicating *M. tuberculosis in vitro* was largely attributable to carryover in one study (30). Among the approved tuberculosis drugs tested in that study, only PA-824 was genuinely and comparably active against *M. tuberculosis* under replicating and nonreplicating conditions (30). Encouragingly, ongoing research is identifying more such compounds among anti-infectives approved for other indications (34) or as new members of drug-like chemical classes.

DIVERSITY IN NONREPLICATION

Sensitivity to an antibiotic is conventionally defined under replicating conditions and reported as an MIC, typically meaning a concentration that restricts growth by at least 90% compared to a culture under the same conditions that is exposed to the vehicle alone for the same period of time. Phenotypically tolerant bacteria of class I are those rare cells that survive exposure to the antibiotic at or above its MIC when tested under these standard, replicating conditions. In contrast, phenotypically tolerant bacteria of class II are the majority of a population that survives exposure to the antibiotic at or above its MIC under different conditions, typically those that impose nonreplication. To distinguish the nonreplication imposed by the test conditions from death imposed by the antibiotic usually requires removing the antibiotic by washing or dilution, reversing the conditions that impose nonreplication, and then detecting recovery or the lack of recovery of the surviving bacteria by allowing survivors to replicate. The hallmark of both class I and class II phenotypic tolerance is that the survivors, when tested again under the standard conditions, display the same MIC as the original population (25).

To fully appreciate the diversity exhibited by nonreplicating cells, it will be useful to start by correcting several misconceptions. First, when Hobby et al. (3) and Bigger (4) discovered what we now call class I persistence, they attributed it to nonreplication of about one bacterium in a million in an otherwise replicating population. They had no direct evidence for this. More than half a century later, it became possible to test this notion, and the results have been mixed. In short, class I phenotypic tolerance sometimes is and sometimes is not associated with nonreplication of a minority of cells in a replicating population. By definition, class II persisters are nonreplicating. Therefore, class I and class II persisters should not be grouped together as "nonreplicating cells." Second, just because a bacterial population has stopped changing in number over a period of time, this does not exclude the occurrence of balanced replication and death. For simplicity, we use the term "nonreplication" to describe a population of static size, but without implying the degree of turnover. Third, just because one population of bacteria has entered a nonreplicating state in response to one condition, this does not mean that it has the same phenotype as another population that has entered a nonreplicating state in response to another condition.

Single-cell analyses of persister populations are now feasible. For example, cell division can be monitored by dilution of a fluorescent signal from a chromosomal copy of mCherry (35, 36) and metabolism monitored using redox sensor green, which generates a fluorescent signal upon reduction by bacterial reductases.

The fates of individual cells can be tracked over time by microfluidics and time-lapse microscopy (36–39). Replicating and nonreplicating cells, and metabolically active and metabolically inactive cells, may be sorted using a fluorescence-activated cell sorter. For example, Brynildsen and colleagues found that while nongrowing cells were enriched for class I persisters, 20% of the persisters were replicating, and slow metabolism correlated with, but was not required for, persistence (36).

Persister diversity may result from heterogeneity in such bacterial processes as maintenance of membrane potential, DNA replication, and ribosomal translation (40, 41) or in host environments, where bacteria may be extracellular in connective tissue or caseum or intracellular in phagosomes or cytosol (42). The transcriptome of M. tuberculosis class I persisters enriched by D-cycloserine treatment to kill replicating cells overlapped very little with the transcriptomes of class II phenotypically tolerant cells generated by incubating M. tuberculosis under conditions of hypoxia (43, 44), stationary phase (12, 44, 45), or nutrient starvation (12). Moreover, only five genes were identified as commonly upregulated in the four nonreplicating models (46), and there was little overlap of M. tuberculosis's differentially regulated genes in the three class II nonreplicating models (43, 44, 46). Another comprehensive comparison found a poor correlation of transcriptomes of M. tuberculosis rendered nonreplicating in multiple models, including removing streptomycin from the streptomycin-addicted strain SS18b; exposing wild-type M. tuberculosis to reactive nitrogen intermediates; depriving it of phosphate, nutrients, or oxygen; or combining a variety of stresses (47). On the other hand, Voskuil et al. found a correlation among the transcriptomes of M. tuberculosis exposed to hypoxia, the nitric oxide donor DETA-NO, and cyanide (48), and the transcriptional changes were similar to those seen during infection by M. tuberculosis of IFN-γ-activated bone marrow-derived macrophages (49). While these transcriptomics experiments were insightful, we do not know the relevance of transcriptional regulation of individual genes to the survival of mycobacteria as class I or class II phenotypically tolerant. Transcriptomics profiles are time-dependent, making it difficult to compare transcriptomes studied at different times. Moreover, many key regulatory steps are posttranslational.

Another indication of the diversity of nonreplicating mycobacteria is that the same compounds are differentially active against M. tuberculosis rendered nonreplicating in different ways, such as nutrient starvation, stationary phase, hypoxia, and a combination of acidic pH and reactive nitrogen intermediates (50–52). In the multistress model (acidic pH, reactive nitrogen interme- diates, hypoxia, and a fatty acid carbon source), some compounds specifically required reactive nitrogen inter- mediates for their activity (28, 53). Grant et al. found that of 52 molecules active against *M. tuberculosis* in a carbon starvation model, only 33% were also active against bacilli rendered nonreplicating by hypoxia (54). The same study found diversity of the activity profiles of four compounds, from three chemical classes, in a class I persister model and three class II models: hy- poxia, starvation, and removal of streptomycin from the addicted strain, SS18b (54, 55).

Very few compounds have been demonstrated to kill *M. tuberculosis* rendered nonreplicating in more than one way. This may be because such "pan-actives" are rare in chemical space or because investigators do not routinely test "actives" from one model in other models. We describe pan-actives in the section "Proof- of-Concept Molecules."

CLASS I PERSISTERS: RARE, DRUG-TOLERANT CELLS

Long before the work of Bigger, Hobby, and colleagues was rediscovered (3, 4) and the term "phenotypic toler- ance" became widely used (56), researchers had ob- served evidence of class I persisters *in vitro* and *in vivo*. Kill curves, in which the *x* axis of the graph represents time and the *y* axis represents the number of viable bacteria recovered on agar plates using a CFU-based assay, often have a biphasic, or "hockey stick," shape (25). Following a sharp, logarithmic decrease in viable CFUs at early time points, the CFUs plateau or de- crease at a reduced rate. Notably, compounds fail to reduce CFUs below the limit of detection at any con- centration tested (46, 55). Put differently, the CFU assay reveals a small population of cells that are refrac- tory to killing by the antibiotic. Biphasic kill curves have been observed for *M. tuberculosis* and other my- cobacterial species treated with dapsone, ciprofloxacin, isoniazid, D-cycloserine, rifampin, streptomycin, and various combinations of these antibiotics (30, 46, 54, 55, 57, 58). Class I persisters appear to play a role in phenotypic drug tolerance during human infections caused by *Pseudomonas aeruginosa*, *Escherichia coli*, and *Candida albicans* (57, 59–61). Evidence of class I persisters was observed in murine and guinea pig models of tuberculosis (62–64) and in the human dis- ease (57).

By definition, class I mycobacterial persisters are re- versibly tolerant to one or another of the standard antibiotics (46, 55, 65) but not necessarily to their combinations. There is no reason to expect class I phe- notypically tolerant bacteria to be more resistant than their siblings to molecules that have multiple targets, such as hydroxyl radicals (55, 66). Unlike in *E. coli* (67), there is conflicting evidence whether class I myco- bacterial persisters are cross-tolerant to other anti- biotics. In one study, *Mycobacterium smegmatis* and *M. tuberculosis* persisters that survived exposure to a combination of ciprofloxacin and isoniazid were toler- ant to a bactericidal concentration of rifampin (55). However, a different study found persister populations of $\sim 1.7 \times 10^{-5}$ to isoniazid, $\sim 7.0 \times 10^{-4}$ to rifampin, and $>10^{-1}$ to pyrazinamide (65). The persister popula- tion resistant to the combination of isoniazid, rifampin, and pyrazinamide was $\sim 2.8 \times 10^{-7}$, indicating that in- dividual persisters were not broadly resistant to other an- tibiotics (65). While strategies to target class I persisters have been proposed (40, 41, 68), to our knowledge, high-throughput screens targeting class I mycobacterial persisters have not been undertaken. Conversely, most compounds known to have activity against mycobacteria have not been tested for activity against mycobacteria displaying class I phenotypic tolerance to other com- pounds. Compound 57, identified in a class II pheno- typic screen against carbon-starved *M. tuberculosis*, serves as an illustrative example of a compound whose ability to additionally kill class I phenotypically toler- ant *M. tuberculosis* was discovered postscreening (54). Compound 57 is described in more detail in the section "Carbon Starvation" (54).

In vitro, genetic mutations in *hipA* and *hipB* (high persister genes) lead to approximately 10- to 10,000- fold more class I drug-tolerant persisters in *E. coli*, *Salmonella*, and other species (57, 69–73). Use of *hip* mutants permitted the observation of persisters by time-lapse studies in microfluidic devices (39). High- persister mutants that survived treatment with strepto- mycin and rifampin were recently identified in an ethyl methanesulfonate-mutagenized auxotrophic strain of *M. tuberculosis* and were characterized by genome resequencing and transcriptomics (57). Genetic control over the size of a class I phenotypically tolerant popula- tion should not be confused with heritable resistance. The survivors, when grown without antibiotic and exposed again, have the same MIC as the population from which they were derived. Even a mutant strain of *E. coli* with a 10,000-fold increase in the wild-type proportion of class I phenotypically tolerant persisters to ampicillin will display a 99% reduction in survival at the same concentration of ampicillin as the wild-type strain if the proportion of class I persisters has in- creased from 1×10^{-6} to 1×10^{-2}.

Numerous mechanisms can impel a cell to display class I phenotypic tolerance (39, 74–79). Mycobacterial asymmetric division results in differential antibiotic sensitivity of daughter cells (80, 81). As in *E. coli* (82, 83), mycobacteria may depend on toxin-antitoxin genes (46, 65, 84) to induce class I tolerance. Javid and colleagues found that mistranslation of two amino acids, glutamate for glutamine, and aspartate for asparagine, resulted in modified RNA polymerase (RpoB, encoded by *rv0667*) that was more resistant to rifampin (85). Only a minority of cells in a wild-type population accumulated enough mutant copies of RpoB with Asp in place of Asn at position 434 to survive rifampin at its MIC (85, 86). When these cells were expanded, the MIC remained the same.

Analogous to the situation with *hip* genes in *E. coli*, mutation in the GatCAB aminotransferase that normally corrects mistranslation of the Asn codon increased the frequency of these class I phenotypically tolerant mycobacteria, but the MIC was no greater in progeny of these cells than in the population from which they were selected (86). Rendering *M. smegmatis* nonreplicating by acidic pH or nutrient starvation led to protein mistranslation and phenotypic kanamycin resistance (85). Isoniazid is a prodrug that requires oxidation by a catalase-peroxidase (KatG, encoded by *rv1908c*) and forms an NAD-isoniazid adduct that targets NADH-dependent enoyl-ACP reductase (InhA, encoded by *rv1484*). Isoniazid kills multiple $\log_{10}$ CFU of replicating mycobacteria within days; yet isoniazid dosed by itself takes weeks to months to achieve a modest reduction in the *M. tuberculosis* bacterial burden in mice (87). Stochastic gene expression has been described in eukaryotes and prokaryotes (88, 89) and provides one potential explanation for the appearance of class I phenotypic tolerance in a small subpopulation of bacteria. For example, Wakamoto et al. found that stochastic expression of *katG* explains some mycobacterial tolerance to isoniazid (90). In *E. coli*, fluoroquinolones can damage DNA and induce an SOS response protein, TisB, which transforms cells to a persister phenotype by depolarizing the membrane and depleting ATP (91–93).

CLASS II PERSISTERS: A MAJORITY POPULATION OF NONREPLICATING, DRUG-TOLERANT CELLS

Class II persisters are defined as a population of cells displaying phenotypic drug tolerance under externally applied conditions that halt net replication. As noted, nonreplication in this sense is a terminologic simpli-

fication that encompasses balanced bacterial growth and death. In some models of nonreplication, there is a slow reduction in viable bacteria over the period of observation that may be difficult to detect by a CFU assay (28, 94). Conditions that arrest growth are associated with resistance to a large number of antibiotics. Some investigators have assumed that failure to grow is synonymous with shutdown of the bacterial machinery that synthesizes macromolecules and that the lack of need for macromolecules explains the lack of sensitivity to drugs that inhibit their synthesis (30, 50–52, 95, 96). However, *M. tuberculosis* adapts to the stresses that impose nonreplication with a robust transcriptional response (46, 49, 97) and cell wall remodeling (98, 99) and maintains metabolic activity, although with a different profile of metabolites than during replication (K. Rhee, personal communication). Nonreliance on biosynthetic processes is an unsatisfactory explanation for class II phenotypic tolerance.

The rate at which *M. tuberculosis* achieves stasis may impact the bacilli's biology and sensitivity to certain compounds. For example, some models of nonreplication, such as hypoxia or starvation, require preadaptation periods of 1 to 2 weeks or more (12, 54, 95). In contrast, reactive nitrogen intermediates cause immediate growth arrest (48, 100). In addition, exogenously applied stresses may be perceived at different rates by mycobacteria at different locations within a clump.

Designing High-Throughput Screens To Target Phenotypically Tolerant Mycobacteria

There have been numerous whole-cell screens to identify small molecules in academic and industrial collections that kill nonreplicating mycobacteria (29, 53, 54, 94, 96, 101–105). Compounds arising from whole-cell screening are presumably taken up into the cell to exert bactericidal activity, without any preconceptions about suitable targets. An alternative approach is to postulate which enzymes play a role in nonreplicating persistence based on informatics or biochemical or genetic studies, set up relevant biochemical assays, identify inhibitors, and then assay those inhibitors for whole-cell activity in nonreplicating models (100, 106–115). The limitation of biochemical screening, however, is that the majority of enzyme inhibitors so identified lack activity against intact *M. tuberculosis* due to poor uptake, the sufficiency of residual enzyme activity for cell survival, intracellular metabolism, or redundant pathways (116). Translating biochemical screening hits to whole-cell activity is hampered by using a binary readout of the life/death of a bacterial cell as a surrogate to monitor target engagement (117).

In screens carried out against nonreplicating bacteria, a failure to increase in optical density over time cannot be used as a measure of antibacterial activity since, by definition, the optical density does not change for the duration of a nonreplicating experiment. There are limited examples of screening by recording fluorescence from nonreplicating mycobacteria (29, 118, 119). While most replicating assays use an inoculum of ~A_{580} of 0.01 or lower, use of a fluorescent readout can require a larger inoculum (upwards of ~50-fold) to achieve a sufficient signal (119). Using a high inoculum of cells may preclude identifying active molecules from compound classes such as beta-lactams, which are highly sensitive to inoculum effects (120). Moreover, nonreplicating screens employing fluorescent readouts often depend on subtle differences in the fluorescence of compound-treated versus vehicle-treated cells (often less than 2-fold), which in turn requires exceptional Z′ scores (29). In some nonreplicating assays, the drug-exposure phase of the assay is coupled to a drug-free secondary phase that permits bacterial growth and allows one to make a semiquantitative estimation of the number of surviving cells (Fig. 1) (53, 54, 96). The two-stage assay, while effective, can take 14 to 17 days (a 7-day drug exposure and a 7- to 10-day outgrowth) and runs a risk of evaporation, edge effects, and contamination with mold (30, 94).

One must carefully weigh the relative importance of potential variables when designing a high-throughput screen against nonreplicating mycobacteria (Fig. 2). Table 2 provides a nonexhaustive list of potential microenvironments encountered by *M. tuberculosis* during infections that may lead to suboptimal growth or nonreplication. The numerous nonreplicating models and technical variables lead to a staggering number of possible combinations.

The most commonly used models for nonreplicating mycobacteria are hypoxia (the Wayne model) and the low oxygen recovery assay (LORA) (29, 95, 96); carbon starvation (54, 121); nutrient starvation (12, 52); stationary phase (105); maintenance of intrabacterial pH under acidic culture conditions (119, 122–126); biofilms (102, 127–130); depleting strain SS18b of streptomycin (103, 104, 131, 132); and a multistress model

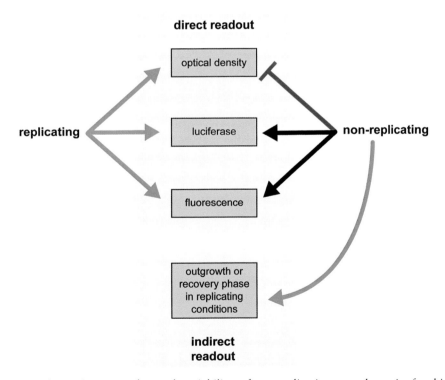

Figure 1 Strategies to evaluate the viability of nonreplicating mycobacteria for high-throughput screening. The arrow color indicates the quality of each readout strategy (considering robustness, ease of use, dynamic range, etc.) as excellent (green arrows), average to poor (black arrows), or infeasible (red line). Compound carryover may result from compound transfer from the nonreplicating assay to replicating assay bacteriologic growth medium or by compound adherence to the bacterial cell wall.

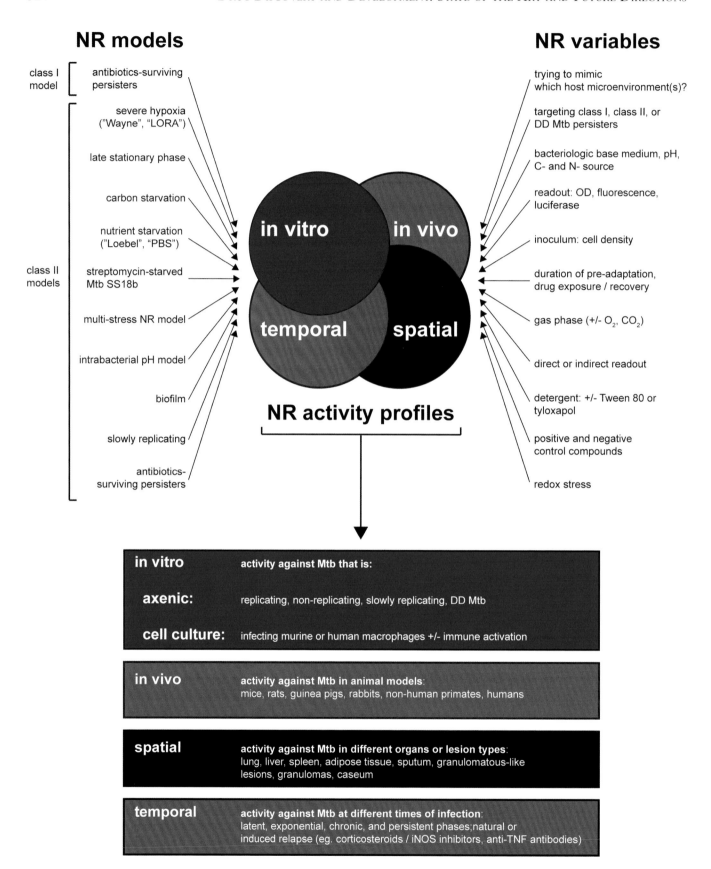

that combines acidic pH (pH 5.0), mild hypoxia (1% O_2), nitric oxide and other reactive nitrogen intermediates (0.5 mM $NaNO_2$), and a fatty acid carbon source (0.05% butyrate) (28, 53, 94, 100, 133). There are variations of these models, including an acidic Wayne model that combines hypoxia with mild acidity (130) and a nutrient-poor, multistress model in which cells are cultured at low pH (pH 5.0) under mild hypoxia or tissue-level normoxia (5% O_2) and supraphysiologic levels of CO_2 (10% CO_2) (134). Sublethal doses of antibiotics targeting translation can also arrest growth (135). Potassium starvation has been reported to lead to the formation of differentially detectable mycobacteria (also called "viable but not culturable") (136, 137).

High-throughput screening typically identifies many molecules with properties unsuitable for further progression, including those whose structures contain toxicophores and/or metabolic liabilities (138, 139). Comprehensive postscreening characterization of compounds from primary screens is extremely expensive in terms of time and resources. In Table 3, we summarize postscreening assays that are suitable for molecules with activity against replicating and/or nonreplicating mycobacteria. Table 4 summarizes assays used to characterize the action of compounds on nonreplicating mycobacteria. A hit progression flowchart for a nonreplicating active compound should attempt to include the assays described in both Tables 3 and 4.

Potential Compound Transformation during Screening and Secondary Assays

As molecules progress from the initial high-throughput screen to *in vivo* models, there are mounting risks of wasting progressively larger amounts of time and money. Meticulous analysis of physicochemical and metabolic properties (138) of compounds is the norm in pharmaceutical companies and, unfortunately, is often pursued insufficiently in academia due to lack of experience, personnel, funds, or access to expert chemistry advice, experimental analysis, and synthesis (139).

Chemical structures can be misidentified as a result of inaccurate assembly of the compound library, erroneous dispensing of compounds, incorrect structure as-

signment, splashing of compounds between microtiter wells, compound degradation, and incomplete removal of reagents or catalysts used to synthesize the original compound, such as organotin, which can have antiseptic properties (140). For these reasons, it is critical to validate a molecule's structure after cherry-pick confirmation and prior to initiating downstream hit characterization. Validation studies include testing a subset of screening hits for correct molecular mass, structure, and purity by liquid chromatography/mass spectrophotometry and nuclear magnetic resonance. Prioritized molecules should be resynthesized and re-evaluated in the original assay to confirm that they recapitulate the activity of the original hits. A surprisingly large number of screening compounds fail to meet these criteria.

Compound solubility is a problem at the forefront of high-throughput screening. The real and assumed concentrations of drug stocks can differ by several orders of magnitude (141–143). Dimethyl sulfoxide is hygroscopic and can absorb water from room air, leading to precipitation of water-insoluble compounds. Some dimethyl sulfoxide-soluble compounds precipitate immediately or over time when transferred to assay plates containing aqueous media or buffers. Antimycobacterial compounds often have high logP values (144) that favor their precipitation in aqueous solution. Compound precipitation can lead to false-negative activity or to false-positive activity in optical density-based assays.

As scientists explore more diverse bacteriologic media for whole-cell screening to mimic *in vivo* microenvironments and stresses, another issue arises: the chemical stability of the compounds in the assay conditions. Careful determination of the structure of a molecule under the nonreplicating assay conditions is a critical, and often overlooked, step. As illustrated in Fig. 3a, structures may be transformed by conditions found in nonreplicating assays, including acidic pH, reactive oxygen intermediates, and reactive nitrogen species. If specific transformation products can be identified, they should be tested for activity in the original model of nonreplication and for their potential toxicity to eukaryotic cells. For example, oxyphenbutazone was chemically transformed in cell-free medium used in the multistress assay of nonreplication (Fig. 3b) (53).

Figure 2 Selecting and designing nonreplicating (NR) models. (Left) Nonexhaustive list of models of class I and class II nonreplication. (Right) Variables to consider when designing models. (Center, bottom) Potential activity profiles of nonreplicating actives. The success of compounds targeting nonreplicating mycobacteria is dependent on the interactions among models, variables, and activity profiles. The term "DD Mtb" (differentially detectable *M. tuberculosis*) is used interchangeably with "viable-but-nonculturable" (VBNC) *M. tuberculosis*.

Table 2 Conditions encountered by *M. tuberculosis* that may contribute to suboptimal replication rates or complete growth stasis[a]

Condition(s)	Chemical mediator(s), examples	Location or situation, example(s)	Responsible for microenvironmental condition	References
Acidic pH	H^+	*M. tuberculosis*-containing phagosome	Immune-stimulated macrophages	231, 232
		Lactate in extracellular fluid at inflammatory sites	Crowding of stromal and parenchymal cells by macrophages, monocytes, dendritic cells, lymphocytes, neutrophils leading to enhanced reliance on glycolysis	299
Hypoxia	Limiting O_2	Succinate	Secreted by *M. tuberculosis* under hypoxic conditions	168, 300
		Necrotic granulomas	Poor vascularization of necrotic granuloma that has a surrounding rim composed of epithelioid macrophages, T cells, B cells, and neutrophils; phagosomes of human macrophages infected with wild-type *M. tuberculosis*	17, 21, 301–303
Reactive nitrogen intermediates	$\bullet NO$, $ONOO^-$, $ONOOH$, $\bullet NO_2$, N_2O_3, N_2O_5	Macrophage phagosomes	Human blood, human interstitial fluid, diet, enterosalivary nitrite cycle, inducible and constitutive nitric oxide synthases in macrophages, fibroblasts, vascular smooth muscle, endothelium, and bronchial epithelium, *M. tuberculosis* under hypoxic conditions or in human macrophages	27, 232, 304–308
Reactive oxygen intermediates	$\bullet O_2^-$, H_2O_2, $ROOH$, $\bullet OH$, $^1O_2$, O_3, $HOCl$, $HOBr$, HOI	Macrophage phagosomes, antibiotics	Activated macrophages and polymorphonuclear leukocytes, the respiratory chain, catabolism (enzymatic and nonenzymatic), response of *M. tuberculosis* to antibiotics	66, 309–312
Metal deficiency	Iron	Animal models, humans	Iron sequestration by host iron-binding proteins such as lactoferrin	229, 313
	Magnesium	Macrophage phagosome, mycobacterial membrane lipids	NRAMP (natural resistance-associated macrophage protein) ion transporter	243, 314
Metal intoxication	Cu(I)	Macrophage phagosome, blood, lungs	Copper transporter ATP7A, copper importer CTR1, ceruloplasmin, NO-dependent release of copper from Cu(I)-protein complexes	140, 230, 315–319
Osmolarity	Chloride ion	Macrophage phagosome, airway surface liquid	Chloride channels, such as chloride channel protein 1	320–323
Carbon sources that support slow growth or survival; growth rate less than maximal	Fatty acids (short/long chain; saturated/unsaturated), cholesterol, amino acids, CO_2	Macrophage phagosomes, caseum, granulomas, adipose tissue	Krebs cycle, glycolysis	233, 236, 237, 324–328
Nutritional starvation	Use of *M. tuberculosis* metabolic reserves: trehalose, glycogen, fatty acids, glutamate	Unlikely to occur	Krebs cycle, glyoxylate shunt	12, 216, 329
Amino acid or vitamin deficiency	Methionine, lysine, leucine, panthothenate	Macrophage phagosomes	Limited quantities *in vivo*, or amino acids and vitamins are not in a form accessible for mycobacterial uptake	238–240, 330, 331
Nitrogen metabolism	Amino acids, inorganic NH_4^+, urea, NO_3^- (nitrate)	Hypoxic lesions and/or hypoxic-acidic phagosomes	*M. tuberculosis* respiring nitrate as an alternative electron acceptor, acid resistance, nutrient starvation	21, 332, 333

[a]Individual conditions, or combinations of them, that are anticipated to lead to phenotypic tolerance observed in animal models of tuberculosis and in human patients.

Table 3 Postscreening assays for molecules active on replicating and/or nonreplicating *M. tuberculosis*

Hit triage assay/study	Description and/or techniques used	Function
Validate chemical identity and purity	LC-MS, nuclear magnetic resonance	Sometimes overlooked, this is an essential component of high-throughput screening that can prevent heartbreak after years of work. It is imperative to confirm that the proposed structure is the molecule responsible for the observed activity.
Confirm activity with resupplied compound; confirm activity with resynthesized compound	Reorder from trusted supplier and conduct *de novo* chemical synthesis	
Medical chemist analysis for structural alerts or toxicophores	Organic, physical, and medical chemistry; cheminformatics; experience	Identification of structural alerts or toxicophores may predict alternative mechanisms of action (often general reactivity) and *in vivo* liabilities, such as liver toxicity or metabolism.
Glutathione reactivity	Mix compound with reduced glutathione and look for possible glutathione-compound adducts	Highly unstable transformation products may be difficult to observe due to their transient nature. Glutathione, with a cysteine nucleophile, reacts avidly with electrophilic molecules and can form stable glutathione-compound adducts.
Toxicity to HepG2 and/or Vero cells	EC_{50} determination by correlating ATP levels with cellular viability	Both the human hepatocellular carcinoma cell lines (HepG2) and monkey kidney epithelial cell lines (Vero) are used to test for cellular toxicity; HepG2 cells also assay for possible bioactivation in the liver.
Determine the selectivity index (SI)	EC_{50} in Vero or HepG2 cells divided by the MIC_{90} against *M. tuberculosis*	Helps prioritize compounds that are more potent against *M. tuberculosis* than against eukaryotic cells. Typically, an SI of >10 is used as a threshold for structure-activity relationship analysis, and an SI of >50 is required to advance to lead candidacy. The duration of compound exposure to *M. tuberculosis* and HepG2/Vero cells and equivalence of serum proteins in the two assays should be taken into account.
Serum shift	Determine MIC_{90} in screening medium ±10% heat inactivated mouse or human serum	A serum shift may indicate if a compound is highly protein bound and provide a warning that eukaryotic toxicity results, typically performed with 10% serum, may have underestimated toxicity.
Inoculum effect	Determine MIC_{90} at an OD_{580} of 0.01 and 0.10	Some compounds such as beta-lactams are well known for inoculum effects, in which their potency decreases as the inoculum increases.
Microbiologic spectrum	Test activity against representative Gram-positive and Gram-negative bacteria and fungi	To determine if a compound has broad- or narrow-spectrum activity
Frequency of resistance (FOR)	Plate 10^6 to 10^9 *M. tuberculosis* on agar plates containing 1–20× the broth MIC_{90} of compound	Determine the number of pre-existing mutants in a population that are naturally resistant to a drug or determine if the drug itself is mutagenic. Acceptable FORs are $\leq 1 \times 10^{-6}$ (the FOR of isoniazid).
Test activity against drug-resistant *M. tuberculosis* strains	Determine the MIC_{90} of a drug against *M. tuberculosis* strains resistant to isoniazid, rifampin, streptomycin, ethionamide, ethambutol, etc.	A new agent should have activity against drug-resistant strains.
Test activity against clinical isolates of *M. tuberculosis*	Determine the MIC_{90} of a drug against clinical isolates from tuberculosis patients	A new agent should have activity against strains of *M. tuberculosis* with diverse genotypes.
Genotoxicity	Ames and micronucleus	Compound series with genotoxicity may be mutagenic. SAR campaigns may find analogues that are not mutagenic; if not, series should be deprioritized or terminated.
Activity against intracellular *M. tuberculosis*	Examples include *M. tuberculosis* infecting human blood monocytes, human macrophage cell lines such as THP-1, or murine J774 and RAW macrophage cell lines	This assay usually omits immunological stimulation of the macrophages. Consequently, *M. tuberculosis* is predominantly replicating.
Activity against *M. tuberculosis* grown with different carbon sources	Test acetate, propionate, dextrose, glutamate, glycerol (without dextrose)	It is essential to confirm that the activity of a molecule is not strictly dependent on the carbon source.
CFU assays: time- and dose-dependency	Test for CFU reduction at multiples of MIC_{90} and at different times of compound exposure	

Table 4 Postscreening assays specific for nonreplicating active or candidate dual-active molecules (active on both replicating and nonreplicating bacilli)[a]

Assay/method	Function/description	References
Charcoal agar resazurin assay	(i) To distinguish replicating-, nonreplicating-, and dual-active molecules; (ii) to distinguish replicating bacteriostatic and replicating bactericidal activity; (iii) to serve as a semiquantitative pretest prior to CFU assays; (iv) to permit testing of the impact of a compound over a wide range of concentrations and time points	30, 145
Cell-free stability assay	To determine if a compound undergoes structural modification in the cell-free medium used for the nonreplicating high-throughput screening model	28, 53
Pre-nonreplicating assay	To determine if any potential transformation products have activity against replicating *M. tuberculosis*. Compounds are preincubated for ~24 hours in cell-free nonreplicating medium and then added to replicating culture of *M. tuberculosis* to determine if any potential transformation products have bacteriostatic or bactericidal activity.	28, 53
Membrane depolarization assays: membrane potential (Δψ) and transmembrane proton concentration gradient (ΔpH)	To identify if the mechanism of action is related to inhibition of an enzymatic target or nonspecific depolarization of the bacterial membrane	157, 258
Intrabacterial pH	To determine if a compound impacts the ability of *M. tuberculosis* to regulate intrabacterial pH. Compounds active in acidic nonreplicating models often function as protonophores and decrease intrabacterial pH. This assay employs a pH-sensitive green fluorescent protein variant.	119, 122, 124
Activity against intracellular *M. tuberculosis*: IFN-γ-activated, bone marrow-derived murine macrophages	To determine if a compound has bactericidal activity against intracellular *M. tuberculosis*. Immunological stimulation of macrophages adapts the *M. tuberculosis*-containing phagosome to a microenvironment that is no longer conducive for exponential replication. Such conditions include acidic pH, a shift to using fatty acid carbon sources, mild hypoxia, reactive oxygen and nitrogen intermediates, itaconic acid production, metal starvation, metal intoxication, etc.	49, 156, 231, 232
CFU-based time-kill curves under both replicating and nonreplicating conditions	To enumerate viable *M. tuberculosis* after exposure to a test agent. The CFU assay is widely considered the gold standard to experimentally demonstrate a compound's activity on replicating and nonreplicating bacteria.	28, 34, 53, 100
Inclusion of 0.4% (wt/vol) activated charcoal or 5% bovine serum albumin (wt/vol) in bacteriologic agar plates used to enumerate CFU assays	To avoid carryover effects when enumerating viable *M. tuberculosis* by a CFU assay. Dual-active molecules, and potent replicating active molecules, may artifactually display activity due to compound carryover in agar plates. Activated charcoal or bovine serum albumin can sequester carryover compound. Activated charcoal is preferred due to its ability to bind a wider range of compounds.	30–33
Deconvolution of nonreplicating assay conditions	To determine which stress, or combination of stresses, is required for a compound to kill nonreplicating *M. tuberculosis*	28, 53
Test activity in alternative class I and/or class II models	To identify candidate molecules with pan-activity against nonreplicating mycobacteria	50, 51, 54, 100
Determination of the Wayne Cidal Concentration (WCC₉₀) and Loebel Cidal Concentration (LCC₉₀)	To determine the concentration of compound that leads to killing ≥90% of the starting inoculum under hypoxic (Wayne) or nutrient starvation (Loebel) conditions	51, 157
Test for activity against nonreplicating Gram-positive and/or Gram-negative bacteria	To determine if a compound kills nonmycobacterial bacterial species under nonreplicating conditions. This is an adaptation of the standard "microbial spectrum" typically run under replicating conditions.	28
Most probable number assay	To quantitate "viable-but-not-culturable," otherwise known as "differentially detectable," *M. tuberculosis* that fails to grow on standard agar-based bacteriologic media. The ability to kill differentially detectable *M. tuberculosis* is considered a highly desirable property of compounds targeting nonreplicating persisters.	10

[a]These assays are used in addition to the standard postscreening assays (Table 3).

In acidic medium containing reactive nitrogen species, the carbon on which the butyl chain attaches to the pyrazolidinedione ring was hydroxylated to form 4-hydroxy-oxyphenbutazone. This oxidation was followed by the pyrazolidinedione ring opening and formation of a quinoneimine. 4-Hydroxy-oxyphenbutazone's quinoneimine, a Michael acceptor, reacted *in vitro* with glutathione and mycothiol (Fig. 3b). In live *M. tuberculosis*, intracellular covalent adducts formed between 4-hydroxy-oxyphenbutazone and mycothiol, *N*-acetyl cysteine, and other uncharacterized metabolites. 4-Hydroxy-oxyphenbutazone killed replicating *M. tuberculosis* and mediated some of oxyphenbutazone's activity against nonreplicating mycobacteria. In another example, three cephalosporin analogues (one of which was compound 68) with equipotent activity against *M. tuberculosis* rendered nonreplicating in the multistress model had different stability profiles: two were stable, and one was unstable (145). These results suggested that their uptake into *M. tuberculosis* occurred more rapidly than their extracellular transformation. As this example indicates, the relevance of cell-free stability should be evaluated on a case-by-case basis.

Evaluating Bactericidal Action against Nonreplicating Mycobacteria

Replicating bacterial cultures fail to increase in biomass when treated with effective concentrations of either bacteriostatic or bactericidal molecules. This makes it relatively straightforward to recognize when compounds are active on replicating mycobacteria. Assays can be short in duration; there are many ways to assess viability; and false-positives are unlikely.

In contrast, determining the impact of compounds on nonreplicating cells is technically challenging. Nonreplicating conditions are themselves bacteriostatic, precluding the detection of viability using methods suitable for replicating cells. By coupling nonreplicating assays to a recovery phase under replicating conditions, one only obtains a rough estimation of a compound's activity (Fig. 1) (28, 53, 54, 94, 96). In the case of dual-active molecules, one must ensure *bona fide* activity against the nonreplicating cells or, alternatively, determine if the nonreplicating activity is an artifact of compound carryover from the nonreplicating phase of the assay into the replicating phase of the assay (Fig. 1) (30). Carryover need not be via the fluid phase; compounds can absorb to mycobacterial components and be carried over to the replicating phase of the assay (30). As noted, drug carry-over was shown to be particularly troublesome for the extremely potent and extremely hydrophobic compound TMC207 (30, 32, 146). This is

not to deny that TMC207 has utility in animal (146, 147) and human (148) tuberculosis, and in fact, drug adsorption to mycobacteria may be a useful property. For example, compounds that associate with the bacterial cell wall may deliver a potent postantibiotic effect (30) as they are slowly released into the intrabacterial cytosol. *In vitro* assays have arbitrary time points that are far shorter than clinical regimens and as such may grossly underestimate a drug's bactericidal potential.

We and others have attempted to minimize carry-over effects from enumerating bacilli from *in vitro* assays or from organs harvested from antibiotic-treated, *M. tuberculosis*-infected animals (31–33). One solution was to include 0.4% (wt/vol) activated charcoal in bacteriologic agar plates to rapidly and completely bind the majority of first- and second-line antimycobacterial antibiotics (30).

Many compounds with nonreplicating activity were originally identified as highly potent replicating actives. Only a few studies confirmed their nonreplicating activity with a CFU assay, and almost never in the presence of activated charcoal or bovine serum albumin in the agar plates. Given the challenge of testing large numbers of candidate dual-active molecules by the CFU assay, the charcoal agar resazurin assay was developed to rapidly categorize molecules as replicating-bacteriostatic, replicating-bactericidal, nonreplicating-bactericidal, or dual-active (that is, replicating bacteriostatic or bactericidal and nonreplicating bactericidal) (30). The charcoal agar resazurin assay helps indicate which compounds should be explored by CFU assays and at which concentrations.

Killing Class II Persisters

Molecules that reportedly kill class II phenotypically tolerant mycobacteria are structurally diverse. We have grouped approximately 100 such compounds according to core structure, potential targets, and/or method of discovery (Fig. 4, 6 to 11, and 13).

The list of compounds was assembled with the intent of demonstrating both diversity and common themes. However, this is by no means a complete catalog. Additional actives can be found in databases such as SciFinder (https://scifinder.cas.org), PubChem (https://pubchem.ncbi.nlm.nih.gov), and Collaborative Drug Discovery (https://www.collaborativedrug.com) (149). Many other actives found in screening do not have their structures in scientific reports or deposited in public databases.

A relatively small number of compounds described to have bacteriostatic or bactericidal activity against replicating mycobacteria have also been tested for activity against nonreplicating bacteria. At best, most

a.

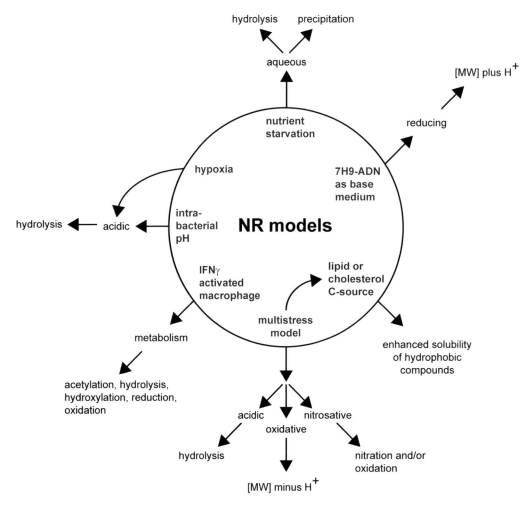

b.

compounds were tested against mycobacteria in a single model of nonreplication. Many studies did not test the activity of the reported compounds with the gold standard CFU-based assay to determine viability.

Highly potent replicating actives may register as false-positives in nonreplicating assays due to compound carryover from the nonreplicating phase to a replicating phase (see the section "Evaluating Bactericidal Action against Nonreplicating Mycobacteria"). TMC207, which is active in multiple nonreplicating models, is an example of a compound that has a high propensity for carryover, clouding interpretation of results (30, 150). Some molecules are listed under more than one classification. For example, TMC207 is in three figures depicting structures: Fig. 4, Fig. 7, and Fig. 12.

The distinction between bactericidal and bacteriostatic varies significantly in the literature. For this review, we define bacteriostatic as preventing growth and affording <99% bacterial kill (<2 $\log_{10}$ CFU) in ≤15 days (30, 151).

Proof-of-concept molecules

A major hurdle for large-scale commitment of resources toward identifying compounds that target nonreplicating bacteria is the paucity of examples that demonstrate the success of this approach. ADEP4 (compound 49), a synthetic acyldepsipeptide that dysregulates ClpP proteolysis, may serve as a prototype (152). ADEP4 killed both *S. aureus* class I persisters surviving ciprofloxacin exposure and bacteria in three class II models of nonreplication: stationary phase, chemically defined minimal medium, and biofilms (153). ADEP4, when dosed with rifampin, eradicated *S. aureus* in a mouse thigh infection. It is unknown to what extent the activity of ADEP4 against the replicating and nonreplicating populations contributes to its *in vivo* efficacy (153). In the following sections we explore examples of proof-of-concept molecules active on mycobacteria.

Selective nonreplicating activity

There are few examples of molecules that fail to kill replicating mycobacteria and that kill those rendered nonreplicating in one or more *in vitro* models of nonreplication (Fig. 4a). Although a limited number of molecules with pan-activity against nonreplicating mycobacteria have been identified, it is likely that more would emerge if the appropriate tests were performed. Since there is a paucity of common transcriptional responses among *M. tuberculosis* populations rendered nonreplicating in different *in vitro* models, such experiments are critical. The first example of a molecule with pan-activity against nonreplicating mycobacteria was published in 2008 (100). Bryk et al. identified a rhodanine, D157070 (compound 1), from a structure activity relationship campaign to develop a prodrug inhibitor of dihydrolipoamide acyltransferase, DlaT (100, 154, 155). D157070 selectively killed *Mycobacterium bovis* bacillus Calmette-Guérin (BCG) and *M. tuberculosis* rendered nonreplicating by acidic pH and reactive nitrogen intermediates (34); hypoxia (95); a multistress model of nonreplication combining acidic pH, reactive nitrogen intermediates, hypoxia, and restriction of the carbon source to a fatty acid (53, 94); human tissue culture medium (Dulbecco's modified Eagle medium containing 10% fetal bovine serum); and infection of bone marrow-derived macrophages activated with IFN-γ (100, 156).

Dual actives with *in vivo* efficacy

Dual-active molecules are defined as possessing bacteriostatic or bactericidal activity against replicating bacteria and bactericidal activity against nonreplicating bacteria. Of the dual actives, moxifloxacin (compound 2 [30, 50, 51, 96, 131, 157]), PA-824 (compound 3 [30, 50, 51, 96, 131, 150, 158]), rifampin (compound 4 [30, 50, 51, 95, 96, 131, 150, 157–162]), and TCM207 (compound 5, bedaquiline [30, 50, 51, 131, 148, 150, 157, 163, 164]) are reported to kill mycobacteria rendered nonreplicating in diverse ways, including hypoxia, nutrient starvation, stationary phase, multistress, and deprivation of streptomycin from an addicted strain (Fig. 4b). Moxifloxacin, PA-824, rifampin, and TMC207 target DNA gyrase, lipid/protein biosynthesis, RNA polymerase, and ATP synthase, respectively.

While none of the available *in vitro* or *in vivo* assays (including those described in Tables 3 and 4) can pre-

Figure 3 Compound transformation during screening assays. (a) Predicted, and experimentally validated, points of compound modification that may occur during phenotypic screening. (b) In cell-free, nonreplicating conditions imposed by the multistress model, oxyphenbutazone (left) rapidly transforms in acidic and nitrosative conditions to the intermediate, 4-hydroxy-oxyphenbutazone (center), which further transforms to 4-hydroxy-oxyphenbutazone quinoneimine (right). The electrophilic quinoneimine (red) can react at carbon atoms (green) with intrabacterial nucleophiles such as *N*-acetyl cysteine (NAC) and/or mycothiol (MSH).

dict the efficacy of a compound in human tuberculosis, it is reasonable to prioritize compounds that have dual activity and potency against mycobacteria infecting macrophages and mice. A combination of three compounds in Fig. 4b—PA-824, moxifloxacin, and PZA (PaMZ)—showed promise in the NC001 clinical trial in tuberculosis patients (165). The 14-day NC001 early bactericidal activity study was too brief to evaluate the impact of PaMZ on eradicating persisters and decreasing relapse rates (165). The Nix-TB clinical trial is evaluating the combination of TMC207, PZA, and linezolid on multidrug-resistant and extensively drug-resistant tuberculosis and may shed light on this question by increasing the duration of treatment up to 6 to 9 months (http://www.tballiance.org/portfolio/trials).

Nonreplicating actives with *in vivo* efficacy

Of the molecules with selective activity against slowly replicating or nonreplicating mycobacteria, only metronidazole (compound 6) (95) and pyrazinamide (compound 7) (166) have been shown to be effective in animal models of tuberculosis (Fig. 4c). As described in the introduction, metronidazole is bactericidal to hypoxic mycobacteria, but this was only demonstrated under conditions in which no alternative electron acceptor was provided; killing was attenuated by inclusion of nitrate, a physiologic electron acceptor used by hypoxic *M. tuberculosis* and present in body fluids (167, 168). Activity of metronidazole did not correlate with evidence of lesion hypoxia (Table 1). Pyrazinamide is the sole representative of the nonreplicating-active class of compounds that is known to kill *M. tuberculosis* in humans, but pyrazinamide also kills slowly replicating mycobacteria *in vitro*. Pyrazinamide's activity on *M. tuberculosis* under acidic conditions was enhanced by additionally including hypoxia (23) or a 3- to 10-day period of preadaptation to nutrient starvation in phosphate-buffered saline (169). While its complete set of targets is still under investigation, pyrazinamide inhibits fatty acid biosynthesis by targeting FAS-I (170–172), trans-translation by targeting ribosomal protein S1 (RpsA, encoded by *rv1630*) (173), and pantothenate and coenzyme A by targeting aspartate decarboxylase (PanD, encoded by *rv3601c*) (174, 175).

Molecules anticipated to engage canonical antibiotic targets and pathways

The potency of many dual-active molecules in Fig. 4 was lower against nonreplicating bacilli than against mycobacteria replicating in a standard bacteriologic medium. This could be due to less reliance on these processes during nonreplication, decreased uptake of the compounds due to a change in membrane composition and/or permeability (176), compound modification by the assay conditions (Fig. 3) (28, 53), increased or altered intrabacterial metabolism of the compound (116), or sequestration of the compound into lipid bodies that accumulate in mycobacteria in some *in vitro* models of nonreplication (28, 53, 134). Moreover, dual actives may kill nonreplicating mycobacteria by engaging noncanonical targets, or they may have a nonspecific mechanism of action (Fig. 5).

The canonical targets of many compounds that kill nonreplicating mycobacteria are in pathways for the biosynthesis of the cell wall, lipids, RNA, DNA, protein, or peptidoglycan (Fig. 6). These compounds build a compelling case that nonreplicating mycobacteria engage in turnover of macromolecules. It is particularly encouraging that numerous antibiotic classes, some of whose members are approved for use in humans, including fluoroquinolones, rifamycins, macrolides, tetracyclines, and beta-lactams, have representatives that kill nonreplicating *M. tuberculosis*. This suggests that the antimycobacterial members of these families may likewise be tailored to display the pharmacokinetic and pharmacodynamic properties and low toxicities that allowed approval of the family members in clinical use (177).

Compounds that generate reactive oxygen species or reactive nitrogen species likely impact the function of numerous targets, including lipids, DNA, and the membrane. For example, PA-824 donates reactive nitrogen species (158). Sublethal nitric oxide induced a specific set of genes in the *dos* regulon, but higher concentrations of nitric oxide induced the expression of hundreds of other genes and implicated reactive nitrogen species in interfering with numerous processes (48, 178). In addition to engaging high-affinity targets, compounds like PA-824 are probably promiscuous when they achieve higher intrabacterial concentrations.

High-affinity targets may exist that have an essential function unique to mycobacteria in a nonreplicating state. However, to date, we know of no instance in which differential expression or differential essentiality of a target has been shown to explain how a compound selectively kills nonreplicating mycobacteria.

Lipid synthesis

A tetrahydrobenzothienopyrimidine (compound 8) targeting InhA killed *M. tuberculosis* rendered nonreplicating by hypoxia (179) (Fig. 6a). That InhA might be an essential target during hypoxia is surprising. Isoniazid, which targets InhA, does not kill hypoxic *M. tuberculosis* or *M. tuberculosis* rendered nonreplicating in other conditions. Isoniazid is even used experimentally

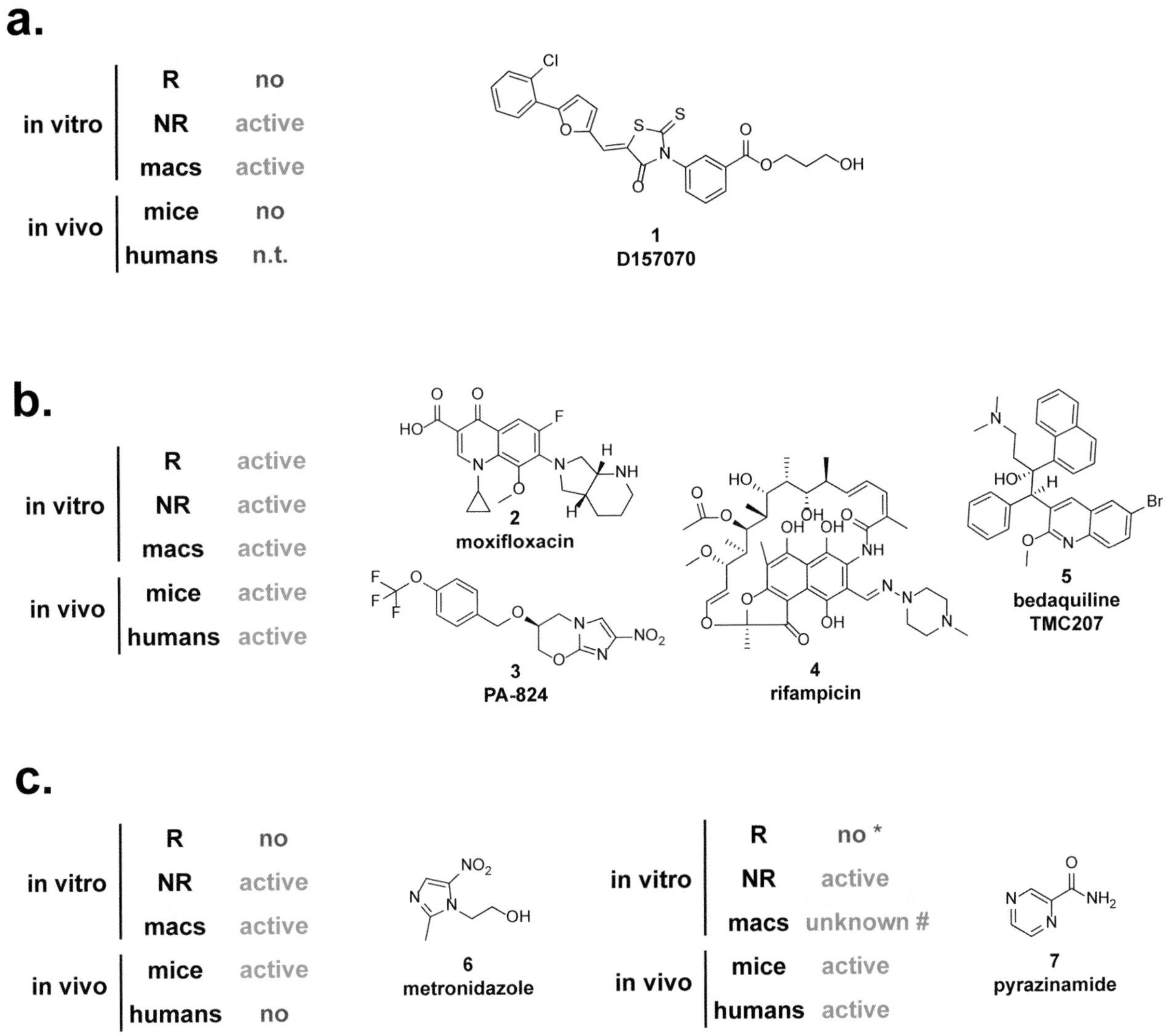

a.

		R	no
in vitro	NR	active
	macs	active
in vivo	mice	no
	humans	n.t.

1
D157070

b.

		R	active
in vitro	NR	active
	macs	active
in vivo	mice	active
	humans	active

2
moxifloxacin

3
PA-824

4
rifampicin

5
bedaquiline
TMC207

c.

		R	no
in vitro	NR	active
	macs	active
in vivo	mice	active
	humans	no

6
metronidazole

		R	no *
in vitro	NR	active
	macs	unknown #
in vivo	mice	active
	humans	active

7
pyrazinamide

Figure 4 Proof-of-concept molecules. Molecules with nonreplicating activity that serve as proof of concept include those that (a) selectively kill nonreplicating mycobacteria; (b) have dual activity, kill mycobacteria in the majority of nonreplicating models, and are effective at treating tuberculosis in animal models; and (c) have selective activity against slowly replicating or nonreplicating mycobacteria and are efficacious in tuberculosis models. n.t., not tested; *, pyrazinamide has activity against slowly replicating mycobacteria; #, experimental data indicate that pyrazinamide is inactive against intracellular mycobacteria *in vitro* (292, 293). However, pyrazinamide's dependency on an acidic environment for activity, and potent *in vivo* activity, suggests that it kills intracellular mycobacteria during animal and human tuberculosis.

as a control compound to confirm that cells have achieved a state of nonreplication. This raises an important question of why isoniazid fails to kill hypoxic, nonreplicating mycobacteria. The structure of isoniazid (likely the hydrazide moiety) may be unstable in hypoxia and/or other nonreplicating conditions (Fig. 3a). Perhaps KatG fails to activate isoniazid under nonreplicating conditions. To test this hypothesis, InhA inhibitors that do not require KatG activation could be tested against nonreplicating bacilli (180). Another possibility is that

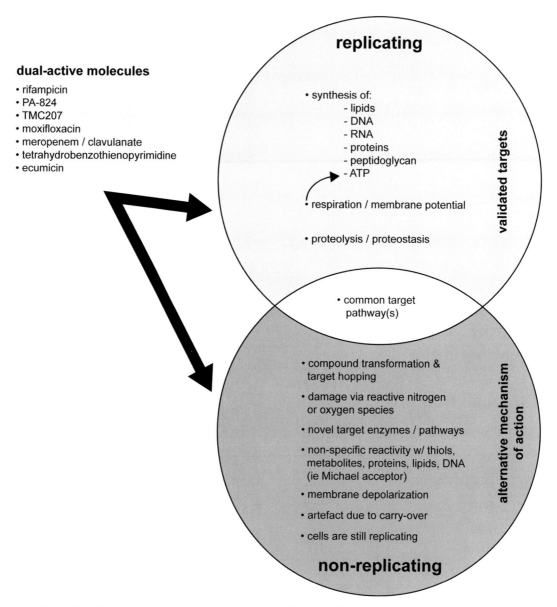

Figure 5   Canonical and noncanonical targets of dual-active molecules. Dual-active molecules, which have bacteriostatic or bactericidal activity against replicating *M. tuberculosis* and bactericidal activity against nonreplicating *M. tuberculosis*, are often presumed to engage the same target under both conditions. Dual-active molecules may exert activity against nonreplicating mycobacteria via novel targets or nonspecific mechanisms. The list of dual-active molecules is not exhaustive.

compound 8, like isoniazid itself, may have more than one target, but unlike isoniazid, one of the alternate targets of compound 8 may be essential in hypoxia.

PA-824 is an inhibitor of lipid and protein synthesis (181, 182). While it has multiple targets, pyrazinamide is an inhibitor of lipid biosynthesis (170–172). Both PA-824 and pyrazinamide are described in the section "Proof-of-Concept Molecules."

DNA synthesis
Nonreplicating conditions may lead to oxidative stress, as may antibiotics with diverse primary targets (55, 66). DNA damage may result and survival may require DNA repair. Compounds that target DNA synthesis and kill nonreplicating mycobacteria are shown in Fig. 6b. Inhibitors of topoisomerase I (TopA, encoded by *rv3646*) (compound 9) (113) and DNA gyrase B

(GyrB, encoded by *rv0005*) (compounds 10 and 11) (108, 112) killed *M. tuberculosis* rendered nonreplicating by nutrient starvation, redox stress, or hypoxia. Cyclohexyl griselimycin (compound 12), which targets the DnaN (encoded by *rv0002*) sliding clamp of DNA polymerase, is anticipated to kill nonreplicating *M. tuberculosis* due to its ability to reduce CFUs during the persistent phase of murine tuberculosis (183–185). To our knowledge, the activity of cyclohexyl griselimycin against *M. tuberculosis* rendered nonreplicating by *in vitro* models has not been explored. Multiple fluoroquinolones, whose canonical targets are DNA gyrase and/or topoisomerase IV (186), including ciprofloxacin (compound 13) (51), gatifloxacin (compound 14) (51), levofloxacin (compound 15) (51), moxifloxacin (30, 50, 51, 96, 131, 157), and sparfloxacin (compound 16) (51), killed nonreplicating *M. tuberculosis* (also described in the section "Quinolones and Their Derivatives").

RNA synthesis

The transcriptomic adaptations of mycobacteria in nonreplicating conditions imply a requirement for RNA synthesis for their survival. Inhibitors of RNA polymerase (RpoB, encoded by *rv0667*) (Fig. 6c), including rifampin (described in the section "Proof-of-Concept Molecules") (30, 50, 51, 95, 96, 131, 150, 157–159), rifabutin (compound 17), and rifapentine (compound 18), killed nutrient-starved and hypoxic *M. tuberculosis* (51, 96).

Protein synthesis

Mycobacteria are killed by a large number of compounds belonging to different structural classes and targeting diverse steps in protein biosynthesis (Fig. 6d). The newly synthesized proteins may help mycobacteria detoxify or compensate for the stresses imposed by nonreplication. In mycobacteria, protein translation is vastly decreased, but not abrogated, during the first 40 days of nonreplication (187). Numerous compounds targeting the 30S and 50S components of the ribosomal machinery killed *M. tuberculosis* in multiple models of nonreplication, including deprivation of strain SS18b for streptomycin, hypoxia, and nutrient starvation. The protein synthesis inhibitors included the oxazolidinones linezolid (compound 19) (103) and sutezolid (compound 20) (103); the tetracycline minocycline (compound 21) (96); the aminoglycosides amikacin (compound 22) (51, 96), streptomycin (compound 23) (50, 51, 96), and kanamycin (compound 24) (51); an aminocyclitol antibiotic, the spectinamycin analogue 1599 (compound 25) (188); the cyclic peptide antibiotic capreomycin

(compound 26) (50, 51, 96); the quinoline macrolide RU66252 (compound 27) (96); and fusidic acid, which prevents elongation factor G turnover and translocation (compound 28) (96). *M. tuberculosis* rendered nonreplicating by incubation for 2 months in stationary phase and then acidified to pH 5.5 under mild hypoxia (1% O$_2$) was susceptible to methionine aminopeptidase inhibitors (compounds 29 [114, 115] and 30 [114]). PA-824, previously described as disrupting lipid biosynthesis, was also shown to inhibit protein synthesis (181).

Peptidoglycan synthesis

Until recently, the dogma in the tuberculosis field was that *M. tuberculosis* was naturally resistant to beta-lactams. The two leading hypotheses were that beta-lactams failed to cross the mycobacterial outer membrane and that beta-lactams were susceptible to beta-lactamase cleavage (189–193). Unexpectedly, there are now multiple examples of beta-lactams and other molecules targeting steps in peptidoglycan biosynthesis that kill nonreplicating mycobacteria (Fig. 6e).

The canonical targets of beta-lactam antibiotics are enzymes catalyzing steps in peptidoglycan biosynthesis. The correlation between the bacterial replication rate and beta-lactam activity fostered the assumption that beta-lactams selectively target replicating bacteria (194). The choice of compounds for these studies led to the belief that activity was restricted to replicating cells, although some beta-lactams were identified that killed both replicating and nonreplicating *Streptococcus pneumoniae* and *E. coli* (56). The basis of dual activity remained a mystery for many years. Most bacteria contain murein predominantly composed of 4→3 transpeptides (195, 196). *M. tuberculosis* in stationary phase, or in hypoxia, had peptidoglycan enriched for 80% and 68% 3→3 cross-links, respectively (98, 99). These studies suggest that the peptidoglycan layer in nonreplicating cells may be different than that of replicating cells, and if so, it offers an underexplored set of target enzymes, such as the L,D-transpeptidases (197). A caveat to this conclusion, however, is that 3→3 cross-links were also enriched in replicating *M. tuberculosis* (~62%) and may not be unique to nonreplicating mycobacteria (99).

A landmark paper in 2009 by Hugonnet et al. demonstrated that meropenem (compound 31), when paired with the beta-lactamase inhibitor clavulanic acid (compound 32), killed replicating *M. tuberculosis* (193). The Hugonnet study made a critical, and unanticipated, discovery—that the combination of meropenem and clavulanate also killed hypoxic, nonreplicating *M. tuberculosis* (193). A 14-day trial demonstrated that

a. lipid synthesis

8

3
PA-824

7
pyrazinamide

b. DNA synthesis

9

10

11

12
cyclohexyl griselimycin

13
ciprofloxacin

14
gatifloxacin

15
levofloxacin

2
moxifloxacin

16
sparfloxacin

c. RNA synthesis

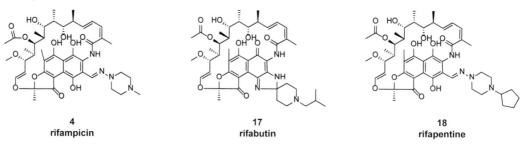

4
rifampicin

17
rifabutin

18
rifapentine

Figure 6 Replicating and nonreplicating mycobacteria may share common targets. Examples of compounds that engage standard antibiotic target pathways under replicating conditions, and also kill nonreplicating mycobacteria, include inhibitors of the biosynthesis of (a) lipids, (b) DNA, (c) RNA, (d) protein, and (e) peptidoglycan.

Figure 6 continues on next page

d. protein synthesis

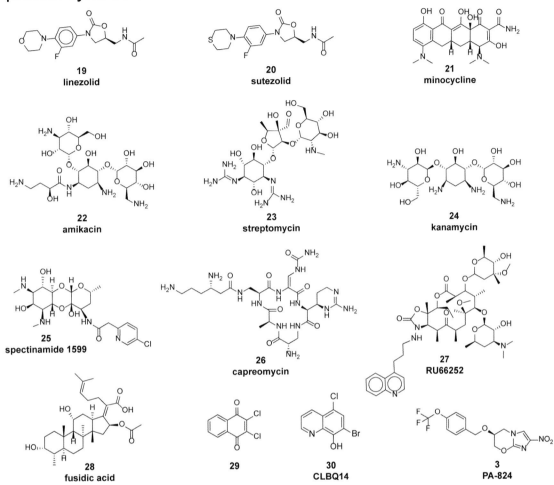

19 linezolid

20 sutezolid

21 minocycline

22 amikacin

23 streptomycin

24 kanamycin

25 spectinamide 1599

26 capreomycin

27 RU66252

28 fusidic acid

29

30 CLBQ14

3 PA-824

e. peptidoglycan synthesis

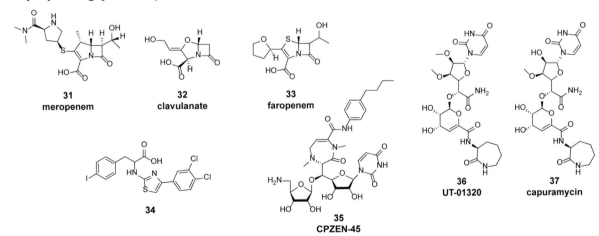

31 meropenem

32 clavulanate

33 faropenem

34

35 CPZEN-45

36 UT-01320

37 capuramycin

Figure 6 _continued_

meropenem, amoxicillin, and clavulanate had marked early bactericidal activity in human tuberculosis (198).

A number of other molecules have been reported to target nonreplicating mycobacteria by disrupting steps of peptidoglycan biosynthesis. These include inhibition of the L,D-transpeptidases by faropenem (compound 33) (38, 199), UDP-galactopyranose mutase by compound 34 (200), phospho-N-acetylmuramoyl-pentapeptidetransferase (MurX) by CPZEN-45 (compound 35) (201), and the capuramycin analogue UT-01320 (compound 36) (202). CPZEN-45 may additionally target decaprenyl-phosphate-GlcNAc-1-transferase (WecA, encoded by *rv1302*), which has a role in synthesizing teichoic acid in *Bacillus subtilis* and mycoylarabinogalactan in mycobacteria (203). UT-01320 (compound 36) was bactericidal to both hypoxic and nutrient-starved *M. tuberculosis* (202). The structure of capuramycin (compound 37) illustrates an example in which replacing a hydroxyl group with an *O*-methyl (UT-01320, yellow highlighted carbon atom in Fig. 6e) confers nonreplicating activity on a molecule whose activity was restricted to replicating mycobacteria. However, UT-01320's activity profile change was accompanied by the failure to inhibit MurX *in vitro* and

suggests that its ability to kill nonreplicating *M. tuberculosis* may have been due to engaging a different target (202).

Folate synthesis
We did not find reports of nonreplicating mycobacteria being killed by inhibitors of folate biosynthesis.

Quinolines and Their Derivatives
There are numerous examples of quinolines and their derivatives that kill nonreplicating mycobacteria (Fig. 7).

Quinolines
Maintaining ATP levels is critical for mycobacteria to survive the nonreplicating state (164). TMC207, which has a quinoline core, is bacteriostatic to replicating mycobacteria and has been reported to kill those rendered nonreplicating by hypoxia, nutrient starvation, and streptomycin removal from the addicted strain SS18b (30, 50, 51, 131, 148, 150, 157, 163, 164). Due to its hydrophobic nature (logP of 7.3) and nanomolar potency, TMC207 is subject to carryover artifacts that make it challenging to evaluate its activity in non-

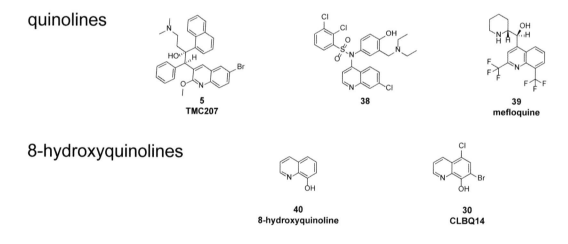

Figure 7 Quinolines.

replicating models (30). To our knowledge, TMC207's activity against mycobacteria in nonreplicating models has not been established by CFU enumeration under conditions that prevent drug carryover, such as the presence of 0.4% (wt/vol) activated charcoal in the bacteriologic agar (described above in "Evaluating Bactericidal Action against Nonreplicating Mycobacteria"). In our own studies, the use of activated charcoal eliminated most of the apparent activity of TMC207 against *M. tuberculosis* in a multistress model of nonreplication (30).

Another ATP synthase inhibitor, the substituted chloroquinoline compound 38 (159, 204), was reported to be bactericidal to hypoxic *M. tuberculosis*. The antimalarial drug mefloquine (compound 39) was reported to kill *M. tuberculosis* rendered nonreplicating by hypoxia and nutrient starvation (51). Mefloquine targets ATP synthase in *S. pneumoniae* (205, 206), but its target in *M. tuberculosis* is currently not known.

8-Hydroxyquinolines

8-Hydroxyquinolines have antibacterial activities on *M. tuberculosis in vitro* and *in vivo* (207, 208). The unsubstituted 8-hydroxyquinoline (compound 40) killed replicating *M. tuberculosis* and was bactericidal to *M. tuberculosis* rendered nonreplicating by mild hypoxia (1% O$_2$), acid (pH 5.5), and nitrosative conditions (pH 5.5 with 0.5 mM NaNO$_2$) (101). Compound 30, a 5-chloro, 7-bromo-substituted 8-hydroxyquinoline inhibitor of methionine aminopeptidase, killed *M. tuberculosis* that had been in stationary phase for 2 months (114). Some 8-hydroxyquinolines may mediate toxicity by chelating metals essential for mycobacterial survival or by forming metal-quinoline complexes that engage target enzymes (209).

4-Hydroxyquinolines

Phenotypic screening led to the discovery of mefloquine-like molecules with a 4-hydroxyquinoline core (compounds 41 and 42) that killed both replicating and hypoxic, nonreplicating *M. tuberculosis* (210–213). Nontoxic isoxazolecarboxylic acid ethyl

ester analogues of compounds 41 and 42, represented by compound 43, killed replicating and nonreplicating hypoxic *M. tuberculosis* (213, 214). 2-Substituted 4-hydroxyquinoline (compounds 44 and 45) inhibitors of triacylglycerol lipase LipY (encoded by *rv3097c*) killed hypoxic *M. tuberculosis* (215). The activity of compounds 44 and 45 was specific to recovery of dormant *M. tuberculosis*, in which LipY plays an essential role in triacylglycerol breakdown (216). With our colleagues at Sanofi, the University of North Carolina, Memorial Sloan Kettering, and the Lankenau Institute, we identified and characterized 4-hydroxyquinolines with bactericidal activity against mycobacteria in the multistress model of nonreplication (data not shown).

Fluoroquinolones

Numerous fluoroquinolones kill nonreplicating *M. tuberculosis* (Fig. 8). As mentioned, moxifloxacin kills mycobacteria in numerous nonreplicating models (30, 50, 51, 96, 131, 157). Similar to moxifloxacin, other fluoroquinolones possess activity against hypoxic, nonreplicating *M. tuberculosis*, including ciprofloxacin (51), gatifloxacin (51), levofloxacin (51), and sparfloxacin (51).

The Proteolysis/Proteostasis Pathway

Inhibitors of the mycobacterial proteolysis and proteostasis pathways are selectively active against bacilli that are nonreplicating or have dual activity (Fig. 9). In addition to turnover of undamaged proteins, the proteolysis pathway also degrades damaged or misfolded proteins that result from exposure to stresses such as reactive nitrogen intermediates or oxidative damage (55, 217). The proteostasis pathway helps ensure proper folding of nascent, misfolded, or damaged proteins with the aid of chaperone proteins and refoldases (218). Some stresses that contribute to nonreplicating persistence engage the proteolysis and proteostasis pathways (Table 2) (55, 66, 217). As described previously, the acyldepsipeptide ADEP4 (compound 49) forces a bacterium to eat itself by unregulated digestion of intrabacterial proteins (153). Unlike the PrcBA proteasome (encoded by *rv2109c* and *rv2110c*), the ClpP1P2 pro-

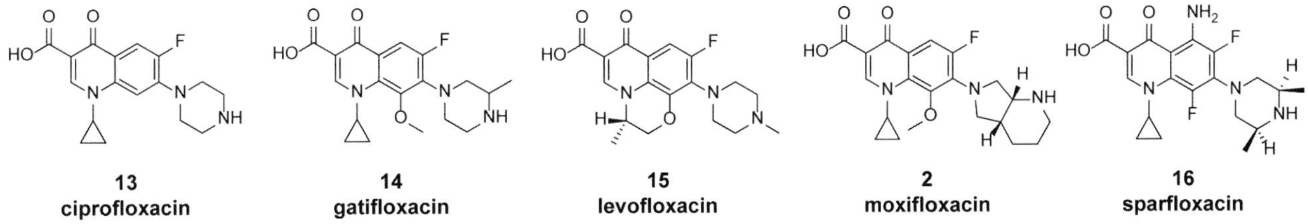

Figure 8 Quinolones.

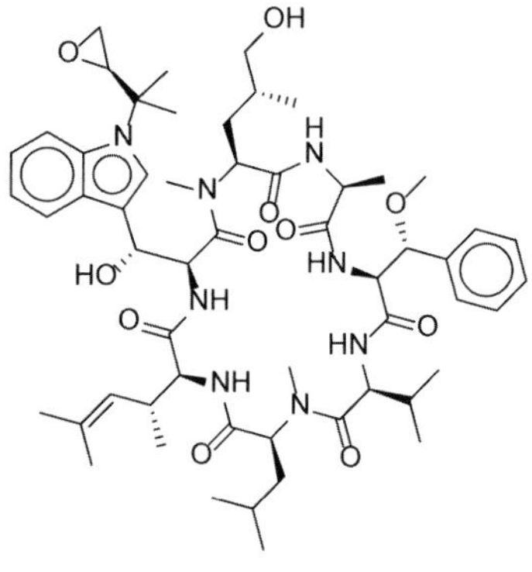

46
cyclomarin A

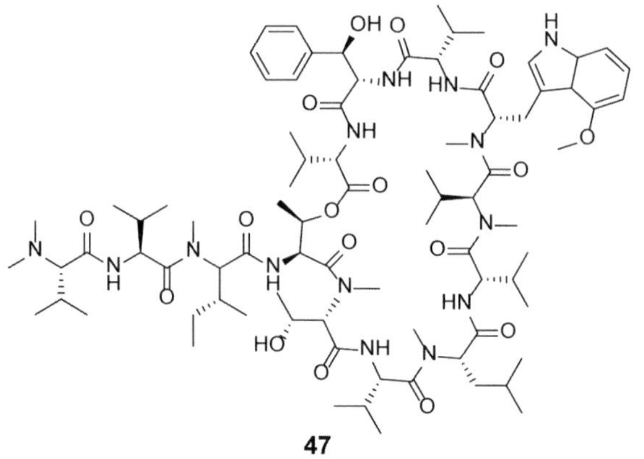

47
ecumicin

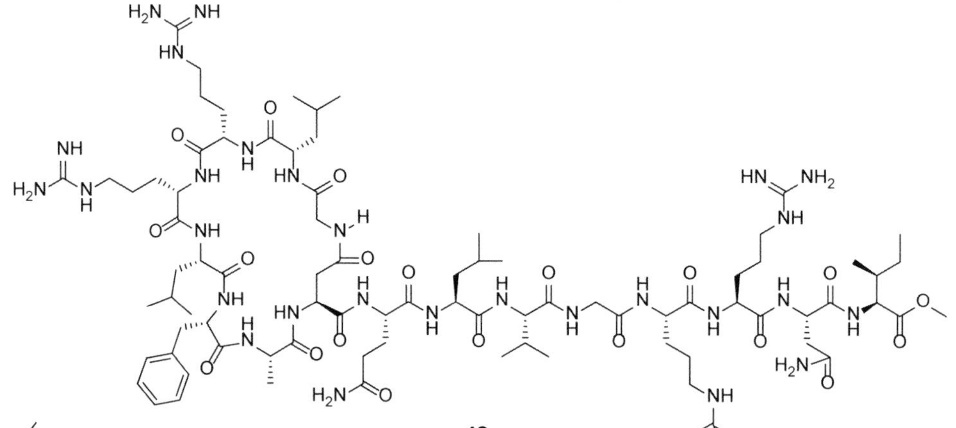

48
lassomycin

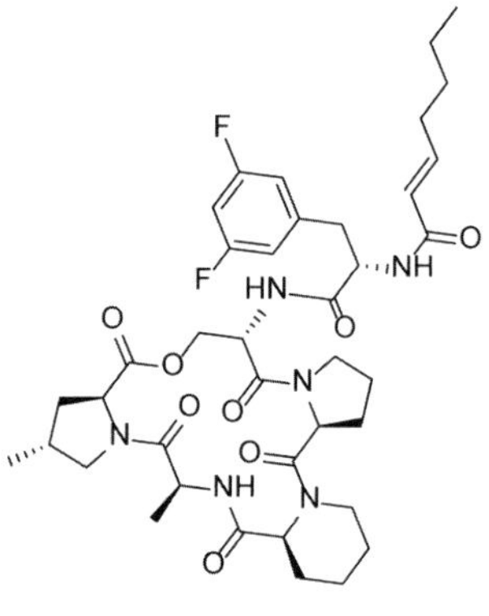

49
ADEP-4

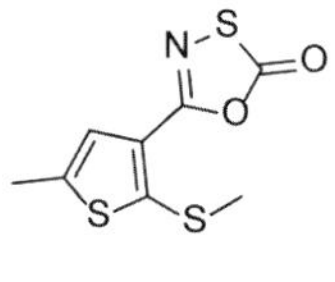

50
GL-5

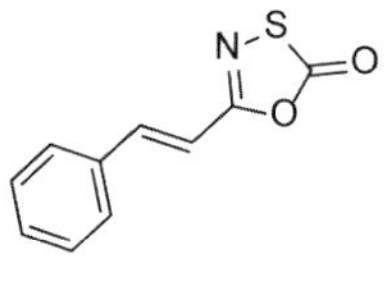

51

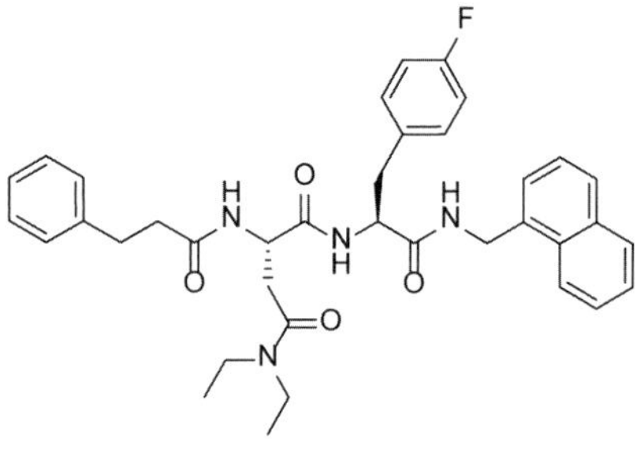

52
DPLG-2

Figure 9 Compounds targeting the proteostasis and proteolysis pathways.

teolytic machinery (encoded by *rv2461c* and *rv2460c*) is essential for *M. tuberculosis* to survive under replicating conditions (219). The dual-active molecules cyclomarin A (compound 46) (220), ecumicin (compound 47) (51, 131, 157, 164, 220, 221), and lassomycin (compound 48, [cyclic(GLRRLFAD)]-QLVGRRNI-CO_2CH_3) (221–223), target the ClpP1P2 pathway by engaging ClpC, and kill *M. tuberculosis* rendered nonreplicating by hypoxia or stationary phase (220, 221, 223, 224). Ecumicin stimulates ClpC's ATPase and impairs its activator activity, while sparing ClpP1P2's proteolytic activity (221, 224). This results in depletion of cellular ATP (see the section "Membrane Depolarizers"). While not essential for logarithmic growth, the *M. tuberculosis* proteasome is required to survive stationary phase and long-term nutrient starvation (225, 226). Small-molecule inhibitors targeting the proteasome, such as GL-5 (compound 50, an irreversible inhibitor) (106) and

DPLG-2 (compound 52, a reversible inhibitor) (227), killed *M. tuberculosis* rendered nonreplicating with acidified nitrite. Compound 51, an analogue of GL-5, had bactericidal activity against a 2-week nutrient-starved culture of *M. tuberculosis* (228). These studies suggest that targeting the ClpP1P2 and PrcAB proteolysis pathways may be good strategies to kill nonreplicating persisters.

Screening Hits
There have been a limited number of phenotypic high-throughput screens to discover molecules that kill nonreplicating mycobacteria (Fig. 10). The following nonexhaustive set of examples illustrates screening methods and the molecular diversity of the hits.

Carbon starvation
Grant et al. identified compounds that killed carbon-starved, nonreplicating *M. tuberculosis* (54) (Fig. 10a). The screen was notable for testing a set of confirmed actives against *M. tuberculosis* in different class I and class II models of phenotypic tolerance. This strategy revealed that the hits had diverse activities: some molecules were active only in the carbon starvation model used for the screen (compounds 53 and 54); others were active in carbon starvation and hypoxia models (compounds 55, 56, and 57); compound 58 was bactericidal to *M. tuberculosis* rendered nonreplicating by carbon starvation or hypoxia as well as to *M. tuberculosis* in a class I persister model.

Hypoxia
As noted, metronidazole kills hypoxic *M. tuberculosis in vitro* and can reduce CFUs in some animal models of tuberculosis (Table 1). Mak et al. set out to identify more molecules that killed nonreplicating, hypoxic *M. bovis* BCG (29) (Fig. 10b). The hypoxia screen was performed using a recombinant *M. bovis* BCG strain expressing the *M. tuberculosis narGHJI* operon. This strategy artificially increased ATP levels by augmenting BCG's use of nitrate as an electron acceptor and made it easier to identify active molecules by their ability to decrease cellular ATP content. Active molecules of the benzamidazole, imidazopyridine, and thiophene classes were confirmed by a CFU assay (compounds 59, 60, and 61).

Multiple physiological stresses
One strategy to identify molecules that kill nonreplicating mycobacteria is to combine various stresses encountered by *M. tuberculosis* during infections of macrophages, animals, and humans (49, 53, 124, 229–

245). A combination of stresses is anticipated to capture a greater diversity of screening hits than a single stress. This strategy requires a secondary hit deconvolution to identify which stress(es) are essential for a given compound's activity. Our laboratory used this strategy to develop a multistress assay of nonreplication, in which replication of *M. tuberculosis* was halted by mild acidity (pH 5.0), nitric oxide, and other reactive nitrogen intermediates generated by NaNO$_2$ at acidic pH, a fatty acid carbon source (butyrate), and mild hypoxia (1% O$_2$). Examples of molecules active in the multistress model of nonreplication (Fig. 10c) include compounds 62, 63, 64, 65, and 66 (28); oxyphenbutazone (compound 67) (53); nitrofuranyl-calanolide (compound 81) (133) (described further in the section "Nitro-Containing Compounds"); and cephalosporins (compounds 68 and 69 [147]). The cephalosporins, compounds 68 and 69, bearing a C-2 alkyl ester or oxadiazole, had clavulanate-independent bactericidal activity against *M. tuberculosis* in a multistress model of nonreplication (145) and killed *M. tuberculosis* infecting IFN-γ-activated bone marrow mouse macrophages. The unusual structures and activity profiles of compounds 68 and 69 suggest that they may engage noncanonical targets (246–249).

Acidic pH
The intraphagosomal environment of an *M. tuberculosis*-infected, IFN-γ-activated mouse macrophage decreases to approximately pH 4.5 (231). Furthermore, *M. tuberculosis* may create local acidic environments by secreting succinate when cultured under hypoxic conditions (22, 168). Using an intrabacterial pH-sensitive green fluorescent protein, Darby et al. screened for compounds that disrupted the intrabacterial pH of *M. tuberculosis* during incubation in growth-restricting conditions of phosphate-citrate pH 4.5 buffer (119, 122, 124) (Fig. 10d). Compounds 70, 71, 72, 40, and 73, identified in this screen, had acidic-pH-dependent bactericidal activity. High-throughput antibacterial screens, in which bacteria are incubated in an acidic pH, often identify protonophores as nonspecific disrupters of the membrane proton gradient. Monensin (compound 88 [119]) is one such example and is described in more detail in the section "Membrane Depolarizers."

Biofilms
Many pathogenic bacteria form biofilms as a survival strategy to evade host immunity and antibiotics (250, 251). Mycobacteria form drug-tolerant biofilms *in vitro* (128, 252), although the relevance of mycobacterial biofilm formation in human disease is unknown. Wang

a. carbon starvation HTS

53   **54**   **55**

56   **57**   **58**

b. severe hypoxia HTS

59
GNF-NITD82

60
GNF-NITD46

61
GNF-NITD101

c. multistress HTS

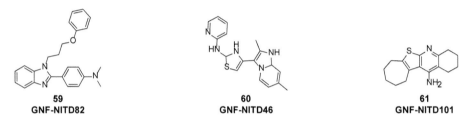

62   **63**   **64**   **65**

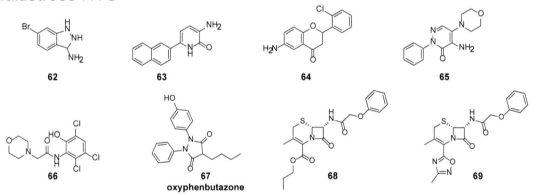

66   **67**
oxyphenbutazone   **68**   **69**

d. acidic pH HTS   **e.** biofilm HTS

70

71

72   **40**
8-hydroxyquinoline   **73**

74
TCA1

et al. screened for compounds that killed nonreplicating *M. smegmatis* that presented as a pellicle at the interface of the bacteriologic medium and air. They identified a replicating-active molecule, TCA1 (compound 74) (Fig. 10e), that potently inhibited biofilm formation by *M. smegmatis*, *M. tuberculosis*, and *M. bovis* BCG and killed *M. tuberculosis* in a nutrient starvation model (102). TCA1 targets both decaprenyl-phosphoryl-β-D-ribose 2-oxidase (DprE1, encoded by *rv3790*), which synthesizes decaprenylphosphoryl-β-D-arabinose, and MoeW (encoded by *rv2338c*), an enzyme involved in the synthesis of a molybdenum-containing prosthetic group, the molybdenum cofactor. Under nutrient starvation conditions, overexpression of MoeW conferred partial resistance to TCA1 (102).

Nitro-Containing Compounds

A number of dual- and nonreplicating-active molecules contain a nitro functional group (Fig. 11). The strongly electronegative nitro moiety has varying degrees of reactivity that depend on its local environment within a molecule. Mycobacterial nitroreductases may catalyze the conversion of the nitro group ($-NO_2$) by first reducing it to a nitroso ($-NO$), then to a hydroxylamine ($-NHOH$), and finally to an amine ($-NH_2$) (253, 254). Nitrofurans and nitroimidazoles undergo intrabacterial bioactivation to metabolites that can redox-cycle and cause oxidative damage and/or dismutate to an electrophilic nitroso intermediate that reacts with intracellular thiols (255, 256). Reactive molecules such as nitrofurantoin may have specific, high-affinity targets such as ribosomal proteins yet become promiscuous at higher intrabacterial concentrations (256). The nitroso radical anion causes DNA oxidation and cell death due to DNA strand breaks (255). PA-824 donates a nitric oxide-like species that may have numerous intrabacterial targets (158, 178).

Examples of nitro-containing molecules that kill nonreplicating mycobacteria include metronidazole (19, 157, 159, 257), furaltadone (compound 75) (257), nitrofurantoin (compound 76) (96, 257), nitrofurazone (compound 77) (257), furazolidone (compound 78) (96), nitazoxanide (compound 79) (34, 50, 258), niclosamide (compound 80) (96), compound 9 (113), nitrofuranylcalanolide (compound 81) (133), OPC-67683 (compound 82) (259, 260), PA-824 (50, 51, 96, 131, 150, 158, 261), TBA-354 (compound 83) (260), and compound 84 (262).

While nitroimidazole-containing molecules such as PA-824 and OPC-67683 are in clinical trials, molecules containing the structurally similar nitrofuran moiety are considered hazardous due to the risk of DNA mutagenicity (263). Even if a molecule is nontoxic to eukaryotic cells, nitroimidazoles, nitrofurans, and nitrothiophenes should be assayed for mutagenicity (Table 4). The nitrofuranylcalanolide (compound 81) has potent MIC_{90} values against replicating and nonreplicating *M. tuberculosis* and kills *M. tuberculosis* infecting human macrophages (133). However, the nitrofuranylcalanolide was genotoxic *in vitro* (133).

Some nitro-containing molecules, such as nitazoxanide and niclosamide, are described in the next section.

Membrane Depolarizers

Nonreplicating mycobacteria maintain an energized membrane (20). During hypoxia, depolarizing the mycobacterial membrane results in the inability to synthesize ATP by disrupting the intracellular to extracellular proton gradient (157, 164). Collapsing the proton motive force, and depleting intrabacterial ATP levels, may be a common feature of molecules that target replicating and nonreplicating mycobacteria (Fig. 12) (264). The structure of a compound may not provide obvious clues that its anti-infective activity results from nonspecific depolarization of the bacterial membrane. For example, some salicylanilides such as niclosamide shuttle protons by forming a stable six-membered ring via hydrogen bonding (Fig. 13) (265–267). The hydrogen-bonded form of salicylanilide has a higher logP than its non-hydrogen-bonded structure, which is predicted to improve penetration across the lipophilic bacterial membrane. After passing into the bacterial cytosol and releasing its proton, the negatively charged salicylanilide anion, which is internally hydrogen bond stabilized, can return across the membrane again to pick up another proton (266).

Compounds that kill nonreplicating mycobacteria by depolarizing the membrane include valinomycin (compound 85) (29, 157), nigericin (compound 86) (29, 131, 157), boromycin (compound 87) (268), nitaz-

Figure 10 Representative compounds identified by whole-cell high-throughput screening (HTS) against mycobacteria rendered nonreplicating by (**a**) carbon starvation (54); (**b**) hypoxia (29); (**c**) multiple stresses, including low pH, nitric oxide and reactive nitrogen intermediates, hypoxia, and a fatty acid carbon source (28, 53, 145); (**d**) acidic pH (119); and (**e**) culture as a biofilm (102).

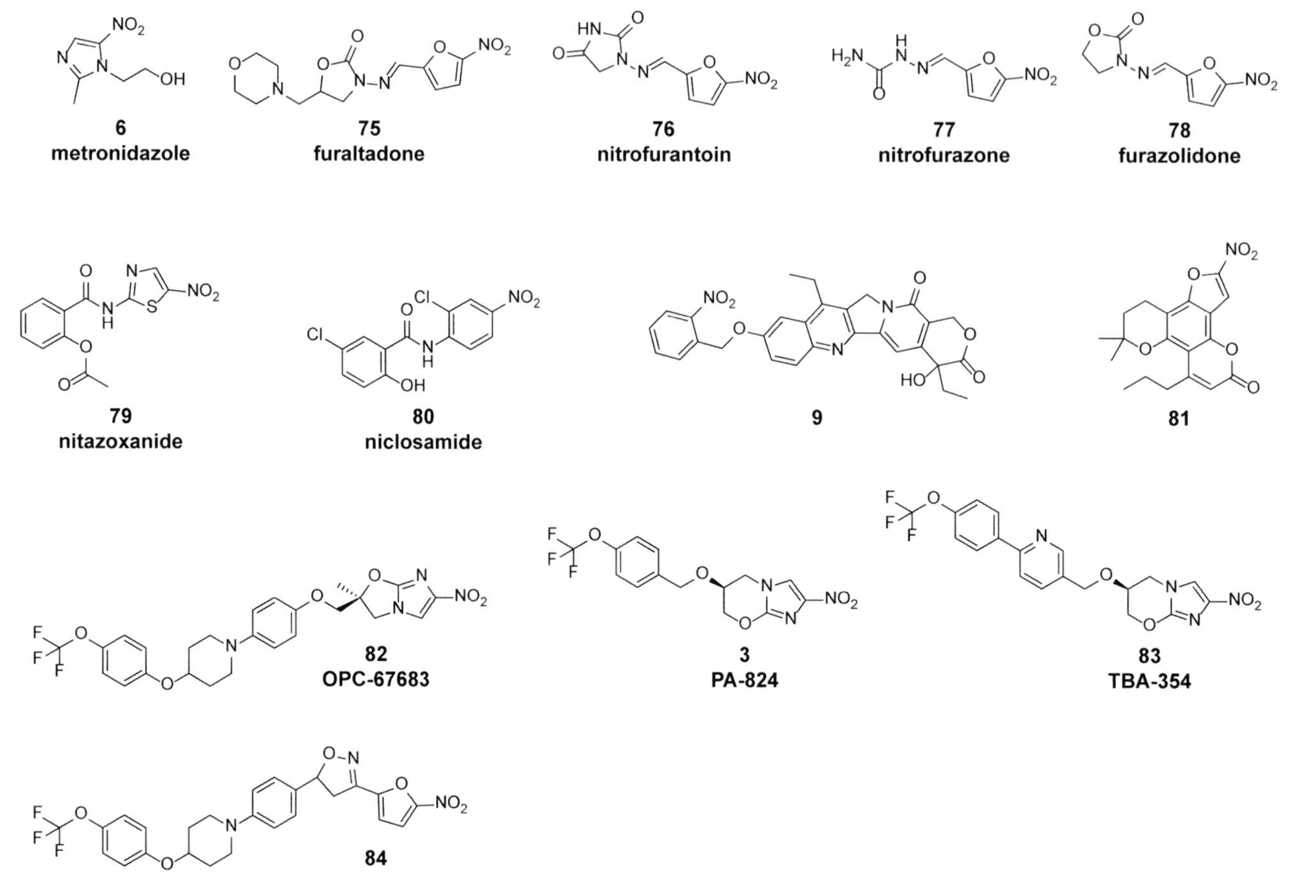

Figure 11 Nitro-containing compounds.

oxanide (34, 50, 258), monensin (compound 88) (119), salinomycin (compound 89) (131), niclosamide (96), a derivative of α-mangostin, A-0016 (compound 90) (269), N,N'-dicyclohexylcarbodiimide (compound 91) (157), clofazimine (compound 92) (50, 55, 96, 270), and thioridazine (compound 93) (29, 51, 157, 159). The prodrug clofazimine is reduced by type 2 NADH-quinone oxidoreductase. Clofazimine likely kills by interfering with mycobacterial respiration by generation of hydroxyl radicals (55, 271). The bactericidal action of clofazimine is reversed by addition of menaquinone-4 (271, 272). The phenothioazines thioridazine and trifluoperazine (compound 94) target the electron transport chain, disrupt membrane potential, and ultimately decrease ATP levels (273). Trifluoperazine was bactericidal to *M. tuberculosis* that was nonreplicating when cultured at acidic pH, in nutrient-starved cultures, or at neutral pH in the presence of the nitric oxide donor DETA-NO (273). As described in the section on quinolines, TMC207 targets ATP synthase (AtpE, encoded by *rv1305*). Compound 95, which kills hypoxic *M. tuberculosis*, targets MenA (encoded by *rv0534c*) (110).

Inhibition of MenA, which catalyzes the prenylation of 1,4-dihydroxy-2-naphthoate to demethylmenaquinone, is anticipated to impact membrane potential and decrease ATP levels (110). *N*-Octanesulfonylacetamide (OSA, compound 96) killed both replicating and hypoxic, nonreplicating *M. tuberculosis* (274–277). The rapid depletion in ATP levels after treating mycobacteria with compound 97 was consistent with inhibition of the ATP synthase and/or the respiratory chain. The compound *n*-decanesulfonylacetamide (similar to compound 96) inhibited ATP synthase and lipid biosynthesis (274, 275, 277), killed hypoxic *M. bovis* BCG, and had bactericidal activity against class I rifampin-tolerant persisters (276). Q203 (compound 97) targets the cytochrome bc_1 complex (QcrB, encoded by *rv2196*), depletes ATP levels, kills replicating and hypoxic *M. tuberculosis*, and has activity in a mouse model of tuberculosis (278).

Dual-active protonophores boast low frequencies of resistance. Membrane depolarization, and ensuing depletion of ATP, has an amplified downstream impact on the cell that cannot be easily compensated for by

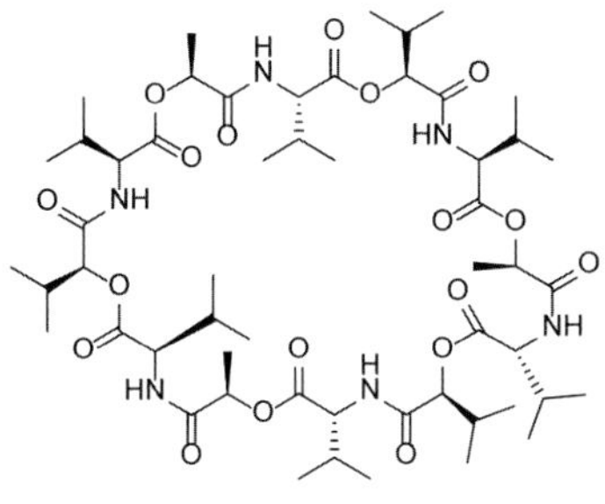

85
valinomycin

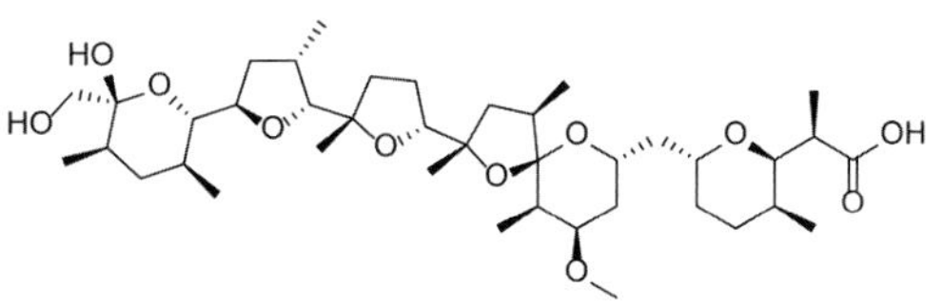

86
nigericin

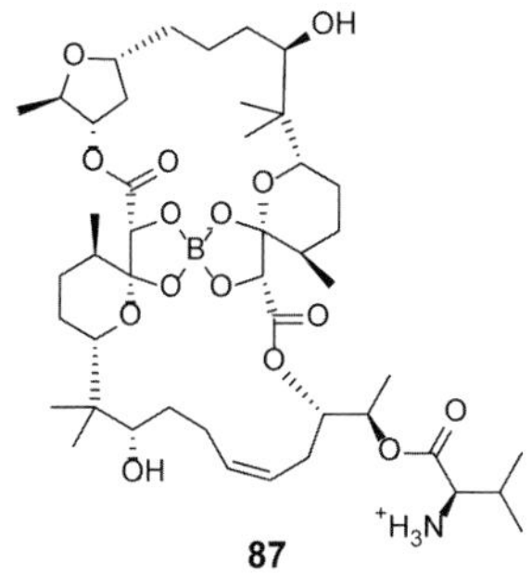

87
boromycin

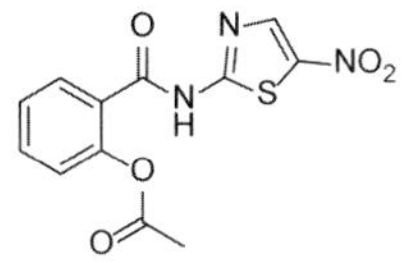

79
nitazoxanide

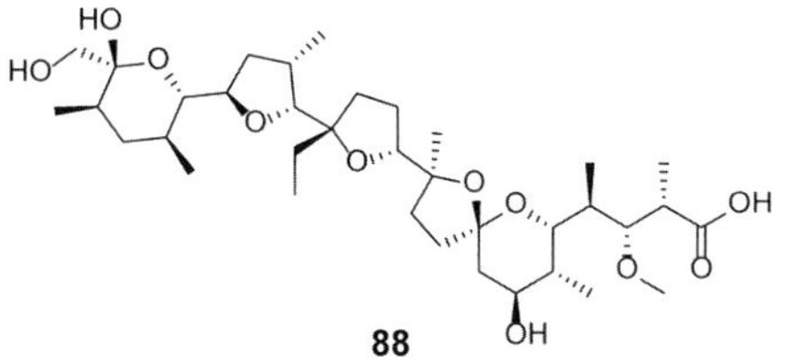

88
monensin

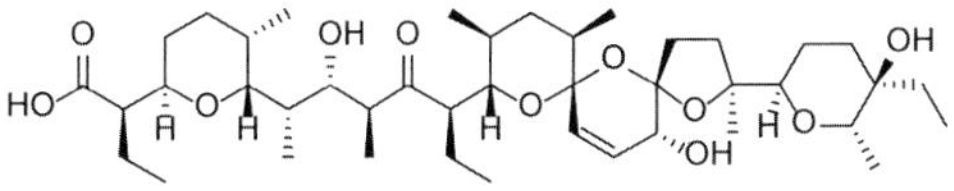

89
salinomycin

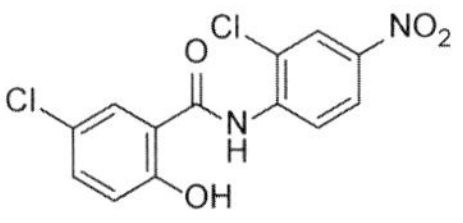

80
niclosamide

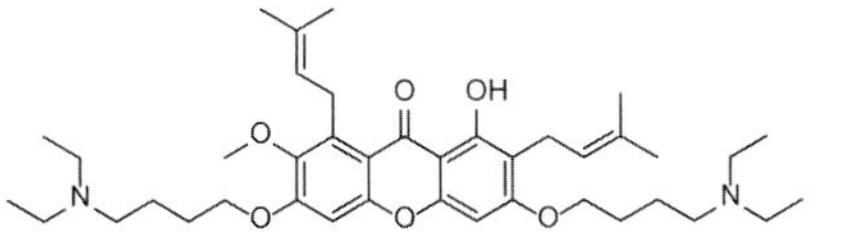

90
AM-0016

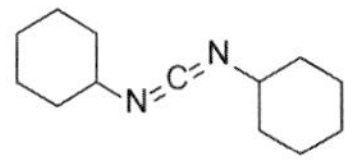

91
DCCD

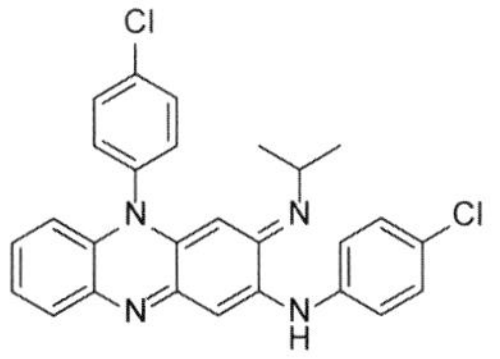

92
clofazimine

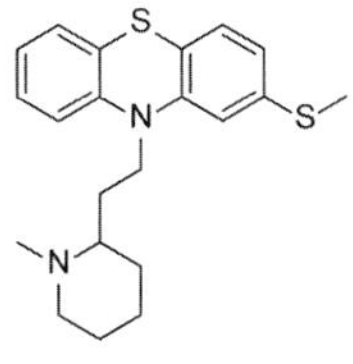

93
thioridazine

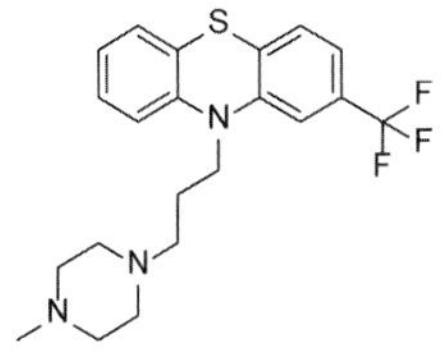

94
trifluoperazine

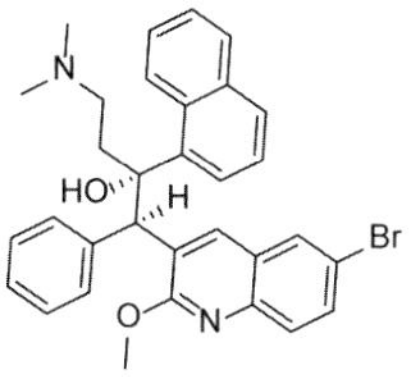

5
TMC207

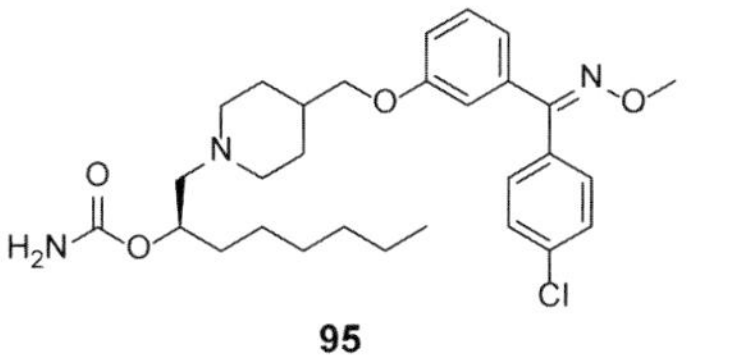

95

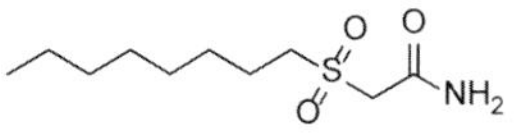

96

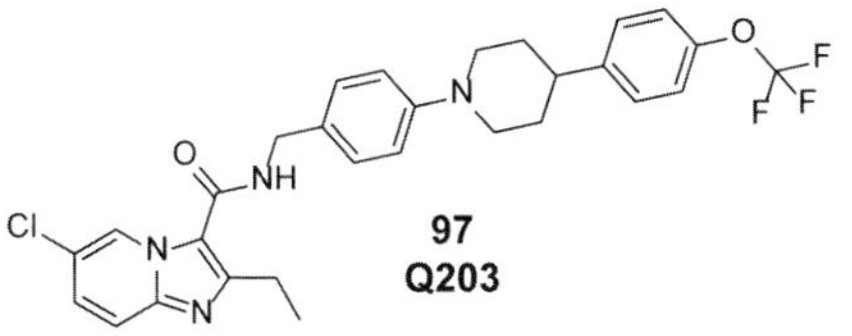

97
Q203

Figure 12 Compounds that depolarize the mycobacterial membrane.

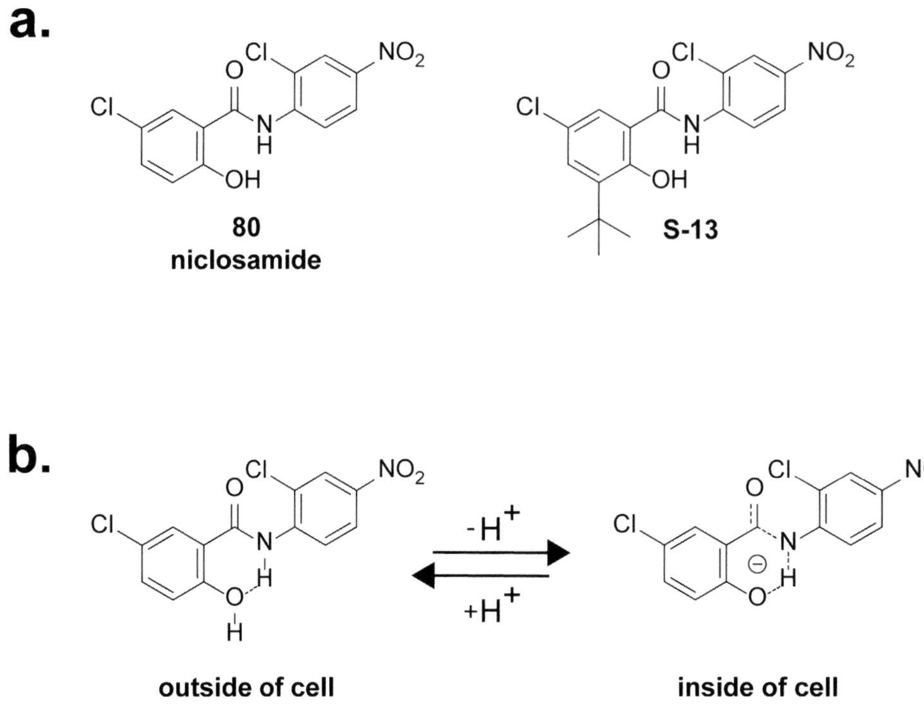

Figure 13 Salicylanilides are protonophores. (a) The commonly drawn structure of niclosamide (left). Compound S-13, which was used for experimental logP calculations (266), is shown for reference (right). (b) As illustrated by niclosamide, salicylanilides capture protons by forming a stable pseudo-6-membered ring via hydrogen bonding. Once inside the bacterial cell and releasing their proton, they maintain a stable anionic form from electron delocalization. Adapted from Terada (266).

mutating a single gene. In the cases of nitazoxanide, boromycin, and AM-0016, the frequencies of resistance were estimated as $<1 \times 10^{-12}$ (34), $<1 \times 10^{-9}$ (268), and $<1 \times 10^{-8}$ (269), respectively. Low frequencies of resistance are consistent with a nonspecific mechanism of action or multiple specific mechanisms of action (279).

ATP depletion can lead to persister formation in *S. aureus* (280). It will be interesting to determine if clinical use of protonophores and membrane-targeting molecules selects for live, ATP-depleted persister populations that are tolerant to other antibiotics.

More Examples of Molecules Targeting Nonreplicating Mycobacteria

Many compounds that are reported to kill nonreplicating mycobacteria do not fall into the categories described above (Fig. 14). Auranofin (compound 98), a drug used to treat rheumatoid arthritis, was recently described as a potent inhibitor of mycobacterial thioredoxin reductase TrxB2 (encoded by *rv3913*) and had bactericidal activity against nutrient-starved *M. tuberculosis* (281). While auranofin probably forms an Au(I) adduct with the cysteine active site of thioredoxin re-

ductase, it has additional thiol targets (274, 281, 282). Compound 99 inhibits CysM (encoded by *rv1336*), which has a critical role in mycobacterial cysteine biosynthesis, and killed nutrient-starved *M. tuberculosis* (107). DevR (also called DosR, encoded by *rv3133c*) controls expression of genes in response to hypoxia (109, 283). A DevR inhibitor, compound 100, killed *M. tuberculosis* that was cultured under hypoxic conditions but spared the bacilli when they were nonreplicating during nutrient starvation (284). A 2-thiopyridine, compound 101, killed both replicating and nonreplicating hypoxic and nutrient-starved *M. tuberculosis* (285). The 2-thiopyridines were bactericidal to viable-but-not-culturable *M. tuberculosis* in a potassium starvation model (285). Compound 102, an inhibitor of pantothenate synthase (PanC, encoded by *rv3602c*), killed *M. tuberculosis* in a nutrient starvation model and killed *Mycobacterium marinum* infecting zebrafish (111). Compound 103 killed hypoxic *M. tuberculosis* (286). A quinoxaline 1,4-di-*N*-oxide, compound 104, displayed potent activity against replicating and hypoxic nonreplicating *M. tuberculosis* and was active in an acute mouse model (287).

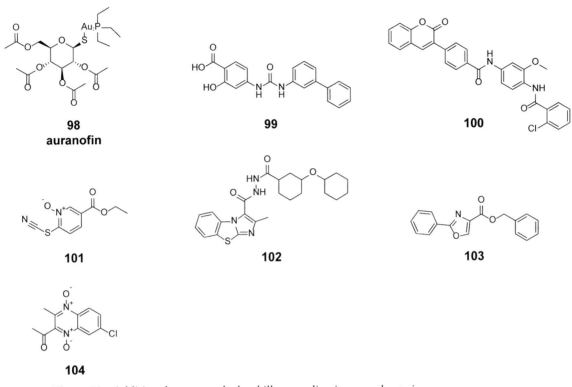

Figure 14 Additional compounds that kill nonreplicating mycobacteria.

FUTURE STUDIES AND CONCLUSIONS

Phenotypic tolerance is complex. We must refrain from projecting the biology deciphered in one persistence model to other persistence models, for fear that we oversimplify phenotypic tolerance, much as Jacques Monod oversimplified biochemical unity when he declared, "Anything found to be true of *E. coli* must also be true of elephants" (288). We need to focus time and resources on developing antibiotics that target mycobacteria in *in vitro* states that have relevance to persisters found during human tuberculosis—antibiotics whose structures are accurately understood under the conditions of the assays, that exert *bona fide* bactericidal activity against nonreplicating mycobacteria, and that have a structure-activity relationship which enables at least one of its derivative compounds to make it through the gauntlet of drug development, or at least to become an informative tool for chemical biology to guide our understanding of bacterial persistence (289, 290).

The challenges are formidable. Our confidence in *in vitro* screens is shaken by the dissociation between the high value of pyrazinamide in the clinic and its lack of activity *in vitro* at the highest concentrations typically considered appropriate for screening. We know many ways to put *M. tuberculosis* into a nonreplicating state *in vitro* but are not confident which states model the class II phenotypic tolerance that is hypothesized to contribute to the inefficiency of conventional drugs against tuberculosis in the human host. We need to validate compounds in animal models but are not sure which animal models (if any) qualitatively and quantitatively mimic which aspects of the human disease (42, 291). It is commonly noted that all current tuberculosis drugs work in mice, but compounds inactive in mouse models of tuberculosis have, to our knowledge, not been tested in primates or humans. A number of compounds active against replicating or nonreplicating *M. tuberculosis in vitro* and displaying suitable pharmacokinetics for studies in mice have failed to show efficacy in mice, but unless they were toxic, we almost never learn why they failed, or if the question is answered, the answer is almost never published. Such failures fail again when little or no insight is gained from the investment that led to the *in vivo* tests.

Two recent developments nonetheless justify optimism. First, academic microbiologists, immunologists, biochemists, structural biologists and physicians interested in these challenges are now working alongside professional medical chemists and pharmacologists. Second, these partnerships involve multiple academic institutions and multiple pharmaceutical companies, and the participants share their questions, hypotheses, failures, and successes as they go along.

SUMMARY OF KEY RECOMMENDATIONS

- Numerous variables need to be considered when designing high-throughput screens against nonreplicating bacteria, including postscreening assays and how to test molecules in animal models of tuberculosis.
- When compounds are reported to kill nonreplicating, phenotypically tolerant mycobacteria, the conditions need to be specified and the assumption of generalizability to other conditions avoided. Whether the compounds kill in more than one model of nonreplication needs to be determined. The structure of the compounds under the test conditions needs to be verified. That the killing took place under nonreplicating conditions, rather than upon removal of the cells from those conditions, needs to be validated.
- When compounds kill bacteria under both replicating and nonreplicating conditions, it should not be assumed that the targets are the same in both cases. Conversely, it should not be assumed that a lack of killing under nonreplicating conditions means that the target of a compound that is active in replicating conditions has become dispensable when the bacteria are no longer replicating.
- The field will experience substantial advances when we can test large numbers of nonreplicating-active molecules in diverse animal models and analyze and publish negative as well as positive results.

Acknowledgments. We are thankful to Drs. Thulasi Warrier, Selin Somersan, Landys Lopez-Quezada, Kristin Burns-Huang, and Kyu Rhee (Weill Cornell Medicine, New York, NY); Drs. Christine Roubert, Laurent Gouilleux, Laurent Fraisse, Sophie Lagrange, and Cédric Couturier (Sanofi, Lyon, France); and Alfonso Mendoza-Losana, David Barros, and Robert Bates (GlaxoSmithKline, Tres Cantos, Spain) for insightful discussions and ideas. We are grateful to Drs. Steven Brickner (SJ Bricker Consulting, LLC), Jeff Aubé (University of North Carolina), and Ouathek Ouerfelli (Memorial Sloan Kettering, New York, NY) for invaluable discussions, ideas, and chemistry expertise. We thank S.B. for bringing the chemistry of salicylanilides to our attention. We thank T.W., S.S., K.B.H., L.L.Q., K.R., and S.B. for careful editing of the manuscript. We thank our colleagues (C.R., L.G., L.F., and C.C. at Sanofi [Lyon, France], J.A. at the University of North Carolina [Chapel Hill], O.O. and G.Y. at Memorial Sloan Kettering, and Mel Reichman at the Lankenau Institute [Wynnewood, PA]) for sharing preliminary data on 4-hydroxyquinolines. The work fostering these ideas was supported by the TB Drug Accelerator of the Bill & Melinda Gates Foundation, the Abby and Howard P.

Milstein Program in Chemical Biology and Translational Medicine, and NIH TB Research Unit grant U19 AI11143. The Department of Microbiology and Immunology is supported by the William Randolph Hearst Foundation.

Citation. Gold B, Nathan C. 2017. Targeting phenotypically tolerant *Mycobacterium tuberculosis*. Microbiol Spectrum 5(1):TBTB2-0031-2016.

References

1. **Nathan C.** 2011. Making space for anti-infective drug discovery. *Cell Host Microbe* **9:**343–348.
2. **Davies J, Davies D.** 2010. Origins and evolution of antibiotic resistance. *Microbiol Mol Biol Rev* **74:**417–433.
3. **Hobby GL, Meyer K, Chaffee E.** 1942. Observations on the mechanism of action of penicillin. *Exp Biol Med* **50:**281–285.
4. **Bigger J.** 1944. Treatment of staphylococcal infections with penicillin by intermittent sterilisation. *Lancet* **244:**497–500.
5. **Hobby GL, Lenert TF.** 1957. The in vitro action of antituberculous agents against multiplying and non-multiplying microbial cells. *Am Rev Tuberc* **76:**1031–1048.
6. **Koul A, Arnoult E, Lounis N, Guillemont J, Andries K.** 2011. The challenge of new drug discovery for tuberculosis. *Nature* **469:**483–490.
7. **McCune RM, Feldmann FM, Lambert HP, McDermott W.** 1966. Microbial persistence. I. The capacity of tubercle bacilli to survive sterilization in mouse tissues. *J Exp Med* **123:**445–468.
8. **Scanga CA, Mohan VP, Joseph H, Yu K, Chan J, Flynn JL.** 1999. Reactivation of latent tuberculosis: variations on the Cornell murine model. *Infect Immun* **67:**4531–4538.
9. **Pai SR, Actor JK, Sepulveda E, Hunter RL Jr, Jagannath C.** 2000. Identification of viable and non-viable *Mycobacterium tuberculosis* in mouse organs by directed RT-PCR for antigen 85B mRNA. *Microb Pathog* **28:**335–342.
10. **Mukamolova GV, Turapov O, Malkin J, Woltmann G, Barer MR.** 2010. Resuscitation-promoting factors reveal an occult population of tubercle bacilli in sputum. *Am J Respir Crit Care Med* **181:**174–180.
11. **Chengalroyen MD, Beukes GM, Gordhan BG, Streicher EM, Churchyard G, Hafner R, Warren R, Otwombe K, Martinson N, Kana BD.** 2016. Detection and quantification of differentially culturable tubercle bacteria in sputum from tuberculosis patients. *Am J Respir Crit Care Med* [Epub ahead of print].
12. **Betts JC, Lukey PT, Robb LC, McAdam RA, Duncan K.** 2002. Evaluation of a nutrient starvation model of *Mycobacterium tuberculosis* persistence by gene and protein expression profiling. *Mol Microbiol* **43:**717–731.
13. **Brooks JV, Furney SK, Orme IM.** 1999. Metronidazole therapy in mice infected with tuberculosis. *Antimicrob Agents Chemother* **43:**1285–1288. PMCID: PMC89261
14. **Carroll MW, Jeon D, Mountz JM, Lee JD, Jeong YJ, Zia N, Lee M, Lee J, Via LE, Lee S, Eum SY, Lee SJ,**

Goldfeder LC, Cai Y, Jin B, Kim Y, Oh T, Chen RY, Dodd LE, Gu W, Dartois V, Park SK, Kim CT, Barry CE III, Cho SN. 2013. Efficacy and safety of metronidazole for pulmonary multidrug-resistant tuberculosis. *Antimicrob Agents Chemother* 57:3903–3909.

15. Hoff DR, Caraway ML, Brooks EJ, Driver ER, Ryan GJ, Peloquin CA, Orme IM, Basaraba RJ, Lenaerts AJ. 2008. Metronidazole lacks antibacterial activity in guinea pigs infected with *Mycobacterium tuberculosis*. *Antimicrob Agents Chemother* 52:4137–4140.

16. Lin PL, Dartois V, Johnston PJ, Janssen C, Via L, Goodwin MB, Klein E, Barry CE III, Flynn JL. 2012. Metronidazole prevents reactivation of latent *Mycobacterium tuberculosis* infection in macaques. *Proc Natl Acad Sci USA* 109:14188–14193.

17. Via LE, Lin PL, Ray SM, Carrillo J, Allen SS, Eum SY, Taylor K, Klein E, Manjunatha U, Gonzales J, Lee EG, Park SK, Raleigh JA, Cho SN, McMurray DN, Flynn JL, Barry CE III. 2008. Tuberculous granulomas are hypoxic in guinea pigs, rabbits, and nonhuman primates. *Infect Immun* 76:2333–2340.

18. Wayne LG. 1994. Dormancy of *Mycobacterium tuberculosis* and latency of disease. *Eur J Clin Microbiol Infect Dis* 13:908–914.

19. Wayne LG, Sramek HA. 1994. Metronidazole is bactericidal to dormant cells of *Mycobacterium tuberculosis*. *Antimicrob Agents Chemother* 38:2054–2058.

20. Boshoff HI, Barry CE III. 2005. Tuberculosis: metabolism and respiration in the absence of growth. *Nat Rev Microbiol* 3:70–80.

21. Cunningham-Bussel A, Zhang T, Nathan CF. 2013. Nitrite produced by *Mycobacterium tuberculosis* in human macrophages in physiologic oxygen impacts bacterial ATP consumption and gene expression. *Proc Natl Acad Sci USA* 110:E4256–E4265.

22. Watanabe S, Zimmermann M, Goodwin MB, Sauer U, Barry CE III, Boshoff HI. 2011. Fumarate reductase activity maintains an energized membrane in anaerobic *Mycobacterium tuberculosis*. *PLoS Pathog* 7:e1002287.

23. Wade MM, Zhang Y. 2004. Anaerobic incubation conditions enhance pyrazinamide activity against *Mycobacterium tuberculosis*. *J Med Microbiol* 53:769–773.

24. Coates A, Hu Y, Bax R, Page C. 2002. The future challenges facing the development of new antimicrobial drugs. *Nat Rev Drug Discov* 1:895–910.

25. Nathan C. 2012. Fresh approaches to anti-infective therapies. *Sci Transl Med* 4:140sr2.

26. Nathan C. 2015. Cooperative development of antimicrobials: looking back to look ahead. *Nat Rev Microbiol* 13:651–657.

27. Nathan C, Barry CE III. 2015. TB drug development: immunology at the table. *Immunol Rev* 264:308–318.

28. Warrier T, et al. 2015. Identification of novel antimycobacterial compounds by screening a pharmaceutical small-molecule library against nonreplicating Mycobacterium tuberculosis. *ACS Infect Dis* 1:580–585. 10.1021/acsinfecdis.5b00025.

29. Mak PA, Rao SP, Ping Tan M, Lin X, Chyba J, Tay J, Ng SH, Tan BH, Cherian J, Duraiswamy J, Bifani P,

Lim V, Lee BH, Ling Ma N, Beer D, Thayalan P, Kuhen K, Chatterjee A, Supek F, Glynne R, Zheng J, Boshoff HI, Barry CE III, Dick T, Pethe K, Camacho LR. 2012. A high-throughput screen to identify inhibitors of ATP homeostasis in non-replicating *Mycobacterium tuberculosis*. *ACS Chem Biol* 7:1190–1197.

30. Gold B, Roberts J, Ling Y, Quezada LL, Glasheen J, Ballinger E, Somersan-Karakaya S, Warrier T, Warren JD, Nathan C. 2015. Rapid, semi-quantitative assay to discriminate among compounds with activity against replicating or non-replicating *Mycobacterium tuberculosis*. *Antimicrob Agents Chemother* 59:6521–6538.

31. Grosset JH, Tyagi S, Almeida DV, Converse PJ, Li SY, Ammerman NC, Bishai WR, Enarson D, Trébucq A. 2013. Assessment of clofazimine activity in a second-line regimen for tuberculosis in mice. *Am J Respir Crit Care Med* 188:608–612.

32. Lounis N, Gevers T, Van Den Berg J, Verhaeghe T, van Heeswijk R, Andries K. 2008. Prevention of drug carryover effects in studies assessing antimycobacterial efficacy of TMC207. *J Clin Microbiol* 46:2212–2215.

33. Tasneen R, Williams K, Amoabeng O, Minkowski A, Mdluli KE, Upton AM, Nuermberger EL. 2015. Contribution of the nitroimidazoles PA-824 and TBA-354 to the activity of novel regimens in murine models of tuberculosis. *Antimicrob Agents Chemother* 59:129–135.

34. de Carvalho LP, Lin G, Jiang X, Nathan C. 2009. Nitazoxanide kills replicating and nonreplicating *Mycobacterium tuberculosis* and evades resistance. *J Med Chem* 52:5789–5792.

35. Roostalu J, Jõers A, Luidalepp H, Kaldalu N, Tenson T. 2008. Cell division in *Escherichia coli* cultures monitored at single cell resolution. *BMC Microbiol* 8:68.

36. Orman MA, Brynildsen MP. 2013. Dormancy is not necessary or sufficient for bacterial persistence. *Antimicrob Agents Chemother* 57:3230–3239.

37. Vega NM, Allison KR, Khalil AS, Collins JJ. 2012. Signaling-mediated bacterial persister formation. *Nat Chem Biol* 8:431–433.

38. Dhar N, Dubée V, Ballell L, Cuinet G, Hugonnet JE, Signorino-Gelo F, Barros D, Arthur M, McKinney JD. 2015. Rapid cytolysis of *Mycobacterium tuberculosis* by faropenem, an orally bioavailable β-lactam antibiotic. *Antimicrob Agents Chemother* 59:1308–1319.

39. Balaban NQ, Merrin J, Chait R, Kowalik L, Leibler S. 2004. Bacterial persistence as a phenotypic switch. *Science* 305:1622–1625.

40. Allison KR, Brynildsen MP, Collins JJ. 2011. Metabolite-enabled eradication of bacterial persisters by aminoglycosides. *Nature* 473:216–220.

41. Allison KR, Brynildsen MP, Collins JJ. 2011. Heterogeneous bacterial persisters and engineering approaches to eliminate them. *Curr Opin Microbiol* 14:593–598.

42. Prideaux B, Via LE, Zimmerman MD, Eum S, Sarathy J, O'Brien P, Chen C, Kaya F, Weiner DM, Chen PY, Song T, Lee M, Shim TS, Cho JS, Kim W, Cho SN, Olivier KN, Barry CE III, Dartois V. 2015. The association between sterilizing activity and drug distribution into tuberculosis lesions. *Nat Med* 21:1223–1227.

43. Muttucumaru DG, Roberts G, Hinds J, Stabler RA, Parish T. 2004. Gene expression profile of *Mycobacterium tuberculosis* in a non-replicating state. *Tuberculosis (Edinb)* 84:239–246.

44. Voskuil MI, Visconti KC, Schoolnik GK. 2004. *Mycobacterium tuberculosis* gene expression during adaptation to stationary phase and low-oxygen dormancy. *Tuberculosis (Edinb)* 84:218–227.

45. Talaat AM, Howard ST, Hale W IV, Lyons R, Garner H, Johnston SA. 2002. Genomic DNA standards for gene expression profiling in *Mycobacterium tuberculosis*. *Nucleic Acids Res* 30:e104.

46. Keren I, Minami S, Rubin E, Lewis K. 2011. Characterization and transcriptome analysis of *Mycobacterium tuberculosis* persisters. *MBio* 2:e00100–e00111.

47. Benjak A, Uplekar S, Zhang M, Piton J, Cole ST, Sala C. 2016. Genomic and transcriptomic analysis of the streptomycin-dependent *Mycobacterium tuberculosis* strain 18b. *BMC Genomics* 17:190.

48. Voskuil MI, Schnappinger D, Visconti KC, Harrell MI, Dolganov GM, Sherman DR, Schoolnik GK. 2003. Inhibition of respiration by nitric oxide induces a *Mycobacterium tuberculosis* dormancy program. *J Exp Med* 198:705–713.

49. Schnappinger D, Ehrt S, Voskuil MI, Liu Y, Mangan JA, Monahan IM, Dolganov G, Efron B, Butcher PD, Nathan C, Schoolnik GK. 2003. Transcriptional adaptation of *Mycobacterium tuberculosis* within macrophages: insights into the phagosomal environment. *J Exp Med* 198:693–704.

50. Franzblau SG, DeGroote MA, Cho SH, Andries K, Nuermberger E, Orme IM, Mdluli K, Angulo-Barturen I, Dick T, Dartois V, Lenaerts AJ. 2012. Comprehensive analysis of methods used for the evaluation of compounds against *Mycobacterium tuberculosis*. *Tuberculosis (Edinb)* 92:453–488.

51. Lakshminarayana SB, Huat TB, Ho PC, Manjunatha UH, Dartois V, Dick T, Rao SP. 2015. Comprehensive physicochemical, pharmacokinetic and activity profiling of anti-TB agents. *J Antimicrob Chemother* 70:857–867.

52. Xie Z, Siddiqi N, Rubin EJ. 2005. Differential antibiotic susceptibilities of starved *Mycobacterium tuberculosis* isolates. *Antimicrob Agents Chemother* 49:4778–4780.

53. Gold B, Pingle M, Brickner SJ, Shah N, Roberts J, Rundell M, Bracken WC, Warrier T, Somersan S, Venugopal A, Darby C, Jiang X, Warren JD, Fernandez J, Ouerfelli O, Nuermberger EL, Cunningham-Bussel A, Rath P, Chidawanyika T, Deng H, Realubit R, Glickman JF, Nathan CF. 2012. Nonsteroidal anti-inflammatory drug sensitizes *Mycobacterium tuberculosis* to endogenous and exogenous antimicrobials. *Proc Natl Acad Sci USA* 109:16004–16011.

54. Grant SS, Kawate T, Nag PP, Silvis MR, Gordon K, Stanley SA, Kazyanskaya E, Nietupski R, Golas A, Fitzgerald M, Cho S, Franzblau SG, Hung DT. 2013. Identification of novel inhibitors of nonreplicating *Mycobacterium tuberculosis* using a carbon starvation model. *ACS Chem Biol* 8:2224–2234.

55. Grant SS, Kaufmann BB, Chand NS, Haseley N, Hung DT. 2012. Eradication of bacterial persisters with antibiotic-generated hydroxyl radicals. *Proc Natl Acad Sci USA* 109:12147–12152.

56. Tuomanen E. 1986. Phenotypic tolerance: the search for beta-lactam antibiotics that kill nongrowing bacteria. *Rev Infect Dis* 8(Suppl 3):S279–S291.

57. Torrey HL, Keren I, Via LE, Lee JS, Lewis K. 2016. High persister mutants in *Mycobacterium tuberculosis*. *PLoS One* 11:e0155127.

58. Pattyn SR, Dockx P, Rollier MT, Rollier R, Saerens EJ. 1976. *Mycobacterium leprae* persisters after treatment with dapsone and rifampicin. *Int J Lepr Other Mycobact Dis* 44:154–158.

59. Mulcahy LR, Burns JL, Lory S, Lewis K. 2010. Emergence of *Pseudomonas aeruginosa* strains producing high levels of persister cells in patients with cystic fibrosis. *J Bacteriol* 192:6191–6199.

60. Lafleur MD, Qi Q, Lewis K. 2010. Patients with long-term oral carriage harbor high-persister mutants of *Candida albicans*. *Antimicrob Agents Chemother* 54:39–44.

61. Schumacher MA, Balani P, Min J, Chinnam NB, Hansen S, Vulić M, Lewis K, Brennan RG. 2015. HipBA-promoter structures reveal the basis of heritable multidrug tolerance. *Nature* 524:59–64.

62. Ahmad Z, Klinkenberg LG, Pinn ML, Fraig MM, Peloquin CA, Bishai WR, Nuermberger EL, Grosset JH, Karakousis PC. 2009. Biphasic kill curve of isoniazid reveals the presence of drug-tolerant, not drug-resistant, *Mycobacterium tuberculosis* in the guinea pig. *J Infect Dis* 200:1136–1143.

63. Ahmad Z, Pinn ML, Nuermberger EL, Peloquin CA, Grosset JH, Karakousis PC. 2010. The potent bactericidal activity of streptomycin in the guinea pig model of tuberculosis ceases due to the presence of persisters. *J Antimicrob Chemother* 65:2172–2175.

64. Driver ER, Ryan GJ, Hoff DR, Irwin SM, Basaraba RJ, Kramnik I, Lenaerts AJ. 2012. Evaluation of a mouse model of necrotic granuloma formation using C3HeB/FeJ mice for testing of drugs against *Mycobacterium tuberculosis*. *Antimicrob Agents Chemother* 56:3181–3195.

65. Singh R, Barry CE III, Boshoff HI. 2010. The three RelE homologs of *Mycobacterium tuberculosis* have individual, drug-specific effects on bacterial antibiotic tolerance. *J Bacteriol* 192:1279–1291.

66. Nandakumar M, Nathan C, Rhee KY. 2014. Isocitrate lyase mediates broad antibiotic tolerance in *Mycobacterium tuberculosis*. *Nat Commun* 5:4306.

67. Wiuff C, Zappala RM, Regoes RR, Garner KN, Baquero F, Levin BR. 2005. Phenotypic tolerance: antibiotic enrichment of noninherited resistance in bacterial populations. *Antimicrob Agents Chemother* 49:1483–1494.

68. Kim JS, Heo P, Yang TJ, Lee KS, Cho DH, Kim BT, Suh JH, Lim HJ, Shin D, Kim SK, Kweon DH. 2011. Selective killing of bacterial persisters by a single chemical compound without affecting normal antibiotic-sensitive cells. *Antimicrob Agents Chemother* 55:5380–5383.

69. Black DS, Irwin B, Moyed HS. 1994. Autoregulation of hip, an operon that affects lethality due to inhibition

of peptidoglycan or DNA synthesis. *J Bacteriol* **176:**4081–4091.

70. **Black DS, Kelly AJ, Mardis MJ, Moyed HS.** 1991. Structure and organization of *hip*, an operon that affects lethality due to inhibition of peptidoglycan or DNA synthesis. *J Bacteriol* **173:**5732–5739.

71. **Moyed HS, Bertrand KP.** 1983. *hipA*, a newly recognized gene of *Escherichia coli* K-12 that affects frequency of persistence after inhibition of murein synthesis. *J Bacteriol* **155:**768–775.

72. **Moyed HS, Broderick SH.** 1986. Molecular cloning and expression of *hipA*, a gene of *Escherichia coli* K-12 that affects frequency of persistence after inhibition of murein synthesis. *J Bacteriol* **166:**399–403.

73. **Slattery A, Victorsen AH, Brown A, Hillman K, Phillips GJ.** 2013. Isolation of highly persistent mutants of *Salmonella enterica* serovar *typhimurium* reveals a new toxin-antitoxin module. *J Bacteriol* **195:**647–657.

74. **Maisonneuve E, Gerdes K.** 2014. Molecular mechanisms underlying bacterial persisters. *Cell* **157:**539–548.

75. **Lewis K.** 2012. Persister cells: molecular mechanisms related to antibiotic tolerance. *Handbook Exp Pharmacol* **211:**121–133.

76. **Lewis K.** 2010. Persister cells. *Annu Rev Microbiol* **64:**357–372.

77. **Lewis K.** 2008. Multidrug tolerance of biofilms and persister cells. *Curr Top Microbiol Immunol* **322:**107–131.

78. **Lewis K.** 2007. Persister cells, dormancy and infectious disease. *Nat Rev Microbiol* **5:**48–56.

79. **Conlon BP, Rowe SE, Lewis K.** 2015. Persister cells in biofilm associated infections. *Adv Exp Med Biol* **831:**1–9.

80. **Aldridge BB, Fernandez-Suarez M, Heller D, Ambravaneswaran V, Irimia D, Toner M, Fortune SM.** 2012. Asymmetry and aging of mycobacterial cells lead to variable growth and antibiotic susceptibility. *Science* **335:**100–104.

81. **Vaubourgeix J, Lin G, Dhar N, Chenouard N, Jiang X, Botella H, Lupoli T, Mariani O, Yang G, Ouerfelli O, Unser M, Schnappinger D, McKinney J, Nathan C.** 2015. Stressed mycobacteria use the chaperone ClpB to sequester irreversibly oxidized proteins asymmetrically within and between cells. *Cell Host Microbe* **17:**178–190.

82. **Keren I, Shah D, Spoering A, Kaldalu N, Lewis K.** 2004. Specialized persister cells and the mechanism of multidrug tolerance in *Escherichia coli*. *J Bacteriol* **186:**8172–8180.

83. **Maisonneuve E, Shakespeare LJ, Jørgensen MG, Gerdes K.** 2011. Bacterial persistence by RNA endonucleases. *Proc Natl Acad Sci USA* **108:**13206–13211.

84. **Sala A, Bordes P, Genevaux P.** 2014. Multiple toxin-antitoxin systems in *Mycobacterium tuberculosis*. *Toxins (Basel)* **6:**1002–1020.

85. **Javid B, Sorrentino F, Toosky M, Zheng W, Pinkham JT, Jain N, Pan M, Deighan P, Rubin EJ.** 2014. Mycobacterial mistranslation is necessary and sufficient for rifampicin phenotypic resistance. *Proc Natl Acad Sci USA* **111:**1132–1137.

86. **Su HW, Zhu JH, Li H, Cai RJ, Ealand C, Wang X, et al.** 2016. The essential mycobacterial amidotransferase GatCAB is a modulator of specific translational fidelity. *Nat Microbiol* **1:**16147. PMID: 27564922.

87. **Dhar N, McKinney JD.** 2010. *Mycobacterium tuberculosis* persistence mutants identified by screening in isoniazid-treated mice. *Proc Natl Acad Sci USA* **107:**12275–12280.

88. **Raj A, Peskin CS, Tranchina D, Vargas DY, Tyagi S.** 2006. Stochastic mRNA synthesis in mammalian cells. *PLoS Biol* **4:**e309.

89. **Maamar H, Raj A, Dubnau D.** 2007. Noise in gene expression determines cell fate in Bacillus subtilis. *Science* **317:**526–529.

90. **Wakamoto Y, Dhar N, Chait R, Schneider K, Signorino-Gelo F, Leibler S, McKinney JD.** 2013. Dynamic persistence of antibiotic-stressed mycobacteria. *Science* **339:**91–95.

91. **Debbia EA, Roveta S, Schito AM, Gualco L, Marchese A.** 2001. Antibiotic persistence: the role of spontaneous DNA repair response. *Microb Drug Res* **7:**335–342. PMID: 11822773.

92. **Theodore A, Lewis K, Vulic M.** 2013. Tolerance of *Escherichia coli* to fluoroquinolone antibiotics depends on specific components of the SOS response pathway. *Genetics* **195:**1265–1276.

93. **Dörr T, Lewis K, Vulić M.** 2009. SOS response induces persistence to fluoroquinolones in *Escherichia coli*. *PLoS Genet* **5:**e1000760.

94. **Gold B, Warrier T, Nathan C.** 2015. A multi-stress model for high throughput screening against non-replicating *Mycobacterium tuberculosis*. *In* Parish T, Roberts D (ed), *Mycobacteria Protocols*. Methods Mol Biol **1285:**293–315.

95. **Wayne LG, Hayes LG.** 1996. An in vitro model for sequential study of shiftdown of *Mycobacterium tuberculosis* through two stages of nonreplicating persistence. *Infect Immun* **64:**2062–2069.

96. **Cho SH, Warit S, Wan B, Hwang CH, Pauli GF, Franzblau SG.** 2007. Low-oxygen-recovery assay for high-throughput screening of compounds against non-replicating *Mycobacterium tuberculosis*. *Antimicrob Agents Chemother* **51:**1380–1385.

97. **Schnappinger D, Schoolnik GK, Ehrt S.** 2006. Expression profiling of host pathogen interactions: how *Mycobacterium tuberculosis* and the macrophage adapt to one another. *Microbes Infect* **8:**1132–1140.

98. **Lavollay M, Arthur M, Fourgeaud M, Dubost L, Marie A, Veziris N, Blanot D, Gutmann L, Mainardi JL.** 2008. The peptidoglycan of stationary-phase *Mycobacterium tuberculosis* predominantly contains cross-links generated by L,D-transpeptidation. *J Bacteriol* **190:**4360–4366.

99. **Kumar P, Arora K, Lloyd JR, Lee IY, Nair V, Fischer E, Boshoff HI, Barry CE III.** 2012. Meropenem inhibits D,D-carboxypeptidase activity in *Mycobacterium tuberculosis*. *Mol Microbiol* **86:**367–381.

100. **Bryk R, Gold B, Venugopal A, Singh J, Samy R, Pupek K, Cao H, Popescu C, Gurney M, Hotha S, Cherian J,**

Rhee K, Ly L, Converse PJ, Ehrt S, Vandal O, Jiang X, Schneider J, Lin G, Nathan C. 2008. Selective killing of nonreplicating mycobacteria. *Cell Host Microbe* **3**: 137–145.

101. Darby CM, Nathan CF. 2010. Killing of non-replicating *Mycobacterium tuberculosis* by 8-hydroxyquinoline. *J Antimicrob Chemother* **65**:1424–1427.

102. Wang F, Sambandan D, Halder R, Wang J, Batt SM, Weinrick B, Ahmad I, Yang P, Zhang Y, Kim J, Hassani M, Huszar S, Trefzer C, Ma Z, Kaneko T, Mdluli KE, Franzblau S, Chatterjee AK, Johnsson K, Mikusova K, Besra GS, Fütterer K, Robbins SH, Barnes SW, Walker JR, Jacobs WR Jr, Schultz PG. 2013. Identification of a small molecule with activity against drug-resistant and persistent tuberculosis. *Proc Natl Acad Sci USA* **110**: E2510–E2517.

103. Zhang M, Sala C, Dhar N, Vocat A, Sambandamurthy VK, Sharma S, Marriner G, Balasubramanian V, Cole ST. 2014. In vitro and in vivo activities of three oxazolidinones against nonreplicating *Mycobacterium tuberculosis*. *Antimicrob Agents Chemother* **58**:3217–3223.

104. Zhang M, Sala C, Hartkoorn RC, Dhar N, Mendoza-Losana A, Cole ST. 2012. Streptomycin-starved *Mycobacterium tuberculosis* 18b, a drug discovery tool for latent tuberculosis. *Antimicrob Agents Chemother* **56**: 5782–5789.

105. Bassett IM, Lun S, Bishai WR, Guo H, Kirman JR, Altaf M, O'Toole RF. 2013. Detection of inhibitors of phenotypically drug-tolerant *Mycobacterium tuberculosis* using an in vitro bactericidal screen. *J Microbiol* **51**:651–658.

106. Lin G, Li D, de Carvalho LP, Deng H, Tao H, Vogt G, et al. 2009. Inhibitors selective for mycobacterial versus human proteasomes. *Nature* **461**(7264):621–626.

107. Brunner K, Maric S, Reshma RS, Almqvist H, Seashore-Ludlow B, Gustavsson AL, Poyraz Ö, Yogeeswari P, Lundbäck T, Vallin M, Sriram D, Schnell R, Schneider G. 2016. Inhibitors of the cysteine synthase CysM with antibacterial potency against dormant *Mycobacterium tuberculosis*. *J Med Chem* **59**:6848–6859.

108. Chopra S, Matsuyama K, Tran T, Malerich JP, Wan B, Franzblau SG, Lun S, Guo H, Maiga MC, Bishai WR, Madrid PB. 2012. Evaluation of gyrase B as a drug target in *Mycobacterium tuberculosis*. *J Antimicrob Chemother* **67**:415–421.

109. Dasgupta N, Kapur V, Singh KK, Das TK, Sachdeva S, Jyothisri K, Tyagi JS. 2000. Characterization of a two-component system, devR-devS, of *Mycobacterium tuberculosis*. *Tuber Lung Dis* **80**:141–159.

110. Debnath J, Siricilla S, Wan B, Crick DC, Lenaerts AJ, Franzblau SG, Kurosu M. 2012. Discovery of selective menaquinone biosynthesis inhibitors against *Mycobacterium tuberculosis*. *J Med Chem* **55**:3739–3755.

111. Samala G, Devi PB, Saxena S, Meda N, Yogeeswari P, Sriram D. 2016. Design, synthesis and biological evaluation of imidazo[2,1-b]thiazole and benzo[d]imidazo[2,1-b]thiazole derivatives as *Mycobacterium tuberculosis* pantothenate synthetase inhibitors. *Bioorg Med Chem* **24**:1298–1307.

112. Shirude PS, Madhavapeddi P, Tucker JA, Murugan K, Patil V, Basavarajappa H, Raichurkar AV, Humnabadkar V, Hussein S, Sharma S, Ramya VK, Narayan CB, Balganesh TS, Sambandamurthy VK. 2013. Amino-pyrazinamides: novel and specific GyrB inhibitors that kill replicating and nonreplicating *Mycobacterium tuberculosis*. *ACS Chem Biol* **8**:519–523.

113. Sridevi JP, Suryadevara P, Janupally R, Sridhar J, Soni V, Anantaraju HS, et al. 2015. Identification of potential *Mycobacterium tuberculosis* topoisomerase I inhibitors: a study against active, dormant and resistant tuberculosis. *Eur J Pharm Sci* **72**:81–92. PMID: 25769524.

114. Olaleye O, Raghunand TR, Bhat S, Chong C, Gu P, Zhou J, Zhang Y, Bishai WR, Liu JO. 2011. Characterization of clioquinol and analogues as novel inhibitors of methionine aminopeptidases from *Mycobacterium tuberculosis*. *Tuberculosis (Edinb)* **91**(Suppl 1):S61–S65.

115. Olaleye O, Raghunand TR, Bhat S, He J, Tyagi S, Lamichhane G, Gu P, Zhou J, Zhang Y, Grosset J, Bishai WR, Liu JO. 2010. Methionine aminopeptidases from *Mycobacterium tuberculosis* as novel antimycobacterial targets. *Chem Biol* **17**:86–97.

116. Chakraborty S, Gruber T, Barry CE III, Boshoff HI, Rhee KY. 2013. Para-aminosalicylic acid acts as an alternative substrate of folate metabolism in *Mycobacterium tuberculosis*. *Science* **339**:88–91.

117. Chakraborty S, Rhee KY. 2015. Tuberculosis drug development: history and evolution of the mechanism-based paradigm. *Cold Spring Harb Perspect Med* **5**: a021147.

118. Vocat A, Hartkoorn RC, Lechartier B, Zhang M, Dhar N, Cole ST, Sala C. 2015. Bioluminescence for assessing drug potency against nonreplicating *Mycobacterium tuberculosis*. *Antimicrob Agents Chemother* **59**: 4012–4019.

119. Darby CM, Ingólfsson HI, Jiang X, Shen C, Sun M, Zhao N, Burns K, Liu G, Ehrt S, Warren JD, Andersen OS, Brickner SJ, Nathan C. 2013. Whole cell screen for inhibitors of pH homeostasis in *Mycobacterium tuberculosis*. *PLoS One* **8**:e68942.

120. Brook I. 1989. Inoculum effect. *Rev Infect Dis* **11**: 361–368.

121. Dahl JL, Kraus CN, Boshoff HI, Doan B, Foley K, Avarbock D, Kaplan G, Mizrahi V, Rubin H, Barry CE III. 2003. The role of RelMtb-mediated adaptation to stationary phase in long-term persistence of *Mycobacterium tuberculosis* in mice. *Proc Natl Acad Sci USA* **100**:10026–10031.

122. Zhao N, Darby CM, Small J, Bachovchin DA, Jiang X, Burns-Huang KE, Botella H, Ehrt S, Boger DL, Anderson ED, Cravatt BF, Speers AE, Fernandez-Vega V, Hodder PS, Eberhart C, Rosen H, Spicer TP, Nathan CF. 2015. Target-based screen against a periplasmic serine protease that regulates intrabacterial pH homeostasis in *Mycobacterium tuberculosis*. *ACS Chem Biol* **10**:364–371.

123. Vandal OH, Nathan CF, Ehrt S. 2009. Acid resistance in *Mycobacterium tuberculosis*. *J Bacteriol* **191**:4714–4721.

124. Vandal OH, Pierini LM, Schnappinger D, Nathan CF, Ehrt S. 2008. A membrane protein preserves intrabacterial pH in intraphagosomal *Mycobacterium tuberculosis*. *Nat Med* 14:849–854. [pii] 10.1038/nm.1795.

125. Vandal OH, Roberts JA, Odaira T, Schnappinger D, Nathan CF, Ehrt S. 2009. Acid-susceptible mutants of *Mycobacterium tuberculosis* share hypersusceptibility to cell wall and oxidative stress and to the host environment. *J Bacteriol* 191:625–631.

126. Miesenböck G, De Angelis DA, Rothman JE. 1998. Visualizing secretion and synaptic transmission with pH-sensitive green fluorescent proteins. *Nature* 394:192–195.

127. Ackart DF, Hascall-Dove L, Caceres SM, Kirk NM, Podell BK, Melander C, Orme IM, Leid JG, Nick JA, Basaraba RJ. 2014. Expression of antimicrobial drug tolerance by attached communities of *Mycobacterium tuberculosis*. *Pathog Dis* 70:359–369.

128. Recht J, Kolter R. 2001. Glycopeptidolipid acetylation affects sliding motility and biofilm formation in *Mycobacterium smegmatis*. *J Bacteriol* 183:57185724.

129. Recht J, Martínez A, Torello S, Kolter R. 2000. Genetic analysis of sliding motility in *Mycobacterium smegmatis*. *J Bacteriol* 182:4348–4351.

130. Piccaro G, Giannoni F, Filippini P, Mustazzolu A, Fattorini L. 2013. Activities of drug combinations against *Mycobacterium tuberculosis* grown in aerobic and hypoxic acidic conditions. *Antimicrob Agents Chemother* 57:1428–1433.

131. Sala C, Dhar N, Hartkoorn RC, Zhang M, Ha YH, Schneider P, Cole ST. 2010. Simple model for testing drugs against nonreplicating *Mycobacterium tuberculosis*. *Antimicrob Agents Chemother* 54:4150–4158.

132. Hartkoorn RC, Ryabova OB, Chiarelli LR, Riccardi G, Makarov V, Cole ST. 2014. Mechanism of action of 5-nitrothiophenes against *Mycobacterium tuberculosis*. *Antimicrob Agents Chemother* 58:2944–2947.

133. Zheng P, Somersan-Karakaya S, Lu S, Roberts J, Pingle M, Warrier T, Little D, Guo X, Brickner SJ, Nathan CF, Gold B, Liu G. 2014. Synthetic calanolides with bactericidal activity against replicating and nonreplicating *Mycobacterium tuberculosis*. *J Med Chem* 57:3755–3772.

134. Deb C, Lee CM, Dubey VS, Daniel J, Abomoelak B, Sirakova TD, Pawar S, Rogers L, Kolattukudy PE. 2009. A novel in vitro multiple-stress dormancy model for *Mycobacterium tuberculosis* generates a lipid-loaded, drug-tolerant, dormant pathogen. *PLoS One* 4:e6077.

135. Deris JB, Kim M, Zhang Z, Okano H, Hermsen R, Groisman A, Hwa T. 2013. The innate growth bistability and fitness landscapes of antibiotic-resistant bacteria. *Science* 342:1237435.

136. Salina EG, Waddell SJ, Hoffmann N, Rosenkrands I, Butcher PD, Kaprelyants AS. 2014. Potassium availability triggers *Mycobacterium tuberculosis* transition to, and resuscitation from, non-culturable (dormant) states. *Open Biol* 4:140106.

137. Ignatov DV, Salina EG, Fursov MV, Skvortsov TA, Azhikina TL, Kaprelyants AS. 2015. Dormant non-culturable *Mycobacterium tuberculosis* retains stable low-abundant mRNA. *BMC Genomics* 16:954.

138. Kazius J, McGuire R, Bursi R. 2005. Derivation and validation of toxicophores for mutagenicity prediction. *J Med Chem* 48:312–320.

139. Baell JB. 2010. Observations on screening-based research and some concerning trends in the literature. *Future Med Chem* 2:1529–1546.

140. Gold B, Deng H, Bryk R, Vargas D, Eliezer D, Roberts J, et al. 2008. Identification of a copper-binding metallothionein in pathogenic mycobacteria. *Nat Chem Biol* 4:609–616. [pii] 10.1038/nchembio.109.

141. Kozikowski BA, Burt TM, Tirey DA, Williams LE, Kuzmak BR, Stanton DT, Morand KL, Nelson SL. 2003. The effect of freeze/thaw cycles on the stability of compounds in DMSO. *J Biomol Screen* 8:210–215.

142. Baillargeon P, Scampavia L, Einsteder R, Hodder P. 2011. Monitoring of HTS compound library quality via a high-resolution image acquisition and processing instrument. *J Lab Autom* 16:197–203.

143. Di L, Kerns EH. 2006. Biological assay challenges from compound solubility: strategies for bioassay optimization. *Drug Discov Today* 11:446–451.

144. Ekins S, Kaneko T, Lipinski CA, Bradford J, Dole K, Spektor A, Gregory K, Blondeau D, Ernst S, Yang J, Goncharoff N, Hohman MM, Bunin BA. 2010. Analysis and hit filtering of a very large library of compounds screened against *Mycobacterium tuberculosis*. *Mol Biosyst* 6:2316–2324.

145. Gold B, Smith R, Nguyen Q, Roberts J, Ling Y, Lopez Quezada L, Somersan S, Warrier T, Little D, Pingle M, Zhang D, Ballinger E, Zimmerman M, Dartois V, Hanson P, Mitscher LA, Porubsky P, Rogers S, Schoenen FJ, Nathan C, Aubé J. 2016. Novel cephalosporins selectively active on non-replicating *Mycobacterium tuberculosis*. *J Med Chem* 59:6027–6044.

146. Williams K, Minkowski A, Amoabeng O, Peloquin CA, Taylor D, Andries K, Wallis RS, Mdluli KE, Nuermberger EL. 2012. Sterilizing activities of novel combinations lacking first- and second-line drugs in a murine model of tuberculosis. *Antimicrob Agents Chemother* 56:3114–3120.

147. Ibrahim M, Truffot-Pernot C, Andries K, Jarlier V, Veziris N. 2009. Sterilizing activity of R207910 (TMC207)-containing regimens in the murine model of tuberculosis. *Am J Respir Crit Care Med* 180:553–557.

148. Diacon AH, Pym A, Grobusch M, Patientia R, Rustomjee R, Page-Shipp L, Pistorius C, Krause R, Bogoshi M, Churchyard G, Venter A, Allen J, Palomino JC, De Marez T, van Heeswijk RP, Lounis N, Meyvisch P, Verbeeck J, Parys W, de Beule K, Andries K, Mc Neeley DF. 2009. The diarylquinoline TMC207 for multidrug-resistant tuberculosis. *N Engl J Med* 360:2397–2405.

149. Hohman M, Gregory K, Chibale K, Smith PJ, Ekins S, Bunin B. 2009. Novel web-based tools combining chemistry informatics, biology and social networks for drug discovery. *Drug Discov Today* 14:261–270.

150. Koul A, Vranckx L, Dendouga N, Balemans W, Van den Wyngaert I, Vergauwen K, Göhlmann HW, Willebrords R, Poncelet A, Guillemont J, Bald D, Andries K. 2008. Diarylquinolines are bactericidal for dormant mycobacteria as a result of disturbed ATP homeostasis. *J Biol Chem* 283:25273–25280.

151. Heifets LB, Cynamon MH. 1991. *Drug Susceptibility in the Chemotherapy of Mycobacterial Infections*. CRC Press, Boca Raton, FL.

152. Brötz-Oesterhelt H, Beyer D, Kroll HP, Endermann R, Ladel C, Schroeder W, Hinzen B, Raddatz S, Paulsen H, Henninger K, Bandow JE, Sahl HG, Labischinski H. 2005. Dysregulation of bacterial proteolytic machinery by a new class of antibiotics. *Nat Med* 11:1082–1087.

153. Conlon BP, Nakayasu ES, Fleck LE, LaFleur MD, Isabella VM, Coleman K, Leonard SN, Smith RD, Adkins JN, Lewis K. 2013. Activated ClpP kills persisters and eradicates a chronic biofilm infection. *Nature* 503:365–370.

154. Tian J, Bryk R, Shi S, Erdjument-Bromage H, Tempst P, Nathan C. 2005. *Mycobacterium tuberculosis* appears to lack alpha-ketoglutarate dehydrogenase and encodes pyruvate dehydrogenase in widely separated genes. *Mol Microbiol* 57:859–868.

155. Bryk R, Lima CD, Erdjument-Bromage H, Tempst P, Nathan C. 2002. Metabolic enzymes of mycobacteria linked to antioxidant defense by a thioredoxin-like protein. *Science* 295:1073–1077.

156. Ehrt S, Schnappinger D, Bekiranov S, Drenkow J, Shi S, Gingeras TR, Gaasterland T, Schoolnik G, Nathan C. 2001. Reprogramming of the macrophage transcriptome in response to interferon-gamma and *Mycobacterium tuberculosis*: signaling roles of nitric oxide synthase-2 and phagocyte oxidase. *J Exp Med* 194:1123–1140.

157. Rao SP, Alonso S, Rand L, Dick T, Pethe K. 2008. The protonmotive force is required for maintaining ATP homeostasis and viability of hypoxic, nonreplicating *Mycobacterium tuberculosis*. *Proc Natl Acad Sci USA* 105:11945–11950.

158. Singh R, Manjunatha U, Boshoff HI, Ha YH, Niyomrattanakit P, Ledwidge R, Dowd CS, Lee IY, Kim P, Zhang L, Kang S, Keller TH, Jiricek J, Barry CE III. 2008. PA-824 kills nonreplicating *Mycobacterium tuberculosis* by intracellular NO release. *Science* 322:1392–1395.

159. Khan SR, Singh S, Roy KK, Akhtar MS, Saxena AK, Krishnan MY. 2013. Biological evaluation of novel substituted chloroquinolines targeting mycobacterial ATP synthase. *Int J Antimicrob Agents* 41:41–46.

160. Herbert D, Paramasivan CN, Venkatesan P, Kubendiran G, Prabhakar R, Mitchison DA. 1996. Bactericidal action of ofloxacin, sulbactam-ampicillin, rifampin, and isoniazid on logarithmic- and stationary-phase cultures of *Mycobacterium tuberculosis*. *Antimicrob Agents Chemother* 40:2296–2299.

161. Hu Y, Coates AR, Mitchison DA. 2003. Sterilizing activities of fluoroquinolones against rifampin-tolerant populations of *Mycobacterium tuberculosis*. *Antimicrob Agents Chemother* 47:653–657.

162. Hu Y, Coates A. 2012. Nonmultiplying bacteria are profoundly tolerant to antibiotics. *Handbook Exp Pharmacol* 211:99–119.

163. Andries K, Verhasselt P, Guillemont J, Göhlmann HW, Neefs JM, Winkler H, Van Gestel J, Timmerman P, Zhu M, Lee E, Williams P, de Chaffoy D, Huitric E, Hoffner S, Cambau E, Truffot-Pernot C, Lounis N, Jarlier V. 2005. A diarylquinoline drug active on the ATP synthase of *Mycobacterium tuberculosis*. *Science* 307:223–227.

164. Gengenbacher M, Rao SP, Pethe K, Dick T. 2010. Nutrient-starved, non-replicating *Mycobacterium tuberculosis* requires respiration, ATP synthase and isocitrate lyase for maintenance of ATP homeostasis and viability. *Microbiology* 156:81–87.

165. Diacon AH, Dawson R, von Groote-Bidlingmaier F, Symons G, Venter A, Donald PR, van Niekerk C, Everitt D, Winter H, Becker P, Mendel CM, Spigelman MK. 2012. 14-day bactericidal activity of PA-824, bedaquiline, pyrazinamide, and moxifloxacin combinations: a randomised trial. *Lancet* 380:986–993.

166. Zhang Y. 2005. The magic bullets and tuberculosis drug targets. *Annu Rev Pharmacol Toxicol* 45:529–564.

167. Tan MP, Sequeira P, Lin WW, Phong WY, Cliff P, Ng SH, Lee BH, Camacho L, Schnappinger D, Ehrt S, Dick T, Pethe K, Alonso S. 2010. Nitrate respiration protects hypoxic *Mycobacterium tuberculosis* against acid- and reactive nitrogen species stresses. *PLoS One* 5:e13356.

168. Eoh H, Rhee KY. 2013. Multifunctional essentiality of succinate metabolism in adaptation to hypoxia in *Mycobacterium tuberculosis*. *Proc Natl Acad Sci USA* 110:6554–6559.

169. Huang Q, Chen ZF, Li YY, Zhang Y, Ren Y, Fu Z, Xu SQ. 2007. Nutrient-starved incubation conditions enhance pyrazinamide activity against *Mycobacterium tuberculosis*. *Chemotherapy* 53:338–343.

170. Zimhony O, Vilchèze C, Arai M, Welch JT, Jacobs WR Jr. 2007. Pyrazinoic acid and its n-propyl ester inhibit fatty acid synthase type I in replicating tubercle bacilli. *Antimicrob Agents Chemother* 51:752–754.

171. Zimhony O, Cox JS, Welch JT, Vilchèze C, Jacobs WR Jr. 2000. Pyrazinamide inhibits the eukaryotic-like fatty acid synthetase I (FASI) of *Mycobacterium tuberculosis*. *Nat Med* 6:1043–1047.

172. Boshoff HI, Mizrahi V, Barry CE III. 2002. Effects of pyrazinamide on fatty acid synthesis by whole mycobacterial cells and purified fatty acid synthase I. *J Bacteriol* 184:2167–2172.

173. Shi W, Zhang X, Jiang X, Yuan H, Lee JS, Barry CE III, Wang H, Zhang W, Zhang Y. 2011. Pyrazinamide inhibits trans-translation in *Mycobacterium tuberculosis*. *Science* 333:1630–1632.

174. Shi W, Chen J, Feng J, Cui P, Zhang S, Weng X, Zhang W, Zhang Y. 2014. Aspartate decarboxylase (PanD) as a new target of pyrazinamide in *Mycobacterium tuberculosis*. *Emerg Microbes Infect* 3:e58.

175. Dillon NA, Peterson ND, Rosen BC, Baughn AD. 2014. Pantothenate and pantetheine antagonize the antitubercular activity of pyrazinamide. *Antimicrob Agents Chemother* 58:7258–7263.

176. Sarathy J, Dartois V, Dick T, Gengenbacher M. 2013. Reduced drug uptake in phenotypically resistant nutrient-starved nonreplicating *Mycobacterium tuberculosis*. *Antimicrob Agents Chemother* 57:1648–1653.

177. Payne DJ, Gwynn MN, Holmes DJ, Pompliano DL. 2007. Drugs for bad bugs: confronting the challenges of antibacterial discovery. *Nat Rev Drug Discov* 6:29–40.

178. Rhee KY, Erdjument-Bromage H, Tempst P, Nathan CF. 2005. S-nitroso proteome of *Mycobacterium tuberculosis*: enzymes of intermediary metabolism and antioxidant defense. *Proc Natl Acad Sci USA* 102:467–472.

179. Vilchèze C, Baughn AD, Tufariello J, Leung LW, Kuo M, Basler CF, Alland D, Sacchettini JC, Freundlich JS, Jacobs WR Jr. 2011. Novel inhibitors of InhA efficiently kill *Mycobacterium tuberculosis* under aerobic and anaerobic conditions. *Antimicrob Agents Chemother* 55:3889–3898.

180. Martínez-Hoyos M, Perez-Herran E, Gulten G, Encinas L, Álvarez-Gómez D, Alvarez E, Ferrer-Bazaga S, García-Pérez A, Ortega F, Angulo-Barturen I, Rullas-Trincado J, Blanco Ruano D, Torres P, Castañeda P, Huss S, Fernández Menéndez R, González Del Valle S, Ballell L, Barros D, Modha S, Dhar N, Signorino-Gelo F, McKinney JD, García-Bustos JF, Lavandera JL, Sacchettini JC, Jimenez MS, Martín-Casabona N, Castro-Pichel J, Mendoza-Losana A. 2016. Antitubercular drugs for an old target: GSK693 as a promising InhA direct inhibitor. *EBioMedicine* 8:291–301.

181. Stover CK, Warrener P, VanDevanter DR, Sherman DR, Arain TM, Langhorne MH, Anderson SW, Towell JA, Yuan Y, McMurray DN, Kreiswirth BN, Barry CE, Baker WR. 2000. A small-molecule nitroimidazopyran drug candidate for the treatment of tuberculosis. *Nature* 405:962–966.

182. Manjunatha U, Boshoff HI, Barry CE. 2009. The mechanism of action of PA-824: novel insights from transcriptional profiling. *Commun Integr Biol* 2:215–218.

183. Machaba KE, Cele FN, Mhlongo NN, Soliman ME. 2016. Sliding clamp of DNA polymerase III as a drug target for TB therapy: comprehensive conformational and binding analysis from molecular dynamic simulations. *Cell Biochem Biophys* [Epub ahead of print].

184. Kling A, Lukat P, Almeida DV, Bauer A, Fontaine E, Sordello S, Zaburannyi N, Herrmann J, Wenzel SC, König C, Ammerman NC, Barrio MB, Borchers K, Bordon-Pallier F, Brönstrup M, Courtemanche G, Gerlitz M, Geslin M, Hammann P, Heinz DW, Hoffmann H, Klieber S, Kohlmann M, Kurz M, Lair C, Matter H, Nuermberger E, Tyagi S, Fraisse L, Grosset JH, Lagrange S, Müller R. 2015. Antibiotics. Targeting DnaN for tuberculosis therapy using novel griselimycins. *Science* 348:1106–1112.

185. Herrmann J, Lukežič T, Kling A, Baumann S, Hüttel S, Petković H, Müller R. 2016. Strategies for the discovery and development of new antibiotics from natural products: three case studies. *Curr Top Microbiol Immunol* [Epub ahead of print].

186. Higgins PG, Fluit AC, Schmitz FJ. 2003. Fluoroquinolones: structure and target sites. *Curr Drug Targets* 4:181–190.

187. Hu YM, Butcher PD, Sole K, Mitchison DA, Coates AR. 1998. Protein synthesis is shutdown in dormant *Mycobacterium tuberculosis* and is reversed by oxygen or heat shock. *FEMS Microbiol Lett* 158:139–145.

188. Lee RE, Hurdle JG, Liu J, Bruhn DF, Matt T, Scherman MS, Vaddady PK, Zheng Z, Qi J, Akbergenov R, Das S, Madhura DB, Rathi C, Trivedi A, Villellas C, Lee RB, Rakesh, Waidyarachchi SL, Sun D, McNeil MR, Ainsa JA, Boshoff HI, Gonzalez-Juarrero M, Meibohm B, Böttger EC, Lenaerts AJ. 2014. Spectinamides: a new class of semisynthetic antituberculosis agents that overcome native drug efflux. *Nat Med* 20:152–158.

189. Jarlier V, Nikaido H. 1990. Permeability barrier to hydrophilic solutes in *Mycobacterium chelonei*. *J Bacteriol* 172:1418–1423.

190. Kasik JE. 1965. The nature of mycobacterial penicillinase. *Am Rev Respir Dis* 91:117–119.

191. Jarlier V, Gutmann L, Nikaido H. 1991. Interplay of cell wall barrier and beta-lactamase activity determines high resistance to beta-lactam antibiotics in *Mycobacterium chelonae*. *Antimicrob Agents Chemother* 35:1937–1939.

192. Finch R. 1986. Beta-lactam antibiotics and mycobacteria. *J Antimicrob Chemother* 18:6–8.

193. Hugonnet JE, Tremblay LW, Boshoff HI, Barry CE III, Blanchard JS. 2009. Meropenem-clavulanate is effective against extensively drug-resistant *Mycobacterium tuberculosis*. *Science* 323:1215–1218.

194. Tuomanen E, Cozens R, Tosch W, Zak O, Tomasz A. 1986. The rate of killing of *Escherichia coli* by beta-lactam antibiotics is strictly proportional to the rate of bacterial growth. *J Gen Microbiol* 132:1297–1304 10.1099/00221287-132-5-1297.

195. Schoonmaker MK, Bishai WR, Lamichhane G. 2014. Nonclassical transpeptidases of Mycobacterium tuberculosis alter cell size, morphology, the cytosolic matrix, protein localization, virulence, and resistance to β-lactams. *J Bacteriol* 196:1394–1402.

196. Vollmer W, Höltje JV. 2004. The architecture of the murein (peptidoglycan) in gram-negative bacteria: vertical scaffold or horizontal layer(s)? *J Bacteriol* 186:5978–5987.

197. Gupta R, Lavollay M, Mainardi JL, Arthur M, Bishai WR, Lamichhane G. 2010. The *Mycobacterium tuberculosis* protein LdtMt2 is a nonclassical transpeptidase required for virulence and resistance to amoxicillin. *Nat Med* 16:466–469.

198. Diacon AH, van der Merwe L, Barnard M, von Groote-Bidlingmaier F, Lange C, García-Basteiro AL, Sevene E, Ballell L, Barros-Aguirre D. 2016. β-Lactams against tuberculosis—new trick for an old dog? *N Engl J Med* 375:393–394.

199. Solapure S, Dinesh N, Shandil R, Ramachandran V, Sharma S, Bhattacharjee D, Ganguly S, Reddy J, Ahuja V, Panduga V, Parab M, Vishwas KG, Kumar N, Balganesh M, Balasubramanian V. 2013. In vitro and in vivo efficacy of β-lactams against replicating and slowly growing/nonreplicating *Mycobacterium tuberculosis*. *Antimicrob Agents Chemother* 57:2506–2510.

200. Borrelli S, Zandberg WF, Mohan S, Ko M, Martinez-Gutierrez F, Partha SK, Sanders DA, Av-Gay Y, Pinto BM. 2010. Antimycobacterial activity of UDP-galactopyranose mutase inhibitors. *Int J Antimicrob Agents* 36:364–368.

201. Engohang-Ndong J. 2012. Antimycobacterial drugs currently in Phase II clinical trials and preclinical phase

for tuberculosis treatment. *Expert Opin Investig Drugs* 21:1789–1800.

202. Siricilla S, Mitachi K, Wan B, Franzblau SG, Kurosu M. 2015. Discovery of a capuramycin analog that kills nonreplicating *Mycobacterium tuberculosis* and its synergistic effects with translocase I inhibitors. *J Antibiot (Tokyo)* 68:271–278.

203. Ishizaki Y, Hayashi C, Inoue K, Igarashi M, Takahashi Y, Pujari V, Crick DC, Brennan PJ, Nomoto A. 2013. Inhibition of the first step in synthesis of the mycobacterial cell wall core, catalyzed by the GlcNAc-1-phosphate transferase WecA, by the novel caprazamycin derivative CPZEN-45. *J Biol Chem* 288:30309–30319.

204. Singh S, Roy KK, Khan SR, Kashyap VK, Sharma A, Jaiswal S, Sharma SK, Krishnan MY, Chaturvedi V, Lal J, Sinha S, Dasgupta A, Srivastava R, Saxena AK. 2015. Novel, potent, orally bioavailable and selective mycobacterial ATP synthase inhibitors that demonstrated activity against both replicating and non-replicating M. tuberculosis. *Bioorg Med Chem* 23:742–752.

205. Danelishvili L, Wu M, Young LS, Bermudez LE. 2005. Genomic approach to identifying the putative target of and mechanisms of resistance to mefloquine in mycobacteria. *Antimicrob Agents Chemother* 49: 3707–3714.

206. Martín-Galiano AJ, Gorgojo B, Kunin CM, de la Campa AG. 2002. Mefloquine and new related compounds target the F(0) complex of the F(0)F(1) H (+)-ATPase of *Streptococcus pneumoniae*. *Antimicrob Agents Chemother* 46:1680–1687.

207. Hongmanee P, Rukseree K, Buabut B, Somsri B, Palittapongarnpim P. 2007. In vitro activities of cloxyquin (5-chloroquinolin-8-ol) against *Mycobacterium tuberculosis*. *Antimicrob Agents Chemother* 51: 1105–1106.

208. Tison F. 1952. [The remarkable effect of a combination of iodochloroxyquinoline with a subactive dose of streptomycin on experimental tuberculosis in guinea pigs]. *Ann Inst Pasteur (Paris)* 83:275–276.

209. Shah S, Dalecki AG, Malalasekera AP, Crawford CL, Michalek SM, Kutsch O, Sun J, Bossmann SH, Wolschendorf F. 2016. 8-Hydroxyquinolines are boosting-agents of copper related toxicity in *Mycobacterium tuberculosis*. *Antimicrob Agents Chemother* 60:5765–5776.

210. Mao J, Wang Y, Wan B, Kozikowski AP, Franzblau SG. 2007. Design, synthesis, and pharmacological evaluation of mefloquine-based ligands as novel antituberculosis agents. *ChemMedChem* 2:1624–1630.

211. Mao J, Yuan H, Wang Y, Wan B, Pieroni M, Huang Q, van Breemen RB, Kozikowski AP, Franzblau SG. 2009. From serendipity to rational antituberculosis drug discovery of mefloquine-isoxazole carboxylic acid esters. *J Med Chem* 52:6966–6978.

212. Jayaprakash S, Iso Y, Wan B, Franzblau SG, Kozikowski AP. 2006. Design, synthesis, and SAR studies of mefloquine-based ligands as potential antituberculosis agents. *ChemMedChem* 1:593–597.

213. Lilienkampf A, Mao J, Wan B, Wang Y, Franzblau SG, Kozikowski AP. 2009. Structure-activity relationships for a series of quinoline-based compounds active

against replicating and nonreplicating *Mycobacterium tuberculosis*. *J Med Chem* 52:2109–2118.

214. Lilienkampf A, Pieroni M, Wan B, Wang Y, Franzblau SG, Kozikowski AP. 2010. Rational design of 5-phenyl-3-isoxazolecarboxylic acid ethyl esters as growth inhibitors of *Mycobacterium tuberculosis*. a potent and selective series for further drug development. *J Med Chem* 53:678–688.

215. Saxena AK, Roy KK, Singh S, Vishnoi SP, Kumar A, Kashyap VK, Kremer L, Srivastava R, Srivastava BS. 2013. Identification and characterisation of small-molecule inhibitors of Rv3097c-encoded lipase (LipY) of *Mycobacterium tuberculosis* that selectively inhibit growth of bacilli in hypoxia. *Int J Antimicrob Agents* 42:27–35.

216. Low KL, Rao PS, Shui G, Bendt AK, Pethe K, Dick T, Wenk MR. 2009. Triacylglycerol utilization is required for regrowth of in vitro hypoxic nonreplicating *Mycobacterium bovis* bacillus Calmette-Guerin. *J Bacteriol* 191:5037–5043.

217. Darwin KH, Ehrt S, Gutierrez-Ramos JC, Weich N, Nathan CF. 2003. The proteasome of *Mycobacterium tuberculosis* is required for resistance to nitric oxide. *Science* 302:1963–1966.

218. Fay A, Glickman MS. 2014. An essential nonredundant role for mycobacterial DnaK in native protein folding. *PLoS Genet* 10:e1004516.

219. Raju RM, Unnikrishnan M, Rubin DH, Krishnamoorthy V, Kandror O, Akopian TN, Goldberg AL, Rubin EJ. 2012. *Mycobacterium tuberculosis* ClpP1 and ClpP2 function together in protein degradation and are required for viability in vitro and during infection. *PLoS Pathog* 8:e1002511.

220. Schmitt EK, Riwanto M, Sambandamurthy V, Roggo S, Miault C, Zwingelstein C, Krastel P, Noble C, Beer D, Rao SP, Au M, Niyomrattanakit P, Lim V, Zheng J, Jeffery D, Pethe K, Camacho LR. 2011. The natural product cyclomarin kills *Mycobacterium tuberculosis* by targeting the ClpC1 subunit of the caseinolytic protease. *Angew Chem Int Ed Engl* 50:5889–5891.

221. Lee H, Suh JW. 2016. Anti-tuberculosis lead molecules from natural products targeting *Mycobacterium tuberculosis* ClpC1. *J Ind Microbiol Biotechnol* 43: 205–212.

222. Lear S, Munshi T, Hudson AS, Hatton C, Clardy J, Mosely JA, Bull TJ, Sit CS, Cobb SL. 2016. Total chemical synthesis of lassomycin and lassomycin-amide. *Org Biomol Chem* 14:4534–4541.

223. Gavrish E, Sit CS, Cao S, Kandror O, Spoering A, Peoples A, Ling L, Fetterman A, Hughes D, Bissell A, Torrey H, Akopian T, Mueller A, Epstein S, Goldberg A, Clardy J, Lewis K. 2014. Lassomycin, a ribosomally synthesized cyclic peptide, kills mycobacterium tuberculosis by targeting the ATP-dependent protease ClpC1P1P2. *Chem Biol* 21:509–518.

224. Gao W, Kim JY, Anderson JR, Akopian T, Hong S, Jin YY, Kandror O, Kim JW, Lee IA, Lee SY, McAlpine JB, Mulugeta S, Sunoqrot S, Wang Y, Yang SH, Yoon TM, Goldberg AL, Pauli GF, Suh JW, Franzblau SG, Cho S. 2015. The cyclic peptide ecumicin targeting

ClpC1 is active against *Mycobacterium tuberculosis* in vivo. *Antimicrob Agents Chemother* 59:880–889.

225. Gandotra S, Schnappinger D, Monteleone M, Hillen W, Ehrt S. 2007. In vivo gene silencing identifies the *Mycobacterium tuberculosis* proteasome as essential for the bacteria to persist in mice. *Nat Med* 13:1515–1520. [pii] 10.1038/nm1683. PMID: 18059281.

226. Gandotra S, Lebron MB, Ehrt S. 2010. The *Mycobacterium tuberculosis* proteasome active site threonine is essential for persistence yet dispensable for replication and resistance to nitric oxide. *PLoS Pathog* 6: e1001040.

227. Lin G, Chidawanyika T, Tsu C, Warrier T, Vaubourgeix J, Blackburn C, Gigstad K, Sintchak M, Dick L, Nathan C. 2013. N,C-Capped dipeptides with selectivity for mycobacterial proteasome over human proteasomes: role of S3 and S1 binding pockets. *J Am Chem Soc* 135: 9968–9971.

228. Russo F, Gising J, Åkerbladh L, Roos AK, Naworyta A, Mowbray SL, Sokolowski A, Henderson I, Alling T, Bailey MA, Files M, Parish T, Karlén A, Larhed M. 2015. Optimization and evaluation of 5-styryl-oxathiazol-2-one *Mycobacterium tuberculosis* proteasome inhibitors as potential antitubercular agents. *ChemistryOpen* 4:342–362.

229. Timm J, Post FA, Bekker LG, Walther GB, Wainwright HC, Manganelli R, Chan WT, Tsenova L, Gold B, Smith I, Kaplan G, McKinney JD. 2003. Differential expression of iron-, carbon-, and oxygen-responsive mycobacterial genes in the lungs of chronically infected mice and tuberculosis patients. *Proc Natl Acad Sci USA* 100:14321–14326.

230. Wolschendorf F, Ackart D, Shrestha TB, Hascall-Dove L, Nolan S, Lamichhane G, Wang Y, Bossmann SH, Basaraba RJ, Niederweis M. 2011. Copper resistance is essential for virulence of *Mycobacterium tuberculosis*. *Proc Natl Acad Sci USA* 108:1621–1626.

231. MacMicking JD, Taylor GA, McKinney JD. 2003. Immune control of tuberculosis by IFN-gamma-inducible LRG-47. *Science* 302:654–659.

232. MacMicking JD, North RJ, LaCourse R, Mudgett JS, Shah SK, Nathan CF. 1997. Identification of nitric oxide synthase as a protective locus against tuberculosis. *Proc Natl Acad Sci USA* 94:5243–5248.

233. Marrero J, Rhee KY, Schnappinger D, Pethe K, Ehrt S. 2010. Gluconeogenic carbon flow of tricarboxylic acid cycle intermediates is critical for *Mycobacterium tuberculosis* to establish and maintain infection. *Proc Natl Acad Sci USA* 107:9819–9824.

234. Gomez JE, McKinney JD. 2004. *M. tuberculosis* persistence, latency, and drug tolerance. *Tuberculosis (Edinb)* 84(1-2):29–44. [pii]. PMID: 14670344.

235. Manina G, Dhar N, McKinney JD. 2015. Stress and host immunity amplify *Mycobacterium tuberculosis* phenotypic heterogeneity and induce nongrowing metabolically active forms. *Cell Host Microbe* 17:32–46.

236. Munoz-Elias EJ, McKinney JD. 2005. *Mycobacterium tuberculosis* isocitrate lyases 1 and 2 are jointly required for in vivo growth and virulence. *Nat Med* 11:638–644. [pii] 10.1038/nm1252. PMID: 15895072.

237. Munoz-Elias EJ, McKinney JD. 2006. Carbon metabolism of intracellular bacteria. *Cell Microbiol* 8:10–22. [pii] 10.1111/j.1462-5822.2005.00648.x. PMID: 16367862.

238. Berney M, Berney-Meyer L, Wong KW, Chen B, Chen M, Kim J, Wang J, Harris D, Parkhill J, Chan J, Wang F, Jacobs WR Jr. 2015. Essential roles of methionine and S-adenosylmethionine in the autarkic lifestyle of *Mycobacterium tuberculosis*. *Proc Natl Acad Sci USA* 112:10008–10013.

239. Hondalus MK, Bardarov S, Russell R, Chan J, Jacobs WR Jr, Bloom BR. 2000. Attenuation of and protection induced by a leucine auxotroph of *Mycobacterium tuberculosis*. *Infect Immun* 68:2888–2898.

240. Sambandamurthy VK, Wang X, Chen B, Russell RG, Derrick S, Collins FM, Morris SL, Jacobs WR Jr. 2002. A pantothenate auxotroph of *Mycobacterium tuberculosis* is highly attenuated and protects mice against tuberculosis. *Nat Med* 8:1171–1174.

241. Rodriguez GM, Smith I. 2003. Mechanisms of iron regulation in mycobacteria: role in physiology and virulence. *Mol Microbiol* 47:1485–1494.

242. Gould TA, van de Langemheen H, Munoz-Elias EJ, McKinney JD, Sacchettini JC. 2006. Dual role of isocitrate lyase 1 in the glyoxylate and methylcitrate cycles in *Mycobacterium tuberculosis*. *Mol Microbiol* 61:940–947. [pii] 10.1111/j.1365-2958.2006.05297.x. PMID: 16879647.

243. Walters SB, Dubnau E, Kolesnikova I, Laval F, Daffe M, Smith I. 2006. The *Mycobacterium tuberculosis* PhoPR two-component system regulates genes essential for virulence and complex lipid biosynthesis. *Mol Microbiol* 60:312–330. [pii] 10.1111/j.1365-2958. 2006.05102.x. PMID: 16573683.

244. Miner MD, Chang JC, Pandey AK, Sassetti CM, Sherman DR. 2009. Role of cholesterol in *Mycobacterium tuberculosis* infection. *Indian J Exp Biol* 47: 407–411.

245. Belton M, Brilha S, Manavaki R, Mauri F, Nijran K, Hong YT, Patel NH, Dembek M, Tezera L, Green J, Moores R, Aigbirhio F, Al-Nahhas A, Fryer TD, Elkington PT, Friedland JS. 2016. Hypoxia and tissue destruction in pulmonary TB. *Thorax* [Epub ahead of print] thoraxjnl-2015-207402.

246. Sperka T, Pitlik J, Bagossi P, Tözsér J. 2005. Beta-lactam compounds as apparently uncompetitive inhibitors of HIV-1 protease. *Bioorg Med Chem Lett* 15: 3086–3090.

247. Powers JC, Asgian JL, Ekici OD, James KE. 2002. Irreversible inhibitors of serine, cysteine, and threonine proteases. *Chem Rev* 102:4639–4750.

248. Paetzel M, Dalbey RE, Strynadka NC. 1998. Crystal structure of a bacterial signal peptidase in complex with a beta-lactam inhibitor. *Nature* 396:186–190.

249. Baranowski C, Rubin EJ. 2016. Could killing bacterial subpopulations hit tuberculosis out of the park? *J Med Chem* 59:6025–6026.

250. Costerton JW, Stewart PS, Greenberg EP. 1999. Bacterial biofilms: a common cause of persistent infections. *Science* 284:1318–1322.

251. Hall-Stoodley L, Costerton JW, Stoodley P. 2004. Bacterial biofilms: from the natural environment to infectious diseases. *Nat Rev Microbiol* **2**:95–108.

252. Ojha AK, Baughn AD, Sambandan D, Hsu T, Trivelli X, Guerardel Y, Alahari A, Kremer L, Jacobs WR Jr, Hatfull GF. 2008. Growth of *Mycobacterium tuberculosis* biofilms containing free mycolic acids and harbouring drug-tolerant bacteria. *Mol Microbiol* **69**:164–174.

253. Purkayastha A, McCue LA, McDonough KA. 2002. Identification of a *Mycobacterium tuberculosis* putative classical nitroreductase gene whose expression is coregulated with that of the acr aene within macrophages, in standing versus shaking cultures, and under low oxygen conditions. *Infect Immun* **70**:1518–1529.

254. Williams EM, Little RF, Mowday AM, Rich MH, Chan-Hyams JV, Copp JN, Smaill JB, Patterson AV, Ackerley DF. 2015. Nitroreductase gene-directed enzyme prodrug therapy: insights and advances toward clinical utility. *Biochem J* **471**:131–153.

255. Viodé C, Bettache N, Cenas N, Krauth-Siegel RL, Chauvière G, Bakalara N, Périé J. 1999. Enzymatic reduction studies of nitroheterocycles. *Biochem Pharmacol* **57**:549–557.

256. McOsker CC, Fitzpatrick PM. 1994. Nitrofurantoin: mechanism of action and implications for resistance development in common uropathogens. *J Antimicrob Chemother*. **33**(Suppl A):23–30. PMID: 7928834.

257. Murugasu-Oei B, Dick T. 2000. Bactericidal activity of nitrofurans against growing and dormant *Mycobacterium bovis* BCG. *J Antimicrob Chemother* **46**:917–919.

258. de Carvalho LP, Darby CM, Rhee KY, Nathan C. 2011. Nitazoxanide disrupts membrane potential and intrabacterial pH homeostasis of *Mycobacterium tuberculosis*. *ACS Med Chem Lett* **2**:849–854.

259. Matsumoto M, Hashizume H, Tomishige T, Kawasaki M, Tsubouchi H, Sasaki H, Shimokawa Y, Komatsu M. 2006. OPC-67683, a nitro-dihydro-imidazooxazole derivative with promising action against tuberculosis in vitro and in mice. *PLoS Med* **3**:e466.

260. Upton AM, Cho S, Yang TJ, Kim Y, Wang Y, Lu Y, Wang B, Xu J, Mdluli K, Ma Z, Franzblau SG. 2015. *In vitro* and *in vivo* activities of the nitroimidazole TBA-354 against *Mycobacterium tuberculosis*. *Antimicrob Agents Chemother* **59**:136–144.

261. Upton AM, McKinney JD. 2007. Role of the methylcitrate cycle in propionate metabolism and detoxification in *Mycobacterium smegmatis*. *Microbiology* **153** (Pt 12):3973–3982. [pii] 10.1099/mic.0.2007/011726-0. PMID: 18048912.

262. Rakesh, Bruhn DF, Scherman MS, Woolhiser LK, Madhura DB, Maddox MM, et al. 2014. Pentacyclic nitrofurans with in vivo efficacy and activity against non-replicating *Mycobacterium tuberculosis*. *PLoS One* **9** (2):e87909. PMID: 24505329; Central PMCID: PMC3914891.

263. Debnath AK, Lopez de Compadre RL, Debnath G, Shusterman AJ, Hansch C. 1991. Structure-activity relationship of mutagenic aromatic and heteroaromatic nitro compounds. Correlation with molecular orbital energies and hydrophobicity. *J Med Chem* **34**:786–797.

264. Feng X, Zhu W, Schurig-Briccio LA, Lindert S, Shoen C, Hitchings R, Li J, Wang Y, Baig N, Zhou T, Kim BK, Crick DC, Cynamon M, McCammon JA, Gennis RB, Oldfield E. 2015. Antiinfectives targeting enzymes and the proton motive force. *Proc Natl Acad Sci USA* **112**:E7073–E7082 10.1073/pnas.1521988112.

265. Lee IY, Gruber TD, Samuels A, Yun M, Nam B, Kang M, Crowley K, Winterroth B, Boshoff HI, Barry CE III. 2013. Structure-activity relationships of antitubercular salicylanilides consistent with disruption of the proton gradient via proton shuttling. *Bioorg Med Chem* **21**:114–126.

266. Terada H. 1990. Uncouplers of oxidative phosphorylation. *Environ Health Perspect* **87**:213–218.

267. Williamson RL, Metcalf RL. 1967. Salicylanilides: a new group of active uncouplers of oxidative phosphorylation. *Science* **158**:1694–1695.

268. Moreira W, Aziz DB, Dick T. 2016. Boromycin kills mycobacterial persisters without detectable resistance. *Front Microbiol* **7**:199.

269. Mukherjee D, Zou H, Liu S, Beuerman R, Dick T. 2016. Membrane-targeting AM-0016 kills mycobacterial persisters and shows low propensity for resistance development. *Future Microbiol* **11**:643–650.

270. Tyagi S, Ammerman NC, Li SY, Adamson J, Converse PJ, Swanson RV, Almeida DV, Grosset JH. 2015. Clofazimine shortens the duration of the first-line treatment regimen for experimental chemotherapy of tuberculosis. *Proc Natl Acad Sci USA* **112**:869–874.

271. Yano T, Kassovska-Bratinova S, Teh JS, Winkler J, Sullivan K, Isaacs A, Schechter NM, Rubin H. 2011. Reduction of clofazimine by mycobacterial type 2 NADH: quinone oxidoreductase: a pathway for the generation of bactericidal levels of reactive oxygen species. *J Biol Chem* **286**:10276–10287.

272. Lechartier B, Cole ST. 2015. Mode of action of clofazimine and combination therapy with benzothiazinones against *Mycobacterium tuberculosis*. *Antimicrob Agents Chemother* **59**:4457–4463.

273. Advani MJ, Siddiqui I, Sharma P, Reddy H. 2012. Activity of trifluoperazine against replicating, non-replicating and drug resistant M. tuberculosis. *PLoS One* **7**:e44245.

274. Jones PB, Parrish NM, Houston TA, Stapon A, Bansal NP, Dick JD, Townsend CA. 2000. A new class of antituberculosis agents. *J Med Chem* **43**:3304–3314.

275. Parrish NM, Houston T, Jones PB, Townsend C, Dick JD. 2001. In vitro activity of a novel antimycobacterial compound, N-octanesulfonylacetamide, and its effects on lipid and mycolic acid synthesis. *Antimicrob Agents Chemother* **45**:1143–1150. PMID: 11257028; Central PMCID: PMC90437.

276. Parrish NM, Ko CG, Dick JD. 2009. Activity of DSA against anaerobically adapted *Mycobacterium bovis* BCG in vitro. *Tuberculosis (Edinb)* **89**:325–327.

277. Parrish NM, Ko CG, Hughes MA, Townsend CA, Dick JD. 2004. Effect of n-octanesulphonylacetamide (OSA) on ATP and protein expression in *Mycobacterium bovis* BCG. *J Antimicrob Chemother* **54**:722–729.

278. Pethe K, et al. 2013. Discovery of Q203, a potent clinical candidate for the treatment of tuberculosis. *Nat Med* 19:1157–1160.

279. Wallace KB, Starkov AA. 2000. Mitochondrial targets of drug toxicity. *Annu Rev Pharmacol Toxicol* 40:353–388.

280. Conlon BP, Rowe SE, Gandt AB, Nuxoll AS, Donegan NP, Zalis EA, et al. 2016. Persister formation in *Staphylococcus aureus* is associated with ATP depletion. *Nat Microbiol* 1. PMID: 27398229; Central PMCID: PMC4932909.

281. Harbut MB, Vilchèze C, Luo X, Hensler ME, Guo H, Yang B, Chatterjee AK, Nizet V, Jacobs WR Jr, Schultz PG, Wang F. 2015. Auranofin exerts broad-spectrum bactericidal activities by targeting thiol-redox homeostasis. *Proc Natl Acad Sci USA* 112:4453–4458.

282. Lin K, O'Brien KM, Trujillo C, Wang R, Wallach JB, Schnappinger D, Ehrt S. 2016. *Mycobacterium tuberculosis* thioredoxin reductase is essential for thiol redox homeostasis but plays a minor role in antioxidant defense. *PLoS Pathog* 12:e1005675.

283. Malhotra V, Sharma D, Ramanathan VD, Shakila H, Saini DK, Chakravorty S, Das TK, Li Q, Silver RF, Narayanan PR, Tyagi JS. 2004. Disruption of response regulator gene, *devR*, leads to attenuation in virulence of *Mycobacterium tuberculosis*. *FEMS Microbiol Lett* 231:237–245.

284. Gupta RK, Thakur TS, Desiraju GR, Tyagi JS. 2009. Structure-based design of DevR inhibitor active against nonreplicating *Mycobacterium tuberculosis*. *J Med Chem* 52:6324–6334.

285. Salina E, Ryabova O, Kaprelyants A, Makarov V. 2014. New 2-thiopyridines as potential candidates for killing both actively growing and dormant *Mycobacterium tuberculosis* cells. *Antimicrob Agents Chemother* 58:55–60.

286. Moraski GC, Chang M, Villegas-Estrada A, Franzblau SG, Möllmann U, Miller MJ. 2010. Structure-activity relationship of new anti-tuberculosis agents derived from oxazoline and oxazole benzyl esters. *Eur J Med Chem* 45:1703–1716.

287. Villar R, Vicente E, Solano B, Pérez-Silanes S, Aldana I, Maddry JA, Lenaerts AJ, Franzblau SG, Cho SH, Monge A, Goldman RC. 2008. In vitro and in vivo antimycobacterial activities of ketone and amide derivatives of quinoxaline 1,4-di-N-oxide. *J Antimicrob Chemother* 62:547–554.

288. Friedmann HC. 2004. From "butyribacterium" to "E. coli": an essay on unity in biochemistry. *Perspect Biol Med* 47:47–66.

289. Schnappinger D. 2015. Genetic approaches to facilitate antibacterial drug development. *Cold Spring Harb Perspect Med* 5:a021139.

290. Kim JH, O'Brien KM, Sharma R, Boshoff HI, Rehren G, Chakraborty S, Wallach JB, Monteleone M, Wilson DJ, Aldrich CC, Barry CE III, Rhee KY, Ehrt S, Schnappinger D. 2013. A genetic strategy to identify targets for the development of drugs that prevent bacterial persistence. *Proc Natl Acad Sci USA* 110:19095–19100.

291. Russell DG, Barry CE III, Flynn JL. 2010. Tuberculosis: what we don't know can, and does, hurt us. *Science* 328:852–856.

292. Heifets L, Higgins M, Simon B. 2000. Pyrazinamide is not active against *Mycobacterium tuberculosis* residing in cultured human monocyte-derived macrophages. *Int J Tuberc Lung Dis* 4:491–495.

293. Rastogi N, Potar MC, David HL. 1988. Pyrazinamide is not effective against intracellularly growing *Mycobacterium tuberculosis*. *Antimicrob Agents Chemother* 32:287.

294. Tsai MC, Chakravarty S, Zhu G, Xu J, Tanaka K, Koch C, Tufariello J, Flynn J, Chan J. 2006. Characterization of the tuberculous granuloma in murine and human lungs: cellular composition and relative tissue oxygen tension. *Cell Microbiol* 8:218–232.

295. Dhillon J, Allen BW, Hu YM, Coates AR, Mitchison DA. 1998. Metronidazole has no antibacterial effect in Cornell model murine tuberculosis. *Int J Tuberc Lung Dis* 2:736–742.

296. Lanoix JP, Lenaerts AJ, Nuermberger EL. 2015. Heterogeneous disease progression and treatment response in a C3HeB/FeJ mouse model of tuberculosis. *Dis Model Mech* 8:603–610.

297. Harper J, Skerry C, Davis SL, Tasneen R, Weir M, Kramnik I, Bishai WR, Pomper MG, Nuermberger EL, Jain SK. 2012. Mouse model of necrotic tuberculosis granulomas develops hypoxic lesions. *J Infect Dis* 205:595–602.

298. Desai CR, Heera S, Patel A, Babrekar AB, Mahashur AA, Kamat SR. 1989. Role of metronidazole in improving response and specific drug sensitivity in advanced pulmonary tuberculosis. *J Assoc Physicians India* 37:694–697.

299. Lardner A. 2001. The effects of extracellular pH on immune function. *J Leukoc Biol* 69:522–530.

300. Eoh H, Rhee KY. 2014. Methylcitrate cycle defines the bactericidal essentiality of isocitrate lyase for survival of *Mycobacterium tuberculosis* on fatty acids. *Proc Natl Acad Sci USA* 111:4976–4981.

301. Dartois V, Barry CE III. 2013. A medicinal chemists' guide to the unique difficulties of lead optimization for tuberculosis. *Bioorg Med Chem Lett* 23:4741–4750.

302. Dannenberg AM Jr. 1993. Immunopathogenesis of pulmonary tuberculosis. *Hosp Pract (Off Ed)* 28:51–58.

303. Aly S, Wagner K, Keller C, Malm S, Malzan A, Brandau S, Bange FC, Ehlers S. 2006. Oxygen status of lung granulomas in *Mycobacterium tuberculosis*-infected mice. *J Pathol* 210:298–305.

304. Schön T, Elmberger G, Negesse Y, Pando RH, Sundqvist T, Britton S. 2004. Local production of nitric oxide in patients with tuberculosis. *Int J Tuberc Lung Dis* 8:1134–1137.

305. Nicholson S, Bonecini-Almeida MG, Lapa e Silva JR, Nathan C, Xie QW, Mumford R, Weidner JR, Calaycay J, Geng J, Boechat N, Linhares C, Rom W, Ho JL. 1996. Inducible nitric oxide synthase in pulmonary alveolar macrophages from patients with tuberculosis. *J Exp Med* 183:2293–2302.

306. Facchetti F, Vermi W, Fiorentini S, Chilosi M, Caruso A, Duse M, Notarangelo LD, Badolato R. 1999. Expression of inducible nitric oxide synthase in human granu-

lomas and histiocytic reactions. *Am J Pathol* **154:** 145–152.

307. **Choi HS, Rai PR, Chu HW, Cool C, Chan ED.** 2002. Analysis of nitric oxide synthase and nitrotyrosine expression in human pulmonary tuberculosis. *Am J Respir Crit Care Med* **166:**178–186.

308. **Nathan C.** 2002. Inducible nitric oxide synthase in the tuberculous human lung. *Am J Respir Crit Care Med* **166:**130–131.

309. **Nathan C, Cunningham-Bussel A.** 2013. Beyond oxidative stress: an immunologist's guide to reactive oxygen species. *Nat Rev Immunol* **13:**349–361.

310. **Nathan C, Shiloh MU.** 2000. Reactive oxygen and nitrogen intermediates in the relationship between mammalian hosts and microbial pathogens. *Proc Natl Acad Sci USA* **97:**8841–8848. PMID: 10922044; Central PMCID: PMC34021.

311. **Kohanski MA, Dwyer DJ, Hayete B, Lawrence CA, Collins JJ.** 2007. A common mechanism of cellular death induced by bactericidal antibiotics. *Cell* **130:**797–810.

312. **Ng VH, Cox JS, Sousa AO, MacMicking JD, McKinney JD.** 2004. Role of KatG catalase-peroxidase in mycobacterial pathogenesis: countering the phagocyte oxidative burst. *Mol Microbiol* **52:**1291–1302.

313. **Skaar EP.** 2010. The battle for iron between bacterial pathogens and their vertebrate hosts. *PLoS Pathog* **6:** e1000949.

314. **Goodsmith N, Guo XV, Vandal OH, Vaubourgeix J, Wang R, Botella H, Song S, Bhatt K, Liba A, Salgame P, Schnappinger D, Ehrt S.** 2015. Disruption of an M. tuberculosis membrane protein causes a magnesium-dependent cell division defect and failure to persist in mice. *PLoS Pathog* **11:**e1004645.

315. **Wolschendorf F, Ackart D, Shrestha TB, Hascall-Dove L, Nolan S, Lamichhane G, Wang Y, Bossmann SH, Basaraba RJ, Niederweis M.** 2010. Copper resistance is essential for virulence of *Mycobacterium tuberculosis*. *Proc Natl Acad Sci USA* **108:**1621–1626. [pii] 10.1073/pnas.1009261108. PMID: 21205886.

316. **Rowland JL, Niederweis M.** 2013. A multicopper oxidase is required for copper resistance in *Mycobacterium tuberculosis*. *J Bacteriol* **195:**3724–3733.

317. **Rowland JL, Niederweis M.** 2012. Resistance mechanisms of *Mycobacterium tuberculosis* against phagosomal copper overload. *Tuberculosis (Edinb)* **92:**202–210.

318. **Darwin KH.** 2015. *Mycobacterium tuberculosis* and copper: a newly appreciated defense against an old foe? *J Biol Chem* **290:**18962–18966.

319. **White C, Lee J, Kambe T, Fritsche K, Petris MJ.** 2009. A role for the ATP7A copper-transporting ATPase in macrophage bactericidal activity. *J Biol Chem* **284:** 33949–33956.

320. **Tan S, Sukumar N, Abramovitch RB, Parish T, Russell DG.** 2013. *Mycobacterium tuberculosis* responds to chloride and pH as synergistic cues to the immune status of its host cell. *PLoS Pathog* **9:**e1003282.

321. **Larrouy-Maumus G, Marino LB, Madduri AV, Ragan TJ, Hunt DM, Bassano L, Gutierrez MG, Moody DB, Pavan FR, de Carvalho LP.** 2016. Cell-envelope re-

modeling as a determinant of phenotypic antibacterial tolerance in *Mycobacterium tuberculosis*. *ACS Infect Dis* **2:**352–360.

322. **Scott CC, Gruenberg J.** 2011. Ion flux and the function of endosomes and lysosomes: pH is just the start: the flux of ions across endosomal membranes influences endosome function not only through regulation of the luminal pH. *BioEssays* **33:**103–110.

323. **Jiang L, Salao K, Li H, Rybicka JM, Yates RM, Luo XW, Shi XX, Kuffner T, Tsai VW, Husaini Y, Wu L, Brown DA, Grewal T, Brown LJ, Curmi PM, Breit SN.** 2012. Intracellular chloride channel protein CLIC1 regulates macrophage function through modulation of phagosomal acidification. *J Cell Sci* **125:**5479–5488.

324. **McKinney JD, Höner zu Bentrup K, Muñoz-Elías EJ, Miczak A, Chen B, Chan WT, Swenson D, Sacchettini JC, Jacobs WR Jr, Russell DG.** 2000. Persistence of *Mycobacterium tuberculosis* in macrophages and mice requires the glyoxylate shunt enzyme isocitrate lyase. *Nature* **406:**735–738.

325. **Munoz-Elias EJ, Upton AM, Cherian J, McKinney JD.** 2006. Role of the methylcitrate cycle in *Mycobacterium tuberculosis* metabolism, intracellular growth, and virulence. *Mol Microbiol* **60:**1109–1122. [pii] 10.1111/j.1365-2958.2006.05155.x. PMID: 16689789.

326. **Beste DJ, Nöh K, Niedenführ S, Mendum TA, Hawkins ND, Ward JL, Beale MH, Wiechert W, McFadden J.** 2013. 13C-flux spectral analysis of host-pathogen metabolism reveals a mixed diet for intracellular *Mycobacterium tuberculosis*. *Chem Biol* **20:**1012–1021.

327. **Pandey AK, Sassetti CM.** 2008. Mycobacterial persistence requires the utilization of host cholesterol. *Proc Natl Acad Sci USA* **105:**4376–4380.

328. **Baek SH, Li AH, Sassetti CM.** 2011. Metabolic regulation of mycobacterial growth and antibiotic sensitivity. *PLoS Biol* **9:**e1001065.

329. **Shi L, Sohaskey CD, Pheiffer C, Datta P, Parks M, McFadden J, North RJ, Gennaro ML.** 2010. Carbon flux rerouting during *Mycobacterium tuberculosis* growth arrest. *Mol Microbiol* **78:**1199–1215.

330. **Larsen MH, Biermann K, Chen B, Hsu T, Sambandamurthy VK, Lackner AA, Aye PP, Didier P, Huang D, Shao L, Wei H, Letvin NL, Frothingham R, Haynes BF, Chen ZW, Jacobs WR Jr.** 2009. Efficacy and safety of live attenuated persistent and rapidly cleared *Mycobacterium tuberculosis* vaccine candidates in non-human primates. *Vaccine* **27:**4709–4717.

331. **Sambandamurthy VK, Derrick SC, Jalapathy KV, Chen B, Russell RG, Morris SL, Jacobs WR Jr.** 2005. Long-term protection against tuberculosis following vaccination with a severely attenuated double lysine and pantothenate auxotroph of *Mycobacterium tuberculosis*. *Infect Immun* **73:**1196–1203.

332. **Gouzy A, Poquet Y, Neyrolles O.** 2014. Nitrogen metabolism in *Mycobacterium tuberculosis* physiology and virulence. *Nat Rev Microbiol* **12:**729–737.

333. **Cunningham-Bussel A, Bange FC, Nathan CF.** 2013. Nitrite impacts the survival of *Mycobacterium tuberculosis* in response to isoniazid and hydrogen peroxide. *MicrobiologyOpen* **2:**901–911.

Biomarkers and Diagnostics

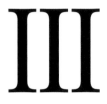

Tuberculosis and the Tubercle Bacillus, 2nd ed.
Edited by William R. Jacobs, Jr., Helen McShane, Valerie Mizrahi, and Ian M. Orme
© 2018 American Society for Microbiology, Washington, DC
doi:10.1128/microbiolspec.TBTB2-0019-2016

Tuberculosis Diagnostics: State of the Art and Future Directions

16

Madhukar Pai[1], Mark P. Nicol[2], and Catharina C. Boehme[3]

INTRODUCTION

Despite the progress made in global tuberculosis (TB) control, TB remains a major global health problem, and drug-resistant TB is a growing threat (1). Early diagnosis of TB including universal drug susceptibility testing (DST), and systematic screening of contacts and high-risk groups are key components of the End TB Strategy by WHO and partners (2).

Rapid, accurate diagnosis is critical for timely initiation of anti-TB treatment, but many people with TB (or TB symptoms) do not have access to adequate initial diagnosis. For example, 37% of the 9.6 million new cases globally are either undiagnosed or not reported. These "missing" 3.6 million people with TB are at the root of ongoing TB transmission, including of multidrug-resistant TB (MDR-TB) (1). Seventy-five percent of the 480,000 cases of MDR-TB are either not detected or not reported (1). Even among previously treated patients at risk of drug resistance, 40% were not tested for drug resistance, and 50% of TB patients have no documented HIV test result (1).

In this article, we provide an overview of current diagnostics for active TB and drug susceptibility testing, and review the unmet needs and gaps. Latent TB diagnostics are covered elsewhere (69). We also describe the pipeline of new diagnostics, and review lessons learned from implementation research on how to deploy new tools for maximum impact.

CURRENT DIAGNOSTICS FOR ACTIVE TB

Currently, there are three main validated methods for the detection of active TB: microscopy, nucleic acid amplification tests (NAATs), and cultures. In addition,

antigen detection tests are commercially available with limited WHO endorsement. For screening of active TB, imaging with chest X ray is a widely used method and may become of increased utility with the emergence of digital radiology and computer-aided interpretation (3). Table 1 shows the technologies that have undergone WHO review, in each category.

Smear Microscopy

Stains that are taken up by the lipid-rich cell wall of *Mycobacterium tuberculosis* resist decolorization with acid-containing reagents. Acid-fast organisms can then be visualized on microscopic examination of smears prepared from sputum or other biological specimens. The most widely used method in low-resource settings involves examination of Ziehl-Neelsen-stained slides under light microscopy. However, fluorescent microscopy, with stains such as Auramine, is 10% more sensitive and permits more rapid screening (at lower magnification) of large numbers of smears (4). Until recently, fluorescent microscopy was relatively expensive, with costly microscopes requiring frequent maintenance (e.g., bulb changes). The replacement of conventional fluorescent light sources with light-emitting diodes (LED fluorescent microscopy) has substantially reduced cost, power (LED microscopes can be battery powered), and maintenance requirements, and has eliminated the need for a darkroom, while retaining sensitivity (5).

The benefit of concentrating sputum prior to microscopy, by centrifugation or sedimentation of sputum that has been liquefied using bleach or NaOH (with or without *N*-acetyl-l-cysteine [NALC]) remains unclear. A systematic review demonstrated that concentration, on average, increased sensitivity, with no loss in specificity, but results varied widely between studies (6); in

[1]McGill International TB Centre, McGill University, Montreal, QC H3A 1A2, Canada; [2]University of Cape Town, Cape Town 7700, South Africa; [3]FIND, 1202 Geneva, Switzerland.

Table 1 Technologies reviewed by WHO for TB case detection

Year	Method	Technology reviewed by WHO
2007	Culture (growth-based)	Commercial liquid culture and rapid speciation strip tests
2010	Microscopy	LED microscopy
2010	NAAT	Xpert MTB/RIF
2016	Antigen detection test	Urine LAM rapid test
2016	NAAT	Loop-mediated amplification test (LAMP)
2017	NAAT	Xpert MTB/RIF Ultra

the case of LED microscopy, concentration appears to significantly decrease sensitivity (5).

The major limitation of smear microscopy is lack of sensitivity, which varies widely (20 to 80%) and is particularly poor in patients with paucibacillary TB including children, patients with extrapulmonary TB, or those who are HIV coinfected. It is estimated that 5,000 to 10,000 bacilli are required per milliliter of sputum for a positive direct (unconcentrated) smear. Specificity is likely to vary considerably depending on the local prevalence of infections with nontuberculous mycobacteria. In regions with a high incidence of tuberculosis, specificity of smear microscopy is high (95 to 98%), although there is some evidence that concentration by centrifugation is associated with variable reduction in specificity.

In summary, the key WHO recommendations (5) for smear microscopy are:

- LED microscopy should replace conventional fluorescent and light microscopy.
- There is insufficient generalizable evidence that microscopy of concentrated sputum specimens provides results that are superior to direct smear microscopy.

Commercial Liquid Culture and Rapid Speciation Strip Tests

Mycobacterial culture on solid agar (e.g., Lowenstein-Jensen [LJ]) or in liquid culture (e.g., Mycobacterial Growth Indicator Tube [MGIT; Becton Dickinson, Franklin Lakes, NJ] or BacT/ALERT MB [bioMérieux, Durham, NC]) remains the gold standard test for diagnosis of tuberculosis. A culture isolate of *M. tuberculosis* is still currently required for detailed DST and for genotyping to identify transmission events or outbreaks. Solid culture is less expensive than liquid culture and less prone to contamination by other bacteria or fungi, but liquid culture is faster, more sensitive (10% increased case detection), and convenient

(growth is detected automatically by monitoring fluorescence) (7).

Samples that are contaminated with normal flora (such as sputum) must first undergo decontamination (typically using NaOH together with NALC), which kills rapidly growing bacteria and fungi, but which has a limited effect on mycobacterial viability. Importantly, high concentrations or prolonged exposure of mycobacteria to NaOH will reduce recovery, and so there is a fine balance between overdecontamination (which reduces the yield of mycobacterial culture) and underdecontamination (which leads to failed cultures because of high rates of bacterial or fungal overgrowth).

Cross contamination occurs when *M. tuberculosis* from one sample or culture is carried over, during batch processing, to another sample. To minimize this risk, cultures should be manipulated in biosafety cabinets separate from those used for specimen processing, specimens with high bacterial load (smear-positive samples) should be processed before those with lower loads (smear-negative samples, samples from children), and single-aliquot reagents should be used.

There are several constraints to widespread implementation of mycobacterial culture, including the need for infrastructure and maintenance to support the appropriate level of biosafety, uninterrupted power supply, training, rapid transport of samples to the laboratory (maximum of 4 days if samples are refrigerated), and cost (7).

In order to take advantage of the more rapid turnaround of liquid culture, rapid identification of positive cultures should be used. Biochemical testing has largely been replaced by molecular or immunochromatographic lateral flow testing. High-throughput laboratories may be able to run frequent batches of line probe assays (see "Current diagnostics for Drug-Resistant TB," below), which confirm the identification as *M. tuberculosis* complex. Alternatively, lateral flow assays incorporating monoclonal antibodies against the *M. tuberculosis* protein MPB64 have been demonstrated to be highly sensitive and specific for *M. tuberculosis* complex, and are simple, rapid, and inexpensive (8).

In summary, the key WHO recommendations (7) on mycobacterial cultures are:

- Liquid culture is feasible for implementation in lower-income settings.
- Liquid culture has a higher rate of mycobacterial isolation and a shorter time to detection compared with solid culture.
- Rapid differentiation of *M. tuberculosis* from other acid-fast organisms recovered in culture is essential.

Xpert MTB/RIF

This cartridge-based molecular assay enables rapid detection of *M. tuberculosis* and simultaneous identification of rifampin resistance directly from clinical specimens, with minimal operator dependence. Sputum (or other suitable sample) is liquefied and inactivated using a fixed ratio of NaOH and isopropanol-containing sample reagent. The liquefied sample is then added to a cartridge where the sample is automatically filtered (to capture *M. tuberculosis* bacilli), sonicated (to release bacterial DNA), and hemi-nested real-time PCR is performed (9). The PCR targets an 81-bp region of the *rpoB* gene of *M. tuberculosis* where more than 95% of mutations associated with rifampin resistance occur. Five molecular probes are designed to bind to the wild-type (sensitive) gene of *M. tuberculosis*; binding is detected by fluorescent signals from each of these probes. Signal from at least two of these probes indicates the presence of *M. tuberculosis*, while delay in binding, or failure to bind, of at least one probe indicates rifampin resistance (9).

The limit of detection of the Xpert MTB/RIF assay in spiked sputum samples has been measured at 131 bacilli per ml of sputum (10). Pooled estimates of sensitivity and specificity of the assay for tuberculosis detection from studies of patients with presumed pulmonary tuberculosis are 89% and 99%, respectively (11). As with smear microscopy, sensitivity is lower in patients with HIV infection (79%) and in children (66%) (12). For extrapulmonary samples, sensitivity varies with sample type. Sensitivity is highest for lymph node biopsies/aspirates and cerebrospinal fluid but poor for pleural fluid (13, 14).

An important limitation of Xpert MTB/RIF is its inability to distinguish between live and dead bacilli. The assay may remain positive even after treatment completion and should not be used to monitor response to treatment (15). Constraints to widespread rollout include cost, need for continuous power supply, sensitivity to high temperatures, and assay throughput. A more sensitive assay, Xpert MTB/RIF Ultra, is currently under clinical evaluation, and is likely to be as sensitive as liquid culture. A more robust, point-of-care, portable, battery-operated GeneXpert platform is also being developed. This device, called GeneXpert Omni, will be available in 2017.

In summary, the key WHO recommendations (16) on Xpert MTB/RIF are:

- Xpert MTB/RIF should be used as the initial diagnostic test in adults or children suspected of having MDR-TB or HIV-associated TB.

- Xpert MTB/RIF may be used as the initial diagnostic test in all adults or children suspected of having TB (conditional recommendation acknowledging resource implications).
- Xpert MTB/RIF should be used as the initial diagnostic test for cerebrospinal fluid specimens from patients suspected of having TB meningitis.
- Xpert MTB/RIF may be used as a replacement test for usual practice for testing specific nonrespiratory specimens (lymph nodes and other tissues) from patients suspected of having extrapulmonary TB.

In January 2017, WHO convened a Technical Expert Consultation to assess the performance of the new Ultra assay compared with the Xpert MTB/RIF assay. The Technical Expert Group found that the Ultra assay is non-inferior to the Xpert MTB/RIF assay for the detection of *M. tuberculosis* and for the detection of rifampin resistance. The Ultra cartridge showed better performance for the detection of *M. tuberculosis* in smear-negative culture-positive specimens, pediatric specimens, and extrapulmonary specimens and in testing smear-negative culture-positive specimens from HIV-positive individuals.

The current WHO recommendations for the use of Xpert MTB/RIF now also apply to the use of Ultra as the initial diagnostic test for all adults and children with signs and symptoms of TB and in the testing of selected extrapulmonary specimens (CSF, lymph nodes, and tissue specimens) (70).

Loop-Mediated Amplification Test

Apart from Xpert MTB/RIF, several other NAATs for TB are at various stages of development. The TB-Loop-Mediated Amplification Test (LAMP) assay (Eiken Chemical Co., Japan) is based on an isothermal amplification protocol (using a simple heating block) and produces a result that can be seen with the naked eye. It therefore offers advantages in terms of cost and suitability for implementation in peripheral settings (17). However, recent data suggest that to achieve acceptable performance of LAMP at the microscopy center level, significant training and infrastructure requirements are necessary (17).

An earlier version of LAMP was reviewed by WHO in 2013 (18). The sensitivity of LAMP was found to be good for smear-positive samples (97%) and lower for smear-negative samples (53 to 62%). Specificity was suboptimal (95 to 97%); low specificity may be due to failure to follow the manufacturer's recommendations precisely. Low specificity may result in unacceptably low positive predictive value of a positive test in low

TB prevalence countries. An updated WHO policy on LAMP, based on an improved assay with new evidence, is expected in 2016.

Urine Lipoarabinomannan Rapid Test

An alternative to detection of whole *M. tuberculosis* bacilli or DNA is detection of structural or secreted *M. tuberculosis*-specific biomolecules in patient samples. Lipoarabinomannan (LAM) is a component of the cell wall of *M. tuberculosis* that may be found in urine of patients with TB. It is not clear whether circulating LAM is filtered by the glomeruli (this may be less likely because LAM typically circulates in an immune complex or associated with high-density lipoprotein carrier molecules) (19) or whether the presence of LAM in urine is due to (subclinical) urinary tract infection with *M. tuberculosis* (20). The initial enzyme-linked immunosorbent assay-based test for LAM has now been replaced with a lateral flow assay suitable for implementation at, or close to, the point of care.

Urine LAM testing lacks sensitivity for diagnosis of TB in HIV-uninfected patients, and should only be used for diagnosis of HIV-associated TB in patients with low CD4 counts (<100 cells/µl), or HIV-infected patients who are seriously ill. Even in this patient group, sensitivity is suboptimal (pooled sensitivity 56%) (21). Reported specificity of the test varies; however, this is likely due to differences between studies in the effort taken to establish a reference standard diagnosis. When extensive investigation is done for TB, and when band intensity of grade 2 on the test strip is used as a cut point for a positive result, it appears that specificity of the LAM test is high (22). The test is not able to distinguish between infection with *M. tuberculosis* and other mycobacterial species; however, the positive predictive value is likely to be high in countries endemic for TB. A positive test is therefore sufficient grounds to start treatment for TB in such countries; however, a negative test cannot be used to rule out TB. While the clinical applicability of this test may be limited, LAM testing and rapid initiation of TB treatment among HIV-infected inpatients suspected to have TB in high-burden countries may reduce early mortality (23).

In summary, the key WHO recommendations (21) on LAM are:

- LAM testing should only be used to assist in the diagnosis of TB in persons with HIV infection with low CD4 counts (<100 cells/µl) or HIV infected patients who are seriously ill.
- LAM testing should not be used as a screening test for TB.

CURRENT DIAGNOSTICS FOR DRUG-RESISTANT TB

Currently, DST is performed using either phenotypic methods or genotypic methods. Table 2 shows the technologies that have undergone WHO review in each category.

Phenotypic Tests for DST

Methods used for phenotypic DST include the absolute concentration, resistance ratio, or proportion methods. Testing on solid agar using the proportion method is still regarded as the reference standard method. This is performed by counting the number of *M. tuberculosis* colonies that grow on agar without antibiotics compared with agar in which a critical concentration of antibiotic has been incorporated; if the number of colonies on antibiotic-containing media is >1% of that on the antibiotic-free media, the isolate is regarded as resistant. The critical concentration is primarily derived by epidemiological cutoff, as the concentration of antibiotic that best discriminates between a population of wild-type bacteria (which have never been exposed to antibiotic) and resistant bacteria (which have persisted in the presence of treatment). While for some antibiotics there is an identifiable concentration that discriminates well between these groups, for some others (e.g., ethambutol) there is considerable overlap between wild-type and resistant organisms, and this limits the applicability of phenotypic DST for these drugs.

Commercial Liquid Culture-Based DST

Commercial automated liquid culture systems (e.g., MGIT, above) use a modification of the proportion method and offer reliable results for isoniazid and rifampin, as well as for fluoroquinolones, aminoglycosides, and polypeptides. Testing for resistance to other first-line (ethambutol and pyrazinamide) and second-

Table 2 Technologies reviewed by WHO for drug-susceptibility testing

Year	Method	Technology reviewed by WHO
2007	Phenotypic	Commercial liquid culture and DST
2008	Genotypic	Molecular LPAs for first-line anti-TB drug resistance detection
2010	Phenotypic	Selected noncommercial DST methods (MODS, CRI, NRA)
2010	Genotypic	Xpert MTB/RIF
2016	Genotypic	Molecular LPAs for second-line anti-TB drug resistance detection
2017	Genotypic	Xpert MTB/RIF Ultra

line drugs is less reliable and reproducible; automated liquid systems are recommended for testing (24).

A limitation of many current commercial systems is the inclusion of only one (or sometimes two) critical concentrations of each antibiotic. The result given is qualitative rather than a semiquantitative minimum inhibitory concentration (MIC). This may be of relevance; for example, recent data suggest that clinically relevant "low-level" resistance to rifampin is missed by testing only one concentration of rifampin (1 µg/ml) (25). An alternative approach is to perform detailed MIC testing for specific antibiotics, particularly in difficult-to-treat highly resistant cases, where individually tailored drug treatment may be required, for example, using the commercial Sensititre *M. tuberculosis* MIC Plate (ThermoFisher, Waltham, MA).

In summary, the key WHO recommendations (7, 24) on liquid culture-based DST are:

- As a minimum, national TB control programs should establish laboratory capacity to detect MDR-TB.
- Automated liquid systems and molecular line probe assays (see "Genotypic Tests for DST," below) for first-line DST are recommended as the current gold standard.
- DST for aminoglycosides, polypeptides, and fluoroquinolones has been shown to have relatively good reliability and reproducibility.

Noncommercial DST Methods

Several noncommercial methods have been developed as alternatives to the automated commercial systems for DST. These methods may be less expensive, but are generally less well standardized, are highly operator dependent, and may have local variation in methodology. They therefore need to be supported by strong quality assurance mechanisms, and should be performed only in reference, centralized laboratories (26). These methods include:

- Microscopic observation of drug susceptibility (MODS), which relies on microscopic observation of microcolonies of *M. tuberculosis* in liquid media (with and without antibiotics). Microtiter plates may be inoculated with sputum specimen (direct testing) or cultured isolates (indirect testing).
- Nitrate reductase assay (NRA), which is based on colorimetric change in solid agar caused by reduction of nitrate by *M. tuberculosis*, and is suitable for direct or indirect testing.
- Colorimetric redox indicator (CRI) methods, which are based on color change due to reduction of an

indicator dye that is added to liquid media containing viable *M. tuberculosis* that has been exposed to antibiotics (indirect testing only).

There is insufficient evidence to recommend other noncommercial methods, such as phage-based assays and thin-layer agar for use (26). In summary, key WHO recommendations (26) on noncommercial DST methods are:

- MODS, CRI, and NRA methods may be used under clearly defined program and operational conditions, in reference laboratories, and as an interim solution while capacity for genotypic or automated liquid culture is being developed.

Genotypic Tests for DST

The genetic basis for acquired drug resistance in *M. tuberculosis* is change (single-nucleotide polymorphisms, deletions, insertions) in the mycobacterial chromosome. Such changes may be detected by interrogating the relevant gene sequence, either directly by DNA sequencing, or indirectly, using probe-based methods or methods that rely on the effect of such mutations on the melting temperature of double-stranded DNA.

Line Probe Assays for Detection of Resistance to First-Line Anti-TB Drugs (Isoniazid and Rifampin)

Line probe assays (LPAs) (e.g., GenoType MTBDR*plus*, Hain Lifescience, Nehren, Germany; and NTM+MDRTB Detection Kit 2, Nipro Corporation, Japan) identify drug-resistance mutations by detecting the binding of PCR-amplified fragments of *M. tuberculosis* DNA to probes targeting the most common mutations conferring resistance to isoniazid and rifampin or to wild-type probes. Resistance is identified by detecting hybridization of DNA from the patient isolate to a mutant (resistant) probe and/or by detecting failure of hybridization to a wild-type (sensitive) probe. Mutations in the *inhA* promoter and *katG* regions (responsible for most isoniazid resistance) and the rifampin-resistance-determining region of the *rpoB* gene (responsible for most rifampin resistance) are targeted. Molecular testing using LPA is significantly more rapid than phenotypic DST, presents lower biosafety risk, and increases throughput.

In meta-analysis, the pooled sensitivity of Hain MTBDR*plus* was 98% (95% CI, 96 to 99%) for detection of resistance to rifampin but more variable for isoniazid (pooled sensitivity 84%; 95% CI, 77 to 90%). Specificity for both was excellent (99%) (27).

LPA testing may be done on cultured isolates or directly from smear-positive sputum samples. Limited data (28) suggest that LPA can also be done directly from smear-negative sputum samples (i.e., for both diagnosis of tuberculosis as well as resistance testing); however, there are insufficient data to recommend the use of LPA in this patient group. A significant limitation of LPA is that the test requires "open" manipulation of PCR amplicons, so the risk of cross contamination between samples is high. Meticulous attention to unidirectional workflow, well-trained staff, and a strong quality assurance program are required to reduce this risk.

In 2008, WHO endorsed the use of Version 1 of the GenoType MTBDR*plus* assay for rapid detection of isoniazid and rifampin resistance on smear-positive samples. In 2015, WHO published an update of the LPA policy where GenoType MTBDR*plus* Version 2 and the Nipro Corporation (Japan) NTM+MDRTB Detection Kit 2 were endorsed. Either tool can be used to detect TB and to genotype alleles that confer resistance to rifampin and isoniazid from either smear-positive sputum samples or from culture-derived isolates.

In summary, the key WHO recommendations (29) on molecular LPAs are:

- LPAs are validated for direct testing of sputum in smear-positive specimens and on isolates of *M. tuberculosis*. They are not recommended for use on smear-negative samples.
- Adoption of LPAs does not eliminate the need for conventional culture and DST capability (for diagnosis of patients with smear-negative TB and for further DST for patients with MDR-TB).
- Appropriate laboratory infrastructure and appropriately trained staff are necessary to ensure adequate precautions for biosafety and prevention of contamination.

Xpert MTB/RIF for Rifampin Resistance

The principle of the Xpert MTB/RIF assay for detection of rifampin resistance has been described in "Xpert MTB/RIF," see above. The pooled sensitivity for detection of resistance to rifampin in meta-analysis was 94% and specificity was 98% (11). The interpretation of these findings is somewhat complicated by different assay versions being tested in different studies; however, in countries with a low prevalence of rifampin resistance, the positive predictive value of Xpert MTB/RIF for rifampin resistance is likely to be relatively low. A rifampin-resistant Xpert MTB/RIF result should therefore be confirmed with a second (different) test.

Furthermore, the correlation between genotypic and phenotypic testing is sometimes complex (30). For example, as described above ("Commercial Liquid Culture-Based DST"), liquid culture-based phenotypic tests may miss low-level rifampin resistance, but these are usually detected by genotypic (Xpert MTB/RIF or LPA) testing (25). The reverse may also be true; Xpert MTB/RIF may miss some locally prevalent rifampin resistance-conferring mutations, which are detectable by phenotypic testing. Detailed understanding of the limitations of the various testing methods is required, as is knowledge of the local distribution of resistance-conferring mutations.

LPAs for detecting resistance to second-line anti-TB drugs

At present, the reference standard for DST for second-line TB drugs is phenotypic testing (liquid or agar proportion). However, in patients in whom a rapid diagnosis of rifampin-resistant TB has been made by molecular testing (Xpert MTB/RIF or LPA), there is often considerable delay before results of phenotypic tests are available. Uncertainty on the most appropriate treatment regimen may delay effective treatment and result in amplified resistance (acquisition of resistance to additional drugs). Rapid genotypic tests for resistance to second-line drugs may reduce this delay. Second-line LPA (MTBDR*sl*, Hain Lifescience) provides information on resistance to injectable drugs and fluoroquinolones. The current version of this assay includes *gyrA* and *gyrB* for detection of resistance to fluoroquinolones and *rrs* and *eis* for detection of resistance to injectable drugs. The previous version of this assay (which did not include *gyrB* nor *eis* but included *embB* for ethambutol resistance) was estimated to have a pooled sensitivity of 83% for detection of resistance to fluoroquinolones and 77% for injectable resistance (31) (this varied by specific drug, since there is incomplete cross-resistance among injectable drugs). Specificity for both was good (>98%). Therefore, this test is useful as a rule-in test for extensively drug-resistant (XDR) or pre-XDR tuberculosis, but, because of suboptimal sensitivity, it cannot be used to completely rule out resistance. Detailed understanding of the local distribution of drug-resistance mutations is required to interpret results of this assay in the local context. In 2016, WHO published an updated policy on second-line LPA (32).

In summary, the key WHO recommendations (32) on second-line molecular line probe assays are:

- For patients with confirmed rifampin-resistant TB or MDR-TB, SL-LPA may be used as the initial test, instead of phenotypic culture-based DST, to detect resistance to fluoroquinolones

• For patients with confirmed rifampin-resistant TB or MDR-TB, SL-LPA may be used as the initial test, instead of phenotypic culture-based DST, to detect resistance to the second-line injectable drugs

Unmet Needs and Gaps

A recently published study of various stakeholders helped establish the most important unmet needs, and helped identify tools that are of highest importance. Kik and colleagues conducted a priority-setting exercise to identify the highest-priority tests for target product profile (TPP) development and investment in research and development (33). For each of the potential TPPs, 10 criteria were used to set priorities, including prioritization by key stakeholders (e.g., National TB Program [NTP] managers), potential impact of the test on TB transmission, morbidity and mortality, market potential and implementation, and scalability of the test. Based on this analysis, the following were identified as the highest priorities (33):

1. A point-of-care sputum-based test as a replacement for smear microscopy;
2. A point-of-care, non-sputum-based test capable of detecting all forms of TB;
3. A point-of-care triage test, which should be a simple, low-cost test for use by first-contact health care providers as a rule-out test;
4. Rapid DST at microscopy center level.

The second and third tests are especially critical also for improved diagnosis in children, who make up an estimated 10% of the global TB burden (34), people living with HIV, and those who have extrapulmonary TB. In the longer term, TB elimination cannot be achieved without identifying those with latent infection who are at the highest risk of progressing to active TB disease. A new test for cure will also be needed to monitor TB treatment (35).

Given the variety of unmet needs and the diversity of sites where testing can occur, it is important for product developers to have access to: (i) a clearly identified list of diagnostics that are considered high priority by the TB community; (ii) well-developed, detailed TPPs for priority diagnostics, based on a consensus-building process; and (iii) up-to-date market size estimations for the priority TPPs.

In 2014, WHO published a consensus document with TPPs for priority diagnostics (36), with elaborations (37, 38). A series of new publications have summarized the served available market in select countries, and the data suggest a sizeable annual TB diagnostics market worth an estimated US$ 480 million in Brazil, China, India, and South Africa combined (39–42). Market projections for future TB diagnostics have also been made (43). These market analyses will, hopefully, encourage greater investments in new product development. All these resources are now available at www.tbfaqs.org.

Pipeline of Future Diagnostics

Figure 1 shows the pipeline of new TB diagnostics, classified by level of complexity and stage of development. At first glance, the pipeline appears well populated. Most products in the pipeline are molecular based, making use of the only proven TB bacterial nucleic acid sequences. Although these tests hold promise for smear replacement and expanded DST, they are unlikely to meet affordability and ease-of-use requirements for integration into primary care. To meet these needs, we need new biomarkers and approaches. Although investment and activity in biomarker research has increased, translation from basic biomarker discovery to clinical applications has been poor (35).

Biomarker discovery efforts focus on host and pathogen markers and we see promising leads in some of the biomarker classes shown in Fig. 2 (44–47). For example, improved detection of the lipoglycan biomarker lipoarabinomannan (LAM) could lead to a breakthrough in urine-based antigen detection (35). An area that gets a lot of attention is TB detection in breath to identify volatile organic compounds (VOCs) (48). Early indications suggest that prototypes fall short of required sensitivity and specificity, and lack independent evaluation. Serological tests detecting antibody responses such as lateral flow assays are appealing because of their simplicity, cost, and lack of specimen processing. However, existing serological assays have failed, and WHO has recommended against their use (49). Ongoing research might help overcome existing challenges. A lot of research is currently focused on host transcriptional markers, notably mRNA signatures to differentiate active from latent TB in both children and adults (44–47). Regardless of promise, none of these findings will yield a policy-endorsed product in the next 3 to 5 years.

In addition to rapid case detection, we need to identify new tools with expanded DST capabilities to help countries reach the post-2015 target of universal DST for all TB patients at the time of diagnosis. With the anticipated introduction of new TB drug regimens, we need to be able to test sensitivity to all critical regimen

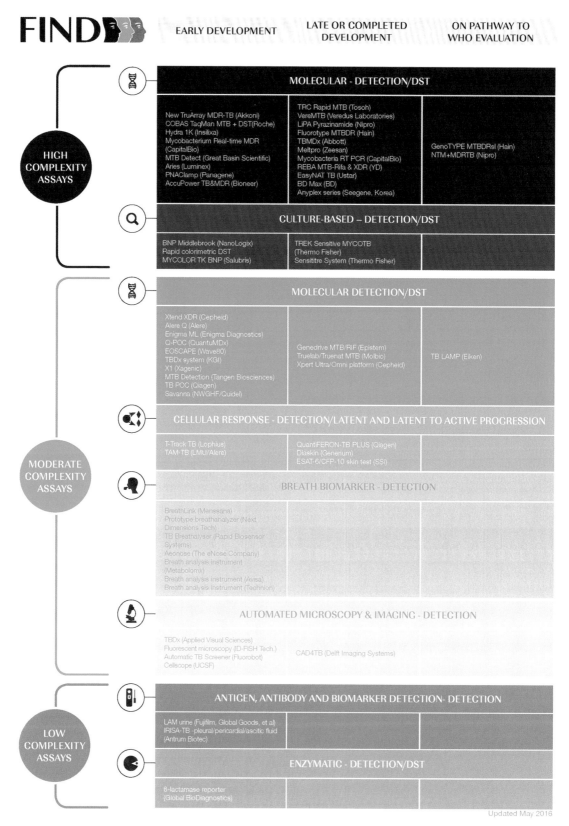

Figure 1 Pipeline of TB diagnostics (source: FIND, Geneva; www.finddx.org).

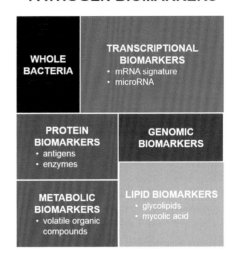

Figure 2 Classes of TB biomarkers under development and validation (source: FIND, Geneva; www.finddx.org).

components (50). Many of the molecular assays in the pipeline aim to expand the drug menu. However, since drug resistance in *M. tuberculosis* can occur as a result of mutations in many different regions of the genome, targeted molecular testing for detection of drug resistance will always be constrained by the need for highly multiplexed assays (51).

In this context, next-generation sequencing tools are showing great promise and may become the method of choice for detailed DST of resistant isolates in the next 5 to 10 years (52, 53). While not WHO endorsed or yet widely used, feasibility has been shown, and the advantages of this approach are the ability to screen broadly for mutations conferring resistance to a range of different anti-TB drugs as well as obtain genotype information useful for tracking transmission and outbreaks (54). However, the paucity of good data on the correlation of mutations with phenotypic DST results and clinical outcomes, and the association with cross-resistance are preventing translation into routine use for clinical decision making. Before sequencing can become more widely used in high-burden settings, there is much work to be done to further simplify and automate procedures and equipment to reduce the need for highly skilled staff, notably improvements in specimen processing and software-based data interpretation support. In addition, the price will have to come down, although cost is becoming competitive with detailed DST (52).

While the TB diagnostics research and development (R&D) space has managed to attract over 50 compa-

nies and product developers, they will require technical and funding support to overcome the translational challenges shown in Table 3 (adapted from reference 55). While many manufacturers remain interested in the development of biomarker-based point-of-care tests, they face significant challenges with identification and validation. Many of the gaps in prioritized diagnostics will not be filled by the current pipeline, which is heavily weighted toward molecular smear replacement and DST, but not true point-of-care tests, ideally non-sputum-based, or tests to determine disease progression or cure. Increased investments are necessary to support biomarker discovery, validation, and translation into clinical tools. Unfortunately, a recent analysis of the TB R&D funding landscape by the Treatment Action Group showed a big gap between the investment needed and actual expenditure on diagnostics R&D (56). Donors and governments must work together to commit sustained funds toward agreed priorities in TB R&D, and the Stop TB Partnership will need to devise creative strategies to advocate for these funds.

How To Maximize the Impact of New Diagnostics, Based on Lessons from Xpert MTB/RIF Rollout

New TB technologies should have a significant impact on patient outcomes. However, as shown in Fig. 3 (57), the technical performance of tests is essential but, on its own, not sufficient. Operational weaknesses and underfunded TB programs hamper effective diagnostic uptake

Table 3 Translational challenges for developing innovative TB technologies that can meet the needs

Indication for testing	Currently used tools	Limitations of existing tools	Desirable new tools	Translational challenges for new tool development
Triage test to identify individuals with presumed TB who need confirmatory testing	1. TB symptoms (e.g., 2 weeks of cough) 2. Chest X rays	1. Symptoms lack sensitivity and specificity, especially in HIV-infected populations and children. 2. Chest X rays are sensitive, but not specific for TB.	A simple, low-cost triage test for use by first-contact health care providers as a rule-out test, ideally suitable for use by community health workers	Lack of validated biomarkers
Diagnosis of active pulmonary TB	1. Sputum smear microscopy 2. Nucleic acid amplification tests (NAATs) 3. Cultures	1. Smear microscopy lacks sensitivity and cannot detect drug resistance. 2. NAATs are expensive and not easily deployable at the peripheral level. 3. Cultures are expensive and require biosafety level 3 (BSL3) laboratories, and results take time.	A sputum-based replacement test for smear microscopy A non-sputum-based biomarker test for all forms of TB, ideally suitable for use at levels below microscopy centers	While several NAATs are being developed for microscopy centers, they will need to be evaluated in field conditions for policy. For the nonsputum TB test, the biggest challenge is lack of validated biomarkers.
Diagnosis of extrapulmonary (EPTB) and childhood TB	1. Smear microscopy 2. Nucleic acid amplification tests 3. Cultures	1. Children and patients with EPTB often do not produce sputum. Invasive samples are usually necessary. Microscopy lacks sensitivity and cannot detect drug resistance. 2. NAATs are expensive and not easily deployable at the peripheral level. Sensitivity in EPTB samples is low. 3. Cultures are expensive and require BSL3 laboratories, and results take time.	A non-sputum-based biomarker test for all forms of TB, ideally suitable for use at levels below microscopy centers	For the nonsputum TB test, the biggest challenge is lack of validated biomarkers.
Drug susceptibility testing	1. Nucleic acid amplification tests 2. Cultures	1. Current NAATs cannot reliably detect all mutations and sensitivity for drugs other than rifampin is poor. 2. Cultures are expensive and require BSL3 laboratories, and results take time. Reliability of phenotypic is poor for second-line drugs.	A new molecular DST for use at a microscopy center level, which can evaluate for resistance to rifampin, fluoroquinolones, isoniazid, and pyrazinamide, and enable the selection of the best drug regimen	Lack of good data on the correlation of mutations with phenotypic results and clinical outcomes and the association with cross-resistance. There is also a need to align emerging TB drug regimens with companion diagnostics.
Diagnosis of latent TB infection (LTBI)	1. Tuberculin skin test (TST) 2. Interferon-gamma release assays (IGRA)	Neither TST nor IGRA can separate latent infection from active disease. Neither test can accurately identify those at highest risk of progression to active disease.	A test that can resolve the spectrum of TB, and identify the subset of latently infected individuals who are at highest risk of progressing to active disease and will benefit from preventive therapy	Lack of validated biomarkers
Test of cure (treatment monitoring)	1. Serial smear microscopy 2. Serial cultures	1. Smears lack sensitivity, and cannot distinguish between live and dead bacilli. 2. Serial cultures are expensive and time consuming.	An accurate test for cure that can be used to make changes in management (e.g., changes in regimens, or DST)	Lack of validated biomarkers

Adapted from Pai (55).

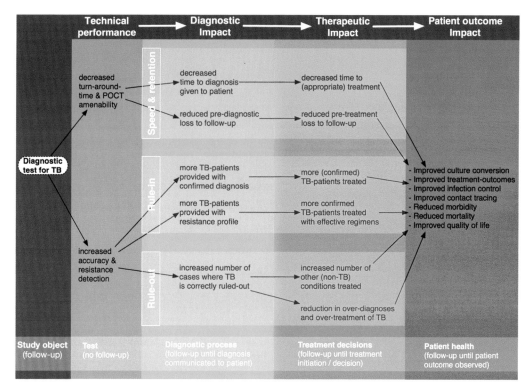

Figure 3 How TB tests can potentially impact patient outcomes (source: Schumacher et al. [57]).

in many countries with high TB burdens. New tests must be paired with actions that ensure rapid—and, where possible, same-day—test results that drive appropriate and prompt clinical and treatment decisions. Good technologies and interventions must be effectively implemented to enable their full potential health impact.

In a recent article, Albert and colleagues reviewed the development, rollout, and impact of Xpert MTB/RIF, and described the lessons learned and identified areas for improvement with new tools (58). The global rollout of Xpert MTB/RIF has changed the TB diagnostic landscape. More than 16 million tests have been performed in 122 countries since 2011, and 6 million were performed in 2015 alone. This remains a small proportion of all TB tests conducted compared with conventional smear microscopy (some 30 million per year in the 22 high-burden countries) (59), and only eight countries have made it the initial diagnostic test for all people suspected of having TB or are in the process of doing so. However, it has become an important method for the detection of drug-resistant TB, which has seen a tripling in the number of cases detected globally since its introduction (1). The rollout has galvanized stakeholders, from donors to civil society, and paved the way for universal DST. It has also attracted

new-product developers to tuberculosis, resulting in a robust molecular diagnostics pipeline.

However, as the first widely used near-patient molecular platform in global health, the rollout of Xpert has highlighted major implementation gaps that have constrained scale-up and limited Xpert's impact on the outcomes of patients with drug-susceptible TB, although significant impact on time to treatment and mortality related to drug-resistant TB has been shown. The rollout has been hampered by high costs for underfunded programs in high-burden countries and lack of a complete diagnostic package for TB (Fig. 4) that includes comprehensive training, quality assurance, implementation plans, service and maintenance support, and impact assessment (58, 60). Clinical impact has been blunted by weak health systems, resulting in prolonged time to diagnosis and treatment (61, 62). In India, an average TB patient is diagnosed after a delay of nearly 2 months and after seeing three providers (63), and even though South Africa has scaled up rapid molecular testing, there are data showing long delays between sample collection and initiation of TB treatment (64, 65). In many countries the private sector plays a dominant role in TB control, yet this sector has limited access to subsidized Xpert MTB/RIF pricing (60).

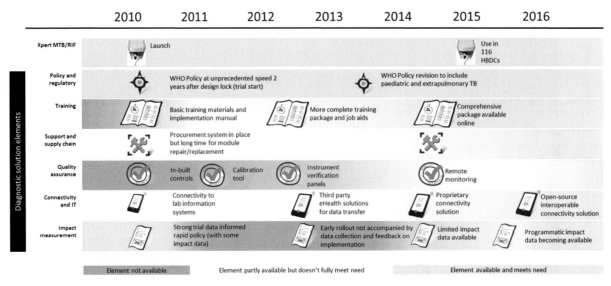

Figure 4 Timeline of availability of required elements for Xpert MTB/RIF implementation (from reference 58 with permission).

A recent report called "Out of Step" by Doctors without Borders and the Stop TB Partnership surveyed eight countries with high TB burdens to see how existing TB policies and interventions were being implemented (59). This survey also found major implementation gaps in the diagnosis and treatment of MDR-TB. For example, in five of six countries providing data on drug susceptibility testing, fewer than 40% of previously treated cases were tested for first-line DST and fewer than 15% were tested for second-line DST. In four of eight surveyed countries, fewer than 75% of MDR-TB cases detected were enrolled in treatment. At the primary care level, TB testing is rare, even for patients with classic TB symptoms, and most patients are managed with repeated cycles of empirical broad-spectrum antibiotic therapies (66, 67). This has shown that an increased focus on same-day return of test results and effective linkage to care of diagnosed patients is required to maximize the potential impact of any new diagnostic tool.

In addition, in many countries the private sector plays a dominant role in TB control. New data suggest that Xpert MTB/RIF is very highly priced in the private sector in high-burden countries, and access is quite limited (60). The Initiative for Promotion of Affordable, Quality TB tests (IPAQT) intervention in India, which is bringing preferential pricing for new TB diagnostic tools to the private sector, is a first step in expanding access to rapid diagnosis in the places where many patients seek care (60).

In light of these lessons learned, the authors advocate for a comprehensive approach to the implementation of diagnostics, including pricing strategies for the private sector, broader health systems strengthening in preparation for new technologies, including greater linkages across the TB and HIV care continuum, and systematic and high-quality data collection from all programs.

While we wait for next-generation technologies, national TB programs must scale up the current best diagnostics, and use implementation science to get the maximum impact (68). Using Xpert MTB/RIF as the example, programs could achieve greater impact if they used Xpert as the initial test among all patients with suspected TB, reduced empiric treatment, and fostered decentralized implementation, guided by operational modeling to maximize cost effectiveness. In particular, programs can maximize impact by implementing Xpert in areas where routine diagnostic capacity is limited and by increasing access to private and informal sector providers who often see patients first.

CONCLUSIONS

Although TB diagnosis in many countries still relies on sputum microscopy, new diagnostics are starting to change the landscape. Stimulated, in part, by the success and rollout of Xpert MTB/RIF, there is now considerable interest in new technologies, but R&D funding commitments now need to catch up to the interest expressed. The landscape looks promising with a pipeline of new tools, particularly molecular diagnostics, and well over 50 companies actively engaged in product development. However, new diagnostics are yet to reach scale, and there needs to be greater convergence between diagnostics development and the development of shorter TB drug regimens. Another concern is the relative absence of non-sputum-based diagnostics in the pipeline for children and of biomarker tests for triage, cure, and latent TB progression. Increased investments are necessary to support biomarker discovery, validation, and translation into clinical tools. In the meantime, high-burden countries will need to improve the efficiency of their health care delivery systems, ensure better uptake of new technologies, and achieve greater linkages across the TB and HIV care continuum. While we wait for next-generation technologies, national TB programs must scale up the current best diagnostics and use implementation science to get the maximum impact.

Acknowledgments. M.P. has no financial or industry disclosures. He serves as a consultant to the Bill & Melinda Gates Foundation. He also serves on the Scientific Advisory Committee of FIND, Geneva. M.P.N. has received funding from the Foundation for Innovative New Diagnostics (Geneva, Switzerland) to do studies to assess the performance and effect of MTB/RIF. C.C.B. is employed by FIND, Geneva. FIND is a nonprofit organization that collaborates with several industry partners on the development, assessment, and demonstration of new diagnostic tests.

Citation. Pai M, Nicol MP, Boehme CC. 2016. Tuberculosis diagnostics: state of the art and future directions. Microbiol Spectrum 4(5):TBTB2-0019-2016.

References

1. **World Health Organization.** 2015. *Global Tuberculosis Report 2015.* WHO, Geneva, Switzerland.

2. **World Health Organization.** *The End TB Strategy. Global strategy and targets for tuberculosis prevention, care and control after 2015.* WHO, Geneva, Switzerland.

3. **Pande T, Pai M, Khan FA, Denkinger CM.** 2015. Use of chest radiography in the 22 highest tuberculosis burden countries. *Eur Respir J* 46:1816–1819.

4. **Steingart KR, Henry M, Ng V, Hopewell PC, Ramsay A, Cunningham J, Urbanczik R, Perkins M, Aziz MA, Pai M.** 2006. Fluorescence versus conventional sputum smear microscopy for tuberculosis: a systematic review. *Lancet Infect Dis* 6:570–581.

5. **World Health Organization.** 2011. *Fluorescent light-emitting diode (LED) microscopy for diagnosis of tuberculosis: policy statement.* WHO, Geneva, Switzerland.

6. **Steingart KR, Ng V, Henry M, Hopewell PC, Ramsay A, Cunningham J, Urbanczik R, Perkins MD, Aziz MA, Pai M.** 2006. Sputum processing methods to improve the sensitivity of smear microscopy for tuberculosis: a systematic review. *Lancet Infect Dis* 6:664–674.

7. **World Health Organization.** *The use of liquid medium for culture and DST, 2007.* WHO, Geneva, Switzerland.

8. **Chikamatsu K, Aono A, Yamada H, Sugamoto T, Kato T, Kazumi Y, et al.** 2014. Comparative evaluation of three immunochromatographic identification tests for culture

9. **Lawn SD, Nicol MP.** 2011. Xpert MTB/RIF assay: development, evaluation and implementation of a new rapid molecular diagnostic for tuberculosis and rifampin resistance. *Future Microbiol* 6:1067–1082.

10. **Helb D, Jones M, Story E, Boehme C, Wallace E, Ho K, Kop J, Owens MR, Rodgers R, Banada P, Safi H, Blakemore R, Lan NT, Jones-López EC, Levi M, Burday M, Ayakaka I, Mugerwa RD, McMillan B, Winn-Deen E, Christel L, Dailey P, Perkins MD, Persing DH, Alland D.** 2010. Rapid detection of *Mycobacterium tuberculosis* and rifampin resistance by use of on-demand, near-patient technology. *J Clin Microbiol* 48:229–237.

11. **Steingart KR, Schiller I, Horne DJ, Pai M, Boehme CC, Dendukuri N.** 2014. Xpert MTB/RIF assay for pulmonary tuberculosis and rifampin resistance in adults. *Cochrane Database Syst Rev* (1):CD009593.

12. **Detjen AK, DiNardo AR, Leyden J, Steingart KR, Menzies D, Schiller I, Dendukuri N, Mandalakas AM.** 2015. Xpert MTB/RIF assay for the diagnosis of pulmonary tuberculosis in children: a systematic review and meta-analysis. *Lancet Respir Med* 3:451–461.

13. **Denkinger CM, Schumacher SG, Boehme CC, Dendukuri N, Pai M, Steingart KR.** 2014. Xpert MTB/RIF assay for the diagnosis of extrapulmonary tuberculosis: a systematic review and meta-analysis. *Eur Respir J* 44:435–446.

14. **Maynard-Smith L, Larke N, Peters JA, Lawn SD.** 2014. Diagnostic accuracy of the Xpert MTB/RIF assay for extrapulmonary and pulmonary tuberculosis when testing non-respiratory samples: a systematic review. *BMC Infect Dis* 14:709.

15. **Friedrich SO, Rachow A, Saathoff E, Singh K, Mangu CD, Dawson R, Phillips PP, Venter A, Bateson A, Boehme CC, Heinrich N, Hunt RD, Boeree MJ, Zumla A, McHugh TD, Gillespie SH, Diacon AH, Hoelscher M, Pan African Consortium for the Evaluation of Anti-tuberculosis Antibiotics (PanACEA).** 2013. Assessment of the sensitivity and specificity of Xpert MTB/RIF assay as an early sputum biomarker of response to tuberculosis treatment. *Lancet Respir Med* 1:462–470.

16. **World Health Organization.** 2013. *Automated real-time nucleic acid amplification technology for rapid and simultaneous detection of tuberculosis and rifampin resistance: Xpert MTB/RIF system for the diagnosis of pulmonary and extrapulmonary TB in adults and children. Policy update.* WHO, Geneva, Switzerland.

17. **Gray CM, Katamba A, Narang P, Giraldo J, Zamudio C, Joloba M, Narang R, Paramasivan CN, Hillemann D, Nabeta P, Amisano D, Alland D, Cobelens F, Boehme CC.** 2016. Feasibility and operational performance of tuberculosis detection by loop-mediated isothermal amplification platform in decentralized settings: results from a multicenter study. *J Clin Microbiol* 54:1984–1991.

18. **World Health Organization.** 2013. *The use of a commercial loop-mediated isothermal amplification assay (TB-LAMP) for the detection of tuberculosis. Expert Group Meeting Report.* WHO, Geneva, Switzerland.

19. **Sakamuri RM, Price DN, Lee M, Cho SN, Barry CE 3rd, Via LE, et al.** 2013. Association of lipoarabino-

mannan with high density lipoprotein in blood: implications for diagnostics. *Tuberculosis (Edinb)* **93**:301–307.

20. **Lawn SD, Gupta-Wright A.** 2016. Detection of lipo-arabinomannan (LAM) in urine is indicative of disseminated TB with renal involvement in patients living with HIV and advanced immunodeficiency: evidence and implications. *Trans R Soc Trop Med Hyg* **110**:180–185.

21. **World Health Organization.** 2015. *The Use of Lateral Flow Urine Lipoarabinomannan Assay (LF-LAM) for the Diagnosis and Screening of Active Tuberculosis in People Living with HIV. Policy Update.* WHO, Geneva, Switzerland.

22. **Lawn SD.** 2012. Point-of-care detection of lipoarabinomannan (LAM) in urine for diagnosis of HIV-associated tuberculosis: a state of the art review. *BMC Infect Dis* **12**:103.

23. **Peter JG, Zijenah LS, Chanda D, Clowes P, Lesosky M, Gina P, Mehta N, Calligaro G, Lombard CJ, Kadzirange G, Bandason T, Chansa A, Liusha N, Mangu C, Mtafya B, Msila H, Rachow A, Hoelscher M, Mwaba P, Theron G, Dheda K.** 2016. Effect on mortality of point-of-care, urine-based lipoarabinomannan testing to guide tuberculosis treatment initiation in HIV-positive hospital inpatients: a pragmatic, parallel-group, multicountry, open-label, randomised controlled trial. *Lancet* **387**: 1187–1197.

24. **World Health Organization.** 2014. *TB Diagnostics and Laboratory Services. Information Note.*

25. **Rigouts L, Gumusboga M, de Rijk WB, Nduwamahoro E, Uwizeye C, de Jong B, et al.** 2013. Rifampin resistance missed in automated liquid culture system for *Mycobacterium tuberculosis* isolates with specific rpoB mutations. *J Clin Microbiol* **51**:2641–2645.

26. **World Health Organization.** 2011. *Noncommercial culture and drug-susceptibility testing methods for screening of patients at risk of multidrug-resistant tuberculosis. Policy statement.* WHO, Geneva, Switzerland.

27. **Ling DI, Zwerling AA, Pai M.** 2008. GenoType MTBDR assays for the diagnosis of multidrug-resistant tuberculosis: a meta-analysis. *Eur Respir J* **32**:1165–1174.

28. **Barnard M, Gey van Pittius NC, van Helden PD, Bosman M, Coetzee G, Warren RM.** 2012. The diagnostic performance of the GenoType MTBDRplus version 2 line probe assay is equivalent to that of the Xpert MTB/RIF assay. *J Clin Microbiol* **50**:3712–3716.

29. **World Health Organization.** 2008. *Molecular line probe assays for rapid screening of patients at risk of multidrug-resistant tuberculosis (MDR-TB). Policy statement.* WHO, Geneva, Switzerland.

30. **Mokaddas E, Ahmad S, Eldeen HS, Al-Mutairi N.** 2015. Discordance between Xpert MTB/RIF assay and Bactec MGIT 960 Culture System for detection of rifampin-resistant Mycobacterium tuberculosis isolates in a country with a low tuberculosis (TB) incidence. *J Clin Microbiol* **53**:1351–1354.

31. **Theron G, Peter J, Richardson M, Barnard M, Donegan S, Warren R, et al.** 2014. The diagnostic accuracy of the GenoType((R)) MTBDRsl assay for the detection of resistance to second-line anti-tuberculosis drugs. *Cochrane Database Syst Rev* **10**:CD010705.

32. **World Health Organization.** 2016. *The use of molecular line probe assays for the detection of resistance to second-line anti-tuberculosis drugs. Policy guidance.* WHO, Geneva, Switzerland.

33. **Kik SV, Denkinger CM, Casenghi M, Vadnais C, Pai M.** 2014. Tuberculosis diagnostics: which target product profiles should be prioritised? *Eur Respir J* **44**: 537–540.

34. **Swaminathan S, Rekha B.** 2010. Pediatric tuberculosis: global overview and challenges. *Clin Infect Dis* **50** (Suppl 3):S184–S194.

35. **Gardiner JL, Karp CL.** 2015. Transformative tools for tackling tuberculosis. *J Exp Med* **212**:1759–1769.

36. **World Health Organization.** 2014. *High-priority target product profiles for new tuberculosis diagnostics: report of a consensus meeting. Meeting report.* WHO, Geneva, Switzerland.

37. **Denkinger CM, Dolinger D, Schito M, Wells W, Cobelens F, Pai M, Zignol M, Cirillo DM, Alland D, Casenghi M, Gallarda J, Boehme CC, Perkins MD.** 2015. Target product profile of a molecular drug-susceptibility test for use in microscopy centers. *J Infect Dis* **211**(S2): S39–S49.

38. **Denkinger CM, Kik SV, Cirillo DM, Casenghi M, Shinnick T, Weyer K, Gilpin C, Boehme CC, Schito M, Kimerling M, Pai M.** 2015. Defining the needs for next generation assays for tuberculosis. *J Infect Dis* **211** (Suppl 2):S29–S38.

39. **TB Diagnostics Market Analysis Consortium.** 2014. Market assessment of tuberculosis diagnostics in Brazil in 2012. *PLoS One* **9**:e104105. (Erratum, **9**: e107651.)

40. **TB Diagnostics Market Analysis Consortium.** 2015. Market assessment of tuberculosis diagnostics in South Africa, 2012–2013. *Int J Tuberc Lung Dis* **19**:216–222.

41. **Maheshwari P, Chauhan K, Kadam R, Pujani A, Kaur M, Chitalia M, Dabas H, Perkins MD, Boehme CC, Denkinger CM, Raizada N, Ginnard J, Jefferson C, Pantoja A, Rupert S, Kik SV, Cohen C, Chedore P, Satyanarayana S, Pai M, TB Diagnostics Market Analysis Consortium.** 2016. Market assessment of tuberculosis diagnostics in India in 2013. *Int J Tuberc Lung Dis* **20**: 304–313.

42. **Zhao YL, Pang Y, Xia H, Du X, Chin D, Huan ST, Dong HY, Zhang ZY, Ginnard J, Perkins MD, Boehme CC, Jefferson C, Pantoja A, Qin ZZ, Chedore P, Denkinger CM, Pai M, Kik SV, TB Diagnostics Market Analysis Consortium.** 2016. Market assessment of tuberculosis diagnostics in China in 2012. *Int J Tuberc Lung Dis* **20**:295–303.

43. **Kik SV, Denkinger CM, Jefferson C, Ginnard J, Pai M.** 2015. Potential market for novel tuberculosis diagnostics: worth the investment? *J Infect Dis* **211**(Suppl 2): S58–S66.

44. **Berry MP, Graham CM, McNab FW, Xu Z, Bloch SA, Oni T, et al.** 2010. An interferon-inducible neutrophil-driven blood transcriptional signature in human tuberculosis. *Nature* **466**:973–977.

45. **Zak DE, Penn-Nicholson A, Scriba TJ, Thompson E, Suliman S, Amon LM, Mahomed H, Erasmus M,**

Whatney W, Hussey GD, Abrahams D, Kafaar F, Hawkridge T, Verver S, Hughes EJ, Ota M, Sutherland J, Howe R, Dockrell HM, Boom WH, Thiel B, Ottenhoff TH, Mayanja-Kizza H, Crampin AC, Downing K, Hatherill M, Valvo J, Shankar S, Parida SK, Kaufmann SH, Walzl G, Aderem A, Hanekom WA, ACS and GC6-74 cohort study groups. 2016. A blood RNA signature for tuberculosis disease risk: a prospective cohort study. *Lancet* 387:2312–2322.

46. Sweeney TE, Braviak L, Tato CM, Khatri P. 2016. Genome-wide expression for diagnosis of pulmonary tuberculosis: a multicohort analysis. *Lancet Respir Med* 4: 213–224.

47. Anderson ST, Kaforou M, Brent AJ, Wright VJ, Banwell CM, Chagaluka G, Crampin AC, Dockrell HM, French N, Hamilton MS, Hibberd ML, Kern F, Langford PR, Ling L, Mlotha R, Ottenhoff TH, Pienaar S, Pillay V, Scott JA, Twahir H, Wilkinson RJ, Coin LJ, Heyderman RS, Levin M, Eley B, ILULU Consortium, KIDS TB Study Group. 2014. Diagnosis of childhood tuberculosis and host RNA expression in Africa. *N Engl J Med* 370: 1712–1723.

48. Phillips M, Basa-Dalay V, Blais J, Bothamley G, Chaturvedi A, Modi KD, Pandya M, Natividad MP, Patel U, Ramraje NN, Schmitt P, Udwadia ZF. 2012. Point-of-care breath test for biomarkers of active pulmonary tuberculosis. *Tuberculosis (Edinb)* 92:314–320.

49. World Health Organization. 2011. *Commercial serodiagnostic tests for diagnosis of tuberculosis. Policy statement.* WHO, Geneva, Switzerland.

50. Wells WA, Boehme CC, Cobelens FG, Daniels C, Dowdy D, Gardiner E, Gheuens J, Kim P, Kimerling ME, Kreiswirth B, Lienhardt C, Mdluli K, Pai M, Perkins MD, Peter T, Zignol M, Zumla A, Schito M. 2013. Alignment of new tuberculosis drug regimens and drug susceptibility testing: a framework for action. *Lancet Infect Dis* 13:449–458.

51. Salamon H, Yamaguchi KD, Cirillo DM, Miotto P, Schito M, Posey J, Starks AM, Niemann S, Alland D, Hanna D, Aviles E, Perkins MD, Dolinger DL. 2015. Integration of published information into a resistance-associated mutation database for *Mycobacterium tuberculosis. J Infect Dis* 211(Suppl 2):S50–S57.

52. Pankhurst LJ, Del Ojo Elias C, Votintseva AA, Walker TM, Cole K, Davies J, et al. 2016. Rapid, comprehensive, and affordable mycobacterial diagnosis with whole-genome sequencing: a prospective study. *Lancet Respir Med* 4:49–58.

53. Walker TM, Kohl TA, Omar SV, Hedge J, Del Ojo Elias C, Bradley P, et al. 2015. Whole-genome sequencing for prediction of *Mycobacterium tuberculosis* drug susceptibility and resistance: a retrospective cohort study. *Lancet Infect Dis* 15:1193–1202.

54. Domínguez J, Boettger EC, Cirillo D, Cobelens F, Eisenach KD, Gagneux S, Hillemann D, Horsburgh R, Molina-Moya B, Niemann S, Tortoli E, Whitelaw A, Lange C, TBNET, RESIST-TB networks. 2016. Clinical implications of molecular drug resistance testing for *Mycobacterium tuberculosis*: a TBNET/RESIST-TB consensus statement. *Int J Tuberc Lung Dis* 20:24–42.

55. Pai M. 2015. Innovations in tuberculosis diagnostics: progress and translational challenges. *EBioMedicine* 2: 182–183.

56. Treatment Action Group & Stop TB Partnership. 2015. *2015 Report on Tuberculosis Research Funding: 2005–2014.* Treatment Action Group, New York, NY.

57. Schumacher SG, Sohn H, Qin ZZ, Gore G, Davis JL, Denkinger CM, et al. 2016. Impact of molecular diagnostics for tuberculosis on patient-important outcomes: a systematic review of study methodologies. *PLoS One* 11: e0151073.

58. Albert H, Nathavitharana R, Isaacs C, Pai M, Denkinger C, Boehme C. 2016. Development, roll-out, and impact of Xpert MTB/RIF for tuberculosis: what lessons have we learnt, and how can we do better? *Eur Respir J* 48: 516–525.

59. Medicins Sans Frontieres and Stop TB Partnership. *Out of Step 2015 – TB policies in 24 countries.* http://www. stoptb.org/assets/documents/news/report_out_of_step_2015_11_pdf_with_interactive_links.pdf. Accessed 3 August 2016.

60. Puri L, Oghor C, Denkinger CM, Pai M. 2016. Xpert MTB/RIF for tuberculosis testing: access and price in highly privatised health markets. *Lancet Glob Health* 4: e94–e95.

61. Theron G, Zijenah L, Chanda D, Clowes P, Rachow A, Lesosky M, Bara W, Mungofa S, Pai M, Hoelscher M, Dowdy D, Pym A, Mwaba P, Mason P, Peter J, Dheda K, TB-NEAT team. 2014. Feasibility, accuracy, and clinical effect of point-of-care Xpert MTB/RIF testing for tuberculosis in primary-care settings in Africa: a multicentre, randomised, controlled trial. *Lancet* 383: 424–435.

62. Churchyard GJ, Stevens WS, Mametja LD, McCarthy KM, Chihota V, Nicol MP, Erasmus LK, Ndjeka NO, Mvusi L, Vassall A, Sinanovic E, Cox HS, Dye C, Grant AD, Fielding KL. 2015. Xpert MTB/RIF versus sputum microscopy as the initial diagnostic test for tuberculosis: a cluster-randomised trial embedded in South African roll-out of Xpert MTB/RIF. *Lancet Glob Health* 3:e450– e457.

63. Sreeramareddy CT, Qin ZZ, Satyanarayana S, Subbaraman R, Pai M. 2014. Delays in diagnosis and treatment of pulmonary tuberculosis in India: a systematic review. *Int J Tuberc Lung Dis* 18:255–266.

64. Jacobson KR, et al. 2012. Implementation of Geno-Type MTBDR*plus* reduces time to multidrug-resistant tuberculosis therapy initiation in South Africa. *Clin Infect Dis* 56:503–508.

65. Naidoo P, du Toit E, Dunbar R, Lombard C, Caldwell J, Detjen A, et al. 2014. A comparison of multidrug-resistant tuberculosis treatment commencement times in MDRTBPlus line probe assay and Xpert(R) MTB/RIF-based algorithms in a routine operational setting in Cape Town. *PLoS One* 9:e103328.

66. Das J, Kwan A, Daniels B, Satyanarayana S, Subbaraman R, Bergkvist S, Das RK, Das V, Pai M. 2015. Use of standardised patients to assess quality of tuberculosis care: a pilot, cross-sectional study. *Lancet Infect Dis* 15:1305– 1313.

67. **McDowell A, Pai M.** 2016. Treatment as diagnosis and diagnosis as treatment: empirical management of presumptive tuberculosis in India. *Int J Tuberc Lung Dis* **20:** 536–543.

68. **Pai M, Temesgen Z.** 2 March 2016. Mind the gap: time to address implementation gaps in tuberculosis diagnosis and treatment. *J Clin Tuberc Other Mycobact Dis.*

69. **Pai M, Behr M.** 2016. Latent *Mycobacterium tuberculosis* infection and interferon-gamma release assays. *Microbiol Spectrum* **4**(5):TBTB2-0023-2016.

70. **World Health Organization.** 2017. *WHO Meeting Report of a Technical Expert Consultation: Non-inferiority analysis of Xpert MTB/RIF Ultra compared to Xpert MTB/RIF.* WHO, Geneva, Switzerland.

Tuberculosis and the Tubercle Bacillus, 2nd ed.
Edited by William R. Jacobs, Jr., Helen McShane, Valerie Mizrahi, and Ian M. Orme
© 2018 American Society for Microbiology, Washington, DC
doi:10.1128/microbiolspec.TBTB2-0023-2016

Latent *Mycobacterium tuberculosis* Infection and Interferon-Gamma Release Assays

17

Madhukar Pai and Marcel Behr

INTRODUCTION

Diagnosis and treatment of latent tuberculosis infection (LTBI) is one of the interventions recommended by the World Health Organization (WHO) to end the TB epidemic worldwide and is one of the elements of the post-2015 End TB Strategy (1). While several high-income countries, notably the United States and Canada, have implemented and scaled up programs to detect and treat LTBI, developing countries have mostly focused on active TB disease control, a much bigger priority in these settings.

In high-income countries, guidelines from agencies such as the U.S. Centers for Disease Control and Prevention (CDC) (2), Canadian Tuberculosis Standards (3), and the United Kingdom's National Institute for Health and Care Excellence (4) provide recommendations on LTBI management. For high-TB-burden countries, the WHO guidelines for the programmatic management of LTBI provide a blueprint for implementing targeted LTBI diagnosis and treatment, specifically in key affected populations such as people living with HIV/AIDS, adult and child contacts of pulmonary TB cases, patients initiating anti-tumor necrosis factor therapy, patients with end-stage renal failure, patients preparing for organ or hematologic transplantation, and patients with silicosis (5, 6). These populations are at high risk of TB exposure or at high risk of progressing from latency to active TB disease. With preventive therapy, it is possible to prevent the future occurrence of active TB disease (7), and a variety of drug regimens are WHO-endorsed for LTBI (6).

THE SPECTRUM OF *MYCOBACTERIUM TUBERCULOSIS* INFECTION

In a majority of individuals who inhale *M. tuberculosis* bacilli, the infection is eliminated by innate immune responses or subsequently contained by poorly understood host defenses, and infection remains latent. Basic research suggests there is a continuum from exposure to infection, and infection to disease, and individuals in each of these classes can transition, either advance or reverse positions, depending on modulators of host immunity (8, 9). Figure 1, from Esmail, Barry, and Wilkinson, provides a helpful illustration of this proposed spectrum of TB (9). However, for clinical and public health decisions, TB is simplistically and pragmatically separated into three groups: (i) those with no evidence of infection, (ii) those with LTBI, and (iii) those with TB disease. In some populations, especially children, these simplistic classifications may be inadequate and misleading (10).

Although latency and active (i.e., symptomatic, infectious) TB disease are likely part of the same dynamic spectrum (8, 9, 11), people with LTBI are typically considered to be asymptomatic and not infectious to others. However, people classified as having LTBI may harbor viable *M. tuberculosis* bacilli that can reactivate later, causing active TB disease. Studies suggest that 5 to 15% of individuals recently infected with *M. tuberculosis* progress rapidly (within 2 years) to active disease (12), whereas the remainder are considered to have LTBI and retain a persistent risk of reactivation (13). Identification and treatment of people with LTBI

McGill International TB Center and Department of Epidemiology and Biostatistics, McGill University, Montreal, Canada.

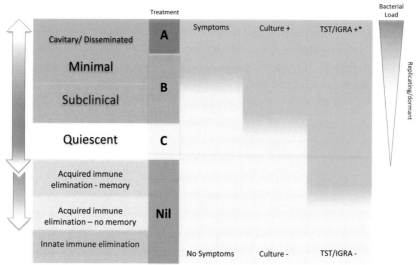

Figure 1 A proposed framework for considering tuberculosis (TB) infection as a spectrum. In this model, from Esmail, Barry, and Wilkinson, after initial exposure, TB bacteria can be eliminated by innate immune mechanisms. Once infection is established and an acquired, adaptive immune response has been generated, interferon-gamma release assay (IGRA) or tuberculin skin test (TST) might become positive. Infection can be eliminated by the acquired immune response, but if antigen-specific effector T-cell memory persists, TST or IGRA might remain positive, even though infection is cleared. Over time, T-cell memory responses can wane, resulting in TST or IGRA reversions. If *M. tuberculosis* is controlled but not eliminated by the acquired immune response, the individual might enter a state of quiescent infection, in which both symptoms and culturable bacilli are absent and with a greater proportion of bacilli in a dormant rather than replicative state. Immunosuppression (e.g., HIV or drugs such as tumor necrosis factor blockers) during this state might lead to rapid progression to active disease. If bacilli are grown on culture and symptoms and signs are absent, this might be a subclinical state. If bacilli are grown on culture and symptoms appear, then this reflects active TB disease (which can range from smear-negative TB to advanced cavitary/miliary TB). (Reproduced from reference 9 with permission.)

can help us understand the pathogenesis of disease, support ongoing efforts to develop new TB vaccines, and reduce the risk of development of disease via preventive therapy (also called chemoprophylaxis) (7, 14, 15).

TESTING METHODS FOR LTBI

The primary purpose of LTBI screening is to identify people who have evidence of *M. tuberculosis* infection and are at increased risk for the development of active TB. A key guiding principle is that only those who would benefit from treatment should be tested. This translates to the well-known dictum, "a decision to test should presuppose a decision to treat if the test is positive" (16).

In general, testing for LTBI is indicated when the risk of development of disease from latent infection (if present) is increased; examples include likely recent infection (e.g., close contact with a TB patient) or decreased capacity to contain latent infection (e.g., because of immunosuppression). In contrast, screening

for LTBI in people who are healthy and have a low risk of progressing to active disease is considered inappropriate, since the positive predictive value of LTBI testing for development of clinical disease is low and the risks of LTBI treatment (e.g., serious hepatotoxicity) can outweigh any potential benefits (7).

With regard to acceptable modalities of LTBI diagnosis, the WHO guidelines recommend that either a tuberculin skin test (TST) or an interferon-gamma release assay (IGRA) be used to detect LTBI in high-income and upper middle-income countries with estimated TB incidences less than 100 per 100,000 population (6). TST is preferred and IGRA should not replace TST in low- and middle-income countries whose TB incidence is ≥100 per 100,000 population (5, 6). This is primarily because IGRAs are more expensive to implement in such settings and do not add much more value compared to TST. In high-income countries, IGRAs are now quite widely used, although they have yet to replace TST entirely.

PURIFIED PROTEIN DERIVATIVE (PPD)-BASED TST

In many settings, the century-old TST, using PPD as the antigen, continues to be the frontline test for LTBI and, thus, the main driver of the LTBI preventive therapy. The TST is usually performed using the Mantoux method (17, 18) (Fig. 2). This consists of the intradermal injection of 5 tuberculin units (5 TU) of PPD-S or 2 TU of PPD RT23 (16). In a person with intact cellular immunity to these antigens, a delayed-type hypersensitivity reaction will occur within 48 to 72 hours. This delayed-type hypersensitivity reaction will cause erythema (redness) and induration of the skin at the injection site. Only the transverse induration is measured (as millimeters of induration) and interpreted using risk-stratified cut-offs (14, 18). PPD administration and reading require training and skill. It is important to note that cellular immunity to PPD antigens can sometimes reflect exposure to similar antigens from environmental, nontuberculous mycobacteria or bacillus Calmette-Guérin (BCG) vaccination or to a previous infection that has been cleared (through immunological mechanisms or treatment) (19).

Interpretation of a TST result is not simple and involves much more than just the size of the induration. A TST result should be interpreted with the probability of prior infection in mind and the likely risk of disease if the person were truly infected (i.e., predictive value) (20). Menzies and coworkers have developed a user-friendly, online, interactive calculator—the Online TST/IGRA Interpreter (Version 3.0, www.tstin3d.com)—that incorporates all these dimensions (20). This risk calculator computes the probability of active TB development, given a TST or IGRA result, and accounts for other risk factors (e.g., history of contact or HIV), as well as BCG vaccination. The calculator also computes the risk of serious adverse events (e.g., hepatotoxicity) due to LTBI treatment.

While the TST has several advantages in low-resource settings, including low reagent cost, no hardware costs, limited skill requirement, and no requirement for laboratories, it does suffer from two big limitations: specificity of PPD-based TST is compromised by late (i.e., after the first year of life) or repeated BCG vaccination (i.e., boosters) and, to a limited extent, by exposure to nontuberculous mycobacteria (19). The BCG World Atlas is available (www.bcgatlas.org) to provide information on when and how many times countries give BCG (21). The second limitation is the limited predictive value for TB disease (15). In other words, a majority of individuals with positive TST results do not progress to active TB disease, so overtreatment is inevitable, since there is no way to know which individual with a positive TST result will actually benefit from LTBI therapy. The TST is also known to have limitations in reproducibility, and challenges such as interreader variability, boosting, conversions, and reversions are well documented (22). TST also has operational drawbacks, including the need for the patient to return for the reading.

IGRAs

IGRAs are *ex vivo* blood tests of T-cell immune response; they measure T-cell release of interferon-gamma

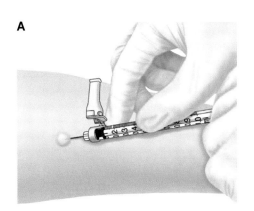
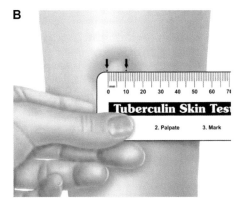

Figure 2 How to (**A**) administer and (**B**) read the tuberculin skin test (TST). TST involves an intradermal injection of 5 tuberculin units (5-TU) of PPD-S (purified protein derivative) or 2 TU of PPD RT23. A delayed-type hypersensitivity reaction might occur within 48 to 72 hours. This reaction will cause erythema (redness) and induration of the skin at the injection site. Only the transverse induration is measured as shown above and interpreted using risk-stratified cut-offs. (Adapted from reference 18.)

(IFN-gamma), an inflammatory cytokine, following stimulation by antigens specific to the *M. tuberculosis* complex (with the exception of BCG vaccines and several exotic species, such as *Mycobacterium microti* and the Dassie bacillus). These antigens include early secreted antigenic target 6 (ESAT-6) and culture filtrate protein 10 (CFP-10), both encoded by genes located within the region of difference 1 locus of the *M. tuberculosis* genome (23, 24). They are considered more specific for *M. tuberculosis* than PPD because they are not produced by BCG vaccine strains, and only a few species of nontuberculous mycobacteria have been shown to produce these antigens (*Mycobacterium marinum*, *Mycobacterium kansasii*, *Mycobacterium szulgai*, and *Mycobacterium flavescens* [25]). There is some evidence of cross-reactivity between ESAT-6 and CFP-10 of *M. tuberculosis* and *Mycobacterium leprae* (26, 27), but the clinical significance of this in leprosy and TB-endemic countries (e.g., India and Brazil) is poorly understood and researched.

Two commercial IGRAs are available in many countries: the QuantiFERON-TB (QFT) Gold In-Tube assay (Qiagen, Valencia, CA) and the T-SPOT.TB assay (Oxford Immunotec, Abingdon, United Kingdom). Both tests are approved by the U.S. Food and Drug Administration (FDA), Health Canada, and Conformité Européenne marked for use in Europe. Figure 3 provides an overview of the immunological basis of commercial IGRAs (28).

The QuantiFERON technology has been through several iterations, with the first version using PPD as the stimulating antigen. The current QFT-Gold In-Tube assay is an enzyme-linked immunosorbent assay-based, whole-blood test that uses peptides from ESAT-6 and CFP-10 as well as peptides from TB7.7 [Rv2654c] (not a region of difference 1 antigen) in an in-tube format in which peptides are coated to the inner surface of the tubes into which venous whole blood is drawn. After incubation, an enzyme-linked immunosorbent assay is conducted to quantify the amount of IFN-gamma in international units per milliliter produced in the antigen

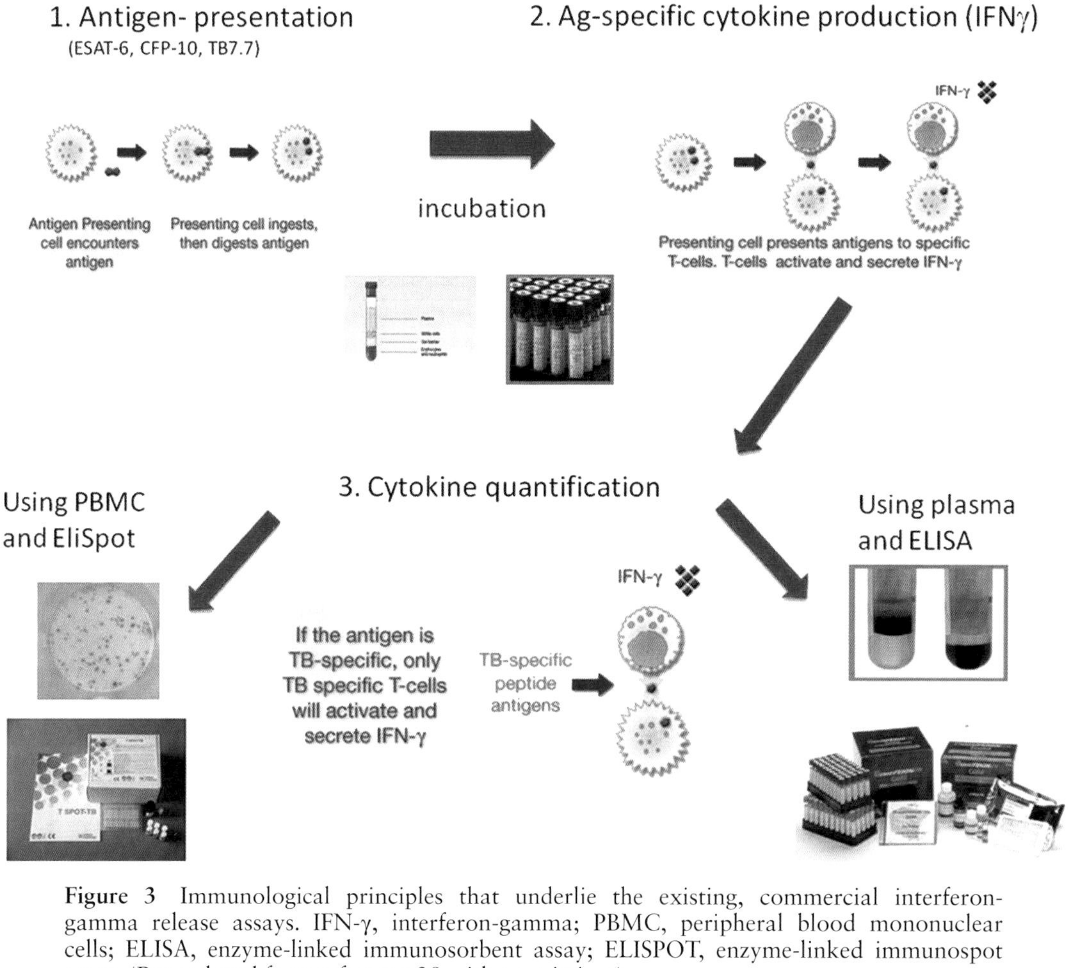

1. Antigen- presentation
(ESAT-6, CFP-10, TB7.7)

2. Ag-specific cytokine production (IFNγ)

Antigen Presenting cell encounters antigen   Presenting cell ingests, then digests antigen

incubation

Presenting cell presents antigens to specific T-cells. T-cells activate and secrete IFN-γ

Using PBMC and EliSpot

3. Cytokine quantification

Using plasma and ELISA

If the antigen is TB-specific, only TB specific T-cells will activate and secrete IFN-γ

TB-specific peptide antigens

Figure 3 Immunological principles that underlie the existing, commercial interferon-gamma release assays. IFN-γ, interferon-gamma; PBMC, peripheral blood mononuclear cells; ELISA, enzyme-linked immunosorbent assay; ELISPOT, enzyme-linked immunospot assay. (Reproduced from reference 28 with permission.)

tubes compared to the control tubes. An individual is considered positive for *M. tuberculosis* infection if the IFN-gamma response to TB antigens is above the test cut-off (after subtracting the background IFN-gamma response in the negative control).

QuantiFERON-TB Gold-Plus (QFT-Plus) is the next-generation IGRA launched by Qiagen in 2015. QFT-Plus uses two TB antigen tubes (TB1 and TB2). Both antigen tubes include peptides from ESAT-6 and CFP-10. While peptides in TB1 are designed to elicit an IFN-gamma response from CD4+ helper T cells, TB2 contains additional peptides to elicit a response from CD8+ cytotoxic T cells. The aim is to increase the assay sensitivity. The test is interpreted as positive when either antigen tube result is positive. Published data on this newer assay are limited (29), but studies are ongoing. There is no policy guidance on QFT-Plus yet.

T-SPOT.TB is an enzyme-linked immunospot assay performed on separated and counted peripheral blood mononuclear cells that are incubated with ESAT-6 and CFP-10 peptides. The result is reported as the number of IFN-gamma-producing T cells (spot-forming cells). An individual is considered positive for *M. tuberculosis*

infection if the spot counts in the TB antigen wells exceed a specific threshold relative to the negative control wells.

What is the evidence on IGRAs? A decade ago, early data raised the hope that the TST could be replaced by an *in vitro* assay with better performance (30). A decade later, after a large number of research studies, evidence shows that both TST and IGRA are acceptable but imperfect tests for LTBI screening (15). Table 1 provides a comparison of TST and IGRA (31). Both tests are indirect markers of *M. tuberculosis* exposure, and neither test is able to accurately differentiate between LTBI and active TB (32) or to resolve the various phases within the *M. tuberculosis* infection continuum (8, 15).

Studies show that both TST and IGRA cannot distinguish individuals who have successfully cleared *M. tuberculosis* infection (i.e., no longer need therapy) from those who have true infection (which is amenable to therapy) (33). This inability to differentiate results in overtreatment with increased costs and adverse events. Both TST and IGRA have reduced sensitivity in immunocompromised patients, particularly in those with a

Table 1 A comparison of available diagnostics for latent TB infection[a]

Characteristic	PPD-based tuberculin skin tests	Newer, specific skin tests (under development or validation)	Interferon-gamma release assays
Examples of products in the category	Tubersol, Aplisol, PPD RT23	C-Tb, Diaskintest	QuantiFERON-TB Gold In-Tube; T-SPOT.TB
Testing format	Intradermal skin test (*in vivo*)	Intradermal skin test (*in vivo*)	*Ex vivo* assay (ELISA or ELISPOT)
Antigens used	Purified protein derivative	ESAT-6 and CFP-10	ESAT-6 and CFP-10
Intended use	Screening for LTBI	Screening for LTBI	Screening for LTBI
Sensitivity	High	Modest	Modest
Sensitivity in immunocompromised populations	Reduced	Reduced	Reduced
Specificity	Modest	High	High
Impact of BCG on specificity	High (when BCG is given after infancy or multiple times)	None	None
Ability to distinguish latent from active TB	Low	Low	Low
Ability to predict progression to active TB disease	Modest	Unknown (but likely to be modest based on indirect evidence from IGRAs)	Modest
Ability to resolve the various stages within the spectrum of *M. tuberculosis* infection	Low	Low	Low
Reagent costs	Low	Unknown (but likely to be low based on indirect evidence from PPD-based TST)	High
Requirement for laboratories	No	No	Yes

[a]Data from reference 31. BCG, bacillus Calmette-Guérin; CFP-10, culture filtrate protein; ELISA, enzyme-linked immunosorbent assay; ESAT-6, early secreted antigen target; IGRA, interferon-gamma release assay; LTBI, latent tuberculosis infection; PPD, purified protein derivative.

severe immune depression, and have low predictive value for progression to active TB (15, 34). As in the case of PPD-based TST, a majority of individuals (i.e., over 95%) with positive IGRA results do not progress to active TB disease. This has been seen in several longitudinal studies and reviewed systematically by Rangaka and colleagues (34) and by WHO (5). Compared to the PPD-based TST, IGRAs have overcome the limited specificity problem, because BCG vaccination does not impact the test results, but they have not overcome the problem of limited predictive value (34).

Another emerging concern with IGRAs is their highly dynamic nature, with inconsistent results and high rates of conversions and reversions, when repeated tests are performed. Some of this dynamism could reflect transitions within the LTBI spectrum, while some is likely related to poor assay reproducibility. Several

serial testing studies of low-risk health care workers have revealed higher false conversion rates with IGRAs than with TSTs (35–38). Reproducibility studies have identified various sources of variability that contribute to nonreproducible results, and these studies have been systematically reviewed elsewhere (39). As reviewed by Banaei and colleagues, sources of variability can be broadly classified as preanalytical, analytical, postanalytical, manufacturing, and immunological (40). Figure 4 provides an overview of the major sources of variation with the QFT assay (15, 40). Similar challenges also affect the reproducibility of the T-SPOT.TB assay.

It is therefore important to note that both TSTs and IGRAs have reproducibility challenges, and dichotomous cut-offs are inadequate for interpretation. Further, extensive efforts need to be made to ensure adequate

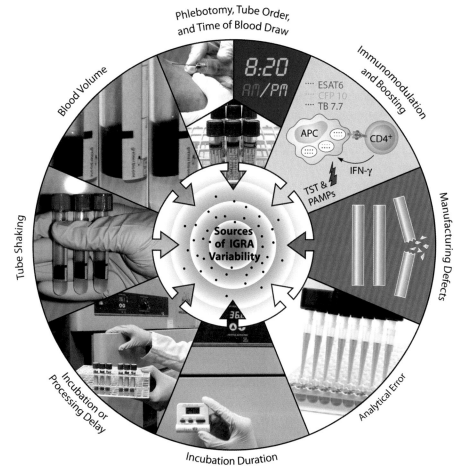

Figure 4   Sources of variability in the QuantiFERON-TB (QFT) Gold In-Tube assay. This graphic illustrates the sources of variability that affect the reproducibility of the QFT-Gold In-Tube assay. Variability can be due to preanalytical, analytical, postanalytical, manufacturing, and immunological factors. (Reproduced from reference 15 with permission.)

training and standardization. Table 2 lists suggestions to better standardize IGRAs and reduce the amount of test variability (40). When IGRAs are used for serial testing of health care workers, simplistic cut-offs (e.g., change from negative to positive) should not be used, because this results in very high conversion rates (41). There is no clear consensus on the best cut-off to use for serial testing with IGRAs (42), and many hospitals tend to repeat an IGRA test among low-risk individuals to check if the repeat test stays positive.

NEWER, SPECIFIC SKIN TESTS

These newer skin tests replace PPD with more specific antigens but in the same intradermal test format. C-Tb, a novel *M. tuberculosis*-specific skin test containing ESAT-6 and CFP-10 antigens, is one such new skin test, developed by Statens Serum Institut, Denmark (43, 44). Another product, Diaskintest (Generium Pharmaceutical, Moscow, Russia), is available commercially in Russia, Ukraine, and Kazakhstan (45), and an ESAT-6-based skin test from China is in clinical trials (46). There is currently no policy guidance on these newer skin tests, because the evidence base is weak.

By substituting PPD with ESAT-6 and CFP-10, these newer skin tests appear to overcome the specificity limitations of the PPD-based TST (43, 44). But this improvement in specificity might come at the cost of reduced sensitivity. One recent trial from South Africa suggests that the sensitivity of PPD-based TSTs is comparable to that of QFT-Gold In-Tube but lower than that of PPD-based TSTs (47). In this trial, the sensitivity of all LTBI tests was compromised in immunosuppressed HIV-infected patients (47).

Although further validation is required, it appears that newer skin tests do offer higher specificity than PPD-based TSTs, but this might compromise sensitivity (Table 1) (31). While there are no data on the predictive value of the newer skin tests, it is highly likely that the predictive value will be modest, based on what is already known about IGRAs based on ESAT-6 and CFP10 peptides (34). Thus, when compared to the PPD-based TST, IGRAs and newer skin tests might offer some incremental advantages, primarily, improved specificity. However, if reagents can be produced at scale and at affordable prices, newer skin tests may help resolve PPD shortages that have been reported in many settings (48).

CONCLUSIONS

Both TSTs and IGRAs are now a part of the LTBI testing landscape, and current guidelines allow the use of both tools, although guidelines vary considerably across countries (49). There are situations where neither test is appropriate (e.g., diagnosis of active TB in adults), and situations where both tests may be necessary to detect *M. tuberculosis* infection (e.g., immunocompromised

Table 2 Some suggested approaches to reduce test variability with IGRAs[a]

Step during the assay	Suggestions for best practices
Disinfection	Standardize skin and tube septum disinfection, akin to that done for blood cultures.
Tube order	Standardize the order of the GFT-GIT tubes during phlebotomy per the package insert (in the order purge tube, nil tube, antigen tube, and mitogen tube).
Blood volume	Standardize blood volume drawn into the QFT-GIT tubes, particularly for the antigen tube. Filling the tubes up to the 1-ml mark is practical. Collecting blood using a syringe and transferring 1 ml to each of the tubes is more accurate.
Tube shaking	Standardize gentle shaking of the QFT-GIT tubes per the package insert. Avoid separate shaking of the nil and antigen tubes, because differential shaking can result in a false-positive or false-negative result.
Processing delay	Minimize delays in incubation of cells. For the QFT-GIT assay, this can be achieved by placing an incubator at the collection site or by using a portable incubator to transport the tubes from the clinic to the laboratory. Further studies are needed to determine whether the T-Cell Xtend reagent can prolong processing time for the T-SPOT assay.
Analytical error	Use automated ELISA and ELISPOT instruments to reduce analytical variability.
Manufacturing defect	Institute a quality assurance program to monitor positivity and indeterminate rates. When rates cross a preset threshold and persist, halt utilization of potentially faulty lots and alert the manufacturer.
Immune boosting	When a two-step testing procedure (TST followed by IGRA) is used, TST boosting of the IGRA result can be avoided by drawing the blood sample for IGRA within 72 h of TST placement.

[a]Data from reference 40. ELISA, enzyme-linked immunosorbent assay; ELISPOT, enzyme-linked immunospot assay; IGRA, interferon-gamma release assay; QFT-GIT, QuantiFERON-TB Gold In-Tube; TST, tuberculin skin test.

populations), since no single test is adequate. And there are situations where one test might offer clear advantages over the other. For example, IGRAs would be preferable to the TST in populations where BCG is given after infancy or given multiple times (19, 21). In contrast, TST is preferable to the IGRAs for serial testing of health care workers, because IGRAs produce high rates of conversions and reversions and are harder to interpret for occupational health programs (3, 41, 50).

Unfortunately, none of the available LTBI tests meet a big felt need in the TB field—a highly predictive test that can help target those who will benefit most from LTBI therapy. To develop such predictive tests, we need transformative research that will enable us to identify biomarkers or biosignatures that can resolve the LTBI spectrum (8) and help target those at highest risk of progressing to active disease (51). Some promising biomarkers have been identified, especially gene expression signatures (52), but much more validation work is required.

A target product profile for such a predictive LTBI test has been developed by the New Diagnostics Working Group of the Stop TB Partnership (53), FIND, and other partners, and recent TB diagnostics market analyses and projections (54) might also help increase industry and donor interest in research and development that will result in the development of such innovative products that make an impact. Ideally, a more predictive LTBI test will also serve as a marker of cure after LTBI therapy.

Until we have substantially improved tools for LTBI, to maximize the predictive value of existing tests, LTBI screening should be selectively used for those who are at sufficiently high risk of progressing to disease. Such high-risk individuals may be identifiable via multivariable risk prediction models that incorporate test results with traditional risk factors (e.g., using risk calculators such as www.tstin3d.com) and via serial testing to resolve underlying phenotypes (15). Needless to say, LTBI testing should be followed by adequate counseling to ensure completion of LTBI therapy.

Acknowledgments. M.P. has no financial conflicts to declare. He serves as a consultant for the Bill & Melinda Gates Foundation and on advisory committees of FIND, Geneva, and TB Alliance, New York. M.B. receives royalties for an antigen used in one of the IGRA tests (QuantiFERON). He serves on the Vaccine Advisory Committee for Aeras. This chapter draws upon previous reviews published by the authors, in particular, the reviews published in Clinical Microbiology Reviews *and* European Respiratory Journal.

Citation. Pai M, Behr M. 2016. Latent *Mycobacterium tuberculosis* infection and interferon-gamma release assays. Microbiol Spectrum 4(5):TBTB2-0023-2016.

References

1. **World Health Organization.** 2014. *The End TB Strategy. Global strategy and targets for tuberculosis prevention, care and control after 2015.*

2. **Mazurek GH, Jereb J, Vernon A, LoBue P, Goldberg S, Castro K, IGRA Expert Committee, Centers for Disease Control and Prevention (CDC).** 2010. Updated guidelines for using interferon gamma release assays to detect *Mycobacterium tuberculosis* infection: United States, 2010. *MMWR Recomm Rep* **59**(RR-5):1–25.

3. **Pai M, Kunimoto D, Jamieson F, Menzies D.** 2013. Diagnosis of latent tuberculosis infection. In Canadian Tuberculosis Standards, 7th Edition. *Can Respir J* **20**:23A–34A.

4. **National Institute for Health and Care Excellence.** 2016. *Tuberculosis. NICE guideline NG33.*

5. **World Health Organization.** 2014. *Guidelines on the Management of Latent Tuberculosis Infection.* WHO, Geneva, Switzerland.

6. **Getahun H, et al.** 2015. Management of latent *Mycobacterium tuberculosis* infection: WHO guidelines for low tuberculosis burden countries. *Eur Respir J* **46**: 1563–1576.

7. **Landry J, Menzies D.** 2008. Preventive chemotherapy. Where has it got us? Where to go next? *Int J Tuberc Lung Dis* **12**:1352–1364.

8. **Barry CE III, Boshoff HI, Dartois V, Dick T, Ehrt S, Flynn J, Schnappinger D, Wilkinson RJ, Young D.** 2009. The spectrum of latent tuberculosis: rethinking the biology and intervention strategies. *Nat Rev Microbiol* **7**:845–855.

9. **Esmail H, Barry CE III, Wilkinson RJ.** 2012. Understanding latent tuberculosis: the key to improved diagnostic and novel treatment strategies. *Drug Discov Today* **17**: 514–521.

10. **Seddon JA.** 2016. Two sizes do not fit all: the terms infection and disease are inadequate for the description of children with tuberculosis. *Arch Dis Child* **101**:594–595.

11. **Dheda K, Schwander SK, Zhu B, van Zyl-Smit RN, Zhang Y.** 2010. The immunology of tuberculosis: from bench to bedside. *Respirology* **15**:433–450.

12. **Vynnycky E, Fine PE.** 1997. The natural history of tuberculosis: the implications of age-dependent risks of disease and the role of reinfection. *Epidemiol Infect* **119**:183–201.

13. **Andrews JR, Noubary F, Walensky RP, Cerda R, Losina E, Horsburgh CR.** 2012. Risk of progression to active tuberculosis following reinfection with *Mycobacterium tuberculosis*. *Clin Infect Dis* **54**:784–791.

14. **American Thoracic Society.** 2000. Targeted tuberculin testing and treatment of latent tuberculosis infection. This official statement of the American Thoracic Society was adopted by the ATS Board of Directors, July 1999. This is a Joint Statement of the American Thoracic Society (ATS) and the Centers for Disease Control and Prevention (CDC). This statement was endorsed by the Council of the Infectious Diseases Society of America. (IDSA), September 1999, and the sections of this statement. *Am J Respir Crit Care Med* **161**:S221–S247.

15. Pai M, Denkinger CM, Kik SV, Rangaka MX, Zwerling A, Oxlade O, Metcalfe JZ, Cattamanchi A, Dowdy DW, Dheda K, Banaei N. 2014. Gamma interferon release assays for detection of *Mycobacterium tuberculosis* infection. *Clin Microbiol Rev* 27:3–20.

16. Menzies RI. 2000. Tuberculin skin testing, p 279–322. *In* Reichman LB, Hershfield ES (ed), *Tuberculosis: a Comprehensive International Approach.* Marcel Dekker, New York, NY.

17. Deck F, Guld J. 1964. The WHO tuberculin test. *Bull Int Union Tuberc* 34:53–70.

18. CDC (ed). 2013. *Core Curriculum on Tuberculosis: What the Clinician Should Know.* CDC, Atlanta, GA.

19. Farhat M, Greenaway C, Pai M, Menzies D. 2006. False-positive tuberculin skin tests: what is the absolute effect of BCG and non-tuberculous mycobacteria? *Int J Tuberc Lung Dis* 10:1192–1204.

20. Menzies D, Gardiner G, Farhat M, Greenaway C, Pai M. 2008. Thinking in three dimensions: a web-based algorithm to aid the interpretation of tuberculin skin test results. *Int J Tuberc Lung Dis* 12:498–505.

21. Zwerling A, Behr MA, Verma A, Brewer TF, Menzies D, Pai M. 2011. The BCG World Atlas: a database of global BCG vaccination policies and practices. *PLoS Med* 8: e1001012.

22. Menzies D. 1999. Interpretation of repeated tuberculin tests. Boosting, conversion, and reversion. *Am J Respir Crit Care Med* 159:15–21.

23. Mahairas GG, Sabo PJ, Hickey MJ, Singh DC, Stover CK. 1996. Molecular analysis of genetic differences between *Mycobacterium bovis* BCG and virulent *M. bovis*. *J Bacteriol* 178:1274–1282.

24. Sørensen AL, Nagai S, Houen G, Andersen P, Andersen AB. 1995. Purification and characterization of a low-molecular-mass T-cell antigen secreted by *Mycobacterium tuberculosis*. *Infect Immun* 63:1710–1717.

25. Andersen P, Munk ME, Pollock JM, Doherty TM. 2000. Specific immune-based diagnosis of tuberculosis. *Lancet* 356:1099–1104.

26. Geluk A, van Meijgaarden KE, Franken KL, Subronto YW, Wieles B, Arend SM, Sampaio EP, de Boer T, Faber WR, Naafs B, Ottenhoff TH. 2002. Identification and characterization of the ESAT-6 homologue of *Mycobacterium leprae* and T-cell cross-reactivity with *Mycobacterium tuberculosis*. *Infect Immun* 70:2544–2548.

27. Geluk A, van Meijgaarden KE, Franken KL, Wieles B, Arend SM, Faber WR, Naafs B, Ottenhoff TH. 2004. Immunological crossreactivity of the *Mycobacterium leprae* CFP-10 with its homologue in *Mycobacterium tuberculosis*. *Scand J Immunol* 59:66–70.

28. Pollock L, Basu Roy R, Kampmann B. 2013. How to use: interferon γ release assays for tuberculosis. *Arch Dis Child Educ Pract Ed* 98:99–105.

29. Hoffmann H, Avsar K, Göres R, Mavi SC, Hofmann-Thiel S. 2016. Equal sensitivity of the new generation QuantiFERON-TB Gold plus in direct comparison with the previous test version QuantiFERON-TB Gold IT. *Clin Microbiol Infect* 22:701–703.

30. Pai M, Riley LW, Colford JM Jr. 2004. Interferon-gamma assays in the immunodiagnosis of tuberculosis: a systematic review. *Lancet Infect Dis* 4:761–776.

31. Pai M, Sotgiu G. 2016. Diagnostics for latent TB infection: incremental, not transformative progress. *Eur Respir J* 47:704–706

32. Sester M, Sotgiu G, Lange C, Giehl C, Girardi E, Migliori GB, Bossink A, Dheda K, Diel R, Dominguez J, Lipman M, Nemeth J, Ravn P, Winkler S, Huitric E, Sandgren A, Manissero D. 2011. Interferon-γ release assays for the diagnosis of active tuberculosis: a systematic review and meta-analysis. *Eur Respir J* 37:100–111.

33. Mack U, Migliori GB, Sester M, Rieder HL, Ehlers S, Goletti D, Bossink A, Magdorf K, Hölscher C, Kampmann B, Arend SM, Detjen A, Bothamley G, Zellweger JP, Milburn H, Diel R, Ravn P, Cobelens F, Cardona PJ, Kan B, Solovic I, Duarte R, Cirillo DM, C Lange for the TBNET. 2009. LTBI: latent tuberculosis infection or lasting immune responses to *M. tuberculosis*? A TBNET consensus statement. *Eur Respir J* 33:956–973.

34. Rangaka MX, Wilkinson KA, Glynn JR, Ling D, Menzies D, Mwansa-Kambafwile J, Fielding K, Wilkinson RJ, Pai M. 2012. Predictive value of interferon-γ release assays for incident active tuberculosis: a systematic review and meta-analysis. *Lancet Infect Dis* 12:45–55.

35. Slater ML, Welland G, Pai M, Parsonnet J, Banaei N. 2013. Challenges with QuantiFERON-TB Gold assay for large-scale, routine screening of U.S. healthcare workers. *Am J Respir Crit Care Med* 188:1005–1010.

36. Dorman SE, Belknap R, Graviss EA, Reves R, Schluger N, Weinfurter P, Wang Y, Cronin W, Hirsch-Moverman Y, Teeter LD, Parker M, Garrett DO, Daley CL, Tuberculosis Epidemiologic Studies Consortium. 2014. Interferon-γ release assays and tuberculin skin testing for diagnosis of latent tuberculosis infection in healthcare workers in the United States. *Am J Respir Crit Care Med* 189: 77–87.

37. Zwerling A, Benedetti A, Cojocariu M, McIntosh F, Pietrangelo F, Behr MA, Schwartzman K, Menzies D, Pai M. 2013. Repeat IGRA testing in Canadian health workers: conversions or unexplained variability? *PLoS One* 8:e54748.

38. Joshi M, Monson TP, Joshi A, Woods GL. 2014. IFN-γ release assay conversions and reversions: challenges with serial testing in U.S. health care workers. *Ann Am Thorac Soc* 11:296–302.

39. Tagmouti S, Slater M, Benedetti A, Kik SV, Banaei N, Cattamanchi A, Metcalfe J, Dowdy D, van Zyl Smit R, Dendukuri N, Pai M, Denkinger C. 2014. Reproducibility of interferon gamma (IFN-γ) release assays: a systematic review. *Ann Am Thorac Soc* 11:1267–1276.

40. Banaei N, Gaur RL, Pai M. 2016. Interferon-gamma release assays for latent tuberculosis: what are the sources of variability? *J Clin Microbiol* 54:845–850.

41. Pai M, Banaei N. 2013. Occupational screening of health care workers for tuberculosis infection: tuberculin skin testing or interferon-γ release assays? *Occup Med (Lond)* 63:458–460.

42. Daley CL, Reves RR, Beard MA, Boyle J, Clark RB, Beebe JL, Catanzaro A, Chen L, Desmond E, Dorman

SE, Hudson TW, Lardizabal AA, Kapoor H, Marder DC, Miranda C, Narita M, Reichman L, Schwab D, Seaworth BJ, Terpeluk P, Thanassi W, Kawamura LM. 2013. A summary of meeting proceedings on addressing variability around the cut point in serial interferon-γ release assay testing. *Infect Control Hosp Epidemiol* **34**:625–630.

43. Aggerbeck H, Giemza R, Joshi P, Tingskov PN, Hoff ST, Boyle J, Andersen P, Lewis DJ. 2013. Randomised clinical trial investigating the specificity of a novel skin test (C-Tb) for diagnosis of *M. tuberculosis* infection. *PLoS One* **8**:e64215.

44. Bergstedt W, Tingskov PN, Thierry-Carstensen B, Hoff ST, Aggerbeck H, Thomsen VO, Andersen P, Andersen AB. 2010. First-in-man open clinical trial of a combined rdESAT-6 and rCFP-10 tuberculosis specific skin test reagent. *PLoS One* **5**:e11277.

45. Kiselev VI, Baranovskii PM, Rudykh IV, Shuster AM, Mart'ianov VA, Mednikov BL, Demin AV, Aleksandrov AN, Mushkin AI, Levi DT, Slogotskaia LV, Ovsiankina ES, Medunitsin NV, Litvinov VI, Perel'man MI, Pal'tsev MA. 2009. Clinical trials of the new skin test Diaskintest for the diagnosis of tuberculosis. *Probl Tuberk Bolezn Legk* **2009**(2):11–16. [In Russian.]

46. Sun QF, Xu M, Wu JG, Chen BW, Du WX, Ding JG, Shen XB, Su C, Wen JS, Wang GZ. 2013. Efficacy and safety of recombinant *Mycobacterium tuberculosis* ESAT-6 protein for diagnosis of pulmonary tuberculosis: a phase II trial. *Med Sci Monit* **19**:969–977.

47. Hoff ST, Peter JG, Theron G, Pascoe M, Tingskov PN, Aggerbeck H, Kolbus D, Ruhwald M, Andersen P, Dheda K. 2016. Sensitivity of C-Tb: a novel RD-1-specific skin test for the diagnosis of tuberculosis infection. *Eur Respir J* **47**:919–928

48. Centers for Disease Control and Prevention (CDC). 2013. Extent and effects of recurrent shortages of purified-protein derivative tuberculin skin test antigen solutions: United States, 2013. *MMWR Morb Mortal Wkly Rep* **62**:1014–1015.

49. Denkinger CM, Dheda K, Pai M. 2011. Guidelines on interferon-γ release assays for tuberculosis infection: concordance, discordance or confusion? *Clin Microbiol Infect* **17**:806–814.

50. Pai M, Elwood K. 2012. Interferon-gamma release assays for screening of health care workers in low tuberculosis incidence settings: dynamic patterns and interpretational challenges. *Can Respir J* **19**:81–83.

51. Gardiner JL, Karp CL. 2015. Transformative tools for tackling tuberculosis. *J Exp Med* **212**:1759–1769.

52. Zak DE, Penn-Nicholson A, Scriba TJ, Thompson E, Suliman S, Amon LM, Mahomed H, Erasmus M, Whatney W, Hussey GD, Abrahams D, Kafaar F, Hawkridge T, Verver S, Hughes EJ, Ota M, Sutherland J, Howe R, Dockrell HM, Boom WH, Thiel B, Ottenhoff TH, Mayanja-Kizza H, Crampin AC, Downing K, Hatherill M, Valvo J, Shankar S, Parida SK, Kaufmann SH, Walzl G, Aderem A, Hanekom WA, ACS and GC6-74 cohort study groups. 2016. A blood RNA signature for tuberculosis disease risk: a prospective cohort study. *Lancet* **387**: 2312–2322.

53. Stop TB Partnership's New Diagnostics Working Group. 2016. *Draft target product profile: test for progression of tuberculosis infection.*

54. FIND, McGill International TB Centre, UNITAID. 2015. *TB Diagnostics Market in Select High-Burden Countries: Current Market and Future Opportunities for Novel Diagnostics.* UNITAID, Geneva, Switzerland.

Tuberculosis and the Tubercle Bacillus, 2nd ed.
Edited by William R. Jacobs, Jr., Helen McShane, Valerie Mizrahi, and Ian M. Orme
© 2018 American Society for Microbiology, Washington, DC
doi:10.1128/microbiolspec.TBTB2-0040-2016

Impact of the GeneXpert MTB/RIF Technology on Tuberculosis Control

18

Wendy Susan Stevens,[1] Lesley Scott,[2] Lara Noble,[2]
Natasha Gous,[1] and Keertan Dheda[3]

INTRODUCTION TO THE GLOBAL TUBERCULOSIS EPIDEMIC

Tuberculosis (TB) remains a global health security risk and a major cause of morbidity and mortality. The TB epidemic continues unabated, with 9.6 million infections occurring globally in 2014, coupled with an overall 1.5 million deaths (1). Of these infected individuals, 12% were found to have concomitant human immunodeficiency virus (HIV) infection. While prevalence and incidence vary significantly across countries, the annual global incidence has decreased year after year since 2000 by an average of 1.5%. Twenty-two high-burden countries (HBCs) are responsible for 80% of all estimated incident TB cases. Alarmingly, one-third of all TB cases remain undiagnosed (or underreported), and the statistics are significantly worse for drug-resistant TB (2). Reported multidrug-resistant TB (MDR-TB) and extensively drug-resistant TB (XDR-TB) cases are inevitably on the rise as increased numbers of individuals are being diagnosed and treated, adherence remains unchecked or unsuccessful, and infection control practices remain suboptimal. Nearly half a million MDR-TB cases are diagnosed annually, representing less than a quarter of estimated incident cases (2). There is significant work to be done to improve detection of drug-resistant TB and to ensure linkage to appropriate care of patients.

The control of TB, once unchecked, is extremely difficult to contain and manage, requiring a multidisciplinary, coordinated set of activities. The cornerstones of classic TB control approaches include early diagnosis, novel ways of case finding beyond health care facilities, shorter and simpler successful treatment regimens for both drug-susceptible and drug-resistant TB, a greater focus on prevention strategies, and steps to reduce mortality and transmission in both adults and children. In high HIV coinfection settings, this needs to go hand in hand with scaling up access to antiretroviral therapy (ART) and continuous treatment monitoring. In 2015, the deadline for the Millennium Development Goals established for both HIV and TB infections, was reached, with varying degrees of success reported across countries. The Millennium Development Goals were transitioned into what are now referred to as the sustainable development goals. The process resulted in the development and announcement of the World Health Organization (WHO) END-TB strategy, which has the overall goal of achieving zero deaths, disease, and suffering due to TB by 2035 (3).

Important pillars of this strategy include the institution of bold policies, strengthened health support systems, integrated patient-centered management, and finally, ongoing research and innovation into new drugs, vaccines, and pertinent to this paper, diagnostics (4). These are not new strategies, but the added complexity of HIV, vaccination failure, the potential for lifelong latency, and continued poor understanding of pathogenic pathways leading to infection makes the achievement of these goals challenging.

Sophisticated modeling has been conducted by several research groups to ascertain the contribution of various strategies that will lead to successful outcomes

[1]Department of Molecular Medicine and Haematology, Faculty of Health Sciences, University of the Witwatersrand, and National Health Laboratory Service and National Priority Program of the National Health Laboratory Service, Johannesburg, South Africa; [2]Department of Molecular Medicine and Haematology, Faculty of Health Sciences, University of the Witwatersrand, Johannesburg, Gauteng, South Africa; [3]Lung Infection and Immunity Unit, Division of Pulmonology and UCT Lung Institute, Department of Medicine, University of Cape Town, Cape Town, South Africa.

within the defined time frame. The WHO recommends baseline and intensified screening of all individuals infected with HIV, knowing that the effectiveness of this case finding depends to a large degree on the epidemiologic setting, regional TB prevalence, and screening strategy (5).

BACKGROUND TO TB DIAGNOSTICS

Mycobacterium tuberculosis was discovered and described by Robert Koch in 1882, for which he received a Nobel Prize in 1905. The first diagnostic assays, such as the Ziehl-Neelsen stain performed on sputum smears, have remained largely unchanged or unchallenged since the early 1850s. The sensitivity of this assay is between 20 and 80% depending on the population within which the assay is applied, but the HIV epidemic alone has reduced the diagnostic value significantly in recent times (6–11).

Culture has been considered the "gold standard" for TB diagnosis for decades, initially using solid-based agar plates and more recently, liquid-based culture that can be automated using Mycobacterial Growth Indicator Tubes (Becton Dickinson, NJ). These assays frequently become clinically irrelevant due to the time taken for growth to occur, which is generally 2 to 6 weeks or much longer if culture is used for drug susceptibility assays (12). The inadequacies of these diagnostic approaches are particularly evident in the paucibacillary nature of cases associated with HIV infection, in the diagnosis of pediatric infections, in extrapulmonary TB (EPTB) (not insignificant in many countries; estimates of 15% in South Africa), in the ever-increasing rates of drug resistance, and in the health care systems that fail to retain patients in care between diagnosis and treatment initiation.

For these and other reasons, there has been a strong drive to seek alternative approaches for earlier, proactive screening and diagnosis of TB and, more recently, to meet the ambitious goals of the END-TB strategy (3). Following the long reign of smear and culture, numerous approaches were sought using new diagnostic targets such as TB DNA, RNA, total nucleic acid (TNA), protein, and lipids using different technological approaches and platforms. More recently, new biomarkers are being investigated using gene expression profiling of both the organism and the susceptible host, with varying success. A recent research paper highlighted the diagnostic potential of a 51-transcript signature or transcriptome in children, which was shown to have increased value as an earlier biomarker for disease diagnosis (13). This remains a highly supported area of research in the TB research roadmap.

Enhanced sputum collection procedures have also been extensively evaluated, and a massive exploration undertaken of more affordable, rapid screens using dipstick formats for both blood and urine. The desirable characteristics of such an assay are no different from those for HIV diagnostics, with affordability, speed, sensitivity, specificity, simplicity, safety, and clinical relevance remaining the major goals. We cannot, however, ignore that sputum, as opposed to blood, is a more difficult sample with which to work; the extrapulmonary nature of TB in many cases poses diagnostic dilemmas, and no predictor for the activation of latent infection is available. The imperfect nature of all these assays results in the ongoing development of complex algorithms for screening and diagnosis, which are confusing clinically, particularly where task-shifting of care to lower echelons of the health care worker sector has occurred, and are therefore not implemented effectively or appropriately (14).

The use of nucleic acid amplification (NAA)-based formats was initiated as far back as the early 1990s. At that time, various DNA-based assays were introduced but, upon evaluation, failed dismally, with poor sensitivity undoubtedly related to the difficulties in extraction of nucleic acid due to the intracellular nature of the organism in macrophages and the hard exterior wall of *M. tuberculosis* itself. The first assays were frequently used in low-burden TB settings to confirm smear-positive TB assays. These include, among others, the COBAS TaqMan MTB Test (Roche Molecular Systems, CA; FDA approved in 1995) (15, 16), the amplified MDT test (Gen-Probe, CA) (17), and the ProbeTec DTB assay (Becton Dickinson, NJ) (18). During this period, numerous publications appeared describing in-house assays on generic platforms such as the Roche LightCycler Mycobacterium Detection kit (Roche Applied Science, IN) and ABI TaqMan analyzers, with similar success rates but poor sensitivity in smear-negative samples (19).

The first molecular test ever endorsed by the WHO, in 2008, was for the detection of TB and MDR-TB: the Genotype MTBDR*plus* version 1 (Hain Life Sciences GmbH, Nehren, Germany), frequently referred to as the line-probe assay (LPA) (20). This assay used conventional DNA PCR with hybridization probes to identify specific mutations for both rifampin (*rpoB* gene) and isoniazid (*katG* and *inhA* genes) and was quite revolutionary for its time. This was followed by the endorsement of the Xpert MTB/RIF (Cepheid Inc, Sunnyvale, CA) assay in 2010 (21). Later an improved MTBDR*plus* version 2 (22–24), as well as the same assay design applied to second-line drug resistance testing in a first version of the MTBDRsl to identify resistance to fluoroquinolones and second-line injectable drugs using probe hybridization to *gyrA*, *rrs*, and ethambutol (*embB*) (25), received WHO endorsement. The MTBDRsl has been modified to version 2, which includes hybridization probes to identify *gyrA*, *gyrB*, *rrs*, and *eis*, and *embB* has been removed (26, 27). The WHO has recommended version 2 as an initial test to detect resistance directly off sputum diagnosed with resistance to rifampin or MDR-TB (28). Since these landmarks, numerous other molecular assays have been developed, are in evaluation or demonstration studies, or are in early market entry and validation stages (Table 1) (29). However, despite these numerous advancements, TB diagnosis remains problematic for certain subpopulations, such as pediatric populations, and for the diagnosis of EPTB. Implementation is also difficult in settings where molecular testing is not routine and infrastructure is poor.

BACKGROUND TO THE GeneXpert TECHNOLOGY

The Xpert MTB/RIF assay, used on the GeneXpert analyzer (Cepheid, Sunnyvale, CA) launched in 2004, underwent extensive validations in the period before demonstration data were presented to the WHO in September 2010, and with unprecedented speed, received endorsement in December of the same year (30). The recommendation by the WHO in 2010 for Xpert MTB/RIF's use as the initial diagnostic test was for the detection of HIV-associated TB and where high rates of drug resistance were suspected (30). The assay was first in class for a number of reasons: (i) improved sensitivity over prior attempts at using NAA testing (NAAT) strategies, (ii) the simultaneous detection of rifampin resistance, (iii) a modular format allowing testing across a spectrum of volume needs, (iv) the possibility of automation (Infinity group of analyzers), (v) simplicity, (vi) speed, and (vii) safety (single room, no biohazard hoods required, and testing available even to the clinic setting) (31–36). Additional advances were that the cartridge contained all relevant components ("lab-in-a-cartridge" is a term frequently used to describe the platform format), there was no need for a cold-chain, and the analyzer with its modular format was random access in nature and had connectivity capabilities to various laboratory information systems and to a remote connectivity platform for the monitoring of instrument performance at a central level (37). This assay has set the bar high for fast followers. The FDA subsequently approved the assay in 2013 as a medium complexity test (38). In the same year, the test use was expanded further to include pediatrics and EPTB, and its use as a smear replacement strategy was given strong support (38).

South Africa, with an ever-increasing incidence and prevalence of TB, elected to take a bold and aggressive smear replacement approach to facilitate earlier diagnosis and treatment with the decision to roll out the Xpert MTB/RIF assay nationally in March 2011. The decision was undertaken based on high smear-negative rates using light emitting diode microscopy (8 to 10% referred cases positive nationally) (National Health Laboratory Service [NHLS]; W. Stevens, personal communication) and based on concern over looming, undiagnosed drug-resistant TB cases and high rates of HIV coinfection (65 to 70% of HIV-positive people are TB coinfected) (39). In addition, diagnosis of EPTB, which accounted for an estimated 15% of cases (40), was complex, as was the diagnosis in pediatrics (41). The length of time to culture diagnosis was becoming clinically irrelevant, and many patients were lost to follow-up. The molecular paradigm and skill required were already accepted in-country, having been used successfully in HIV for expansion of PCR for HIV viral load testing and early infant diagnosis of HIV on a national scale (42).

HISTORICAL CONTEXT OF THE FIRST SCALED NATIONAL IMPLEMENTATION OF THE Xpert ASSAY

While a number of countries have now incorporated or are planning to incorporate the Xpert assay in their national TB programs, there were few willing to implement immediately post-WHO approval in 2010, because there were no available implementation models or guidelines at that time. In addition, there were uncertainties around field performance and overall program cost and no guidance on how to operationalize the assay in complex clinical algorithms already available for TB. These guidance documents, along with training, maintenance, and procurement guidelines and policies, came later and are now facilitating implementation of operational plans.

TB in South Africa

South Africa remains one of the HBCs, with the second-highest estimated incidence rate of TB and number of diagnosed MDR-TB cases. The TB prevalence, while it appears to be declining, is estimated at 380/100,000 population with a wide confidence interval (210 to 590), and the TB incidence is 450/100,000 (400 to 510) (1).

Table 1 NAAT-based TB technologies in the pipeline[a]

NAAT Technology	Assay	Intended placement			Target[b]		Polyvalency		Anticipated release date
		Microscopy	Intermediate	Reference	MTBC	DST	Yes	No	
GeneXpert (Cepheid, Inc.)	MTB/RIF ULTRA assay		✓	✓	✓		✓		2017
	MTB/RIF XDR assays		✓	✓		✓	✓		2017
Abbott m2000sp and m2000rt (Abbott Molecular)	MDR-TB companion assay			✓		✓	✓		2017
BD Max platform (Becton Dickinson)	Multiplexed TB assay			✓	✓		✓		2017
	DST assay			✓		✓	✓		
Fluorocycler 96 (Hain LifeScience)	Fluorotype MDR-TB		✓		✓	✓	✓		2016
	Fluorotype XDR-TB		✓		✓	✓	✓		2017
Savanna platform (Northwestern Global Health Foundation in partnership with Quidel)	MTBC assay	✓			✓		✓		2016
	MDR-TB assay	✓				✓	✓		
EOSCAPE Systems (Wave-80 Biosciences)	EOSCAPE TB	✓			✓		✓		2016
	RIF-FQ assays	✓				✓	✓		
Alere q (Alere Inc.)	MTB/DST assay	✓			✓	✓	✓		2016 for performance assessments
GeneXpert Omni (Cepheid, Inc)	MTB/RIF or ULTRA assays and XDR assay[c]	✓			✓	✓	✓		2017
Q-POC (QuantuMDx)	MTBC/MDR-TB	✓			✓	✓	✓		2017
TBDx System (Keck Graduate Institute in collaboration with various partners)	MTBC assay	✓			✓			✓	2018
GenePOC Diagnostic Platform (Canada)	TB assay	✓			✓		Unknown		2018
Point of Need platform (Qiagen)	TB, MDR-TB assays	✓			✓	✓	Unknown		2018–2019

[a]Adapted from reference 84.
[b]MTBC, M. tuberculosis complex; DST, drug susceptibility testing.
[c]And potentially the XDR assay.

Coupled with the highest global TB and HIV coinfection rates, with up to 70% of all TB cases being HIV positive, an aggressive approach to early diagnostic strategies was taken (43). This was strongly supported against a backdrop of approximately 6.3 million HIV-infected individuals, with only half these cases on appropriate ART (44).

The diagnosis of rifampin resistance and its use as a surrogate marker for MDR-TB, bringing with it a whole new set of new challenges such as linkage to MDR and XDR treatment and care, has been one of the most successful outcomes of the TB program in South Africa (45).

South African National Implementation of the Xpert MTB/RIF Assay

The national implementation rollout was conducted in a phased approach between March 2011 and September 2013, through the networked NHLS (265 laboratories), which was responsible for close to 90% of national public health diagnostic testing.

The process was accelerated by selecting sites where routine TB microscopy was being conducted in 2011 (Fig. 1). Based on reasonably predictable smear averages conducted per site using retrospective data, and assuming South Africans received an average of 1.8 smears per diagnostic and treatment cycle, the national

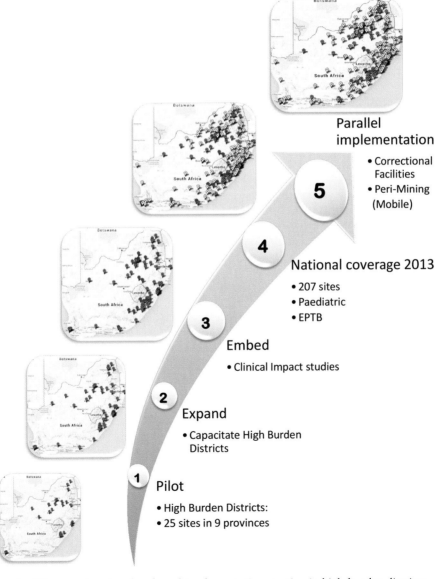

Figure 1 Diagram showing the phased implementation starting in high-burden districts.

estimates for Xpert assays were forecast (46). This process enabled selection of the instrumentation with the appropriate throughput for each site (43) (NHLS; W. Stevens, personal communication). Using this crude information together with the available clinical data, different research teams were able to cost and model the national needs that, with time, achieved a very high level of sophistication, currently culminating in the South African TB and HIV investment case (47). To date, over 8 million assays have been conducted in South Africa, still accounting for over half the global usage of cartridges (http://apps.who.int/tb/laboratory/xpertmap/).

For maximum impact, 25 microscopy centers in the highest-TB-burden districts were identified and the GeneXpert analyzers were implemented. The average *M. tuberculosis* positivity in these microscopy centers was 8% at program inception, but this quickly rose to positivity rates of 16% as detection was doubled using the Xpert MTB/RIF assay (48). The second phase involved fully capacitating laboratories established in phase I, with additional instrumentation to meet the needs of a particular center, and was followed quickly by full capacitation of these high-burden districts.

Embedded in the third rollout phase was the XTEND study, a randomized controlled trial which created much debate (49). This study highlighted the strengthening of health systems that is required to make a diagnostic intervention successful early on in the program, but it was considered harsh in its assessment in that this outcome is not really different from the expected diagnostic lag postintroduction of any new assay.

The remaining microscopy centers were capacitated once full financial commitment was obtained, resulting in 207 microscopy centers distributed across all nine provinces (Fig. 2). There are currently 314 GeneXpert instruments in the field: 115 GX4, 190 GX16, 1 GX48, and 8 GX80. As testing volumes began to rise, the placement of seven Infinity analyzers (7 GX80) was undertaken at the highest-volume microscopy centers. The political will and the success of both treasury-funded and donor-funded support we believe emanate from having a single plan, forecasted and managed by the National TB program and the NHLS.

Challenges and Opportunities Encountered during National Implementation Efforts

As with any large-scale implementation of new technology, there are always challenges (Table 2): those that could be predicted and those that were unexpected. A level of confidence in the technology needs to be established within the laboratory as well as by the clinical users. Acceptable error rate/invalid calculations need to be defined. The development of the clinical algorithm was perhaps one of the most highly debated compo-

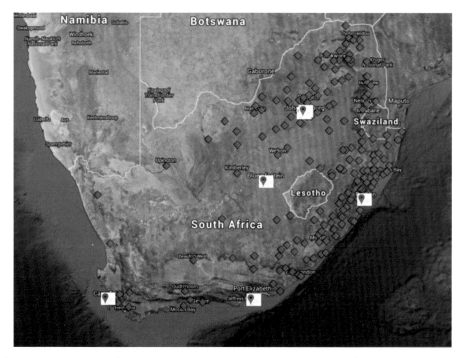

Figure 2 GeneXpert placement in 207 microscopy centers in South Africa.

Table 2 Challenges experienced with large-scale implementation of GeneXpert technology and mitigation strategies[a]

Challenges	Solutions
Programmatic	
National TB Costing Model, national plan, treasury support	Donor and NDoH funding received (treasury support gained)
Forecasting difficult; global fund projects delayed	Global forecasting
Equity issues	Phased implementation of algorithm: high-burden districts first and then full capacitation
Clinical training (MDR especially) lagged behind laboratory implementation	Trainers employed by NHLS and Global Fund
	Linkage to Care program initiated (funded by CDC, NHLS, JHU, NDoH)
Traditional and molecular algorithms used simultaneously; nonadherence to diagnostic algorithm	Complex algorithm included expansion of culture testing
	Improvement in adherence over time from 20 to 41%. In 2015 this improved to closer to 50%.
LPA inadequate for confirmation	Simplification needed, especially for second-line testing
	Still requires a rapid TB test
	Sequencing: new gold standard?
Clinical data collection poor	TB link to HIV database is imminent
High-risk populations: Department of Correctional Services, mines, MDR-TB	Programs initiated
Impact studies needed	Training initiated
	Linkage to Care projects initiated (EXIT-RIF, Gates XTEND studies)
	Linkage coordinators
Monopoly	Pipeline improving
	Investment not wasted with new assays at Cepheid; 2012 onward: 50 new products
Quality	
Verification of analyzer needed on site	Development of DCS verification program
	DCS received WHO/CDC approval
Need to monitor performance and quality testing; EQA program nonexistent	Developed the DCS EQA program
	Trialed successfully in South Africa and ACTG sites
Massive scale-up of quality assurance material required	Business plan reviewed
	Innovation awards and patent
Extended warranty	For South Africa, an extended warranty was 30% more expensive. Implemented a change in the procurement model
Laboratory considerations	
Stock shortages	Stabilized over time
	Focused utility and lab capacity, stock and workflow management
	Global forecasting useful
Module failures; errors	Replacement of modules
	Dust, temperature, user, refurbished
	RemoteCHEK calibration
Sensitivity lower in HIV-positive presumptive TB cases	MTB ULTRA undergoing evaluation in 2016
	Other assays being investigated
Reporting, real-time monitoring	Monthly reports
	Remote connectivity system (Cepheid, NHLS)
Testing of EPTB specimens	In-country study, WHO meta-analysis
	SOPs and policy developed for EPTB
Pediatric diagnosis	Policy developed, although compared with culture, two Xperts better than one
	Alternative samples being investigated

[a]Abbreviations: ACTG, AIDS Clinical Trials Group; DCS, dried culture spots; JHU, Johns Hopkins University; NDoH, National Department of Health; SOP, standard operating procedure.

nents of the program and remains a dilemma under constant review, which was also divided across the nine provinces in South Africa (the Western Cape is the only province that implemented the receipt of two sputum specimens at presentation, unlike the remaining eight provinces, which only received one). Instrumentation had to be interfaced with the laboratory information system across all sites for result reporting and for internal monitoring of quality. Staff training at a laboratory, followed by that in a clinical program, is arduous and still ongoing 5 years postimplementation. One of the lessons learned from training in the field was not so much the need for technical training on the Xpert MTB/RIF assay workflow process, but rather, that more attention is needed for computer literacy and Windows-based training and support, because the GeneXpert instrumentation is PC powered.

The major challenges encountered relatively early in the implementation process included (i) cartridge shortages due to supplier manufacturing issues and early cartridge version change (G3 to G4), (ii) difficulty posed by phased implementation using both Xpert and microscopy for reasons of equity and difficulties at the laboratory or clinical level, (iii) nonadherence to the clinical algorithm (which remains a constant concern), (iv) pediatric and extrapulmonary sample testing uncertainties, and (v) the constant debate about the level of placement, initially resolved simply by costs and later by complexity of the analyzer maintenance (at the time defined by the FDA as a medium-complexity instrument which was commensurate with laboratory experience). Further challenges realized were the need to interface with donors and manage expectations (50). In addition, through the maturity of the South African program, the TIME impact epidemiological transmission model (http://www.TIMEmodelling.com; a component of TIME, a set of modeling tools) (50), as well as other modeling tools (35, 51, 52), highlight further aspects such as the need to include latent stratification by HIV and ART status, MDR, treatment history and age, as well as changes that need to be built in over time: change in disease burden (prevalence, incidence, and mortality), changes in TB dynamics (proportion latently infected, recent infections, annual risk of infection) and programmatic outputs (notifications, numbers screened, positive predictive value of diagnostic algorithm), socio-economic trends, and structural determinants in the population (53) which are needed to further inform the investment case and improve diagnostic algorithms.

Several studies have highlighted the current performance of the analyzer for pediatric and/or extrapul-

monary samples. This resulted in South Africa rapidly implementing its own recommendations for use in managing sites, permissible samples, and ongoing training and relevant research and development. The final outreach established using the laboratory technology platform and footprint was the expansion of testing to support vulnerable populations such as offenders in correctional services (242 sites) and miners and peri-mining communities in two large global fund projects that are ongoing.

IMPACT OF THE Xpert MTB/RIF ON NATIONAL TB PROGRAMS

The national coverage of testing led to consequences that were perhaps not completely expected (Fig. 3), other than the routine, earlier diagnosis of TB and rifampin resistance. Words such as "disruptive" or "a game changer" were particularly apt for the program. The performance of the assay beyond those original demonstration studies has been confirmed, evaluated, and explored in virtually every clinical setting, in every country, and there are now volumes of data that speak to its successes and failures in both low- and high-burden countries with differing epidemiological trends (33), including more recent reports of point mutations affecting results (54, 55).

Perhaps what is not as obvious, unless one has been intimately involved with the national rollout of the Xpert assay on a scale as has occurred in South Africa, was how many areas of the national TB control program the Xpert program affected to allow for a transitioning of practice. Information gathered in this program has further reinforced the approaches required in implementation models for large scale-up of testing programs in South Africa and elsewhere and for other assays and, we believe, has increased awareness of implementation science as a new discipline, particularly in the diagnostics arena. The assay faced widespread skepticism from individuals where conventional microbiologic diagnostic methods had been entrenched in practice for decades. Thus, the assay had to interface within the context of other molecular assays and the prevailing culture paradigm. This legacy remains, and thus the complexity of algorithms frequently confuses the user or clinician and the assay is not used optimally.

Interfacing with clinical diagnostics and relevant clinical treatment guidelines is needed at program inception. This needs to integrate into HIV treatment programs where coinfection rates are high. Empiric treatment appears to undermine the value of the Xpert assay in high-burden HIV settings, especially with respect to presentation of extremely ill patients. The

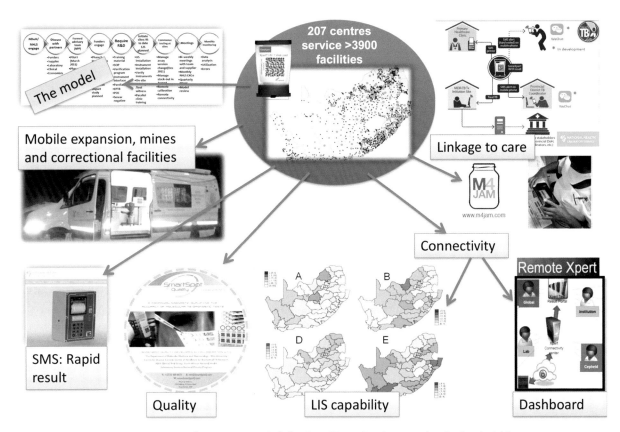

Figure 3   Innovations that accompanied the GeneXpert implementation in South Africa.

polyvalency of the platform does, however, assist with better integration of HIV and TB services. The roles of digital X rays and screening tests, such as the urine lipoarabinomannan, are additional considerations as we move forward. Numerous studies have expressed concern about the sensitivity of the assay in paucibacillary, HIV-infected individuals that may be addressed in the future with the newer cartridge planned for the Xpert assay, namely the ULTRA assay, or other assays in development such as the Abbott MTB assay (Abbott Molecular) (29).

In countries where laboratory information systems exist, the analyzers need to be interfaced for actionable resulting. These systems assist with the development of innovative solutions with respect to linking patients to care. The result from the Xpert assay is simple and can be reported in fewer than 160 characters, allowing various mHealth strategies such as smartphones and SMS printers to be used.

The collection of all results from all analyzers into a central data warehouse has enabled accountability at all levels of the health care system: on the laboratory side, information such as turnaround times, laboratory sites, and even instrument modules can be monitored.

On the clinical side, since all clinics are GIS (geographic information system)-mapped to all laboratories, accountability can be introduced at the national, regional, facility, and individual patient level. Nowhere has this been more evident than in the monitoring of rifampin resistance, a marker for MDR, but a tracker too of program success and treatment success facilitating targeted interventions. In addition, when unique identifiers are used, one can ascertain whether the clinical algorithm is followed; e.g., if no follow-up sample for confirmation of MDR and XDR is received, then adherence to clinical practice can be monitored further (37, 56).

It is difficult to monitor 314 analyzers across the programs, and since the Xpert assay exists in a modular format, one is essentially monitoring 4,180 separate instruments. An interface for monitoring the analyzer performance in real time is thus needed, and a process of continuous, internal quality monitoring has been developed. Establishing the requirements for a full quality assurance program was a huge task and included capability for continuous monitoring of quality indicators off the analyzer and an external quality assurance program (EQA) in the laboratories, together with ensuring that simple, appropriate sample collection and processing were followed (57, 58). Since whole TB bacteria are required for quality assurance material for the Xpert analyzer and TB is biohazardous to transport, a novel quality assurance product was developed in the form of a dried culture spot (DCS) (58). Thus, one will discover that the assay needs to interface with current laboratory quality management systems and EQA and highlights the weaknesses in these programs very quickly.

FINANCIAL MODELING, COSTING AND FORECASTING, AND PROCUREMENT STRATEGIES

The initial modeling exercises in South Africa prior to and in concert with the rollout were undertaken (i) to estimate implementation costs for the NHLS, (ii) to inform national-level budget requirements (2011 to 2017), and (iii) to estimate the incremental national health service cost of replacing the existing pulmonary TB diagnostic algorithm with a new algorithm incorporating GeneXpert costs, under routine care conditions and at costs incurred by the government and focused on the entire process from TB suspects to TB cases and treatment (referred to as the National TB Costing Model). In addition, the XTEND study described previously contained a component to verify modeling and evaluate the cost-effectiveness and impact of the Xpert assay. Early decisions were made on the National TB Costing Model for timing reasons alone.

What did we discover? A model is just that, and flexibility is needed with constant revision and re-evaluation (59, 60). Inputs that are likely to be important include (i) the number of suspects, (ii) background prevalence of TB and MDR-TB, (iii) extent of loss to follow-up, (iv) extent of clinical diagnosis and empirical treatment, (v) costs and models for TB treatment of individuals diagnosed, (vi) costs and models of MDR-TB treatment, (vii) HIV and effects of antiretroviral intervention, (viii) age, and (ix) rates of EPTB. All these inputs need to be placed in the context of the geographical variation that is present. We were able to conclude that mathematical modeling is extremely useful, particularly in resource-constrained settings, but not always accessible. In addition, the introduction of a new intervention stimulated the development and reassessment of national TB costing and model strategies. For purposes of long-term program sustainability and country ownership, increased access to and training with respect to modeling is essential, with limitations being clearly understood (35, 50). Models assisted interac-

tions with the National TB Program, treasury, donors, laboratory services, provincial and district health care workers, and clinicians. The TB investment model is now reaching a greater level of maturity in South Africa, following a great deal of experience gained with the ARV investment model. There are now a number of user-friendly tools available to assist in bridging the gap between scientific evidence and policy (evidence-based decision-making) (60). It is important that programmatic achievements can be tested against modeled projection.

Menzies and colleagues estimated that health system costs would increase by approximately $460,000 over a 10-year period and highlighted substantial additional costs related to the provision of long-term ART to HIV-infected people and treating MDR-TB (52). Langley and colleagues used an integrated model to assess the effects of different algorithms using GeneXpert MTB/RIF and light-emitting diode microscopy in Tanzania (61). Their integrated modeling approach predicted that full rollout of GeneXpert in Tanzania would be cost-effective and has the potential to substantially reduce the national TB burden (62, 63). Like Menzies and colleagues, they also highlighted the substantial level of funding that would be required to translate this into clinical practice. Dowdy and colleagues highlight the need for impact and cost-effectiveness modeling studies to gain further insight into potential impact (63). Collectively, these data using predictive mathematical modeling suggest that Xpert is likely to be cost-effective but accompanied by substantial downstream implementation costs and is also likely to impact disease burden and mortality.

INTERFACE WITH PROCUREMENT, SUPPLIERS, AND SERVICE-LEVEL AGREEMENTS

Procurement strategies were negotiated at a high-level-donor meeting at the time of Xpert MTB/RIF recommendation (21). The agreement was to subsidize the cost of cartridges in the public sector for HBCs at a fixed rate, and then the purchase of analyzers was required. This model of procurement was not standard practice in South Africa, where equipment is generally leased for high-volume assays through strict tender negotiations (64). We are of the impression that this model of purchase is the reason for poorer uptake in many countries because the cost of the analyzers may be prohibitive. The nature of the analyzer where every module is a stand-alone entity, a new molecular design paradigm, also complicates maintenance contracts.

SERIOUS FAILURES IN THE MOLECULAR DIAGNOSTIC ARMAMENTARIUM

Tools for Adequately Confirming First- and Second-Line-Drug Resistance

The status quo for many MDR patients is a severe systemic illness characterized by significant lung damage and high mycobacterial bacillary burden. Early identification and screening may facilitate the detection and allow for a less advanced clinical phenotype to facilitate better treatment outcomes, less transmission, and/or the need for complex MDR preventative treatment regimens (65). Whole-genome sequencing may lead to the next generation of assays to rapidly detect resistance and evaluate transmission patterns (4, 66). Some caution has been expressed by groups highlighting the current limitations of its use in transmission investigation, which include prevalence of TB (likelihood of reinfection, mixed infection), depth of sequencing, and diversity, among others. In addition to whole-genome sequencing, which may have limited access for a time to come due to ongoing developing techniques supported by the appropriate bioinformatics, there are creative, real-time approaches currently under investigation. The molecular characteristics of the Xpert MTB/RIF assay (the cycle threshold value of each hybridization probe), together with GIS mapping of the location where the specimen was received and tested, could be used as a crude epidemiological tool to identify hot spots of TB transmission and changes in patterns of circulating MDR-TB strains (67).

EXPANSION OF THE GeneXpert TECHNOLOGY IN OTHER COUNTRIES

The limitations of many of the studies in resource-limited contexts are that (i) culture is not available to deal with potential misclassifications, (ii) a lack of intensive bacteriological confirmation is common, and (iii) neither Xpert nor sputum microscopy can always be performed with same-day results.

While the Xpert assay appears to have expanded quite rapidly compared to the slow movement of recommendations for prior diagnostic assays, South Africa still purchases almost half the global cartridges. In a recent evaluation, 86% of HBCs had responses to or national plans for the rollout of the Xpert assay. At the time of writing, only four countries (South Africa, Brazil, Russia, and India) recommend Xpert for all presumptive TB cases. For purposes of drug resistance screening, four countries recommend first-line screening using Xpert. The remainder of countries use Xpert largely for diagnosis in HIV-infected patients.

IMPACT

The field of diagnostics is good at validation, monitoring, and assay performance but not very good at measuring impact or outcome because this requires longer-term patient cohorts (frequently a 5- to 10-year lag between introduction of a new diagnostic and its appropriate use in the clinic).

Diagnostic impact can be measured in several ways:

- Classic randomized controlled trials
- Pragmatic trials that aim to assess whether interventions work in settings more appropriate to routine practice (68)
- Implementation setting and resource implications, which are important to consider (69)
- Xpert cost-effectiveness studies, which have generally been favorable. The limitation to much of this work is that it remains based on accuracy and not clinical outcome data (35).

In consideration of the above, empiric treatment is a major factor that may overestimate the population-level effect of new tests such as GeneXpert MTB/RIF. We have previously outlined the relevant considerations in detail (70). To date, study designs evaluating disease burden or outcome have measured variables before and after the introduction of Xpert (prospective cohort design) or used pragmatic or cluster randomized control trial designs. These studies evaluated GeneXpert against the status quo of smear microscopy. Patients for whom smear microscopy was negative were treated empirically, as has been the practice in TB-endemic countries for many decades. Thus, the incremental diagnostic yield of Xpert (which translates into true-positive treatment initiation) is frequently negated by empiric treatment (true- and false-positive treatment initiation) within a few days of a negative smear microscopy result. Often this empirical treatment is either same-day or rapidly instituted. It also needs to be borne in mind that in some subpopulations, such as in HIV-infected individuals, a false-negative Xpert result may erroneously result in the withholding of treatment in someone who would have otherwise received empiric treatment.

Thus, the assumption that the GeneXpert scale-up will have large population-level effects on TB incidence or mortality, over and above smear microscopy, may be heavily compromised by empiric treatment practices in TB-endemic settings. More studies are now needed to accurately assess the impact of new TB tests and the role and drivers of empiric treatment in real-world settings. More data are also required about community-based patient and clinician attitudes to empiric treatment after the introduction of GeneXpert MTB/RIF and about how many false-positive treatments would be tolerated to treat one true-positive or false-negative patient in different clinical settings.

Current Evidence of Impact on Disease Burden and Morbidity

In evaluating whether GeneXpert MTB/RIF is likely to impact TB control and disease burden, it is useful to review the key drivers of TB. The attributable risk of TB due to HIV, biomass fuel exposure, smoking, alcohol abuse, and diabetes is 11%, 22%, 16%, 10%, and 8%, respectively (71). Although difficult to quantify precisely, it is well accepted that poverty and overcrowding, which is a surrogate for poor nutrition, substance abuse, and transmission, is a major driver of TB in addition to lack of an effective vaccine and several health system issues. It is also well known that the majority of transmission occurs several weeks or months prior to diagnosis due to the programmatic practice of passive rather than active case finding. We also know that approximately 30 to 40% of TB remains undiagnosed in the community, and in some settings such as Nigeria up to 80% of this burden remains undiagnosed in a community-based setting (1). Many of these individuals have atypical or minimal symptoms and either never seek health care or seek care some time after developing symptoms. A significant minority of these individuals may be smear positive (30% in the XACT I study performed in Harare and Cape Town; 111). Because the diagnosis by GeneXpert occurs fairly late in the disease cycle, and given the other considerations outlined above including that a diagnostic test does not impact the major drivers of TB, intuitively, it seems that Xpert is likely to have a minimal impact on transmission and, hence, on burden of disease and TB control. Table 3 outlines many of the studies addressing the impact of Xpert on TB control.

Impact on Burden of Disease and Patient-Important Outcomes

The potential impact on cost, program efficacy, and capacity has already been outlined, but impact on disease burden and patient-important outcomes must be discussed. The key objective of any new TB intervention is to impact TB control and patient-important outcomes. For policy makers, public health costs and hence disease burden are important, and the potential of a new intervention to impact disease burden through reduced transmission while also treating larger numbers of patients is attractive. For policy makers, and particularly for patients and their families, reduction in morbidity, organ damage, complication rates, and reduced death are crucial. Intuitively, it could be reasoned that more

rapid diagnosis of TB would result in reduced transmission because of earlier diagnosis. Similarly, earlier diagnosis would reduce cumulative immunopathological and structural lung damage (morbidity) and potentially reduce mortality. On the other hand, it could be argued that a new diagnostic intervention would have minimal impact on disease burden and mortality because most transmission would have occurred prior to diagnosis. Similarly, given the relatively late phase of the disease in which the diagnosis is made, morbidity and mortality reduction may be negligible. However, impact will also depend on the extent to which the time to treatment initiation is shortened within the specific clinical context. For example, subgroups with a poorer prognosis such as HIV-infected people would be perceived to have a greater potential benefit from more rapid diagnosis. Indeed, earlier treatment by even several days may make a difference in those with advanced HIV coinfection. In the case of MDR-TB, for which earlier diagnosis may precede a culture-based diagnosis by several months, earlier diagnosis could potentially have a substantial impact on disease burden, morbidity, and mortality. The equipoise and evidence surrounding these considerations are outlined below.

Current Evidence of the Impact of GeneXpert MTB/RIF on Mortality

In addition to the studies in Table 3, John Metcalfe and colleagues conducted an individual patient data meta-analysis of controlled studies to collectively evaluate the impact of GeneXpert on mortality in the context of passive case finding (preliminary analysis has been published in abstract format as part of conference proceedings) (72). The analysis was conducted in two stages: (i) to rederive effect estimates from the individual patient data for each trial, and (ii) to combine the effect estimates using methods similar to those used for aggregated data. As of the beginning of 2016, 137 publications were screened, of which 10 met the criteria for full publication screening. Five randomized control trials were identified, and four, with 8,567 participants, were included in the final mortality analysis (49, 73–75). In a period-based time-to-event analysis, the rate ratio of mortality in the Xpert versus smear microscopy arm in the aggregated cohort was 0.84 (95% confidence intervals: 0.65 to 1.09; $P = 0.2$). Thus, there was no significant effect of GeneXpert on overall mortality. However, in HIV-infected people the rate ratio was 0.76 (0.6 to 0.97; $P = 0.03$), suggesting that Xpert had a mortality benefit in these patients. Mortality data from the individual studies are outlined in Fig. 4. While three of the four randomized control trials evaluated patients with symptoms presenting to primary care clinics for evaluation, the study by Mupfumi and colleagues evaluated HIV-infected patients who were screened prior to initiating ART (74). Not surprisingly, the most substantial mortality benefit was seen in this population. In summary, the available data suggest that Xpert does not have a mortality benefit, except in HIV-infected people. In the latter subgroup, missing the diagnosis will likely have deleterious consequences over a short-term period of several days to weeks. Thus, introduction of Xpert in HIV-endemic settings is likely to have a significant impact on mortality reduction, but this requires confirmation in larger studies in different settings.

Impact on Outcomes in Drug-Resistant TB

The considerations for drug-resistant TB are substantially different. In the era of smear microscopy, culture-based readouts were generally only requested in endemic countries when patients were failing treatment, and consequently, the diagnosis of MDR-TB or XDR-TB was only made several months later compared to GeneXpert MTB/RIF. Indeed, the introduction of GeneXpert MTB/RIF in South Africa has resulted in a substantial increase in the detection of MDR-TB. For example, in 2013 there were 26,023 laboratory-confirmed rifampin-resistant cases reported in South Africa (76). By contrast, 2 years earlier in 2011 only 10,085 laboratory-confirmed MDR-TB cases were reported. Stagg and coworkers showed a substantially decreased time to treatment initiation for MDR-TB patients based on Xpert MTB/RIF usage (77). Similarly, in Kazakhstan, the time to testing from initiation of MDR treatment was reduced to approximately 1 week (78). In South Africa, from 2003 to 2006, the time to treatment initiation for MDR-TB was on average 71 days (range of 49 to 134 days). Decentralization together with GeneXpert was associated with a reduction in time to treatment initiation to only 7 days in 2013. The authors concluded that Xpert implementation significantly reduced the time to treatment initiation and therefore has the potential to reduce transmission of drug-resistant TB (79).

In a mathematical model evaluating TB transmission, Sachdeva and colleagues found that widespread public sector deployment of a rapid molecular test like GeneXpert MTB/RIF could substantially impact MDR-TB in India and could potentially avert over 180,000 MDR-TB cases between 2015 and 2025 (80). Thus, widespread deployment of Xpert MTB/RIF could have a substantial impact on the MDR epidemic in India. In another modeling study, Salje and coworkers found that access of public sector patients to Xpert MTB/RIF could significantly reduce MDR-TB incidence in India (81). It has also been shown that delayed diagnosis of MDR-TB is associated with higher morbidity and radiographic disease extent (82).

Although there are no published studies, introduction of GeneXpert MTB/RIF is likely to have significant impact on the incidence and burden of MDR-TB and on the morbidity and mortality associated with MDR-TB. Confirmatory evidence is awaited. However, even with the widespread introduction of GeneXpert MTB/RIF, the impact will be limited in the absence of a strategy incorporating active case finding given that approximately 50% or more of MDR-TB cases remain undiagnosed within the community. Thus, the diagnostic gap in MDR-TB is even more substantial than in drug-sensitive TB, and this underscores the need to move toward an active case finding approach for MDR-TB in targeted populations and MDR-TB hotspots. However, the current paradigm for TB diagnosis is one of passive rather than active case finding, and the Xpert assay could have substantial mortality benefits if used in the context of active finding. There are, however, hardly any data about the feasibility and impact of GeneXpert in this context. We await a randomized controlled trial in which community-based participants from Cape Town and Harare with TB symptoms, or HIV coinfection, are screened in community-based congregate settings (e.g., outside shopping centers etc.) using sputum induction-equipped mobile clinics staffed by three health care workers (Calligaro and Dheda, submitted). Making the Xpert MTB/RIF assay even more mobile with implementation options such as the Xpert Omni could further revolutionize TB control measures and impact patient care.

WHAT DOES THE FUTURE HOLD?

It is important to stress that health systems strengthening is essential to optimize the impact of GeneXpert testing. For example, of 320 patients microbiologically proven (based on culture and Xpert) to have MDR-TB in Kwazulu-Natal, South Africa, 16% were untraceable, 40% were initiated on treatment after 1 month, 21% after 2 months, 8% after 3 months, and 3% were never initiated on treatment (83). Future directions include reassessing the impact of Xpert in the context of active case finding.

The new Xpert ULTRA cartridge, which uses higher-resolution melt detection technology, is being marketed as a slightly more sensitive and specific assay, though clinical trial data are awaited in 2016. This will complement the release of a single-cartridge-use point-of-care

Table 3 GeneXpert impact on treatment outcomes: review of studies

Authors	Setting[a]	Impact on time to treatment (TTT)	Impact on treatment	Key outcome
Hanrahan et al. (86)	Uganda, 8 onsite and 10 offsite Xpert facilities, routine TB testing facilities	Not significant	Not significant because many patients were empirically treated; no difference in TTT	Xpert highly underutilized, indicating that new programs require ongoing support at all levels to impact on patient health
Opota et al. (87)	Switzerland, Lausanne University Hospital, TB laboratory (retrospective)	Faster than culture	Semiquantitative Xpert results allowed for faster and more accurate patient management	In low-prevalence settings, Xpert impacts positively on patient management
Stagg et al. (77)	Latvia, MDR-TB surveillance data (retrospective)	Significant decrease (MDR-TB)	Median delay to MDR-TB treatment was 6 days for patients who tested RIF-positive with Xpert and 40 days for those without Xpert testing. NB: for 12% of patients with negative RIF result, MDR-TB treatment lagged to a median of 57 days	Xpert decreases TTT for patients with RIF-resistant MDR-TB
Mbonze et al. (88)	Kinshasa, Democratic Republic of Congo	Not discussed	Not significant	Xpert as a follow-up to smear microscopy did not significantly increase case notification
Churchyard et al. (49)	South Africa, 20 laboratories in medium-burden districts (XTEND study)	No difference	No significant difference in the proportion of patients treated for TB in microscopy and Xpert arms (10.8% vs. 12.5%)	No difference in mortality at 6 months (3.9% for Xpert vs. 5% for microscopy)
Lorent et al. (89)	Cambodia, referral hospital	Significant decrease (MDR-TB)	Presumptive screening enabled more rapid diagnosis (2 days with Xpert vs. 8 with confirmatory LPA) and treatment of MDR-TB	More rapid diagnosis and treatment of MDR-TB; confirmatory LPA testing added little to clinical decisions
Schumacher et al. (90)	India, tertiary hospital, POC vs. routine laboratory Xpert	Decreased at POC	Only 6% incremental value of one Xpert vs. two smears for diagnosis → treatment	Xpert at POC reduced time to diagnosis to 5.5 days; no difference in time in routine laboratory (vs. smear microscopy)
Van Kampen et al. (91)	Kazakhstan	Significant reduction in time to both first- and second-line treatment (MDR-TB)	Patients treated more rapidly for MDR-TB using Xpert results	TTT for MDR-TB was reduced to ~1 week with Xpert
Hanrahan et al. (92)	South Africa, primary care clinic	Decreased at POC	Treatment started at a median of 0 vs. 5 days for POC Xpert-positive, but empiric treatment resulted in no difference in treated numbers	Positive Xpert at POC led to increased treatment of confirmed TB, but samples sent to laboratory increased empirical treatment
Cox et al. (79)	South Africa, Khayelitsha decentralized RIF-R TB care program (retrospective)	Significant decrease (MDR-TB)	No significant change in treatment initiation with use of Xpert, but treatment could be started after 8 rather than 40 days (time at initial decentralization)	Xpert significantly decreased TTT and has potential to decrease transmission of TB/MDR-TB. Decentralization of services is important
Manabe et al. (93)	Uganda, 10 intervention mid-level facilities	Not discussed	More patients started on treatment, more patients completed treatment, fewer patients lost to follow-up using the bundled (fluorescent microscopy and Xpert) diagnostics at mid-level centers. Xpert only used for 6 months of study; further evaluation required	Decentralization of services to mid-level providers has a positive impact on TB treatment and prevention; further Xpert studies needed, particularly with stock-outs and interrupted electricity

Study	Setting	TTT	Treatment initiation	Findings
Sachdeva et al. (94)	India, 14 subdistrict TB treatment units	Not discussed	Decreased proportion of clinically diagnosed cases when Xpert is positive, negating need for antibiotic trial in these patients. Bacteriological confirmation and RIF-sensitivity results were available sooner	First-line MTB/RIF increased confirmed TB case notification by 39% and increased RIF-resistant TB case notification 5-fold. Xpert could potentially avert >180,000 MDR-TB cases by 2025
Trajman et al. (95)	Brazil	Not discussed	No impact on successful treatment or loss to follow-up	Xpert implementation resulted in a 35% decrease in TB-related mortality but did not increase treatment completion or decrease loss to follow-up
Cresswell et al. (96)	Nepal, 16 districts (TB case finding)	Not discussed	Reduced empirical treatment of smear-negative TB; almost doubled treatment initiation for MDR-TB	Bacteriologically confirmed TB notifications increased, but PTB notifications decreased due to less empirical treatment. Significant increase in MDR-TB treatment initiation
Van Den Handel et al. (97)	Central Karoo, South Africa (one site SOC, one centralized Xpert, one decentralized Xpert)	Fastest using decentralized Xpert	Reduced time to treatment initiation (1 day with POC, 6 days with centralized Xpert, and 11.5 days with SOC)	In remote areas, initial diagnosis with Xpert increases proportion of bacteriologically confirmed cases and decreases TTT, but it was cautioned that POC placement may have reduced the numbers of people tested
Alvarez et al. (98)	Canada, remote area (high TB prevalence in selected population)	Significantly shortened	Treatment initiation at 1.8 days vs. 7.7 days (smear-positive) or 37.1 days (smear-negative)	In remote areas with high TB burden and no TB facilities, onsite Xpert shortened TTT
Moyenga et al. (99)	Burkina Faso (centralized Xpert)	Shortened	Shortened TTT in TB centers	Xpert impacts positively on patients in TB treatment centers but not in other facilities, indicating that increased service coordination is needed
Mupfumi et al. (74)	Harare, Zimbabwe, Beatrice Road Infectious Diseases Hospital	No difference between FM and Xpert	No difference in treatment initiation times or numbers because most patients were treated empirically	With empirical treatment prevalent, there was no difference in treatment initiation. No differences between FM and Xpert for diagnosis
Durovni et al. (100)	Brazil, 14 primary care laboratories in 2 cities, enrolling ~24,000 patients	Shortened	Treatment was initiated earlier, with RIF sensitivity information	Shorter TTT and increased PTB confirmation, but no difference in overall notification rates (empirical treatment)
Cox et al. (101)	Khayelitsha, South Africa, large primary health care center	Shortened	Proportionally more patients, notably HIV-positive patients, initiated on treatment in the Xpert vs. smear arm. Proportion of patients treated without confirmed PTB was halved	Increased treatment of confirmed PTB by 3 months and decreased TTT, especially in HIV-positive patients, but potential confounders were present
Chaisson et al. (102)	U.S., San Francisco General Hospital	Shortened	Patients could be treated earlier, but more significantly, up to 35 days of isolation could be avoided after a negative Xpert result	Replacing serial sputum smear microscopy with a single sputum Xpert could eliminate most unnecessary isolation
Davis et al. (103)	San Francisco, U.S., Department of Public Health TB Clinic	Shortened	Hypothetical 94% reduction in overtreatment (unnecessary empirical treatment)	Reduced overtreatment with negative impact on early TB detection. Similar benefits projected for contact investigations
Theron et al. (70)		Not discussed		No difference in morbidity

(Continued)

Table 3   GeneXpert impact on treatment outcomes: review of studies *(Continued)*

Authors	Setting[a]	Impact on time to treatment (TTT)	Impact on treatment	Key outcome
Ramirez et al. (104)	**Four African countries (controlled study: TB-NEAT)**		Minimal: by day 56, 42% of patients in smear arm initiated on treatment vs. 43% of patients in Xpert arm	Positive Xpert results led to shorter treatment initiation delays and may assist in breaking the transmission chain
	Oviedo, Spain, Hospital Universitario Central de Asturias	Significantly shortened	Xpert enabled same-day diagnosis and rapid treatment initiation in 67% of smear-negative patients	
Balcha et al. (105)	**Ethiopia, all centers providing ART in Adama Town**	Significantly shortened	Xpert-positive, smear-negative HIV-positive patients accessed treatment faster, but there was no difference in 2-month mortality	Xpert increased TB detection, particularly in patients with advanced immunosuppression
Omrani et al. (106)	Saudi Arabia, single, large, tertiary center, retrospective review	No difference vs. smear	Very limited impact	Xpert was underutilized for patient management. Further investigations on use of testing all smear-negatives warranted
Sohn et al. (107)	Canada, Montreal Chest Hospital Tuberculosis Clinic	Not significant	Very little difference in treatment initiation time within the current routine diagnostics	Limited impact in low-incidence, high-resource setting
Al-Darraji (108)	Malaysia, Kajang Prison (HIV, prisoners)	Not described	Increased detection of active TB at an early stage of disease → earlier treatment	Increased active TB detection by single Xpert (vs. smear microscopy). Sensitivity still low (53.3%) in HIV-infected people, indicating intensified screening protocols are warranted
Theron et al. (109)	**South Africa**	Significantly shortened	Increased detection of TB using bronchoalveolar lavage fluid and decreased empirical treatment	Xpert outperformed smear microscopy; Xpert using bronchoalveolar lavage fluid decreased empirical treatment
Hanrahan et al. (110)	**Johannesburg, South Africa, Witkoppen Health and Welfare Center**	Significantly shortened	Same-day treatment initiation for Xpert-positive patients (<50% of all patients started on treatment)	Single Xpert had no impact on treatment initiation or mortality in a high HIV-positive cohort
Yoon et al. (36)	Kampala, Uganda, Mugalo Hospital	No difference	Earlier detection, but not earlier treatment	More accurate TB diagnosis with Xpert, but no difference in TTT or 2-month mortality
Menzies et al. (52)	Dynamic modeling of TB in Botswana, Lesotho, Namibia, South Africa, and Swaziland	Not applicable	Not applicable	Estimated that Xpert implementation could reduce TB morbidity and mortality, but only modestly reduce TB incidence

[a]Boldface indicates areas of high TB prevalence.

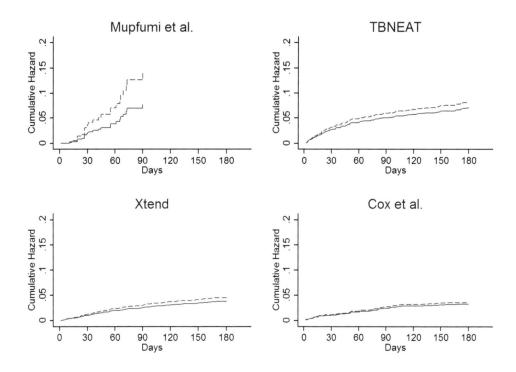

Figure 4 Cumulative risk curves based on Cox models using individual patient data for the key randomized control trials evaluating mortality associated with GeneXpert compared to smear microscopy.

(POC) version of the GeneXpert assay called the Xpert Omni, which is anticipated in mid-2017, with the idea that Xpert Omni could be placed within primary care TB clinics at the POC to minimize patient drop-out (test-positive patients not returning to initiate treatment). In the TB-NEAT study we found that POC GeneXpert within the clinic significantly reduced drop-out (75). However, if Xpert Omni is situated at the POC, several technical and logistical issues will need to be addressed including funding streams, quality control, space requirements, human resources and training, patient workflow, and systems to integrate test readouts with patient recall. Furthermore, several other POC molecular diagnostic platforms are currently in development (see Table 1) (84). However, the real attractiveness of POC systems is their ability to facilitate active case finding.

In addition to these Xpert developments is the development of an XDR cartridge, which would incorporate genotypic resistance readouts for isoniazid, the aminoglycosides, and fluoroquinolones. This is anticipated to be an immediate rule-in test to provide direction to clinicians for therapy toward either pre-XDR (fluoroquinolone- or aminoglycoside-resistant MDR-TB) or XDR-TB. How-

ever, this tool will not individualize or optimize therapy for MDR-TB, for which the successful treatment outcome rate is only ~50% (1), and developments will be required for newer and repurposed drugs that are becoming available (85). The advent of next-generation whole-genome sequencing is now available to the clinical laboratory and can enable such a strategy. However, the impact and feasibility of such a strategy as well as processing directly off sputum will need to be proven as well as models for implementation at national levels.

CONCLUSION

Ultimately, a change in health systems functioning and quality, poverty alleviation, and political will will be required for any new tool to have a substantial impact and to meet the goals of the WHO END-TB strategy. Thus, greater emphasis and resources need to be channeled toward training health care workers, better drug availability, patient retention, improvement of laboratory infrastructure, and so forth, all interlinking to improve program efficiency. Diagnostics can only be effective if other components of the health care system are functional and working efficiently. Alleviation of global poverty and overcrowding, and political will, are critical because diagnostic tools on their own will have little impact if these factors, including other major drivers of TB (smoking, diabetes, use of biomass fuels, etc.), are not addressed.

Acknowledgments. We wish to thank Dr. Leigh Berrie and the National Priority Program staff of the NHLS.

Citation. Stevens WS, Scott L, Noble L, Gous N, Dheda K. 2017. Impact of the GeneXpert MTB/RIF technology on tuberculosis control. Microbiol Spectrum 5(1):TBTB2-0040-2016.

References

1. World Health Organization. 2015. *Global Tuberculosis Report*. World Health Organization, Geneva, Switzerland.

2. World Health Organization. 2013. *Global Tuberculosis Report*. World Health Organization, Geneva, Switzerland.

3. World Health Organization. 2014. *WHO End TB Strategy*. World Health Organization, Geneva, Switzerland.

4. Abubakar I, Lipman M, McHugh TD, Fletcher H. 2016. Uniting to end the TB epidemic: advances in disease control from prevention to better diagnosis and treatment. *BMC Med* 14:47

5. Kranzer K, Houben RM, Glynn JR, Bekker LG, Wood R, Lawn SD. 2010. Yield of HIV-associated tuberculosis during intensified case finding in resource-limited settings: a systematic review and meta-analysis. *Lancet Infect Dis* 10:93–102.

6. Apers L, Mutsvangwa J, Magwenzi J, Chigara N, Butterworth A, Mason P, Van der Stuyft P. 2003. A comparison of direct microscopy, the concentration method and the Mycobacteria Growth Indicator Tube for the examination of sputum for acid-fast bacilli. *Int J Tuberc Lung Dis* 7:376–381.

7. Cattamanchi A, Dowdy DW, Davis JL, Worodria W, Yoo S, Joloba M, Matovu J, Hopewell PC, Huang L. 2009. Sensitivity of direct versus concentrated sputum smear microscopy in HIV-infected patients suspected of having pulmonary tuberculosis. *BMC Infect Dis* 9:53

8. Crampin AC, Floyd S, Mwaungulu F, Black G, Ndhlovu R, Mwaiyeghele E, Glynn JR, Warndorff DK, Fine PE. 2001. Comparison of two versus three smears in identifying culture-positive tuberculosis patients in a rural African setting with high HIV prevalence. *Int J Tuberc Lung Dis* 5:994–999.

9. Scott CP, Dos Anjos Filho L, De Queiroz Mello FC, Thornton CG, Bishai WR, Fonseca LS, Kritski AL, Chaisson RE, Manabe YC. 2002. Comparison of C (18)-carboxypropylbetaine and standard N-acetyl-L-cysteine-NaOH processing of respiratory specimens for increasing tuberculosis smear sensitivity in Brazil. *J Clin Microbiol* 40:3219–3222.

10. Selvakumar N, Rahman F, Garg R, Rajasekaran S, Mohan NS, Thyagarajan K, Sundaram V, Santha T, Frieden TR, Narayanan PR. 2002. Evaluation of the phenol ammonium sulfate sedimentation smear microscopy method for diagnosis of pulmonary tuberculosis. *J Clin Microbiol* 40:3017–3020.

11. Swai HF, Mugusi FM, Mbwambo JK. 2011. Sputum smear negative pulmonary tuberculosis: sensitivity and specificity of diagnostic algorithm. *BMC Res Notes* 4:475.

12. World Health Organization. 2010. *Policy Framework for Implementing New Tuberculosis Diagnostics*. World Health Organization, Geneva, Switzerland.

13. Anderson ST, Kaforou M, Brent AJ, Wright VJ, Banwell CM, Chagaluka G, Crampin AC, Dockrell HM, French N, Hamilton MS, Hibberd ML, Kern F, Langford PR, Ling L, Mlotha R, Ottenhoff TH, Pienaar S, Pillay V, Scott JA, Twahir H, Wilkinson RJ, Coin LJ, Heyderman RS, Levin M, Eley B, ILULU Consortium, KIDS TB Study Group. 2014. Diagnosis of childhood tuberculosis and host RNA expression in Africa. *N Engl J Med* 370:1712–1723.

14. Black A. 2013. A new algorithm for the diagnosis of all forms of tuberculosis is required for South Africa. *S Afr Med J* 103:355–356.

15. Jönsson B, Lönnermark E, Ridell M. 2015. Evaluation of the Cobas TaqMan MTB test for detection of *Mycobacterium tuberculosis* complex. *Infect Dis (Lond)* 47:231–236.

16. Lee MR, Chung KP, Wang HC, Lin CB, Yu CJ, Lee JJ, Hsueh PR. 2013. Evaluation of the Cobas TaqMan MTB real-time PCR assay for direct detection of *Mycobacterium tuberculosis* in respiratory specimens. *J Med Microbiol* 62:1160–1164.

17. Dalovisio JR, Montenegro-James S, Kemmerly SA, Genre CF, Chambers R, Greer D, Pankey GA, Failla DM, Haydel KG, Hutchinson L, Lindley MF, Nunez BM, Praba A, Eisenach KD, Cooper ES. 1996. Comparison of the amplified *Mycobacterium tuberculosis* (MTB) direct test, Amplicor MTB PCR, and IS6110-PCR for detection of MTB in respiratory specimens. *Clin Infect Dis* 23:1099–1106, discussion 1107–1108.

18. Wang JY, Lee LN, Chou CS, Huang CY, Wang SK, Lai HC, Hsueh PR, Luh KT. 2004. Performance assessment of a nested-PCR assay (the RAPID BAP-MTB) and the BD ProbeTec ET system for detection of *Mycobacterium tuberculosis* in clinical specimens. *J Clin Microbiol* 42:4599–4603.

19. Scott LE, McCarthy K, Gous N, Nduna M, Van Rie A, Sanne I, Venter WF, Duse A, Stevens W. 2011. Comparison of Xpert MTB/RIF with other nucleic acid technologies for diagnosing pulmonary tuberculosis in a high HIV prevalence setting: a prospective study. *PLoS Med* 8:e1001061.

20. World Health Organization. 2008. *Molecular line probe assays for rapid screening of patients at risk of multidrug-resistant tuberculosis (MDR-TB)*. World Health Organization, Geneva, Switzerland.

21. World Health Organization. 2010. WHO endorses new rapid tuberculosis test. A major milestone for global TB diagnosis and care. http://www.who.int/mediacentre/news/releases/2010/tb_test_20101208/en/.

22. Barnard M, Gey van Pittius NC, van Helden PD, Bosman M, Coetzee G, Warren RM. 2012. The diagnostic performance of the GenoType MTBDRplus version 2 line probe assay is equivalent to that of the Xpert MTB/RIF assay. *J Clin Microbiol* 50:3712–3716.

23. Crudu V, Stratan E, Romancenco E, Allerheiligen V, Hillemann A, Moraru N. 2012. First evaluation of an improved assay for molecular genetic detection of tuberculosis as well as rifampin and isoniazid resistances. *J Clin Microbiol* **50:**1264–1269.

24. Matabane MM, Ismail F, Strydom KA, Onwuegbuna O, Omar SV, Ismail N. 2015. Performance evaluation of three commercial molecular assays for the detection of *Mycobacterium tuberculosis* from clinical specimens in a high TB-HIV-burden setting. *BMC Infect Dis* **15:**508.

25. Theron G, Peter J, Richardson M, Barnard M, Donegan S, Warren R, Steingart KR, Dheda K. 2014. The diagnostic accuracy of the GenoType() MTBDRsl assay for the detection of resistance to second-line anti-tuberculosis drugs. *Cochrane Database Syst Rev* (10):CD010705 10.1002/14651858.CD010705.pub2:CD010705.

26. Brossier F, Guindo D, Pham A, Reibel F, Sougakoff W, Veziris N, Aubry A. 2016. Performance of the new version (v2.0) of the GenoType MTBDRsl test for detection of resistance to second-line drugs in multidrug-resistant *Mycobacterium tuberculosis* complex strains. *J Clin Microbiol* **54:**1573–1580.

27. Tagliani E, Cabibbe AM, Miotto P, Borroni E, Toro JC, Mansjö M, Hoffner S, Hillemann D, Zalutskaya A, Skrahina A, Cirillo DM. 2015. Diagnostic performance of the new version (v2.0) of GenoType MTBDRsl assay for detection of resistance to fluoroquinolones and second-line injectable drugs: a multicenter study. *J Clin Microbiol* **53:**2961–2969.

28. World Health Organization. 2016. *The Use of Molecular Line Probe Assays for the Detection of Resistance to Second-Line Anti-Tuberculosis Drugs.* World Health Organization, Geneva, Switzerland.

29. UNITAID. 2015. *Tuberculosis Diagnostics Technology and Market Landscape.* World Health Organization, Geneva, Switzerland.

30. World Health Organization. 2011. *Policy Statement: Automated Real-Time Nucleic Acid Amplification Technology for Rapid and Simultaneous Detection of Tuberculosis and Rifampicin Resistance: Xpert MTB/RIF System.* World Health Organization, Geneva, Switzerland.

31. Lawn SD, Nicol MP. 2011. Xpert MTB/RIF assay: development, evaluation and implementation of a new rapid molecular diagnostic for tuberculosis and rifampicin resistance. *Future Microbiol* **6:**1067–1082.

32. O'Grady J, Bates M, Chilukutu L, Mzyece J, Cheelo B, Chilufya M, Mukonda L, Mumba M, Tembo J, Chomba M, Kapata N, Maeurer M, Rachow A, Clowes P, Hoelscher M, Mwaba P, Zumla A. 2012. Evaluation of the Xpert MTB/RIF assay at a tertiary care referral hospital in a setting where tuberculosis and HIV infection are highly endemic. *Clin Infect Dis* **55:**1171–1178.

33. Steingart KR, Sohn H, Schiller I, Kloda LA, Boehme CC, Pai M, Dendukuri N. 2013. Xpert MTB/RIF assay for pulmonary tuberculosis and rifampicin resistance in adults. *Cochrane Database Syst Rev* (1):CD009593 10.1002/14651858.CD009593.pub2:CD009593.

34. Theron G, Peter J, van Zyl-Smit R, Mishra H, Streicher E, Murray S, Dawson R, Whitelaw A, Hoelscher M,

Sharma S, Pai M, Warren R, Dheda K. 2011. Evaluation of the Xpert MTB/RIF assay for the diagnosis of pulmonary tuberculosis in a high HIV prevalence setting. *Am J Respir Crit Care Med* **184:**132–140.

35. Vassall A, van Kampen S, Sohn H, Michael JS, John KR, den Boon S, Davis JL, Whitelaw A, Nicol MP, Gler MT, Khaliqov A, Zamudio C, Perkins MD, Boehme CC, Cobelens F. 2011. Rapid diagnosis of tuberculosis with the Xpert MTB/RIF assay in high burden countries: a cost-effectiveness analysis. *PLoS Med* **8:**e1001120.

36. Yoon C, Cattamanchi A, Davis JL, Worodria W, den Boon S, Kalema N, Katagira W, Kaswabuli S, Miller C, Andama A, Albert H, Nabeta P, Gray C, Ayakaka I, Huang L. 2012. Impact of Xpert MTB/RIF testing on tuberculosis management and outcomes in hospitalized patients in Uganda. *PLoS One* **7:**e48599.

37. Stevens WS, Cunningham B, Cassim N, Gous N, Scott L. 2016. Cloud-based surveillance, connectivity, and distribution of the GeneXpert analyzers for diagnosis of tuberculosis (TB) and multiple-drug-resistant TB in South Africa. *In* Persing DH (ed), *Molecular Microbiology: Diagnostic Principles and Practice*, 3rd ed. ASM Press, Washington DC.

38. World Health Organization. 2013. *Xpert MTB/RIF Assay for the Diagnosis of Pulmonary and Extrapulmonary TB in Adults and Children. Policy update.* World Health Organization, Geneva, Switzerland.

39. South African National Department of Health. 2014. *National Department of Health Annual Performance Plan 2014/15-2016/17.* http://www.hst.org.za/publications/national-department-health-annual-performance-plan-201415-201617.

40. Directorate Drug-Resistant TB TB and HIV. 2011. *Management of Drug-Resistant Tuberculosis: Policy Guidelines.* http://www.hst.org.za/publications/management-drug-resistant-tuberculosis-policy-guidelines.

41. Nhu NT, Ha DT, Anh ND, Thu DD, Duong TN, Quang ND, Lan NT, Quyet TV, Tuyen NT, Ha VT, Giang DC, Dung NH, Wolbers M, Farrar J, Caws M. 2013. Evaluation of Xpert MTB/RIF and MODS assay for the diagnosis of pediatric tuberculosis. *BMC Infect Dis* **13:**31.

42. Stevens WS, Marshall TM. 2010. Challenges in implementing HIV load testing in South Africa. *J Infect Dis* **201**(Suppl 1):S78–S84.

43. Qin ZZ, Pai M, Van Gemert W, Sahu S, Ghiasi M, Creswell J. 2015. How is Xpert MTB/RIF being implemented in 22 high tuberculosis burden countries? *Eur Respir J* **45:**549–554.

44. UNAIDS. 2013. *South Africa: HIV and AIDS estimates 2013.* http://www.unaids.org/en/regionscountries/countries/southafrica.

45. Nicol MP. 2013. Xpert MTB/RIF: monitoring response to tuberculosis treatment. *Lancet Respir Med* **1:**427–428.

46. Schnippel K, Meyer-Rath G, Long L, Stevens WS, Sanne I, Rosen S. 2013. Diagnosing Xpert MTB/RIF negative TB: impact and cost of alternative algorithms for South Africa. *S Afr Med J* **103:**101–106.

47. **South African National AIDS Council.** 2016. *South African HIV and TB Investment Case Phase 1 Reference Report.* Department of Health, South Africa.

48. **National Health Laboratory Service.** 2014. *GeneXpert MTB/RIF progress report to the National Department of Health.* http://www.nhls.ac.za/assets/files/GeneXpert%20Progress%20Report%20July%202014_Final.pdf.

49. **Churchyard GJ, Stevens WS, Mametja LD, McCarthy KM, Chihota V, Nicol MP, Erasmus LK, Ndjeka NO, Mvusi L, Vassall A, Sinanovic E, Cox HS, Dye C, Grant AD, Fielding KL.** 2015. Xpert MTB/RIF versus sputum microscopy as the initial diagnostic test for tuberculosis: a cluster-randomised trial embedded in South African roll-out of Xpert MTB/RIF. *Lancet Glob Health* **3:** e450–e457.

50. **Houben RM, Lalli M, Sumner T, Hamilton M, Pedrazzoli D, Bonsu F, Hippner P, Pillay Y, Kimerling M, Ahmedov S, Pretorius C, White RG.** 2016. TIME Impact: a new user-friendly tuberculosis (TB) model to inform TB policy decisions. *BMC Med* **14:**56

51. **Basu S, Andrews JR, Poolman EM, Gandhi NR, Shah NS, Moll A, Moodley P, Galvani AP, Friedland GH.** 2007. Prevention of nosocomial transmission of extensively drug-resistant tuberculosis in rural South African district hospitals: an epidemiological modelling study. *Lancet* **370:**1500–1507.

52. **Menzies NA, Cohen T, Lin HH, Murray M, Salomon JA.** 2012. Population health impact and cost-effectiveness of tuberculosis diagnosis with Xpert MTB/RIF: a dynamic simulation and economic evaluation. *PLoS Med* **9:** e1001347

53. **Uplekar M.** 2015. Implementing the End TB Strategy: well begun will be half done. *Indian J Tuberc* **62:**61–63.

54. **Rufai SB, Kumar P, Singh A, Prajapati S, Balooni V, Singh S.** 2014. Comparison of Xpert MTB/RIF with line probe assay for detection of rifampin-monoresistant *Mycobacterium tuberculosis. J Clin Microbiol* **52:** 1846–1852.

55. **Sanchez-Padilla E, Merker M, Beckert P, Jochims F, Dlamini T, Kahn P, Bonnet M, Niemann S.** 2015. Detection of drug-resistant tuberculosis by Xpert MTB/RIF in Swaziland. *N Engl J Med* **372:**1181–1182.

56. **Theron G, Jenkins HE, Cobelens F, Abubakar I, Khan AJ, Cohen T, Dowdy DW.** 2015. Data for action: collection and use of local data to end tuberculosis. *Lancet* **386:**2324–2333.

57. **Scott L, Albert H, Gilpin C, Alexander H, DeGruy K, Stevens W.** 2014. Multicenter feasibility study to assess external quality assessment panels for Xpert MTB/RIF assay in South Africa. *J Clin Microbiol* **52:**2493–2499.

58. **Scott LE, Gous N, Cunningham BE, Kana BD, Perovic O, Erasmus L, Coetzee GJ, Koornhof H, Stevens W.** 2011. Dried culture spots for Xpert MTB/RIF external quality assessment: results of a phase 1 pilot study in South Africa. *J Clin Microbiol* **49:**4356–4360.

59. **Garnett GP, Cousens S, Hallett TB, Steketee R, Walker N.** 2011. Mathematical models in the evaluation of health programmes. *Lancet* **378:**515–525.

60. **Knight GM, Dharan NJ, Fox GJ, Stennis N, Zwerling A, Khurana R, Dowdy DW.** 2016. Bridging the gap

between evidence and policy for infectious diseases: how models can aid public health decision-making. *Int J Infect Dis* **42:**17–23.

61. **Langley I, Lin HH, Egwaga S, Doulla B, Ku CC, Murray M, Cohen T, Squire SB.** 2014. Assessment of the patient, health system, and population effects of Xpert MTB/RIF and alternative diagnostics for tuberculosis in Tanzania: an integrated modelling approach. *Lancet Glob Health* **2:**e581–e591.

62. **Dheda K, Theron G, Welte A.** 2014. Cost-effectiveness of Xpert MTB/RIF and investing in health care in Africa. *Lancet Glob Health* **2:**e554–e556.

63. **Dowdy DW, Houben R, Cohen T, Pai M, Cobelens F, Vassall A, Menzies NA, Gomez GB, Langley I, Squire SB, White R, TB MAC meeting participants.** 2014. Impact and cost-effectiveness of current and future tuberculosis diagnostics: the contribution of modelling. *Int J Tuberc Lung Dis* **18:**1012–1018.

64. **World Health Organization.** 2014. *WHO Monitoring of Xpert MTB/RIF Rollout.* World Health Organization, Geneva, Switzerland.

65. **Moore DA.** 2016. What can we offer to 3 million MDRTB household contacts in 2016? *BMC Med* **14:**64

66. **Witney AA, Cosgrove CA, Arnold A, Hinds J, Stoker NG, Butcher PD.** 2016. Clinical use of whole genome sequencing for *Mycobacterium tuberculosis. BMC Med* **14:**46

67. **Scott L, Schnippel K, Ncayiyana J, Berrie L, Berhanu R, Van Rie A.** 2015. The use of national Xpert MTB/RIF's cycle threshold (Ct) as an audit indicator for program and laboratory performance. 46th Union World Conference on Lung Health. Cape Town, South Africa. 2–6 December 2015.

68. **Bratton DJ, Nunn AJ.** 2011. Alternative approaches to tuberculosis treatment evaluation: the role of pragmatic trials. *Int J Tuberc Lung Dis* **15:**440–446.

69. **Luoto J, Maglione MA, Johnsen B, Chang C, Higgs ES, Perry T, Shekelle PG.** 2013. A comparison of frameworks evaluating evidence for global health interventions. *PLoS Med* **10:**e1001469

70. **Theron G, Peter J, Dowdy D, Langley I, Squire SB, Dheda K.** 2014. Do high rates of empirical treatment undermine the potential effect of new diagnostic tests for tuberculosis in high-burden settings? *Lancet Infect Dis* **14:**527–532.

71. **Dheda K, Barry CE III, Maartens G.** 2016. Tuberculosis. *Lancet* **387:**1211–1226.

72. **Luca Di Tanna G, Theron G, McCarthy K, Cox H, Mupfumil L, Sohn A, Weyer K, Zijenah L, Mason P, Hoelscher M, Clowes P, Mangu C, Chanda D, Pym A, Mwaba P, Khaki AR, Cobelens F, Nicol K, Dheda K, Churchyard G, Fielding K, Metcalfe J.** 2015. The effect of nucleic acid amplification assays on patient important outcomes in routine care settings: meta-analysis of individual participant data. 46th Union World Conference on Lung Health. Cape Town, South Africa. 2–6 December 2015.

73. **Cox H, McDermid C.** 2008. XDR tuberculosis can be cured with aggressive treatment. *Lancet* **372:**1363–1365.

74. Mupfumi L, Makamure B, Chirehwa M, Sagonda T, Zinyowera S, Mason P, Metcalfe JZ, Mutetwa R. 2014. Impact of Xpert MTB/RIF on antiretroviral therapy-associated tuberculosis and mortality: a pragmatic randomized controlled trial. *Open Forum Infect Dis* **1**: ofu038

75. Theron G, Zijenah L, Chanda D, Clowes P, Rachow A, Lesosky M, Bara W, Mungofa S, Pai M, Hoelscher M, Dowdy D, Pym A, Mwaba P, Mason P, Peter J, Dheda K. 2013. Feasibility, accuracy, and clinical effect of point-of-care Xpert MTB/RIF testing for tuberculosis in primary-care settings in Africa: a multicentre, randomised, controlled trial. *Lancet* **383**:424–435 10.1016/S0140-6736(13)62073-5.

76. World Health Organization. 2014. *Global Tuberculosis Report*. World Health Organization, Geneva, Switzerland.

77. Stagg HR, White PJ, Riekstiņa V, Cīrule A, Šķenders Ģ, Leimane V, Kuksa L, Dravniece G, Brown J, Jackson C. 2016. Decreased time to treatment initiation for multidrug-resistant tuberculosis patients after use of Xpert MTB/RIF test, Latvia. *Emerg Infect Dis* **22**: 482–490.

78. van Kampen SC, Susanto NH, Simon S, Astiti SD, Chandra R, Burhan E, Farid MN, Chittenden K, Mustikawati DE, Alisjahbana B. 2015. Effects of introducing Xpert MTB/RIF on diagnosis and treatment of drug-resistant tuberculosis patients in Indonesia: a pre-post intervention study. *PLoS One* **10**:e0123536.

79. Cox HS, Daniels JF, Muller O, Nicol MP, Cox V, van Cutsem G, Moyo S, De Azevedo V, Hughes J. 2015. Impact of decentralized care and the Xpert MTB/RIF test on rifampicin-resistant tuberculosis treatment initiation in Khayelitsha, South Africa. *Open Forum Infect Dis* **2**:ofv014.

80. Sachdeva KS, Raizada N, Gupta RS, Nair SA, Denkinger C, Paramasivan CN, Kulsange S, Thakur R, Dewan P, Boehme C, Arinaminpathy N. 2015. The potential impact of up-front drug sensitivity testing on India's epidemic of multi-drug resistant tuberculosis. *PLoS One* **10**:e0131438.

81. Salje H, Andrews JR, Deo S, Satyanarayana S, Sun AY, Pai M, Dowdy DW. 2014. The importance of implementation strategy in scaling up Xpert MTB/RIF for diagnosis of tuberculosis in the Indian health-care system: a transmission model. *PLoS Med* **11**:e1001674.

82. Singla N, Singla R, Fernandes S, Behera D. 2009. Post treatment sequelae of multi-drug resistant tuberculosis patients. *Indian J Tuberc* **56**:206–212.

83. Dlamini-Mvelase NR, Werner L, Phili R, Cele LP, Mlisana KP. 2014. Effects of introducing Xpert MTB/RIF test on multi-drug resistant tuberculosis diagnosis in KwaZulu-Natal South Africa. *BMC Infect Dis* **14**:442

84. UNITAID. 2014. *Tuberculosis diagnostic technology landscape*. World Health Organization, Geneva, Switzerland. http://unitaid.org/images/marketdynamics/publications/UNITAID_TB_Diagnostics_Landscape_3rd-edition.pdf.

85. World Health Organization. 2016. *WHO Treatment Guidelines for Drug-Resistant Tuberculosis: 2016 Update*. World Health Organization, Geneva, Switzerland.

86. Hanrahan CF, Haguma P, Ochom E, Kinera I, Cobelens F, Cattamanchi A, Davis L, Katamba A, Dowdy D. 2016. Implementation of Xpert MTB/RIF in Uganda: missed opportunities to improve diagnosis of tuberculosis. *Open Forum Infect Dis* **3**:ofw068

87. Opota O, Senn L, Prod'hom G, Mazza-Stalder J, Tissot F, Greub G, Jaton K. 2016. Added value of molecular assay Xpert MTB/RIF compared to sputum smear microscopy to assess the risk of tuberculosis transmission in a low-prevalence country. *Clin Microbiol Infect* **22**:613–619 10.1016/j.cmi.2016.04.010.

88. Mbonze NB, Tabala M, Wenzi LK, Bakoko B, Brouwer M, Creswell J, Van Rie A, Behets F, Yotebieng M. 2016. Xpert MTB/RIF for smear-negative presumptive TB: impact on case notification in DR Congo. *Int J Tuberc Lung Dis* **20**:240–246.

89. Lorent N, Kong C, Kim T, Sam S, Thai S, Colebunders R, Rigouts L, Lynen L. 2015. Systematic screening for drug-resistant tuberculosis with Xpert MTB/RIF in a referral hospital in Cambodia. *Int J Tuberc Lung Dis* **19**:1528–1535.

90. Schumacher SG, Thangakunam B, Denkinger CM, Oliver AA, Shakti KB, Qin ZZ, Michael JS, Luo R, Pai M, Christopher DJ. 2015. Impact of point-of-care implementation of Xpert MTB/RIF: product vs. process innovation. *Int J Tuberc Lung Dis* **19**:1084–1090.

91. van Kampen SC, Tursynbayeva A, Koptleuova A, Murzabekova Z, Bigalieva L, Aubakirova M, Pak S, van den Hof S. 2015. Effect of introducing Xpert MTB/RIF to test and treat individuals at risk of multidrug-resistant tuberculosis in Kazakhstan: a prospective cohort study. *PLoS One* **10**:e0132514 [Erratum, **10**: e0136368.]

92. Hanrahan CF, Clouse K, Bassett J, Mutunga L, Selibas K, Stevens W, Scott L, Sanne I, Van Rie A. 2015. The patient impact of point-of-care vs. laboratory placement of Xpert MTB/RIF. *Int J Tuberc Lung Dis* **19**:811–816.

93. Manabe YC, Zawedde-Muyanja S, Burnett SM, Mugabe F, Naikoba S, Coutinho A. 2015. Rapid improvement in passive tuberculosis case detection and tuberculosis treatment outcomes after implementation of a bundled laboratory diagnostic and on-site training intervention targeting mid-level providers. *Open Forum Infect Dis* **2**: ofv030.

94. Sachdeva KS, Raizada N, Sreenivas A, Van't Hoog AH, van den Hof S, Dewan PK, Thakur R, Gupta RS, Kulsange S, Vadera B, Babre A, Gray C, Parmar M, Ghedia M, Ramachandran R, Alavadi U, Arinaminpathy N, Denkinger C, Boehme C, Paramasivan CN. 2015. Use of Xpert MTB/RIF in decentralized public health settings and its effect on pulmonary TB and DR-TB case finding in India. *PLoS One* **10**:e0126065

95. Trajman A, Durovni B, Saraceni V, Menezes A, Cordeiro-Santos M, Cobelens F, Van den Hof S. 2015. Impact on patients' treatment outcomes of XpertMTB/RIF implementation for the diagnosis of tuberculosis: follow-up of a stepped-wedge randomized clinical trial. *PLoS One* **10**:e0123252 [Erratum, **11**:e0156471.]

96. Creswell J, Rai B, Wali R, Sudrungrot S, Adhikari LM, Pant R, Pyakurel S, Uranw D, Codlin AJ. 2015. Intro-

ducing new tuberculosis diagnostics: the impact of Xpert MTB/RIF testing on case notifications in Nepal. *Int J Tuberc Lung Dis* **19**:545–551.

97. Van Den Handel T, Hampton KH, Sanne I, Stevens W, Crous R, Van Rie A. 2015. The impact of Xpert MTB/RIF in sparsely populated rural settings. *Int J Tuberc Lung Dis* **19**:392–398.

98. Alvarez GG, Van Dyk DD, Desjardins M, Yasseen AS III, Aaron SD, Cameron DW, Obed N, Baikie M, Pakhale S, Denkinger CM, Sohn H, Pai M. 2015. The feasibility, accuracy, and impact of Xpert MTB/RIF testing in a remote aboriginal community in Canada. *Chest* **148**:767–773.

99. Moyenga I, Roggi A, Sulis G, Diande S, Tamboura D, Tagliani E, Castelli F, Matteelli A. 2015. The impact of Xpert MTB/RIF depends on service coordination: experience in Burkina Faso. *Int J Tuberc Lung Dis* **19**:285–287.

100. Durovni B, Saraceni V, van den Hof S, Trajman A, Cordeiro-Santos M, Cavalcante S, Menezes A, Cobelens F. 2014. Impact of replacing smear microscopy with Xpert MTB/RIF for diagnosing tuberculosis in Brazil: a stepped-wedge cluster-randomized trial. *PLoS Med* **11**:e1001766 [Erratum, **12**:e1001928.]

101. Cox HS, Mbhele S, Mohess N, Whitelaw A, Muller O, Zemanay W, Little F, Azevedo V, Simpson J, Boehme CC, Nicol MP. 2014. Impact of Xpert MTB/RIF for TB diagnosis in a primary care clinic with high TB and HIV prevalence in South Africa: a pragmatic randomised trial. *PLoS Med* **11**:e1001760.

102. Chaisson LH, Roemer M, Cantu D, Haller B, Millman AJ, Cattamanchi A, Davis JL. 2014. Impact of GeneXpert MTB/RIF assay on triage of respiratory isolation rooms for inpatients with presumed tuberculosis: a hypothetical trial. *Clin Infect Dis* **59**:1353–1360.

103. Davis JL, Kawamura LM, Chaisson LH, Grinsdale J, Benhammou J, Ho C, Babst A, Banouvong H, Metcalfe JZ, Pandori M, Hopewell PC, Cattamanchi A. 2014. Impact of GeneXpert MTB/RIF on patients and tuberculosis programs in a low-burden setting: a hypothetical trial. *Am J Respir Crit Care Med* **189**:1551–1559.

104. Ramirez HL, García-Clemente MM, Alvarez-Álvarez C, Palacio-Gutierrez JJ, Pando-Sandoval A, Gagatek S, Arias-Guillén M, Quezada-Loaiza CA, Casan-Clará P.

2014. Impact of the Xpert MTB/RIF molecular test on the late diagnosis of pulmonary tuberculosis. *Int J Tuberc Lung Dis* **18**:435–437

105. Balcha TT, Sturegård E, Winqvist N, Skogmar S, Reepalu A, Jemal ZH, Tibesso G, Schön T, Björkman P. 2014. Intensified tuberculosis case-finding in HIV-positive adults managed at Ethiopian health centers: diagnostic yield of Xpert MTB/RIF compared with smear microscopy and liquid culture. *PLoS One* **9**:e85478.

106. Omrani AS, Al-Otaibi MF, Al-Ateah SM, Al-Onazi FM, Baig K, El-Khizzi NA, Albarrak AM. 2014. GeneXpert MTB/RIF testing in the management of patients with active tuberculosis: a real life experience from Saudi Arabia. *Infect Chemother* **46**:30–34.

107. Sohn H, Aero AD, Menzies D, Behr M, Schwartzman K, Alvarez GG, Dan A, McIntosh F, Pai M, Denkinger CM. 2014. Xpert MTB/RIF testing in a low tuberculosis incidence, high-resource setting: limitations in accuracy and clinical impact. *Clin Infect Dis* **58**:970–976.

108. Al-Darraji HA, Abd Razak H, Ng KP, Altice FL, Kamarulzaman A. 2013. The diagnostic performance of a single GeneXpert MTB/RIF assay in an intensified tuberculosis case finding survey among HIV-infected prisoners in Malaysia. *PLoS One* **8**:e73717.

109. Theron G, Peter J, Meldau R, Khalfey H, Gina P, Matinyena B, Lenders L, Calligaro G, Allwood B, Symons G, Govender U, Setshedi M, Dheda K. 2013. Accuracy and impact of Xpert MTB/RIF for the diagnosis of smear-negative or sputum-scarce tuberculosis using bronchoalveolar lavage fluid. *Thorax* **68**:1043–1051.

110. Hanrahan CF, Selibas K, Deery CB, Dansey H, Clouse K, Bassett J, Scott L, Stevens W, Sanne I, Van Rie A. 2013. Time to treatment and patient outcomes among TB suspects screened by a single point-of-care Xpert MTB/RIF at a primary care clinic in Johannesburg, South Africa. *PLoS One* **8**:e65421.

111. Calligaro GL, Zijenah LS, Peter JG, Theron G, Buser V, McNerney R, Bara W, Bandason T, Govender U, Tomasicchio M, Smith L, Mayosi BM, Dheda K. 2017. Effect of new tuberculosis diagnostic technologies on community-based intensified case finding: a multicentre randomised controlled trial. *Lancet Infect Dis* (epub ahead of print)

Host and Strain Diversity

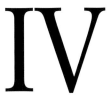

Tuberculosis and the Tubercle Bacillus, 2nd ed.
Edited by William R. Jacobs, Jr., Helen McShane, Valerie Mizrahi, and Ian M. Orme
© 2018 American Society for Microbiology, Washington, DC
doi:10.1128/microbiolspec.TBTB2-0011-2016

The Role of Host Genetics (and Genomics) in Tuberculosis

19

Vivek Naranbhai

INTRODUCTION

Familial risk of tuberculosis (TB) has been recognized for centuries; indeed, Greek, Arabic, Chinese, and Sanskrit texts are said to include descriptions of the familial nature of disease as early as 600 BCE, and many scholars, including Aristotle (300 BCE), Francastoro (1546), and Marten (1720), explicitly conjectured that this may be because the disease is contagious. However, largely through studies of mono- and dizygotic twin concordance rates, studies of families with Mendelian susceptibility to mycobacterial disease (MSMD), and candidate gene studies performed in the 20th century, it was recognized that susceptibility to TB disease has a substantial host genetic component. Limitations in candidate gene studies and early linkage studies made robust identification of specific loci associated with disease challenging, and few loci have been convincingly associated across multiple populations. Genome-wide association studies (GWAS) and transcriptome-wide association studies, based on microarray (commonly known as genechip) technologies, conducted in the past decade have helped shed some light on pathogenesis, but only a handful of new pathways have been identified. This apparent paradox, of high heritability but few replicable associations, has spurred current large-scale collaborative projects, such as the International Tuberculosis Host Genetics Consortium (ITHGC), that aim to take into account heterogeneity in both host and pathogen genetics, variation in exposure rates, and outcome definitions (referred to as phenotypes by geneticists). Recent studies that also leverage low-cost, high-throughput sequencing to interrogate genetic, transcriptomic, and epigenetic changes in the context of TB are also beginning to be reported.

This review aims to comprehensively assess the heritability of TB, critically review the genetic correlates of disease, and highlight current studies and future prospects in the study of host genomics in TB. Since this is the first edition of this book in which host genetics has been dealt with, the schematic and accompanying text in Fig. 1 serves to refresh the reader's understanding of terminology, concepts, and methods in host genomic research. An implicit goal of elucidating host genetic correlates of susceptibility to *Mycobacterium tuberculosis* infection or TB disease is to identify pathophysiological features amenable to translation to new preventive, diagnostic, or therapeutic interventions. The translation of genomic insights into new clinical tools is therefore also discussed.

In animal models of TB, genetic manipulation has made it possible to probe the mechanistic role of specific genes and pathways in TB disease, and these approaches are largely dealt with in other reviews (530–535). Similarly, although genomic tools such as genome editing and T-cell and B-cell receptor repertoire sequencing are at the forefront of basic science enquiries that link host genetics and immunology, these are dealt with elsewhere also (536).

THE HERITABILITY OF TUBERCULOSIS SUSCEPTIBILITY

Twin Studies

Twin studies aim to partition the proportion of variance in risk or liability of TB disease into that which can be attributed to additive genetic effects (A), shared or common (C) environmental effects (events that

Wellcome Trust Centre for Human Genetics, Nuffield Department of Medicine, University of Oxford, Oxford, Oxfordshire OX37BN, United Kingdom; Centre for the AIDS Programme of Research in South Africa, University of KwaZulu Natal, Durban, South Africa.

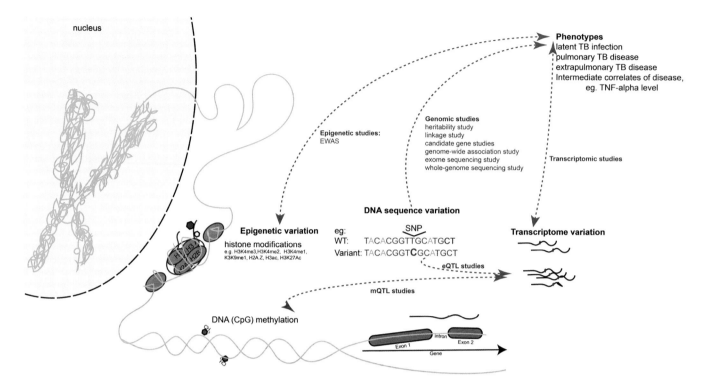

Figure 1 Host "omics" in tuberculosis. The haploid human genome consists of 3 billion bp, encoding 20,687 expressed functional units (genes), the majority of which are translated into protein products. Most (98.86%) of the genome does not code for any specific gene or protein product, but these intergenic or intronic regions may act as enhancers and repressors and modify gene expression. The small proportion of coding sequence, collectively known as the exome, is responsible for protein coding. Each gene undergoes variable splicing of exons to form a full-length transcript leading to transcript variation; on average, each gene has about four different isoforms, but this varies considerably by gene. Approximately 90% of all DNA sequence variation is in the form of single-nucleotide change known as a single-nucleotide polymorphism (SNP); about 10,000 SNPs have been reported, and these occur approximately every 100 to 300 bp, clustered around genes. Other forms of sequence variation include insertions, deletions, and copy number variation. The major force generating diversity is homologous recombination during meiosis, when crossing-over of segments of maternal and paternal chromosomes occurs. Because contiguous blocks of DNA between recombination hot spots recombine, genetic variants tend to be coinherited, resulting in linkage disequilibrium between variants. DNA sequence variation can be studied in a per gene manner (a candidate gene approach), using microsatellites that recur frequently across the genome in the context of pedigrees (linkage mapping), studying specific genes (candidate gene studies), genotyping >0.5M variants across the genome (as in a GWAS) and leveraging linkage disequilibrium to infer additional variants (imputation), or sequencing the exome (exome sequencing) or entire genome (whole-genome sequencing). DNA sequence variation may bear its effect through any variety of different mechanisms including altering the quantity of, or type of, transcript leading to transcriptomic variation, or by altering the resulting protein. Genetic loci that affect expression are known as expression quantitative loci (eQTL), and those that affect transcription only in response to stimulation, for example, with *M. tuberculosis*, are known as response QTL (reQTL). Additional epigenetic features that may affect the quantity of a gene expression are methylation of cytosine nucleotides in DNA (studying in methylation QTL [mQTL] studies) and methylation or acetylation of lysine residues of histone proteins that together make up a nucleosome.

affect both twins), and unshared environmental (E) effects (events that affect each twin differentially). Since monozygotic (MZ, identical) and dizygotic (DZ, nonidentical) twins share approximately 100 and 50% of genetic variation, all the shared environmental effects (C, for twins reared together), and none of the unshared effects (E), comparison of disease or biomarker concordance estimates between MZ and DZ twin pairs allows inference about the relative contribution of genetic factors to the outcome of interest when the zygosity of twin pairs and their outcomes is known but without need for any further genetic measurements.

Three twin studies of TB disease susceptibility have been reported (1–3). As shown in Table 1, the concordance rates among MZ twins are consistently higher than among DZ twins, consistent with the presence of additive genetic factors that associate with risk of disease. Although varying by the differing underlying concordance rate estimates, the narrow-sense heritability is up to 80%. Van der Eijik and colleagues have argued that, in the case of infectious diseases where exposure is a necessary cause, greater concordance among MZ twins may be explained by greater environmental sharing among MZ versus DZ twins and consequent greater exposure of an uninfected twin to an infected MZ twin (4). There is, however, no empirical evidence of discordant environmental sharing between MZ and DZ twins raised in the same household. Nevertheless, their argument highlights the challenges of ascribing etiological roles to host genetics in a condition such as TB.

Based on insights gleaned from studies of individuals with MSMD (further discussed below) and immune-correlate studies, heritability of intermediate traits has been of recent interest. Twin and family studies of the heritability of gamma interferon (IFN-γ), tumor necrosis factor alpha (TNF-α), and transforming growth factor beta (TGF-β) production after *in vitro* antigen stimulation of whole blood demonstrate that TNF-α response is the most heritable of the three at 69% (5, 6). Twin studies of the heritability of tuberculin reactivity after *Mycobacterium bovis* BCG vaccination estimate heritability at 28% (7). Understanding the genetic correlates of intermediate traits may therefore be an additional approach to delineating susceptibility pathways.

Mendelian Susceptibility to Mycobacterial Disease

MSMD is an established clinical disorder described in more than 100 individuals (8) in whom familial susceptibility to mycobacterial disease is observed.

About half of all cases of MSMD have an identifiable genetic cause. The pattern of heritability differs according to the gene affected and the specific genetic lesion (these have been reviewed in detail elsewhere [9]). There are nine genes in which one or more causal mutations have been described in individuals with MSMD: *IFNGR1* (OMIM 209950, 615978, 600263, 610424, 607948; 6q23.3), *IFNGR2* (OMIM 614889; Chr21q22.11), *STAT1* (OMIM 614892, 613796, 614162; Chr2q32.2), *IL12RB1* (OMIM 614891, Chr19q13.11), *IL12B* (5q33.3), IRF8 (OMIM 614893-4; Chr16q24.1), *ISG15* (OMIM 61626; Chr1p36.33), *TYK2* (OMIM 611521, Chr19p13.2) and two on the X-chromosome, *IKBG/NEMO* (OMIM 300636, ChrXq28) and *CYBB* (also known as p91-phox, OMIM 306400, 300545; ChrXp21.1-p11.4). As illustrated in Fig. 2, these genes implicate the IFN-γ/interleukin-12 (IL-12) pathway as central to protection from mycobacterial disease in general, but, because many individuals with MSMD do not appear to be at elevated risk of TB disease *per se*, it is possible that either protection from *M. tuberculosis* requires multiple redundant pathways and disabling a single node is insufficient to cause disease, or alternative pathways are important. In many cases of MSMD, susceptibility is to poorly virulent, nontuberculous mycobacterial disease as opposed to disease with *M. tuberculosis*. Although MSMD may therefore not explain the familial tendency toward *M. tuberculosis* infection in most humans, the genes implicated in MSMD have frequently been studied through linkage and candidate gene studies which cumulatively indicate that genes involved in MSMD do not appear to account for nonfamilial cases of TB (10).

Table 1 Twin studies of TB susceptibility

No. of MZ twin pairs	Concordance in MZ twin pairs (R$_{MZ}$)[a]	No. of DZ twin pairs	Concordance in DZ twin pairs (R$_{DZ}$)[a]	Heritability estimate	Reference(s)
80	0.65	125	0.25	80%	2
78	0.88	230	0.28	>100% (suggesting nonadditive effects)	3
54	0.33	148	0.14	38%	1, 2

[a]R$_{MZ}$ and R$_{DZ}$ refer to concordance estimates of the phenotype among monozygotic and dizygotic twins, respectively.

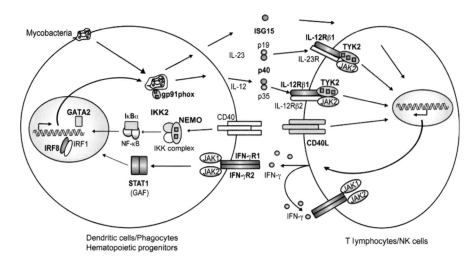

Figure 2 Mendelian susceptibility to mycobacterial disease (MSMD) affects the IFN-γ/ IL-12 pathway, focused on interaction between phagocytes/dendritic cells and lymphocytes/ natural killer cells during mycobacterial infection. Molecules in blue are mutated in patients with a broad infectious phenotype including mycobacterial diseases. Molecules in red are mutated in patients with isolated mycobacterial diseases. Molecules in blue with red dots indicate that specific mutations in the corresponding genes are responsible for isolated mycobacterial diseases. Patients with acquired or inherited profound T-cell deficiency are also susceptible to mycobacterial infections. Adapted from reference 9 with permission from the publisher.

Revisiting Heritability in the Post-GWAS Era

Twin studies are limited because the heritability estimates generated may not be generalizable beyond studies that share the same genetic background and exposure rates and to the current era. Because individuals in a family may share stretches of genetic code due to shared descent (referred to as identity by descent [IBD]), family studies may also be used to infer the heritability of TB disease risk, but there are no reported family-based heritability estimates. Large population-based studies of individuals with and without TB infection or disease that measure hundreds of thousands of genetic markers across the genome, such as GWAS, may also be used to estimate heritability based on comparison between the genetic and phenotypic correlations to generate "polygenic heritability" estimates (11). Although none of the published GWAS have reported polygenic heritability estimates from their studies, analyses by the ITHGC, further described under "Current and Future Prospects" below, are reportedly yielding heritability estimates of between 25 and 50% (ITHGC, personal communication).

IDENTIFICATION OF SPECIFIC GENETIC VARIANTS ASSOCIATED WITH TB DISEASE

Studies to define specific genetic determinants of host susceptibility to TB have been ongoing for about 2 de-

cades contemporaneously with advancements in molecular biology: typing of polymorphisms in candidate genes by restriction-fragment length polymorphism (RFLP), PCR, and sequencing and microsatellite-based linkage studies, and genotyping of hundreds of thousands of variants by microarray-based genotyping in GWAS. Here, I present a comprehensive summary of the published candidate gene studies, systematic reviews thereof, and published GWAS. In Fig. 3, the aggregate of genetic associations with TB susceptibility that have been reported is schematically shown on a karyogram.

Linkage Studies

In a pedigree or collection of pedigrees, the pattern of phenotype segregation can be compared with genotype, historically assessed by typing microsatellites across the genome, to infer genetic loci that are in linkage with that phenotype and thereby identify regions of the genome that may harbor variation that alters disease risk. This approach yielded some of the earliest genome-scale maps of loci that may be associated with TB. Shaw and colleagues studied 98 pedigrees in Brazil and identified a TB-linked locus surrounding *SLC11A1* (formerly known as *NRAMP1*) that includes *CXCR2* (*IL8RA*) but neither *SLC11A1* itself nor the *TNF* gene cluster (12). In contrast, the *SCL11A1* locus around Chr2q35 was significantly linked to TB disease susceptibility in a multicase Aboriginal Canadian family, that

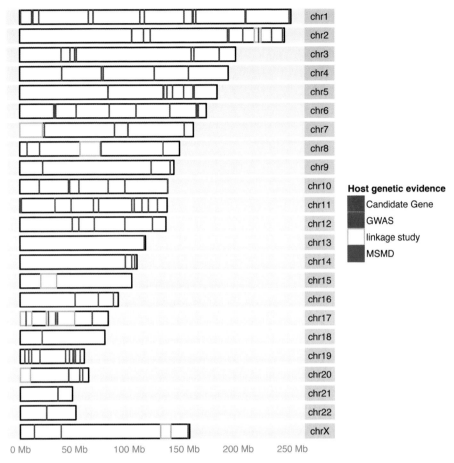

Figure 3 Karyogram highlighting host-genetic correlates of tuberculosis susceptibility according to the type of study from which evidence arose.

also ruled out linkage to the MHC locus (13). Bellamy and colleagues studied 92 Gambian and South African sib-pairs and replicated their findings in a further set of 81 sib-pairs to identify loci around Chr15q11-q13 and the Xq26 chromosome that were in linkage with disease (14, 15). Baghdadi and colleagues used a similar approach in studying 96 Moroccan families to identify the Chr8q12-13 locus as in linkage with TB (16), as did Stein and colleagues in studying 193 Ugandan pedigrees to identify the Chr7p22-p21 as in linkage with TB (17). Stein and colleagues additionally assessed individuals with a persistent lack of tuberculin skin test reactivity and reported two loci (Chr2q21-24 and Chr5p13-5q22) associated with this phenotype. In an observation returned to later, Mahasirimongkol and colleagues studied 93 Thai pedigrees and reported that two regions in possible linkage were identified only when age of TB onset was taken into account (Chr17p13.3-13.1 and Chr20p13-12.3), highlighting possible age-specific variation in underlying pathophysiology.

Some investigators have used the linkage-study approach to attempt to identify specific regions within an extended region that may be associated with disease and hence focused on specific regions as opposed to the entire genome, referred to as fine-mapping. Jamieson and colleagues used this approach to study the 17q11-21 locus that includes many chemokine genes such as *CCL2* and *CCL5* in 92 Brazilian pedigrees, and reported independent linkage of loci around *NOS2A*, *CCL18*, *CCL4*, and *STAT5B* with TB (18).

The lack of replication of loci across populations in linkage studies, in retrospect, presaged the lack of replication of findings seen in the candidate gene studies that have formed the majority of genetic enquiries into TB susceptibility.

Candidate Gene Studies

The study of variants within a specific gene, usually a gene implicated in pathogenesis through animal studies, involvement in MSMD, or basic immunology studies, is referred to as a candidate gene study. These studies have tended to study genes with known immunological importance, comparing cases with TB disease or infection with controls that have either TB infection or no infection.

Candidate gene studies have three important limitations: confounding due to unadjusted population stratification (systematic differences between cases and controls due to differences in ancestry), elevated type I error due to multiple hypothesis testing, and publication bias through which the effects of a variant tend to be biased away from the null. These challenges can be addressed through adjusting for ancestry differences measured by ancestry-informative markers (AIMs) with principal components or linear-mixed models, as is now the norm in GWAS, and through correction of multiple comparisons by any of a wide variety of accepted methods.

Table 2 provides a directory of published candidate gene studies. In total, more than 120 genes have been implicated in TB susceptibility by more than 390 independent reports published at the time of writing (January 2016). As the candidate gene era draws to a close, this directory of published candidate gene studies is, therefore, a compendium of genes and pathways that have been implicated in host genetic studies and been subject of specific study, but cannot be taken to indicate evidence that these genes are truly associated with TB.

The most well-known and well-studied candidate genes in TB include *SCL11A1* (formerly known as *NRAMP1*) (55 reports), *HLADRB1* (45 reports), *IFN-* (42 studies), *VDR* (40 reports), *IL-10* (36 reports), and *TNFA* (30 reports). Systematic review and meta-analysis (SR/MA) of 24 genes has also been reported, largely of the most widely studied genes, allowing assessment of the presence of publication bias and the robustness of association (see Table 3 for specific findings). In general, for most variants, meta-analyses suggest that if the association truly exists, it is likely to be present in only select ethnic groups. For example, four variants in *SLC11A1* have been studied in many populations because this gene is a homologue to a locus linked to TB susceptibility in mice and in some human linkage studies. In the largest meta-analysis of the candidate gene studies of *SLC11A1*, all four variants were nominally associated with TB risk, but when stratified further, the D543N coding variant was significantly associated among Asians, but neither African, European, nor South American populations. Similar observations of heterogeneity between ethnic groups have been observed for *CCL2*, *CCL5*, *CD209*, *HLADRB1*, *IFN-*,

IFNGR1, *IL1B*, *IL-6*, *IL10*, *MBL*, *P2RX7*, *TLR1*, *TL2*, and *VDR*. Although variation in sample sizes across the different ethnic groups may account for the observed heterogeneity, the apparent pervasiveness of interethnic heterogeneity regardless of gene and sample size is consistent with alternative reasons for variation in effects that are discussed further below. Moreover, many of the candidate gene studies reported are small, are subject to publication bias, and may be confounded by population structure.

GWAS that adjust for population structure and multiple comparisons are therefore likely to enhance resolution of these reported candidate gene variants.

Genome-Wide Association Studies

Subsequent to the development of microarrays spotted with hundreds of thousands of oligonucleotides homologous to regions harboring sequence variation, the comparison of DNA sequence variant frequency, typically between cases with a phenotype and controls without the phenotype, became feasible on a large scale. The use of these so-called genome-wide association studies (GWAS, also known as whole genome association studies) to identify disease-associated genes has exploded since the first was reported in 2005, with >1,200 GWAS on hundreds of different diseases and traits now having been reported (19). A typical GWAS measures more than half a million variants in several hundreds or thousands of cases and controls and is powered to identify variants that have a frequency of >5% (so-called common variants) and have moderate to large effect sizes. Availability of a large reference panel of sequenced humans from different ethnicities through the 1,000 genomes and International Hapmap projects has enabled imputation of additional variation by leveraging linkage disequilibrium (20, 21). The GWAS approach can also be used to study continuous outcomes, for example, immune measures, and can be applied in a prospective study setting. In addition to the classical limitations of the case-control epidemiological design, case-control GWAS studies have several additional challenges. First, if cases and controls are drawn from a different risk distribution, this may confound analyses: for example, if cases with TB disease (who *de facto* have experienced exposure) are compared with controls who have no exposure to TB, spurious findings may ensue. Systematic differences attributable to differences in ancestry may be addressed through adjusting for ancestry with principal components built on genetic markers that reflect ethnic differences, or in a linear-mixed model in which relatedness is treated as a random effect. However, careful case-control selection remains prudent. The second challenge is that of multiple comparisons, because typically >0.5M variants are assessed. Reducing the α proportionate to the number of effective comparisons is therefore necessary (hence, a P value of $<5 \times 10^{-8}$ is the accepted level for "genome-wide" statistical significance [GWS]), as is replication of findings in additional cohorts from the same or another population (with replication of GWS variants typically requiring P values of <0.05). The third challenge is that inferring a causal allele can be challenging due to the linkage disequilibrium between variants resulting in variants "tagging" one another. *In vitro* and *in vivo* functional follow-up of loci may help; however, as discussed later, *in silico* analyses play an appreciable role in prioritizing variants for functional assessment.

Five GWAS for pulmonary TB (pTB) have been reported (22–27) and several additional GWAS are under way. In total, GWAS have identified three genome-wide significant loci associated with TB disease (Table 3).

The first published GWAS of TB was of HIV-negative adults with pTB and healthy controls in The Gambia and Ghana. Following replication in additional cohorts resulted in a total of 3,632 cases and 7,501 controls; this study confirmed that a variant, rs4331426 Chr18q 11.2, was associated with pTB at GWS (22).

The Gambian-Ghanaian groups later identified a second variant associated with TB following imputation (see Fig. 1) and genotyping in additional Indonesian and Russian cohorts, resulting in a total of 13,859 cases and 8,821 controls, namely, rs2057178, a variant on Chr11p13 near *WT1* (25). The function of both variants identified in the Gambian-Ghanaian studies is not known. The Chr11p13 variant association was replicated by a GWAS performed among the South African Colored population, in which 642 cases with pulmonary TB and 91 controls were genotyped and an association study was performed (27). The study in South Africa did not identify any GWS loci associated with disease.

Finally, a GWAS of 5,530 cases and 5,607 controls performed among Russian adults identified a variant in an intron of *ASAP1* (rs4733781) that was shown to be associated (26) with TB disease and was demonstrated to alter *ASAP1* expression in dendritic cells. The Russian study also replicated the Chr11p13 finding.

Two additional GWAS have been reported. A GWAS of 393 cases and 1,255 controls from Thailand and Japan suggested that at least one new region tagged by rs6071980 in *HSPEP/MAFB* was associated with pTB among individuals <40 years of age (23), but this did not achieve GWS. This study's failure to identify many

replicable associations, even among a population with less sparse linkage disequilibrium than Africans, confirms that many common variants with large effect sizes are unlikely to explain pTB risk and that larger sample sizes are necessary. These findings are also interesting because the association was observed only in individuals <40 years of age, but not among a further 906 cases and 1,786 controls older than 40 years, potentially because of a gene-environment interaction such as exposure to TB. A small two-stage genome-wide scan was reported in which 108 cases and 115 Indonesian controls were genotyped at ±100,000 single-nucleotide polymorphisms (SNPs) (24), then 2,453 SNPs with the lowest P value for association were replicated in 1,189 further Indonesians and 3,760 Russians. These results suggested that variants at eight novel loci could be involved in TB susceptibility—*JAG1*, *DYNLRB2*, *EBF1*, *TMEFF2*, *CCL17*, *HAUS6*, *PENK*, and *TXNDC4*—but none of the eight reported associations achieved GWS.

Collectively, these genome-wide studies demonstrated that there are likely few common variants with large effect sizes that explain TB susceptibility across different populations.

Transcriptomic Studies of TB

An alternative approach to identify genes and pathways involved in TB is to directly assess whether expression of specific genes is associated with different TB disease states or outcomes. Array technology similar to that used in GWAS is available to quantify mRNA (or cDNA) levels. In contrast to sequence variation, which cannot be altered by disease state and can therefore be compared between individuals with TB and those without to identify susceptibility loci, gene expression is sensitive to subtle differences even in age, sex, timing, and season of venipuncture, as well as disease status. Accordingly, the majority of transcriptomic studies have studied individuals with or without disease to identify genes whose expression is modified during disease. Quantification of these genes is suggesting new diagnostic approaches for TB.

Studies have searched for transcriptomic signals of response to *in vitro* M. *tuberculosis* infection such as M. *tuberculosis* stimulation of macrophages from 12 individuals (28) to identify *CCL1* as differentially expressed according to case-control status. Another study evaluated M. *tuberculosis*-stimulated peripheral blood mononuclear cells (PBMCs) (29) and suggested that a set of 127 probes could classify individuals into one of four groups: BCG-vaccinated, latently infected, active disease, or healthy control. A more recent study

TABLE 2 Directory of published candidate gene studies

Gene	Function[a]	Studies	Reference(s)	Systematic review/ meta-analysis finding	Systematic review or meta-analysis reference(s)
ABCB1 (MDR)	ATP-dependent drug efflux pump for xenobiotic compounds	1	69	–	–
AIM2	Cytosolic dsDNA sensor. IFN-γ-inducible gene component of inflammasome; affects IL-1β responses in fungal containment and in animal models	1	70	–	–
AKT1	Serine-threonine protein kinase activated by PDGF	1	71	–	–
ALOX5	Lipoxygenase family member involved in synthesis of leukotrienes	1	72	–	–
APOE	Major component of chylomicrons	1	73	–	–
	Control inbuilt breakdown of cellular and pathogen components	1	74	–	–
Autophagy-related genes: ATG10, ATG16L2, ATG2B, ATG5, ATG9B, IRGM, LAMP1, LAMP3, WIPI1, MTOR, and ATG4C					
BAG6	Within MHC-III region. Encodes a nuclear protein involved in apoptosis, and required for p53 acetylation	1	75	–	–
BTNL2	HLA-II-related gene within which variants are known to be associated with sarcoidosis, also a pulmonary disease with granulomas	2	76, 77	–	–
CARD8	Member of CARD family, part of inflammasome, and involved in negative regulation of NFκB and caspase activation	1	70	–	–
CASP1	Centrally involved in apoptosis and responsible for cleavage of IL-1 to IL-1B	1	70	–	–
CTSZ	Lysosomal cysteine proteinase	3	78–80	–	–
CCL2 (MCP-1)	Involved in recruitment of monocytes and probable granuloma formation	18	81–98	3 SR/MA: Nominally significant association of CCL2 –2518G>A allele with TB in Asians and Americans but not Africans	99–101
CCL3L1	Ligand for CCR5 and several other chemokine receptors	2	102, 103	–	–
CCL5 (RANTES)	Chemokine for T cells, monocytes, eosinophils, and basophils. In animal models, CCL5 appears to be important for granuloma formation	7	85, 91, 104–108	2 SR/MA: CCL5 –403G>A allele not associated with TB CCL5 –28C>G nominally associated with TB in Asian and Middle Eastern groups	–

Gene	Function	No.	Meta-analysis	References	
CCR2	Receptor for CCL2 (MCP-1) responsible for monocyte chemotaxis	2	—	81, 91	—
CCR5	Receptor for CCL5 and CCL2, MIP1-α, MIP1-β, and RANTES	4	—	85, 91, 102, 103	—
CD1a	Mediates presentation of lipid and glycolipid antigens to T cells	1	—	109	—
CD14	LPS receptor and monocyte marker	8	2 SR/MA: CD14 −159T>C nominally associated with risk in Asians	110–117	118, 119
CD40	Member of the TNF superfamily of receptors, crucial to immunoglobulin class switch, memory B-cell and germinal center development	1	—	120	—
TNFRSF1B (CD120b)	Member of TNF superfamily of receptors and probably responsible for antiapoptotic signaling	1	—	121	—
MRC1 (CD206)	Receptor for mannose and partially regulates M. tuberculosis uptake. Modulates phagosome-lysosome fusion	2	—	122, 123	—
CD209 (DC-SIGN)	Recognizes wide range of pathogens as binds carbohydrate ligands. Mediates phagocytosis of M. tuberculosis by DCs and is involved in receptor signaling and trafficking of ligand particles	12	3 SR/MA: Discrepant results: −336G>A nominally associated with risk in Asians only in two MA, not associated in other; −871A>G nominally associated in one MA, not associated in other	81, 124–134	135–137
CISH	Cytokine-responsive gene and one of many suppressors of cytokine signaling (SOCS)	4	—	138–141	—
Complement genes (several)	Involved in complement cascade leading to opsonization	2	—	142, 143	—
CR1 (Knops)	Complement component C3b/4b receptor involved in immune complex binding	1	—	144	—
CSF2	Cytokine responsible for production, differentiation, and function of granulocytes and macrophages	1	—	145	—
CTDSP1 (NLIIF)	Nuclear phosphatase involved in transcriptional regulation	1	—	146	—
CTLA4	Inhibitory signaling to T cells	1	—	147	—
CXCL10 (IP-10)	Chemokine for multiple cell types and involved in NK cell and T-cell recruitment. Binds CXCR3	1	—	148	—
CXCL12 (SDF-1)	Antimicrobial gene, ligand for CXCR4 and involved in inflammation, tissue homeostasis, immune surveillance	1	—	148	—
CXCL14 (MIP-2g)	Antimicrobial chemokine for monocytes	1	—	145	—
CYBB (gp91-PHOX)	Transmembrane transporter responsible for NADPH-mediated oxygen reduction to generate superoxides. Involved in MSMD and chronic granulomatous disease	1	—	149	—

(Continued)

Table 2 Directory of published candidate gene studies (*Continued*)

Gene	Function[a]	Studies	Reference(s)	Systematic review/ meta-analysis finding	Systematic review or meta-analysis reference(s)
CYP genes (several)	Cytochrome P450 enzymes involved in toxin and drug metabolism typically by terminal oxidase in electron transfer	3	69, 150, 151	—	—
DEFB1	Antimicrobial peptide involved in epithelial protection	1	152	—	—
EBI3	Heterodimerizes with IL-27 to regulate T-cell and inflammatory responses	1	145	—	—
EREG	Secreted peptide hormone ligand to EGFR and ERBB4 and involved in inflammation, cell proliferation, wound healing	2	153, 154	—	—
FAM46A	Unknown but associated with several eye and bowel conditions	1	75	—	—
FCGR2A (CD32) and FCGR3A (CD16)	Binds Fc fragment of immunoglobulins with low affinity. Expressed on wide array of innate immune cells	1	155	—	—
FCN2	Member of ficolin family of proteins, binds carbohydrates, and opsonizes pathogens	2	156, 157	—	—
SLC40A1 (Ferroportin)	Involved in iron export from cells	1	158	—	—
FUT1	Part of Golgi apparatus and involved in blood group antigen synthesis	1	159	—	—
G6PD	Cytosolic enzyme involved in NADPH production to protect from oxidizing agents	1	160	—	—
GSTT1, GSTM1	Cytosolic glutathione-S-transferases responsible for ligation of reduced glutathione to electrophilic compounds	2	69, 161	—	—
HP (haptoglobin)	Forms tetramer that binds free hemoglobin allowing breakdown and preventing free renal loss. Possesses antimicrobial properties	1	162	—	—
HLA (mainly HLADRB1)	Known pleiotropic locus for infectious disease, presents peptide antigens to T and NK cells	45	163–207	1 SR/MA: No overall association between HLA*DRB1 alleles and TB, possible association in Asians	208
HSP70 and HSP90 genes (several)	Molecular chaperone proteins involved in stabilizing proteins during folding. Encoded in MHC-III cluster	2	70, 209	—	—
IFITM3	Interferon-inducible protein involved in immunity against influenza, West Nile virus, and dengue	1	210	—	—
IFNB1	Member of type 1 interferon family involved in cell differentiation, antiviral and antibacterial responses, and responsible for induction of many genes	1	145	—	—

Gene	Function	n	References	SR/MA association	Ref
IFNG	Cytokine crucial for protection against intracellular organisms	42	90, 105, 142, 211–248	3 SR/MA: −+874T>A nominally associated with TB in Asians, not Caucasians	249–251
IFNGR1	Receptor for IFN-γ. Mutations described in MSMD	10	217, 221, 223, 225, 235, 240, 252–255	1 SR/MA: −56C>T nominally associated with risk in Africans, not Asians or Caucasians	256
NFKB1L	Encoded in MHC1 region, function unclear	1	257	–	–
IL1B	Proinflammatory cytokine secreted in pro-protein form that is cleaved by caspase 1 and triggers multiple additional inflammatory responses	13	70, 159, 216, 243, 257–265	1 SR/MA: −511T>C nominally associated with TB in Africans only	266
IL1R1	Receptor for IL-1α, IL-1β, and IL-1RA	5	70, 159, 216, 258, 264	–	–
IL2	Key cytokine responsible for T- and B-cell proliferation	2	242, 263	–	–
IL4	Cytokine involved in inducing Th0→Th2 differentiation	7	145, 216, 242, 243, 246, 258, 263	–	–
IL6 (IFNB2)	Proinflammatory and pyrogenic cytokine. Also anti-inflammatory in inhibiting TNF-α and IL-1	6	90, 212, 224, 242, 258, 267	2 SR/MA: No overall association; 174C>G nominally associated with TB in Asians only	266, 268
CXCL8 (IL8)	Chemotactic cytokine involved in recruitment of inflammatory cells (especially neutrophils) to sites of inflammation and angiogenesis	3	269–271	–	–
IL10	Suppresses proinflammatory responses but may also block phagosome maturation in macrophages permitting latency. Downregulates Th1 cytokines and NFκB activity	36	106, 142, 159, 163, 212, 213, 224, 230, 234, 236, 242, 243, 248, 258, 260, 261, 263, 264, 270, 272–288	4 SR/MA: −1082G>A and −592A>C: No overall association; nominally associated in European subgroup −819T>C: No overall association; associated with TB in Asians only	249, 268, 289, 290
IL10RA and IL10RB	Receptor components of IL-10. Activation leads to TYK2 phosphorylation	1	274	–	–
IL12A and IL12B	Induces IFN-γ production by T cells via IL-12 receptor signaling. Involved in MSMD. Responsible for maintaining memory Th1 cells (IL-12B)	13	216, 232, 240, 242, 244, 247, 263, 282, 291–295	–	–
IL12RB1 (CD212)	Subunit component of IL-12R. Mutations in IL-12RB1 described in MSMD	9	232, 240, 242, 247, 263, 291, 296–298	–	–
IL17A	Proinflammatory cytokine produced by activated T cells and activates NFκB	1	299	–	–
IL-18	Proinflammatory cytokine involved in IFN-γ production in synergy with IL-12	4	300–303	–	–

(Continued)

Table 2   Directory of published candidate gene studies (*Continued*)

Gene	Function[a]	Studies	Reference(s)	Systematic review/ meta-analysis finding	Systematic review or meta-analysis reference(s)
IL23R	Heterodimerizes with IL-12RB1 to mediate I-L23 binding	2	291, 304	—	—
NOS2	Involved in synthesis of nitric oxide (NO), an effector molecule against TB. Probably more important in mice than humans because of differences in macrophage NO production	6	92, 226, 255, 305–307	—	—
IRF1	Transcription factor; activator of IFN-α, IFN-β, and genes induced by type 1 interferons	2	308, 309	—	—
IRF8	Transcription factor; involved in lineage commitment and type 1 IFN expression. Mutations described in MSMD	1	308	—	—
IRGM	Involved in autophagy of intracellular pathogens	3	310–312	—	—
KIR	Ligands for HLA expressed on NK (and some T cells) and responsible for identifying malignant cells or cells with intracellular infection	6	313–318	—	—
LTA4H	Involved in leukotriene B4 synthesis and modulates inflammatory TNF production	4	264, 319–321	—	—
LY96 (MD2)	Associated with TLR4 to bind LPS	1	322	—	—
NR1H3 (LXRA) and *NR1H2* (LXRB)	Transcription factors, responsible for oxysterol binding and macrophage function. Heterodimerize with retinoid X receptors	1	323	—	—
MARCO	Binds bacteria	2	324, 325	—	—
MASP2	Complement-dependent bactericidal factor that binds polysaccharides	3	156, 326, 327	—	—
MBL2	Soluble lectin receptor produced as an acute-phase protein by the liver. Recognizes surface carbohydrates and results in opsonization that enhances complement-dependent and -independent phagocytosis	22	112, 142, 229, 277, 326–343	2 SR/MA: No overall association in one SR, possible association in Chinese only	344, 345
MC3R	Melanocortin receptor	2	78, 80	—	—
MCL1	Antiapoptotic protein	1	346	—	—
MICA	Stress ligand for NKG2D	1	200	—	—
MIF	Macrophage chemokine	4	155, 347–349	—	—
miRNA genes (several): *miR-146a, miR-499, miR-149, miR-196a2*	22-nucleotide RNA responsible for posttranscriptional RNA silencing	4	350–353	—	—
MMP1	Metalloproteinase responsible for extracellular matrix breakdown	1	87	—	—
MMP9	Metalloproteinase responsible for collagen type IV and V degradation and in neutrophil chemotaxis	1	354	—	—

Gene	Function	N	References	Notes	Ref.
MYD88	Adaptor protein involved in TLR and IL-1 signaling	2	145, 355	—	—
NAT2	Acetyltransferase gene involved in drug metabolism	2	69, 161	—	—
NLRP1 and NLRP3	Components of inflammasome and regulator of NFκB signaling. NLRP1 involved in apoptosis	1	70	—	—
NOD2 (CARD15)	Cytoplasmic sensor protein that binds strongly to N-glycolyl muramyl dipeptide (MDP) in M. tuberculosis and other bacterial cell walls	5	356–360	1 SR/MA: nominally significant association of Arg702Trp coding change and TB, no association with other variants	361
SLC11A1 (NRAMP)	Proton-coupled divalent metal transporter of Fe and Mn	55	69, 105, 112, 142, 205, 229, 260, 273, 280, 295, 306, 307, 339, 341, 343, 362–401	4 SR/MA: Variable association with apparent nominally significant association in Asians dependent on variant: D543N coding; stronger in Asians for EPTB change, 3′ TGTG indel INT4 and 5′ (GT)n repeat	402–405
P2RX7	Ligand-gated ion channel responsible for ATP-dependent macrophage lysis. Linked to interferon signaling	14	74, 264, 390, 406–416	5 SR/MA: 1513A>C: no overall association, possible association in Indians in one SR, or Asians and Americans in another. −762T>C: no overall association	417–421
PACRG	Adjacent to PARK2 and reportedly associated with leprosy disease	1	422	—	—
PADI4	Key enzyme involved in citrullination of arginine residues during neutrophil extracellular trap formation	1	423	—	—
PARK2	Component of E3 ubiquitin ligase complex	1	422	—	—
PTPN22	Protein-tyrosine-phosphate that is associated with CBL and may be involved in T-cell receptor signaling. Pleiotropic association with many autoimmune diseases	2	424, 425	—	—
PTX3	Binds C1q TNFAIP6 and many pathogens and is secreted in response to inflammatory signals	1	130	—	—
SRFP1	Soluble mediator of Wnt signaling	1	426	—	—
SIGIRR	Modulator of immune responses by negatively regulating TLR1 signaling	2	150, 427	—	—
SP110	Nuclear protein possibly involved in myeloid cell differentiation. Able to activate gene transcription	8	278, 428–434	1 SR/MA: No overall association	435
SFTPA1 and SFTPA2	Surfactant lectin proteins that bind glycolipids on microorganisms	3	436, 437438	—	—
TAP/LMP	Involved in antigen processing	4	257, 439–441	—	—
TGFB1	Multifunction peptide involved in proliferation, differentiation, adhesion, etc., of cells	5	224, 248, 258, 264, 442	—	—

(Continued)

Table 2 Directory of published candidate gene studies *(Continued)*

Gene	Function[a]	Studies	Reference(s)	Systematic review/meta-analysis finding	Systematic review or meta-analysis reference(s)
TIRAP	Adaptor protein involved in TLR4 signaling pathway	10	264, 355, 443–450	1 SR/MA: No association	451
TLR1 (CD281)	Forms a heterodimer with TLR2 to bind bacterial lipoproteins and peptidoglycan	9	279, 445, 449, 452–457	2 SR/MA: 1805G>T: No overall association, nominally significant association in Africans and American Hispanics	458, 459
TLR2 (CD282)	Recognizes wide variety of pathogen peptidoglycans	18	262, 279, 307, 355, 449, 452, 454, 456, 460–469	4 SR/MA: 2258G>A: nominally associated overall and in Asians, not Caucasians; 597T>C: no association	458, 459, 470, 471
TLR4 (CD384)	Recognizes LPS as well as many viral and polysaccharide proteins	11	255, 355, 449, 454, 469, 472–477	2 SR/MA: Asp299Gly and Thr399Ile coding changes: no association	459, 478
TLR6 (CD286)	Recognizes bacterial lipoprotein	1	454	3 SR/MA: −745C>T: nominally associated in all groups	458, 459, 471
TLR8	Recognizes ssRNA and phagocytosed bacterial RNA	3	456, 479, 480	1 SR/MA: several variants nominally associated with TB	471
TLR9	Recognizes methylated DNA	8	355, 449, 456, 467, 481–484	1 SR/MA: nominally associated all groups	459
TLR10	Ligand unknown.	2	454, 456	–	–
TNF	Involved in protective responses against TB through many different mechanisms and as a proinflammatory cytokine. Meta-analysis does not support presence of association (249)	30	90, 142, 212, 216, 236, 243, 248, 258, 260, 264, 270, 272, 275, 279, 281, 283, 287, 306, 320, 363, 389, 400, 476, 485–491	6 SR/MA: −308G>A: not overall associated, nominally associated in Asians, not Caucasians, in 3 SR −238G>A: no overall association in 4 SR −863 C>A and −857C>T: no overall association in 2 SR, nominally associated in Asians	249, 492–496
TOLLIP	Interacts with several TLR signaling components	1	497	–	–
TCIRG1 (V-ATPase A3)	Vacuolar ATPase involved in acidification of lysosomes	2	154, 498	–	–
VDR	Vitamin D has been shown to suppress *M. tuberculosis* growth *in vitro* through production of the antimicrobial peptide cathelicidin and possibly via modulation of TLR signaling polymorphisms associated with TB in meta-analysis (527)	40	90, 130, 142, 181, 205, 229, 260, 262, 339, 343, 374, 383, 385, 389, 395, 499–523	7 SR/MA: FokI: nominally associated overall in 1 SR, probably only in Asians according to 4 SR TaqI: Not associated in 3 SR, associated in Asians in 1 SR BsmI: Not associated in 1 SR ApaI: Not associated in 1 SR	FokI: 524, 525, 526527 TaqI: 525, 528, 527, 529526 BsmI: 525, 526 ApaI: 525, 526

[a]dsDNA, double-stranded DNA; LPS, lipopolysaccharide; PDGF, platelet-derived growth factor; ssRNA, single-stranded RNA.

Table 3 Loci associated with TB susceptibility through genome-wide association studies

Locus	Function	First identified	Replication studies, outcome:details
Chr18q11.2, rs4331426	Unknown, nearest genes: *CTAGE1* and *RBBP8*	Gambia and Ghana GWAS and replication in Ghana and Malawi: total 3,632 cases, 7,501 controls: OR 1.19, $P = 1.6 \times 10^{-8}$	Yes: Taiwanese candidate SNP study in 200 cases, 188 controls No: Chinese candidate SNP study in 578 cases, 756 controls analysis No: Russian GWAS
Chr11p13, rs2057178	Unknown Downstream of WT1	Gambia and Ghana GWAS and imputation, replication in Indonesia and Russia: total 13,858 cases, 8,821 controls: OR 0.77, 0.80, 0.84, and 0.91 in Ghanaians, Gambians, Indonesians, and Russians, respectively; $P = 2.57 \times 10^{-11}$ overall	Yes: South African GWAS of 91 cases, 642 controls Russian GWAS: 5,539 cases and 5,607 controls
Chr8q24, rs4733781	Fine-mapped association to rs10956514, shown to reduce ASAP1 expression in dendritic cells	Russian GWAS and imputation: Total 6,432 cases, 8,082 controls. OR 0.84, $P = 2.6 \times 10^{-11}$	Partial: reanalysis of Gambia and Ghana GWAS

examined *in vitro* response to infection with *M. tuberculosis* of monocytes from cases with TB and controls according to age and found that although there was no difference in transcriptomic response due to age, monocytes from healthy controls reduced expression of IL-26 following *in vitro* infection, consistent with reduced *in vivo* levels in cases. These data suggest that IL-26 downregulation may be an advantageous response to infection (30).

In vivo studies have also been performed, and these have yielded many new insights into TB pathogenesis. Berry et al. (31) identified an 86-gene transcript signature in peripheral blood that differentiated adults infected with TB from other inflammatory diseases (32). The signature was shown to plausibly arise from neutrophils and was markedly enriched for genes involved in type I and type II interferon pathways. These transcriptomic results were confirmed by a second independent study (33) and an additional independent study that delineated novel transethnic transcriptomic signatures of active TB disease, such as activation of the FcGR1 signaling pathway (34). Recent evidence in mouse models and in humans demonstrates that IL-1 induces eicosanoids that inhibit type 1 interferons, leading to enhanced bacterial containment, and confirms a role for type 1 interferons in risk of TB (35). In many of these studies, the transcriptomic signature was also shown to associate with the severity of disease and to dissipate with response to anti-TB therapy (31, 33), as was also specifically shown in a study of patients on treatment (36). Some studies have also identified transcriptomic signatures that differentiate those with active versus latent TB infection (37). Although these studies were performed in adults, often in high-prevalence settings, only one study has addressed the question of

whether similar diagnostic signatures may exist in children. Anderson and colleagues identified a 51-transcript set that differentiated South African and Malawian children with TB and those without TB and confirmed the validity in Kenyan children (38). Taken together, these studies offer exciting new prospects for the ability of transcriptomic signatures to diagnose TB in adults and children. A caveat is that these studies often differ in whether the transcriptome of mixed populations of cells in blood, PBMCs, or purified cell subsets is considered. Moreover, studies suggest that peripheral markers may not reflect pulmonary events (39), and hence, transcriptomic measures from pulmonary samples may provide additional insights.

Prospects for identifying signatures that differentiate those who subsequently develop TB and those who do not are likewise promising but less advanced. Two studies, of infants (40) and of adolescents (41) at risk for TB, have gained much attention at recent conferences and suggest that transcriptomic differences may predict disease susceptibility. In addition, a published study suggests that TB relapse among individuals who had experienced an episode of TB can be predicted by transcriptomic measures (42) that demarcate excessive cytolytic responses.

CURRENT STUDIES AND FUTURE PROSPECTS

Identification of genetic variants replicably associated with TB susceptibility across populations has proven to be challenging despite the high heritability estimates of TB. This problem is referred to as the "missing heritability" issue and has been explored in the context of many other diseases (43). This section addresses the question of why identifying TB-susceptibility-associated genetic variants has proven to be so challenging and how current and future studies are responding to this.

Large-Scale Collaborative Meta-Analyses To Resolve Population-Specific Associations

Common genetic variants may individually contribute only weak effects; the effect sizes observed in candidate gene and GWAS studies have typically been small. Larger studies, or meta-analyses, may therefore be required to confidently identify whether these variants are associated across populations as is suggested by concordant directions of effect. Taking advantage of differences between linkage disequilibrium among ethnic groups may fine-map associations to identify causal alleles and yield novel loci associated with disease due to enhanced statistical power. The ITHGC, a consortium of a dozen cohorts across 10 countries that includes primary GWAS data from individuals with pTB, is coordinating efforts in this regard. Similar approaches have proven to be rewarding in studying other complex diseases such as type 2 diabetes mellitus (44). Furthermore, meta-analytical approaches applied in the study of malaria (45, 46), which faces challenges similar to TB studies in accounting for variable exposure, have demonstrated that meta-analytical efforts, at the very least, allow careful study of patterns of heterogeneity to give insights into population-specific associations.

Sequence-Based Approaches To Identify Loci Associated with Disease: The Role of Exome, Whole-Genome, and RNA Sequencing

An alternative explanation for missing heritability is that rare variants (typically those with frequency <1%), or variants not captured by GWAS genotyping and imputation, may explain a greater proportion of heritability. Newer methods, which are becoming more cost-effective, such as exome and whole-genome sequencing, allow assessment of the contribution of rare variants to TB susceptibility. A small pilot study of exome sequencing to identify susceptibility loci demonstrated the feasibility of this approach (47) in TB, but large sample sizes are likely required (43). Whole-genome sequencing is rapidly becoming the first-line approach to identification of causative mutations in individuals with Mendelian disorders once known mutations are excluded.

Similarly, array-based transcriptomics is limited to interrogation of a limited set of transcripts, whereas RNA-sequencing approaches now offer enhanced resolution of transcripts and transcript variants. The cost of RNA sequencing remains relatively high, however, and

only a handful of current studies have made use of this approach. Future studies will likely make greater use of RNA-sequencing technologies.

Host-Pathogen Coevolution

Studies in which sequencing of *M. tuberculosis* isolates from diverse geographic locations was performed suggest that *M. tuberculosis* likely followed the human migration out of Africa ~70,000 years ago and has remained a primary human pathogen (48). The evolution of *M. tuberculosis* strains and what impact this has on its biology is discussed in detail elsewhere (532, 537, 538). For host genetic studies, the significance of host-pathogen coevolution is that it is plausible that *M. tuberculosis* may have been a powerful selective force over the course of human history, and conversely that host restriction may have been a powerful selective force on *M. tuberculosis* evolution. There are few detailed studies of *M. tuberculosis* as a human selective force (49). *Mycobacterium leprae*, in contrast, has been shown to have likely influenced human evolution, resulting in selection of loci that may protect from leprosy but increase the risk of Crohn's disease (50). Conversely, evidence for immune responses as a selective force on *M. tuberculosis* evolution is illustrated by the hyperconservation of *M. tuberculosis* antigenic epitopes presented by HLA, suggesting that *M. tuberculosis* may have adapted and indeed acquired an ability to subvert T-cell responses (51). Future studies that leverage the growing volume of whole-genome sequences from global populations and *M. tuberculosis* sequences to identify the nature of host-pathogen coevolution and selection are on the horizon.

Host-pathogen coevolution may also potentially explain population-specific associations on the basis that if geographic differentiation between mycobacteria into distinct lineages occurred together with evolution of host defense mechanisms, susceptibility associations may be seen only in the context of infection with a specific lineage or human population. Therefore, heterogeneity in association between susceptibility variants and disease among different populations may plausibly be due to differences in lineage evolution. This may explain the relative absence of host genetic correlates in candidate gene and GWAS studies that replicate across different population groups. A further implication is that host-pathogen coevolution may explain the relative success of a lineage that is newly introduced into a population that coevolved with a heterologous lineage. The next generation of host genetic studies is therefore carefully examining pathogen genetics contemporaneously with host genetics.

Systems Biology of TB: Integration of TB Host Genetics with Broader Genomics Data Sets

There is now a plethora of data sets giving insights into the genomic regulation of immunologically relevant genes, and standards in genomics research require data sharing. This provides the opportunity to assess findings in a systemic way so as to assemble a systems-based understanding of TB pathogenesis. For example, integrating cell-type-specific methylation, histone modification, and gene expression maps from diverse sources may help fine-map disease-associated loci to identify likely causative variants and prioritize mechanistic experiments (52).

At least one group has attempted to unite host genetic data with transcriptomic data in TB by performing expression quantitative loci (eQTL) and methylation QTL (mQTL) studies. Barreiro et al. (53) identified 198 SNPs that were associated with variation in gene expression levels in either untreated or *M. tuberculosis*-treated DC but not both. These eQTL studies were overrepresented among nominally significant GWAS results of pTB relative to expectations. Moreover, these data helped identify the likely mechanism behind the association of variants in ASAP1 and TB disease identified in a GWAS in Russia, illustrating how combined analyses can be used. The same group of investigators recently also reported how *M. tuberculosis* remodels the epigenetic landscape in human dendritic cells (54), consistent with mechanistic studies that identify *M. tuberculosis* proteins such as Rv1988 as modifiers of histone methylation (55).

Host Genetic Studies Responding to the Epidemiology of TB

The global burden of TB disease is characterized by geographic disparities as well as variation according to underlying risk factors such as HIV, diabetes mellitus, age, and gender. An extraordinary strength in host genetic studies thus far is the geographic representativeness of these studies, including studies from most regions of the world. The majority of candidate gene studies and all the GWAS recruited HIV-negative volunteers to avoid confounding. One GWAS, discussed above, examined whether host genetic correlates differed according to age (23); together with another *in vitro* transcriptomic study (30) that asked a similar question, this study suggests that there may be pathophysiological differences between TB in younger adults and that in older or elderly adults. A few candidate gene studies have studied HIV-infected volunteers specifically to ascertain whether host genetic factors affect risk, but few convincing findings have been observed.

Similarly, transcriptomic studies are beginning to study individuals with additional risk factors including diabetes mellitus (56), and a consortium to study TB in patients with diabetes, the TANDEM consortium, will include aspects of host genetic studies (57). Some epidemiological observations suggest a sex-specific difference in TB risk, and a few host genetic studies have explored this (e.g., reference 15), but the large-scale GWAS studies have yet to address this fully.

Further studies that take on the specific epidemiology of TB in risk groups, or explicitly address concurrent environmental risks, would assist in establishing the generalizability of pathophysiological mechanisms of disease and potentially lead to new tools applicable in risk groups: so-called precision medicine.

Refining and Expanding Phenotype Definitions

The majority of host genetic studies have focused on comparisons between individuals with pulmonary TB and either healthy controls or individuals with latent TB infection. In contrast, transcriptomic studies have been careful to examine these three groups separately. Because of the complexity of diagnosing TB, many studies have performed sensitivity analyses to ascertain the influence of diagnostic uncertainty. Future studies will likely address this issue by differentiation of individuals with latent TB infection, those with active disease (pulmonary or extrapulmonary), those with proven exposure who have remained uninfected, and those who may never have been exposed to TB.

In this review, I have not highlighted the differences between studies that focus on extrapulmonary TB and those that focus on pulmonary TB because there have been only a handful of candidate gene studies, and one *in vitro* transcriptomic study (28), that examine this topic. The pathophysiology of susceptibility to extrapulmonary TB and pTB may intuitively be expected to differ somewhat, and host genetic studies that examine this issue in detail may prove to be valuable in testing this intuition formally. Likewise, studies that take into account the severity of disease (as some transcriptomic studies have) and intermediate phenotypes that may be associated with TB may advance understanding of the role of host genetics in TB.

Clinical Translation of Host Genomic Insights

Predictive tools: developing risk-score estimates

If genetic markers that predicted risk were confidently identified, they might be used to generate risk estimates that could be used to stratify preventive interventions. Such approaches are being applied to a few diseases (58, 59), but, like many of these other disorders, the evidence for individual susceptibility loci in TB is as yet insufficient to predict risk accurately. Nevertheless, the high heritability estimates may themselves, in principle, be used to predict risk, and future studies will likely exploit this further.

Predictive biomarker validation using genetics: the role of Mendelian randomization studies

Several biomarkers or risk factors for TB risk have been identified, such as vitamin D levels or T-cell immunity. A major problem in modern biomarker research is biomarker validation and differentiating causal from noncausal predictors. Mendelian randomization (MR) studies that test whether genetic correlates of a biomarker are associated with the outcome of interest (TB) are a powerful way to validate the causal association between a biomarker and disease risk (60). MR studies are akin to the randomized control trial because both study designs involve randomization of exposure categories, genetic exposure through meiosis, and intervention exposure though random assignment. Hence, MR studies are a potential gold standard for biomarker validation. Application of this approach helped to refute the notion that high-density lipoprotein levels were independently and causally associated with myocardial infarction risk (61) and to show that vitamin D levels are likely causally associated with multiple sclerosis disease risk (62). MR studies in TB may be instrumental in establishing causal associations between biomarkers and disease risk.

Host genomics to advance vaccine development

An area that has received much deserved attention has been the role host genomics is playing in vaccine development; this is covered in greater detail elsewhere (532, 536). Transcriptomic studies are playing a leading role in identifying immune correlates of vaccine and adjuvant response, predictive signatures of disease, and nodes for intervention (63, 64). Similarly aligning basic immunological and host genomic studies has helped identify possible mechanisms that may underlie the apparent nonspecific effectiveness of BCG for preventing mortality (65).

Diagnosing active tuberculosis using transcriptomic assays

A major advancement arising from host transcriptomic studies is diagnostic biomarkers based on differentially expressed gene sets. These diagnostic signatures have been replicated across multiple settings, and studies identifying and replicating a signature for use in children have also been reported. Efforts are under way to simplify assays so that they may be deployed cheaply in the field and their robustness in real-world settings may be tested.

Therapeutic tools to stratify therapy: a role for pharmacogenomics and host genetics in host-directed immunotherapy

Genetic predictors of isoniazid-induced hepatotoxicity have been widely studied. A NAT2 polymorphism has been shown to confer reduced acetylation of isoniazid, resulting in higher drug levels, and stratifying therapy by NAT2 status reduces adverse outcomes (66). Although not addressed in this review, identifying genetic correlates of adverse reactions to other anti-TB drugs would greatly advance the ability to stratify therapy and could ease efforts to repurpose drugs associated with high toxicity to patients with drug-resistant TB. Crucially, future pharmacogenomics studies should not omit the key populations (67).

Efforts to identify new therapeutic approaches to TB include consideration of host-directed therapy (68). In this regard, host genomics may play a major role in identifying which immunological nodes to target, in monitoring response (e.g., through transcriptomic downstream target measurement), and in identifying hosts most likely to benefit from therapy.

CONCLUSIONS

Host genetic factors play a major role in TB disease risk, accounting for a large proportion of risk variance. Identifying specific loci that mediate this effect has proven challenging, but host genetics have played a substantial role in our understanding of host-pathogen interactions in TB, and the new wave of enquiries is likely to assist further in this regard.

Citation. Naranbhai V. 2016. The role of host genetics (and genomics) in tuberculosis. Microbiol Spectrum 4(5):TBTB2-0011-2016.

References

1. **Comstock GW.** 1978. Tuberculosis in twins: a re-analysis of the Prophit survey. *Am Rev Respir Dis* 117:621–624.
2. **Diehl K, von Verschner OF.** 1933. *Zwillingsforschung und erbliche Tuberkulosedisposition, Zwillingstuberkulose: Zwillingsforschung und erbliche Tuberkulosedisposition.* 1.
3. **Kallmann FJ, Reisner D.** 1943. Twin studies on genetic variations in resistance to tuberculosis. *J Hered* 34: 269–276.

4. van der Eijk EA, van de Vosse E, Vandenbroucke JP, van Dissel JT. 2007. Heredity versus environment in tuberculosis in twins: the 1950s United Kingdom Prophit Survey Simonds and Comstock revisited. *Am J Respir Crit Care Med* **176**:1281–1288

5. Cobat A, Gallant CJ, Simkin L, Black GF, Stanley K, Hughes J, Doherty TM, Hanekom WA, Eley B, Beyers N, Jaïs JP, van Helden P, Abel L, Hoal EG, Alcaic A, Schurr E. 2010. High heritability of antimycobacterial immunity in an area of hyperendemicity for tuberculosis disease. *J Infect Dis* **201**:15–19.

6. Stein CM, Guwatudde D, Nakakeeto M, Peters P, Elston RC, Tiwari HK, Mugerwa R, Whalen CC. 2003. Heritability analysis of cytokines as intermediate phenotypes of tuberculosis. *J Infect Dis* **187**:1679–1685.

7. Sepulveda RL, Heiba IM, Navarrete C, Elston RC, Gonzalez B, Sorensen RU. 1994. Tuberculin reactivity after newborn BCG immunization in mono- and dizygotic twins. *Tuber Lung Dis* **75**:138–143.

8. Cottle LE. 2011. Mendelian susceptibility to mycobacterial disease. *Clin Genet* **79**:17–22.

9. Boisson-Dupuis S, Bustamante J, El-Baghdadi J, Camcioglu Y, Parvaneh N, El Azbaoui S, Agader A, Hassani A, El Hafidi N, Mrani NA, Jouhadi Z, Ailal F, Najib J, Reisli I, Zamani A, Yosunkaya S, Gulle-Girit S, Yildiran A, Cipe FE, Torun SH, Metin A, Atikan BY, Hatipoglu N, Aydogmus C, Kilic SS, Dogu F, Karaca N, Aksu G, Kutukculer N, Keser-Emiroglu M, Somer A, Tanir G, Aytekin C, Adimi P, Mahdaviani SA, Mamishi S, Bousfiha A, Sanal O, Mansouri D, Casanova JL, Abel L. 2015. Inherited and acquired immunodeficiencies underlying tuberculosis in childhood. *Immunol Rev* **264**:103–120.

10. Meyer CG, Intemann CD, Förster B, Owusu-Dabo E, Franke A, Horstmann RD, Thye T. 2016. No significant impact of IFN-γ pathway gene variants on tuberculosis susceptibility in a West African population. *Eur J Hum Genet* **24**:748–755.

11. Yang J, Lee SH, Goddard ME, Visscher PM. 2011. GCTA: a tool for genome-wide complex trait analysis. *Am J Hum Genet* **88**:76–82.

12. Shaw MA, Collins A, Peacock CS, Miller EN, Black GF, Sibthorpe D, Lins-Lainson Z, Shaw JJ, Ramos F, Silveira F, Blackwell JM. 1997. Evidence that genetic susceptibility to *Mycobacterium tuberculosis* in a Brazilian population is under oligogenic control: linkage study of the candidate genes NRAMP1 and TNFA. *Tuber Lung Dis* **78**:35–45.

13. Greenwood CM, Fujiwara TM, Boothroyd LJ, Miller MA, Frappier D, Fanning EA, Schurr E, Morgan K. 2000. Linkage of tuberculosis to chromosome 2q35 loci, including NRAMP1, in a large aboriginal Canadian family. *Am J Hum Genet* **67**:405–416.

14. Bellamy R. 2000. Identifying genetic susceptibility factors for tuberculosis in Africans: a combined approach using a candidate gene study and a genome-wide screen. *Clin Sci (Lond)* **98**:245–250.

15. Bellamy R, Beyers N, McAdam KP, Ruwende C, Gie R, Samaai P, Bester D, Meyer M, Corrah T, Collin M, Camidge DR, Wilkinson D, Hoal-Van Helden E, Whittle HC, Amos W, van Helden P, Hill AV. 2000. Genetic susceptibility to tuberculosis in Africans: a genome-wide scan. *Proc Natl Acad Sci USA* **97**:8005–8009.

16. Baghdadi JE, Orlova M, Alter A, Ranque B, Chentoufi M, Lazrak F, Archane MI, Casanova JL, Benslimane A, Schurr E, Abel L. 2006. An autosomal dominant major gene confers predisposition to pulmonary tuberculosis in adults. *J Exp Med* **203**:1679–1684.

17. Stein CM, Zalwango S, Malone LL, Won S, Mayanja-Kizza H, Mugerwa RD, Leontiev DV, Thompson CL, Cartier KC, Elston RC, Iyengar SK, Boom WH, Whalen CC. 2008. Genome scan of *M. tuberculosis* infection and disease in Ugandans. *PLoS One* **3**:e4094

18. Jamieson SE, Miller EN, Black GF, Peacock CS, Cordell HJ, Howson JM, Shaw MA, Burgner D, Xu W, Lins-Lainson Z, Shaw JJ, Ramos F, Silveira F, Blackwell JM. 2004. Evidence for a cluster of genes on chromosome 17q11-q21 controlling susceptibility to tuberculosis and leprosy in Brazilians. *Genes Immun* **5**:46–57.

19. Welter D, MacArthur J, Morales J, Burdett T, Hall P, Junkins H, Klemm A, Flicek P, Manolio T, Hindorff L, Parkinson H. 2014. The NHGRI GWAS Catalog, a curated resource of SNP-trait associations. *Nucleic Acids Res* **42**(D1):D1001–D1006.

20. Auton A, Brooks LD, Durbin RM, Garrison EP, Kang HM, Korbel JO, Marchini JL, McCarthy S, McVean GA, Abecasis GR, 1000 Genomes Project Consortium. 2015. A global reference for human genetic variation. *Nature* **526**:68–74.

21. Altshuler DM, et al, International HapMap 3 Consortium. 2010. Integrating common and rare genetic variation in diverse human populations. *Nature* **467**:52–58.

22. Thye T, Vannberg FO, Wong SH, Owusu-Dabo E, Osei I, Gyapong J, Sirugo G, Sisay-Joof F, Enimil A, Chinbuah MA, Floyd S, Warndorff DK, Sichali L, Malema S, Crampin AC, Ngwira B, Teo YY, Small K, Rockett K, Kwiatkowski D, Fine PE, Hill PC, Newport M, Lienhardt C, Adegbola RA, Corrah T, Ziegler A, Morris AP, Meyer CG, Horstmann RD, Hill AV, African TB Genetics Consortium, Wellcome Trust Case Control Consortium. 2010. Genome-wide association analyses identifies a susceptibility locus for tuberculosis on chromosome 18q11.2. *Nat Genet* **42**:739–741.

23. Mahasirimongkol S, Yanai H, Mushiroda T, Promphittayarat W, Wattanapokayakit S, Phromjai J, Yuliwulandari R, Wichukchinda N, Yowang A, Yamada N, Kantipong P, Takahashi A, Kubo M, Sawanpanyalert P, Kamatani N, Nakamura Y, Tokunaga K. 2012. Genome-wide association studies of tuberculosis in Asians identify distinct at-risk locus for young tuberculosis. *J Hum Genet* **57**:363–367.

24. Png E, Alisjahbana B, Sahiratmadja E, Marzuki S, Nelwan R, Balabanova Y, Nikolayevskyy V, Drobniewski F, Nejentsev S, Adnan I, van de Vosse E, Hibberd ML, van Crevel R, Ottenhoff TH, Seielstad M. 2012. A genome wide association study of pulmonary tuberculosis susceptibility in Indonesians. *BMC Med Genet* **13**:5

25. Thye T, Owusu-Dabo E, Vannberg FO, van Crevel R, Curtis J, Sahiratmadja E, Balabanova Y, Ehmen C, Muntau B, Ruge G, Sievertsen J, Gyapong J, Nikolayevskyy V, Hill PC, Sirugo G, Drobniewski F, van de Vosse E, Newport M, Alisjahbana B, Nejentsev S, Ottenhoff TH, Hill AV, Horstmann RD, Meyer CG. 2012. Common variants at 11p13 are associated with susceptibility to tuberculosis. *Nat Genet* **44:**257–259.

26. Curtis J, Luo Y, Zenner HL, Cuchet-Lourenço D, Wu C, Lo K, Maes M, Alisaac A, Stebbings E, Liu JZ, Kopanitsa L, Ignatyeva O, Balabanova Y, Nikolayevskyy V, Baessmann I, Thye T, Meyer CG, Nürnberg P, Horstmann RD, Drobniewski F, Plagnol V, Barrett JC, Nejentsev S. 2015. Susceptibility to tuberculosis is associated with variants in the ASAP1 gene encoding a regulator of dendritic cell migration. *Nat Genet* **47:**523–527.

27. Chimusa ER, Zaitlen N, Daya M, Möller M, van Helden PD, Mulder NJ, Price AL, Hoal EG. 2014. Genome-wide association study of ancestry-specific TB risk in the South African Coloured population. *Hum Mol Genet* **23:**796–809.

28. Thuong NT, Dunstan SJ, Chau TT, Thorsson V, Simmons CP, Quyen NT, Thwaites GE, Thi Ngoc Lan N, Hibberd M, Teo YY, Seielstad M, Aderem A, Farrar JJ, Hawn TR. 2008. Identification of tuberculosis susceptibility genes with human macrophage gene expression profiles. *PLoS Pathog* **4:**e1000229

29. Lesho E, Forestiero FJ, Hirata MH, Hirata RD, Cecon L, Melo FF, Paik SH, Murata Y, Ferguson EW, Wang Z, Ooi GT. 2011. Transcriptional responses of host peripheral blood cells to tuberculosis infection. *Tuberculosis (Edinb)* **91:**390–399.

30. Guerra-Laso JM, Raposo-García S, García-García S, Diez-Tascón C, Rivero-Lezcano OM. 2015. Microarray analysis of *Mycobacterium tuberculosis*-infected monocytes reveals IL26 as a new candidate gene for tuberculosis susceptibility. *Immunology* **144:**291–301.

31. Berry MP, Graham CM, McNab FW, Xu Z, Bloch SA, Oni T, Wilkinson KA, Banchereau R, Skinner J, Wilkinson RJ, Quinn C, Blankenship D, Dhawan R, Cush JJ, Mejias A, Ramilo O, Kon OM, Pascual V, Banchereau J, Chaussabel D, O'Garra A. 2010. An interferon-inducible neutrophil-driven blood transcriptional signature in human tuberculosis. *Nature* **466:**973–977.

32. Bloom CI, Graham CM, Berry MP, Rozakeas F, Redford PS, Wang Y, Xu Z, Wilkinson KA, Wilkinson RJ, Kendrick Y, Devouassoux G, Ferry T, Miyara M, Bouvry D, Valeyre D, Gorochov G, Blankenship D, Saadatian M, Vanhems P, Beynon H, Vancheeswaran R, Wickremasinghe M, Chaussabel D, Banchereau J, Pascual V, Ho LP, Lipman M, O'Garra A. 2013. Transcriptional blood signatures distinguish pulmonary tuberculosis, pulmonary sarcoidosis, pneumonias and lung cancers. *PLoS One* **8:**e70630. (Erratum: 8[8])

33. Ottenhoff TH, Dass RH, Yang N, Zhang MM, Wong HE, Sahiratmadja E, Khor CC, Alisjahbana B, van Crevel R, Marzuki S, Seielstad M, van de Vosse E, Hibberd ML. 2012. Genome-wide expression profiling identifies type 1 interferon response pathways in active tuberculosis. *PLoS One* **7:**e45839

34. Maertzdorf J, Ota M, Repsilber D, Mollenkopf HJ, Weiner J, Hill PC, Kaufmann SH. 2011. Functional correlations of pathogenesis-driven geneexpression signatures in tuberculosis. *PLoS One* **6:**e26938

35. Mayer-Barber KD, Andrade BB, Oland SD, Amaral EP, Barber DL, Gonzales J, Derrick SC, Shi R, Kumar NP, Wei W, Yuan X, Zhang G, Cai Y, Babu S, Catalfamo M, Salazar AM, Via LE, Barry CE III, Sher A. 2014. Host-directed therapy of tuberculosis based on interleukin-1 and type I interferon crosstalk. *Nature* **511:**99–103.

36. Cliff JM, Lee JS, Constantinou N, Cho JE, Clark TG, Ronacher K, King EC, Lukey PT, Duncan K, Van Helden PD, Walzl G, Dockrell HM. 2013. Distinct phases of blood gene expression pattern through tuberculosis treatment reflect modulation of the humoral immune response. *J Infect Dis* **207:**18–29.

37. Kaforou M, Wright VJ, Oni T, French N, Anderson ST, Bangani N, Banwell CM, Brent AJ, Crampin AC, Dockrell HM, Eley B, Heyderman RS, Hibberd ML, Kern F, Langford PR, Ling L, Mendelson M, Ottenhoff TH, Zgambo F, Wilkinson RJ, Coin LJ, Levin M. 2013. Detection of tuberculosis in HIV-infected and -uninfected African adults using whole blood RNA expression signatures: a case-control study. *PLoS Med* **10:**e1001538

38. Anderson ST, Kaforou M, Brent AJ, Wright VJ, Banwell CM, Chagaluka G, Crampin AC, Dockrell HM, French N, Hamilton MS, Hibberd ML, Kern F, Langford PR, Ling L, Mlotha R, Ottenhoff TH, Pienaar S, Pillay V, Scott JA, Twahir H, Wilkinson RJ, Coin LJ, Heyderman RS, Levin M, Eley B, ILULU Consortium, KIDS TB Study Group. 2014. Diagnosis of childhood tuberculosis and host RNA expression in Africa. *N Engl J Med* **370:**1712–1723.

39. Gideon HP, Phuah J, Myers AJ, Bryson BD, Rodgers MA, Coleman MT, Maiello P, Rutledge T, Marino S, Fortune SM, Kirschner DE, Lin PL, Flynn JL. 2015. Variability in tuberculosis granuloma T cell responses exists, but a balance of pro- and anti-inflammatory cytokines is associated with sterilization. *PLoS Pathog* **11:**e1004603

40. Fletcher HA, Filali-Mouhim A, Nemes E, Hawkridge A, Keyser A, Njikan S, Hatherill M, Scriba TJ, Abel B, Kagina BM, Veldsman A, Agudelo NM, Kaplan G, Hussey GD, Sekaly RP, Hanekom WA; BCG study team. 2016. Human newborn bacille Calmette-Guérin vaccination and risk of tuberculosis disease: a case-control study. *BMC Med* **14:**76.

41. Zak DE et al; ACS and GC6-74 cohort study groups. 2016. A blood RNA signature for tuberculosis disease risk: a prospective cohort study. *Lancet* **387**(10035):2312–2322.

42. Cliff JM, Cho JE, Lee JS, Ronacher K, King EC, van Helden P, Walzl G, Dockrell HM. 2016. Excessive cytolytic responses predict tuberculosis relapse after apparently successful treatment. *J Infect Dis* **213:**485–495.

43. Zuk O, Hechter E, Sunyaev SR, Lander ES. 2012. The mystery of missing heritability: genetic interactions

create phantom heritability. *Proc Natl Acad Sci USA* 109:1193–1198

44. Mahajan A, et al, DIAbetes Genetics Replication And Meta-analysis (DIAGRAM) Consortium, Asian Genetic Epidemiology Network Type 2 Diabetes (AGEN-T2D) Consortium, South Asian Type 2 Diabetes (SAT2D) Consortium, Mexican American Type 2 Diabetes (MAT2D) Consortium, Type 2 Diabetes Genetic Exploration by Next-generation sequencing in multi-Ethnic Samples (T2D-GENES) Consortium. 2014. Genome-wide trans-ancestry meta-analysis provides insight into the genetic architecture of type 2 diabetes susceptibility. *Nat Genet* 46:234–244.

45. Band G, Rockett KA, Spencer CC, Kwiatkowski DP, Malaria Genomic Epidemiology Network. 2015. A novel locus of resistance to severe malaria in a region of ancient balancing selection. *Nature* 526:253–257.

46. Malaria Genomic Epidemiology Network. 2014. Reappraisal of known malaria resistance loci in a large multicenter study. *Nat Genet* 46:1197–1204.

47. Duncan C, Jamieson F, Mehaffy C. 2015. Preliminary evaluation of exome sequencing to identify genetic markers of susceptibility to tuberculosis disease. *BMC Res Notes* 8:750

48. Comas I, Coscolla M, Luo T, Borrell S, Holt KE, Kato-Maeda M, Parkhill J, Malla B, Berg S, Thwaites G, Yeboah-Manu D, Bothamley G, Mei J, Wei L, Bentley S, Harris SR, Niemann S, Diel R, Aseffa A, Gao Q, Young D, Gagneux S. 2013. Out-of-Africa migration and Neolithic coexpansion of *Mycobacterium tuberculosis* with modern humans. *Nat Genet* 45:1176–1182.

49. Lipsitch M, Sousa AO. 2002. Historical intensity of natural selection for resistance to tuberculosis. *Genetics* 161:1599–1607.

50. Jostins L, et al, International IBD Genetics Consortium (IIBDGC). 2012. Host-microbe interactions have shaped the genetic architecture of inflammatory bowel disease. *Nature* 491:119–124.

51. Comas I, Chakravartti J, Small PM, Galagan J, Niemann S, Kremer K, Ernst JD, Gagneux S. 2010. Human T cell epitopes of *Mycobacterium tuberculosis* are evolutionarily hyperconserved. *Nat Genet* 42:498–503.

52. Trynka G, Sandor C, Han B, Xu H, Stranger BE, Liu XS, Raychaudhuri S. 2013. Chromatin marks identify critical cell types for fine mapping complex trait variants. *Nat Genet* 45:124–130.

53. Barreiro LB, Tailleux L, Pai AA, Gicquel B, Marioni JC, Gilad Y. 2012. Deciphering the genetic architecture of variation in the immune response to *Mycobacterium tuberculosis* infection. *Proc Natl Acad Sci USA* 109:1204–1209

54. Pacis A, Tailleux L, Morin AM, Lambourne J, MacIsaac JL, Yotova V, Dumaine A, Danckaert A, Luca F, Grenier JC, Hansen KD, Gicquel B, Yu M, Pai A, He C, Tung J, Pastinen T, Kobor MS, Pique-Regi R, Gilad Y, Barreiro LB. 2015. Bacterial infection remodels the DNA methylation landscape of human dendritic cells. *Genome Res* 25:1801–1811.

55. Yaseen I, Kaur P, Nandicoori VK, Khosla S. 2015. Mycobacteria modulate host epigenetic machinery by Rv1988 methylation of a non-tail arginine of histone H3. *Nat Commun* 6:8922

56. Qu HQ, Rentfro AR, Lu Y, Nair S, Hanis CL, McCormick JB, Fisher-Hoch SP. 2012. Host susceptibility to tuberculosis: insights from a longitudinal study of gene expression in diabetes. *Int J Tuberc Lung Dis* 16:370–372.

57. van Crevel R, Dockrell HM, TANDEM Consortium. 2014. TANDEM: understanding diabetes and tuberculosis. *Lancet Diabetes Endocrinol* 2:270–272.

58. Goldstein BA, Knowles JW, Salfati E, Ioannidis JP, Assimes TL. 2014. Simple, standardized incorporation of genetic risk into non-genetic risk prediction tools for complex traits: coronary heart disease as an example. *Front Genet* 5:254

59. Jostins L, Barrett JC. 2011. Genetic risk prediction in complex disease. *Hum Mol Genet* 20(R2):R182–R188.

60. Evans DM, Davey Smith G. 2015. Mendelian randomization: new applications in the coming age of hypothesis-free causality. *Annu Rev Genomics Hum Genet* 16:327–350.

61. Voight BF, et al. 2012. Plasma HDL cholesterol and risk of myocardial infarction: a mendelian randomisation study. *Lancet* 380:572–580.

62. Mokry LE, Ross S, Ahmad OS, Forgetta V, Smith GD, Leong A, Greenwood CM, Thanassoulis G, Richards JB. 2015. Vitamin D and risk of multiple sclerosis: a mendelian randomization study. *PLoS Med* 12:e1001866

63. Matsumiya M, Stylianou E, Griffiths K, Lang Z, Meyer J, Harris SA, Rowland R, Minassian AM, Pathan AA, Fletcher H, McShane H. 2013. Roles for Treg expansion and HMGB1 signaling through the TLR1-2-6 axis in determining the magnitude of the antigen-specific immune response to MVA85A. *PLoS One* 8:e67922

64. Matsumiya M, Harris SA, Satti I, Stockdale L, Tanner R, O'Shea MK, Tameris M, Mahomed H, Hatherill M, Scriba TJ, Hanekom WA, McShane H, Fletcher HA. 2014. Inflammatory and myeloid-associated gene expression before and one day after infant vaccination with MVA85A correlates with induction of a T cell response. *BMC Infect Dis* 14:314

65. Kleinnijenhuis J, Quintin J, Preijers F, Joosten LA, Ifrim DC, Saeed S, Jacobs C, van Loenhout J, de Jong D, Stunnenberg HG, Xavier RJ, van der Meer JW, van Crevel R, Netea MG. 2012. Bacille Calmette-Guerin induces NOD2-dependent nonspecific protection from reinfection via epigenetic reprogramming of monocytes. *Proc Natl Acad Sci USA* 109:17537–17542.

66. Matsumoto T, Ohno M, Azuma J. 2014. Future of pharmacogenetics-based therapy for tuberculosis. *Pharmacogenomics* 15:601–607.

67. McIlleron H, Abdel-Rahman S, Dave JA, Blockman M, Owen A. 2015. Special populations and pharmacogenetic issues in tuberculosis drug development and clinical research. *J Infect Dis* 211(Suppl 3):S115–S125.

68. Wallis RS, Hafner R. 2015. Advancing host-directed therapy for tuberculosis. *Nat Rev Immunol* 15:255–263.

69. Gra OA, Kozhekbaeva ZM, Litvinov VI. 2010. [Analysis of genetic predisposition to pulmonary tuberculosis in native Russians]. *Genetika* 46:262–271.

70. Pontillo A, Carvalho MS, Kamada AJ, Moura R, Schindler HC, Duarte AJ, Crovella S. 2013. Susceptibility to *Mycobacterium tuberculosis* infection in HIV-positive patients is associated with CARD8 genetic variant. *J Acquir Immune Defic Syndr* 63:147–151.

71. Wang X, Cao Z, Jiang J, Zhu Y, Dong M, Tong A, Cheng X. 2010. AKT1 polymorphisms are associated with tuberculosis in the Chinese population. *Int J Immunogenet* 37:97–101

72. Herb F, Thye T, Niemann S, Browne EN, Chinbuah MA, Gyapong J, Osei I, Owusu-Dabo E, Werz O, Rüsch-Gerdes S, Horstmann RD, Meyer CG. 2008. ALOX5 variants associated with susceptibility to human pulmonary tuberculosis. *Hum Mol Genet* 17:1052–1060.

73. Wozniak MA, Maude RJ, Innes JA, Hawkey PM, Itzhaki RF. 2009. Apolipoprotein E-ε2 confers risk of pulmonary tuberculosis in women from the Indian subcontinent–a preliminary study. *J Infect* 59:219–222.

74. Songane M, Kleinnijenhuis J, Alisjahbana B, Sahiratmadja E, Parwati I, Oosting M, Plantinga TS, Joosten LA, Netea MG, Ottenhoff TH, van de Vosse E, van Crevel R. 2012. Polymorphisms in autophagy genes and susceptibility to tuberculosis. *PLoS One* 7:e41618

75. Etokebe GE, Bulat-Kardum L, Munthe LA, Balen S, Dembic Z. 2014. Association of variable number of tandem repeats in the coding region of the FAM46A gene, FAM46A rs11040 SNP and BAG6 rs3117582 SNP with susceptibility to tuberculosis. *PLoS One* 9:e91385

76. Lian Y, Yue J, Han M, Liu J, Liu L. 2010. Analysis of the association between BTNL2 polymorphism and tuberculosis in Chinese Han population. *Infect Genet Evol* 10:517–521.

77. Moller M, Kwiatkowski R, Nebel A, van Helden PD, Hoal EG, Schreiber S. 2007. Allelic variation in BTNL2 and susceptibility to tuberculosis in a South African population. *Microbes Infect* 9:522–528.

78. Adams LA, Möller M, Nebel A, Schreiber S, van der Merwe L, van Helden PD, Hoal EG. 2011. Polymorphisms in MC3R promoter and CTSZ 3'UTR are associated with tuberculosis susceptibility. *Eur J Hum Genet* 19:676–681.

79. Baker AR, Zalwango S, Malone LL, Igo RP Jr, Qiu F, Nsereko M, Adams MD, Supelak P, Mayanja-Kizza H, Boom WH, Stein CM. 2011. Genetic susceptibility to tuberculosis associated with cathepsin Z haplotype in a Ugandan household contact study. *Hum Immunol* 72:426–430.

80. Cooke GS, Campbell SJ, Bennett S, Lienhardt C, McAdam KP, Sirugo G, Sow O, Gustafson P, Mwangulu F, van Helden P, Fine P, Hoal EG, Hill AV. 2008. Mapping of a novel susceptibility locus suggests a role for MC3R and CTSZ in human tuberculosis. *Am J Respir Crit Care Med* 178:203–207.

81. Alagarasu K, Selvaraj P, Swaminathan S, Raghavan S, Narendran G, Narayanan PR. 2009. CCR2, MCP-1, SDF-1a & DC-SIGN gene polymorphisms in HIV-1 infected patients with & without tuberculosis. *Indian J Med Res* 130:444–450.

82. Arji N, Busson M, Iraqi G, Bourkadi JE, Benjouad A, Boukouaci W, Lahlou O, Ben Amor J, Krishnamoorthy R, Charron D, El Aouad R, Tamouza R. 2012. The MCP-1 (CCL2) -2518 GG genotype is associated with protection against pulmonary tuberculosis in Moroccan patients. *J Infect Dev Ctries* 6:73–78.

83. Ben-Selma W, Harizi H, Boukadida J. 2011. MCP-1 -2518 A/G functional polymorphism is associated with increased susceptibility to active pulmonary tuberculosis in Tunisian patients. *Mol Biol Rep* 38:5413–5419.

84. Buijtels PC, van de Sande WW, Parkinson S, Petit PL, van der Sande MA, van Soolingen D, Verbrugh HA, van Belkum A. 2008. Polymorphism in CC-chemokine ligand 2 associated with tuberculosis in Zambia. *Int J Tuberc Lung Dis* 12:1485–1488.

85. Chu SF, Tam CM, Wong HS, Kam KM, Lau YL, Chiang AK. 2007. Association between RANTES functional polymorphisms and tuberculosis in Hong Kong Chinese. *Genes Immun* 8:475–479.

86. Flores-Villanueva PO, Ruiz-Morales JA, Song CH, Flores LM, Jo EK, Montaño M, Barnes PF, Selman M, Granados J. 2005. A functional promoter polymorphism in monocyte chemoattractant protein-1 is associated with increased susceptibility to pulmonary tuberculosis. *J Exp Med* 202:1649–1658.

87. Ganachari M, Ruiz-Morales JA, Gomez de la Torre Pretell JC, Dinh J, Granados J, Flores-Villanueva PO. 2010. Joint effect of MCP-1 genotype GG and MMP-1 genotype 2G/2G increases the likelihood of developing pulmonary tuberculosis in BCG-vaccinated individuals. *PLoS One* 5:e8881

88. Gao Q, Du Q, Zhang H, Guo C, Lu S, Deng A, Tang M, Liu S, Wang Y, Huang J, Guo Q. 2014. Monocyte chemotactic protein-1 -2518 gene polymorphism and susceptibility to spinal tuberculosis. *Arch Med Res* 45:183–187

89. Hussain R, Ansari A, Talat N, Hasan Z, Dawood G. 2011. CCL2/MCP-I genotype-phenotype relationship in latent tuberculosis infection. *PLoS One* 6:e25803

90. Larcombe LA, Orr PH, Lodge AM, Brown JS, Dembinski IJ, Milligan LC, Larcombe EA, Martin BD, Nickerson PW. 2008. Functional gene polymorphisms in Canadian aboriginal populations with high rates of tuberculosis. *J Infect Dis* 198:1175–1179.

91. Mishra G, Poojary SS, Raj P, Tiwari PK. 2012. Genetic polymorphisms of CCL2, CCL5, CCR2 and CCR5 genes in Sahariya tribe of North Central India: an association study with pulmonary tuberculosis. *Infect Genet Evol* 12:1120–1127.

92. Möller M, Nebel A, Valentonyte R, van Helden PD, Schreiber S, Hoal EG. 2009. Investigation of chromosome 17 candidate genes in susceptibility to TB in a South African population. *Tuberculosis (Edinb)* 89:189–194.

93. Naderi M, Hashemi M, Karami H, Moazeni-Roodi A, Sharifi-Mood B, Kouhpayeh H, Taheri M, Ghavami S. 2011. Lack of association between rs1024611 (-2581 A/G) polymorphism in CC-chemokine Ligand 2 and susceptibility to pulmonary tuberculosis in Zahedan, Southeast Iran. *Prague Med Rep* 112:272–278.

94. Tamouza R, Labie D. 2006. [A promotor polymorphism in monocyte chemoattractant is associated with increased susceptibility to pulmonary tuberculosis]. *Med Sci (Paris)* **22:**571–572.

95. Thye T, Nejentsev S, Intemann CD, Browne EN, Chinbuah MA, Gyapong J, Osei I, Owusu-Dabo E, Zeitels LR, Herb F, Horstmann RD, Meyer CG. 2009. MCP-1 promoter variant -362C associated with protection from pulmonary tuberculosis in Ghana, West Africa. *Hum Mol Genet* **18:**381–388.

96. Velez Edwards DR, Tacconelli A, Wejse C, Hill PC, Morris GA, Edwards TL, Gilbert JR, Myers JL, Park YS, Stryjewski ME, Abbate E, Estevan R, Rabna P, Novelli G, Hamilton CD, Adegbola R, Østergaard L, Williams SM, Scott WK, Sirugo G. 2012. MCP1 SNPs and pulmonary tuberculosis in cohorts from West Africa, the USA and Argentina: lack of association or epistasis with IL12B polymorphisms. *PLoS One* **7:**e32275

97. Xu ZE, Xie YY, Chen JH, Xing LL, Zhang AH, Li BX, Zhu CM. 2009. [Monocyte chemotactic protein-1 gene polymorphism and monocyte chemotactic protein-1 expression in Chongqing Han children with tuberculosis]. *Zhonghua Er Ke Za Zhi* **47:**200–203.

98. Yang BF, Zhuang B, Li F, Zhang CZ, Song AQ. 2009. [The relationship between monocyte chemoattractant protein-1 gene polymorphisms and the susceptibility to pulmonary tuberculosis]. *Zhonghua Jie He He Hu Xi Za Zhi* **32:**454–456.

99. Feng WX, Flores-Villanueva PO, Mokrousov I, Wu XR, Xiao J, Jiao WW, Sun L, Miao Q, Shen C, Shen D, Liu F, Jia ZW, Shen A. 2012. CCL2-2518 (A/G) polymorphisms and tuberculosis susceptibility: a meta-analysis. *Int J Tuberc Lung Dis* **16:**150–156.

100. Gong T, Yang M, Qi L, Shen M, Du Y. 2013. Association of MCP-1 -2518A/G and -362G/C variants and tuberculosis susceptibility: a meta-analysis. *Infect Genet Evol* **20:**1–7

101. VÁsquez-Loarte T, Trubnykova M, Guio H. 2015. Genetic association meta-analysis: a new classification to assess ethnicity using the association of MCP-1 -2518 polymorphism and tuberculosis susceptibility as a model. *BMC Genet* **16:**128

102. Carpenter D, Taype C, Goulding J, Levin M, Eley B, Anderson S, Shaw MA, Armour JA. 2014. CCL3L1 copy number, CCR5 genotype and susceptibility to tuberculosis. *BMC Med Genet* **15:**5

103. Mamtani M, Mummidi S, Ramsuran V, Pham MH, Maldonado R, Begum K, Valera MS, Sanchez R, Castiblanco J, Kulkarni H, Ndung'u T, He W, Anaya JM, Ahuja SK. 2011. Influence of variations in CCL3L1 and CCR5 on tuberculosis in a northwestern Colombian population. *J Infect Dis* **203:**1590–1594.

104. Ben-Selma W, Harizi H, Bougmiza I, Ben Kahla I, Letaief M, Boukadida J. 2011. Polymorphisms in the RANTES gene increase susceptibility to active tuberculosis in Tunisia. *DNA Cell Biol* **30:**789–800.

105. de Wit E, van der Merwe L, van Helden PD, Hoal EG. 2011. Gene-gene interaction between tuberculosis candidate genes in a South African population. *Mamm Genome* **22:**100–110.

106. Mhmoud N, Fahal A, van de Sande WJ. 2013. Association of IL-10 and CCL5 single nucleotide polymorphisms with tuberculosis in the Sudanese population. *Trop Med Int Health* **18:**1119–1127.

107. Sanchez-Castanon M, Baquero IC, Sanchez-Velasco P, Farinas MC, Ausin F, Leyva-Cobian F, Ocejo-Vinyals JG. 2009. Polymorphisms in CCL5 promoter are associated with pulmonary tuberculosis in northern Spain. *Int J Tuberc Lung Dis* **13:**480–485.

108. Selvaraj P, Alagarasu K, Singh B, Afsal K. 2011. CCL5 (RANTES) gene polymorphisms in pulmonary tuberculosis patients of south India. *Int J Immunogenet* **38:** 397–402.

109. Seshadri C, Thuong NT, Yen NT, Bang ND, Chau TT, Thwaites GE, Dunstan SJ, Hawn TR. 2014. A polymorphism in human CD1A is associated with susceptibility to tuberculosis. *Genes Immun* **15:**195–198.

110. Alavi-Naini R, Salimi S, Sharifi-Mood B, Davoodikia AA, Moody B, Naghavi A. 2012. Association between the CD14 gene C-159T polymorphism and serum soluble CD14 with pulmonary tuberculosis. *Int J Tuberc Lung Dis* **16:**1383–1387.

111. Ayaslioglu E, Kalpaklioglu F, Kavut AB, Erturk A, Capan N, Birben E. 2013. The role of CD14 gene promoter polymorphism in tuberculosis susceptibility. *J Microbiol Immunol Infect* **46:**158–163.

112. Druszczynska M, Strapagiel D, Kwiatkowska S, Kowalewicz-Kulbat M, Rozalska B, Chmiela M, Rudnicka W. 2006. Tuberculosis bacilli still posing a threat. Polymorphism of genes regulating anti-mycobacterial properties of macrophages. *Pol J Microbiol* **55:**7–12.

113. Kang YA, Lee HW, Kim YW, Han SK, Shim YS, Yim JJ. 2009. Association between the -159C/T CD14 gene polymorphism and tuberculosis in a Korean population. *FEMS Immunol Med Microbiol* **57:**229–235.

114. Pacheco E, Fonseca C, Montes C, Zabaleta J, García LF, Arias MA. 2004. CD14 gene promoter polymorphism in different clinical forms of tuberculosis. *FEMS Immunol Med Microbiol* **40:**207–213.

115. Rosas-Taraco AG, Revol A, Salinas-Carmona MC, Rendon A, Caballero-Olin G, Arce-Mendoza AY. 2007. CD14 C(-159)T polymorphism is a risk factor for development of pulmonary tuberculosis. *J Infect Dis* **196:** 1698–1706.

116. Xue Y, Zhao ZQ, Chen F, Zhang L, Li GD, Ma KW, Bai XF, Zuo YJ. 2012. Polymorphisms in the promoter of the CD14 gene and their associations with susceptibility to pulmonary tuberculosis. *Tissue Antigens* **80:** 437–443.

117. Zhao MY, Xue Y, Zhao ZQ, Li FJ, Fan DP, Wei LL, Sun XJ, Zhang X, Wang XC, Zhang YX, Li JC. 2012. Association of CD14 G(-1145)A and C(-159)T polymorphisms with reduced risk for tuberculosis in a Chinese Han population. *Genet Mol Res* **11:**3425–3431.

118. Zhao J, Lin G, Zhang WH, Ge M, Zhang Y. 2013. Contribution of CD14-159C/T polymorphism to tuberculosis susceptibility: a meta-analysis. *Int J Tuberc Lung Dis* **17:**1472–1478

119. Miao R, Ge H, Xu L, Xu F. 2014. CD14 -159C/T polymorphism contributes to the susceptibility to tuberculo-

sis: evidence from pooled 1,700 cases and 1,816 controls. *Mol Biol Rep* **41:**3481–3486.

120. Campbell SJ, Sabeti P, Fielding K, Sillah J, Bah B, Gustafson P, Manneh K, Lisse I, Sirugo G, Bellamy R, Bennett S, Aaby P, McAdam KP, Bah-Sow O, Lienhardt C, Hill AV. 2003. Variants of the CD40 ligand gene are not associated with increased susceptibility to tuberculosis in West Africa. *Immunogenetics* **55:**502–507.

121. Möller M, Flachsbart F, Till A, Thye T, Horstmann RD, Meyer CG, Osei I, van Helden PD, Hoal EG, Schreiber S, Nebel A, Franke A. 2010. A functional haplotype in the 3'untranslated region of TNFRSF1B is associated with tuberculosis in two African populations. *Am J Respir Crit Care Med* **181:**388–393.

122. Zhang X, Jiang F, Wei L, Li F, Liu J, Wang C, Zhao M, Jiang T, Xu D, Fan D, Sun X, Li JC. 2012. Polymorphic allele of human MRC1 confer protection against tuberculosis in a Chinese population. *Int J Biol Sci* **8:**375–382.

123. Zhang X, Li X, Zhang W, Wei L, Jiang T, Chen Z, Meng C, Liu J, Wu F, Wang C, Li F, Sun X, Li Z, Li JC. 2013. The novel human MRC1 gene polymorphisms are associated with susceptibility to pulmonary tuberculosis in Chinese Uygur and Kazak populations. *Mol Biol Rep* **40:**5073–5083.

124. Barreiro LB, Neyrolles O, Babb CL, Tailleux L, Quach H, McElreavey K, Helden PD, Hoal EG, Gicquel B, Quintana-Murci L. 2006. Promoter variation in the DC-SIGN-encoding gene CD209 is associated with tuberculosis. *PLoS Med* **3:**e20

125. Ben-Ali M, Barreiro LB, Chabbou A, Haltiti R, Braham E, Neyrolles O, Dellagi K, Gicquel B, Quintana-Murci L, Barbouche MR. 2007. Promoter and neck region length variation of DC-SIGN is not associated with susceptibility to tuberculosis in Tunisian patients. *Hum Immunol* **68:**908–912

126. Gómez LM, Anaya JM, Sierra-Filardi E, Cadena J, Corbí A, Martín J. 2006. Analysis of DC-SIGN (CD209) functional variants in patients with tuberculosis. *Hum Immunol* **67:**808–811.

127. Kobayashi K, Yuliwulandari R, Yanai H, Lien LT, Hang NT, Hijikata M, Keicho N, Tokunaga K. 2011. Association of CD209 polymorphisms with tuberculosis in an Indonesian population. *Hum Immunol* **72:**741–745.

128. Naderi M, Hashemi M, Taheri M, Pesarakli H, Eskandari-Nasab E, Bahari G. 2014. CD209 promoter -336 A/G (rs4804803) polymorphism is associated with susceptibility to pulmonary tuberculosis in Zahedan, southeast Iran. *J Microbiol Immunol Infect* **47:**171–175.

129. Ogarkov O, Mokrousov I, Sinkov V, Zhdanova S, Antipina S, Savilov E. 2012. 'Lethal' combination of *Mycobacterium tuberculosis* Beijing genotype and human CD209 -336G allele in Russian male population. *Infect Genet Evol* **12:**732–736.

130. Olesen R, Wejse C, Velez DR, Bisseye C, Sodemann M, Aaby P, Rabna P, Worwui A, Chapman H, Diatta M, Adegbola RA, Hill PC, Østergaard L, Williams SM, Sirugo G. 2007. DC-SIGN (CD209), pentraxin 3 and

vitamin D receptor gene variants associate with pulmonary tuberculosis risk in West Africans. *Genes Immun* **8:**456–467.

131. Sadki K, Lamsyah H, Rueda B, Lahlou O, El Aouad R, Martin J. 2009. CD209 promoter single nucleotide polymorphism -336A/G and the risk of susceptibility to tuberculosis disease in the Moroccan population. *Int J Hum Genet* **9:**239–243.

132. Selvaraj P, Alagarasu K, Swaminathan S, Harishankar M, Narendran G. 2009. CD209 gene polymorphisms in South Indian HIV and HIV-TB patients. *Infect Genet Evol* **9:**256–262.

133. Vannberg FO, Chapman SJ, Khor CC, Tosh K, Floyd S, Jackson-Sillah D, Crampin A, Sichali L, Bah B, Gustafson P, Aaby P, McAdam KP, Bah-Sow O, Lienhardt C, Sirugo G, Fine P, Hill AV. 2008. CD209 genetic polymorphism and tuberculosis disease. *PLoS One* **3:**e1388

134. Zheng R, Zhou Y, Qin L, Jin R, Wang J, Lu J, Wang W, Tang S, Hu Z. 2011. Relationship between polymorphism of DC-SIGN (CD209) gene and the susceptibility to pulmonary tuberculosis in an eastern Chinese population. *Hum Immunol* **72:**183–186.

135. Chang K, Deng S, Lu W, Wang F, Jia S, Li F, Yu L, Chen M. 2012. Association between CD209 -336A/G and -871A/G polymorphisms and susceptibility of tuberculosis: a meta-analysis. *PLoS One* **7:**e41519

136. Miao R, Li J, Sun Z, Li C, Xu F. 2012. Association between the CD209 promoter -336A/G polymorphism and susceptibility to tuberculosis: a meta-analysis. *Respirology* **17:**847–853.

137. Yi L, Zhang K, Mo Y, Zhen G, Zhao J. 2015. The association between CD209 gene polymorphisms and pulmonary tuberculosis susceptibility: a meta-analysis. *Int J Clin Exp Pathol* **8:**12437–12445.

138. Ji LD, Xu WN, Chai PF, Zheng W, Qian HX, Xu J. 2014. Polymorphisms in the CISH gene are associated with susceptibility to tuberculosis in the Chinese Han population. *Infect Genet Evol* **28:**240–244.

139. Khor CC, Vannberg FO, Chapman SJ, Guo H, Wong SH, Walley AJ, Vukcevic D, Rautanen A, Mills TC, Chang KC, Kam KM, Crampin AC, Ngwira B, Leung CC, Tam CM, Chan CY, Sung JJ, Yew WW, Toh KY, Tay SK, Kwiatkowski D, Lienhardt C, Hien TT, Day NP, Peshu N, Marsh K, Maitland K, Scott JA, Williams TN, Berkley JA, Floyd S, Tang NL, Fine PE, Goh DL, Hill AV. 2010. CISH and susceptibility to infectious diseases. *N Engl J Med* **362:**2092–2101.

140. Sun L, Jin YQ, Shen C, Qi H, Chu P, Yin QQ, Li JQ, Tian JL, Jiao WW, Xiao J, Shen AD. 2014. Genetic contribution of CISH promoter polymorphisms to susceptibility to tuberculosis in Chinese children. *PLoS One* **9:**e92020

141. Zhao L, Chu H, Xu X, Yue J, Li H, Wang M. 2014. Association between single-nucleotide polymorphism in CISH gene and susceptibility to tuberculosis in Chinese Han population. *Cell Biochem Biophys* **68:**529–534.

142. Fitness J, Floyd S, Warndorff DK, Sichali L, Malema S, Crampin AC, Fine PE, Hill AV. 2004. Large-scale candidate gene study of tuberculosis susceptibility in the

Karonga district of northern Malawi. *Am J Trop Med Hyg* 71:341–349.

143. Senbagavalli P, Kumar N, Kaur G, Mehra NK, Geetha ST, Ramanathan VD. 2011. Major histocompatibility complex class III (C2, C4, factor B) and C3 gene variants in patients with pulmonary tuberculosis. *Hum Immunol* 72:173–178

144. Noumsi GT, Tounkara A, Diallo H, Billingsley K, Moulds JJ, Moulds JM. 2011. Knops blood group polymorphism and susceptibility to *Mycobacterium tuberculosis* infection. *Transfusion* 51:2462–2469.

145. Zheng R, Liu H, Song P, Feng Y, Qin L, Huang X, Chen J, Yang H, Liu Z, Cui Z, Hu Z, Ge B. 2015. Epstein-Barr virus-induced gene 3 (EBI3) polymorphisms and expression are associated with susceptibility to pulmonary tuberculosis. *Tuberculosis (Edinb)* 95:497–504.

146. Ma X, Wright J, Dou S, Olsen P, Teeter L, Adams G, Graviss E. 2002. Ethnic divergence and linkage disequilibrium of novel SNPs in the human NLI-IF gene: evidence of human origin and lack of association with tuberculosis susceptibility. *J Hum Genet* 47:140–145.

147. Wang C, Jiang T, Wei L, Li F, Sun X, Fan D, Liu J, Zhang X, Xu D, Chen Z, Li Z, Fu X, Li JC. 2012. Association of CTLA4 gene polymorphisms with susceptibility and pathology correlation to pulmonary tuberculosis in Southern Han Chinese. *Int J Biol Sci* 8:945–952.

148. Tang NL, Fan HP, Chang KC, Ching JK, Kong KP, Yew WW, Kam KM, Leung CC, Tam CM, Blackwell J, Chan CY. 2009. Genetic association between a chemokine gene CXCL-10 (IP-10, interferon gamma inducible protein 10) and susceptibility to tuberculosis. *Clin Chim Acta* 406:98–102.

149. Liu Q, Wang J, Sandford AJ, Wu J, Wang Y, Wu S, Ji G, Chen G, Feng Y, Tao C, He JQ. 2015. Association of CYBB polymorphisms with tuberculosis susceptibility in the Chinese Han population. *Infect Genet Evol* 33:169–175.

150. Feng WX, Liu F, Gu Y, Jiao WW, Sun L, Xiao J, Wu XR, Miao Q, Shen C, Shen D, Shen A. 2012. Functional polymorphisms in CYP2C19 & CYP3A5 genes associated with decreased susceptibility for paediatric tuberculosis. *Indian J Med Res* 135:642–649.

151. Qrafli M, Amar Y, Bourkadi J, Ben Amor J, Iraki G, Bakri Y, Amzazi S, Lahlou O, Seghrouchni F, El Aouad R, Sadki K. 2014. The CYP7A1 gene rs3808607 variant is associated with susceptibility of tuberculosis in Moroccan population. *Pan Afr Med J* 18:1

152. Wu XM, Gong LY, Lin J, Wang HH. 2012. [Association between human beta defensin-1 single nucleotide polymorphisms and susceptibility to pulmonary tuberculosis]. *Zhonghua Yu Fang Yi Xue Za Zhi* 46:912–915.

153. Thuong NT, Hawn TR, Chau TT, Bang ND, Yen NT, Thwaites GE, Teo YY, Seielstad M, Hibberd M, Lan NT, Caws M, Farrar JJ, Dunstan SJ. 2012. Epiregulin (EREG) variation is associated with susceptibility to tuberculosis. *Genes Immun* 13:275–281.

154. White MJ, Tacconelli A, Chen JS, Wejse C, Hill PC, Gomes VF, Velez-Edwards DR, Østergaard LJ, Hu T,

155. Moore JH, Novelli G, Scott WK, Williams SM, Sirugo G. 2014. Epiregulin (EREG) and human V-ATPase (TCIRG1): genetic variation, ethnicity and pulmonary tuberculosis susceptibility in Guinea-Bissau and The Gambia. *Genes Immun* 15:370–377.

155. Sadki K, Lamsyah H, Rueda B, Akil E, Sadak A, Martin J, El Aouad R. 2010. Analysis of MIF, FCGR2A and FCGR3A gene polymorphisms with susceptibility to pulmonary tuberculosis in Moroccan population. *J Genet Genomics* 37:257–264.

156. Chalmers JD, Matsushita M, Kilpatrick DC, Hill AT. 2015. No strong relationship between components of the lectin pathway of complement and susceptibility to pulmonary tuberculosis. *Inflammation* 38:1731–1737.

157. Xu DD, Wang C, Jiang F, Wei LL, Shi LY, Yu XM, Liu CM, Liu XH, Feng XM, Ping ZP, Jiang TT, Chen ZL, Li ZJ, Li JC. 2015. Association of the FCN2 gene single nucleotide polymorphisms with susceptibility to pulmonary tuberculosis. *PLoS One* 10:e0138356

158. Baker MA, Wilson D, Wallengren K, Sandgren A, Iartchouk O, Broodie N, Goonesekera SD, Sabeti PC, Murray MB. 2012. Polymorphisms in the gene that encodes the iron transport protein ferroportin 1 influence susceptibility to tuberculosis. *J Infect Dis* 205:1043–1047.

159. Bellamy R, Ruwende C, Corrah T, McAdam KP, Whittle HC, Hill AV. 1998. Assessment of the interleukin 1 gene cluster and other candidate gene polymorphisms in host susceptibility to tuberculosis. *Tuber Lung Dis* 79:83–89.

160. Insanov AB, Abdullaev FM, Ragimov AA, Talybova AM, Umniashkin AA. 1989. [Pulmonary tuberculosis in patients with hereditary glucose-6-phosphate dehydrogenase deficiency]. *Ter Arkh* 61:75–77.

161. Adams CH, Werely CJ, Victor TC, Hoal EG, Rossouw G, van Helden PD. 2003. Allele frequencies for glutathione S-transferase and N-acetyltransferase 2 differ in African population groups and may be associated with oesophageal cancer or tuberculosis incidence. *Clin Chem Lab Med* 41:600–605.

162. Kasvosve I, Gomo ZA, Mvundura E, Moyo VM, Saungweme T, Khumalo H, Gordeuk VR, Boelaert JR, Delanghe JR, De Bacquer D, Gangaidzo IT. 2000. Haptoglobin polymorphism and mortality in patients with tuberculosis. *Int J Tuberc Lung Dis* 4:771–775.

163. Akgunes A, Coban AY, Durupinar B. 2011. Human leucocyte antigens and cytokine gene polymorphisms and tuberculosis. *Indian J Med Microbiol* 29:28–32.

164. Amirzargar AA, Yalda A, Hajabolbaghi M, Khosravi F, Jabbari H, Rezaei N, Niknam MH, Ansari B, Moradi B, Nikbin B. 2004. The association of HLA-DRB, DQA1, DQB1 alleles and haplotype frequency in Iranian patients with pulmonary tuberculosis. *Int J Tuberc Lung Dis* 8:1017–1021.

165. Balamurugan A, Sharma SK, Mehra NK. 2004. Human leukocyte antigen class I supertypes influence susceptibility and severity of tuberculosis. *J Infect Dis* 189:805–811.

166. Chandanayingyong D, Maranetra N, Bovornkitti S. 1988. HLA antigen profiles in Thai tuberculosis patients. *Asian Pac J Allergy Immunol* 6:77–80.

167. Delgado JC, Baena A, Thim S, Goldfeld AE. 2006. Aspartic acid homozygosity at codon 57 of HLA-DQ beta is associated with susceptibility to pulmonary tuberculosis in Cambodia. *J Immunol* **176**:1090–1097.

168. Duarte R, Carvalho C, Pereira C, Bettencourt A, Carvalho A, Villar M, Domingos A, Barros H, Marques J, Pinho Costa P, Mendonça D, Martins B. 2011. HLA class II alleles as markers of tuberculosis susceptibility and resistance. *Rev Port Pneumol* **17**:15–19.

169. Dubaniewicz A, Dubaniewicz-Wybieralska M, Moszkowska G, Sternau A. 2006. Comparative analysis of DR and DQ alleles occurrence in sarcoidosis and tuberculosis in the same ethnic group: preliminary study. *Sarcoidosis Vasc Diffuse Lung Dis* **23**:180–189.

170. Dubaniewicz A, Lewko B, Moszkowska G, Zamorska B, Stepinski J. 2000. Molecular subtypes of the HLA-DR antigens in pulmonary tuberculosis. *Int J Infectious Dis* **4**:129–133.

171. Dubaniewicz A, Moszkowska G. 2007. [Analysis of occurrence of DRB and DQ alleles in sarcoidosis and tuberculosis from Northern Poland]. *Pneumonol Alergol Pol* **75**:13–21.

172. Figueiredo JF, Rodrigues Mde L, Deghaide NH, Donadi EA. 2008. HLA profile in patients with AIDS and tuberculosis. *Braz J Infect Dis* **12**:278–280.

173. Goldfeld AE, Delgado JC, Thim S, Bozon MV, Uglialoro AM, Turbay D, Cohen C, Yunis EJ. 1998. Association of an HLA-DQ allele with clinical tuberculosis. *JAMA* **279**:226–228

174. Hafez M, el-Fiky A, Bassiouny MR, el-Hafez SA, el-Morsy A, Khaled A, el-Ziny M, al-Tonbary Y, Settein A. 1992. Clinico-immunogenetic study on Egyptian multicase tuberculous families. *Dis Markers* **10**:143–149.

175. Hafez M, el-Salab S, el-Shennawy F, Bassiony MR. 1985. HLA-antigens and tuberculosis in the Egyptian population. *Tubercle* **66**:35–40

176. Harfouch-Hammoud EI, Daher NA. 2008. Susceptibility to and severity of tuberculosis is genetically controlled by human leukocyte antigens. *Saudi Med J* **29**:1625–1629.

177. Jagannathan L, Chaturvedi M, Satish B, Satish KS, Desai A, Subbakrishna DK, Satishchandra P, Pitchappan R, Balakrishnan K, Kondaiah P, Ravi V. 2011. HLA-B57 and gender influence the occurrence of tuberculosis in HIV infected people of south India. *Clin Dev Immunol* **2011**:549023

178. John GT, Murugesan K, Jeyaseelan L, Pulimood RB, Jacob CK, Shastry JC. 1995. HLA phenotypes in Asians developing tuberculosis on dialysis or after renal transplantation. *Natl Med J India* **8**:144, 146.

179. Khomenko AG, Pospelov LE, Malenko AF, Chukanova VP, Romanov VV. 1985. [HLA antigens in lung diseases]. *Ter Arkh* **57**:77–80.

180. Kim HS, Park MH, Song EY, Park H, Kwon SY, Han SK, Shim YS. 2005. Association of HLA-DR and HLA-DQ genes with susceptibility to pulmonary tuberculosis in Koreans: preliminary evidence of associations with drug resistance, disease severity, and disease recurrence. *Hum Immunol* **66**:1074–1081.

181. Lombard Z, Dalton DL, Venter PA, Williams RC, Bornman L. 2006. Association of HLA-DR, -DQ, and vitamin D receptor alleles and haplotypes with tuberculosis in the Venda of South Africa. *Hum Immunol* **67**:643–654

182. Louie LG, Hartogensis WE, Jackman RP, Schultz KA, Zijenah LS, Yiu CH, Nguyen VD, Sohsman MY, Katzenstein DK, Mason PR. 2004. *Mycobacterium tuberculosis*/HIV-1 coinfection and disease: role of human leukocyte antigen variation. *J Infect Dis* **189**:1084–1090.

183. Lucena-Silva N, Baliza MD, Martins AE, Deghaide NH, Teixeira KM, Rodrigues LC, Ximenes R, Donadi EA, de Albuquerque M. 2010. Relatedness and HLA-DRB1 typing may discriminate the magnitude of the genetic susceptibility to tuberculosis using a household contact model. *J Epidemiol Community Health* **64**:513–517.

184. Lugo-Zamudio GE, Yamamoto-Furusho JK, Delgado-Ochoa D, Nunez-Farfan RM, Vargas-Alarcon G, Barbosa-Cobos RE, Granados J. 2010. Human leukocyte antigen typing in tuberculous rheumatism: Poncet's disease. *Int J Tuberc Lung Dis* **14**:916–920.

185. Magira EE, Papasteriades C, Kanterakis S, Toubis M, Roussos C, Monos DS. 2012. HLA-A and HLA-DRB1 amino acid polymorphisms are associated with susceptibility and protection to pulmonary tuberculosis in a Greek population. *Hum Immunol* **73**:641–646.

186. Mahmoudzadeh-Niknam H, Khalili G, Fadavi P. 2003. Allelic distribution of human leukocyte antigen in Iranian patients with pulmonary tuberculosis. *Hum Immunol* **64**:124–129.

187. Mehra NK. 1990. Role of HLA linked factors in governing susceptibility to leprosy and tuberculosis. *Trop Med Parasitol* **41**:352–354.

188. Pospelov LE, Matrakshin AG, Chernousova LN, Tsoi KN, Afanasjev KI, Rubtsova GA, Yeremeyev VV. 1996. Association of various genetic markers with tuberculosis and other lung diseases in Tuvinian children. *Tuber Lung Dis* **77**:77–80.

189. Pospelova LE, Matrashkin AG, Larionova EE, Eremeev VV, Mes'ko EM. 2005. [The association of tuberculosis with the specificities of the HLA gene DRB1 in different regions of Tuva]. *Probl Tuberk Bolezn Legk* (7):23–25.

190. Raghavan S, Selvaraj P, Swaminathan S, Alagarasu K, Narendran G, Narayanan PR. 2009. Haplotype analysis of HLA-A, -B antigens and -DRB1 alleles in south Indian HIV-1-infected patients with and without pulmonary tuberculosis. *Int J Immunogenet* **36**:129–133.

191. Rakhimov AK, Pospelov LE. 1990. [Study of genetic markers in families of patients with tuberculosis]. *Probl Tuberk* (9):7–8.

192. Rojas-Alvarado Mde L, Diaz-Mendoza ML, Said-FernÁndez S, Caballero-Olín G, Cerda-Flores RM. 2008. [Association of pulmonary tuberculosis with HLA system antigens in Northeastern Mexico.] *Gac Med Mex* **144**:233–238.

193. Sanjeevi CB, Narayanan PR, Prabakar R, Charles N, Thomas BE, Balasubramaniam R, Olerup O. 1992. No association or linkage with HLA-DR or -DQ genes in

south Indians with pulmonary tuberculosis. *Tuber Lung Dis* 73:280–284.

194. Selvaraj P, Kurian SM, Uma H, Reetha AM, Narayanan PR. 2000. Influence of non-MHC genes on lymphocyte response to *Mycobacterium tuberculosis* antigens & tuberculin reactive status in pulmonary tuberculosis. *Indian J Med Res* 112:86–92.

195. Selvaraj P, Raghavan S, Swaminathan S, Alagarasu K, Narendran G, Narayanan PR. 2008. HLA-DQB1 and -DPB1 allele profile in HIV infected patients with and without pulmonary tuberculosis of south India. *Infect Genet Evol* 8:664–671.

196. Sharma SK, Turaga KK, Balamurugan A, Saha PK, Pandey RM, Jain NK, Katoch VM, Mehra NK. 2003. Clinical and genetic risk factors for the development of multi-drug resistant tuberculosis in non-HIV infected patients at a tertiary care center in India: a case-control study. *Infect Genet Evol* 3:183–188.

197. Shi GL, Hu XL, Yang L, Rong CL, Guo YL, Song CX. 2011. Association of HLA-DRB alleles and pulmonary tuberculosis in North Chinese patients. *Genet Mol Res* 10:1331–1336.

198. Singh SP, Mehra NK, Dingley HB, Pande JN, Vaidya MC. 1983. Human leukocyte antigen (HLA)-linked control of susceptibility to pulmonary tuberculosis and association with HLA-DR types. *J Infect Dis* 148:676–681.

199. Sinch SP, Mehra NK, Dingley HB, Pande JN, Vaidya MC. 1984. HLA haplotype segregation study in multiple case families of pulmonary tuberculosis. *Tissue Antigens* 23:84–86.

200. Souza CF, Noguti EN, Visentainer JE, Cardoso RF, Petzl-Erler ML, Tsuneto LT. 2012. HLA and MICA genes in patients with tuberculosis in Brazil. *Tissue Antigens* 79:58–63.

201. Terán-Escandón D, Terán-Ortiz L, Camarena-Olvera A, González-Avila G, Vaca-Marín MA, Granados J, Selman M. 1999. Human leukocyte antigen-associated susceptibility to pulmonary tuberculosis: molecular analysis of class II alleles by DNA amplification and oligonucleotide hybridization in Mexican patients. *Chest* 115:428–433

202. Vasilca V, Oana R, Munteanu D, Zugun F, Constantinescu D, Carasevici E. 2004. HLA-A and -B phenotypes associated with tuberculosis in population from north-eastern Romania. *Roum Arch Microbiol Immunol* 63:209–221.

203. Vejbaesya S, Chierakul N, Luangtrakool K, Srinak D, Stephens HA. 2002. Associations of HLA class II alleles with pulmonary tuberculosis in Thais. *Eur J Immunogenet* 29:431–434.

204. Vijaya Lakshmi V, Rakh SS, Anu Radha B, Hari Sai Priya V, Pantula V, Jasti S, Suman Latha G, Murthy KJ. 2006. Role of HLA-B51 and HLA-B52 in susceptibility to pulmonary tuberculosis. *Infect Genet Evol* 6:436–439.

205. Wu F, Zhang W, Zhang L, Wu J, Li C, Meng X, Wang X, He P, Zhang J. 2013. NRAMP1, VDR, HLA-DRB1, and HLA-DQB1 gene polymorphisms in susceptibility to tuberculosis among the Chinese Kazakh population: a case-control study. *BioMed Res Int* 2013:484535

206. Yuliwulandari R, Sachrowardi Q, Nakajima H, Kashiwase K, Hirayasu K, Mabuchi A, Sofro AS, Tokunaga K. 2010. Association of HLA-A, -B, and -DRB1 with pulmonary tuberculosis in western Javanese Indonesia. *Hum Immunol* 71:697–701.

207. Zhang NR, Fan G, Deng YF, Wang XF, Lu C, Zhang CZ, Dong ZF, Zhang J, Li L, Zhao SM, Lu ZM. 2012. [A preliminary study on the relationship between HLA-Cw polymorphism and susceptibility to pulmonary tuberculosis]. *Zhonghua Jie He He Hu Xi Za Zhi* 35:120–124.

208. Li CP, Zhou Y, Xiang X, Zhou Y, He M. 2015. Relationship of HLA-DRB1 gene polymorphism with susceptibility to pulmonary tuberculosis: updated meta-analysis. *Int J Tuberc Lung Dis* 19:841–849.

209. Raja lingam R, Mehra NK, Singal DP. 2000. Polymorphism in heat-shock protein 70-1 (HSP70-1) gene promoter region and susceptibility to tuberculoid leprosy and pulmonary tuberculosis in Asian Indians. *Indian J Exp Biol* 38:658–662.

210. Shen C, Wu XR, Jiao WW, Sun L, Feng WX, Xiao J, Miao Q, Liu F, Yin QQ, Zhang CG, Guo YJ, Shen AD. 2013. A functional promoter polymorphism of IFITM3 is associated with susceptibility to pediatric tuberculosis in Han Chinese population. *PLoS One* 8:e67816

211. Amim LH, Pacheco AG, Fonseca-Costa J, Loredo CS, Rabahi MF, Melo MH, Ribeiro FC, Mello FC, Oliveira MM, Lapa e Silva JR, Ottenhoff TH, Kritski AL, Santos AR. 2008. Role of IFN-gamma +874 T/A single nucleotide polymorphism in the tuberculosis outcome among Brazilians subjects. *Mol Biol Rep* 35:563–566.

212. Ansari A, Hasan Z, Dawood G, Hussain R. 2011. Differential combination of cytokine and interferon-γ +874 T/A polymorphisms determines disease severity in pulmonary tuberculosis. *PLoS One* 6:e27848

213. Ansari A, Talat N, Jamil B, Hasan Z, Razzaki T, Dawood G, Hussain R. 2009. Cytokine gene polymorphisms across tuberculosis clinical spectrum in Pakistani patients. *PLoS One* 4:e4778

214. Awomoyi AA, Nejentsev S, Richardson A, Hull J, Koch O, Podinovskaia M, Todd JA, McAdam KP, Blackwell JM, Kwiatkowski D, Newport MJ. 2004. No association between interferon-gamma receptor-1 gene polymorphism and pulmonary tuberculosis in a Gambian population sample. *Thorax* 59:291–294.

215. Ben Selma W, Harizi H, Bougmiza I, Hannachi N, Ben Kahla I, Zaieni R, Boukadida J. 2011. Interferon gamma +874T/A polymorphism is associated with susceptibility to active pulmonary tuberculosis development in Tunisian patients. *DNA Cell Biol* 30:379–387.

216. Abhimanyu, Bose M, Jha P, Indian Genome Variation Consortium. 2012. Footprints of genetic susceptibility to pulmonary tuberculosis: cytokine gene variants in north Indians. *Indian J Med Res* 135:763–770.

217. Cooke GS, Campbell SJ, Sillah J, Gustafson P, Bah B, Sirugo G, Bennett S, McAdam KP, Sow O, Lienhardt C, Hill AV. 2006. Polymorphism within the interferon-gamma/receptor complex is associated with pulmonary tuberculosis. *Am J Respir Crit Care Med* 174:339–343.

218. de Albuquerque AC, Rocha LQ, de Morais Batista AH, Teixeira AB, Dos Santos DB, Nogueira NA. 2012. Association of polymorphism +874 A/T of interferon-gamma and susceptibility to the development of tuberculosis: meta-analysis. *Eur J Clin Microbiol Infect Dis* **31:**2887–2895.

219. Ding S, Li L, Zhu X. 2008. Polymorphism of the interferon-gamma gene and risk of tuberculosis in a southeastern Chinese population. *Hum Immunol* **69:** 129–133

220. Etokebe GE, Bulat-Kardum L, Johansen MS, Knezevic J, Balen S, Matakovic-Mileusnic N, Matanic D, Flego V, Pavelic J, Beg-Zec Z, Dembic Z. 2006. Interferon-gamma gene (T874A and G2109A) polymorphisms are associated with microscopy-positive tuberculosis. *Scand J Immunol* **63:**136–141

221. Fraser DA, Bulat-Kardum L, Knezevic J, Babarovic P, Matakovic-Mileusnic N, Dellacasagrande J, Matanic D, Pavelic J, Beg-Zec Z, Dembic Z. 2003. Interferon-gamma receptor-1 gene polymorphism in tuberculosis patients from Croatia. *Scand J Immunol* **57:**480–484.

222. Hashemi M, Sharifi-Mood B, Nezamdoost M, Moazeni-Roodi A, Naderi M, Kouhpayeh H, Taheri M, Ghavami S. 2011. Functional polymorphism of interferon-γ (IFN-γ) gene +874T/A polymorphism is associated with pulmonary tuberculosis in Zahedan, Southeast Iran. *Prague Med Rep* **112:**38–43.

223. He J, Wang J, Lei D, Ding S. 2010. Analysis of functional SNP in ifng/ifngr1 in Chinese Han population with tuberculosis. *Scand J Immunol* **71:**452–458.

224. Henao MI, Montes C, París SC, García LF. 2006. Cytokine gene polymorphisms in Colombian patients with different clinical presentations of tuberculosis. *Tuberculosis (Edinb)* **86:**11–19.

225. Hwang JH, Kim EJ, Kim SY, Lee SH, Suh GY, Kwon OJ, Ji Y, Kang M, Kim DH, Koh WJ. 2007. Polymorphisms of interferon-gamma and interferon-gamma receptor 1 genes and pulmonary tuberculosis in Koreans. *Respirology* **12:**906–910.

226. Leandro AC, Rocha MA, Lamoglia-Souza A, VandeBerg JL, Rolla VC, Bonecini-Almeida MG. 2013. No association of IFNG+874T/A SNP and NOS2A-954G/C SNP variants with nitric oxide radical serum levels or susceptibility to tuberculosis in a Brazilian population subset. *BioMed Res Int* **2013:**901740

227. Lee SW, Chuang TY, Huang HH, Lee KF, Chen TT, Kao YH, Wu LS. 2015. Interferon gamma polymorphisms associated with susceptibility to tuberculosis in a Han Taiwanese population. *J Microbiol Immunol Infect* **48:**376–380

228. Lio D, Marino V, Serauto A, Gioia V, Scola L, Crivello A, Forte GI, Colonna-Romano G, Candore G, Caruso C. 2002. Genotype frequencies of the +874T->A single nucleotide polymorphism in the first intron of the interferon-gamma gene in a sample of Sicilian patients affected by tuberculosis. *Eur J Immunogenet* **29:**371–374

229. Liu YD, Zheng RJ, Xiao HP, Sha W, Zhang Q, Wu FR, Sun H, Zhang ZS, Cui HY, Liu ZB, Tang SJ. 2011. [Study on the correlation between polymorphisms of genes with susceptibility to tuberculosis and drug-resistant tuberculosis in Chinese Han population]. *Zhonghua Liu Xing Bing Xue Za Zhi* **32:**279–284.

230. López-Maderuelo D, Arnalich F, Serantes R, GonzÁlez A, Codoceo R, Madero R, VÁzquez JJ, Montiel C. 2003. Interferon-gamma and interleukin-10 gene polymorphisms in pulmonary tuberculosis. *Am J Respir Crit Care Med* **167:**970–975.

231. Mirsaeidi SM, Houshmand M, Tabarsi P, Banoei MM, Zargari L, Amiri M, Mansouri SD, Sanati MH, Masjedi MR. 2006. Lack of association between interferon-gamma receptor-1 polymorphism and pulmonary TB in Iranian population sample. *J Infect* **52:**374–377.

232. Möller M, Nebel A, van Helden PD, Schreiber S, Hoal EG. 2010. Analysis of eight genes modulating interferon gamma and human genetic susceptibility to tuberculosis: a case-control association study. *BMC Infect Dis* **10:**154

233. Moran A, Ma X, Reich RA, Graviss EA. 2007. No association between the +874T/A single nucleotide polymorphism in the IFN-gamma gene and susceptibility to TB. *Int J Tuberc Lung Dis* **11:**113–115.

234. Mosaad YM, Soliman OE, Tawhid ZE, Sherif DM. 2010. Interferon-gamma +874 T/A and interleukin-10 -1082 A/G single nucleotide polymorphism in Egyptian children with tuberculosis. *Scand J Immunol* **72:** 358–364

235. Onay H, Ekmekci AY, Durmaz B, Sayin E, Cosar H, Bayram N, Can D, Akin H, Ozkinay C, Ozkinay F. 2010. Interferon-gamma gene and interferon-gamma receptor-1 gene polymorphisms in children with tuberculosis from Turkey. *Scand J Infect Dis* **42:**39–42.

236. Oral HB, Budak F, Uzaslan EK, BaŞtürk B, Bekar A, Akalin H, Ege E, Ener B, Göral G. 2006. Interleukin-10 (IL-10) gene polymorphism as a potential host susceptibility factor in tuberculosis. *Cytokine* **35:**143–147.

237. Park GY, Im YH, Ahn CH, Park JW, Jeong SW, Ahn JY, Hwang YJ. 2004. Functional and genetic assessment of IFN-gamma receptor in patients with clinical tuberculosis. *Int J Tuberc Lung Dis* **8:**1221–1227.

238. Rosenzweig SD, Schäffer AA, Ding L, Sullivan R, Enyedi B, Yim JJ, Cook JL, Musser JM, Holland SM. 2004. Interferon-gamma receptor 1 promoter polymorphisms: population distribution and functional implications. *Clin Immunol* **112:**113–119.

239. Rossouw M, Nel HJ, Cooke GS, van Helden PD, Hoal EG. 2003. Association between tuberculosis and a polymorphic NFkappaB binding site in the interferon gamma gene. *Lancet* **361:**1871–1872.

240. Sahiratmadja E, Baak-Pablo R, de Visser AW, Alisjahbana B, Adnan I, van Crevel R, Marzuki S, van Dissel JT, Ottenhoff TH, van de Vosse E. 2007. Association of polymorphisms in IL-12/IFN-gamma pathway genes with susceptibility to pulmonary tuberculosis in Indonesia. *Tuberculosis (Edinb)* **87:**303–311.

241. Sallakci N, Coskun M, Berber Z, Gürkan F, Kocamaz H, Uysal G, Bhuju S, Yavuzer U, Singh M, Yeğin O. 2007. Interferon-gamma gene+874T-A polymorphism is associated with tuberculosis and gamma interferon response. *Tuberculosis (Edinb)* **87:**225–230.

242. Selvaraj P, Alagarasu K, Harishankar M, Vidyarani M, Nisha Rajeswari D, Narayanan PR. 2008. Cytokine gene polymorphisms and cytokine levels in pulmonary tuberculosis. *Cytokine* 43:26–33.

243. Trajkov D, Trajchevska M, Arsov T, Petlichkovski A, Strezova A, Efinska-Mladenovska O, Sandevski A, Spiroski M. 2009. Association of 22 cytokine gene polymorphisms with tuberculosis in Macedonians. *Indian J Tuberc* 56:117–131.

244. Tso HW, Lau YL, Tam CM, Wong HS, Chiang AK. 2004. Associations between IL12B polymorphisms and tuberculosis in the Hong Kong Chinese population. *J Infect Dis* 190:913–919.

245. Vallinoto AC, Graça ES, Araújo MS, Azevedo VN, Cayres-Vallinoto I, Machado LF, Ishak MO, Ishak R. 2010. IFNG +874T/A polymorphism and cytokine plasma levels are associated with susceptibility to *Mycobacterium tuberculosis* infection and clinical manifestation of tuberculosis. *Hum Immunol* 71:692–696.

246. Vidyarani M, Selvaraj P, Prabhu Anand S, Jawahar MS, Adhilakshmi AR, Narayanan PR. 2006. Interferon gamma (IFNgamma) & interleukin-4 (IL-4) gene variants & cytokine levels in pulmonary tuberculosis. *Indian J Med Res* 124:403–410.

247. Wang J, Tang S, Shen H. 2010. Association of genetic polymorphisms in the IL12-IFNG pathway with susceptibility to and prognosis of pulmonary tuberculosis in a Chinese population. *Eur J Clin Microbiol Infect Dis* 29:1291–1295.

248. Wu F, Qu Y, Tang Y, Cao D, Sun P, Xia Z. 2008. Lack of association between cytokine gene polymorphisms and silicosis and pulmonary tuberculosis in Chinese iron miners. *J Occup Health* 50:445–454.

249. Pacheco AG, Cardoso CC, Moraes MO. 2008. IFNG +874T/A, IL10 -1082G/A and TNF -308G/A polymorphisms in association with tuberculosis susceptibility: a meta-analysis study. *Hum Genet* 123:477–484.

250. Tian C, Zhang Y, Zhang J, Deng Y, Li X, Xu D, Huang H, Huang J, Fan H. 2011. The +874T/A polymorphism in the interferon-γ gene and tuberculosis risk: an update by meta-analysis. *Hum Immunol* 72:1137–1142.

251. de Albuquerque AC, Rocha LQ, de Morais Batista AH, Teixeira AB, Dos Santos DB, Nogueira NA. 2012. Association of polymorphism +874 A/T of interferon-γ and susceptibility to the development of tuberculosis: meta-analysis. *Eur J Clin Microbiol Infect Dis* 31:2887–2895.

252. Bulat-Kardum L, Etokebe GE, Knezevic J, Balen S, Matakovic-Mileusnic N, Zaputovic L, Pavelic J, Beg-Zec Z, Dembic Z. 2006. Interferon-gamma receptor-1 gene promoter polymorphisms (G-611A; T-56C) and susceptibility to tuberculosis. *Scand J Immunol* 63:142–150.

253. Ding S, Li F, Wang J, Xu K, Li L. 2008. Interferon gamma receptor 1 gene polymorphism in patients with tuberculosis in China. *Scand J Immunol* 68:140–144.

254. Newport MJ, Awomoyi AA, Blackwell JM. 2003. Polymorphism in the interferon-gamma receptor-1 gene and susceptibility to pulmonary tuberculosis in The Gambia. *Scand J Immunol* 58:383–385

255. Velez DR, Hulme WF, Myers JL, Weinberg JB, Levesque MC, Stryjewski ME, Abbate E, Estevan R, Patillo SG, Gilbert JR, Hamilton CD, Scott WK. 2009. NOS2A, TLR4, and IFNGR1 interactions influence pulmonary tuberculosis susceptibility in African-Americans. *Hum Genet* 126:643–653.

256. Wang W, Ren W, Zhang X, Liu Y, Li C. 2014. Association between interferon gamma receptor 1-56C/T gene polymorphism and tuberculosis susceptibility: a meta-analysis. *Chin Med J (Engl)* 127:3782–3788.

257. Gomez LM, Camargo JF, Castiblanco J, Ruiz-Narváez EA, Cadena J, Anaya JM. 2006. Analysis of IL1B, TAP1, TAP2 and IKBL polymorphisms on susceptibility to tuberculosis. *Tissue Antigens* 67:290–296.

258. Amirzargar AA, Rezaei N, Jabbari H, Danesh AA, Khosravi F, Hajabdolbaghi M, Yalda A, Nikbin B. 2006. Cytokine single nucleotide polymorphisms in Iranian patients with pulmonary tuberculosis. *Eur Cytokine Netw* 17:84–89.

259. Awomoyi AA, Charurat M, Marchant A, Miller EN, Blackwell JM, McAdam KP, Newport MJ. 2005. Polymorphism in IL1B: IL1B-511 association with tuberculosis and decreased lipopolysaccharide-induced IL-1beta in IFN-gamma primed ex-vivo whole blood assay. *J Endotoxin Res* 11:281–286.

260. Delgado JC, Baena A, Thim S, Goldfeld AE. 2002. Ethnic-specific genetic associations with pulmonary tuberculosis. *J Infect Dis* 186:1463–1468.

261. Meenakshi P, Ramya S, Shruthi T, Lavanya J, Mohammed HH, Mohammed SA, Vijayalakshmi V, Sumanlatha G. 2013. Association of IL-1β +3954 C/T and IL-10-1082 G/A cytokine gene polymorphisms with susceptibility to tuberculosis. *Scand J Immunol* 78:92–97.

262. Motsinger-Reif AA, Antas PR, Oki NO, Levy S, Holland SM, Sterling TR. 2010. Polymorphisms in IL-1beta, vitamin D receptor Fok1, and Toll-like receptor 2 are associated with extrapulmonary tuberculosis. *BMC Med Genet* 11:37

263. Naslednikova IO, Urazova OI, Voronkova OV, Strelis AK, Novitsky VV, Nikulina EL, Hasanova RR, Kononova TE, Serebryakova VA, Vasileva OA, Suhalentseva NA, Churina EG, Kolosova AE, Fedorovich TV. 2009. Allelic polymorphism of cytokine genes during pulmonary tuberculosis. *Bull Exp Biol Med* 148:175–180.

264. Taype CA, Shamsuzzaman S, Accinelli RA, Espinoza JR, Shaw MA. 2010. Genetic susceptibility to different clinical forms of tuberculosis in the Peruvian population. *Infect Genet Evol* 10:495–504.

265. Zhang G, Zhou B, Li S, Yue J, Yang H, Wen Y, Zhan S, Wang W, Liao M, Zhang M, Zeng G, Feng CG, Sassetti CM, Chen X. 2014. Allele-specific induction of IL-1β expression by C/EBPβ and PU.1 contributes to increased tuberculosis susceptibility. *PLoS Pathog* 10:e1004426

266. Mao X, Ke Z, Liu S, Tang B, Wang J, Huang H, Chen S. 2015. IL-1β+3953C/T, -511T/C and IL-6 -174C/G polymorphisms in association with tuberculosis susceptibility: a meta-analysis. *Gene* 573:75–83.

267. Zhang G, Zhou B, Wang W, Zhang M, Zhao Y, Wang Z, Yang L, Zhai J, Feng CG, Wang J, Chen X. 2012. A

functional single-nucleotide polymorphism in the promoter of the gene encoding interleukin 6 is associated with susceptibility to tuberculosis. *J Infect Dis* **205**: 1697–1704.

268. Ke Z, Yuan L, Ma J, Zhang X, Guo Y, Xiong H. 2015. IL-10 polymorphisms and tuberculosis susceptibility: an updated meta-analysis. *Yonsei Med J* **56**:1274–1287.

269. Cooke GS, Campbell SJ, Fielding K, Sillah J, Manneh K, Sirugo G, Bennett S, McAdam KP, Lienhardt C, Hill AV. 2004. Interleukin-8 polymorphism is not associated with pulmonary tuberculosis in the gambia. *J Infect Dis* **189**:1545–1546, author reply 1546

270. Lindenau JD, Guimarães LS, Friedrich DC, Hurtado AM, Hill KR, Salzano FM, Hutz MH. 2014. Cytokine gene polymorphisms are associated with susceptibility to tuberculosis in an Amerindian population. *Int J Tuberc Lung Dis* **18**:952–957.

271. Ma X, Reich RA, Wright JA, Tooker HR, Teeter LD, Musser JM, Graviss EA. 2003. Association between interleukin-8 gene alleles and human susceptibility to tuberculosis disease. *J Infect Dis* **188**:349–355.

272. Ates O, Musellim B, Ongen G, Topal-Sarikaya A. 2008. Interleukin-10 and tumor necrosis factor-alpha gene polymorphisms in tuberculosis. *J Clin Immunol* **28**: 232–236.

273. Awomoyi AA, Marchant A, Howson JM, McAdam KP, Blackwell JM, Newport MJ. 2002. Interleukin-10, polymorphism in SLC11A1 (formerly NRAMP1), and susceptibility to tuberculosis. *J Infect Dis* **186**:1808–1814.

274. Ben-Selma W, Ben-Abderrahmen Y, Boukadida J, Harizi H. 2012. IL-10R1 S138G loss-of-function polymorphism is associated with extrapulmonary tuberculosis risk development in Tunisia. *Mol Biol Rep* **39**: 51–56.

275. Ben-Selma W, Harizi H, Boukadida J. 2011. Association of TNF-α and IL-10 polymorphisms with tuberculosis in Tunisian populations. *Microbes Infect* **13**: 837–843.

276. García-Elorriaga G, Vera-Ramírez L, del Rey-Pineda G, GonzÁlez-Bonilla C. 2013. -592 and -1082 interleukin-10 polymorphisms in pulmonary tuberculosis with type 2 diabetes. *Asian Pac J Trop Med* **6**:505–509.

277. Garcia-Laorden MI, Pena MJ, Caminero JA, Garcia-Saavedra A, Campos-Herrero MI, Caballero A, Rodriguez-Gallego C. 2006. Influence of mannose-binding lectin on HIV infection and tuberculosis in a Western-European population. *Mol Immunol* **43**:2143–2150.

278. Liang L, Zhao YL, Yue J, Liu JF, Han M, Wang H, Xiao H. 2011. Association of SP110 gene polymorphisms with susceptibility to tuberculosis in a Chinese population. *Infect Genet Evol* **11**:934–939.

279. Ma MJ, Xie LP, Wu SC, Tang F, Li H, Zhang ZS, Yang H, Chen SL, Liu N, Liu W, Cao WC. 2010. Toll-like receptors, tumor necrosis factor-α, and interleukin-10 gene polymorphisms in risk of pulmonary tuberculosis and disease severity. *Hum Immunol* **71**:1005–1010.

280. Meilang Q, Zhang Y, Zhang J, Zhao Y, Tian C, Huang J, Fan H. 2012. Polymorphisms in the SLC11A1 gene and tuberculosis risk: a meta-analysis update. *Int J Tuberc Lung Dis* **16**:437–446

281. Oh JH, Yang CS, Noh YK, Kweon YM, Jung SS, Son JW, Kong SJ, Yoon JU, Lee JS, Kim HJ, Park JK, Jo EK, Song CH. 2007. Polymorphisms of interleukin-10 and tumour necrosis factor-alpha genes are associated with newly diagnosed and recurrent pulmonary tuberculosis. *Respirology* **12**:594–598.

282. Prabhu Anand S, Selvaraj P, Jawahar MS, Adhilakshmi AR, Narayanan PR. 2007. Interleukin-12B & interleukin-10 gene polymorphisms in pulmonary tuberculosis. *Indian J Med Res* **126**:135–138.

283. Scola L, Crivello A, Marino V, Gioia V, Serauto A, Candore G, Colonna-Romano G, Caruso C, Lio D. 2003. IL-10 and TNF-alpha polymorphisms in a sample of Sicilian patients affected by tuberculosis: implication for ageing and life span expectancy. *Mech Ageing Dev* **124**:569–572

284. Shin HD, Park BL, Kim YH, Cheong HS, Lee IH, Park SK. 2005. Common interleukin 10 polymorphism associated with decreased risk of tuberculosis. *Exp Mol Med* **37**:128–132.

285. Thye T, Browne EN, Chinbuah MA, Gyapong J, Osei I, Owusu-Dabo E, Brattig NW, Niemann S, Rüsch-Gerdes S, Horstmann RD, Meyer CG. 2009. IL10 haplotype associated with tuberculin skin test response but not with pulmonary TB. *PLoS One* **4**:e5420

286. Ulger M, EmekdaŞ G, Aslan G, TaŞ D, Ilvan A, Tezcan S, Calıkoğlu M, Erdal ME, Kartaloğlu Z. 2013. [Determination of the cytokine gene polymorphism and genetic susceptibility in tuberculosis patients]. *Mikrobiyol Bul* **47**:250–264.

287. Yang H, Liang ZH, Liu XL, Wang F. 2010. [Association between polymorphisms of interleukin-10, interferon-γ gene and the susceptibility to pulmonary tuberculosis]. *Zhonghua Liu Xing Bing Xue Za Zhi* **31**:155–158.

288. Zembrzuski VM, Basta PC, Callegari-Jacques SM, Santos RV, Coimbra CE, Salzano FM, Hutz MH. 2010. Cytokine genes are associated with tuberculin skin test response in a native Brazilian population. *Tuberculosis (Edinb)* **90**:44–49.

289. Zhang J, Chen Y, Nie XB, Wu WH, Zhang H, Zhang M, He XM, Lu JX. 2011. Interleukin-10 polymorphisms and tuberculosis susceptibility: a meta-analysis. *Int J Tuberc Lung Dis* **15**:594–601.

290. Gao X, Chen J, Tong Z, Yang G, Yao Y, Xu F, Zhou J. 2015. Interleukin-10 promoter gene polymorphisms and susceptibility to tuberculosis: a meta-analysis. *PLoS One* **10**:e0127496

291. Kusuhara K, Yamamoto K, Okada K, Mizuno Y, Hara T. 2007. Association of IL12RB1 polymorphisms with susceptibility to and severity of tuberculosis in Japanese: a gene-based association analysis of 21 candidate genes. *Int J Immunogenet* **34**:35–44.

292. Ma X, Reich RA, Gonzalez O, Pan X, Fothergill AK, Starke JR, Teeter LD, Musser JM, Graviss EA. 2003. No evidence for association between the polymorphism in the 3′ untranslated region of interleukin-12B and human susceptibility to tuberculosis. *J Infect Dis* **188**: 1116–1118.

293. Morahan G, Kaur G, Singh M, Rapthap CC, Kumar N, Katoch K, Mehra NK, Huang D. 2007. Association of

variants in the IL12B gene with leprosy and tuberculosis. *Tissue Antigens* 69(Suppl 1):234–236.

294. Morris GA, Edwards DR, Hill PC, Wejse C, Bisseye C, Olesen R, Edwards TL, Gilbert JR, Myers JL, Stryjewski ME, Abbate E, Estevan R, Hamilton CD, Tacconelli A, Novelli G, Brunetti E, Aaby P, Sodemann M, Østergaard L, Adegbola R, Williams SM, Scott WK, Sirugo G. 2011. Interleukin 12B (IL12B) genetic variation and pulmonary tuberculosis: a study of cohorts from The Gambia, Guinea-Bissau, United States and Argentina. *PLoS One* 6:e16656

295. Puzyrev VP, Freĭdin MB, Rudko AA, Strelis AK, Kolokolova OV. 2002. [Polymorphisms of the candidate genes for genetic susceptibility to tuberculosis in the Slavic population of Siberia: a pilot study]. *Mol Biol (Mosk)* 36:788–791.

296. Akahoshi M, Nakashima H, Miyake K, Inoue Y, Shimizu S, Tanaka Y, Okada K, Otsuka T, Harada M. 2003. Influence of interleukin-12 receptor beta1 polymorphisms on tuberculosis. *Hum Genet* 112:237–243.

297. Lee HW, Lee HS, Kim DK, Ko DS, Han SK, Shim YS, Yim JJ. 2005. Lack of an association between interleukin-12 receptor beta1 polymorphisms and tuberculosis in Koreans. *Respiration* 72:365–368.

298. Remus N, El Baghdadi J, Fieschi C, Feinberg J, Quintin T, Chentoufi M, Schurr E, Benslimane A, Casanova JL, Abel L. 2004. Association of IL12RB1 polymorphisms with pulmonary tuberculosis in adults in Morocco. *J Infect Dis* 190:580–587

299. Peng R, Yue J, Han M, Zhao Y, Liu L, Liang L. 2013. The IL-17F sequence variant is associated with susceptibility to tuberculosis. *Gene* 515:229–232.

300. Han M, Yue J, Lian YY, Zhao YL, Wang HX, Liu LR. 2011. Relationship between single nucleotide polymorphism of interleukin-18 and susceptibility to pulmonary tuberculosis in the Chinese Han population. *Microbiol Immunol* 55:388–393.

301. Harishankar M, Selvaraj P, Rajeswari DN, Anand SP, Narayanan PR. 2007. Promoter polymorphism of IL-18 gene in pulmonary tuberculosis in South Indian population. *Int J Immunogenet* 34:317–320.

302. Zhang J, Zheng L, Zhu D, An H, Yang Y, Liang Y, Zhao W, Ding W, Wu X. 2014. Polymorphisms in the interleukin 18 receptor 1 gene and tuberculosis susceptibility among Chinese. *PLoS One* 9:e110734

303. Zhou C, Ouyang N, Li QH, Luo SX, He Q, Lei H, Liu Q. 2015. The -137G/C single nucleotide polymorphism in IL-18 gene promoter contributes to tuberculosis susceptibility in Chinese Han population. *Infect Genet Evol* 36:376–380.

304. Jiang D, Wubuli A, Hu X, Ikramullah S, Maimaiti A, Zhang W, Wushouer Q. 2015. The variations of IL-23R are associated with susceptibility and severe clinical forms of pulmonary tuberculosis in Chinese Uygurs. *BMC Infect Dis* 15:550

305. Gómez LM, Anaya JM, Vilchez JR, Cadena J, Hinojosa R, Vélez L, Lopez-Nevot MA, Martín J. 2007. A polymorphism in the inducible nitric oxide synthase gene is associated with tuberculosis. *Tuberculosis (Edinb)* 87:288–294.

306. Qu Y, Tang Y, Cao D, Wu F, Liu J, Lu G, Zhang Z, Xia Z. 2007. Genetic polymorphisms in alveolar macrophage response-related genes, and risk of silicosis and pulmonary tuberculosis in Chinese iron miners. *Int J Hyg Environ Health* 210:679–689.

307. Velez DR, Hulme WF, Myers JL, Stryjewski ME, Abbate E, Estevan R, Patillo SG, Gilbert JR, Hamilton CD, Scott WK. 2009. Association of SLC11A1 with tuberculosis and interactions with NOS2A and TLR2 in African-Americans and Caucasians. *Int J Tuberc Lung Dis* 13:1068–1076.

308. Ding S, Jiang T, He J, Qin B, Lin S, Li L. 2012. Tagging single nucleotide polymorphisms in the IRF1 and IRF8 genes and tuberculosis susceptibility. *PLoS One* 7:e42104

309. Vollstedt S, Yuliwulandari R, Okamoto K, Lien LT, Keicho N, Rochani JT, Wikaningrum R, Tokunaga K. 2009. No evidence for association between the interferon regulatory factor 1 (IRF1) gene and clinical tuberculosis. *Tuberculosis (Edinb)* 89:71–76.

310. Bahari G, Hashemi M, Taheri M, Naderi M, Eskandari-Nasab E, Atabaki M. 2012. Association of IRGM polymorphisms and susceptibility to pulmonary tuberculosis in Zahedan, Southeast Iran. *Scientific World Journal* 2012:950801

311. Che N, Li S, Gao T, Zhang Z, Han Y, Zhang X, Sun Y, Liu Y, Sun Z, Zhang J, Ren W, Tian M, Li Y, Li W, Cheng J, Li C. 2010. Identification of a novel IRGM promoter single nucleotide polymorphism associated with tuberculosis. *Clin Chim Acta* 411:1645–1649.

312. King KY, Lew JD, Ha NP, Lin JS, Ma X, Graviss EA, Goodell MA. 2011. Polymorphic allele of human IRGM1 is associated with susceptibility to tuberculosis in African Americans. *PLoS One* 6:e16317

313. Braun K, Larcombe L, Orr P, Nickerson P, Wolfe J, Sharma M. 2013. Killer immunoglobulin-like receptor (KIR) centromeric-AA haplotype is associated with ethnicity and tuberculosis disease in a Canadian First Nations cohort. *PLoS One* 8:e67842

314. Lu C, Bai XL, Deng YF, Wang CY, Fan G, Shen YJ, Liu YQ, Zhang BC, Zhao YR, Huan C, Zhang CZ, Lu ZM. 2014. Killer cell immunoglobulin-like receptor genotypes and haplotypes with susceptibility to pulmonary tuberculosis infection. *Clin Lab* 60:821–825.

315. Lu C, Shen YJ, Deng YF, Wang CY, Fan G, Liu YQ, Zhao SM, Zhang BC, Zhao YR, Wang ZE, Zhang CZ, Lu ZM. 2012. Association of killer cell immunoglobulin-like receptors with pulmonary tuberculosis in Chinese Han. *Genet Mol Res* 11:1370–1378.

316. Salie M, Daya M, Möller M, Hoal EG. 2015. Activating KIRs alter susceptibility to pulmonary tuberculosis in a South African population. *Tuberculosis (Edinb)* 95:817–821.

317. Shahsavar F, Mousavi T, Azargon A, Entezami K. 2012. Association of KIR3DS1+HLA-B Bw4Ile80 combination with susceptibility to tuberculosis in Lur population of Iran. *Iran J Immunol* 9:39–47.

318. Tajik N, Shah-hosseini A, Mohammadi A, Jafari M, Nasiri M, Radjabzadeh MF, Farnia P, Jalali A. 2012. Susceptibility to pulmonary tuberculosis in Iranian

individuals is not affected by compound KIR/HLA genotype. *Tissue Antigens* 79:90–96.

319. Curtis J, Kopanitsa L, Stebbings E, Speirs A, Ignatyeva O, Balabanova Y, Nikolayevskyy V, Hoffner S, Horstmann R, Drobniewski F, Nejentsev S. 2011. Association analysis of the LTA4H gene polymorphisms and pulmonary tuberculosis in 9115 subjects. *Tuberculosis (Edinb)* 91:22–25.

320. García-Elorriaga G, Carrillo-Montes G, Mendoza-Aguilar M, GonzÁlez-Bonilla C. 2010. Polymorphisms in tumor necrosis factor and lymphotoxin A in tuberculosis without and with response to treatment. *Inflammation* 33:267–275.

321. Tobin DM, Vary JC Jr, Ray JP, Walsh GS, Dunstan SJ, Bang ND, Hagge DA, Khadge S, King MC, Hawn TR, Moens CB, Ramakrishnan L. 2010. The lta4h locus modulates susceptibility to mycobacterial infection in zebrafish and humans. *Cell* 140:717–730.

322. Xue Y, Zhao ZQ, Hong D, Zhao MY, Zhang YX, Wang HJ, Wang Y, Li JC. 2010. Lack of association between MD-2 promoter gene variants and tuberculosis. *Genet Mol Res* 9:1584–1590.

323. Han M, Liang L, Liu LR, Yue J, Zhao YL, Xiao HP. 2014. Liver X receptor gene polymorphisms in tuberculosis: effect on susceptibility. *PLoS One* 9:e95954

324. Bowdish DM, Sakamoto K, Lack NA, Hill PC, Sirugo G, Newport MJ, Gordon S, Hill AV, Vannberg FO. 2013. Genetic variants of MARCO are associated with susceptibility to pulmonary tuberculosis in a Gambian population. *BMC Med Genet* 14:47

325. Ma MJ, Wang HB, Li H, Yang JH, Yan Y, Xie LP, Qi YC, Li JL, Chen MJ, Liu W, Cao WC. 2011. Genetic variants in MARCO are associated with the susceptibility to pulmonary tuberculosis in Chinese Han population. *PLoS One* 6:e24069

326. Chen M, Deng J, Su C, Li J, Wang M, Abuaku BK, Hu S, Tan H, Wen SW. 2014. Impact of passive smoking, cooking with solid fuel exposure, and MBL/MASP-2 gene polymorphism upon susceptibility to tuberculosis. *Int J Infect Dis* 29:1–6.

327. Chen M, Liang Y, Li W, Wang M, Hu L, Abuaku BK, Huang X, Tan H, Wen SW. 2015. Impact of MBL and MASP-2 gene polymorphism and its interaction on susceptibility to tuberculosis. *BMC Infect Dis* 15:151

328. Alagarasu K, Selvaraj P, Swaminathan S, Raghavan S, Narendran G, Narayanan PR. 2007. Mannose binding lectin gene variants and susceptibility to tuberculosis in HIV-1 infected patients of South India. *Tuberculosis (Edinb)* 87:535–543.

329. Bellamy R, Ruwende C, McAdam KP, Thursz M, Sumiya M, Summerfield J, Gilbert SC, Corrah T, Kwiatkowski D, Whittle HC, Hill AV. 1998. Mannose binding protein deficiency is not associated with malaria, hepatitis B carriage nor tuberculosis in Africans. *QJM* 91:13–18

330. Capparelli R, Iannaccone M, Palumbo D, Medaglia C, Moscariello E, Russo A, Iannelli D. 2009. Role played by human mannose-binding lectin polymorphisms in pulmonary tuberculosis. *J Infect Dis* 199:666–672.

331. Cosar H, Ozkinay F, Onay H, Bayram N, Bakiler AR, Anil M, Can D, Ozkinay C. 2008. Low levels of mannose-binding lectin confers protection against tuberculosis in Turkish children. *Eur J Clin Microbiol Infect Dis* 27:1165–1169.

332. da Cruz HL, da Silva RC, Segat L, de Carvalho MS, Brandão LA, Guimarães RL, Santos FC, de Lira LA, Montenegro LM, Schindler HC, Crovella S. 2013. MBL2 gene polymorphisms and susceptibility to tuberculosis in a northeastern Brazilian population. *Infect Genet Evol* 19:323–329.

333. El Sahly HM, Reich RA, Dou SJ, Musser JM, Graviss EA. 2004. The effect of mannose binding lectin gene polymorphisms on susceptibility to tuberculosis in different ethnic groups. *Scand J Infect Dis* 36:106–108.

334. Feng FM, Guo M, Liu Q, Wang D, Gao BX, Sun YH, An YC, Ji CM. 2006. [Study on mannose-binding protein gene polymorphisms and susceptibility to pulmonary tuberculosis]. *Zhonghua Liu Xing Bing Xue Za Zhi* 27:1082–1085.

335. Mombo LE, Lu CY, Ossari S, Bedjabaga I, Sica L, Krishnamoorthy R, Lapoumeroulie C. 2003. Mannose-binding lectin alleles in sub-Saharan Africans and relation with susceptibility to infections. *Genes Immun* 4:362–367.

336. OzbaŞ-Gerçeker F, Tezcan I, Berkel AI, Ozkara S, Ozcan A, Ersoy F, Sanal O, Ozgüç M. 2003. The effect of mannose-binding protein gene polymorphisms in recurrent respiratory system infections in children and lung tuberculosis. *Turk J Pediatr* 45:95–98.

337. Selvaraj P, Narayanan PR, Reetha AM. 1999. Association of functional mutant homozygotes of the mannose binding protein gene with susceptibility to pulmonary tuberculosis in India. *Tuber Lung Dis* 79:221–227.

338. Singla N, Gupta D, Joshi A, Batra N, Singh J, Birbian N. 2012. Association of mannose-binding lectin gene polymorphism with tuberculosis susceptibility and sputum conversion time. *Int J Immunogenet* 39:10–14.

339. Søborg C, Andersen AB, Range N, Malenganisho W, Friis H, Magnussen P, Temu MM, Changalucha J, Madsen HO, Garred P. 2007. Influence of candidate susceptibility genes on tuberculosis in a high endemic region. *Mol Immunol* 44:2213–2220.

340. Søborg C, Madsen HO, Andersen AB, Lillebaek T, Kok-Jensen A, Garred P. 2003. Mannose-binding lectin polymorphisms in clinical tuberculosis. *J Infect Dis* 188:777–782.

341. Solğun HA, TaŞtemir D, Aksaray N, Inan I, Demirhan O. 2011. Polymorphisms in NRAMP1 and MBL2 genes and their relations with tuberculosis in Turkish children. *Tuberk Toraks* 59:48–53

342. Thye T, Niemann S, Walter K, Homolka S, Intemann CD, Chinbuah MA, Enimil A, Gyapong J, Osei I, Owusu-Dabo E, Rüsch-Gerdes S, Horstmann RD, Ehlers S, Meyer CG. 2011. Variant G57E of mannose binding lectin associated with protection against tuberculosis caused by Mycobacterium africanum but not by M. tuberculosis. *PLoS One* 6:e20908

343. Wu L, Deng H, Zheng Y, Mansjö M, Zheng X, Hu Y, Xu B. 2015. An association study of NRAMP1, VDR, MBL and their interaction with the susceptibility to

tuberculosis in a Chinese population. *Int J Infect Dis* **38**:129–135.

344. Denholm JT, McBryde ES, Eisen DP. 2010. Mannose-binding lectin and susceptibility to tuberculosis: a meta-analysis. *Clin Exp Immunol* **162**:84–90.

345. Shi J, Xie M, Wang JM, Xu YJ, Xiong WN, Liu XS. 2013. Mannose-binding lectin two gene polymorphisms and tuberculosis susceptibility in Chinese population: a meta-analysis. *J Huazhong Univ Sci Technolog Med Sci* **33**:166–171.

346. Shin HD, Cheong HS, Park BL, Kim LH, Han CS, Lee IH, Park SK. 2008. Common MCL1 polymorphisms associated with risk of tuberculosis. *BMB Rep* **41**:334–337.

347. Gómez LM, SÁnchez E, Ruiz-Narvaez EA, López-Nevot MA, Anaya JM, Martín J. 2007. Macrophage migration inhibitory factor gene influences the risk of developing tuberculosis in northwestern Colombian population. *Tissue Antigens* **70**:28–33.

348. Li Y, Zeng Z, Deng S. 2012. Study of the relationship between human MIF level, MIF-794CATT5-8 microsatellite polymorphism, and susceptibility of tuberculosis in Southwest China. *Braz J Infect Dis* **16**:383–386.

349. Liu A, Li J, Bao F, Zhu Z, Feng S, Yang J, Wang L, Shi M, Wen X, Zhao H, Voravuthikunchai SP. 2016. Single nucleotide polymorphisms in cytokine MIF gene promoter region are closely associated with human susceptibility to tuberculosis in a southwestern province of China. *Infect Genet Evol* **39**:219–224 10.1016/j.meegid.2015.12.003.

350. Li D, Wang T, Song X, Qucuo M, Yang B, Zhang J, Wang J, Ying B, Tao C, Wang L. 2011. Genetic study of two single nucleotide polymorphisms within corresponding microRNAs and susceptibility to tuberculosis in a Chinese Tibetan and Han population. *Hum Immunol* **72**:598–602.

351. Naderi M, Hashemi M, Khorgami P, Koshki M, Ebrahimi M, Amininia S, Sharifi-Mood B, Taheri M. 2015. Lack of association between miRNA-146a rs2910164 and miRNA-499 rs3746444 gene polymorphisms and susceptibility to pulmonary tuberculosis. *Int J Mol Cell Med* **4**:40–45.

352. Song X, Li S, QuCuo M, Zhou M, Zhou Y, Hu X, Zhou J, Lu X, Wang J, Hua W, Ye Y, Ying B, Wang L. 2013. Association between SNPs in microRNA-machinery genes and tuberculosis susceptibility in Chinese Tibetan population. *Mol Biol Rep* **40**:6027–6033.

353. Zhang X, Li Y, Li X, Zhang W, Pan Z, Wu F, Wang C, Chen Z, Jiang T, Xu D, Ping Z, Liu J, Liu C, Li Z, Li JC. 2015. Association of the miR-146a, miR-149, miR-196a2 and miR-499 polymorphisms with susceptibility to pulmonary tuberculosis in the Chinese Uygur, Kazak and Southern Han populations. *BMC Infect Dis* **15**:41

354. Lee SH, Han SK, Shim YS, Yim JJ. 2009. Effect of matrix metalloproteinase-9 -1562C/T gene polymorphism on manifestations of pulmonary tuberculosis. *Tuberculosis (Edinb)* **89**:68–70.

355. Sánchez D, Lefebvre C, Rioux J, García LF, Barrera LF. 2012. Evaluation of Toll-like receptor and adaptor

molecule polymorphisms for susceptibility to tuberculosis in a Colombian population. *Int J Immunogenet* **39**:216–223

356. Austin CM, Ma X, Graviss EA. 2008. Common non-synonymous polymorphisms in the NOD2 gene are associated with resistance or susceptibility to tuberculosis disease in African Americans. *J Infect Dis* **197**:1713–1716.

357. Möller M, Nebel A, Kwiatkowski R, van Helden PD, Hoal EG, Schreiber S. 2007. Host susceptibility to tuberculosis: CARD15 polymorphisms in a South African population. *Mol Cell Probes* **21**:148–151.

358. Pan H, Dai Y, Tang S, Wang J. 2012. Polymorphisms of NOD2 and the risk of tuberculosis: a validation study in the Chinese population. *Int J Immunogenet* **39**:233–240

359. Stockton JC, Howson JM, Awomoyi AA, McAdam KP, Blackwell JM, Newport MJ. 2004. Polymorphism in NOD2, Crohn's disease, and susceptibility to pulmonary tuberculosis. *FEMS Immunol Med Microbiol* **41**:157–160

360. Zhao M, Jiang F, Zhang W, Li F, Wei L, Liu J, Xue Y, Deng X, Wu F, Zhang L, Zhang X, Zhang Y, Fan D, Sun X, Jiang T, Li JC. 2012. A novel single nucleotide polymorphism within the NOD2 gene is associated with pulmonary tuberculosis in the Chinese Han, Uygur and Kazak populations. *BMC Infect Dis* **12**:91

361. Wang C, Chen ZL, Pan ZF, Wei LL, Xu DD, Jiang TT, Zhang X, Ping ZP, Li ZJ, Li JC. 2013. NOD2 polymorphisms and pulmonary tuberculosis susceptibility: a systematic review and meta-analysis. *Int J Biol Sci* **10**:103–108.

362. Abe T, Iinuma Y, Ando M, Yokoyama T, Yamamoto T, Nakashima K, Takagi N, Baba H, Hasegawa Y, Shimokata K. 2003. NRAMP1 polymorphisms, susceptibility and clinical features of tuberculosis. *J Infect* **46**:215–220.

363. An YC, Feng FM, Yuan JX, Ji CM, Wang YH, Guo M, Deng XJ, Gao BX, Wang D, Liu Q. 2006. [Study on the association of INT4 and 3'UTR polymorphism of natural-resistance-associated macrophage protein 1 gene with susceptibility to pulmonary tuberculosis]. *Zhonghua Liu Xing Bing Xue Za Zhi* **27**:37–40.

364. Asai S, Abe Y, Fujino T, Masukawa A, Arami S, Furuya H, Miyachi H. 2008. Association of the SLC11A1 gene polymorphisms with susceptibility to Mycobacterium infections in a Japanese population. *Infect Dis Clin Pract* **16**:230–234.

365. Ates O, Dalyan L, Müsellim B, Hatemi G, Türker H, Ongen G, Hamuryudan V, Topal-Sarikaya A. 2009. NRAMP1 (SLC11A1) gene polymorphisms that correlate with autoimmune versus infectious disease susceptibility in tuberculosis and rheumatoid arthritis. *Int J Immunogenet* **36**:15–19.

366. Awomoyi A, Sirugo G, Newport MJ, Tishkoff S. 2006. Global distribution of a novel trinucleotide microsatellite polymorphism (ATA)n in intron 8 of the SLC11A1 gene and susceptibility to pulmonary tuberculosis. *Int J Immunogenet* **33**:11–15.

367. Bellamy R, Ruwende C, Corrah T, McAdam KP, Whittle HC, Hill AV. 1998. Variations in the NRAMP1

gene and susceptibility to tuberculosis in West Africans. *N Engl J Med* **338**:640–644.

368. Ben-Selma W, Harizi H, Letaief M, Boukadida J. 2012. Age- and gender-specific effects on NRAMP1 gene polymorphisms and risk of the development of active tuberculosis in Tunisian populations. *Int J Infect Dis* **16**:e543–e550.

369. Borgdorff MW. 1998. The NRAMP1 gene and susceptibility to tuberculosis. *N Engl J Med* **339**:199–200; author reply 200–201.

370. Cervino AC, Lakiss S, Sow O, Hill AV. 2000. Allelic association between the NRAMP1 gene and susceptibility to tuberculosis in Guinea-Conakry. *Ann Hum Genet* **64**:507–512.

371. Chen XR, Feng YL, Ma Y, Zhang ZD, Li CY, Wen FQ, Tang XY, Su ZG. 2009. [A study on the haplotype of the solute carrier family 11 member 1 gene in Tibetan patients with pulmonary tuberculosis in China]. *Zhonghua Jie He He Hu Xi Za Zhi* **32**:360–364.

372. Duan HF, Zhou XH, Ma Y, Li CY, Chen XY, Gao WW, Zheng SH. 2003. [A study on the association of 3'UTR polymorphisms of NRAMP1 gene with susceptibility to tuberculosis in Hans]. *Zhonghua Jie He Hu Xi Za Zhi* **26**:286–289.

373. El Baghdadi J, Remus N, Benslimane A, El Annaz H, Chentoufi M, Abel L, Schurr E. 2003. Variants of the human NRAMP1 gene and susceptibility to tuberculosis in Morocco. *Int J Tuberc Lung Dis* **7**:599–602.

374. Fernández-Mestre M, Villasmil Á, Takiff H, Alcalá ZF. 2015. NRAMP1 and VDR gene polymorphisms in susceptibility to tuberculosis in Venezuelan population. *Dis Markers* **2015**:860628

375. Gao PS, Fujishima S, Mao XQ, Remus N, Kanda M, Enomoto T, Dake Y, Bottini N, Tabuchi M, Hasegawa N, Yamaguchi K, Tiemessen C, Hopkin JM, Shirakawa T, Kishi F, International Tuberculosis Genetics Team. 2000. Genetic variants of NRAMP1 and active tuberculosis in Japanese populations. *Clin Genet* **58**:74–76.

376. Hatta M, Ratnawati, Tanaka M, Ito J, Shirakawa T, Kawabata M. 2010. NRAMP1/SLC11A1 gene polymorphisms and host susceptibility to *Mycobacterium tuberculosis* and *M. leprae* in South Sulawesi, Indonesia. *Southeast Asian J Trop Med Public Health* **41**:386–394.

377. Hoal EG, Lewis LA, Jamieson SE, Tanzer F, Rossouw M, Victor T, Hillerman R, Beyers N, Blackwell JM, Van Helden PD. 2004. SLC11A1 (NRAMP1) but not SLC11A2 (NRAMP2) polymorphisms are associated with susceptibility to tuberculosis in a high-incidence community in South Africa. *Int J Tuberc Lung Dis* **8**:1464–1471.

378. Hsu YH, Chen CW, Sun HS, Jou R, Lee JJ, Su IJ. 2006. Association of NRAMP 1 gene polymorphism with susceptibility to tuberculosis in Taiwanese aboriginals. *J Formos Med Assoc* **105**:363–369.

379. Jin J, Sun L, Jiao W, Zhao S, Li H, Guan X, Jiao A, Jiang Z, Shen A. 2009. SLC11A1 (Formerly NRAMP1) gene polymorphisms associated with pediatric tuberculosis in China. *Clin Infect Dis* **48**:733–738.

380. Kim JH, Lee SY, Lee SH, Sin C, Shim JJ, In KH, Yoo SH, Kang KH. 2003. NRAMP1 genetic polymorphisms

as a risk factor of tuberculous pleurisy. *Int J Tuberc Lung Dis* **7**:370–375.

381. Leung KH, Yip SP, Wong WS, Yiu LS, Chan KK, Lai WM, Chow EY, Lin CK, Yam WC, Chan KS. 2007. Sex- and age-dependent association of SLC11A1 polymorphisms with tuberculosis in Chinese: a case control study. *BMC Infect Dis* **7**:19

382. Liaw YS, Tsai-Wu JJ, Wu CH, Hung CC, Lee CN, Yang PC, Luh KT, Kuo SH. 2002. Variations in the NRAMP1 gene and susceptibility of tuberculosis in Taiwanese. *Int J Tuberc Lung Dis* **6**:454–460.

383. Liu W, Cao WC, Zhang CY, Tian L, Wu XM, Habbema JD, Zhao QM, Zhang PH, Xin ZT, Li CZ, Yang H. 2004. VDR and NRAMP1 gene polymorphisms in susceptibility to pulmonary tuberculosis among the Chinese Han population: a case-control study. *Int J Tuberc Lung Dis* **8**:428–434.

384. Liu W, Zhang CY, Tian L, Li CZ, Wu XM, Zhao QM, Zhang PH, Yang SM, Yang H, Cao WC. 2003. [A case-control study on natural-resistance-associated macrophage protein 1 gene polymorphisms and susceptibility to pulmonary tuberculosis]. *Zhonghua Yu Fang Yi Xue Za Zhi* **37**:408–411.

385. Liu ZB, Zheng RJ, Xiao HP, Sha W, Zhang Q, Wu FR, Sun H, Zhang ZS, Cui HY, Liu YD, Tang SJ. 2011. [The correlation between polymorphisms of genes with susceptibility to tuberculosis and the clinical characteristics of tuberculosis in 459 Han patients]. *Zhonghua Jie He He Hu Xi Za Zhi* **34**:923–928.

386. Ma X, Dou S, Wright JA, Reich RA, Teeter LD, El Sahly HM, Awe RJ, Musser JM, Graviss EA. 2002. 5' dinucleotide repeat polymorphism of NRAMP1 and susceptibility to tuberculosis among Caucasian patients in Houston, Texas. *Int J Tuberc Lung Dis* **6**:818–823.

387. Malik S, Abel L, Tooker H, Poon A, Simkin L, Girard M, Adams GJ, Starke JR, Smith KC, Graviss EA, Musser JM, Schurr E. 2005. Alleles of the NRAMP1 gene are risk factors for pediatric tuberculosis disease. *Proc Natl Acad Sci USA* **102**:12183–12188.

388. McDermid JM, Prentice AM. 2006. Iron and infection: effects of host iron status and the iron-regulatory genes haptoglobin and NRAMP1 (SLC11A1) on host-pathogen interactions in tuberculosis and HIV. *Clin Sci (Lond)* **110**:503–524.

389. Merza M, Farnia P, Anoosheh S, Varahram M, Kazampour M, Pajand O, Saeif S, Mirsaeidi M, Masjedi MR, Velayati AA, Hoffner S. 2009. The NRAMPI, VDR and TNF-alpha gene polymorphisms in Iranian tuberculosis patients: the study on host susceptibility. *Braz J Infect Dis* **13**:252–256.

390. Niño-Moreno P, Portales-Pérez D, HernÁndez-Castro B, Portales-Cervantes L, Flores-Meraz V, Baranda L, Gómez-Gómez A, Acuña-Alonzo V, Granados J, GonzÁlez-Amaro R. 2007. P2X7 and NRAMP1/SLC11 A1 gene polymorphisms in Mexican mestizo patients with pulmonary tuberculosis. *Clin Exp Immunol* **148**:469–477.

391. Nugraha J, Anggraini R. 2011. NRAMP1 polymorphism and susceptibility to lung tuberculosis in Surabaya, Indonesia. *Southeast Asian J Trop Med Public Health* **42**:338–341.

392. Ryu S, Park YK, Bai GH, Kim SJ, Park SN, Kang S. 2000. 3'UTR polymorphisms in the NRAMP1 gene are associated with susceptibility to tuberculosis in Koreans. *Int J Tuberc Lung Dis* 4:577–580.

393. Sahiratmadja E, Wieringa FT, van Crevel R, de Visser AW, Adnan I, Alisjahbana B, Slagboom E, Marzuki S, Ottenhoff TH, van de Vosse E, Marx JJ. 2007. Iron deficiency and NRAMP1 polymorphisms (INT4, D543N and 3'UTR) do not contribute to severity of anaemia in tuberculosis in the Indonesian population. *Br J Nutr* 98:684–690.

394. Selvaraj P, Chandra G, Kurian SM, Reetha AM, Charles N, Narayanan P. 2002. NRAMP1 gene polymorphism in pulmonary and spinal tuberculosis. *Curr Sci* 82:451–454.

395. Singh A, Gaughan JP, Kashyap VK. 2011. SLC11A1 and VDR gene variants and susceptibility to tuberculosis and disease progression in East India. *Int J Tuberc Lung Dis* 15:1468–1474, i.

396. Søborg C, Andersen AB, Madsen HO, Kok-Jensen A, Skinhøj P, Garred P. 2002. Natural resistance-associated macrophage protein 1 polymorphisms are associated with microscopy-positive tuberculosis. *J Infect Dis* 186:517–521.

397. Stagas MK, Papaetis GS, Orphanidou D, Kostopoulos C, Syriou S, Reczko M, Drakoulis N. 2011. Polymorphisms of the NRAMP1 gene: distribution and susceptibility to the development of pulmonary tuberculosis in the Greek population. *Med Sci Monit* 17:PH1–PH6.

398. Takahashi K, Hasegawa Y, Abe T, Yamamoto T, Nakashima K, Imaizumi K, Shimokata K. 2008. SLC11A1 (formerly NRAMP1) polymorphisms associated with multidrug-resistant tuberculosis. *Tuberculosis (Edinb)* 88:52–57.

399. Taype CA, Castro JC, Accinelli RA, Herrera-Velit P, Shaw MA, Espinoza JR. 2006. Association between SLC11A1 polymorphisms and susceptibility to different clinical forms of tuberculosis in the Peruvian population. *Infect Genet Evol* 6:361–367.

400. Vejbaesya S, Chierakul N, Luangtrakool P, Sermduangprateep C. 2007. NRAMP1 and TNF-alpha polymorphisms and susceptibility to tuberculosis in Thais. *Respirology* 12:202–206.

401. Zhang W, Shao L, Weng X, Hu Z, Jin A, Chen S, Pang M, Chen ZW. 2005. Variants of the natural resistance-associated macrophage protein 1 gene (NRAMP1) are associated with severe forms of pulmonary tuberculosis. *Clin Infect Dis* 40:1232–1236.

402. Li HT, Zhang TT, Huang QH, Lv B, Huang J. 2006. [Meta-analysis on NRAMP1 gene polymorphisms and tuberculosis susceptibility in East-Asia population]. *Zhonghua Liu Xing Bing Xue Za Zhi* 27:428–432.

403. Li HT, Zhang TT, Zhou YQ, Huang QH, Huang J. 2006. SLC11A1 (formerly NRAMP1) gene polymorphisms and tuberculosis susceptibility: a meta-analysis. *Int J Tuberc Lung Dis* 10:3–12.

404. Li X, Yang Y, Zhou F, Zhang Y, Lu H, Jin Q, Gao L. 2011. SLC11A1 (NRAMP1) polymorphisms and tuberculosis susceptibility: updated systematic review and meta-analysis. *PLoS One* 6:e15831

405. Meilang Q, Zhang Y, Zhang J, Zhao Y, Tian C, Huang J, Fan H. 2012. Polymorphisms in the SLC11A1 gene and tuberculosis risk: a meta-analysis update. *Int J Tuberc Lung Dis* 16:437–446.

406. Bahari G, Hashemi M, Taheri M, Naderi M, Moazeni-Roodi A, Kouhpayeh HR, Eskandari-Nasab E. 2013. Association of P2X7 gene polymorphisms with susceptibility to pulmonary tuberculosis in Zahedan, Southeast Iran. *Genet Mol Res* 12:160–166.

407. Ben-Selma W, Ben-Kahla I, Boukadida J, Harizi H. 2011. Contribution of the P2X7 1513A/C loss-of-function polymorphism to extrapulmonary tuberculosis susceptibility in Tunisian populations. *FEMS Immunol Med Microbiol* 63:65–72.

408. Denholm JT, McBryde ES. 2012. P2X7 A1513 polymorphisms and tuberculosis susceptibility. *Respirology* 17:191, author reply 191–192

409. Fernando SL, Saunders BM, Sluyter R, Skarratt KK, Goldberg H, Marks GB, Wiley JS, Britton WJ. 2007. A polymorphism in the P2X7 gene increases susceptibility to extrapulmonary tuberculosis. *Am J Respir Crit Care Med* 175:360–366.

410. Li CM, Campbell SJ, Kumararatne DS, Bellamy R, Ruwende C, McAdam KP, Hill AV, Lammas DA. 2002. Association of a polymorphism in the P2X7 gene with tuberculosis in a Gambian population. *J Infect Dis* 186:1458–1462.

411. Mokrousov I, Sapozhnikova N, Narvskaya O. 2008. Mycobacterium tuberculosis co-existence with humans: making an imprint on the macrophage P2X(7) receptor gene? *J Med Microbiol* 57:581–584.

412. Ozdemir FA, Erol D, Konar V, Yüce H, Kara Şenli E, Bulut F, Deveci F. 2014. Lack of association of 1513 A/C polymorphism in P2X7 gene with susceptibility to pulmonary and extrapulmonary tuberculosis. *Tuberk Toraks* 62:7–11.

413. Sambasivan V, Murthy KJ, Reddy R, Vijayalakshimi V, Hasan Q. 2010. P2X7 gene polymorphisms and risk assessment for pulmonary tuberculosis in Asian Indians. *Dis Markers* 28:43–48.

414. Sharma S, Kumar V, Khosla R, Kajal N, Sarin B, Sehajpal P. 2010. Association of P2X7 receptor +1513 (A->C) polymorphism with tuberculosis in a Punjabi population. *Int J Tuberc Lung Dis* 14:1159–1163.

415. Singla N, Gupta D, Joshi A, Batra N, Singh J. 2012. Genetic polymorphisms in the P2X7 gene and its association with susceptibility to tuberculosis. *Int J Tuberc Lung Dis* 16:224–229.

416. Xiao J, Sun L, Jiao W, Li Z, Zhao S, Li H, Jin J, Jiao A, Guo Y, Jiang Z, Mokrousov I, Shen A. 2009. Lack of association between polymorphisms in the P2X7 gene and tuberculosis in a Chinese Han population. *FEMS Immunol Med Microbiol* 55:107–111.

417. Xiao J, Sun L, Yan H, Jiao W, Miao Q, Feng W, Wu X, Gu Y, Jiao A, Guo Y, Peng X, Shen A. 2010. Meta-analysis of P2X7 gene polymorphisms and tuberculosis susceptibility. *FEMS Immunol Med Microbiol* 60:165–170.

418. Wang X, Xiao H, Lan H, Mao C, Chen Q. 2011. Lack of association between the P2X7 receptor A1513C

polymorphism and susceptibility to pulmonary tuberculosis: a meta-analysis. *Respirology* 16:790–795.

419. Wu G, Zhao M, Gu X, Yao Y, Liu H, Song Y. 2014. The effect of P2X7 receptor 1513 polymorphism on susceptibility to tuberculosis: a meta-analysis. *Infect Genet Evol* 24:82–91

420. Yi L, Cheng D, Shi H, Huo X, Zhang K, Zhen G. 2014. A meta-analysis of P2X7 gene-762T/C polymorphism and pulmonary tuberculosis susceptibility. *PLoS One* 9:e96359

421. Ge HB, Chen S. 2016. A meta-analysis of P2X7 gene-1513A/C polymorphism and pulmonary tuberculosis susceptibility. *Hum Immunol* 77:126–130.

422. Udina IG, Kordicheva SI, Pospelov LE, Malenko AF, Gergert VI, Pospelov AL, Matrashkin AG, Kyzyl-Ool MM, Nachin AA, Zhivotovskiĭ LA. 2007. [Study of the polymorphic markers–the PARK2 and PACRG genes due to the incidence of pulmonary tuberculosis in two districts of the Republic of Tyva]. *Probl Tuberk Bolezn Legk* (7):27–29.

423. Lim MK, Shim TS, Park M, Lee SK, Sohn YH, Sheen DH, Shim SC. 2015. Heterozygote genotypes for PADI4_89 were protectively associated with susceptibility to tuberculosis in Koreans. *Rheumatol Int* 35:651–655.

424. Gomez LM, Anaya JM, Martin J. 2005. Genetic influence of PTPN22 R620W polymorphism in tuberculosis. *Hum Immunol* 66:1242–1247

425. Lamsyah H, Rueda B, Baassi L, Elaouad R, Bottini N, Sadki K, Martin J. 2009. Association of PTPN22 gene functional variants with development of pulmonary tuberculosis in Moroccan population. *Tissue Antigens* 74:228–232.

426. Zhao Z, Peng W, Hu X, Zhang J, Shang M, Zhou J, Zhou Y, Song X, Lu X, Ying B, Chen X. 2016. SFRP1 variations influence susceptibility and immune response to *Mycobacterium tuberculosis* in a Chinese Hanpopulation. *Infect Genet Evol* 37:259–265.

427. Horne DJ, Randhawa AK, Chau TT, Bang ND, Yen NT, Farrar JJ, Dunstan SJ, Hawn TR. 2012. Common polymorphisms in the PKP3-SIGIRR-TMEM16J gene region are associated with susceptibility to tuberculosis. *J Infect Dis* 205:586–594.

428. Abhimanyu, Jha P, Jain A, Arora K, Bose M. 2011. Genetic association study suggests a role for SP110 variants in lymph node tuberculosis but not pulmonary tuberculosis in north Indians. *Hum Immunol* 72:576–580.

429. Babb C, Keet EH, van Helden PD, Hoal EG. 2007. SP110 polymorphisms are not associated with pulmonary tuberculosis in a South African population. *Hum Genet* 121:521–522.

430. Cong J, Li G, Zhou D, Tao Y, Xiong Y. 2010. [Study on relation between Sp110 gene polymorphism and tuberculosis genetic susceptibility of Chongqing Han People]. *Wei Sheng Yan Jiu* 39:540–544.

431. Png E, Alisjahbana B, Sahiratmadja E, Marzuki S, Nelwan R, Adnan I, van de Vosse E, Hibberd M, van Crevel R, Ottenhoff TH, Seielstad M. 2012. Polymorphisms in SP110 are not associated with pulmonary tuberculosis in Indonesians. *Infect Genet Evol* 12:1319–1323.

432. Szeszko JS, Healy B, Stevens H, Balabanova Y, Drobniewski F, Todd JA, Nejentsev S. 2007. Resequencing and association analysis of the SP110 gene in adult pulmonary tuberculosis. *Hum Genet* 121:155–160.

433. Thye T, Browne EN, Chinbuah MA, Gyapong J, Osei I, Owusu-Dabo E, Niemann S, Rüsch-Gerdes S, Horstmann RD, Meyer CG. 2006. No associations of human pulmonary tuberculosis with Sp110 variants. *J Med Genet* 43:e32

434. Tosh K, Campbell SJ, Fielding K, Sillah J, Bah B, Gustafson P, Manneh K, Lisse I, Sirugo G, Bennett S, Aaby P, McAdam KP, Bah-Sow O, Lienhardt C, Kramnik I, Hill AV. 2006. Variants in the SP110 gene are associated with genetic susceptibility to tuberculosis in West Africa. *Proc Natl Acad Sci USA* 103:10364–10368.

435. Lei X, Zhu H, Zha L, Wang Y. 2012. SP110 gene polymorphisms and tuberculosis susceptibility: a systematic review and meta-analysis based on 10 624 subjects. *Infect Genet Evol* 12:1473–1480.

436. Floros J, Lin HM, García A, Salazar MA, Guo X, DiAngelo S, Montaño M, Luo J, Pardo A, Selman M. 2000. Surfactant protein genetic marker alleles identify a subgroup of tuberculosis in a Mexican population. *J Infect Dis* 182:1473–1478.

437. Madan T, Saxena S, Murthy KJ, Muralidhar K, Sarma PU. 2002. Association of polymorphisms in the collagen region of human SP-A1 and SP-A2 genes with pulmonary tuberculosis in Indian population. *Clin Chem Lab Med* 40:1002–1008.

438. Malik S, Greenwood CM, Eguale T, Kifle A, Beyene J, Habte A, Tadesse A, Gebrexabher H, Britton S, Schurr E. 2006. Variants of the SFTPA1 and SFTPA2 genes and susceptibility to tuberculosis in Ethiopia. *Hum Genet* 118:752–759

439. Roh EY, Yoon JH, Shin S, Song EY, Park MH. 2015. Association of TAP1 and TAP2 genes with susceptibility to pulmonary tuberculosis in Koreans. *APMIS* 123:457–464.

440. Sunder SR, Hanumanth SR, Gaddam S, Jonnalagada S, Valluri VL. 2011. Association of TAP 1 and 2 gene polymorphisms with human immunodeficiency virus-tuberculosis co-infection. *Hum Immunol* 72:908–911.

441. Wang D, Zhou Y, Ji L, He T, Lin F, Lin R, Lin T, Mo Y. 2012. Association of LMP/TAP gene polymorphisms with tuberculosis susceptibility in Li population in China. *PLoS One* 7:e33051

442. Mak JC, Leung HC, Sham AS, Mok TY, Poon YN, Ling SO, Wong KC, Chan-Yeung M. 2007. Genetic polymorphisms and plasma levels of transforming growth factor-beta(1) in Chinese patients with tuberculosis in Hong Kong. *Cytokine* 40:177–182.

443. Dissanayeke SR, Levin S, Pienaar S, Wood K, Eley B, Beatty D, Henderson H, Anderson S, Levin M. 2009. Polymorphic variation in TIRAP is not associated with susceptibility to childhood TB but may determine susceptibility to TBM in some ethnic groups. *PLoS One* 4:e6698

444. Hamann L, Kumpf O, Schuring RP, Alpsoy E, Bedu-Addo G, Bienzle U, Oskam L, Mockenhaupt FP,

Schumann RR. 2009. Low frequency of the TIRAP S180L polymorphism in Africa, and its potential role in malaria, sepsis, and leprosy. *BMC Med Genet* 10:65

445. Hawn TR, Dunstan SJ, Thwaites GE, Simmons CP, Thuong NT, Lan NT, Quy HT, Chau TT, Hieu NT, Rodrigues S, Janer M, Zhao LP, Hien TT, Farrar JJ, Aderem A. 2006. A polymorphism in Toll-interleukin 1 receptor domain containing adaptor protein is associated with susceptibility to meningeal tuberculosis. *J Infect Dis* 194:1127–1134.

446. Khor CC, Chapman SJ, Vannberg FO, Dunne A, Murphy C, Ling EY, Frodsham AJ, Walley AJ, Kyrieleis O, Khan A, Aucan C, Segal S, Moore CE, Knox K, Campbell SJ, Lienhardt C, Scott A, Aaby P, Sow OY, Grignani RT, Sillah J, Sirugo G, Peshu N, Williams TN, Maitland K, Davies RJ, Kwiatkowski DP, Day NP, Yala D, Crook DW, Marsh K, Berkley JA, O'Neill LA, Hill AV. 2007. A Mal functional variant is associated with protection against invasive pneumococcal disease, bacteremia, malaria and tuberculosis. *Nat Genet* 39: 523–528.

447. Liu Q, Li W, Li D, Feng Y, Tao C. 2014. TIRAP C539T polymorphism contributes to tuberculosis susceptibility: evidence from a meta-analysis. *Infect Genet Evol* 27:32–39

448. Nejentsev S, Thye T, Szeszko JS, Stevens H, Balabanova Y, Chinbuah AM, Hibberd M, van de Vosse E, Alisjahbana B, van Crevel R, Ottenhoff TH, Png E, Drobniewski F, Todd JA, Seielstad M, Horstmann RD. 2008. Analysis of association of the TIRAP (MAL) S180L variant and tuberculosis in three populations. *Nat Genet* 40:261–262, author reply 262–263

449. Selvaraj P, Harishankar M, Singh B, Jawahar MS, Banurekha VV. 2010. Toll-like receptor and TIRAP gene polymorphisms in pulmonary tuberculosis patients of South India. *Tuberculosis (Edinb)* 90:306–310.

450. Zhang YX, Xue Y, Liu JY, Zhao MY, Li FJ, Zhou JM, Wang HJ, Li JC. 2011. Association of TIRAP (MAL) gene polymorphisms with susceptibility to tuberculosis in a Chinese population. *Genet Mol Res* 10:7–15.

451. Miao R, Li J, Sun Z, Xu F, Shen H. 2011. Meta-analysis on the association of TIRAP S180L variant and tuberculosis susceptibility. *Tuberculosis (Edinb)* 91: 268–272.

452. Caws M, Thwaites G, Dunstan S, Hawn TR, Lan NT, Thuong NT, Stepniewska K, Huyen MN, Bang ND, Loc TH, Gagneux S, van Soolingen D, Kremer K, van der Sande M, Small P, Anh PT, Chinh NT, Quy HT, Duyen NT, Tho DQ, Hieu NT, Torok E, Hien TT, Dung NH, Nhu NT, Duy PM, van Vinh Chau N, Farrar J. 2008. The influence of host and bacterial genotype on the development of disseminated disease with *Mycobacterium tuberculosis*. *PLoS Pathog* 4: e1000034

453. Dittrich N, Berrocal-Almanza LC, Thada S, Goyal S, Slevogt H, Sumanlatha G, Hussain A, Sur S, Burkert S, Oh DY, Valluri V, Schumann RR, Conrad ML. 2015. Toll-like receptor 1 variations influence susceptibility and immune response to *Mycobacterium tuberculosis*. *Tuberculosis (Edinb)* 95:328–335.

454. Ma X, Liu Y, Gowen BB, Graviss EA, Clark AG, Musser JM. 2007. Full-exon resequencing reveals toll-like receptor variants contribute to human susceptibility to tuberculosis disease. *PLoS One* 2:e1318

455. Ocejo-Vinyals JG, Puente de Mateo E, Ausín F, Agüero R, Arroyo JL, Gutiérrez-Cuadra M, Fariñas MC. 2013. Human toll-like receptor 1 T1805G polymorphism and susceptibility to pulmonary tuberculosis in northern Spain. *Int J Tuberc Lung Dis* 17:652–654.

456. Salie M, Daya M, Lucas LA, Warren RM, van der Spuy GD, van Helden PD, Hoal EG, Möller M. 2015. Association of toll-like receptors with susceptibility to tuberculosis suggests sex-specific effects of TLR8 polymorphisms. *Infect Genet Evol* 34:221–229.

457. Uciechowski P, Imhoff H, Lange C, Meyer CG, Browne EN, Kirsten DK, Schröder AK, Schaaf B, Al-Lahham A, Reinert RR, Reiling N, Haase H, Hatzmann A, Fleischer D, Heussen N, Kleines M, Rink L. 2011. Susceptibility to tuberculosis is associated with TLR1 polymorphisms resulting in a lack of TLR1 cell surface expression. *J Leukoc Biol* 90:377–388.

458. Zhang Y, Jiang T, Yang X, Xue Y, Wang C, Liu J, Zhang X, Chen Z, Zhao M, Li JC. 2013. Toll-like receptor -1, -2, and -6 polymorphisms and pulmonary tuberculosis susceptibility: a systematic review and meta-analysis. *PLoS One* 8:e63357

459. Schurz H, Daya M, Möller M, Hoal EG, Salie M. 2015. TLR1, 2, 4, 6 and 9 variants associated with tuberculosis susceptibility: a systematic review and meta-analysis. *PLoS One* 10:e0139711

460. Ben-Ali M, Barbouche MR, Bousnina S, Chabbou A, Dellagi K. 2004. Toll-like receptor 2 Arg677Trp polymorphism is associated with susceptibility to tuberculosis in Tunisian patients. *Clin Diagn Lab Immunol* 11: 625–626.

461. Chen YC, Hsiao CC, Chen CJ, Chin CH, Liu SF, Wu CC, Eng HL, Chao TY, Tsen CC, Wang YH, Lin MC. 2010. Toll-like receptor 2 gene polymorphisms, pulmonary tuberculosis, and natural killer cell counts. *BMC Med Genet* 11:17

462. Dalgic N, Tekin D, Kayaalti Z, Soylemezoglu T, Cakir E, Kilic B, Kutlubay B, Sancar M, Odabasi M. 2011. Arg753Gln polymorphism of the human Toll-like receptor 2 gene from infection to disease in pediatric tuberculosis. *Hum Immunol* 72:440–445.

463. Etokebe GE, Skjeldal F, Nilsen N, Rodionov D, Knezevic J, Bulat-Kardum L, Espevik T, Bakke O, Dembic Z. 2010. Toll-like receptor 2 (P631H) mutant impairs membrane internalization and is a dominant negative allele. *Scand J Immunol* 71:369–381.

464. Khan AU, Aslam MA, Hussain I, Naz AG, Rana IA, Ahmad MM, Ali M, Ahmad S. 2014. Role of Toll-like receptor 2 (-196 to -174) polymorphism in susceptibility to pulmonary tuberculosis in Pakistani population. *Int J Immunogenet* 41:105–111.

465. Ogus AC, Yoldas B, Ozdemir T, Uguz A, Olcen S, Keser I, Coskun M, Cilli A, Yegin O. 2004. The Arg753GLn polymorphism of the human toll-like receptor 2 gene in tuberculosis disease. *Eur Respir J* 23: 219–223.

466. Thuong NT, Hawn TR, Thwaites GE, Chau TT, Lan NT, Quy HT, Hieu NT, Aderem A, Hien TT, Farrar JJ, Dunstan SJ. 2007. A polymorphism in human TLR2 is associated with increased susceptibility to tuberculous meningitis. *Genes Immun* 8:422–428.

467. Velez DR, Wejse C, Stryjewski ME, Abbate E, Hulme WF, Myers JL, Estevan R, Patillo SG, Olesen R, Tacconelli A, Sirugo G, Gilbert JR, Hamilton CD, Scott WK. 2010. Variants in toll-like receptors 2 and 9 influence susceptibility to pulmonary tuberculosis in Caucasians, African-Americans, and West Africans. *Hum Genet* 127:65–73

468. Xue Y, Jin L, Li AZ, Wang HJ, Li M, Zhang YX, Wang Y, Li JC. 2010. Microsatellite polymorphisms in intron 2 of the toll-like receptor 2 gene and their association with susceptibility to pulmonary tuberculosis in Han Chinese. *Clin Chem Lab Med* 48:785–789.

469. Xue Y, Zhao ZQ, Wang HJ, Jin L, Liu CP, Wang Y, Li JC. 2010. Toll-like receptors 2 and 4 gene polymorphisms in a southeastern Chinese population with tuberculosis. *Int J Immunogenet* 37:135–138.

470. Wang JJ, Xia X, Tang SD, Wang J, Deng XZ, Zhang Y, Yue M. 2013. Meta-analysis on the associations of TLR2 gene polymorphisms with pulmonary tuberculosis susceptibility among Asian populations. *PLoS One* 8: e75090

471. Sun Q, Zhang Q, Xiao HP, Bai C. 2015. Toll-like receptor polymorphisms and tuberculosis susceptibility: a comprehensive meta-analysis. *J Huazhong Univ Sci Technolog Med Sci* 35:157–168.

472. Ferwerda B, Kibiki GS, Netea MG, Dolmans WM, van der Ven AJ. 2007. The toll-like receptor 4 Asp299Gly variant and tuberculosis susceptibility in HIV-infected patients in Tanzania. *AIDS* 21:1375–1377.

473. Najmi N, Kaur G, Sharma SK, Mehra NK. 2010. Human Toll-like receptor 4 polymorphisms TLR4 Asp299Gly and Thr399Ile influence susceptibility and severity of pulmonary tuberculosis in the Asian Indian population. *Tissue Antigens* 76:102–109.

474. Newport MJ, Allen A, Awomoyi AA, Dunstan SJ, McKinney E, Marchant A, Sirugo G. 2004. The toll-like receptor 4 Asp299Gly variant: no influence on LPS responsiveness or susceptibility to pulmonary tuberculosis in The Gambia. *Tuberculosis (Edinb)* 84:347–352.

475. Pulido I, Leal M, Genebat M, Pacheco YM, SÁez ME, Soriano-Sarabia N. 2010. The TLR4 ASP299GLY polymorphism is a risk factor for active tuberculosis in Caucasian HIV-infected patients. *Curr HIV Res* 8:253–258.

476. Rosas-Taraco AG, Revol A, Salinas-Carmona MC, Rendon A, Caballero-Olin G, Arce-Mendoza AY. 2007. CD14 C(-159)T polymorphism is a risk factor for development of pulmonary tuberculosis. *J Infect Dis* 196: 1698–1706.

477. Zaki HY, Leung KH, Yiu WC, Gasmelseed N, Elwali NE, Yip SP. 2012. Common polymorphisms in TLR4 gene associated with susceptibility to pulmonary tuberculosis in the Sudanese. *Int J Tuberc Lung Dis* 16:934–940.

478. Tian T, Jin S, Dong J, Li G. 2013. Lack of association between Toll-like receptor 4 gene Asp299Gly and Thr399Ile polymorphisms and tuberculosis susceptibility: a meta-analysis. *Infect Genet Evol* 14:156–160.

479. Dalgic N, Tekin D, Kayaalti Z, Cakir E, Soylemezoglu T, Sancar M. 2011. Relationship between toll-like receptor 8 gene polymorphisms and pediatric pulmonary tuberculosis. *Dis Markers* 31:33–38.

480. Davila S, Hibberd ML, Hari Dass R, Wong HE, Sahiratmadja E, Bonnard C, Alisjahbana B, Szeszko JS, Balabanova Y, Drobniewski F, van Crevel R, van de Vosse E, Nejentsev S, Ottenhoff TH, Seielstad M. 2008. Genetic association and expression studies indicate a role of toll-like receptor 8 in pulmonary tuberculosis. *PLoS Genet* 4:e1000218

481. Bharti D, Kumar A, Mahla RS, Kumar S, Ingle H, Shankar H, Joshi B, Raut AA, Kumar H. 2014. The role of TLR9 polymorphism in susceptibility to pulmonary tuberculosis. *Immunogenetics* 66:675–681.

482. Graustein AD, Horne DJ, Arentz M, Bang ND, Chau TT, Thwaites GE, Caws M, Thuong NT, Dunstan SJ, Hawn TR. 2015. TLR9 gene region polymorphisms and susceptibility to tuberculosis in Vietnam. *Tuberculosis (Edinb)* 95:190–196

483. Kobayashi K, Yuliwulandari R, Yanai H, Naka I, Lien LT, Hang NT, Hijikata M, Keicho N, Tokunaga K. 2012. Association of TLR polymorphisms with development of tuberculosis in Indonesian females. *Tissue Antigens* 79:190–197.

484. Torres-García D, Cruz-Lagunas A, García-Sancho Figueroa MC, Fernández-Plata R, Baez-Saldaña R, Mendoza-Milla C, Barquera R, Carrera-Eusebio A, Ramírez-Bravo S, Campos L, Angeles J, Vargas-Alarcón G, Granados J, Gopal R, Khader SA, Yunis EJ, Zuñiga J. 2013. Variants in toll-like receptor 9 gene influence susceptibility to tuberculosis in a Mexican population. *J Transl Med* 11:220

485. Bikmaeva AR, Sibiriak SV, Valiakhmetova DK, Khusnutdinova EK. 2002. [Polymorphism of the tumor necrosis factor alpha gene in patients with infiltrative tuberculosis and from the Bashkorstan populations]. *Mol Biol (Mosk)* 36:784–787.

486. Correa PA, Gomez LM, Cadena J, Anaya JM. 2005. Autoimmunity and tuberculosis. Opposite association with TNF polymorphism. *J Rheumatol* 32:219–224.

487. Fan HM, Wang Z, Feng FM, Zhang KL, Yuan JX, Sui H, Qiu HY, Liu LH, Deng XJ, Ren JX. 2010. Association of TNF-alpha-238G/A and 308 G/A gene polymorphisms with pulmonary tuberculosis among patients with coal worker's pneumoconiosis. *Biomed Environ Sci* 23:137–145.

488. Kumar V, Khosla R, Gupta V, Sarin BC, Sehajpal PK. 2008. Differential association of tumour necrosis factor-alpha single nucleotide polymorphism (-308) with tuberculosis and bronchial asthma. *Natl Med J India* 21: 120–122.

489. Mokrousov I, Wu XR, Vyazovaya A, Feng WX, Sun L, Xiao J, Miao Q, Jiao WW, Shen A. 2011. Polymorphism of 3′UTR region of TNFR2 coding gene and its role in clinical tuberculosis in Han Chinese pediatric population. *Infect Genet Evol* 11:1312–1318.

490. Selvaraj P, Sriram U, Mathan Kurian S, Reetha AM, Narayanan PR. 2001. Tumour necrosis factor alpha (-238 and -308) and beta gene polymorphisms in pul-

monary tuberculosis: haplotype analysis with HLA-A, B and DR genes. *Tuberculosis (Edinb)* **81**:335–341.

491. Sharma S, Rathored J, Ghosh B, Sharma SK. 2010. Genetic polymorphisms in TNF genes and tuberculosis in North Indians. *BMC Infect Dis* **10**:165

492. Wang Q, Zhan P, Qiu LX, Qian Q, Yu LK. 2012. TNF-308 gene polymorphism and tuberculosis susceptibility: a meta-analysis involving 18 studies. *Mol Biol Rep* **39**:3393–3400.

493. Zhang Z, Zhu H, Pu X, Meng S, Zhang F, Xun L, Liu Q, Wang Y. 2012. Association between tumor necrosis factor alpha-238G/a polymorphism and tuberculosis susceptibility: a meta-analysis study. *BMC Infect Dis* **12**:328

494. Zhu H, Zhang Z, Lei X, Feng J, Zhang F, Wang Y. 2012. Tumor necrosis factor alpha -308G>A, -863C>A, -857C>T gene polymorphisms and tuberculosis susceptibility: a meta-analysis. *Gene* **509**:206–214.

495. Zhang ZJ, Zhu H, Pu XD, Zhang F, Lei X, Zhou WJ, Wang Y. 2013. [Tumor necrosis factor alpha-238G/A polymorphism and tuberculosis susceptibility: a meta-analysis]. *Zhonghua Jie He He Hu Xi Za Zhi* **36**:33–37.

496. Lee YH, Song GG. 2015. Associations between tumor necrosis factor-α polymorphisms and susceptibility to pulmonary tuberculosis: meta-analysis. *Genet Mol Res* **14**:8602–8612

497. Shah JA, Vary JC, Chau TT, Bang ND, Yen NT, Farrar JJ, Dunstan SJ, Hawn TR. 2012. Human TOLLIP regulates TLR2 and TLR4 signaling and its polymorphisms are associated with susceptibility to tuberculosis. *J Immunol* **189**:1737–1746.

498. Capparelli R, Palumbo D, Iannaccone M, Iannelli D. 2009. Human V-ATPase gene can protect or predispose the host to pulmonary tuberculosis. *Genes Immun* **10**:641–646.

499. Alagarasu K, Selvaraj P, Swaminathan S, Narendran G, Narayanan PR. 2009. 5′ regulatory and 3′ untranslated region polymorphisms of vitamin D receptor gene in south Indian HIV and HIV-TB patients. *J Clin Immunol* **29**:196–204

500. Ates O, Dolek B, Dalyan L, Musellim B, Ongen G, Topal-Sarikaya A. 2011. The association between BsmI variant of vitamin D receptor gene and susceptibility to tuberculosis. *Mol Biol Rep* **38**:2633–2636.

501. Babb C, van der Merwe L, Beyers N, Pheiffer C, Walzl G, Duncan K, van Helden P, Hoal EG. 2007. Vitamin D receptor gene polymorphisms and sputum conversion time in pulmonary tuberculosis patients. *Tuberculosis (Edinb)* **87**:295–302.

502. Banoei MM, Mirsaeidi MS, Houshmand M, Tabarsi P, Ebrahimi G, Zargari L, Kashani BH, Masjedi MR, Mansouri SD, Ramirez J. 2010. Vitamin D receptor homozygote mutant tt and bb are associated with susceptibility to pulmonary tuberculosis in the Iranian population. *Int J Infect Dis* **14**:e84–e85.

503. Bellamy R, Ruwende C, Corrah T, McAdam KP, Thursz M, Whittle HC, Hill AV. 1999. Tuberculosis and chronic hepatitis B virus infection in Africans and variation in the vitamin D receptor gene. *J Infect Dis* **179**:721–724.

504. Bornman L, Campbell SJ, Fielding K, Bah B, Sillah J, Gustafson P, Manneh K, Lisse I, Allen A, Sirugo G, Sylla A, Aaby P, McAdam KP, Bah-Sow O, Bennett S, Lienhardt C, Hill AV. 2004. Vitamin D receptor polymorphisms and susceptibility to tuberculosis in West Africa: a case-control and family study. *J Infect Dis* **190**:1631–1641.

505. Cao S, Luo PF, Li W, Tang WQ, Cong XN, Wei PM. 2012. Vitamin D receptor genetic polymorphisms and tuberculosis among Chinese Han ethnic group. *Chin Med J (Engl)* **125**:920–925.

506. Chen XR, Feng YL, Ma Y, Zhang ZD, Li CY, Wen FQ, Tang XY, Su ZG. 2006. [Study on the association of two polymorphisms of the vitamin D receptor (VDR) gene with the susceptibility to pulmonary tuberculosis (PTB) in Chinese Tibetans]. *Sichuan Da Xue Xue Bao Yi Xue* **37**:847–851.

507. Liu W, Zhang CY, Wu XM, Tian L, Li CZ, Zhao QM, Zhang PH, Yang SM, Yang H, Zhang XT, Cao WC. 2003. [A case-control study on the vitamin D receptor gene polymorphisms and susceptibility to pulmonary tuberculosis]. *Zhonghua Liu Xing Bing Xue Za Zhi* **24**:389–392.

508. Marashian SM, Farnia P, Seyf S, Anoosheh S, Velayati AA. 2010. Evaluating the role of vitamin D receptor polymorphisms on susceptibility to tuberculosis among Iranian patients: a case-control study. *Tuberk Toraks* **58**:147–153.

509. Martineau AR, Leandro AC, Anderson ST, Newton SM, Wilkinson KA, Nicol MP, Pienaar SM, Skolimowska KH, Rocha MA, Rolla VC, Levin M, Davidson RN, Bremner SA, Griffiths CJ, Eley BS, Bonecini-Almeida MG, Wilkinson RJ. 2010. Association between Gc genotype and susceptibility to TB is dependent on vitamin D status. *Eur Respir J* **35**:1106–1112.

510. Rashedi J, Asgharzadeh M, Moaddab SR, Sahebi L, Khalili M, Mazani M, Abdolalizadeh J. 2014. Vitamin d receptor gene polymorphism and vitamin d plasma concentration: correlation with susceptibility to tuberculosis. *Adv Pharm Bull* **4**(Suppl 2):607–611.

511. Roth DE, Soto G, Arenas F, Bautista CT, Ortiz J, Rodriguez R, Cabrera L, Gilman RH. 2004. Association between vitamin D receptor gene polymorphisms and response to treatment of pulmonary tuberculosis. *J Infect Dis* **190**:920–927.

512. Selvaraj P, Alagarasu K, Harishankar M, Vidyarani M, Narayanan PR. 2008. Regulatory region polymorphisms of vitamin D receptor gene in pulmonary tuberculosis patients and normal healthy subjects of south India. *Int J Immunogenet* **35**:251–254.

513. Selvaraj P, Chandra G, Jawahar MS, Rani MV, Rajeshwari DN, Narayanan PR. 2004. Regulatory role of vitamin D receptor gene variants of Bsm I, Apa I, Taq I, and Fok I polymorphisms on macrophage phagocytosis and lymphoproliferative response to mycobacterium tuberculosis antigen in pulmonary tuberculosis. *J Clin Immunol* **24**:523–532.

514. Selvaraj P, Kurian SM, Chandra G, Reetha AM, Charles N, Narayanan PR. 2004. Vitamin D receptor gene variants of BsmI, ApaI, TaqI, and FokI polymorphisms in spinal tuberculosis. *Clin Genet* **65**:73–76.

515. Selvaraj P, Narayanan PR, Reetha AM. 2000. Association of vitamin D receptor genotypes with the susceptibility to pulmonary tuberculosis in female patients & resistance in female contacts. *Indian J Med Res* **111:** 172–179.

516. Selvaraj P, Prabhu Anand S, Harishankar M, Alagarasu K. 2009. Plasma 1,25 dihydroxy vitamin D3 level and expression of vitamin d receptor and cathelicidin in pulmonary tuberculosis. *J Clin Immunol* **29:**470–478.

517. Selvaraj P, Vidyarani M, Alagarasu K, Prabhu Anand S, Narayanan PR. 2008. Regulatory role of promoter and 3′ UTR variants of vitamin D receptor gene on cytokine response in pulmonary tuberculosis. *J Clin Immunol* **28:** 306–313

518. Sharma PR, Singh S, Jena M, Mishra G, Prakash R, Das PK, Bamezai RN, Tiwari PK. 2011. Coding and noncoding polymorphisms in VDR gene and susceptibility to pulmonary tuberculosis in tribes, castes and Muslims of Central India. *Infect Genet Evol* **11:**1456–1461.

519. Sinaga BY, Amin M, Siregar Y, Sarumpaet SM. 2014. Correlation between vitamin D receptor gene FOKI and BSMI polymorphisms and the susceptibility to pulmonary tuberculosis in an Indonesian Batak-ethnic population. *Acta Med Indones* **46:**275–282.

520. Vidyarani M, Selvaraj P, Raghavan S, Narayanan PR. 2009. Regulatory role of 1, 25-dihydroxyvitamin D3 and vitamin D receptor gene variants on intracellular granzyme A expression in pulmonary tuberculosis. *Exp Mol Pathol* **86:**69–73.

521. Wilbur AK, Kubatko LS, Hurtado AM, Hill KR, Stone AC. 2007. Vitamin D receptor gene polymorphisms and susceptibility M. *tuberculosis* in native Paraguayans. *Tuberculosis (Edinb)* **87:**329–337.

522. Wilkinson RJ, Llewelyn M, Toossi Z, Patel P, Pasvol G, Lalvani A, Wright D, Latif M, Davidson RN. 2000. Influence of vitamin D deficiency and vitamin D receptor polymorphisms on tuberculosis among Gujarati Asians in west London: a case-control study. *Lancet* **355:**618–621

523. Zhang HQ, Deng A, Guo CF, Wang YX, Chen LQ, Wang YF, Wu JH, Liu JY. 2010. Association between FokI polymorphism in vitamin D receptor gene and susceptibility to spinal tuberculosis in Chinese Han population. *Arch Med Res* **41:**46–49.

524. Sun YP, Cai QS. 2015. Vitamin D receptor FokI gene polymorphism and tuberculosis susceptibility: a meta-analysis. *Genet Mol Res* **14:**6156–6163.

525. Lee YH, Song GG. 2015. Vitamin D receptor gene FokI, TaqI, BsmI, and ApaI polymorphisms and susceptibility to pulmonary tuberculosis: a meta-analysis. *Genet Mol Res* **14:**9118–9129

526. Gao L, Tao Y, Zhang L, Jin Q. 2010. Vitamin D receptor genetic polymorphisms and tuberculosis: updated systematic review and meta-analysis. *Int J Tuberc Lung Dis* **14:**15–23.

527. Zhao ZZ, Zhang TZ, Gao YM, Feng FM. 2009. [Meta-analysis of relationship of vitamin D receptor gene polymorphism and tuberculosis susceptibility]. *Zhonghua Jie He He Hu Xi Za Zhi* **32:**748–751.

528. Cao Y, Wang X, Cao Z, Cheng X. 2015. Association of Vitamin D receptor gene TaqI polymorphisms with tuberculosis susceptibility: a meta-analysis. *Int J Clin Exp Med* **8:**10187–10203.

529. Areeshi MY, Mandal RK, Akhter N, Panda AK, Haque S. 2014. Evaluating the association between TaqI variant of vitamin D receptor gene and susceptibility to tuberculosis: a meta-analysis. *Toxicol Int* **21:**140–147.

530. Allen AR, Minozzi G, Glass EJ, Skuce RA, McDowell SW, Woolliams JA, Bishop SC. 2010. Bovine tuberculosis: the genetic basis of host susceptibility. *Proc Biol Sci* **277:**2737–2745.

531. Di Pietrantonio T, Schurr E. 2005. Mouse models for the genetic study of tuberculosis susceptibility. *Brief Funct Genomics Proteomics* **4:**277–292.

532. Jacobs WR Jr, McShane H, Mizrahi V, Orme IM (ed). *Tuberculosis and the Tubercle Bacillus*, 2nd ed. ASM Press, Washington, DC, in press.

533. Orme IM, Ordway DJ. 2016. Mouse and guinea pig models of tuberculosis. *Microbiol Spectrum* **4(3):**TBTB2-0002-2015.

534. Peña JC, Ho W-Z. 2016. Non-human primate models of tuberculosis. *Microbiol Spectrum* **4(3):**TBTB2-0007-2016.

535. Buddle BM, Vordermeier HM, Hewinson RG. 2016. Experimental infection models of TB in domestic livestock. *Microbiol Spectrum* **4(4):**TBTB2-0017-2016.

536. Scriba TJ, Coussens AK, Fletcher HA. 2016. Human immunology of tuberculosis. *Microbiol Spectrum* **4(1):** TBTB2-0016-2016.

537. Barbier M, Wirth T. 2016. The evolutionary history, demography, and spread of the *Mycobacterium tuberculosis* complex. *Microbiol Spectrum* **4(4):**TBTB2-0008-2016.

538. Niemann S, Merker M, Kohl T, Supply P. 2016. Impact of genetic diversity on the biology of *Mycobacterium tuberculosis* complex strains. *Microbiol Spectrum* **4(6):** TBTB2-0022-2016.

Tuberculosis and the Tubercle Bacillus, 2nd ed.
Edited by William R. Jacobs, Jr., Helen McShane, Valerie Mizrahi, and Ian M. Orme
© 2018 American Society for Microbiology, Washington, DC
doi:10.1128/microbiolspec.TBTB2-0008-2016

The Evolutionary History, Demography, and Spread of the *Mycobacterium tuberculosis* Complex

20

Maxime Barbier and Thierry Wirth

INTRODUCTION

Tuberculosis has plagued mankind over the centuries and probably accompanied modern *Homo sapiens* out of Africa. The epidemiological agent of phthisis, also known as "consumption," reached its epidemic apex during the 18th and 19th centuries. During the industrialization era, the disease was associated with the concentration of labor and poor socioeconomic settings that ultimately favored the spread of this "crowd" pathogen. This high-burden period was then followed by a progressive decline of the death and disease tolls that predated the antibiotic era and the *Mycobacterium bovis* BCG vaccination. The evolutionary histories of the host and its pathogen are intricately associated, implying that tuberculosis can only be fully understood in the light of *H. sapiens* origins, migrations, and demography (1). Excluding these parameters from our analyses might lead us to false conclusions regarding evolution, epidemiology, and pathobiology. In the same line, there is also an urgent need to unravel the genomic features that can explain the contrasted infectivity and transmission observed between *Mycobacterium tuberculosis* complex (MTBC) lineages (2–4), without neglecting the genetic architecture of the host's immune system (5).

Another challenge we have to face is the effect of globalization, i.e., the dramatic increase of population and individual movements that encompass touristic activities, refugee diasporas, and, soon to come, climatic migrants. This ongoing maelstrom has multiple consequences, such as an increasing number of patients infected by nonendemic strains, the spread of multidrug-resistant (MDR) strains from health care-deficient countries, and the frightening specter of the expansion of totally drug-resistant (TDR) strains (6). In this review, we will illustrate how genomic insights driven by whole-genome sequencing and comparative genomics can help us to combat this old foe, and unravel its evolutionary history, spread, and demography. From a more practical point of view, the approaches we will discuss here, combined with selection and population genomics models, might also help us to evaluate the impacts of treatment programs on the relative transmission success, to pinpoint the molecular targets of selection, and, eventually, to develop new drugs.

HISTORICAL CONSIDERATION AND EARLY (MIS)CONCEPTIONS ON TUBERCULOSIS EVOLUTION

Few diseases, with the exception of plague (*Yersinia pestis*), have left such an important written signature as tuberculosis. The first literary traces were detected in Chinese medical texts predating the Xia dynasty and in the Indian Vedas (7), respectively, some 5,700 and 3,500 years ago. Until recently, little was known about tuberculosis origins, evolution, and spread. Thanks to the development of molecular tools, four distinct species were identified as causing the disease: *M. tuberculosis*, the human pathogen; *M. bovis* (8), found primarily in cattle; *Mycobacterium africanum* (9), isolated from African patients; and *Mycobacterium microti*

Laboratoire Biologie Intégrative des Populations, Evolution Moléculaire; Institut de Systématique, Evolution, Biodiversité, UMR-CNRS 7205, Muséum National d'Histoire Naturelle, Univ. Pierre et Marie Curie, EPHE, Sorbonne Universités, 75231 Paris cedex 05, France.

(10), isolated from voles. These species were defined based on the host from which strains had been isolated. However, biochemical analyses, including *in vitro* growth rates, microscopic observations, and differential host-specific pathogenicity, suggested that interspecies borders were less well defined than initially expected (11). All these taxa belong to the MTBC, although their status in terms of taxonomic level (species, subspecies) might be further debated. In this group, *M. tuberculosis* and *M. bovis* are the more prevalent ones, although this might be due to strong sampling biases driven by health-economic priorities, as well as by differences in access to funding. *M. tuberculosis sensu stricto* infects humans and, until recently, the species was divided into five variants based on biochemical properties, namely the classical human, Asian human, bovine, African I, and African II variants (12).

The initial paradigm concerning the evolution of *M. tuberculosis* was that the bacillus evolved from *M. bovis* (13). Thanks to novel molecular data, however, this scenario was revised (14), although the old concept keeps being cited (15). The observations that led to these prime conclusions were the following. First, many diseases afflicting humans are zoonoses, and tuberculosis should be no exception. Famous examples of transmission from animals to humans encompass the Ebola virus, HIV, and Chagas' disease (15). The transmission process can oscillate between sporadic outbreaks with little human-to-human transmission and a more settled coevolution if the bug can adapt to its new niche. Based on this knowledge, the initial hypothesis was that a cattle *M. bovis* strain infected a human and successfully spread in the *H. sapiens* populations. After some millennia of coevolution, the bacterium specialized to its novel host, became human specific, and is now known as *M. tuberculosis*. In fact, it is not unusual to see patients infected by bovine tuberculosis, with transmission occurring via aerosols or the consumption of infected milk. Moreover, until now, no human remains older than 11,000 years have shown traces of tuberculosis disease (16, 17), whereas the most ancient animal case has been found in a 17,000-year-old extinct bison (18). This apparent anteriority of animal infection was used to promote the cattle-to-human transmission route hypothesis. Furthermore, the fact that the earliest human remains carrying tuberculosis date back to the Neolithic revolution (8,000 to 10,000 years ago) is intriguing and suggests some causality with the rise of domestication. It is tempting to think that the concomitant increase of animal stocks and host population size favored the interactions and contacts between these two players. Indeed, in the past,

humans shared their home with bovines to protect them against predators and extreme temperatures (14): a single infected and coughing animal might have been able to transmit the disease to an entire family.

Here we see the dangerous attraction we have for nice, logical, flowing narratives; yet, mycobacterial interspersed repetitive unit genotyping and whole-genome sequencing (WGS) provided strong evidence against such a linear explanation, as we shall see in the next section.

THE PREGENOMIC ERA AND FIRST-GENERATION PHYLOGENETIC ANALYSES

The Fingerprint Era

The advances of molecular biology enabled the study of bacterial DNA, unraveled fine-scale genetic structures, and clearly segregated sister strains, which previously seemed nearly identical, mostly because morphological and biochemical traits provide little information about relatedness and species phylogenies. We will present first the main pre-next-generation sequencing (NGS) methods that enabled us to discriminate the principal MTBC families and to disentangle their evolutionary link, and how these methods shifted our vision of tuberculosis evolution and spread.

One of the first typing techniques applied to *M. tuberculosis* was the restriction fragment length polymorphism (RFLP) method. It is a fingerprint-based approach that relies on the enzymatic digestion of the circular chromosomal DNA, followed by gel electrophoresis revealed with radiolabeled probes targeting a particular sequence, such as an insertion sequence (IS). The IS6100 RFLP analysis (19) has been widely used for *M. tuberculosis* molecular typing. The IS6100 sequence is usually present in multiple copies on the chromosome. Depending on the locations and the copy number of this element, a profile is established that allows for strain discrimination. Such profiles enabled the demonstration that *M. microti* was responsible for human infections (20). Other insertion sequences have been used such as IS1081 (21) and IS986 (22), but they did not reach the success of IS6100. This marker presents a high evolutionary pace and therefore evolves relatively quickly in an otherwise relatively homogeneous genetic background. Therefore, IS6100 proved very useful in epidemiological studies and facilitated the segregation of clusters of closely related strains or, in the best case, of clones (23). A major drawback of this technique comes from its poor portability and laboratory dependency in terms of fingerprint profiles, leading therefore to little insight at larger evolutionary scales (24). Besides, differentiation of strains is strongly dependent on the number of IS6100 copies. Strains with high copy numbers are accurately differentiated from their close variants, while strains with few copies are more difficult to segregate. Numerous other markers have been used in the field of microbiology with more or less the same advantages and flaws (25). Another limitation of RFLP is that it requires mycobacterial culture, lasting from 20 to 40 days. This time frame is very long when studying infection chains in a clinical context. According to a search on the Web of Science database, the topic "IS6100" reached a citation apex in 2012 and now follows a gentle but regular decline.

The Multilocus Era

Next came PCR-based techniques that allowed fast, reproducible, and efficient typing (between 1 day and 1 week) like the spacer oligotyping method, called "spoligotyping" (26). The goal of this technique is to type the direct repeat (DR) locus of *M. tuberculosis*. This locus is an alternation of DRs, composed of a well-conserved sequence of 36 bp, and nonrepetitive spacer sequences, 34 to 41 bp long. *M. tuberculosis* strains can be discriminated based on their number of DRs and the presence or absence of particular spacers (27). Spoligotyping is therefore an efficient typing method (28) that differentiates MTBC strains from other environmental mycobacteria and clearly separates *M. bovis* from *M. tuberculosis*. It has less discriminatory power than IS6100, when present in high copy numbers, but it is present in all strains, unlike IS6100. The principal inconvenience of this method is that spoligo patterns are CRISPR structures that play a role in *Eubacteria* and *Archaebacteria* defense against phages (29). Consequently, this marker is under strong diversifying selection, prone to homoplasy, and of little interest for phylogenetic reconstructions, if any.

The second PCR-based method developed in the early 2000s is a high-resolution typing method based on variable number tandem repeats (VNTRs) of genetic elements named mycobacterial interspersed repetitive units (MIRUs) (30). Those markers resemble the human mini-satellite-like regions developed by Sir Alec Jeffreys and widely used in forensics. MIRU loci are scattered in the genome of *M. tuberculosis* and consist of repetitive patterns 51 to 77 bp long. Only minor indels or polymorphisms occur in these sequences, mostly following the so-called stepwise-mutation model (SMM), meaning that the allelic state changes by the acquisition or the loss of one repetitive unit. The typing of these MIRUs is simply the measure of the number of repetitions at each locus where the number of repetitions varies between 0 and a maximum of 25. The MIRU typing underwent progressive upgrading steps, from 12 to 15 and finally 24 MIRU loci.

A third way used to differentiate strains consisted of the sequencing of a set of structural genes, allowing defining their relatedness based on sequence polymorphisms. Sreevatsan et al. implemented this approach in 1997 (31). They used 26 different genes or gene fragments, in which they observed a lack of neutral mutation, with up to 95% of nonsynonymous mutations associated with antibiotic resistance. However, phylogenetic inferences and evolutionary scenarios inferred from genes under strong positive selection (involved in antibiotic resistance, for example) are generally not reliable. Alternatively, taking into account the sole synonymous single nucleotide polymorphisms (SNPs) might be a solution but this remains very restrictive. The authors ultimately used the only two nonsynonymous mutations that were not involved in antibiotic resistance to define three different groups. We see here that, because of technical barriers, biased locus choice, and little genetic diversity of the MTBC, the pre-NGS area sequencing studies remained tricky and led to partially misleading conclusions.

Yet another simple analytical approach turned out to be far more promising. Thanks to genome-wide comparisons (32), variable regions resulting from insertion-deletion events have been discovered. Approximately 20 such regions are phylogenetically highly informative since they follow a completely parsimonious and non-homoplastic evolutionary path, from presence to definitive loss, turning any change into a marble-engraved event (33). Based on these so-called regions of difference (RDs), a new evolutionary scenario emerged that contradicted previous thoughts (Fig. 1) because it stated that human strains did not derive from *M. bovis*. RD-based analyses even suggested that humans transmitted tuberculosis to cattle and other animals rather than the other way around. One deletion, TbD1, separates "modern strains" from "ancient strains." This latter clade comprises animal strains, *M. africanum*, and some less virulent human strains, whereas "modern strains" exclusively infect humans. An interesting analysis of PhoPR virulence factors provided some novel insights into those splits and might explain how some mutations lowered the virulence of strains belonging to *M. bovis* and *M. africanum* (34). As an alternative to overstep the lack of accuracy or the drawbacks of all markers previously presented, some researchers chose to combine them (35). Such combined analyses have been conducted in numerous surveys and allowed

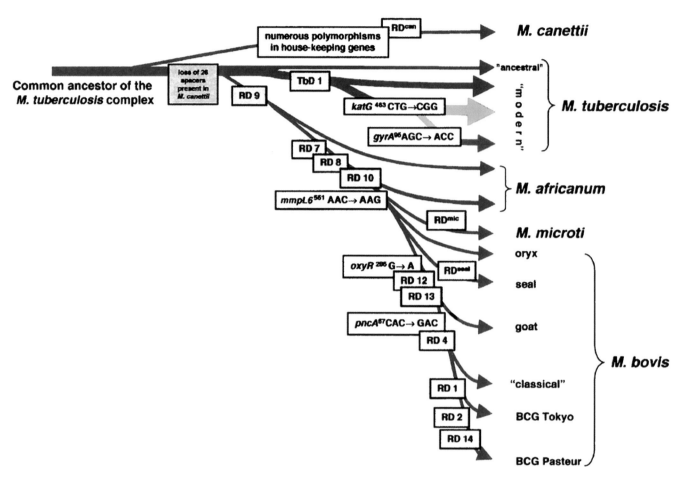

Figure 1 Diagram of the proposed evolutionary pathway of the tubercle bacilli illustrating successive losses of DNA in certain lineages (gray boxes). The diagram is based on the presence or absence of conserved deleted regions and on sequence polymorphisms in five selected genes. The distances between certain branches may not correspond to actual phylogenetic differences calculated by other methods. Blue arrows indicate that strains are characterized by *katG*463. CTG (Leu), *gyrA*95 ACC (Thr), typical for group 1 organisms. Green arrows indicate that strains belong to group 2 characterized by *katG*463 CGG (Arg), *gyrA*95 ACC (Thr). The red arrow indicates that strains belong to group 3, characterized by *katG*463 CGG (Arg), *gyrA*95 AGC (Ser), as defined by Sreevatsan et al. (31). Adapted from Brosch et al. (33).

the separation of *M. tuberculosis* human strains into different clades (Table 1). Those clades were initially named based on the prevalence and geographical source of their members (36, 37). The most remarkable phylogeographical clades belonging to the "modern strains" were Beijing (highly prevalent in East Asia), CAS (central Asia), and Haarlem, X, and LAM (Latin American-Mediterranean). *M. africanum* and EAI (East African Indian) composed the "ancient strains" group. Captivatingly, lineages from neighboring regions are more closely related than randomly chosen lineages, advocating for a strong biogeographical structuring: Haarlem, X, and LAM clades are more prevalent

in Europe and cluster together; the same holds for the Asiatic Beijing and CAS clades. The other lineages form a paraphyletic group of ancient strains, which are essentially restricted to Africa and India. The observed relationships between MTBC lineages are similar to those observed in humans, suggesting that humans could have carried tuberculosis for millennia and that the present-day geographical distribution of tuberculosis has been shaped by ancient if not first human migrations out of Africa. The hypothesis that humans and *M. tuberculosis* coevolved and spread together has been studied and detailed by Wirth et al. (38). Using MIRU genetic markers, the authors identified two ma-

Table 1 Correspondence table of the MTBC human-adapted strains identified by main typing methods and including the latest nomenclature[a]

Evolutionary age (species)	Lineage name based on LSP/SNP[b]	Lineage and sublineage [RD associated]				Spoligotype family
Ancient lineage (M. tuberculosis)	Indo-Oceanic lineage	1 [RD239]	1.1	1.1.1		EAI4 and EAI5
					1.1.1.1	EAI4
				1.1.2		EAI5 and EAI3
				1.1.3		EAI6
			1.2	1.2.1		EAI2
				1.2.2		EAI1
Modern lineages (M. tuberculosis)	East-Asian lineage	2	2.1 (non-Beijing)			MANU ancestor and orphan profile
			2.2 (Beijing) [RD105, RD207]	2.2.1 [RD181]		Beijing
					2.2.1.1 [RD150]	Beijing
					2.2.1.2 [RD142]	Beijing
				2.2.2		Beijing
	East African-Indian lineage	3 [RD750]	3.1			CAS except CAS1-Delhi
				3.1.1		CAS1-Kili
				3.1.2	3.1.2.1	CAS2
					3.1.2.2	CAS
	Euro-American lineage	4	4.1	4.1.1 (X-type)	4.1.1.1 [RD183]	X2
					4.1.1.2	X1
					4.1.1.3 [RD193]	X3 and X1
				4.1.2	4.1.2.1 (Haarlem)	T1 and H1
					[RD182]	T1 and H1
			4.2	4.2.1 (Ural)		H3 and H4
				4.2.2		LAM7-TUR and T1
					4.2.2.1 (TUR)	LAM7-TUR
			4.3 (LAM)	4.3.1	[RD182]	LAM9
				4.3.2		LAM3
					4.3.2.1 [RD761]	LAM3
				4.3.3 [RD115]		LAM9 and T5
				4.3.4 [RD174]	4.3.4.1	LAM1
					4.3.4.2	LAM11-ZWE, LAM9, LAM1, and LAM4
					4.3.4.2.1	LAM11-ZWE
			4.4	4.4.1	4.4.1.1 (S-type)	S
					4.4.1.2	T1
				4.4.2		T1 and T2
			4.5 [RD122]			H3, H4, and T1
			4.6	4.6.1 (Uganda) [RD724]	4.6.1.1	T2-Uganda
					4.6.1.2	T2
				4.6.2 [RD726]	4.6.2.1	T3
					4.6.2.2 (Cameroon)	LAM10-CAM
			4.7			T1 and T5
			4.8 [RD219]			T1, T2, T3, T4 and T5
			4.9 (H37Rv-like)			T1
Ancient lineages (M. africanum)	West-Africa lineage 1	5 [RD711]				AFRI_2 and AFRI_3
	West-Africa lineage 2	6 [RD702]				AFRI_1
Intermediary lineage (M. tuberculosis)	Lineage 7	7				

[a]Regions of deletion (RD) are given in brackets and appear below the lineage/sublineage in which they are present. Synthetic table adapted from Coll et al. (86).
[b]LSP, large sequence polymorphism.

jor clades, one composed of human strains only and one containing both human and animal strains. Interestingly, the basal and genetically more diverse lineage of the second clade infects humans, confirming that animal strains derived from human ones. Moreover, using Bayesian approaches and coalescent-based theory, they estimated the clade ages and inferred the *M. tuberculosis* demographic history. Based on these calculations, the common ancestor of the MTBC appeared some 40,000 years ago. In a second step, the ancestral strains reached the Fertile Crescent where they diversified during and shortly after the onset of domestication, 10,000 years ago. They ultimately spread out of Mesopotamia, accompanying different human migration waves in Africa, Asia, and Europe, and gave rise to locally adapted pathogens. Furthermore, a strong signal of demographic expansion was detected in the past 200 years, concomitant with industrialization. All these clues point toward a strong association and long coevolution between *H. sapiens* and *M. tuberculosis*.

Last, just before the rise of NGS and WGS, some researchers began to use SNP-based approaches to assess lineage relationships and to unravel deep MTBC sublineages. Since mutations are rare in *M. tuberculosis* genomes, they compared the complete genomes of few available reference strains and identified a list of SNPs. Then they sequenced these genes or called the SNPs in a large NGS data set gathered from strain collections (39–41). The authors retrieved the principal clades described above, but all generated phylogenies turned out to be poorly resolved, ending in star-like topologies. At first glance, one might have invoked a sudden radiative burst and a hard polytomy. What we were facing was, in fact, a methodological issue called ascertainment bias, which is often driven by biased taxonomic sampling (42). Indeed, strong ascertainment bias and related phylogenetic reconstructions systematically lead to the collapse of divergent lineages into single points, failing therefore to generate reliable tree topologies. This is exemplified by the Filliol et al. (41) paper, where the authors reached the unrealistic conclusions that *M. tuberculosis* had an Indian origin.

NGS AND TUBERCULOSIS EVOLUTIONARY HISTORY

The Global Picture

The ultimate knowledge that can be gathered using NGS is a complete list of all nucleotides that constitute the circular chromosome of a strain. Our understanding of the evolutionary relationships of the different MTB

lineages, their radiation, and time to the most common ancestor (TMRCA) greatly profited from WGS, resulting in a quantum-leap progress in the field of MTBC phylogenetics (43). NGS favored the characterization of the genetic diversity of an increasing number of strains, covering different lineages and large geographic distributions. Thanks to a high-quality reference genome (44) (Sanger sequenced) gathered from the H37Rv laboratory strain, the scientific community has a template on which Illumina or Roche 454 reads can be mapped. Unraveling the topology of the MTBC tree is also highly dependent on the availability of a reliable outgroup. Fortunately, Supply and colleagues (45) sequenced and analyzed the whole genomes of five strains belonging to the smooth tubercle bacilli (STB), the closest outgroup known so far (46, 47). These strains harbor a unique smooth colony phenotype on culture media, are less persistent and virulent than their *M. tuberculosis* counterpart, and were essentially collected from the Horn of Africa, the cradle of humankind. Furthermore, the so-called "*Mycobacterium canettii*" and/or "*Mycobacterium prototuberculosis*" strains display a unique feature in the MTBC world: they are highly recombinogenic and they are prone to horizontal gene transfer (HGT). Indeed, they possess distinct CRISPR-Cas systems relative to *M. tuberculosis* that are closely related to the genera *Thioalkalivibrio*, *Moorella*, and *Thiorhodovibrio* (45). Interestingly, this latter species is adapted to warm and salty waters, a type of environment that is often encountered in the western part of Djibouti where large saline lakes coexist with hot springs. These scars of past genetic exchanges definitively advocate for an environmental origin of the ancestor of *M. tuberculosis* that might date back 3 million years (46).

Once rooted with *M. canettii*, the first attempt to solve the evolutionary history of the MTBC with full genomes relied on a set of 25 *M. tuberculosis* strains representing the six main human lineages known at that time (48). The molecular diversity of those strains remained rather modest, with only one SNP call for every 3 kb of sequence generated, highlighting the relative youth of this human pathogen, its clonality, and putative rise through a major bottleneck. The neighbor-joining tree proposed by the authors did not add much in terms of branching order but illustrated the power of genomics in terms of bootstrap branch supports (≥99%) and within-lineage resolution. Three major clades could be distinguished, one encompassing lineages 2, 3, and 4; followed by its sister group, lineage 1; and, finally, a marginally more basal group represented by the two *M. africanum* lineages (Table 1). Because the rationale of this first genomic paper was to study *M. tuberculosis* human T-cell epitopes, the absence of animal strains was not surprising. However, in terms of evolutionary history, this no-attendance needed to be corrected in future studies. This was done in a landmark study (49) where genomes of 259 *M. tuberculosis* strains were analyzed. At such scales, with more than 30 strains per major lineage, the likelihood to get much closer to the real picture significantly increases. Comas and colleagues included in this study a new member of the MTBC, the recently described lineage 7 (50), which was only collected from Ethiopian patients, as well as a couple of animal strains. Again, the maximum-likelihood tree confirmed the monophyly of the modern strains (L2, 3, and 4), but also suggested that the animal lineage diverged from the African lineage 6 (*M. africanum*). Another important feature is the strong biogeographical structure of the different lineages; their distribution around the planet is not random at all, and clearly corresponds to well-defined geographic and cultural areas. This observation, coupled with the fact that tree topologies and geographic distribution between MTBC strains and the main human mitochondrial macrohaplogroups were highly similar, prompted the authors to calibrate the tuberculosis evolutionary

tree on its human backbone. More specifically, the striking resemblance and branching order of the Southeast Asian and Oceania tuberculosis strains and the Southeast Asian, Oceanian macrohaplogroup M in humans were used for this purpose (Fig. 2).

This elegant approach, coupled with a coalescent-based approach, indicates that the MTBC emerged at least 70,000 years ago. The demographic success and the timing of the propagation of *M. tuberculosis* were evaluated with Bayesian skyline plots (51–53) that unraveled the effective population size of the bug through time. According to this scenario, MTBC accompanied the migrations of anatomically modern humans out of Africa and started to spread at a higher pace during the Neolithic demographic transition (54). It is tempting to connect a sustainable infectious cycle with the advance of farming and domestication, accompanied by dramatic changes in lifestyle, from hunter-gatherers to farmers, from low-density populations to local crowds. However, the data also show that the conquest of the Indian Ocean areas by lineage 1 largely predated the Fertile Crescent onset, starting as early as 67,000 years ago and followed by a second wave of peopling that reached the Middle East, Europe, and Asia some 46,000 years ago. Overall, WGS highlights the coevolution be-

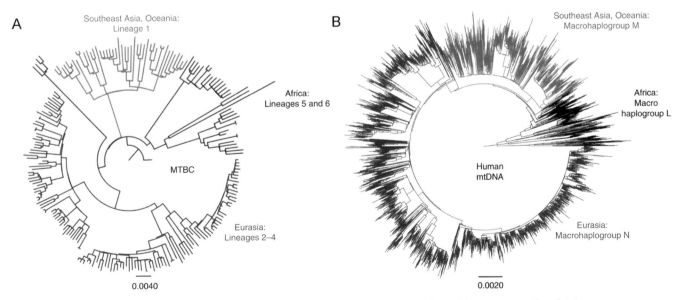

Figure 2 The genome-based phylogeny of MTBC mirrors that of human mitochondrial genomes. Comparison of the MTBC phylogeny (**A**) and a phylogeny derived from 4,955 mitochondrial genomes (mtDNA) representative of the main human haplogroups (**B**). Color-coding highlights the similarities in tree topology and geographic distribution between MTBC strains and the main human mitochondrial macrohaplogroups (black, African clades: MTBC lineages 5 and 6, human mitochondrial macrohaplogroups L0 to L3; pink, Southeast Asian and Oceanian clades: MTBC lineage 1, human mitochondrial macrohaplogroup M; blue, Eurasian clades: MTBC lineage 2 to 4, human mitochondrial macrohaplogroup N). Scale bars indicate substitutions per site. Adapted from Comas et al. (49).

tween a host and its pathogen, *H. sapiens* and *M. tuberculosis*, their intricate evolutionary histories, their African origin, and their adaptation from low to high population densities.

Yet recently a new publication dramatically affected the temporal dimension of the scenario presented above. Bos et al. (55) analyzed three 1,000-year-old mycobacterial genomes from Peruvian skeletons showing stigmata of tuberculosis infection that proved to be *Mycobacterium pinnipedii* (Fig. 3), a type of strain mostly isolated from seal species in the Southern Hemisphere. It is worth mentioning that two of the archeological sites (El Algodonal and Chiribaya Alta) were close to the Rio Algodonal and only 5 to 10 km upstream from the river mouth. The team led by German experts in ancient DNA managed to successfully sequence these genomes by applying DNA capture (56) and genomic assembly of the metagenomic reads. The assembled genomes harbored the typical signature and damage of ancient DNA, and accounted for 2% of the total reads.

The authors then calibrated the molecular clock using the archeological data and the fact that branch lengths are a function of the elapsed time, being longer for strains collected in the 21st century and shorter for much older strains. This Bayesian calibration process, under a relaxed clock model, resulted in a substitution rate of about 5×10^{-8} substitutions per site per year, placing the most recent common ancestor for the MTBC at 4,000 years, which turns to be more than one order of magnitude younger than the age proposed by Comas and colleagues (49). For comparative purposes, we should mention that the substitution rate obtained by Comas et al. was much slower, i.e., 2.6×10^{-9} substitutions per site per year. This MTBC TMRCA dating issue definitively splits the mycobacteriology community into two entities, i.e., the pros and the cons. The more recent dating of the Bos study conflicts with numerous archeological proofs, including evidence of MTBC in a 17,500-year-old bison in Wyoming, United States (18), the presence of a 9,000-year-old modern

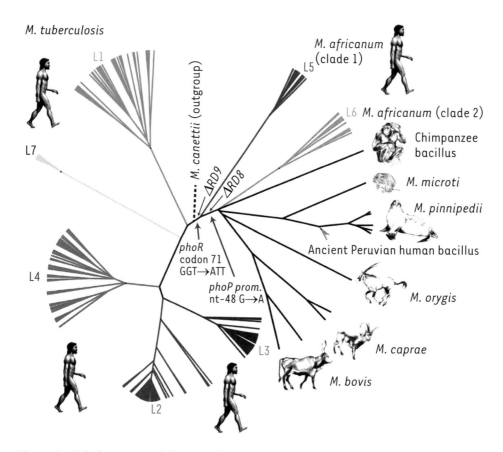

Figure 3 Whole-genome phylogeny of 261 strains belonging to the MTBC. Animal and *M. africanum* specific deletions are indicated, as well as mutations affecting the PhoPR virulence regulator. Adapted from Bos et al. (55) and Gonzalo-Asensio et al. (34).

tuberculosis strain in a Neolithic infant skeleton from Israel (16), and an animal MTBC strain harboring the RD9 deletion some 7,000 years ago (57). The cumulative evidence gathered from amplification of IS6100 and spoligotyping patterns from bones predating the Bos et al. MTBC TMRCA are questioned by some scientists, claiming that these mobile genetic elements and CRISPR systems are not MTBC specific enough and that they might be observed in environmental mycobacteria (58, 59), leading to false positives. The same arguments are used to question the validity of the presence of mycolic acids (60, 61) in biosamples to identify MTBC strains. Other colleagues came to the same molecular clock as Bos et al. (55) using a calibration point based on aboriginal communities in Canada that acquired *M. tuberculosis* via the fur trade in the late 18th century (62). Nearly identical rates were obtained again based on a calibration relying on an 18th-century mummy collected from a Dominican church in Hungary (63). Furthermore, Pepperell et al. (62) did not find statistical support for codivergence of *M. tuberculosis* with its host in formal phylogenetic congruence tests.

Another by-product of this study is that, according to the authors, seals are the source of New World human tuberculosis, therefore predating the likely entry of tuberculosis in South America with the Conquistadores, putatively harboring lineage 4 strains in their lungs. The Bos et al. conclusions based on the sole observation of a couple of ancient Peruvian humans are overinterpreted in the best case if not dubious at all. This scenario possibly transforms the exception into the rule by extrapolating conclusions based on local observations to continental-scale lessons. A more parsimonious setup could be built on a small population of indigenous hunters who incidentally contracted tuberculosis from infected seals that might be part of their natural prey or diet. Such transfers are rare but can be observed in zoos; notably, South American sea lions managed to infect a camel and a Malayan tapir in neighboring enclosures with their *M. pinnipedii* strains (64), and animal keepers were infected in a zoo in the Netherlands (65). The observation made at the southern border of Peru might be therefore anecdotal and may have resulted in an evolutionary dead end. Before claiming that *M. pinnipedii* plagued South and North American indigenous populations, before being completely replaced by the L4 lineage in present days, far more evidence is needed. This includes additional samples from a larger geographic distribution and additional workable skeletons from diverse archeological sites.

Animal-Related MTBC Strains

According to the currently available sampling and population genomics data, the animal lineages emerged from a common ancestor closely related to lineage 6 (*M. africanum*) (55) (Fig. 3). Consequently, multiple mammalian host jumps occurred leading to adaptive processes and genomic erosion (66). Those animal genomes are of particular interest because genes that undergo pseudogenization or get lost are indicative of host specificity, notably here *H. sapiens* specificity. Interestingly, three independent losses of the RD1 region have been observed in *M. microti* (67), the dassie bacillus, (68) and *Mycobacterium mungi* (69). This convergent evolution might underline the key role of the ESX-1 secretion system for infecting *H. sapiens*. Beyond the evolutionary dimension, the adaptive radiation of animal MTBC should attract more attention since animal lineages can tell us a lot about human-specific genes, which are prone to be altered or deleted in genomes belonging to the former lineages. This critical situation is illustrated by the relative paucity of published animal MTBC strains, with the notable exception of *M. bovis*, where veterinary and socioeconomic factors prevail. The few available genomes cover the following members of MTBC, *M. suricattae*, the chimpanzee bacillus, *M. microti*, *M. pinnipedii*, *M. bovis*, and *M. caprae*, but no phylogeny including all these members has been published so far. The likelihood that other ignored animal lineages exist in the field is high; a good hint would be to further investigate in the direction of social or highly promiscuous mammal species where the settlement of epidemic episodes are favored.

Zooming into the Lineages

One of the major advances linked with WGS is the possibility to switch to population genetic approaches in the field of *M. tuberculosis* since enough SNPs can be accumulated in the evolutionary history and the coalescence of local populations. For instance, up to 0.4 mutations per genome per year can be accumulated (70). Applying such an approach, Comas et al. (49) scrutinized the evolutionary history of the Beijing lineage, an important member of lineage 2. The Beijing family attracted much attention because its members are hypervirulent in mouse models, spread quickly in Eurasia and Western Europe, and are associated with multidrug resistance (71). The family TMRCA was estimated at 8,000 years coinciding with the rise of agriculture in the Yangtze River region, the domestication of crops and the onset of Chinese farmer populations. Interestingly, the Bayesian skyline of the Beijing family matched pretty well the one obtained from the human mitochondrial haplogroups from East Asia, confirming this likely scenario. Moreover, the dating of the Beijing family is relatively congruent with former analyses based on MIRU typing (38), but also with more recent data obtained from a large collection of 5,000 Beijing strains (72). In the later publication, Merker et al. (72) unraveled the genetic structure and global spread of the Beijing lineage; this lineage is globally distributed but still entails a fine-scale genetic structuring. The authors detected six clonal complexes (CCs) and one basal lineage; those CCs proved to be strongly associated with geographical entities (Fig. 4). They also confirmed that this lineage initially originated in the Far East 6,600 years ago from where it radiated worldwide in several waves. This was illustrated by a negative correlation (r^2 = 0.626) between the mean allelic richness of the strains and their distance from the Yangtze River. An ancestral East Asian population of strains, mostly endemic, that gave rise to new variants following different migration routes, can explain this pattern. The consequence of this scenario is a stepping-stone propagation of the germs, followed by successive bottlenecks, resulting in genetic erosion with increasing distance from the source. The situation is similar for *H. sapiens* and its little companion *Helicobacter pylori*, where the highest genetic diversity can be observed in Africa and the lowest one in South America (73, 74). Worth mentioning are the contrasted profiles between the ancestral strains (CC6 and BL7) that only marginally dispersed from their area of endemicity and the other derived CCs that successfully spread at continental scales. CC5 is probably the best illustration to show how a minor variant, originating from Southeast Asia, spread some 1,500 years ago into the Pacific and increased its frequency due to drift and successive founder effects, culminating at a more than 90% prevalence in Micronesia and Polynesia. One of the most striking features was the evolutionary history of CC1, also called the central Asian clade, and CC2, the Russian clone. The first CC spread westward, becoming highly predominant in central Asia and around the Black Sea, and the latter one became predominant in Russia and Eastern Europe. Both CCs had the highest clustering rates for MDR strains, indicating population expansion amplified by the recent transmission of MDR strains. The demographic success of CC1 and CC2 was confirmed by coalescent-based analyses, and their expansion dated back some 200 to 250 years ago.

These recent expansions remarkably match known episodes of migration in Asia. Indeed, several waves of Chinese refugees migrated to the Russian empire, especially Kyrgyzstan, Kazakhstan, and Uzbekistan, as a consequence of a series of national uprisings from 1861 to 1877, which might have driven the expansion of the CC1 and CC2 strains in these regions (75). These recent western expansions are probably superimposed on a more historical, continuous flux of the different Beijing sublineages westward along the Silk Road. After a tip-dating calibration, the authors reconstructed the demogenetical changes in the Beijing lineage based on a subset of 110 genomes, and they detected a two-step increase in *M. tuberculosis* population size. The first expansion corresponded with the industrial revolution and the second one took place at the end of the 19th century, fitting the information gathered from historical and medical records. This trend was more pronounced for the most-westward distributed clonal complexes and the combined epidemic growth periods resulted in a 10-fold increase of *M. tuberculosis* Beijing's effective population size. The mild population drop that followed the expansion phase took place in the early 1960s and might be linked to the democratization of the antibiotic use. The analysis also captured a last tiny population growth that matches the rise of the HIV epidemics. To conclude, this study demonstrated the power of NGS to explain past and yet "uncaptured" migratory paths from a single lineage and how societal changes impact tuberculosis demography and epidemics. The sudden success of some lineages can even result in full lineage replacements, as exemplified in other pathogens such as *Salmonella enterica* serovar Typhi (76), highlighting the need for and power of population genomics. In the same year, Luo et al. (77) analyzed a novel data set comprising whole-genome sequences of 358 East Asian strains belonging to the Beijing family. The authors applied the molecular clock of Comas et al. (49), which is much faster than the mutation rate implemented by Merker et al. (72). Consequently, both scientific teams reported a demographic expansion of the Beijing family, similar genetic structure and spread, but strongly disagreed on the timing and TMRCA calculations. This situation might be disturbing for the nonspecialist, and it deserves specific explanations. The molecular clock issue will be addressed in greater detail in "The relativity of the clock" (see below), which might help to clarify the situation and propose analytical improvements.

Another lineage that attracted much attention is lineage 4 (the Euro-American lineage) that circulates in Aboriginal and French Canadian communities (78). Some sublineages were introduced in the indigenous populations in the mid-18th century and spread westward through canoe routes until 1850, illustrating the impact of recent trans-Atlantic migrations on remote

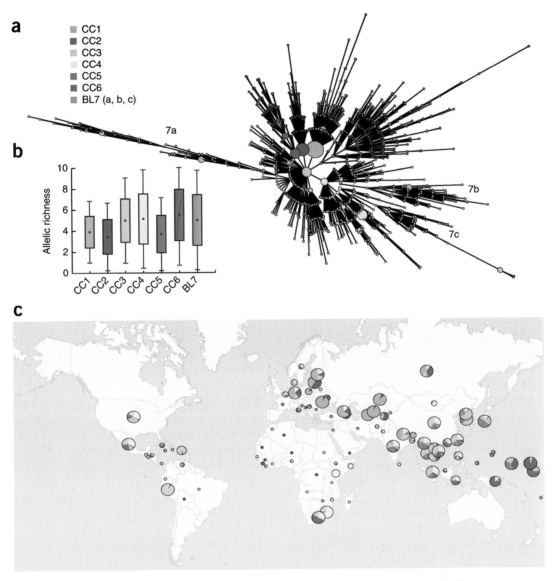

Figure 4 Biogeographical structure of the *M. tuberculosis* Beijing lineage. (a) MStree based on 24 MIRU-VNTR markers delineating the clonal complexes (CCs) gathered from a worldwide collection (n = 4,987). Major nodes and associated multilocus variants were grouped into six CCs and a basal sublineage (BL). (b) Genetic variability in the different Beijing lineage CCs and the BL calculated using a rarefaction procedure. Dots correspond to the mean allelic richness; boxes correspond to mean values ± standard error of the mean and error bars correspond to mean values ± standard deviation. (c) Worldwide distribution of the Beijing CCs and BL. Each circle corresponds to a country, and circle sizes are proportional to the number of strains. Adapted from Merker et al. (72).

North American communities. It is particularly worrying to see that the Inuit living in the Nunavik region of Québec present an incidence 50-fold higher than the Canadian average. In a recent population genomics analysis, Lee et al. (79) disentangled the genetic diver-

sity and population structure of 163 *M. tuberculosis* strains scattered in 11 remote Inuit villages. Their main finding confirmed that all patients harbored either one of two sublineages belonging to lineage 4; the TMRCA of the main sublineage, represented by 94% of the strains, dated back to the early 20th century. This result shows that the spread of tuberculosis was not interrupted after the fur trade decline, but that indigenous communities are still prone to "foreign"-mediated epidemics.

If we focus at microevolutionary scales, we reach the borders of the molecular epidemiology field and identification of transmission chains (80, 81). Lee et al. (79) nicely showed that pairs of isolates within villages had significantly fewer SNPs than pairs from different villages (6 versus 47), hinting toward intravillage chain transmissions.

Toward a Universal Taxonomic Nomenclature?

One of the major difficulties that a nonspecialist faces when he or she goes through the tuberculosis literature is the fluctuating and evolving nomenclature concerning the different lineages (see Table 1). The nomenclature was mainly driven by a couple of leading teams, starting from phage typing (82), regions of difference parsimony analyses (3), MIRU cladograms (35, 38), extended MLST trees (83), SNP sets (41, 84, 85), and ultimately whole-genome-based phylogenies. With the drop of the costs of Illumina and PacBio sequencing, thousands of new genomes became available, leading to the discovery of fine-scale phylogenetic structuring but also to the unearthing of new lineages. To facilitate the navigation in this growing complexity, Coll et al. (86) proposed a novel SNP-based bar code approach and implemented the PhyTB tool related to the PhyloTrack library. This numeric code relies on a subset of 62 canonical SNPs gathered from essential genes under negative selection that resolves all seven lineages and another 55 sublineages (Fig. 5). This approach can be upgraded and can evolve with the ongoing sequencing effort.

THE RELATIVITY OF THE CLOCK

Substitution Rate Estimates

Deciphering the evolutionary history of tuberculosis is highly dependent on a rigorous estimation of the molecular clock. One effective way to estimate the substitution rate is to focus on recent epidemics linked to a clone (70), retrospective observational studies (80, 87, 88), or even better on measuring the pace of mutational events within a host (89). The concept behind such approaches is that *M. tuberculosis* is composed of "measurably evolving populations" (90–92), meaning that whole genomes accumulate novel mutations over time frames of months to years. Convincingly, all these WGS studies reported congruent estimates of 0.3 to 0.5 SNP per genome per year, which translates roughly into 1×10^{-7} substitutions per nucleotide per year, with no notable difference between hosts (human or macaque). This mutation rate places *M. tuberculosis* at the lower bound of bacterial species, compared with *Staphylococcus aureus* displaying a mutation rate of 1 to 2×10^{-6} (93, 94), *Escherichia coli* of 5×10^{-6} (95, 96), and the mismatch repair-lacking *H. pylori* of 1×10^{-5} (97, 98) to 7×10^{-4} substitution per nucleotide per year during the acute phase of infection (99). Another approach to calibrate the clock relies on the high similarity of the human mtDNA-based phylogenies and the MTBC human-specific phylogeny, anchoring the Southeast Asian Oceanian lineage 1 with the human macrohaplogroup M (49). This alternative strategy resulted in a substitution rate estimate of 2.58×10^{-9} substitutions per site per year. These two substitution rates are rather incompatible and divergent. So the question is, how can they be combined into a single model?

A way to present the problem is to invoke the fields of quantum physics and relativity to build a couple of metaphors. For example, the observer effect and the Heisenberg uncertainty principle stipulate that there is trade-off in capturing simultaneously the position and the momentum of a particle, meaning that obtaining the exact position will lower the information concerning the momentum. In the same way, applying a short-term mutation rate to a *M. tuberculosis* data set covering a large temporal scale will likely provide reliable information concerning the terminal nodes and the demogenetic changes in the past century, but will perform poorly in terms of TMRCA and vice versa. The other metaphor concerns the theory of relativity where the faster the relative velocity is, the greater the magnitude of time dilatation will be. Again, here we can imagine that the substitution rate is a function of time and may vary following a yet-to-discover mathematical law.

These concepts have indeed some biological meaning, as we shall see. The substitution rate refers to the rate at which nucleotide changes become fixed in populations. This notion differs from the mutation rate, i.e., the rate at which novel mutations arise. In the latter case, some slightly deleterious mutations will be progressively removed by purifying selection, gradually in large populations and more stochastically in small ones. Accordingly, the mutation rate corresponds to the upper limit of mutational changes acquired per unit of time in a given biological system (100). Therefore, the combination of selective pressure (purifying selection),

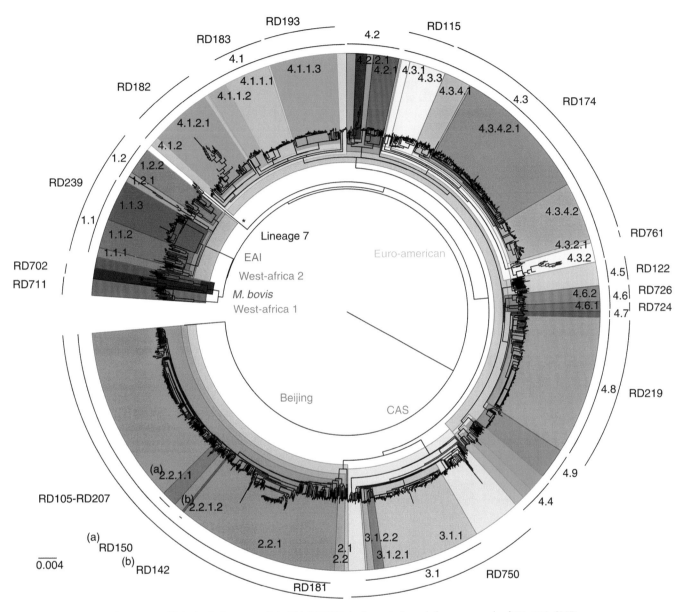

Figure 5 Global phylogeny of 1,601 MTBC isolates inferred from a total of 91,648 SNPs spanning the whole genome. All seven main MTBC lineages are indicated in the inner area of the tree. The main sublineages are annotated at the outer arc along with lineage-specific RDs. Identified clades are color-coded. Adapted from Coll et al. (86).

possible saturation at variable sites, and demographic fluctuations will shape the time dependency of evolutionary rates. This trend was noticed based on strong discrepancies between molecular and paleontological dating (101), reviewed by Ho et al. (102), but also subject to some controversies (103). However, there is growing empirical evidence for an exponential-decay law of the substitution rate, fluctuating between two natural boundaries, the mutation and the long-term substitution rates, as exemplified in New Zealand fish

species (104), birds and primates (105, 106), and *Vibrio cholerae* (107). This pattern might also be more effective and important in the relative short term (over centuries) for bacterial species and viruses, since they possess much shorter generation times than, e.g., large vertebrates. This is exemplified in Fig. 6, where a strong negative linear correlation between the evolutionary rate and time (both log-transformed) could be detected in three bacterial species, based on available complete genomes.

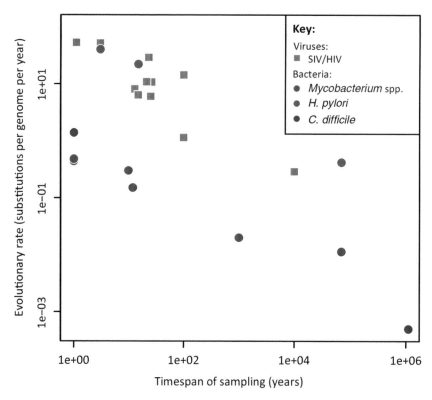

Figure 6   Consistent with a general pattern for measurably evolving populations, the evolutionary rates of microbial pathogens decrease as a function of the time span over which they are estimated. Data shown are selected representative examples, including one group of RNA viruses and several bacterial pathogens. Adapted from Biek et al. (100).

Consequently, there is an urgent need to reunify the analyses obtained from different scientific teams implementing contrasting short- or long-term substitution rates on *M. tuberculosis* data sets (108) under a same mathematical model. To reach this goal, we will have to define the parameters that define the J-shaped curve of the etiological agent of tuberculosis and to develop, and extend, tools like BEAST that will integrate in a unique coalescent framework, a substitution rate dependent on time (109). However, this task remains challenging, since there is a paucity of reliable calibration points for the intermediate time frames.

Other Limitations

Some additional features must be mentioned that possibly complicate the clock estimates. Among them, we have to consider both intrachromosomal and interlineage variations in the ticking rates. The 4.4 Mb *M. tuberculosis* genome presents highly variable repetitive genetic regions, encompassing genes such as the PPE, PE_PGRS, and ESX families. Those gene families are prone to increased mutation rates, are difficult to assemble, and are often removed from the analyses.

Therefore, the accuracy of the trimming step might explain some outliers observed in terms of mutation rate estimates. Furthermore, Martincorena et al. (110) detected mutational hot and cold spots across 2,659 genes from a collection of 34 *E. coli* strains. Lower rates were observed in highly expressed genes and there is no strong argument that *M. tuberculosis* should behave differently. At shorter timescales, mutations affecting genes involved in MTBC DNA repair (111) can inflate the mutation rate, resulting in hypermutator phenotypes. These transient phenotypes are adaptively cardinal and are involved in the fast acquisition of SNPs conferring resistance to second-generation antibiotics. For, example, one copy of the major replicative DNA polymerase, dnaE2, proved to be a mediator of *M. tuberculosis* survival through inducible mutagenesis and contributed to the emergence of drug resistance *in vivo* (112). At a higher hierarchical level, there is growing evidence that some Beijing sublineages undergo faster evolutionary rates relative to other human tuberculosis lineages. Ebrahimi-Rad et al. (113) detected alterations in *mut* genes, mostly missense mutations that improve the adaptability of the W-Beijing clade.

In the same vein, Ford et al. (114) demonstrated that cultured *M. tuberculosis* strains from lineage 2 acquired *in vitro* drug resistance against isoniazid and ethambutol three times faster than *M. tuberculosis* strains from lineage 4, invoking again contrasted mutation rates between lineages. However, this difference remains relatively modest compared with *E. coli* (115) and *Pseudomonas aeruginosa* (116), where mutator phenotypes are orders of magnitude more mutable than the wild-type strains. The latter species harbor a mismatch-repair system whose dysfunction increases mutation and recombination rates; in that respect, they differ from *M. tuberculosis*, which is lacking such a system (117).

A final complication can be called up, linked to the peculiar strategy employed by the tubercle bacillus to survive in the host. During latent infection, which accounts for most of its life history, *M. tuberculosis* is in a dormant state with little to no replication activity. This latent stage dramatically contrasts with the active stage of the disease in which clonal multiplication occurs in the lung. The question can therefore be raised whether mutation rates differ between the two different stages and whether this might impact the evolutionary history of the MTBC and the TMRCA estimates. This problem was targeted by a team at the Harvard School of Public Health (89); the authors were able to show, based on whole-genome sequencing of *M. tuberculosis* isolated from cynomolgus macaques, that the mutation rates were similar during latent and active disease. Since most of the chromosome mutations appear during the replication process, this result was somehow unexpected. One of the explanations proposed relies on the high oxidative stress that the bacilli undergo in the macrophage phagolysosome resulting in cytosine deamination or the formation of 8-oxoguanine (118, 119). Alternatively, *M. tuberculosis* keeps dividing more actively during latency than previously thought.

PERSPECTIVES

High financial investments coupled with novel methodological and analytical approaches have driven human population genomics to the upper edge of scientific excellence. The study of the natural host of *M. tuberculosis* reached a new summit with the rise of the study of ancient DNA (120). In 2006, Svante Pääbo and his colleagues analyzed 1 million bp of a 38,000-year-old Neanderthal fossil using the 454 technology (121) and were able to handle the small degraded DNA molecules. Among the most common "lesions," depurination and deaminated cytosine residues near the fragment ends were reported (122). Four years later, thanks to a methodological switch toward Illumina sequencing, they provided the scientific community with the first draft genome of a Neanderthal gathered from three individuals that lived in the Vindija cave in Croatia (123). This major technological step, accompanied with suites of bioinformatics tools, opened the door to late Pleistocene genomics (124–126) and allowed the discovery of new Hominin lineages, like the Denisovan (127), an extinct relative of Neanderthals.

The first bacterial paleogenomes came just after, notably with the first draft genome of *Y. pestis*, the etiological agent of the plague (128). This ancient genome at an average 30-fold coverage was isolated using targeted capture from Black Death victims in London who died in approximately 1348 to 1350. Even more impressive was the publication of a Bronze Age *Y. pestis* genome from Asia, 3 millennia earlier than any historical records of plague (129). Auspiciously, the bacteria belonging to the MTBC present a complex waxy and hydrophobic cell wall, facilitating therefore the conservation of the DNA molecules. With the development of the field of paleomicrobiology we might soon have the unique opportunity to sample temporal series of skeletons showing stigmata of tuberculosis infection (up to 5% of the patients). Thanks to precise radiocarbon dating, we know that such a material extends through the supposed "life span" of the disease, from the late Pleistocene to the present (17, 130–133). The accumulation of heterochronous *M. tuberculosis* paleopopulation genomics will ultimately solve the molecular clock issue and possibly reunify the fields of evolutionary mycobacteriology, paleoepidemiology, and paleopathology. The first steps have been already accomplished, with 100- (56), 250- (63), and 1,000-year-old (55) genomes made available.

Beyond this rather technical issue, the spread of different lineages through time, lineage replacements, extinct lineages discovery, and eventually a complete revision of current models will be driven by paleomicrobiology. Once Pandora's box is open, we might consider the possibility that Neanderthals may have faced *M. tuberculosis*. If true, two conflicting scenarios can be tested. Neanderthals harbored their own MTBC-like ancestor or they contracted a *H. sapiens*-associated strain during their coexistence with modern humans, some 30,000 years ago in southwestern Europe. Last but not least, ancestral genomes will also improve our understanding of pathogen adaptation and the pace and dynamics of coevolution with its natural host. Studying tuberculosis remains a challenging task, but for sure, we live in interesting times.

Acknowledgments. We gratefully acknowledge the contributions and comments of Jean-Philippe Rasigade, Olivier Dutour, and Jan Willem Dogger on the manuscript. We also thank the Ecole Pratiques des Hautes Etudes for financial support via the priority research action Grant (ARP).

Citation. Barbier M, Wirth T. 2016. The evolutionary history, demography, and spread of the *Mycobacterium tuberculosis* complex. Microbiol Spectrum 4(4):TBTB2-0008-2016.

References

1. Wirth T, Meyer A, Achtman M. 2005. Deciphering host migrations and origins by means of their microbes. *Mol Ecol* 14:3289–3306.

2. Albanna AS, Reed MB, Kotar KV, Fallow A, McIntosh FA, Behr MA, Menzies D. 2011. Reduced transmissibility of East African Indian strains of *Mycobacterium tuberculosis*. *PLoS One* 6:e25075.

3. Gagneux S, DeRiemer K, Van T, Kato-Maeda M, de Jong BC, Narayanan S, Nicol M, Niemann S, Kremer K, Gutierrez MC, Hilty M, Hopewell PC, Small PM. 2006. Variable host-pathogen compatibility in *Mycobacterium tuberculosis*. *Proc Natl Acad Sci USA* 103:2869–2873.

4. Reed MB, Pichler VK, McIntosh F, Mattia A, Fallow A, Masala S, Domenech P, Zwerling A, Thibert L, Menzies D, Schwartzman K, Behr MA. 2009. Major *Mycobacterium tuberculosis* lineages associate with patient country of origin. *J Clin Microbiol* 47:1119–1128.

5. Brites D, Gagneux S. 2015. Co-evolution of *Mycobacterium tuberculosis* and *Homosapiens*. *Immunol Rev* 264:6–24.

6. Velayati AA, Masjedi MR, Farnia P, Tabarsi P, Ghanavi J, Ziazarifi AH, Hoffner SE. 2009. Emergence of new forms of totally drug-resistant tuberculosis bacilli: super extensively drug-resistant tuberculosis or totally drug-resistant strains in Iran. *Chest* 136:420–425.

7. Prasad PV. 2002. General medicine in Atharvaveda with special reference to Yaksma (consumption/tuberculosis). *Bull Indian Inst Hist Med Hyderabad* 32:1–14.

8. Karlson AG, Lessel EW. 1970. *Mycobacterium bovis* nom. nov. *Int J Syst Evol Microbiol* 20:273–282.

9. Castets M, Boisvert H, Grumbach F, Brunel M, Rist N. 1968. [Tuberculosis bacilli of the African type: preliminary note]. *Rev Tuberc Pneumol (Paris)* 32:179–184.

10. Reed GB. 1957. *Mycobacterium microti*, p 703. In Breed RS, Murray EGD, Smith NR (ed), *Bergey's Manual of Determinative Bacteriology*, 7th ed. The Williams and Wilkins Co, Baltimore.

11. Tsukamura M, Mizuno S, Toyama H. 1985. Taxonomic studies on the *Mycobacterium tuberculosis* series. *Microbiol Immunol* 29:285–299.

12. Collins CH, Yates MD, Grange JM. 1982. Subdivision of *Mycobacterium tuberculosis* into five variants for epidemiological purposes: methods and nomenclature. *J Hyg (Lond)* 89:235–242.

13. Smith NH, Hewinson RG, Kremer K, Brosch R, Gordon SV. 2009. Myths and misconceptions: the origin and evolution of *Mycobacterium tuberculosis*. *Nat Rev Microbiol* 7:537–544.

14. Stead WW. 1997. The origin and erratic global spread of tuberculosis. How the past explains the present and is the key to the future. *Clin Chest Med* 18:65–77.

15. Wolfe ND, Dunavan CP, Diamond J. 2007. Origins of major human infectious diseases. *Nature* 447:279–283.

16. Hershkovitz I, Donoghue HD, Minnikin DE, Besra GS, Lee OY, Gernaey AM, Galili E, Eshed V, Greenblatt CL, Lemma E, Bar-Gal GK, Spigelman M. 2008. Detection and molecular characterization of 9,000-year-old *Mycobacterium tuberculosis* from a Neolithic settlement in the Eastern Mediterranean. *PLoS One* 3:e3426.

17. Baker O, Lee OY, Wu HH, Besra GS, Minnikin DE, Llewellyn G, Williams CM, Maixner F, O'Sullivan N, Zink A, Chamel B, Khawam R, Coqueugniot E, Helmer D, Le Mort F, Perrin P, Gourichon L, Dutailly B, Pálfi G, Coqueugniot H, Dutour O. 2015. Human tuberculosis predates domestication in ancient Syria. *Tuberculosis (Edinb)* 95(Suppl 1):S4–S12.

18. Rothschild BM, Martin LD, Lev G, Bercovier H, Bar-Gal GK, Greenblatt C, Donoghue H, Spigelman M, Brittain D. 2001. *Mycobacterium tuberculosis* complex DNA from an extinct bison dated 17,000 years before the present. *Clin Infect Dis* 33:305–311.

19. van Embden JD, Cave MD, Crawford JT, Dale JW, Eisenach KD, Gicquel B, Hermans P, Martin C, McAdam R, Shinnick TM, et al. 1993. Strain identification of *Mycobacterium tuberculosis* by DNA fingerprinting: recommendations for a standardized methodology. *J Clin Microbiol* 31:406–409.

20. van Soolingen D, van der Zanden AG, de Haas PE, Noordhoek GT, Kiers A, Foudraine NA, Portaels F, Kolk AH, Kremer K, van Embden JD. 1998. Diagnosis of *Mycobacterium microti* infections among humans by using novel genetic markers. *J Clin Microbiol* 36:1840–1845.

21. Collins DM, Stephens DM. 1991. Identification of an insertion sequence, IS*1081*, in *Mycobacterium bovis*. *FEMS Microbiol Lett* 67:11–15.

22. van Soolingen D, Hermans PW, de Haas PE, Soll DR, van Embden JD. 1991. Occurrence and stability of insertion sequences in *Mycobacterium tuberculosis* complex strains: evaluation of an insertion sequence-dependent DNA polymorphism as a tool in the epidemiology of tuberculosis. *J Clin Microbiol* 29:2578–2586.

23. Yeh RW, Ponce de Leon A, Agasino CB, Hahn JA, Daley CL, Hopewell PC, Small PM. 1998. Stability of *Mycobacterium tuberculosis* DNA genotypes. *J Infect Dis* 177:1107–1111.

24. Fang Z, Morrison N, Watt B, Doig C, Forbes KJ. 1998. IS*6100* transposition and evolutionary scenario of the direct repeat locus in a group of closely related *Mycobacterium tuberculosis* strains. *J Bacteriol* 180:2102–2109.

25. Achtman M. 1996. A surfeit of YATMs? *J Clin Microbiol* 34:1870.

26. Kamerbeek J, Schouls L, Kolk A, van Agterveld M, van Soolingen D, Kuijper S, Bunschoten A, Molhuizen H, Shaw R, Goyal M, van Embden J. 1997. Simultaneous detection and strain differentiation of *Mycobacterium tuberculosis* for diagnosis and epidemiology. *J Clin Microbiol* 35:907–914.

27. Groenen PM, Bunschoten AE, van Soolingen D, van Embden JD. 1993. Nature of DNA polymorphism in the direct repeat cluster of *Mycobacterium tuberculosis*; application for strain differentiation by a novel typing method. *Mol Microbiol* 10:1057–1065.

28. Gori A, Bandera A, Marchetti G, Degli Esposti A, Catozzi L, Nardi GP, Gazzola L, Ferrario G, van Embden JD, van Soolingen D, Moroni M, Franzetti F. 2005. Spoligotyping and *Mycobacterium tuberculosis*. *Emerg Infect Dis* 11:1242–1248.

29. Barrangou R, Fremaux C, Deveau H, Richards M, Boyaval P, Moineau S, Romero DA, Horvath P. 2007. CRISPR provides acquired resistance against viruses in prokaryotes. *Science* 315:1709–1712.

30. Mazars E, Lesjean S, Banuls AL, Gilbert M, Vincent V, Gicquel B, Tibayrenc M, Locht C, Supply P. 2001. High-resolution minisatellite-based typing as a portable approach to global analysis of *Mycobacterium tuberculosis* molecular epidemiology. *Proc Natl Acad Sci USA* 98:1901–1906.

31. Sreevatsan S, Pan X, Stockbauer KE, Connell ND, Kreiswirth BN, Whittam TS, Musser JM. 1997. Restricted structural gene polymorphism in the *Mycobacterium tuberculosis* complex indicates evolutionarily recent global dissemination. *Proc Natl Acad Sci USA* 94:9869–9874.

32. Brosch R, Pym AS, Gordon SV, Cole ST. 2001. The evolution of mycobacterial pathogenicity: clues from comparative genomics. *Trends Microbiol* 9:452–458.

33. Brosch R, Gordon SV, Marmiesse M, Brodin P, Buchrieser C, Eiglmeier K, Garnier T, Gutierrez C, Hewinson G, Kremer K, Parsons LM, Pym AS, Samper S, van Soolingen D, Cole ST. 2002. A new evolutionary scenario for the *Mycobacterium tuberculosis* complex. *Proc Natl Acad Sci USA* 99:3684–3689.

34. Gonzalo-Asensio J, Malaga W, Pawlik A, Astarie-Dequeker C, Passemar C, Moreau F, Laval F, Daffé M, Martin C, Brosch R, Guilhot C. 2014. Evolutionary history of tuberculosis shaped by conserved mutations in the PhoPR virulence regulator. *Proc Natl Acad Sci USA* 111:11491–11496.

35. Filliol I, Ferdinand S, Negroni L, Sola C, Rastogi N. 2000. Molecular typing of *Mycobacterium tuberculosis* based on variable number of tandem DNA repeats used alone and in association with spoligotyping. *J Clin Microbiol* 38:2520–2524.

36. Sola C, Filliol I, Legrand E, Mokrousov I, Rastogi N. 2001. *Mycobacterium tuberculosis* phylogeny reconstruction based on combined numerical analysis with IS*1081*, IS*6100*, VNTR, and DR-based spoligotyping suggests the existence of two new phylogeographical clades. *J Mol Evol* 53:680–689.

37. Sola C, Filliol I, Legrand E, Lesjean S, Locht C, Supply P, Rastogi N. 2003. Genotyping of the *Mycobacterium tuberculosis* complex using MIRUs: association with VNTR and spoligotyping for molecular epidemiology and evolutionary genetics. *Infect Genet Evol* 3:125–133.

38. Wirth T, Hildebrand F, Allix-Béguec C, Wölbeling F, Kubica T, Kremer K, van Soolingen D, Rüsch-Gerdes S, Locht C, Brisse S, Meyer A, Supply P, Niemann S. 2008. Origin, spread and demography of the *Mycobacterium tuberculosis* complex. *PLoS Pathog* 4:e1000160.

39. Baker L, Brown T, Maiden MC, Drobniewski F. 2004. Silent nucleotide polymorphisms and a phylogeny for *Mycobacterium tuberculosis*. *Emerg Infect Dis* 10:1568–1577.

40. Gutacker MM, Smoot JC, Migliaccio CA, Ricklefs SM, Hua S, Cousins DV, Graviss EA, Shashkina E, Kreiswirth BN, Musser JM. 2002. Genome-wide analysis of synonymous single nucleotide polymorphisms in *Mycobacterium tuberculosis* complex organisms: resolution of genetic relationships among closely related microbial strains. *Genetics* 162:1533–1543.

41. Filliol I, Motiwala AS, Cavatore M, Qi W, Hazbón MH, Bobadilla del Valle M, Fyfe J, García-García L, Rastogi N, Sola C, Zozio T, Guerrero MI, León CI, Crabtree J, Angiuoli S, Eisenach KD, Durmaz R, Joloba ML, Rendón A, Sifuentes-Osornio J, Ponce de León A, Cave MD, Fleischmann R, Whittam TS, Alland D. 2006. Global phylogeny of *Mycobacterium tuberculosis* based on single nucleotide polymorphism (SNP) analysis: insights into tuberculosis evolution, phylogenetic accuracy of other DNA fingerprinting systems, and recommendations for a minimal standard SNP set. *J Bacteriol* 188:759–772.

42. Pearson T, Busch JD, Ravel J, Read TD, Rhoton SD, U'Ren JM, Simonson TS, Kachur SM, Leadem RR, Cardon ML, Van Ert MN, Huynh LY, Fraser CM, Keim P. 2004. Phylogenetic discovery bias in *Bacillus anthracis* using single-nucleotide polymorphisms from whole-genome sequencing. *Proc Natl Acad Sci USA* 101:13536–13541.

43. Galagan JE. 2014. Genomic insights into tuberculosis. *Nat Rev Genet* 15:307–320.

44. Cole ST, Brosch R, Parkhill J, Garnier T, Churcher C, Harris D, Gordon SV, Eiglmeier K, Gas S, Barry CE III, Tekaia F, Badcock K, Basham D, Brown D, Chillingworth T, Connor R, Davies R, Devlin K, Feltwell T, Gentles S, Hamlin N, Holroyd S, Hornsby T, Jagels K, Krogh A, McLean J, Moule S, Murphy L, Oliver K, Osborne J, Quail MA, Rajandream MA, Rogers J, Rutter S, Seeger K, Skelton J, Squares R, Squares S, Sulston JE, Taylor K, Whitehead S, Barrell BG. 1998. Deciphering the biology of *Mycobacterium tuberculosis* from the complete genome sequence. *Nature* 393:537–544.

45. Supply P, Marceau M, Mangenot S, Roche D, Rouanet C, Khanna V, Majlessi L, Criscuolo A, Tap J, Pawlik A, Fiette L, Orgeur M, Fabre M, Parmentier C, Frigui W, Simeone R, Boritsch EC, Debrie AS, Willery E, Walker D, Quail MA, Ma L, Bouchier C, Salvignol G, Sayes F, Cascioferro A, Seemann T, Barbe V, Locht C, Gutierrez MC, Leclerc C, Bentley SD, Stinear TP, Brisse S, Médigue C, Parkhill J, Cruveiller S, Brosch R. 2013. Genomic analysis of smooth tubercle bacilli provides insights into ancestry and pathoadaptation of *Mycobacterium tuberculosis*. *Nat Genet* 45:172–179.

46. Gutierrez MC, Brisse S, Brosch R, Fabre M, Omaïs B, Marmiesse M, Supply P, Vincent V. 2005. Ancient origin and gene mosaicism of the progenitor of *Mycobacterium tuberculosis*. *PLoS Pathog* 1:e5.

47. van Soolingen D, Hoogenboezem T, de Haas PE, Hermans PW, Koedam MA, Teppema KS, Brennan PJ, Besra GS, Portaels F, Top J, Schouls LM, van Embden JD. 1997. A novel pathogenic taxon of the *Mycobacterium tuberculosis* complex, Canetti: characterization of an exceptional isolate from Africa. *Int J Syst Bacteriol* **47**: 1236–1245

48. Comas I, Chakravartti J, Small PM, Galagan J, Niemann S, Kremer K, Ernst JD, Gagneux S. 2010. Human T cell epitopes of *Mycobacterium tuberculosis* are evolutionarily hyperconserved. *Nat Genet* **42**:498–503.

49. Comas I, Coscolla M, Luo T, Borrell S, Holt KE, Kato-Maeda M, Parkhill J, Malla B, Berg S, Thwaites G, Yeboah-Manu D, Bothamley G, Mei J, Wei L, Bentley S, Harris SR, Niemann S, Diel R, Aseffa A, Gao Q, Young D, Gagneux S. 2013. Out-of-Africa migration and Neolithic coexpansion of *Mycobacterium tuberculosis* with modern humans. *Nat Genet* **45**:1176–1182.

50. Firdessa R, Berg S, Hailu E, Schelling E, Gumi B, Erenso G, Gadisa E, Kiros T, Habtamu M, Hussein J, Zinsstag J, Robertson BD, Ameni G, Lohan AJ, Loftus B, Comas I, Gagneux S, Tschopp R, Yamuah L, Hewinson G, Gordon SV, Young DB, Aseffa A. 2013. Mycobacterial lineages causing pulmonary and extrapulmonary tuberculosis, Ethiopia. *Emerg Infect Dis* **19**:460–463.

51. Ho SY, Shapiro B. 2011. Skyline-plot methods for estimating demographic history from nucleotide sequences. *Mol Ecol Resour* **11**:423–434.

52. Drummond AJ, Rambaut A. 2007. BEAST: bayesian evolutionary analysis by sampling trees. *BMC Evol Biol* **7**:214.

53. Drummond AJ, Rambaut A, Shapiro B, Pybus OG. 2005. Bayesian coalescent inference of past population dynamics from molecular sequences. *Mol Biol Evol* **22**: 1185–1192.

54. Bocquet-Appel JP. 2011. When the world's population took off: the springboard of the Neolithic Demographic Transition. *Science* **333**:560–561.

55. Bos KI, Harkins KM, Herbig A, Coscolla M, Weber N, Comas I, Forrest SA, Bryant JM, Harris SR, Schuenemann VJ, Campbell TJ, Majander K, Wilbur AK, Guichon RA, Wolfe Steadman DL, Cook DC, Niemann S, Behr MA, Zumarraga M, Bastida R, Huson D, Nieselt K, Young D, Parkhill J, Buikstra JE, Gagneux S, Stone AC, Krause J. 2014. Pre-Columbian mycobacterial genomes reveal seals as a source of New World human tuberculosis. *Nature* **514**:494–497.

56. Bouwman AS, Kennedy SL, Müller R, Stephens RH, Holst M, Caffell AC, Roberts CA, Brown TA. 2012. Genotype of a historic strain of *Mycobacterium tuberculosis*. *Proc Natl Acad Sci USA* **109**:18511–18516.

57. Nicklisch N, Maixner F, Ganslmeier R, Friederich S, Dresely V, Meller H, Zink A, Alt KW. 2012. Rib lesions in skeletons from early Neolithic sites in Central Germany: on the trail of tuberculosis at the onset of agriculture. *Am J Phys Anthropol* **149**:391–404.

58. Coros A, DeConno E, Derbyshire KM. 2008. IS*6100*, a *Mycobacterium tuberculosis* complex-specific insertion sequence, is also present in the genome of *Mycobacterium smegmatis*, suggestive of lateral gene transfer among mycobacterial species. *J Bacteriol* **190**:3408–3410.

59. Müller R, Roberts CA, Brown TA. 2015. Complications in the study of ancient tuberculosis: non-specificity of IS*6100* PCRs. *Sci Technol Archeol Res* **1**:1–8.

60. Minnikin DE, Minnikin SM, Parlett JH, Goodfellow M, Magnusson M. 1984. Mycolic acid patterns of some species of *Mycobacterium*. *Arch Microbiol* **139**:225–231.

61. Minnikin DE, Parlett JH, Magnusson M, Ridell M, Lind A. 1984. Mycolic acid patterns of representatives of *Mycobacterium bovis* BCG. *J Gen Microbiol* **130**: 2733–2736.

62. Pepperell CS, Casto AM, Kitchen A, Granka JM, Cornejo OE, Holmes EC, Birren B, Galagan J, Feldman MW. 2013. The role of selection in shaping diversity of natural *M. tuberculosis* populations. *PLoS Pathog* **9**:e1003543 (Erratum: **9**[8]).

63. Kay GL, Sergeant MJ, Zhou Z, Chan JZ, Millard A, Quick J, Szikossy I, Pap I, Spigelman M, Loman NJ, Achtman M, Donoghue HD, Pallen MJ. 2015. Eighteenth-century genomes show that mixed infections were common at time of peak tuberculosis in Europe. *Nat Commun* **6**:6717.

64. Moser I, Prodinger WM, Hotzel H, Greenwald R, Lyashchenko KP, Bakker D, Gomis D, Seidler T, Ellenberger C, Hetzel U, Wuennemann K, Moisson P. 2008. *Mycobacterium pinnipedii*: transmission from South American sea lion (*Otaria byronia*) to Bactrian camel (*Camelus bactrianus bactrianus*) and Malayan tapirs (*Tapirus indicus*). *Vet Microbiol* **127**:399–406.

65. Kiers A, Klarenbeek A, Mendelts B, Van Soolingen D, Koëter G. 2008. Transmission of *Mycobacterium pinnipedii* to humans in a zoo with marine mammals. *Int J Tuberc Lung Dis* **12**:1469–1473.

66. Garnier T, Eiglmeier K, Camus JC, Medina N, Mansoor H, Pryor M, Duthoy S, Grondin S, Lacroix C, Monsempe C, Simon S, Harris B, Atkin R, Doggett J, Mayes R, Keating L, Wheeler PR, Parkhill J, Barrell BG, Cole ST, Gordon SV, Hewinson RG. 2003. The complete genome sequence of *Mycobacterium bovis*. *Proc Natl Acad Sci USA* **100**:7877–7882.

67. Pym AS, Brodin P, Brosch R, Huerre M, Cole ST. 2002. Loss of RD1 contributed to the attenuation of the live tuberculosis vaccines *Mycobacterium bovis* BCG and Mycobacterium microti. *Mol Microbiol* **46**:709–717.

68. Mostowy S, Cousins D, Behr MA. 2004. Genomic interrogation of the dassie bacillus reveals it as a unique RD1 mutant within the *Mycobacterium tuberculosis* complex. *J Bacteriol* **186**:104–109.

69. Alexander KA, Laver PN, Michel AL, Williams M, van Helden PD, Warren RM, Gey van Pittius NC. 2010. Novel *Mycobacterium tuberculosis* complex pathogen, *M. mungi*. *Emerg Infect Dis* **16**:1296–1299.

70. Roetzer A, Diel R, Kohl TA, Rückert C, Nübel U, Blom J, Wirth T, Jaenicke S, Schuback S, Rüsch-Gerdes S, Supply P, Kalinowski J, Niemann S. 2013. Whole genome sequencing versus traditional genotyping for investigation of a *Mycobacterium tuberculosis* outbreak: a longitudinal molecular epidemiological study. *PLoS Med* **10**:e1001387.

71. Mokrousov I. 2013. Insights into the origin, emergence, and current spread of a successful Russian clone of *Mycobacterium tuberculosis*. *Clin Microbiol Rev* **26:** 342–360.

72. Merker M, Blin C, Mona S, Duforet-Frebourg N, Lecher S, Willery E, Blum MG, Rüsch-Gerdes S, Mokrousov I, Aleksic E, Allix-Béquec C, Antierens A, Augustynowicz-Kopeć E, Ballif M, Barletta F, et al. 2015. Evolutionary history and global spread of the *Mycobacterium tuberculosis* Beijing lineage. *Nat Genet* **47:**242–249.

73. Linz B, Balloux F, Moodley Y, Manica A, Liu H, Roumagnac P, Falush D, Stamer C, Prugnolle F, van der Merwe SW, Yamaoka Y, Graham DY, Perez-Trallero E, Wadstrom T, Suerbaum S, Achtman M. 2007. An African origin for the intimate association between humans and *Helicobacter pylori*. *Nature* **445:**915–918.

74. Ramachandran S, Deshpande O, Roseman CC, Rosenberg NA, Feldman MW, Cavalli-Sforza LL. 2005. Support from the relationship of genetic and geographic distance in human populations for a serial founder effect originating in Africa. *Proc Natl Acad Sci USA* **102:**15942–15947.

75. Laruelle M, Peyrouse S. 2009. Cross-border minorities as cultural and economic mediators between China and central Asia. *China Eurasia Forum Quarterly* **7:** 93–119.

76. Wirth T. 2015. Massive lineage replacements and cryptic outbreaks of *Salmonella* Typhi in eastern and southern Africa. *Nat Genet* **47:**565–567.

77. Luo T, Comas I, Luo D, Lu B, Wu J, Wei L, Yang C, Liu Q, Gan M, Sun G, Shen X, Liu F, Gagneux S, Mei J, Lan R, Wan K, Gao Q. 2015. Southern East Asian origin and coexpansion of *Mycobacterium tuberculosis* Beijing family with Han Chinese. *Proc Natl Acad Sci USA* **112:** 8136–8141.

78. Pepperell CS, Granka JM, Alexander DC, Behr MA, Chui L, Gordon J, Guthrie JL, Jamieson FB, Langlois-Klassen D, Long R, Nguyen D, Wobeser W, Feldman MW. 2011. Dispersal of *Mycobacterium tuberculosis* via the Canadian fur trade. *Proc Natl Acad Sci USA* **108:** 6526–6531.

79. Lee RS, Radomski N, Proulx JF, Levade I, Shapiro BJ, McIntosh F, Soualhine H, Menzies D, Behr MA. 2015. Population genomics of *Mycobacterium tuberculosis* in the Inuit. *Proc Natl Acad Sci USA* **112:**13609–13614.

80. Walker TM, Ip CL, Harrell RH, Evans JT, Kapatai G, Dedicoat MJ, Eyre DW, Wilson DJ, Hawkey PM, Crook DW, Parkhill J, Harris D, Walker AS, Bowden R, Monk P, Smith EG, Peto TE. 2013. Whole-genome sequencing to delineate *Mycobacterium tuberculosis* outbreaks: a retrospective observational study. *Lancet Infect Dis* **13:**137–146.

81. Eldholm V, Monteserin J, Rieux A, Lopez B, Sobkowiak B, Ritacco V, Balloux F. 2015. Four decades of transmission of a multidrug-resistant *Mycobacterium tuberculosis* outbreak strain. *Nat Commun* **6:**7119.

82. Rado TA, Bates JH, Engel HW, Mankiewicz E, Murohashi T, Mizuguchi Y, Sula L. 1975. World Health Organization studies on bacteriophage typing of mycobacteria.

Subdivision of the species *Mycobacterium tuberculosis*. *Am Rev Respir Dis* **111:**459–468.

83. Hershberg R, Lipatov M, Small PM, Sheffer H, Niemann S, Homolka S, Roach JC, Kremer K, Petrov DA, Feldman MW, Gagneux S. 2008. High functional diversity in *Mycobacterium tuberculosis* driven by genetic drift and human demography. *PLoS Biol* **6:**e311.

84. Homolka S, Projahn M, Feuerriegel S, Ubben T, Diel R, Nübel U, Niemann S. 2012. High resolution discrimination of clinical *Mycobacterium tuberculosis* complex strains based on single nucleotide polymorphisms. *PLoS One* **7:**e39855.

85. Comas I, Homolka S, Niemann S, Gagneux S. 2009. Genotyping of genetically monomorphic bacteria: DNA sequencing in *Mycobacterium tuberculosis* highlights the limitations of current methodologies. *PLoS One* **4:**e7815.

86. Coll F, McNerney R, Guerra-Assunção JA, Glynn JR, Perdigão J, Viveiros M, Portugal I, Pain A, Martin N, Clark TG. 2014. A robust SNP barcode for typing *Mycobacterium tuberculosis* complex strains. *Nat Commun* **5:**4812.

87. Bryant JM, Schürch AC, van Deutekom H, Harris SR, de Beer JL, de Jager V, Kremer K, van Hijum SA, Siezen RJ, Borgdorff M, Bentley SD, Parkhill J, van Soolingen D. 2013. Inferring patient to patient transmission of *Mycobacterium tuberculosis* from whole genome sequencing data. *BMC Infect Dis* **13:**110.

88. Bryant JM, Harris SR, Parkhill J, Dawson R, Diacon AH, van Helden P, Pym A, Mahayiddin AA, Chuchottaworn C, Sanne IM, Louw C, Boeree MJ, Hoelscher M, McHugh TD, Bateson AL, Hunt RD, Mwaigwisya S, Wright L, Gillespie SH, Bentley SD. 2013. Whole-genome sequencing to establish relapse or re-infection with *Mycobacterium tuberculosis*: a retrospective observational study. *Lancet Respir Med* **1:** 786–792.

89. Ford CB, Lin PL, Chase MR, Shah RR, Iartchouk O, Galagan J, Mohaideen N, Ioerger TR, Sacchettini JC, Lipsitch M, Flynn JL, Fortune SM. 2011. Use of whole genome sequencing to estimate the mutation rate of *Mycobacterium tuberculosis* during latent infection. *Nat Genet* **43:**482–486.

90. Ewing G, Nicholls G, Rodrigo A. 2004. Using temporally spaced sequences to simultaneously estimate migration rates, mutation rate and population sizes in measurably evolving populations. *Genetics* **168:** 2407–2420.

91. Gray RR, Pybus OG, Salemi M. 2011. Measuring the temporal structure in serially-sampled phylogenies. *Methods Ecol Evol* **2:**437–445.

92. Drummond AJ, Pybus OG, Rambaut A, Forsberg R, Rodrigo AG. 2003. Measurably evolving populations. *Trends Ecol Evol* **18:**481–488.

93. Nübel U, Dordel J, Kurt K, Strommenger B, Westh H, Shukla SK, Zemlicková H, Leblois R, Wirth T, Jombart T, Balloux F, Witte W. 2010. A timescale for evolution, population expansion, and spatial spread of an emerging clone of methicillin-resistant *Staphylococcus aureus*. *PLoS Pathog* **6:**e1000855.

94. Stegger M, Wirth T, Andersen PS, Skov RL, De Grassi A, Simões PM, Tristan A, Petersen A, Aziz M, Kiil K, Cirković I, Udo EE, del Campo R, Vuopio-Varkila J, Ahmad N, Tokajian S, Peters G, Schaumburg F, Olsson-Liljequist B, Givskov M, Driebe EE, Vigh HE, Shittu A, Ramdani-Bougessa N, Rasigade JP, Price LB, Vandenesch F, Larsen AR, Laurent F. 2014. Origin and evolution of European community-acquired methicillin-resistant *Staphylococcus aureus*. *MBio* 5:e01044-14.

95. Wielgoss S, Barrick JE, Tenaillon O, Cruveiller S, Chane-Woon-Ming B, Médigue C, Lenski RE, Schneider D, Andrews BJ. 2011. Mutation rate inferred from synonymous substitutions in a long-term evolution experiment with *Escherichia coli*. *G3 (Bethesda)* 1:183–186.

96. Lee H, Popodi E, Tang H, Foster PL. 2012. Rate and molecular spectrum of spontaneous mutations in the bacterium *Escherichia coli* as determined by whole-genome sequencing. *Proc Natl Acad Sci USA* 109: E2774–E2783.

97. Kennemann L, Didelot X, Aebischer T, Kuhn S, Drescher B, Droege M, Reinhardt R, Correa P, Meyer TF, Josenhans C, Falush D, Suerbaum S. 2011. *Helicobacter pylori* genome evolution during human infection. *Proc Natl Acad Sci USA* 108:5033–5038.

98. Didelot X, Nell S, Yang I, Woltemate S, van der Merwe S, Suerbaum S. 2013. Genomic evolution and transmission of *Helicobacter pylori* in two South African families. *Proc Natl Acad Sci USA* 110:13880–13885.

99. Linz B, Windsor HM, McGraw JJ, Hansen LM, Gajewski JP, Tomsho LP, Hake CM, Solnick JV, Schuster SC, Marshall BJ. 2014. A mutation burst during the acute phase of *Helicobacter pylori* infection in humans and rhesus macaques. *Nat Commun* 5:4165.

100. Biek R, Pybus OG, Lloyd-Smith JO, Didelot X. 2015. Measurably evolving pathogens in the genomic era. *Trends Ecol Evol* 30:306–313.

101. Ho SY, Larson G. 2006. Molecular clocks: when times are a-changin'. *Trends Genet* 22:79–83.

102. Ho SY, Lanfear R, Bromham L, Phillips MJ, Soubrier J, Rodrigo AG, Cooper A. 2011. Time-dependent rates of molecular evolution. *Mol Ecol* 20:3087–3101.

103. Bandelt HJ. 2008. Clock debate: when times are a-changin': time dependency of molecular rate estimates: tempest in a teacup. *Heredity (Edinb)* 100:1–2.

104. Burridge CP, Craw D, Fletcher D, Waters JM. 2008. Geological dates and molecular rates: fish DNA sheds light on time dependency. *Mol Biol Evol* 25:624–633.

105. Ho SY, Phillips MJ, Cooper A, Drummond AJ. 2005. Time dependency of molecular rate estimates and systematic overestimation of recent divergence times. *Mol Biol Evol* 22:1561–1568.

106. Penny D. 2005. Evolutionary biology: relativity for molecular clocks. *Nature* 436:183–184.

107. Feng L, Reeves PR, Lan R, Ren Y, Gao C, Zhou Z, Ren Y, Cheng J, Wang W, Wang J, Qian W, Li D, Wang L. 2008. A recalibrated molecular clock and independent origins for the cholera pandemic clones. *PLoS One* 3:e4053.

108. Jamrozy D, Kallonen T. 2015. Looking at Beijing's skyline. *Nat Rev Microbiol* 13:528.

109. Rodrigo A, Bertels F, Heled J, Noder R, Shearman H, Tsai P. 2008. The perils of plenty: what are we going to do with all these genes? *Philos Trans R Soc Lond B Biol Sci* 363:3893–3902.

110. Martincorena I, Seshasayee AS, Luscombe NM. 2012. Evidence of non-random mutation rates suggests an evolutionary risk management strategy. *Nature* 485: 95–98.

111. Dos Vultos T, Mestre O, Tonjum T, Gicquel B. 2009. DNA repair in *Mycobacterium tuberculosis* revisited. *FEMS Microbiol Rev* 33:471–487.

112. Boshoff HI, Reed MB, Barry CE III, Mizrahi V. 2003. DnaE2 polymerase contributes to in vivo survival and the emergence of drug resistance in *Mycobacterium tuberculosis*. *Cell* 113:183–193.

113. Ebrahimi-Rad M, Bifani P, Martin C, Kremer K, Samper S, Rauzier J, Kreiswirth B, Blazquez J, Jouan M, van Soolingen D, Gicquel B. 2003. Mutations in putative mutator genes of *Mycobacterium tuberculosis* strains of the W-Beijing family. *Emerg Infect Dis* 9: 838–845.

114. Ford CB, Shah RR, Maeda MK, Gagneux S, Murray MB, Cohen T, Johnston JC, Gardy J, Lipsitch M, Fortune SM. 2013. *Mycobacterium tuberculosis* mutation rate estimates from different lineages predict substantial differences in the emergence of drug-resistant tuberculosis. *Nat Genet* 45:784–790.

115. Giraud A, Matic I, Tenaillon O, Clara A, Radman M, Fons M, Taddei F. 2001. Costs and benefits of high mutation rates: adaptive evolution of bacteria in the mouse gut. *Science* 291:2606–2608.

116. Oliver A, Cantón R, Campo P, Baquero F, Blázquez J. 2000. High frequency of hypermutable *Pseudomonas aeruginosa* in cystic fibrosis lung infection. *Science* 288:1251–1254.

117. Mizrahi V, Andersen SJ. 1998. DNA repair in *Mycobacterium tuberculosis*. What have we learnt from the genome sequence? *Mol Microbiol* 29:1331–1339.

118. Ng VH, Cox JS, Sousa AO, MacMicking JD, McKinney JD. 2004. Role of KatG catalase-peroxidase in mycobacterial pathogenesis: countering the phagocyte oxidative burst. *Mol Microbiol* 52:1291–1302.

119. Sassetti CM, Rubin EJ. 2003. Genetic requirements for mycobacterial survival during infection. *Proc Natl Acad Sci USA* 100:12989–12994.

120. Orlando L, Cooper A. 2014. Using ancient DNA to understand evolutionary and ecological processes. *Annu Rev Ecol Evol Syst* 45:573–598.

121. Green RE, Krause J, Ptak SE, Briggs AW, Ronan MT, Simons JF, Du L, Egholm M, Rothberg JM, Paunovic M, Pääbo S. 2006. Analysis of one million base pairs of Neanderthal DNA. *Nature* 444:330–336.

122. Dabney J, Meyer M, Pääbo S. 2013. Ancient DNA damage. *Cold Spring Harb Perspect Biol* 5:a012567.

123. Green RE, Krause J, Briggs AW, Maricic T, Stenzel U, Kircher M, Patterson N, Li H, Zhai W, Fritz MH-Y, Hansen NF, Durand EY, Malaspinas A-S, Hensen JD, Marques-Bonet T, et al. 2010. A draft sequence of the Neanderthal genome. *Science* 328:710–722.

124. Fu Q, Li H, Moorjani P, Jay F, Slepchenko SM, Bondarev AA, Johnson PL, Aximu-Petri A, Prüfer K, de Filippo C, Meyer M, Zwyns N, Salazar-García DC, Kuzmin YV, Keates SG, Kosintsev PA, Razhev DI, Richards MP, Peristov NV, Lachmann M, Douka K, Higham TF, Slatkin M, Hublin JJ, Reich D, Kelso J, Viola TB, Pääbo S. 2014. Genome sequence of a 45,000-year-old modern human from western Siberia. *Nature* 514:445–449.

125. Pääbo S. 2015. The diverse origins of the human gene pool. *Nat Rev Genet* 16:313–314.

126. Prüfer K, Racimo F, Patterson N, Jay F, Sankararaman S, Sawyer S, Heinze A, Renaud G, Sudmant PH, de Filippo C, Li H, Mallick S, Dannemann M, Fu Q, Kircher M, Kuhlwilm M, Lachmann M, Meyer M, Ongyerth M, Siebauer M, Theunert C, Tandon A, Moorjani P, Pickrell J, Mullikin JC, Vohr SH, Green RE, Hellmann I, Johnson PL, Blanche H, Cann H, Kitzman JO, Shendure J, Eichler EE, Lein ES, Bakken TE, Golovanova LV, Doronichev VB, Shunkov MV, Derevianko AP, Viola B, Slatkin M, Reich D, Kelso J, Pääbo S. 2014. The complete genome sequence of a Neanderthal from the Altai Mountains. *Nature* 505:43–49.

127. Meyer M, Kircher M, Gansauge MT, Li H, Racimo F, Mallick S, Schraiber JG, Jay F, Prüfer K, de Filippo C, Sudmant PH, Alkan C, Fu Q, Do R, Rohland N, Tandon A, Siebauer M, Green RE, Bryc K, Briggs AW, Stenzel U, Dabney J, Shendure J, Kitzman J, Hammer MF, Shunkov MV, Derevianko AP, Patterson N, Andrés AM, Eichler EE, Slatkin M, Reich D, Kelso J, Pääbo S. 2012. A high-coverage genome sequence from an archaic Denisovan individual. *Science* 338:222–226.

128. Bos KI, Schuenemann VJ, Golding GB, Burbano HA, Waglechner N, Coombes BK, McPhee JB, DeWitte SN, Meyer M, Schmedes S, Wood J, Earn DJ, Herring DA, Bauer P, Poinar HN, Krause J. 2011. A draft genome of *Yersinia pestis* from victims of the Black Death. *Nature* 478:506–510.

129. Rasmussen S, Allentoft ME, Nielsen K, Orlando L, Sikora M, Sjögren KG, Pedersen AG, Schubert M, Van Dam A, Kapel CM, Nielsen HB, Brunak S, Avetisyan P, Epimakhov A, Khalyapin MV, Gnuni A, Kriiska A, Lasak I, Metspalu M, Moiseyev V, Gromov A, Pokutta D, Saag L, Varul L, Yepiskoposyan L, Sicheritz-Pontén T, Foley RA, Lahr MM, Nielsen R, Kristiansen K, Willerslev E. 2015. Early divergent strains of *Yersinia pestis* in Eurasia 5,000 years ago. *Cell* 163:571–582.

130. Pálfi G, Dutour O, Perrin P, Sola C, Zink A. 2015. Tuberculosis in evolution. *Tuberculosis (Edinb)* 95(Suppl 1): S1–S3.

131. Pálfi G, Maixner F, Maczel M, Molnár E, Pósa A, Kristóf LA, Marcsik A, Balázs J, Masson M, Paja L, Palkó A, Szentgyörgyi R, Nerlich A, Zink A, Dutour O. 2015. Unusual spinal tuberculosis in an Avar Age skeleton (Csongrád-Felgyő, Ürmös-tanya, Hungary): A morphological and biomolecular study. *Tuberculosis (Edinb)* 95(Suppl 1):S29–S34.

132. Pósa A, Maixner F, Mende BG, Köhler K, Osztás A, Sola C, Dutour O, Masson M, Molnár E, Pálfi G, Zink A. 2015. Tuberculosis in Late Neolithic-Early Copper Age human skeletal remains from Hungary. *Tuberculosis(Edinb)* 95(Suppl 1):S18–S22.

133. Lee OY, Wu HH, Besra GS, Rothschild BM, Spigelman M, Hershkovitz I, Bar-Gal GK, Donoghue HD, Minnikin DE. 2015. Lipid biomarkers provide evolutionary signposts for the oldest known cases of tuberculosis. *Tuberculosis (Edinb)* 95(Suppl 1):S127–S132.

Tuberculosis and the Tubercle Bacillus, 2nd ed.
Edited by William R. Jacobs, Jr., Helen McShane, Valerie Mizrahi, and Ian M. Orme
© 2018 American Society for Microbiology, Washington, DC
doi:10.1128/microbiolspec.TBTB2-0022-2016

Impact of Genetic Diversity on the Biology of *Mycobacterium tuberculosis* Complex Strains

21

Stefan Niemann,[1,2] Matthias Merker,[1]
Thomas Kohl,[1] and Philip Supply[3]

INTRODUCTION

The causative agents of human and animal tuberculosis (TB), *Mycobacterium tuberculosis* and the other members of the *M. tuberculosis* complex, remain a major cause of human mortality and morbidity and have a massive socioeconomic impact (1) (http://www.stoptb.org/assets/documents/events/meetings/amsterdam_conference/ahlburg.pdf). According to the latest estimates, around 100 million new tuberculosis (TB) infections, 8.5 million new notified TB cases, and 1.5 million deaths due to TB occur annually (2, 184).

Particularly worrisome is the global emergence of multidrug-resistant (MDR, defined as resistance to at least isoniazid and rifampin) TB strains, which poses a serious threat to TB control (2–4). As an example of the utmost importance of the problem in some world regions, in a nationwide survey performed in Belarus in 2010–2011, every third new TB patient was found to be infected with an MDR strain (5). Only approximately 20% of the estimated half-million MDR-TB patients are presumably properly diagnosed and treated with adequate second-line treatment regimens (4). Ineffective treatments in the majority of the cases result in high mortality and continued transmission, as well as amplification of resistance leading to tens of thousands of nearly untreatable, extensively drug-resistant (XDR, defined as MDR plus additional resistance to any fluoroquinolone and at least one of three injectable drugs, i.e., amikacin, kanamycin, or capreomycin) TB cases (184). Cases with XDR strains that are even resis-

tant to the two newest anti-TB drugs, delamanid and bedaquiline, have already been reported (6, 7).

Well-known human-related, socioepidemiological factors, ranging from bad living conditions, such as overcrowding, poverty, malnutrition, war, and displacement, to underfunding or even breakdown of TB control systems, contribute to this situation. As one of the earliest recognized contributors to susceptibility to TB disease, malnutrition has been shown to impair anti-TB immunity in infected individuals (8, 9). The key role played by host immunity is also illustrated by the interaction between HIV and TB infection. Coinfection with HIV magnifies the TB burden especially in countries of sub-Saharan Africa (2, 10). The risk of developing a TB disease is 20 to 30 times higher in TB-HIV-coinfected individuals than in HIV-uninfected individuals with a TB infection (11, 12). Accordingly, differences in immune status and other host- and host environment-related factors have thus been considered for a long time as the major drivers of the course and transmission of infection, while the potential influence of pathogen strain variation was considered unimportant (13), despite some early indications for disparities in virulence properties among *M. tuberculosis* complex (MTBC) strains (14–16). This prevalent conception tended to be reinforced by findings from initial molecular exploration, which showed restricted polymorphism in a set of structural genes among MTBC strains (17, 18).

This paradigm has progressively changed as a result of deeper molecular investigation of the diversity and

[1]Molecular Mycobacteriology, Forschungszentrum Borstel, Leibniz-Zentrum für Medizin und Biowissenschaften, 23845 Borstel, Germany;
[2]German Center for Infection Research (DZIF), partner site Borstel, 23845 Borstel, Germany; [3]Univ. Lille, CNRS, Inserm, CHU Lille, Institut Pasteur de Lille, U1019 - UMR 8204 - CIIL - Centre d'Infection et d'Immunité de Lille, F-59000 Lille, France.

structure of the TB strain population and of detailed comparative analyses of biological properties linked to different strain genetic backgrounds. Systematic genotyping, whole-genome sequencing (WGS), and comparative genomics of TB strains from human and animal sources worldwide revealed that the MTBC population is composed of multiple clonal lineages and sublineages (Fig. 1), marked by a variety of specific mutations such as single nucleotide polymorphisms (SNPs)—a majority of which are nonsynonymous—and genomic deletions (19–35). Moreover, a nonclonal and 20- to 30-fold more diversified population of tubercle bacilli was discovered for the sole *Mycobacterium canettii*, representing several early branching lineages that predated the emergence of the common ancestor of the MTBC (36–42).

Most of these lineages are characterized by marked differential distribution, where some are preferentially associated with distinct animal hosts, while others, in-

cluding *M. tuberculosis sensu stricto*, show relatively stable associations with human populations from distinct world regions (43). This pronounced phyloecological and phylogeographical structure suggests parallel evolution and thus potential biological adaptation of individual strain lineages to their preferential host populations (29, 44, 45). Potential (co)adaptation is also suggested by striking parallels in the evolutionary histories and demographic changes between the pathogen and its human host, suggesting a long-lasting association starting from a common African origin (38, 39, 44) followed by episodes of comigration out of Africa and coexpansion at different steps of human population densification (31, 33–35, 46). This hypothesis of coadaptation is supported by multiple lines of evidence indicating covariation between strain genotypes and clinical, epidemiological, or biological correlates of pathogenicity or epidemicity, as measured in human

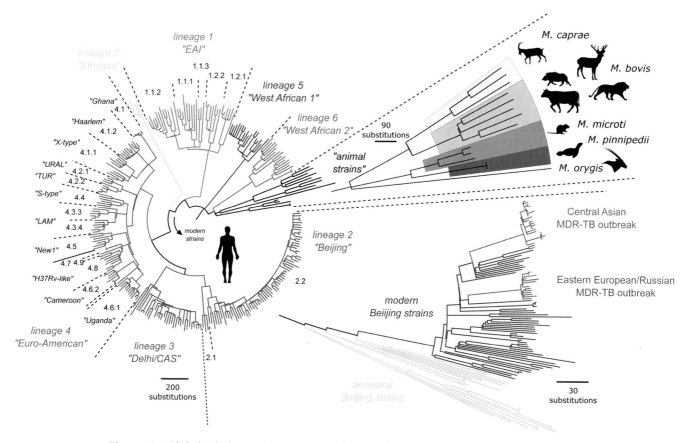

Figure 1 Global phylogenetic structure of *M. tuberculosis* complex (MTBC) strains presented in a neighbor joining tree with 1,000 bootstrap replicates based on 35,577 variable sites. MTBC isolates can be classified into seven major lineages that are often composed of further geographically confined subgroups. So-called "modern" MTBC lineages (lineages 2, 3, 4) are distributed worldwide, whereas infections with "ancestral" MTBC strains are mainly restricted to western and eastern Africa. (Sequence data compiled from Comas et al. [31] and Merker et al. [33]).

populations, or in animal or cellular infection models (reviewed in references 13 and 43).

The following sections will provide an overview of this current knowledge on the pathogen diversity at different population levels and on its links with pathobiology and drug resistance evolution and transmission, with a particular emphasis on cases with experimentally identified molecular determinants.

GLOBAL GENETIC DIVERSITY OF TB BACILLI

A significant part of our current knowledge on the genetic diversity of the TB bacilli has been gained through molecular epidemiological studies, primarily focused on analyzing TB transmission and strain population structures in multiple world regions. Before the progressive deployment of next-generation sequencing, these studies mostly exploited different types of highly polymorphic, repetitive DNA elements as genetic markers to identify and differentiate strains. International standardization of the genotyping methods facilitated gradual acquisition of global pictures of strain distribution, revealing distinct families or groups of closely related strains and genotypes that predominate in different world regions (e.g., references 19, 22, 47, and 48).

IS*6110* fingerprinting, detecting banding patterns associated to the insertion element IS*6110* present in variable copy numbers and positions in MTBC genomes, was used as a first standard for genotyping of clinical isolates for more than a decade (49). Because of its slow time-to-result and labor intensiveness, IS*6110* fingerprinting has been replaced by PCR-based spoligotyping (50) and mostly by MIRU-VNTR typing (51–53). Spoligotyping interrogates the presence or absence of 43 variable spacer sequences in the direct repeat (DR) region of MTBC genomes (50, 54). Although the low-resolution power of spoligotyping precludes its use as a sole tool for identification at strain level, spoligotype signatures reflect, to a certain degree, the main clonal (sub)lineages of the MTBC (19, 21, 55, 56). In its standard format (48), MIRU-VNTR typing analyzes 24 loci containing variable numbers of tandem repeats (VNTR) of genetic elements including mycobacterial interspersed repetitive units (MIRUs) (51, 52, 57–59). Compared with spoligotyping, 24-locus MIRU-VNTR typing generates a higher-resolution power and performs better for identification of phylogenetic lineages as defined by canonical phylogenetic markers (see below) (35, 48, 53, 56, 60). An additional consensus set of four hypervariable MIRU-VNTR loci has been defined, but its use is primarily restricted to focused mo-

lecular epidemiological analysis of large 24-locus-based clusters, especially in cases of prevalent clonal complexes of Beijing or other genotypes (61, 62). The portable barcode-like data sets or 24-number genotypes generated by spoligotyping and standard MIRU-VNTR typing, respectively, allowed the construction of large databases, such as MIRU-VNTR*plus* (63, 64) and the SpolDB/SITVIT databases (20, 22, 23, 65), compiling and classifying genotypes into families or sublineages. As of April 2016, these databases respectively hosted approximately 19,000 different MIRU-VNTR types (based on the 15 most discriminatory loci; http://www.miru-vntrplus.org/MIRU/types15.faces) and more than 7,000 different spoligotypes (http://www.pasteur-guadeloupe.fr:8081/SITVIT_ONLINE/description.jsp#) collected worldwide. As such, they probably give the best qualitative view of the global diversity of TB bacilli.

However, these relatively rapidly evolving DNA repeat-based markers typically show homoplasy, as indicated, for example, for the evolution of a MIRU-VNTR marker in the BCG strain phylogeny (52), and are thus not optimal for phylogenetic reconstruction (56). Therefore, most robust phylogenetic structures of the MTBC strain population have been obtained by analysis of regions of genomic differences (RDs)/large sequence polymorphisms (LSPs) occurring as unique event polymorphisms (MTBC branch-specific) (27–29, 44, 66), and other canonical approaches including multilocus sequence typing (18, 26, 67), SNP typing (32, 68–70), and ultimately WGS (30–32). Despite variable levels of resolution and specific biases inherent to some marker sets, strain groupings into lineages obtained by these different approaches are largely congruent. As a result, a global phylogeny has emerged, which includes seven main lineages of human-associated strains (including *M. tuberculosis sensu stricto*, in lineages 1 to 4 and 7, as well as *Mycobacterium africanum* in lineages 5 and 6) with clear geographic association, as well as at least one branch of strains associated with different mammalian species such as *Mycobacterium bovis*, *M. caprae*, *M. pinnipedii*, and *M. microti*.

Recent studies based on WGS analysis of approximately 260 strains representing the global diversity of the MTBC found a maximum genetic distance of 2,200 SNPs separating any human and animal strains, and a maximum of about 1,800 SNPs between any two human strains in this phylogeny (31, 43, 71). This restricted level of diversity, as well as the vertical inheritance of most RDs/LSPs and SNPs, suggests that the whole MTBC strain population results from recent clonal expansion from few or a single common ancestor(s) (that probably emerged from a *M. canettii*-like pool; see below) (25, 27, 29, 30). Nevertheless, different branches with distinct geographic association are even discernible within some of the main lineages (e.g., in lineages 2 and 4, see below). To designate them, different nomenclature systems, based on naming, color, or hierarchical numbering, have been defined based on branch-defining SNP sets, RDs/LSPs, and/or WGS data (13, 30–32, 72).

In order to provide a synthetic view of the MTBC population structure, we computed a neighbor-joining tree with 1,000 bootstrap replicates based on 35,577 SNPs derived from 283 MTBC strains representing the global strain diversity (Fig. 1), on which the correspondence between different main nomenclatures (including that principally based on spoligotyping [22]) is shown. The most ancestral human-associated lineages (namely, 1, 5, 6, and 7) are all linked to Africa, either to western

(lineages 5 and 6) or eastern Africa (lineages 1 and 7), which is in favor of an African origin of the MTBC (see below). In contrast, the strains of more recently derived "modern" lineages show a distribution rather centered on Asia (lineage 3), or even broader, intercontinental distributions (lineages 2 and 4), but still with strong phylogeographical signatures at sublineage levels. For instance, ancestral branches of lineage 2 (alias Beijing) are mainly associated with patients from East Asia, whereas strains from modern branches of the same lineage are most frequently obtained from patients from Eastern Europe or Central Asia (Fig. 2) (33). Likewise, different sublineages within lineage 4 are connected with distinct regions in Europe (e.g., 4.1.2, alias Haarlem), in western Africa (e.g., 4.1, alias Ghana; 4.6.2, Cameroon), or Latin America/Mediterranean (e.g., 4.3.3 and 4.3.4, alias LAM) (19, 21, 22, 32, 60, 73).

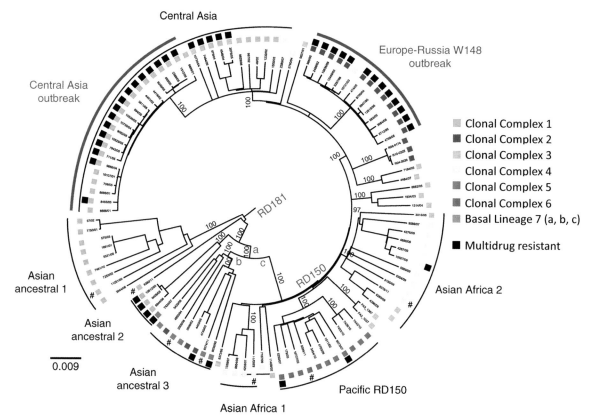

Figure 2 Phylogenetic reconstruction of the MTBC Beijing lineage population. Midpoint-rooted maximum-likelihood tree based on 110 genomes and a total of 6,001 concatenated SNPs. Characteristic mutations differentiating modern and ancestral Beijing strain types are mapped on the tree—*mutT4* encoding p.Arg48Gly (branch a), *ogt* encoding p.Arg37Leu (branch b), and *mutT2* encoding p.Gly58Arg (branch c)—as is the absence of the RD181 and RD150 regions of difference. Black squares correspond to strains with an MDR or XDR phenotype, and a number sign indicates strains lacking drug susceptibility test information. Numbers on branches correspond to bootstrap values. The tree topology remains the same when H37Rv is used as an outgroup (Merker et al. [33]).

Interestingly, such sympatric association between strain genetic lineage and patient's origin is not only visible at a global level, when analyzing isolates from patients living on different continents, but often seen at a local level as well. Indeed, studies showed that in a cosmopolitan urban center, transmission occurs more frequently in sympatric strain-host combinations than in allopatric strain-host pathogen combinations (29, 44). In addition, this sympatric association appears looser in immunodeficient patients, suggesting that impairment in host immunity could increase vulnerability to infection with allopatric strains (44, 74). Along the same lines, a study documented that patients who had TB caused by an allopatric strain were more likely to have pulmonary impairment after TB than patients with TB caused by a sympatric strain (75). Taken together, these observations are suggestive of differential adaptation of *M. tuberculosis* lineages to different human populations, and are thus supporting the hypothesis of coevolution between the pathogen and its host (see below). This hypothesis is also suggested by studies suggesting a correlation between protection against TB caused by strains of a particular lineage and certain human gene variants involved in anti-infective responses (76, 77).

The hypothesis of host-adapted lineages is also supported by the strong association between the different animal-related MTBC branches and their respective host ranges. While *M. bovis* strains can be found in a range of mammalian species (cow, badger, wild boar, deer, lion, etc.), other strain types show a clearly more restricted host range, such as *M. microti* (vole), *M. caprae* (goat), *M. pinnipedii* (seal), and *M. orygis* (oryx) (46). It has been proposed to regard these different MTBC members as a series of host-adapted ecotypes, rather than as different species (45, 78). As indicated in a following section, experimental evidence supportive for such adaptation has been obtained, which links differences in virulence to distinct phylogenetically conserved genomic differences between *M. microti* or *M. bovis* with *M. tuberculosis* (79, 80).

M. canettii strains appear as clear outliers relative to the (classical) MTBC strains. All of the hundred or so *M. canettii* isolates identified so far have been obtained from human TB cases, with an extreme pattern of geographic restriction, because most isolates have been obtained from patients living or having lived in or near the Horn of Africa, especially in the Djibouti region (38–41, 81–83). Despite this strong geographic confinement, the numbers of SNPs found among their genomes, and between them and MTBC genomes, range from approximately 9,000 to 65,000, thus exceeding by far the diversity of the entire MTBC strain population found worldwide. In addition, in contrast to the highly clonal MTBC genomes, *M. canettii* genomes show multiple traces of interstrain horizontal gene transfers, suggesting the potential existence of an environmental reservoir (36, 37, 42). Together with their larger genomes, this diversified and nonclonal population structure positions them in evolutionarily early branching lineages of tubercle bacilli that predated the emergence of the most recent common ancestor of the MTBC (36, 37, 84, 85).

This strong association of these earliest branches of human TB bacilli with East Africa and the systematics links of the deepest branching, human-associated lineages (1, 5–7) of the MTBC with Africa conjointly point to an African origin of the MTBC ancestor shared with its human host (36, 38, 39, 44). Based on dating of the age of the MTBC and its main lineages, several studies proposed that the MTBC then started to differentiate by accompanying human migration out of Africa perhaps between 40,000 and 80,000 years ago, although conflicting evidence exists for such timing (31, 35, 71, 86). The reconstructed MTBC phylogeny suggests that animal-associated lineages then diverged from human-associated strains, perhaps at the time of animal domestication around 10,000 years ago (27, 28, 35, 67). Such stable longitudinal host-pathogen association thus offers favorable conditions for coadaptation to evolve.

As reviewed further below, the latter hypothesis is supported by results from multiple studies indicating lineage-specific pathobiological characteristics, some of which were directly linked to lineage-specific polymorphisms.

Intrapatient Diversity

As a corollary of the general belief in the uniformity of the overall pathogen's population, TB patients have often been assumed to be infected by a single MTBC strain. Repeated reporting of cases of simultaneous (so-called mixed) infection by two strains with clearly independent genetic backgrounds led researchers to reconsider this prevalent dogma of single clonal infection, at least in high TB prevalence settings (87–91). Moreover, an original infecting strain can undergo microevolution in individual patients leading to clonal subpopulations of close genetic variants, especially during prolonged, chronic disease resulting, for example, from delayed diagnostics (92–95). As an illustration, single locus differences in MIRU-VNTR genotypes are occasionally seen among clonal variants from a same patient (48, 96). As a reflection of the higher resolution afforded by WGS, limited genome sequence variation, most often by 1 to 5 SNPs, is more regularly observed among intrapatient variants (95). However, in some cases, intrapatient variants were found to mutually differ by up to 12 to 14 SNPs (97), which exceeds the limit generally considered for defining recent human-to-human transmission events (95, 98, 99). Such examples suggest that strict universal thresholds of genetic drift, as detected by WGS or even by MIRU-VNTR typing, might not be applicable for delimiting TB transmission in all situations (48, 97, 100).

In addition, WGS analyses of serial isolates from patients undergoing longitudinal treatments have shown complex patterns of evolution that can develop under anti-TB drug selective pressure in some cases, leading to stepwise acquisition of drug resistance from a drug sensitive to an MDR or XDR *M. tuberculosis* strain. These patterns are characterized by transient emergence of distinct variants carrying different drug-resistance-conferring mutations in combination with distinct potential compensatory mutations or hitchhiked neutral mutations, leading to fixation of the most fit and resistant mutation combinations and clones (100–102). In addition to also potentially confusing inferences of TB transmission, such simultaneous coexistence of drug-sensitive and (multi)drug-resistant strains or strain/clone variants during the course of infection can complicate the diagnostics of resistance and the definition of the most appropriate treatment at given time points, potentially leading to amplification of resistance and ultimately to unsuccessful therapy (101–104).

Biological Impact of Genetic Diversity

The notion that the influence of the infecting strain type on the outcome of TB infection was unimportant compared with host (e.g., immunity) or environmental factors (indoor air pollution, passive smoking) has long prevailed. However, some historical data have already documented significant pathobiological differences among some MTBC strain types. The known natural attenuation of *M. microti* for humans, leading to its use as an alternative vaccine to *M. bovis* BCG (14), and contrasting to fulminant TB forms caused in voles and shrews (105), represents some of the clearest evidence arguing for different host-adapted types (also termed ecotypes [45]) in the MTBC. Similar inferences could also be made from conclusions of a nationwide population study in Denmark, indicating a much lower risk of progression to pulmonary TB among patients infected with *M. bovis* than *M. tuberculosis* (15). Other old studies investigated potential physiopathological differences among human TB isolates. For instance,

Mitchison and colleagues reported that cultured isolates from South Indian patients were, on the average, of lower virulence, and had a wider range of virulence when infecting the guinea pig than cultured isolates from British patients (16). Moreover, considerable variability was observed in the same study among tuberculin-induced delayed-type hypersensitivity reactions in guinea pigs infected by South Indian isolates, indicating differences in elicited immune responses. These data thus already suggested significant variability in virulence-related properties within the human-adapted, *M. tuberculosis* compartment of the MTBC, potentially even among distinct strain types circulating within a geographic region.

With the use of molecular typing tools and/or WGS, multiple additional hints and indications of the influence of the strain (genetic) background have been obtained, e.g., by field studies looking at clinical or epidemiological correlates of virulence and transmissibility of strains from different MTBC lineages (e.g., references 81, 106–110), or by identifying strain- or (sub)lineage-specific differences in various virulence-related features, mycobacterial transcriptomic responses, or cytokine induction profiles in animal or cellular infection models (e.g., references 36, 111–117). Such multiple indications of consequences of the genomic diversity have been the subject of previous extensive reviews, including recent ones (13, 43, 118–120). Therefore, we will hereafter rather emphasize cases of formally proven and still debated links between biological and genomic differences.

Evidence for the Potential of Biological Variation from Genomics

Predominant patterns of genome sequence variation observed among TB strains independently suggest significant potential for biological disparities, even within the relatively restricted limits of genetic diversity in the MTBC. Indeed, one of the key findings that recurrently resulted from genome comparisons or targeted gene-sequencing analysis of diverse strain collections is that roughly two-thirds of the SNPs found in MTBC genes are nonsynonymous and thus potentially have functional consequences (18, 67, 121, 122). In addition, the different genomic deletion regions, including those specifically marking the different (sub)lineages in the phylogeny and indicating the reductive clonal evolution of the MTBC, can exceed 10 kbp and involve blocks of genes of different functional categories (27–29, 66, 123–125). Furthermore, different massive genomic duplication events, spanning large gene blocks that can exceed 500 kbp and could thus significantly impact biological properties, have been detected in strains from different MTBC (sub)lineages (126, 127). Last, the highly variable distribution of insertion sites of IS*6110* elements linked to dynamic transposition into various coding or gene regulation regions, and also associated with some genomic deletions through homologous recombination between proximal copies, can also translate into significant phenotypic variation at strain level (79, 123, 128–132).

However, a substantial part of these nonsynonymous SNPs and genomic duplications and deletions may not be directly associated with host-imposed selective pressure and adaptation to different animal or human populations, even in the case of fixed, lineage-defining polymorphisms. Indeed, the successive bacterial population bottlenecks encountered during serial TB transmission, characteristically involving few bacilli or even one, predictably favor fixation by genetic drift (random evolution) rather than by natural selection (45, 67). Such conditions of relaxed purifying selection in small successive founder populations may even contribute to fix by chance some slightly deleterious nonsynonymous SNPs or genomic deletions, especially in the highly clonal context of the MTBC (with little to no detectable trace of horizontal transfer) (25, 29, 133). Moreover, as another consequence of clonal evolution, most of such (sub)lineage-defining polymorphisms might be fixed just by linkage to only a few or even one highly selected locus in the original ancestor of the (sub)lineage (hitchhiking effect [45, 134]). In addition, part of the polymorphisms detected among strains likely result from genetic drift or from selective pressure under *in vitro* culture conditions, rather than from selective pressure *in vivo*, as illustrated, for example, for one of the large genomic duplications mentioned above (135).

As a matter of fact, only a limited number of genetic polymorphisms have hitherto been experimentally demonstrated, by mutagenesis and/or genetic complementation, to account for significant virulence differences among TB strains. Such demonstration has been obtained mostly for more prominent variation between *M. tuberculosis* and other MTBC members or *M. canettii*, as illustrated below.

Genomic Differences Linked to Biological Differences Between Animal-Associated and Human-Associated MTBC Lineages

Natural attenuation of *M. microti* has been linked to a specific 14-kbp genomic deletion, called RD1(mic), which partially overlaps the RD1 deletion involved in the attenuation by serial *in vitro* passages of the *M. bovis* BCG vaccine (80, 124, 136–138). This deletion affects the *esx1* locus, which in *M. tuberculosis* en-

codes a type VII secretion system driving the secretion of major T-cell antigens ESAT6 and CFP-10 and is required for virulence (139, 140). Complementation of this deletion by knock-in with the intact *M. tuberculosis* region resulted in increased virulence in infected mice, both for BCG and *M. microti*, and in a change in colony morphotypes linked to cell envelope alteration in the case of BCG (80).

A few other genetic polymorphisms, shared by *M. bovis* and other animal-adapted branches and *M. africanum* (MTBC lineage 6), have been recently demonstrated to contribute to common differences relative to *M. tuberculosis* (79). Different lines of evidence suggest that, as animal-adapted strains, *M. africanum* strains are less virulent in, and/or transmissible among, humans than *M. tuberculosis*. As for *M. bovis* (see above), risk for progression to active disease seems lower in patients infected by lineage 6 *M. africanum* strains than in patients infected with *M. tuberculosis* (107), and the fitness of lineage 6 *M. africanum* strains was found to be lower compared with *M. tuberculosis* strains in mouse infection models (141). Also similarly to *M. bovis*, evidence for inter-human transmission of *M. africanum*, outside and even within West Africa, is limited, which may help explain its geographical restriction to this region. A study suggested transmission in household contexts, but, because molecular clustering analysis was only done at relatively low resolution by using spoligotyping and lineage-defining large sequence polymorphisms, transmission links could have been substantially overestimated (107). A recent WGS-based study on strains from TB cases in Mali found few isolates of lineage 6 *M. africanum* that were separated by fewer than 10 SNPs after WGS, suggesting limited potential transmission (142).

Two SNPs, conserved in *M. bovis* and lineage 6 *M. africanum* strains and creating a missense mutation in the *phoR* gene, can account for these features shared by *M. bovis* and *M. africanum*. Comparative genomics and allelic exchange experiments demonstrated that these SNPs impair functions of the two-component virulence regulation system PhoPR, which results in reduced replication in human macrophages and in mice and lack of production of polyacetyltrehaloses (PATs) and sulfolipids (SLs) specific to *M. tuberculosis*. However, another genetic polymorphism specific to animal-adapted and lineage 6 *M. africanum* strains, namely the genomic deletion RD8, appears to partly compensate for this impairment. By removing a portion of the promoter region of the *espACD* operon, which belongs to the PhoPR regulon, this deletion restored expression of this operon and secretion via EspACD of the important virulence factor ESAT-6, independently of *phoPR*.

These SNPs and this deletion have likely been acquired in a distant past, by common ancestors of the animal-adapted and *M. africanum* strains.

Experimental evidence for an additional compensatory mutation, restricted to a particular (multidrug) *M. bovis* strain, was found by the same study, which consisted of an IS*6110* insertion inserted 75 bp upstream of the *phoPR* operon. This insertion suppresses deficiencies induced by the SNPs in *phoR* by increasing the expression of the operon and of the genes of its regulon, resulting in production of PAT and SL, increased secretion of ESAT-6, and increased virulence in mice (79). This upregulation of the *phoPR* operon probably reflects the presence of an outward-directed promoter in the 3′ end of the IS*6110* element (132, 143). This mutation, necessarily acquired after the divergence and diversification of *M. bovis* strains, may explain in part the uniquely successful inter-human transmission of this strain, responsible for an outbreak with 36 TB cases (144), which contrasts with the apparently low human-to-human transmissibility of the bulk of the *M. bovis* strain population. The latter finding thus represents remarkable evidence of an important pathobiological difference, linked to IS*6110*-mediated genetic variation at intra-MTBC lineage level.

Recent WGS analysis of *M. africanum* strains of lineages 5 and 6 from Mali pinpointed a set of other *M. africanum*-specific mutations in genes encoding, e.g., molybdenum and vitamin B$_{12}$ and B$_3$ cofactors, L,D-transpeptidases, and some adenylate cyclases, which could perhaps additionally contribute to differential host adaptation, slower growth rate, and virulence of *M. africanum* strains (142). These hypotheses are supported by experimental evidence indicating, for instance, a role for vitamin B$_{12}$ in mycobacterial pathogenesis (145, 146), and a role of L,D-transpeptidases in the growth rate and virulence of *M. tuberculosis* (147). Future mutagenesis and genetic complementation approaches in the *M. africanum* background and/or in *M. tuberculosis* should verify the potential causal effects of the mutations found in the *M. africanum* strains.

Genomic Differences Linked to Biological Differences Between *M. canettii* and the MTBC

M. canettii isolates characteristically show a smooth colony phenotype on solid culture (hence, their alternative name of smooth tubercle bacilli [STBs]). They grow faster than MTBC strains and show differences in cell envelope composition, including a lipooligosaccharide (LOS) absent from MTBC strains. Most *M. canettii* isolates have been obtained from patients living or having lived in the Djibouti region in East Africa (36–41, 148). Together with the clear traces of interstrain horizontal gene transfer and the different CRISPR-Cas system-encoding loci detected in their genomes (36, 37, 84, 85), this strong geographical restriction suggests the potential existence of an environmental reservoir for *M. canettii* and potentially lower pathoadaptation to mammalian hosts. Consistent with the latter hypothesis, *M. canettii* isolates showed lower virulence/persistence than *M. tuberculosis* in mouse infection models (36).

A recombination in *pks5* locus has also been recently demonstrated to account for these differences in morphotypes, LOS production, and virulence between *M. canettii* and the MTBC (149). This role was shown by comparative genomics and physiopathological analysis of typically smooth *M. canettii* strains and variants with a stable rough colony morphotype, similar to that of MTBC strains, observed at low frequency on solid culture. In smooth *M. canettii* strains, this locus harbors two proximal *pks5* homologues separated by an associated *pap* gene, similarly to the LOS-producing nontuberculous mycobacteria *M. marinum* and *M. kansasii*. In contrast, in one rough variant, this locus was found to contain a single *pks5* gene, similar to the situation found in MTBC genomes, indicating a homologous recombination between *pks5* copies and removal of the interspaced *pap* gene. This rough variant was deficient in LOS synthesis and showed increased replication rates in human macrophages and in lungs of infected guinea pigs, induced higher levels of inflammatory cytokines interleukin-6 (IL-6) and IL-12p40 in infected phagocytes, and killed SCID mice more rapidly than its parental smooth strain. These phenotypes were all reverted upon complementation with the twin-*pks5* configuration from a smooth strain. These results thus point to a change in bacterial surface, mediated by *pks5* recombination, as an important virulence-determining difference among TB bacilli. This cell surface LOS- and morphotype-related difference in virulence is reminiscent of the covariation of colony morphotypes, cell wall compounds, and virulence linked to complementation of the RD1 region in BCG (80) (see above), which thus convergently points to the key role of the bacterial cell surface-related features in mycobacterial pathogenicity.

Genomic Differences and Biological Differences among *M. tuberculosis* Strains

Differences in pathobiological properties among *M. tuberculosis* strains from different lineages have been documented by multiple studies. However, in contrast to differences seen with more divergent animal-associated or *M. canettii* lineages, these variations have not been directly or unambiguously linked with (sub) lineage-specific polymorphisms yet.

Specific pathobiological properties of the Beijing/ East Asian lineage (alias lineage 2) are the most intensively studied. A variety of molecular epidemiological studies reported rapid emergence and/or high rates of transmission of strains of this lineage in some world regions, frequently (but not systematically) in association with (multi)drug resistance (e.g., references 150 and 151; reviewed in references 120 and 152). These observations have been proposed to result from specific selective advantages such as higher virulence and/or an elicited immune response skewed toward a less protective Th1 response, which were reported for some Beijing strains in animal or cellular infection models (111, 153–156). Conflicting evidence also exists for a potential role of BCG vaccination, which was suggested to be less protective against Beijing strains (111, 157, 158). However, several studies suggested that differences in virulence-related and other properties such

as transmissibility exist even among Beijing strains (115, 155, 159–163), suggesting that the putative selective advantages mentioned above might not be fixed at the overall lineage level. Compatible with this hypothesis are the findings of a recent study, using MIRU-VNTR typing-based screening combined with WGS, which revealed the existence of three ancestral and five modern branches among 5,000 clinical isolates from the Beijing lineage from 99 countries (33) (Fig. 2). In contrast to the dominant association of ancestral strain types with patients from East Asia, corresponding to the likely origin of the Beijing lineage overall, modern types have a much broader distribution (Fig. 3), suggesting a possibly favored propagation. In accordance with this suggestion, strains of modern Beijing sublineages tend to be more virulent in animal and intracellular infection experiments, when compared with strains from ancient Beijing sublineages (115, 161).

However, the molecular determinants of such (sub) lineage-specific pathobiological differences remain speculative. For instance, while the production of a phenolic glycolipid by an intact *pks15-1* gene in Beijing strains

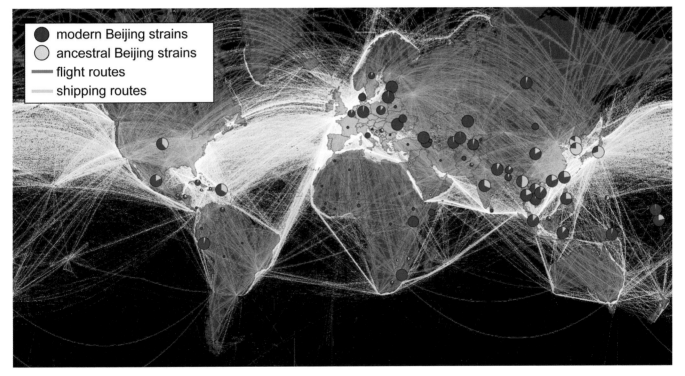

Figure 3 Geographical distribution of nearly 5,000 clinical Beijing (i.e., lineage 2) isolates (data from Merker et al. [33]). Evolutionary ancestral Beijing strains are mainly dominating in East Asia, the likely origin of this MTBC lineage, whereas modern Beijing strains are globally distributed, suggesting a more virulent phenotype. In addition, the effects of globalization also shape the diversity of MTBC strains in different settings, yet with unknown consequences on host-pathogen interactions and tuberculosis progression (world map from flickr.com).

modulates the early host cytokine response *in vitro*, this production does not in itself determine an increased virulence (164). It is also known that Beijing strains classified as "modern" constitutively upregulate the DosR regulon, involved in adaption for periods of nonreplicating persistence *in vitro*, putatively providing selective advantages in conditions encountered during chronic or latent phases of infection (165). A frameshift mutation has been identified in the gene encoding the DosT sensor kinase putatively interacting with the DosR regulator in these Beijing strains, but this mutation is not directly responsible for the phenotype of constitutive upregulation (166). Along the same lines, a massive gene duplication event including the *dosR* region identified in some sublineages of modern Beijing strains (126) was recently shown to result from selective pressure under *in vitro* culture conditions, rather than from host-induced selective pressure *in vivo* (135).

More indications exist on mechanisms likely underlying the association of some genetic backgrounds, from the Beijing lineage (as well as from other *M. tuberculosis* lineages; see below), with drug resistance and high rates of drug resistance transmission. Probable major factors are epistatic interactions between drug resistance mutations, associated with bacterial fitness costs, and compensatory mutations acquired in a different region of the same proteins affected by the drug resistance mutations or in different gene products involved in a same or linked metabolic pathway(s). For example, high fitness costs associated with mutations in *katG*, the 16S rRNA, or *rpoB*, causing resistance to isoniazid, aminoglycosides, or rifampin, respectively, are believed to be compensated by mutations in the regulatory region of *ahpC* (167, 168) or in other regions of the 16S rRNA (169), or by *rpoA* or *rpoC* (170, 171). In accordance with this presumption, coemergence of drug resistance and putative compensatory mutations has been observed by deep sequencing of *M. tuberculosis* genome populations isolated from TB patients during development of drug resistance under treatment (100–102).

Also insightful in this respect is the observation that, in a worldwide collection of Beijing isolates, MDR strains (thus resistant to rifampin) from the Central Asian branch, characterized by high rates of genotypic and genomic clustering suggestive of recent clonal expansion and successful ongoing transmission, were enriched in mutations in *rpoC* (33). Consistently, in Abkhazia/Georgia, Uzbekistan, and Kazakhstan, which are the countries with the highest incidence of MDR TB worldwide and where Central Asian Beijing strains

predominate, approximately one-third of MDR clinical isolates were found to harbor potential compensatory mutations in *rpoA* or *rpoC* (170). A vast study using WGS of 1,000 isolates identified another large group of Beijing strains showing obvious traces of strong clonal expansion and epidemiological success in a southwestern region of Russia, which harbored particular combinations of drug resistance and putative compensatory mutations in *rpoB* (172). However, such mechanisms of epistasis and compensatory evolution of MDR strains are not limited to the Beijing lineage, because they were detected during the evolution reconstructed over four decades of two longitudinal outbreaks involving distinct MDR and/or XDR clones of the Euro-American lineages in South Africa and Argentina (173, 174). Such epistatic interactions, thought to drive the emergence and the transmission of particular MDR and XDR strains, might be promoted in genetic backgrounds of specific (sub)lineages or clones, which could provide more or less favorable arrays of preexisting mutations for compensating the cost of an emerging drug resistance mutation (175).

Of note, a few studies provided evidence for a higher mutation rate of strains of the East Asian/Beijing (sub) lineage leading to increased acquisition of drug resistance *in vitro* and a higher probability of MDR in TB patients infected with these strains, which was proposed to contribute to frequent association of this (sub) lineage with drug resistance. However, this is strongly debated (176–182). As an example of a debated point, one study reported an extremely high mutation rate to rifampin resistance of about 10^{-3} for two Beijing strains, whereas the mutation rate of *M. tuberculosis* strains is normally in the range of 10^{-8} (177). However, as subsequently pointed out (181), one of these two strains was previously tested in another study and found to have a normal mutation rate to rifampin resistance (183). Among other potential technical reasons (181), the lack of use of a proper fluctuation assay, to rule out the potential presence of a preexisting mutant subpopulation in the assayed strain inoculum, was invoked to explain the surprisingly high rate reported in reference 177. In contrast, by using fluctuation analysis, Ford et al. reported an overall much more moderately (10-fold) elevated rate of acquisition of rifampin resistance by Beijing strains when compared with strains of the Euro-American lineage. However, only four strains were compared per lineage, with substantial strain-to-strain variation observed within each group (from 10^{-8} to 7×10^{-8} and 0.1 to 0.7×10^{-8}, respectively). No mechanism has been defined yet for these (potential) variations.

CONCLUDING REMARKS

Findings from contemporary molecular approaches increasingly confirm early, frequently forgotten phenotypic observations suggesting significant biological and genetic heterogeneity among the tubercle bacilli. The world population of TB strains is highly structured into distinct phylogenetic lineages, with differential host (animal or human) and geographical distribution. The use of WGS provides an accurate genetic framework for differentiating clinical isolates from lineage to individual clone level. Moreover, comparative genomics, in combination with genetics and comparative physiopathological experiments, recently revealed some key molecular mechanisms probably involved in the course of pathoadaptive evolution and biological differentiation, at least among *M. canettii*, *M. microti*/*M. bovis* and *M. africanum*, and *M. tuberculosis*. Identification of these mechanisms was probably facilitated by the fact that some of the phenotypic differences involved were clear-cut dissimilarities recognized as fixed in the respective bacterial strain populations, such as the smooth versus rough colony morphotype of *M. canettii* versus classical MTBC strains, or the avirulence of BCG strains relative to *M. tuberculosis*. Identification of the mechanisms underlying more subtle or more complex differences existing among *M. tuberculosis* lineages, for instance, regarding their sympatric association with different human populations or the epidemiological success of particular strain groups in association or not with multidrug resistance, will require large investigations, integrating the variability of both the pathogen and host. Expected challenges will include recruitment of sufficiently large population sizes and standardized collection of high-quality phenotypic data and metadata to empower association analysis, and definition and use of appropriate experimental models to formally test associations between phenotypes and genotypes detected at population levels. Such integrative approaches will be key for the development of new, most effective diagnostics, drugs, and vaccination strategies.

Citation. Niemann S, Merker M, Kohl T, Supply P. 2016. Impact of genetic diversity on the biology of *Mycobacterium tuberculosis* complex strains. Microbiol Spectrum 4(6):TBTB2-0022-2016.

References

1. Diel R, Vandeputte J, de Vries G, Stillo J, Wanlin M, Nienhaus A. 2014. Costs of tuberculosis disease in the European Union: a systematic analysis and cost calculation. *Eur Respir J* 43:554–565.
2. Dye C, Williams BG. 2010. The population dynamics and control of tuberculosis. *Science* 328:856–861.
3. Gandhi NR, Nunn P, Dheda K, Schaaf HS, Zignol M, van Soolingen D, Jensen P, Bayona J. 2010. Multidrug-resistant and extensively drug-resistant tuberculosis: a threat to global control of tuberculosis. *Lancet* 375:1830–1843.
4. Marais BJ. 2016. The global tuberculosis situation and the inexorable rise of drug-resistant disease. *Adv Drug Deliv Rev* 102:3–9.
5. Skrahina A, Hurevich H, Zalutskaya A, Sahalchyk E, Astrauko A, Hoffner S, Rusovich V, Dadu A, de Colombani P, Dara M, van Gemert W, Zignol M. 2013. Multidrug-resistant tuberculosis in Belarus: the size of the problem and associated risk factors. *Bull World Health Organ* 91:36–45.
6. Hoffmann H, Kohl TA, Hofmann-Thiel S, Merker M, Beckert P, Jaton K, Nedialkova L, Sahalchyk E, Rothe T, Keller PM, Niemann S. 2016. Delamanid and bedaquiline resistance in *Mycobacterium tuberculosis* ancestral Beijing genotype causing extensively drug-resistant tuberculosis in a Tibetan refugee. *Am J Respir Crit Care Med* 193:337–340.
7. Bloemberg GV, Keller PM, Stucki D, Trauner A, Borrell S, Latshang T, Coscolla M, Rothe T, Hömke R, Ritter C, Feldmann J, Schulthess B, Gagneux S, Böttger EC. 2015. Acquired resistance to bedaquiline and delamanid in therapy for tuberculosis. *N Engl J Med* 373:1986–1988.
8. Anuradha R, Munisankar S, Bhootra Y, Kumar NP, Dolla C, Kumaran P, Babu S. 2016. Coexistent malnutrition is associated with perturbations in systemic and antigen-specific cytokine responses in latent tuberculosis infection. *Clin Vaccine Immunol* 23:339–345.
9. Chan J, Tian Y, Tanaka KE, Tsang MS, Yu K, Salgame P, Carroll D, Kress Y, Teitelbaum R, Bloom BR. 1996. Effects of protein calorie malnutrition on tuberculosis in mice. *Proc Natl Acad Sci USA* 93:14857–14861.
10. Corbett EL, Watt CJ, Walker N, Maher D, Williams BG, Raviglione MC, Dye C. 2003. The growing burden of tuberculosis: global trends and interactions with the HIV epidemic. *Arch Intern Med* 163:1009–1021.
11. Kwan CK, Ernst JD. 2011. HIV and tuberculosis: a deadly human syndemic. *Clin Microbiol Rev* 24:351–376.
12. Pawlowski A, Jansson M, Sköld M, Rottenberg ME, Källenius G. 2012. Tuberculosis and HIV co-infection. *PLoS Pathog* 8:e1002464.
13. Gagneux S, Small PM. 2007. Global phylogeography of *Mycobacterium tuberculosis* and implications for tuberculosis product development. *Lancet Infect Dis* 7:328–337.
14. Wells AQ. 1949. Vaccination with the murine type of tubercle bacillus (vole bacillus). *Lancet* 254:53–55.
15. Magnus K. 1966. Epidemiological basis of tuberculosis eradication. 3. Risk of pulmonary tuberculosis after human and bovine infection. *Bull World Health Organ* 35:483–508.
16. Bhatia AL, Csillag A, Mitchison DA, Selkon JB, Somasundaram PR, Subbaiah TV. 1961. The virulence in the guinea-pig of tubercle bacilli isolated before treatment from South Indian patients with pulmonary tuber-

culosis. 2. Comparison with virulence of tubercle bacilli from British patients. *Bull World Health Organ* **25:** 313–322.

17. Kapur V, Whittam TS, Musser JM. 1994. Is *Mycobacterium tuberculosis* 15,000 years old? *J Infect Dis* **170:** 1348–1349.

18. Sreevatsan S, Pan X, Stockbauer KE, Connell ND, Kreiswirth BN, Whittam TS, Musser JM. 1997. Restricted structural gene polymorphism in the *Mycobacterium tuberculosis* complex indicates evolutionarily recent global dissemination. *Proc Natl Acad Sci USA* **94:** 9869–9874.

19. Kremer K, van Soolingen D, Frothingham R, Haas WH, Hermans PW, Martín C, Palittapongarnpim P, Plikaytis BB, Riley LW, Yakrus MA, Musser JM, van Embden JD. 1999. Comparison of methods based on different molecular epidemiological markers for typing of *Mycobacterium tuberculosis* complex strains: interlaboratory study of discriminatory power and reproducibility. *J Clin Microbiol* **37:**2607–2618.

20. Sola C, Filliol I, Gutierrez MC, Mokrousov I, Vincent V, Rastogi N. 2001. Spoligotype database of *Mycobacterium tuberculosis*: biogeographic distribution of shared types and epidemiologic and phylogenetic perspectives. *Emerg Infect Dis* **7:**390–396.

21. Sola C, Filliol I, Legrand E, Mokrousov I, Rastogi N. 2001. *Mycobacterium tuberculosis* phylogeny reconstruction based on combined numerical analysis with IS1081, IS6110, VNTR, and DR-based spoligotyping suggests the existence of two new phylogeographical clades. *J Mol Evol* **53:**680–689.

22. Brudey K, et al. 2006. *Mycobacterium tuberculosis* complex genetic diversity: mining the fourth international spoligotyping database (SpolDB4) for classification, population genetics and epidemiology. *BMC Microbiol* **6:**23.

23. Filliol I, Driscoll JR, van Soolingen D, Kreiswirth BN, Kremer K, Valétudie G, Anh DD, Barlow R, Banerjee D, Bifani PJ, Brudey K, Cataldi A, Cooksey RC, Cousins DV, Dale JW, Dellagostin OA, Drobniewski F, Engelmann G, Ferdinand S, Gascoyne-Binzi D, Gordon M, Gutierrez MC, Haas WH, Heersma H, Kassa-Kelembho E, Ly HM, Makristathis A, Mammina C, Martin G, Moström P, Mokrousov I, Narbonne V, Narvskaya O, Nastasi A, Niobe-Eyangoh SN, Pape JW, Rasolofo-Razanamparany V, Ridell M, Rossetti ML, Stauffer F, Suffys PN, Takiff H, Texier-Maugein J, Vincent V, de Waard JH, Sola C, Rastogi N. 2003. Snapshot of moving and expanding clones of *Mycobacterium tuberculosis* and their global distribution assessed by spoligotyping in an international study. *J Clin Microbiol* **41:**1963–1970.

24. Supply P, Lesjean S, Savine E, Kremer K, van Soolingen D, Locht C. 2001. Automated high-throughput genotyping for study of global epidemiology of *Mycobacterium tuberculosis* based on mycobacterial interspersed repetitive units. *J Clin Microbiol* **39:**3563–3571.

25. Supply P, Warren RM, Bañuls AL, Lesjean S, Van Der Spuy GD, Lewis LA, Tibayrenc M, Van Helden PD, Locht C. 2003. Linkage disequilibrium between mini-

26. Baker L, Brown T, Maiden MC, Drobniewski F. 2004. Silent nucleotide polymorphisms and a phylogeny for *Mycobacterium tuberculosis*. *Emerg Infect Dis* **10:** 1568–1577.

27. Brosch R, Gordon SV, Marmiesse M, Brodin P, Buchrieser C, Eiglmeier K, Garnier T, Gutierrez C, Hewinson G, Kremer K, Parsons LM, Pym AS, Samper S, van Soolingen D, Cole ST. 2002. A new evolutionary scenario for the *Mycobacterium tuberculosis* complex. *Proc Natl Acad Sci USA* **99:**3684–3689.

28. Mostowy S, Cousins D, Brinkman J, Aranaz A, Behr MA. 2002. Genomic deletions suggest a phylogeny for the *Mycobacterium tuberculosis* complex. *J Infect Dis* **186:**74–80.

29. Hirsh AE, Tsolaki AG, DeRiemer K, Feldman MW, Small PM. 2004. Stable association between strains of *Mycobacterium tuberculosis* and their human host populations. *Proc Natl Acad Sci USA* **101:**4871–4876.

30. Comas I, Chakravartti J, Small PM, Galagan J, Niemann S, Kremer K, Ernst JD, Gagneux S. 2010. Human T cell epitopes of *Mycobacterium tuberculosis* are evolutionarily hyperconserved. *Nat Genet* **42:**498–503.

31. Comas I, Coscolla M, Luo T, Borrell S, Holt KE, Kato-Maeda M, Parkhill J, Malla B, Berg S, Thwaites G, Yeboah-Manu D, Bothamley G, Mei J, Wei L, Bentley S, Harris SR, Niemann S, Diel R, Aseffa A, Gao Q, Young D, Gagneux S. 2013. Out-of-Africa migration and Neolithic coexpansion of *Mycobacterium tuberculosis* with modern humans. *Nat Genet* **45:** 1176–1182.

32. Coll F, McNerney R, Guerra-Assunção JA, Glynn JR, Perdigão J, Viveiros M, Portugal I, Pain A, Martin N, Clark TG. 2014. A robust SNP barcode for typing *Mycobacterium tuberculosis* complex strains. *Nat Commun* **5:**4812.

33. Merker M, et al. 2015. Evolutionary history and global spread of the *Mycobacterium tuberculosis* Beijing lineage. *Nat Genet* **47:**242–249.

34. Luo T, Comas I, Luo D, Lu B, Wu J, Wei L, Yang C, Liu Q, Gan M, Sun G, Shen X, Liu F, Gagneux S, Mei J, Lan R, Wan K, Gao Q. 2015. Southern East Asian origin and coexpansion of *Mycobacterium tuberculosis* Beijing family with Han Chinese. *Proc Natl Acad Sci USA* **112:**8136–8141.

35. Wirth T, Hildebrand F, Allix-Béguec C, Wölbeling F, Kubica T, Kremer K, van Soolingen D, Rüsch-Gerdes S, Locht C, Brisse S, Meyer A, Supply P, Niemann S. 2008. Origin, spread and demography of the *Mycobacterium tuberculosis* complex. *PLoS Pathog* **4:**e1000160.

36. Supply P, Marceau M, Mangenot S, Roche D, Rouanet C, Khanna V, Majlessi L, Criscuolo A, Tap J, Pawlik A, Fiette L, Orgeur M, Fabre M, Parmentier C, Frigui W, Simeone R, Boritsch EC, Debrie AS, Willery E, Walker D, Quail MA, Ma L, Bouchier C, Salvignol G, Sayes F, Cascioferro A, Seemann T, Barbe V, Locht C, Gutierrez MC, Leclerc C, Bentley SD, Stinear TP, Brisse S, Médigue C, Parkhill J, Cruveiller S, Brosch R. 2013.

Genomic analysis of smooth tubercle bacilli provides insights into ancestry and pathoadaptation of *Mycobacterium tuberculosis*. *Nat Genet* 45:172–179.

37. Blouin Y, Cazajous G, Dehan C, Soler C, Vong R, Hassan MO, Hauck Y, Boulais C, Andriamanantena D, Martinaud C, Martin É, Pourcel C, Vergnaud G. 2014. Progenitor *"Mycobacterium canettii"* clone responsible for lymph node tuberculosis epidemic, Djibouti. *Emerg Infect Dis* 20:21–28.

38. Fabre M, Koeck JL, Le Flèche P, Simon F, Hervé V, Vergnaud G, Pourcel C. 2004. High genetic diversity revealed by variable-number tandem repeat genotyping and analysis of hsp65 gene polymorphism in a large collection of *"Mycobacterium canettii"* strains indicates that the *M. tuberculosis* complex is a recently emerged clone of *"M. canettii"*. *J Clin Microbiol* 42:3248–3255.

39. Gutierrez MC, Brisse S, Brosch R, Fabre M, Omaïs B, Marmiesse M, Supply P, Vincent V. 2005. Ancient origin and gene mosaicism of the progenitor of *Mycobacterium tuberculosis*. *PLoS Pathog* 1:e5.

40. Fabre M, Hauck Y, Soler C, Koeck JL, van Ingen J, van Soolingen D, Vergnaud G, Pourcel C. 2010. Molecular characteristics of *"Mycobacterium canettii"* the smooth *Mycobacterium tuberculosis* bacilli. *Infect Genet Evol* 10:1165–1173.

41. van Soolingen D, Hoogenboezem T, de Haas PE, Hermans PW, Koedam MA, Teppema KS, Brennan PJ, Besra GS, Portaels F, Top J, Schouls LM, van Embden JD. 1997. A novel pathogenic taxon of the *Mycobacterium tuberculosis* complex, Canetti: characterization of an exceptional isolate from Africa. *Int J Syst Bacteriol* 47:1236–1245.

42. Boritsch EC, Supply P, Honoré N, Seeman T, Stinear TP, Brosch R. 2014. A glimpse into the past and predictions for the future: the molecular evolution of the tuberculosis agent. *Mol Microbiol* 93:835–852. (Erratum, 94:742.)

43. Coscolla M, Gagneux S. 2014. Consequences of genomic diversity in *Mycobacterium tuberculosis*. *Semin Immunol* 26:431–444.

44. Gagneux S, DeRiemer K, Van T, Kato-Maeda M, de Jong BC, Narayanan S, Nicol M, Niemann S, Kremer K, Gutierrez MC, Hilty M, Hopewell PC, Small PM. 2006. Variable host-pathogen compatibility in *Mycobacterium tuberculosis*. *Proc Natl Acad Sci USA* 103:2869–2873.

45. Smith NH, Gordon SV, de la Rua-Domenech R, Clifton-Hadley RS, Hewinson RG. 2006. Bottlenecks and broomsticks: the molecular evolution of *Mycobacterium bovis*. *Nat Rev Microbiol* 4:670–681.

46. Niemann S, Supply P. 2014. Diversity and evolution of *Mycobacterium tuberculosis*: moving to whole-genome-based approaches. *Cold Spring Harb Perspect Med* 4:a021188.

47. van Soolingen D, Qian L, de Haas PE, Douglas JT, Traore H, Portaels F, Qing HZ, Enkhsaikan D, Nymadawa P, van Embden JD. 1995. Predominance of a single genotype of *Mycobacterium tuberculosis* in countries of east Asia. *J Clin Microbiol* 33:3234–3238.

48. Supply P, Allix C, Lesjean S, Cardoso-Oelemann M, Rüsch-Gerdes S, Willery E, Savine E, de Haas P, van Deutekom H, Roring S, Bifani P, Kurepina N, Kreiswirth B, Sola C, Rastogi N, Vatin V, Gutierrez MC, Fauville M, Niemann S, Skuce R, Kremer K, Locht C, van Soolingen D. 2006. Proposal for standardization of optimized mycobacterial interspersed repetitive unit-variable-number tandem repeat typing of *Mycobacterium tuberculosis*. *J Clin Microbiol* 44:4498–4510.

49. van Embden JD, et al. 1993. Strain identification of *Mycobacterium tuberculosis* by DNA fingerprinting: recommendations for a standardized methodology. *J Clin Microbiol* 31:406–409.

50. Kamerbeek J, Schouls L, Kolk A, van Agterveld M, van Soolingen D, Kuijper S, Bunschoten A, Molhuizen H, Shaw R, Goyal M, van Embden J. 1997. Simultaneous detection and strain differentiation of *Mycobacterium tuberculosis* for diagnosis and epidemiology. *J Clin Microbiol* 35:907–914.

51. Frothingham R, Meeker-O'Connell WA. 1998. Genetic diversity in the *Mycobacterium tuberculosis* complex based on variable numbers of tandem DNA repeats. *Microbiology* 144:1189–1196.

52. Supply P, Mazars E, Lesjean S, Vincent V, Gicquel B, Locht C. 2000. Variable human minisatellite-like regions in the *Mycobacterium tuberculosis* genome. *Mol Microbiol* 36:762–771.

53. Mazars E, Lesjean S, Banuls AL, Gilbert M, Vincent V, Gicquel B, Tibayrenc M, Locht C, Supply P. 2001. High-resolution minisatellite-based typing as a portable approach to global analysis of *Mycobacterium tuberculosis* molecular epidemiology. *Proc Natl Acad Sci USA* 98:1901–1906.

54. Cowan LS, Diem L, Brake MC, Crawford JT. 2004. Transfer of a *Mycobacterium tuberculosis* genotyping method, Spoligotyping, from a reverse line-blot hybridization, membrane-based assay to the Luminex multi-analyte profiling system. *J Clin Microbiol* 42:474–477.

55. Driscoll JR, Bifani PJ, Mathema B, McGarry MA, Zickas GM, Kreiswirth BN, Taber HW. 2002. Spoligologos: a bioinformatic approach to displaying and analyzing *Mycobacterium tuberculosis* data. *Emerg Infect Dis* 8:1306–1309.

56. Comas I, Homolka S, Niemann S, Gagneux S. 2009. Genotyping of genetically monomorphic bacteria: DNA sequencing in *Mycobacterium tuberculosis* highlights the limitations of current methodologies. *PLoS One* 4:e7815.

57. Cole ST, Supply P, Honoré N. 2001. Repetitive sequences in *Mycobacterium leprae* and their impact on genome plasticity. *Lepr Rev* 72:449–461.

58. Supply P, Magdalena J, Himpens S, Locht C. 1997. Identification of novel intergenic repetitive units in a mycobacterial two-component system operon. *Mol Microbiol* 26:991–1003.

59. Smittipat N, Palittapongarnpim P. 2000. Identification of possible loci of variable number of tandem repeats in *Mycobacterium tuberculosis*. *Tuber Lung Dis* 80:69–74.

60. Cardoso Oelemann M, Gomes HM, Willery E, Possuelo L, Batista Lima KV, Allix-Béguec C, Locht C, Goguet

de la Salmonière YO, Gutierrez MC, Suffys P, Supply P. 2011. The forest behind the tree: phylogenetic exploration of a dominant *Mycobacterium tuberculosis* strain lineage from a high tuberculosis burden country. *PLoS One* 6:e18256.

61. Allix-Béguec C, Wahl C, Hanekom M, Nikolayevskyy V, Drobniewski F, Maeda S, Campos-Herrero I, Mokrousov I, Niemann S, Kontsevaya I, Rastogi N, Samper S, Sng LH, Warren RM, Supply P. 2014. Proposal of a consensus set of hypervariable mycobacterial interspersed repetitive-unit-variable-number tandem-repeat loci for subtyping of *Mycobacterium tuberculosis* Beijing isolates. *J Clin Microbiol* 52:164–172.

62. Trovato A, Tafaj S, Battaglia S, Alagna R, Bardhi D, Kapisyzi P, Bala S, Haldeda M, Borroni E, Hafizi H, Cirillo DM. 2016. Implementation of a consensus set of hypervariable mycobacterial interspersed repetitive-unit-variable-number tandem-repeat loci in *Mycobacterium tuberculosis* molecular epidemiology. *J Clin Microbiol* 54:478–482.

63. Allix-Béguec C, Harmsen D, Weniger T, Supply P, Niemann S. 2008. Evaluation and strategy for use of MIRU-VNTRplus, a multifunctional database for online analysis of genotyping data and phylogenetic identification of *Mycobacterium tuberculosis* complex isolates. *J Clin Microbiol* 46:2692–2699.

64. Weniger T, Krawczyk J, Supply P, Niemann S, Harmsen D. 2010. MIRU-VNTRplus: a web tool for polyphasic genotyping of *Mycobacterium tuberculosis* complex bacteria. *Nucleic Acids Res* 38(Suppl):W326–W331.

65. Demay C, Liens B, Burguière T, Hill V, Couvin D, Millet J, Mokrousov I, Sola C, Zozio T, Rastogi N. 2012. SITVITWEB–a publicly available international multimarker database for studying *Mycobacterium tuberculosis* genetic diversity and molecular epidemiology. *Infect Genet Evol* 12:755–766.

66. Tsolaki AG, Hirsh AE, DeRiemer K, Enciso JA, Wong MZ, Hannan M, Goguet de la Salmoniere YO, Aman K, Kato-Maeda M, Small PM. 2004. Functional and evolutionary genomics of *Mycobacterium tuberculosis*: insights from genomic deletions in 100 strains. *Proc Natl Acad Sci USA* 101:4865–4870.

67. Hershberg R, Lipatov M, Small PM, Sheffer H, Niemann S, Homolka S, Roach JC, Kremer K, Petrov DA, Feldman MW, Gagneux S. 2008. High functional diversity in *Mycobacterium tuberculosis* driven by genetic drift and human demography. *PLoS Biol* 6:e311.

68. Gutacker MM, Mathema B, Soini H, Shashkina E, Kreiswirth BN, Graviss EA, Musser JM. 2006. Single-nucleotide polymorphism-based population genetic analysis of *Mycobacterium tuberculosis* strains from 4 geographic sites. *J Infect Dis* 193:121–128.

69. Gutacker MM, Smoot JC, Migliaccio CA, Ricklefs SM, Hua S, Cousins DV, Graviss EA, Shashkina E, Kreiswirth BN, Musser JM. 2002. Genome-wide analysis of synonymous single nucleotide polymorphisms in *Mycobacterium tuberculosis* complex organisms: resolution of genetic relationships among closely related microbial strains. *Genetics* 162:1533–1543.

70. Filliol I, Motiwala AS, Cavatore M, Qi W, Hazbón MH, Bobadilla del Valle M, Fyfe J, García-García L, Rastogi N, Sola C, Zozio T, Guerrero MI, León CI, Crabtree J, Angiuoli S, Eisenach KD, Durmaz R, Joloba ML, Rendón A, Sifuentes-Osornio J, Ponce de León A, Cave MD, Fleischmann R, Whittam TS, Alland D. 2006. Global phylogeny of *Mycobacterium tuberculosis* based on single nucleotide polymorphism (SNP) analysis: insights into tuberculosis evolution, phylogenetic accuracy of other DNA fingerprinting systems, and recommendations for a minimal standard SNP set. *J Bacteriol* 188:759–772.

71. Bos KI, Harkins KM, Herbig A, Coscolla M, Weber N, Comas I, Forrest SA, Bryant JM, Harris SR, Schuenemann VJ, Campbell TJ, Majander K, Wilbur AK, Guichon RA, Wolfe Steadman DL, Cook DC, Niemann S, Behr MA, Zumarraga M, Bastida R, Huson D, Nieselt K, Young D, Parkhill J, Buikstra JE, Gagneux S, Stone AC, Krause J. 2014. Pre-Columbian mycobacterial genomes reveal seals as a source of New World human tuberculosis. *Nature* 514:494–497.

72. Homolka S, Projahn M, Feuerriegel S, Ubben T, Diel R, Nübel U, Niemann S. 2012. High resolution discrimination of clinical *Mycobacterium tuberculosis* complex strains based on single nucleotide polymorphisms. *PLoS One* 7:e39855.

73. Niobe-Eyangoh SN, Kuaban C, Sorlin P, Thonnon J, Vincent V, Gutierrez MC. 2004. Molecular characteristics of strains of the Cameroon family, the major group of *Mycobacterium tuberculosis* in a country with a high prevalence of tuberculosis. *J Clin Microbiol* 42:5029–5035.

74. Fenner L, Egger M, Bodmer T, Furrer H, Ballif M, Battegay M, Helbling P, Fehr J, Gsponer T, Rieder HL, Zwahlen M, Hoffmann M, Bernasconi E, Cavassini M, Calmy A, Dolina M, Frei R, Janssens JP, Borrell S, Stucki D, Schrenzel J, Böttger EC, Gagneux S, Swiss HIV Cohort and Molecular Epidemiology of Tuberculosis Study Groups. 2013. HIV infection disrupts the sympatric host-pathogen relationship in human tuberculosis. *PLoS Genet* 9:e1003318.

75. Pasipanodya JG, Moonan PK, Vecino E, Miller TL, Fernandez M, Slocum P, Drewyer G, Weis SE. 2013. Allopatric tuberculosis host-pathogen relationships are associated with greater pulmonary impairment. *Infect Genet Evol* 16:433–440.

76. Thye T, Niemann S, Walter K, Homolka S, Intemann CD, Chinbuah MA, Enimil A, Gyapong J, Osei I, Owusu-Dabo E, Rüsch-Gerdes S, Horstmann RD, Ehlers S, Meyer CG. 2011. Variant G57E of mannose binding lectin associated with protection against tuberculosis caused by *Mycobacterium africanum* but not by *M. tuberculosis*. *PLoS One* 6:e20908.

77. Intemann CD, Thye T, Niemann S, Browne EN, Amanua Chinbuah M, Enimil A, Gyapong J, Osei I, Owusu-Dabo E, Helm S, Rüsch-Gerdes S, Horstmann RD, Meyer CG. 2009. Autophagy gene variant IRGM -261T contributes to protection from tuberculosis caused by *Mycobacterium tuberculosis* but not by *M. africanum* strains. *PLoS Pathog* 5:e1000577.

78. Smith NH, Hewinson RG, Kremer K, Brosch R, Gordon SV. 2009. Myths and misconceptions: the origin and evolution of *Mycobacterium tuberculosis*. *Nat Rev Microbiol* 7:537–544.

79. Gonzalo-Asensio J, Malaga W, Pawlik A, Astarie-Dequeker C, Passemar C, Moreau F, Laval F, Daffé M, Martin C, Brosch R, Guilhot C. 2014. Evolutionary history of tuberculosis shaped by conserved mutations in the PhoPR virulence regulator. *Proc Natl Acad Sci USA* 111:11491–11496.

80. Pym AS, Brodin P, Brosch R, Huerre M, Cole ST. 2002. Loss of RD1 contributed to the attenuation of the live tuberculosis vaccines *Mycobacterium bovis* BCG and *Mycobacterium microti*. *Mol Microbiol* 46:709–717.

81. Koeck JL, Fabre M, Simon F, Daffé M, Garnotel E, Matan AB, Gérôme P, Bernatas JJ, Buisson Y, Pourcel C. 2011. Clinical characteristics of the smooth tubercle bacilli '*Mycobacterium canettii*' infection suggest the existence of an environmental reservoir. *Clin Microbiol Infect* 17:1013–1019.

82. Pfyffer GE, Auckenthaler R, van Embden JD, van Soolingen D. 1998. *Mycobacterium canettii*, the smooth variant of *M. tuberculosis*, isolated from a Swiss patient exposed in Africa. *Emerg Infect Dis* 4:631–634.

83. Somoskovi A, Dormandy J, Mayrer AR, Carter M, Hooper N, Salfinger M. 2009. "*Mycobacterium canettii*" isolated from a human immunodeficiency virus-positive patient: first case recognized in the United States. *J Clin Microbiol* 47:255–257.

84. Derbyshire KM, Gray TA. 2014. Distributive conjugal transfer: new insights into horizontal gene transfer and genetic exchange in mycobacteria. *Microbiol Spectr* 2:MGM2-0022-2013.

85. Mortimer TD, Pepperell CS. 2014. Genomic signatures of distributive conjugal transfer among mycobacteria. *Genome Biol Evol* 6:2489–2500.

86. Pepperell CS, Casto AM, Kitchen A, Granka JM, Cornejo OE, Holmes EC, Birren B, Galagan J, Feldman MW. 2013. The role of selection in shaping diversity of natural *M. tuberculosis* populations. *PLoS Pathog* 9:e1003543 (Erratum, 9).

87. Braden CR, Morlock GP, Woodley CL, Johnson KR, Colombel AC, Cave MD, Yang Z, Valway SE, Onorato IM, Crawford JT. 2001. Simultaneous infection with multiple strains of *Mycobacterium tuberculosis*. *Clin Infect Dis* 33:e42–e47.

88. Chaves F, Dronda F, Alonso-Sanz M, Noriega AR. 1999. Evidence of exogenous reinfection and mixed infection with more than one strain of *Mycobacterium tuberculosis* among Spanish HIV-infected inmates. *AIDS* 13:615–620.

89. García de Viedma D, Marín M, Ruiz Serrano MJ, Alcalá L, Bouza E. 2003. Polyclonal and compartmentalized infection by *Mycobacterium tuberculosis* in patients with both respiratory and extrarespiratory involvement. *J Infect Dis* 187:695–699.

90. Shamputa IC, Jugheli L, Sadradze N, Willery E, Portaels F, Supply P, Rigouts L. 2006. Mixed infection and clonal representativeness of a single sputum sample in tuber-culosis patients from a penitentiary hospital in Georgia. *Respir Res* 7:99.

91. Shamputa IC, Rigouts L, Eyongeta LA, El Aila NA, van Deun A, Salim AH, Willery E, Locht C, Supply P, Portaels F. 2004. Genotypic and phenotypic heterogeneity among *Mycobacterium tuberculosis* isolates from pulmonary tuberculosis patients. *J Clin Microbiol* 42:5528–5536.

92. Al-Hajoj SA, Akkerman O, Parwati I, al-Gamdi S, Rahim Z, van Soolingen D, van Ingen J, Supply P, van der Zanden AG. 2010. Microevolution of *Mycobacterium tuberculosis* in a tuberculosis patient. *J Clin Microbiol* 48:3813–3816.

93. de Viedma DG, Marín M, Andrés S, Lorenzo G, Ruiz-Serrano MJ, Bouza E. 2006. Complex clonal features in an mycobacterium tuberculosis infection in a two-year-old child. *Pediatr Infect Dis J* 25:457–459.

94. de Boer AS, Borgdorff MW, de Haas PE, Nagelkerke NJ, van Embden JD, van Soolingen D. 1999. Analysis of rate of change of IS6110 RFLP patterns of *Mycobacterium tuberculosis* based on serial patient isolates. *J Infect Dis* 180:1238–1244.

95. Walker TM, Ip CL, Harrell RH, Evans JT, Kapatai G, Dedicoat MJ, Eyre DW, Wilson DJ, Hawkey PM, Crook DW, Parkhill J, Harris D, Walker AS, Bowden R, Monk P, Smith EG, Peto TE. 2013. Whole-genome sequencing to delineate *Mycobacterium tuberculosis* outbreaks: a retrospective observational study. *Lancet Infect Dis* 13:137–146.

96. Savine E, Warren RM, van der Spuy GD, Beyers N, van Helden PD, Locht C, Supply P. 2002. Stability of variable-number tandem repeats of mycobacterial interspersed repetitive units from 12 loci in serial isolates of *Mycobacterium tuberculosis*. *J Clin Microbiol* 40:4561–4566.

97. Pérez-Lago L, Comas I, Navarro Y, González-Candelas F, Herranz M, Bouza E, García-de-Viedma D. 2014. Whole genome sequencing analysis of intrapatient microevolution in *Mycobacterium tuberculosis*: potential impact on the inference of tuberculosis transmission. *J Infect Dis* 209:98–108.

98. Walker TM, Lalor MK, Broda A, Ortega LS, Morgan M, Parker L, Churchill S, Bennett K, Golubchik T, Giess AP, Del Ojo Elias C, Jeffery KJ, Bowler IC, Laurenson IF, Barrett A, Drobniewski F, McCarthy ND, Anderson LF, Abubakar I, Thomas HL, Monk P, Smith EG, Walker AS, Crook DW, Peto TE, Conlon CP. 2014. Assessment of *Mycobacterium tuberculosis* transmission in Oxfordshire, UK, 2007-12, with whole pathogen genome sequences: an observational study. *Lancet Respir Med* 2:285–292.

99. Roetzer A, Diel R, Kohl TA, Rückert C, Nübel U, Blom J, Wirth T, Jaenicke S, Schuback S, Rüsch-Gerdes S, Supply P, Kalinowski J, Niemann S. 2013. Whole genome sequencing versus traditional genotyping for investigation of a *Mycobacterium tuberculosis* outbreak: a longitudinal molecular epidemiological study. *PLoS Med* 10:e1001387.

100. Eldholm V, Norheim G, von der Lippe B, Kinander W, Dahle UR, Caugant DA, Mannsåker T, Mengshoel AT,

Dyrhol-Riise AM, Balloux F. 2014. Evolution of extensively drug-resistant *Mycobacterium tuberculosis* from a susceptible ancestor in a single patient. *Genome Biol* 15:490.

101. Merker M, Kohl TA, Roetzer A, Truebe L, Richter E, Rüsch-Gerdes S, Fattorini L, Oggioni MR, Cox H, Varaine F, Niemann S. 2013. Whole genome sequencing reveals complex evolution patterns of multidrug-resistant *Mycobacterium tuberculosis* Beijing strains in patients. *PLoS One* 8:e82551.

102. Sun G, Luo T, Yang C, Dong X, Li J, Zhu Y, Zheng H, Tian W, Wang S, Barry CE III, Mei J, Gao Q. 2012. Dynamic population changes in *Mycobacterium tuberculosis* during acquisition and fixation of drug resistance in patients. *J Infect Dis* 206:1724–1733.

103. Niemann S, Richter E, Rüsch-Gerdes S, Schlaak M, Greinert U. 2000. Double infection with a resistant and a multidrug-resistant strain of *Mycobacterium tuberculosis*. *Emerg Infect Dis* 6:548–551.

104. Theisen A, Reichel C, Rüsch-Gerdes S, Haas WH, Rockstroh JK, Spengler U, Sauerbruch T. 1995. Mixed-strain infection with a drug-sensitive and multidrug-resistant strain of *Mycobacterium tuberculosis*. *Lancet* 345:1512–1513.

105. Wells AQ. 1937. Tuberculosis in wild voles. *Lancet* 229:1221.

106. de Jong BC, Hill PC, Brookes RH, Gagneux S, Jeffries DJ, Otu JK, Donkor SA, Fox A, McAdam KP, Small PM, Adegbola RA. 2006. *Mycobacterium africanum* elicits an attenuated T cell response to early secreted antigenic target, 6 kDa, in patients with tuberculosis and their household contacts. *J Infect Dis* 193: 1279–1286.

107. de Jong BC, Hill PC, Aiken A, Awine T, Antonio M, Adetifa IM, Jackson-Sillah DJ, Fox A, Deriemer K, Gagneux S, Borgdorff MW, McAdam KP, Corrah T, Small PM, Adegbola RA. 2008. Progression to active tuberculosis, but not transmission, varies by *Mycobacterium tuberculosis* lineage in The Gambia. *J Infect Dis* 198:1037–1043.

108. Caws M, Thwaites G, Dunstan S, Hawn TR, Lan NT, Thuong NT, Stepniewska K, Huyen MN, Bang ND, Loc TH, Gagneux S, van Soolingen D, Kremer K, van der Sande M, Small P, Anh PT, Chinh NT, Quy HT, Duyen NT, Tho DQ, Hieu NT, Torok E, Hien TT, Dung NH, Nhu NT, Duy PM, van Vinh Chau N, Farrar J. 2008. The influence of host and bacterial genotype on the development of disseminated disease with *Mycobacterium tuberculosis*. *PLoS Pathog* 4:e1000034.

109. Kong Y, Cave MD, Zhang L, Foxman B, Marrs CF, Bates JH, Yang ZH. 2007. Association between *Mycobacterium tuberculosis* Beijing/W lineage strain infection and extrathoracic tuberculosis: insights from epidemiologic and clinical characterization of the three principal genetic groups of *M. tuberculosis* clinical isolates. *J Clin Microbiol* 45:409–414.

110. Rakotosamimanana N, Raharimanga V, Andriamandimby SF, Soares JL, Doherty TM, Ratsitorahina M, Ramarokoto H, Zumla A, Huggett J, Rook G, Richard V, Gicquel B, Rasolofo-Razanamparany V, VACSEL/VACSIS Study Group. 2010. Variation in gamma interferon responses to different infecting strains of *Mycobacterium tuberculosis* in acid-fast bacillus smear-positive patients and household contacts in Antananarivo, Madagascar. *Clin Vaccine Immunol* 17:1094–1103.

111. López B, Aguilar D, Orozco H, Burger M, Espitia C, Ritacco V, Barrera L, Kremer K, Hernandez-Pando R, Huygen K, van Soolingen D. 2003. A marked difference in pathogenesis and immune response induced by different *Mycobacterium tuberculosis* genotypes. *Clin Exp Immunol* 133:30–37.

112. Homolka S, Niemann S, Russell DG, Rohde KH. 2010. Functional genetic diversity among *Mycobacterium tuberculosis* complex clinical isolates: delineation of conserved core and lineage-specific transcriptomes during intracellular survival. *PLoS Pathog* 6:e1000988.

113. Portevin D, Gagneux S, Comas I, Young D. 2011. Human macrophage responses to clinical isolates from the *Mycobacterium tuberculosis* complex discriminate between ancient and modern lineages. *PLoS Pathog* 7: e1001307.

114. Reiling N, Homolka S, Walter K, Brandenburg J, Niwinski L, Ernst M, Herzmann C, Lange C, Diel R, Ehlers S, Niemann S. 2013. Clade-specific virulence patterns of *Mycobacterium tuberculosis* complex strains in human primary macrophages and aerogenically infected mice. *MBio* 4:eDD250-13.

115. Ribeiro SC, Gomes LL, Amaral EP, Andrade MR, Almeida FM, Rezende AL, Lanes VR, Carvalho EC, Suffys PN, Mokrousov I, Lasunskaia EB. 2014. *Mycobacterium tuberculosis* strains of the modern sublineage of the Beijing family are more likely to display increased virulence than strains of the ancient sublineage. *J Clin Microbiol* 52:2615–2624.

116. Krishnan N, Malaga W, Constant P, Caws M, Chau TTH, Salmons J, Lan NT, Bang ND, Daffé M, Young DB, Robertson BD, Guilhot C, Thwaites GE. 2011. *Mycobacterium tuberculosis* lineage influences innate immune response and virulence and is associated with distinct cell envelope lipid profiles. *PLoS One* 6:e23870

117. Rose G, Cortes T, Comas I, Coscolla M, Gagneux S, Young DB. 2013. Mapping of genotype-phenotype diversity among clinical isolates of *Mycobacterium tuberculosis* by sequence-based transcriptional profiling. *Genome Biol Evol* 5:1849–1862.

118. Coscolla M, Gagneux S. 2010. Does M. tuberculosis genomic diversity explain disease diversity? *Drug Discov Today Dis Mech* 7:e43–e59.

119. Gagneux S. 2013. Genetic diversity in *Mycobacterium tuberculosis*. *Curr Top Microbiol Immunol* 374:1–25.

120. Parwati I, van Crevel R, van Soolingen D. 2010. Possible underlying mechanisms for successful emergence of the *Mycobacterium tuberculosis* Beijing genotype strains. *Lancet Infect Dis* 10:103–111.

121. Fleischmann RD, Alland D, Eisen JA, Carpenter L, White O, Peterson J, DeBoy R, Dodson R, Gwinn M, Haft D, Hickey E, Kolonay JF, Nelson WC, Umayam LA, Ermolaeva M, Salzberg SL, Delcher A, Utterback T, Weidman J, Khouri H, Gill J, Mikula A, Bishai W, Jacobs WR Jr, Venter JC, Fraser CM. 2002. Whole-

genome comparison of *Mycobacterium tuberculosis* clinical and laboratory strains. *J Bacteriol* **184**: 5479–5490.

122. Garnier T, Eiglmeier K, Camus JC, Medina N, Mansoor H, Pryor M, Duthoy S, Grondin S, Lacroix C, Monsempe C, Simon S, Harris B, Atkin R, Doggett J, Mayes R, Keating L, Wheeler PR, Parkhill J, Barrell BG, Cole ST, Gordon SV, Hewinson RG. 2003. The complete genome sequence of *Mycobacterium bovis*. *Proc Natl Acad Sci USA* **100**:7877–7882.

123. Gordon SV, Brosch R, Billault A, Garnier T, Eiglmeier K, Cole ST. 1999. Identification of variable regions in the genomes of tubercle bacilli using bacterial artificial chromosome arrays. *Mol Microbiol* **32**:643–655.

124. Mahairas GG, Sabo PJ, Hickey MJ, Singh DC, Stover CK. 1996. Molecular analysis of genetic differences between *Mycobacterium bovis* BCG and virulent M. bovis. *J Bacteriol* **178**:1274–1282.

125. Alland D, Lacher DW, Hazbón MH, Motiwala AS, Qi W, Fleischmann RD, Whittam TS. 2007. Role of large sequence polymorphisms (LSPs) in generating genomic diversity among clinical isolates of *Mycobacterium tuberculosis* and the utility of LSPs in phylogenetic analysis. *J Clin Microbiol* **45**:39–46.

126. Domenech P, Kolly GS, Leon-Solis L, Fallow A, Reed MB. 2010. Massive gene duplication event among clinical isolates of the *Mycobacterium tuberculosis* W/Beijing family. *J Bacteriol* **192**:4562–4570.

127. Weiner B, Gomez J, Victor TC, Warren RM, Sloutsky A, Plikaytis BB, Posey JE, van Helden PD, Gey van Pittius NC, Koehrsen M, Sisk P, Stolte C, White J, Gagneux S, Birren B, Hung D, Murray M, Galagan J. 2012. Independent large scale duplications in multiple M. tuberculosis lineages overlapping the same genomic region. *PLoS One* **7**:e26038.

128. McEvoy CR, Falmer AA, Gey van Pittius NC, Victor TC, van Helden PD, Warren RM. 2007. The role of IS6110 in the evolution of *Mycobacterium tuberculosis*. *Tuberculosis (Edinb)* **87**:393–404.

129. Ho TB, Robertson BD, Taylor GM, Shaw RJ, Young DB. 2000. Comparison of *Mycobacterium tuberculosis* genomes reveals frequent deletions in a 20 kb variable region in clinical isolates. *Yeast* **17**:272–282.

130. Brosch R, Philipp WJ, Stavropoulos E, Colston MJ, Cole ST, Gordon SV. 1999. Genomic analysis reveals variation between *Mycobacterium tuberculosis* H37Rv and the attenuated *M. tuberculosis* H37Ra strain. *Infect Immun* **67**:5768–5774.

131. Casart Y, Turcios L, Florez I, Jaspe R, Guerrero E, de Waard J, Aguilar D, Hérnandez-Pando R, Salazar L. 2008. IS6110 in oriC affects the morphology and growth of *Mycobacterium tuberculosis* and attenuates virulence in mice. *Tuberculosis (Edinb)* **88**:545–552.

132. Soto CY, Menéndez MC, Pérez E, Samper S, Gómez AB, García MJ, Martín C. 2004. IS6110 mediates increased transcription of the phoP virulence gene in a multidrug-resistant clinical isolate responsible for tuberculosis outbreaks. *J Clin Microbiol* **42**:212–219.

133. Felsenstein J. 1974. The evolutionary advantage of recombination. *Genetics* **78**:737–756.

134. Smith JM, Haigh J. 1974. The hitch-hiking effect of a favourable gene. *Genet Res* **23**:23–35.

135. Domenech P, Rog A, Moolji JU, Radomski N, Fallow A, Leon-Solis L, Bowes J, Behr MA, Reed MB. 2014. Origins of a 350-kilobase genomic duplication in *Mycobacterium tuberculosis* and its impact on virulence. *Infect Immun* **82**:2902–2912.

136. Behr MA, Wilson MA, Gill WP, Salamon H, Schoolnik GK, Rane S, Small PM. 1999. Comparative genomics of BCG vaccines by whole-genome DNA microarray. *Science* **284**:1520–1523.

137. Brodin P, Eiglmeier K, Marmiesse M, Billault A, Garnier T, Niemann S, Cole ST, Brosch R. 2002. Bacterial artificial chromosome-based comparative genomic analysis identifies *Mycobacterium microti* as a natural ESAT-6 deletion mutant. *Infect Immun* **70**: 5568–5578.

138. Pym AS, Brodin P, Majlessi L, Brosch R, Demangel C, Williams A, Griffiths KE, Marchal G, Leclerc C, Cole ST. 2003. Recombinant BCG exporting ESAT-6 confers enhanced protection against tuberculosis. *Nat Med* **9**: 533–539.

139. Stanley SA, Raghavan S, Hwang WW, Cox JS. 2003. Acute infection and macrophage subversion by *Mycobacterium tuberculosis* require a specialized secretion system. *Proc Natl Acad Sci USA* **100**:13001–13006.

140. Guinn KM, Hickey MJ, Mathur SK, Zakel KL, Grotzke JE, Lewinsohn DM, Smith S, Sherman DR. 2004. Individual RD1-region genes are required for export of ESAT-6/CFP-10 and for virulence of *Mycobacterium tuberculosis*. *Mol Microbiol* **51**:359–370.

141. Bold TD, Davis DC, Penberthy KK, Cox LM, Ernst JD, de Jong BC. 2012. Impaired fitness of *Mycobacterium africanum* despite secretion of ESAT-6. *J Infect Dis* **205**: 984–990.

142. Winglee K, Manson McGuire A, Maiga M, Abeel T, Shea T, Desjardins CA, Diarra B, Baya B, Sanogo M, Diallo S, Earl AM, Bishai WR. 2016. Whole genome sequencing of *Mycobacterium africanum* strains from Mali provides insights into the mechanisms of geographic restriction. *PLoS Negl Trop Dis* **10**:e0004332.

143. Safi H, Barnes PF, Lakey DL, Shams H, Samten B, Vankayalapati R, Howard ST. 2004. IS6110 functions as a mobile, monocyte-activated promoter in *Mycobacterium tuberculosis*. *Mol Microbiol* **52**:999–1012.

144. Rivero A, Márquez M, Santos J, Pinedo A, Sánchez MA, Esteve A, Samper S, Martín C. 2001. High rate of tuberculosis reinfection during a nosocomial outbreak of multidrug-resistant tuberculosis caused by *Mycobacterium bovis* strain B. *Clin Infect Dis* **32**:159–161.

145. Gopinath K, Moosa A, Mizrahi V, Warner DF. 2013. Vitamin B(12) metabolism in *Mycobacterium tuberculosis*. *Future Microbiol* **8**:1405–1418.

146. Gopinath K, Venclovas C, Ioerger TR, Sacchettini JC, McKinney JD, Mizrahi V, Warner DF. 2013. A vitamin B12 transporter in *Mycobacterium tuberculosis*. *Open Biol* **3**:120175.

147. Schoonmaker MK, Bishai WR, Lamichhane G. 2014. Nonclassical transpeptidases of *Mycobacterium tuberculosis* alter cell size, morphology, the cytosolic

matrix, protein localization, virulence, and resistance to β-lactams. *J Bacteriol* **196:**1394–1402.

148. Koeck JL, Bernatas JJ, Gerome P, Fabre M, Houmed A, Herve V, Teyssou R. 2002. [Epidemiology of resistance to antituberculosis drugs in *Mycobacterium tuberculosis* complex strains isolated from adenopathies in Djibouti. Prospective study carried out in 1999.] (In French.) *Med Trop (Mars)* **62:**70–72.

149. Boritsch EC, Frigui W, Cascioferro A, Malaga W, Etienne G, Laval F, Pawlik A, Le Chevalier F, Orgeur M, Ma L, Bouchier C, Stinear TP, Supply P, Majlessi L, Daffé M, Guilhot C, Brosch R. 2016. *pks5*-recombination-mediated surface remodelling in *Mycobacterium tuberculosis* emergence. *New Microbiol* **1:**15019.

150. Niemann S, Diel R, Khechinashvili G, Gegia M, Mdivani N, Tang YW. 2010. *Mycobacterium tuberculosis* Beijing lineage favors the spread of multidrug-resistant tuberculosis in the Republic of Georgia. *J Clin Microbiol* **48:**3544–3550.

151. Cowley D, Govender D, February B, Wolfe M, Steyn L, Evans J, Wilkinson RJ, Nicol MP. 2008. Recent and rapid emergence of W-Beijing strains of *Mycobacterium tuberculosis* in Cape Town, South Africa. *Clin Infect Dis* **47:**1252–1259.

152. Glynn JR, Whiteley J, Bifani PJ, Kremer K, van Soolingen D. 2002. Worldwide occurrence of Beijing/W strains of *Mycobacterium tuberculosis*: a systematic review. *Emerg Infect Dis* **8:**843–849.

153. Manca C, Reed MB, Freeman S, Mathema B, Kreiswirth B, Barry CE III, Kaplan G. 2004. Differential monocyte activation underlies strain-specific *Mycobacterium tuberculosis* pathogenesis. *Infect Immun* **72:**5511–5514.

154. Reed MB, Domenech P, Manca C, Su H, Barczak AK, Kreiswirth BN, Kaplan G, Barry CE III. 2004. A glycolipid of hypervirulent tuberculosis strains that inhibits the innate immune response. *Nature* **431:**84–87.

155. Dormans J, Burger M, Aguilar D, Hernandez-Pando R, Kremer K, Roholl P, Arend SM, van Soolingen D. 2004. Correlation of virulence, lung pathology, bacterial load and delayed type hypersensitivity responses after infection with different *Mycobacterium tuberculosis* genotypes in a BALB/c mouse model. *Clin Exp Immunol* **137:**460–468.

156. Tsenova L, Ellison E, Harbacheuski R, Moreira AL, Kurepina N, Reed MB, Mathema B, Barry CE III, Kaplan G. 2005. Virulence of selected *Mycobacterium tuberculosis* clinical isolates in the rabbit model of meningitis is dependent on phenolic glycolipid produced by the bacilli. *J Infect Dis* **192:**98–106.

157. Jeon BY, Derrick SC, Lim J, Kolibab K, Dheenadhayalan V, Yang AL, Kreiswirth B, Morris SL. 2008. *Mycobacterium bovis* BCG immunization induces protective immunity against nine different *Mycobacterium tuberculosis* strains in mice. *Infect Immun* **76:**5173–5180.

158. Ordway DJ, Shang S, Henao-Tamayo M, Obregon-Henao A, Nold L, Caraway M, Shanley CA, Basaraba RJ, Duncan CG, Orme IM. 2011. *Mycobacterium bovis* BCG-mediated protection against W-Beijing strains of *Mycobacterium tuberculosis* is diminished concomitant

with the emergence of regulatory T cells. *Clin Vaccine Immunol* **18:**1527–1535.

159. Kato-Maeda M, Kim EY, Flores L, Jarlsberg LG, Osmond D, Hopewell PC. 2010. Differences among sublineages of the East-Asian lineage of *Mycobacterium tuberculosis* in genotypic clustering. *Int J Tuberc Lung Dis* **14:**538–544.

160. Kato-Maeda M, Shanley CA, Ackart D, Jarlsberg LG, Shang S, Obregon-Henao A, Harton M, Basaraba RJ, Henao-Tamayo M, Barrozo JC, Rose J, Kawamura LM, Coscolla M, Fofanov VY, Koshinsky H, Gagneux S, Hopewell PC, Ordway DJ, Orme IM. 2012. Beijing sublineages of *Mycobacterium tuberculosis* differ in pathogenicity in the guinea pig. *Clin Vaccine Immunol* **19:**1227–1237.

161. Aguilar D, Hanekom LM, Mata D, Gey van Pittius NC, van Helden PD, Warren RM, Hernandez-Pando R. 2010. *Mycobacterium tuberculosis* strains with the Beijing genotype demonstrate variability in virulence associated with transmission. *Tuberculosis (Edinb)* **90:**319–325.

162. Hanekom M, van der Spuy GD, Streicher E, Ndabambi SL, McEvoy CR, Kidd M, Beyers N, Victor TC, van Helden PD, Warren RM. 2007. A recently evolved sublineage of the *Mycobacterium tuberculosis* Beijing strain family is associated with an increased ability to spread and cause disease. *J Clin Microbiol* **45:**1483–1490.

163. Mokrousov I. 2013. Insights into the origin, emergence, and current spread of a successful Russian clone of *Mycobacterium tuberculosis*. *Clin Microbiol Rev* **26:**342–360.

164. Sinsimer D, Huet G, Manca C, Tsenova L, Koo MS, Kurepina N, Kana B, Mathema B, Marras SA, Kreiswirth BN, Guilhot C, Kaplan G. 2008. The phenolic glycolipid of *Mycobacterium tuberculosis* differentially modulates the early host cytokine response but does not in itself confer hypervirulence. *Infect Immun* **76:**3027–3036.

165. Reed MB, Gagneux S, Deriemer K, Small PM, Barry CE III. 2007. The W-Beijing lineage of *Mycobacterium tuberculosis* overproduces triglycerides and has the DosR dormancy regulon constitutively upregulated. *J Bacteriol* **189:**2583–2589.

166. Fallow A, Domenech P, Reed MB. 2010. Strains of the East Asian (W/Beijing) lineage of *Mycobacterium tuberculosis* are DosS/DosT-DosR two-component regulatory system natural mutants. *J Bacteriol* **192:**2228–2238.

167. Gagneux S, Long CD, Small PM, Van T, Schoolnik GK, Bohannan BJ. 2006. The competitive cost of antibiotic resistance in *Mycobacterium tuberculosis*. *Science* **312:**1944–1946.

168. Hazbón MH, Brimacombe M, Bobadilla del Valle M, Cavatore M, Guerrero MI, Varma-Basil M, Billman-Jacobe H, Lavender C, Fyfe J, García-García L, León CI, Bose M, Chaves F, Murray M, Eisenach KD, Sifuentes-Osornio J, Cave MD, Ponce de León A, Alland D. 2006. Population genetics study of isoniazid resistance mutations and evolution of multidrug-resistant *Mycobacterium tuberculosis*. *Antimicrob Agents Chemother* **50:**2640–2649.

169. Shcherbakov D, Akbergenov R, Matt T, Sander P, Andersson DI, Böttger EC. 2010. Directed mutagenesis of *Mycobacterium smegmatis* 16S rRNA to reconstruct the in vivo evolution of aminoglycoside resistance in *Mycobacterium tuberculosis*. *Mol Microbiol* 77:830–840.

170. Comas I, Borrell S, Roetzer A, Rose G, Malla B, Kato-Maeda M, Galagan J, Niemann S, Gagneux S. 2011. Whole-genome sequencing of rifampicin-resistant *Mycobacterium tuberculosis* strains identifies compensatory mutations in RNA polymerase genes. *Nat Genet* 44:106–110.

171. Casali N, Nikolayevskyy V, Balabanova Y, Ignatyeva O, Kontsevaya I, Harris SR, Bentley SD, Parkhill J, Nejentsev S, Hoffner SE, Horstmann RD, Brown T, Drobniewski F. 2012. Microevolution of extensively drug-resistant tuberculosis in Russia. *Genome Res* 22:735–745.

172. Casali N, Nikolayevskyy V, Balabanova Y, Harris SR, Ignatyeva O, Kontsevaya I, Corander J, Bryant J, Parkhill J, Nejentsev S, Horstmann RD, Brown T, Drobniewski F. 2014. Evolution and transmission of drug-resistant tuberculosis in a Russian population. *Nat Genet* 46:279–286.

173. Cohen KA, Abeel T, Manson McGuire A, Desjardins CA, Munsamy V, Shea TP, Walker BJ, Bantubani N, Almeida DV, Alvarado L, Chapman SB, Mvelase NR, Duffy EY, Fitzgerald MG, Govender P, Gujja S, Hamilton S, Howarth C, Larimer JD, Maharaj K, Pearson MD, Priest ME, Zeng Q, Padayatchi N, Grosset J, Young SK, Wortman J, Mlisana KP, O'Donnell MR, Birren BW, Bishai WR, Pym AS, Earl AM. 2015. Evolution of extensively drug-resistant tuberculosis over four decades: whole genome sequencing and dating analysis of *Mycobacterium tuberculosis* isolates from KwaZulu-Natal. *PLoS Med* 12:e1001880.

174. Eldholm V, Monteserin J, Rieux A, Lopez B, Sobkowiak B, Ritacco V, Balloux F. 2015. Four decades of transmission of a multidrug-resistant *Mycobacterium tuberculosis* outbreak strain. *Nat Commun* 6:7119.

175. Müller B, Borrell S, Rose G, Gagneux S. 2013. The heterogeneous evolution of multidrug-resistant *Mycobacterium tuberculosis*. *Trends Genet* 29:160–169.

176. de Steenwinkel JE, Soolingen D, Bakker-Woudenberg IA. 2013. *Mycobacterium tuberculosis* Beijing type mutation frequency–author's response. *Emerg Infect Dis* 19:522–523.

177. de Steenwinkel JE, ten Kate MT, de Knegt GJ, Kremer K, Aarnoutse RE, Boeree MJ, Verbrugh HA, van Soolingen D, Bakker-Woudenberg IA. 2012. Drug susceptibility of *Mycobacterium tuberculosis* Beijing genotype and association with MDR TB. *Emerg Infect Dis* 18:660–663.

178. Ford CB, Shah RR, Maeda MK, Gagneux S, Murray MB, Cohen T, Johnston JC, Gardy J, Lipsitch M, Fortune SM. 2013. *Mycobacterium tuberculosis* mutation rate estimates from different lineages predict substantial differences in the emergence of drug-resistant tuberculosis. *Nat Genet* 45:784–790.

179. McGrath M, Gey van Pittius NC, van Helden PD, Warren RM, Warner DF. 2014. Mutation rate and the emergence of drug resistance in *Mycobacterium tuberculosis*. *J Antimicrob Chemother* 69:292–302.

180. Mestre O, Luo T, Dos Vultos T, Kremer K, Murray A, Namouchi A, Jackson C, Rauzier J, Bifani P, Warren R, Rasolofo V, Mei J, Gao Q, Gicquel B. 2011. Phylogeny of *Mycobacterium tuberculosis* Beijing strains constructed from polymorphisms in genes involved in DNA replication, recombination and repair. *PLoS One* 6:e16020.

181. Werngren J. 2013. *Mycobacterium tuberculosis* Beijing type mutation frequency. *Emerg Infect Dis* 19:522.

182. Werngren J, Hoffner SE. 2003. Drug-susceptible *Mycobacterium tuberculosis* Beijing genotype does not develop mutation-conferred resistance to rifampin at an elevated rate. *J Clin Microbiol* 41:1520–1524.

183. Bergval I, Kwok B, Schuitema A, Kremer K, van Soolingen D, Klatser P, Anthony R. 2012. Pre-existing isoniazid resistance, but not the genotype of *Mycobacterium tuberculosis* drives rifampicin resistance codon preference in vitro. *PLoS One* 7:e29108.

184. World Health Organization. 2015. *Global Health Observatory data*. World Health Organization, Geneva, Switzerland. http://www.who.int/gho/tb/en/.

Tuberculosis and the Tubercle Bacillus, 2nd ed.
Edited by William R. Jacobs, Jr., Helen McShane, Valerie Mizrahi, and Ian M. Orme
© 2018 American Society for Microbiology, Washington, DC
doi:10.1128/microbiolspec.TBTB2-0020-2016

Evolution of *Mycobacterium tuberculosis*: New Insights into Pathogenicity and Drug Resistance

22

Eva C. Boritsch and Roland Brosch

INTRODUCTION

The evolution of *Mycobacterium tuberculosis* toward one of the most dangerous human pathogens is of particular interest for the analysis of the continued importance of tuberculosis as a global disease. While the majority of mycobacterial species are harmless environmental bacteria, *M. tuberculosis* is able to induce pulmonary lesions and disease in the human host, which represents an essential step for the aerosol transmission of the bacterium to new individuals. The question of when and where *M. tuberculosis* or one of its progenitors has acquired this faculty has interested scientists for years. It is hypothesized that the ancestors of *M. tuberculosis* once had an environmental reservoir and gradually evolved to adapt to the life within host cells, leading finally to the feature of getting transmitted from one host to another (1, 2). First insights into this issue can be obtained from genomic comparison of *M. tuberculosis* with related nontuberculous mycobacteria (NTM), also known as atypical mycobacteria or mycobacteria other than tuberculosis (MOTT). Based on 16S rRNA sequence similarity, *Mycobacterium marinum* and *Mycobacterium ulcerans* were the currently known closest relatives of *M. tuberculosis* (3). In a later study, based on whole-genome sequencing (WGS), *Mycobacterium kansasii* was found as the closest NTM species of *M. tuberculosis* (4), whereas a different WGS study designated *M. marinum*/*M. ulcerans* as most closely related to *M. tuberculosis*, followed by a subgroup containing *Mycobacterium haemophilum*, *Mycobacterium lepromatosis*, and *Mycobacterium*

leprae (5). However, despite the similarities at the DNA and protein level, the genome size differences between the closest NTM species relative to *M. tuberculosis* are considerable (6). *M. tuberculosis* strains harbor a 4.4 MB genome (7–9), whereas the genomes of *M. marinum*, *M. kansasii*, and *M. ulcerans* are larger in size (6.7, 6.4, and 5.8 MB, respectively) (10–12). In contrast, the genomes of *M. haemophilum*, *M. lepromatosis*, and *M. leprae* are smaller in size (4.2, 3.3, and 3.3 MB, respectively) (5, 13, 14), whereby the strong size reduction of the latter two species is due to a common, extensive phase of reductive evolution (13). It seems conceivable that the individual adaptations of the different mycobacterial species to specific environmental conditions went along with genome downsizing, gene acquisition through horizontal gene transfer, genome rearrangements, and/or recombination.

The emergence of WGS as an affordable, commonly used tool to study bacterial phylogenies at the genus, species, and more recently even at the intrapatient strain level opened the door to a refined appreciation of the evolutionary events that led to a specification of *M. tuberculosis* and related tubercle bacilli and their adaptation to different hosts. This technique is now extensively used to elucidate the factors that contributed to the successful expansion of certain clades within the tubercle bacilli. This review will briefly summarize selected molecular events in the evolution of *M. tuberculosis* toward becoming a professional human pathogen, as well as give an update on the evolution of (drug-resistant) clinical strains in the course of infections and outbreaks.

Institut Pasteur, Unit for Integrated Mycobacterial Pathogenomics, 75015 Paris, France.

FROM ENVIRONMENT TO HOST? LESSONS TO LEARN FROM *MYCOBACTERIUM CANETTII*

From genome comparisons with NTM species, it is clear that *M. tuberculosis* and related tubercle bacilli of the so-called *M. tuberculosis* complex (MTBC) represent a single bacterial species within the mycobacterial genus. The situation with the MTBC is somewhat special because, in previous years, different variants of this complex were characterized with different names, according to the host from which the bacteria were isolated. As such, the *M. tuberculosis* complex comprises *Mycobacterium africanum*, corresponding to strains of two sublineages, named L5 and L6 (15) that cause tuberculosis in humans in West Africa (16), and a growing number of identified variants isolated from different animal species, named lineage L8 (17). The latter strains, which may also be defined as so-called ecotypes (18), comprise *Mycobacterium bovis, Mycobacterium caprae, Mycobacterium microti, Mycobacterium mungi, Mycobacterium orygis, Mycobacterium pinnipedii, Mycobacterium suricattae*, and a chimpanzee isolate, which were named according to the mammalian species from where they were isolated (19–25). The members of this animal lineage share more than 99.9% similarity at the DNA level with *M. tuberculosis* and *M. africanum*, but they may differ with respect to pathogenicity and a limited number of phenotypic and/or genotypic characteristics. The wide distribution of tubercle bacilli among different animal species might have also contributed to the previous hypothesis that *M. tuberculosis* evolved from bovine tubercle bacilli (26), until genome comparisons revealed that the evolution of the human tuberculosis bacillus was more complex, and apparently independent of the evolution of the animal strain lineages (2, 27–30). Indeed, signs of selected genomic deletion events, specifically marked by the absence of region of difference 9 (RD9) and other specific RD regions from *M. bovis* relative to *M. tuberculosis* and *M. canettii*, suggested an evolutionary scenario that places *M. canettii*-like mycobacteria at the origin of the strains that evolved into the different lineages of the MTBC (2, 27, 31).

The isolation and analysis of the rare *M. canettii* strains from pulmonary lesions, lymph nodes, and/or skin lesions of infected patients (1, 32–37) represent crucial steps toward a better understanding of the molecular events that promoted the pathogenic lifestyle of the MTBC members. *M. canettii* strains were shown to have branched from the most recent common ancestor (MRCA) of the MTBC before the clonal emergence of the latter, and even though *M. canettii* strains are able to cause certain types of disease, they seem to be defective in human-to-human transmission. For *M. tuberculosis*, transmission is promoted by the ability of the bacilli to establish acute and/or persistent infections, the latter of which can result in a reactivation and thus spread of the disease to new hosts. Interestingly, *M. canettii* strains were shown to be less virulent and less persistent in mouse infection models (2). *M. canettii* also grows faster than the members of the MTBC, underlining the probable environmental nature of these strains (1, 2). From data on the identification of DNA of MTBC strains in the environment (38) and growth experiments of tubercle bacilli in amoebae (39), a potential scenario emerges in which an MTBC ancestor possibly evolved from a pool of *M. canettii*-like mycobacteria living in soil-, water-, and/or protozoan-associated settings (2). Such a situation would have allowed frequent contact with other microorganisms, facilitating potential genetic exchange and horizontal gene transfer leading to the acquisition of necessary features for a pathogenic lifestyle.

Since the first isolation of unusual tubercle bacilli for a case of pulmonary tuberculosis by the team of Canetti at the Institut Pasteur in Paris in the 1960s, fewer than 100 similar isolates have been recovered, mainly from patients from or with some connection to East Africa (1, 2, 30–33, 35, 37). The most characteristic feature of these strains, named after Georges Canetti by van Soolingen and coworkers (33), is an unusual smooth colony morphology, which also gave rise to their description as smooth tubercle bacilli. Comparative genome sequence analysis of several *M. canettii* strains revealed a high genetic variation and thus a much greater phylogenetic distance among *M. canettii* strains, than among the members of the MTBC, which display a highly clonal population structure (Fig. 1) (2, 40). Hence intriguingly, in the few *M. canettii* strains isolated until now, originating from a geographically restricted region, a much higher genetic variability can be found than in the worldwide population of MTBC strains. This situation points to a scenario where advantageous molecular events helped selected progenitor strains of the MTBC to gain virulence and host specification factors that became fixed in the genomes after the diversification from the *M. canettii*-like strain pool. Smooth tubercle bacilli might thus provide clues for the identification of determinants that drove the global emergence and spread of *M. tuberculosis*. Genome comparison showed that the core genome of the studied *M. canettii* strains was about 20% larger than that of the MTBC members. While most extra genes are specific to individual *M. canettii* isolates, some of them

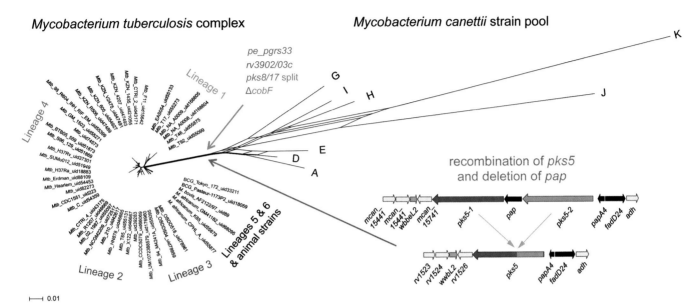

Figure 1 Scheme showing supposed molecular key events in mycobacterial evolution from a recombinogenic *M. canettii* strain pool toward professional pathogens of mammalian hosts. Network phylogeny inferred among eight *M. canettii* strains and 46 selected genome sequences from MTBC members by NeighborNet analysis. Pairwise alignments of whole genome SNP data are the basis of the calculation. Recombination of *pks5* and deletion of *pap* in a potential progenitor of the MTBC strains illustrated in the inset. Figure reproduced from reference 44.

are shared by all *M. canettii* strains (2). One such an example is the precorrin 6A synthase homologue, CobF, which might be involved in vitamin B$_{12}$ synthesis. CobF is common to all *M. canettii* strains, but absent from MTBC members (Fig. 1) (2, 31). Although *M. tuberculosis* possesses the remaining genes necessary for cobalamin biosynthesis, it does not seem to produce vitamin B$_{12}$ *in vitro* or in macrophages (41). In contrast, MTBC members appear to be able to take up exogenous vitamin B$_{12}$ precursors provided by the host (41). The deletion of *cobF* might be a possible explanation for this lack of vitamin B$_{12}$ production in MTBC strains, even though it was also suggested that other enzymes might partially counteract the absence of CobF (41). Yet, it seems likely that adaptation to an intracellular lifestyle of the MTBC members might have gradually abrogated the need for vitamin B$_{12}$ biosynthesis because of its availability from the host. This evolutionary scenario is further supported by the finding of various nonsynonymous single-nucleotide polymorphisms (SNPs) and frameshift mutations in other cobalamin biosynthesis genes, which were discovered in a genomic screen including more than 200 clinical *M. tuberculosis* isolates (42, 43). Whether vitamin B$_{12}$ production in *M. canettii* strains is functional remains to be determined.

An important molecular event in the evolution from a potentially environmental *M. canettii*-like strain toward

highly specialized pathogenic tubercle bacilli was recently found to involve a recombination in two highly homologous gene variants encoding polyketide synthase Pks5 in *M. canettii* (44). Homologous recombination of the two *pks5* genes in a spontaneous smooth-to-rough mutant of an *M. canettii* strain resulted in a single *pks5* configuration with the loss of an interspersed gene coding for a polyketide synthase-associated acyltransferase named Pap. Interestingly, a similar genomic organization of the *pks5* locus is fixed in all members of the MTBC, arguing that such a recombination of two *pks5* genes occurred in the MRCA of the MTBC (Fig. 1). As a consequence, all strains with the truncated, single *pks5* locus were found to be deficient in the synthesis of lipooligosaccharides (LOS), a cell wall component found in numerous slow-growing mycobacteria, with the exception of MTBC members. Importantly, the surface remodeling that went along with LOS biosynthesis deficiency resulted in increased virulence of the rough *M. canettii* morphotypes in cellular and animal infection models compared with their smooth counterparts. Hence, the *pks5* recombination event might represent an important *in vivo* fitness advantage in the evolution of the MTBC (44). In addition, the identification of the molecular mechanism distinguishing smooth from rough tubercle bacilli is also a proof of concept that *M. canettii* strains can serve as tools to define the factors that are driving the emergence of *M. tuberculosis*, which makes them a powerful model for the assessment of pathoadaptation in the evolution of *M. tuberculosis*.

However, genome comparisons not only identified gene deletions in the MTBC members relative to *M. canettii* strains, but, most interestingly, also several MTBC-specific gene insertions, some of which might have had an impact on virulence. One such an example is the protein PE_PGRS33 (Rv1818c), which belongs to the group of *M. tuberculosis* proteins with a characteristic Pro-Glu (PE) N-terminal motif and repetitions encoded by polymorphic GC-rich sequences (PGRS) (7, 45). This protein has been studied extensively in *M. tuberculosis*, and has been described as possessing potent immunomodulatory features putatively playing a role in uptake by macrophages and/or transmission of MTBC strains (46–48). Since the gene encoding PE_PGRS33 is neither present in *M. canettii* strains nor in more distantly related mycobacteria, it seems to represent a specific insertion event into the genomes of MTBC strains (2, 40). Another example is CpnT, a channel protein that induces necrosis through its C-terminal DUF4237 toxin domain (49). While the N-terminal pore domain is highly conserved between *M. canettii* and *M. tuberculosis* strains, a different toxin domain is present in *M. canettii* strains compared with the MTBC members (40). Whether the toxin domain of the *M. canettii* strains exerts a similar function as the MTBC domain needs to be evaluated.

Moreover, some MTBC-specific genes have no homologues in *M. canettii* or other mycobacteria. Representative sequence comparisons showed best hits with proteins from other bacteria, such as *Gordonia otitidis* (Rv0394c), "*Candidatus* Kuenenia stuttgartiensis" (Rv2023c), or *Pseudonocardia dioxanivorans* (Rv3190c), suggesting that these genes might have been acquired by an MTBC progenitor through horizontal gene transfer after the separation from the *M. canettii* strains (2). However, the functions of these genes are unknown, and assessment of whether they had an impact on virulence is awaiting further experimental analyses.

The above-mentioned examples demonstrate that *M. canettii* strains are a potent model to study the early evolution of *M. tuberculosis* becoming a professional pathogen. The finding of an outbreak of lymph node tuberculosis caused by a cluster of *M. canettii* D strains in the geographical region of Djibouti also points to a scenario where favorable mutations in an *M. canettii* strain might have led to higher pathogenicity and epidemiological visibility (31). However, in the case of the *M. canettii* D strains, human-to-human transmis-

sibility does not seem to be the causative factor for the accumulation of cases and none of the identified putative mutations found in the outbreak strains are exclusively present in these strains, but are also common to all other *M. canettii* strains (31). Nonetheless, careful evaluation of *M. canettii* outbreak clusters will be instrumental for our understanding of the determinants that trigger increased case rates and/or transmission. In addition, WGS of clinical *M. tuberculosis* strains during outbreaks, as well as in single patients, now gives precise insights on the processes that promote global spread of certain *M. tuberculosis* clades and thus will be further highlighted in the following paragraphs.

THE *M. TUBERCULOSIS* COMPLEX: PAVING THE WAY TO PROFESSIONAL PATHOGENICITY

The monomorphic *M. tuberculosis* complex does not only contain the human pathogens such as *M. tuberculosis* and *M. africanum*, but as aforementioned, also various animal pathogens (e.g., *M. microti*, *M. pinnipedii*, *M. orygis*, and *M. bovis*). MTBC members of human origin were differentiated into seven main lineages (L1 to L7) based on SNP-derived phylogeny, which can be associated with specific geographic regions (15, 27, 50–54). The fact that Africa is the only continent where strains of all the different lineages have been isolated gave rise to the hypothesis that MTBC emerged in East Africa and that subsequently successful clones migrated out of Africa and spread around the world (15, 27, 55). Because the evolution of *M. tuberculosis* is closely associated with its interaction with the human host, it was further suggested that its separation into the main lineages was linked to human migrations (15, 53, 55). Strains of lineage L1 are predominantly found in East Africa, South India, and Southeast Asia. These strains belong to the *M. tuberculosis* strains with a conserved genomic region containing the *mmpl6S* and *mmpL6* genes, named TbD1 region, which was used to differentiate "ancestral" (TbD1 region preserved) and "modern" (TbD1 region deleted) *M. tuberculosis* strains (27). Moreover, human isolates from other lineages that also have conserved the TbD1 region, namely, *M. africanum* L5 and L6 strains or *M. tuberculosis* L7 strains, are associated with West Africa (L5, L6) or East Africa (L7), respectively (53–56). In contrast, TbD1 region-deleted, "modern" *M. tuberculosis* strains belonging to lineage L2, L3, and L4 are associated with East Asia (L2), North India (L3), as well as Europe and the Americas (L4), respectively (Fig. 2).

The differences between the various lineages mainly consist of a number of SNPs and specific deletions of RDs (27). Interestingly, many of the recently emerging epidemic *M. tuberculosis* strains belong to the lineages L2, L3, and L4, all lacking the TbD1 region, which raises the question whether deletion/truncation of MmpS6 and MmpL6 represents an advantageous molecular event for an increased virulence in selected hosts. A recent study correlates the absence of region TbD1 with increased growth in human macrophages and higher replication rates in lungs of infected mice, endorsing such hypotheses (57), which, however, need more experimental and mechanistic analyses for further confirmation.

A Story of Success: Global Spread of *M. tuberculosis* L2 Beijing and L4 Strains

The fact that different lineages developed varying virulence traits, most probably attributable to interdependence on local hosts, demonstrates that adaptations of tubercle bacilli during infection might play an important role for achieving fine-tuned host-pathogen interaction. Some lineages thus seem to have adapted to particular human populations and are rarely found outside their geographical niches, like, for example, *M. africanum* L5 and L6, which are mainly present in western Africa (50, 58). However, adaptations in other lineages resulted in hypervirulent phenotypes, potentially higher transmission rates, and thus more global spread, as seen for the predominating clinical strains of the modern L2 and L4 lineages (40, 59). In a study conducted in The Gambia, patients infected with L2 or L4 strains were shown to have a higher probability of developing active tuberculosis than those infected with *M. africanum* L6 strains (60). Several other studies also reported a potential fitness advantage of the modern *M. tuberculosis* lineages in selected hosts, because they seem to outcompete L5 and L6 strains even in their geographical niche of western Africa (61–64). Hence, although the genetic variability among the MTBC strains

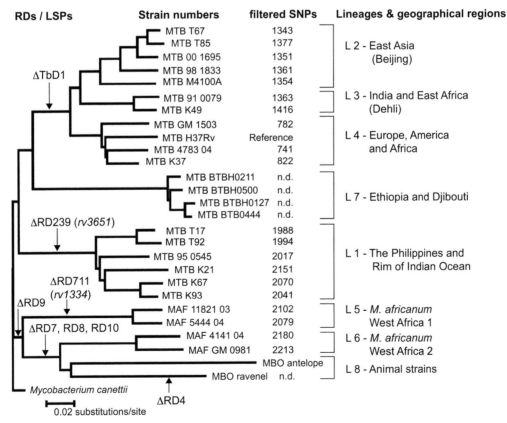

Figure 2 Neighbor-joining phylogeny scheme based on variable nucleotide positions with main focus on tubercle bacilli that have a human host preference, using *M. canettii* as root of the tree (after reference 56). The filtered SNPs refer to the mutations identified between the various strains relative to *M. tuberculosis* H37Rv (15). Figure reproduced from reference 40.

is remarkably low, ongoing evolution still is a major player driving the expansion of the most successful clones. It has previously been suggested that the modern lifestyle of humans may also have changed the lifestyle and infection behavior of the modern *M. tuberculosis* strains (65). In ancient times, in less densely populated societies, where contact with other humans was more scarce, long periods of latency might have been desirable for an effective transmission of the bacilli. The change in human living conditions to urban agglomerations facilitated a frequent inter-human contact and thus the spread of the bacilli. This situation subsequently might have abrogated the need for long phases of persistence and might have led to hypervirulent phenotypes and thus faster and higher transmission rates (65). The following paragraphs will highlight some of the molecular events that might have driven the transition from an ancient to a modern form of disease via the emergence of hypervirulent, globally spread *M. tuberculosis* strains.

Evolution of the *M. tuberculosis* L2 Beijing Sublineage

One of the most pathogenic clades of the *M. tuberculosis* complex with a high tendency to cause outbreaks is the Beijing clade. This L2 sublineage is estimated to originate from the region of northeastern China, Korea, and Japan some 6,000 to 11,000 years ago, during a period that is corresponding to the beginning of agriculture in this area (42, 66). Beijing strains represent an important fraction of multidrug-resistant (MDR) *M. tuberculosis* strains in Asia and parts of Europe, America, and Africa (66). They were first described in 1995 as a predominant strain cluster isolated from patients in the Beijing region in China (67), which subsequently spread to neighboring countries and can now be found worldwide (66, 68, 69). The expansion of the Beijing lineage had two major peaks, coinciding with the Industrial Revolution and the period around the First World War. Later, antituberculosis drug treatment temporarily led to a reduction in the number of cases caused by these strains, yet, resulted in the emergence of MDR strain variants, a process that was strongly enhanced by the breakdown of a functional public health system in the former Soviet Union and by the onset of the HIV epidemic (66). One of the first MDR-TB outbreaks was caused by the Beijing strain W and occurred in the beginning of the 1990s among mainly HIV-infected patients in New York City (70, 71). Since then, multiple MDR tuberculosis and even extensively drug-resistant (XDR) tuberculosis outbreaks have been

attributed to strains of the Beijing genotype, which led to the hypothesis that Beijing strains are more virulent, more transmissible, and more likely to develop drug resistance mutations than other lineages (72–76). In addition, it was hypothesized that BCG vaccination might protect less efficiently against disease caused by Beijing strains, which could as well have contributed to their global dissemination (77, 78). WGS of 110 Beijing strains representing the 7 Beijing sublineages (modern Beijing strains CC1 to CC5 and ancestral Beijing strains CC6 and BL7) identified SNPs in the *mce* (mammalian cell entry) and *vapBC* (virulence-associated protein) gene families in the modern Beijing sublineages as well as a frameshift mutation in the signal transduction system-encoding *kdpDE* operon, which is specific for the European-Russian W148 MDR outbreak cluster (CC2 sublineage) (66). The W148 strains account for about one-fourth of Beijing isolates from patients from different parts of the former Soviet Union as well as from Russian immigrants around the world and were thus hypothesized to possess potential advantageous pathogenic properties (69). Since a partial deletion of the *kdpDE* operon in *M. tuberculosis* was found to result in greater virulence (79), it is likely that the mutation in the W148 strains represents an advantageous molecular event toward a more virulent phenotype.

Another specific feature of the Beijing lineage is an intact *pks15/1* locus, coding for a polyketide synthase involved in phenolic glycolipid (PGL) synthesis. The cell surface molecule PGL is only produced in strains where *pks15/1* corresponds to a single gene and is not divided into *pks1* and *pks15* due to a 7-bp deletion, as is the case for *M. tuberculosis* strains of the phylogenetic lineage 4 (e.g., *M. tuberculosis* H37Rv, Erdman, or CDC1551) (80, 81). Complementation of PGL-deficient strains with the single fused *pks15/1* gene of a PGL producer restored PGL production (82). PGLs were found to inhibit the release of the proinflammatory cytokines tumor necrosis factor alpha (TNF-α), interleukin-6 (IL-6), and interleukin-12 (IL-12), and disruption of PGL synthesis in a hypervirulent strain resulted in the loss of this phenotype (83). The occurrence of PGLs in this highly epidemic Beijing family has raised the question of a contribution of this glycolipid to epidemic spread and drug resistance. However, not all Beijing isolates with an intact *pks15/1* gene produce PGLs; and, even though restored PGL production in L4 *M. tuberculosis* H37Rv had a cytokine-modulatory effect, it did not confer hypervirulence (84). These results suggest that PGLs are not the sole factors that can explain the hypervirulence of the Beijing strains.

Another factor that was suggested to have contributed to an increased virulence of the Beijing strains is the constitutive expression of the transcriptional regulator DosR (dormancy survival regulator) (85). The DosR regulon coordinates a set of genes in response to hypoxia or nitric oxide (NO) treatment and might thus confer an *in vivo* growth advantage in the microaerophilic or anaerobic conditions encountered during infection. The two-component regulatory system DosT/DosS activates DosR transcription upon O_2 depletion or NO binding. A frameshift mutation in the sensor kinase DosT in the modern Beijing lineages seems to circumvent the need for this activation signal. This mutation was further shown to correlate with the constitutive overexpression of DosR, even though it does not seem to be the direct cause for it, as seen in complementation studies (86). Interestingly, subsequent studies with the aim to better understand the mechanism behind the DosR overexpression revealed that modern Beijing lineages possess two *dosR* copies as part of a massive duplication of a 350-kb genomic region that is flanked by two IS*6110* elements (87). This gene duplication seems to be the result of a selective pressure during infection because it was only observed in clinical strains and is unstable in *in vitro* cultures (87).

Furthermore, modern Beijing strains display missense mutations in the mutator genes *mutT2* and *mutT4*, which were suggested, as well, to aid in the acquisition of mutations favoring adaptation within the host (88). Because of their ability to increase virulence and develop drug resistance, it was initially speculated whether mutations present in the mutator genes *mutT2* and *mutT4* evoke a mutator phenotype in the Beijing strains (88). However, several studies comparing whole genomes of a large number of outbreak strains from different regions around the globe revealed that mutations leading to enhanced pathogenicity or drug resistance are more likely a consequence of positive selection, because mutator phenotypes would result in a more general, genome-wide accumulation of nonsynonymous as well as synonymous SNPs, which does not seem to be the case in Beijing strains compared with other lineages (66, 73, 74, 89, 90). Furthermore, mutations in *mutT2* and *mutT4* are only fixed in the most recent Beijing lineages, yet, extensive emergence of drug resistance also appears in more ancestral Beijing strains as well as in strains belonging to the Euro-American lineage 4 (66, 73, 88, 91, 92).

Altogether, it is little surprising that the hypervirulence phenotype of Beijing outbreak strains does not seem to be attributable to one single mutation but is the result of several, probably synergistically acting genomic events. The use of WGS to follow the evolution of strains during outbreaks will certainly allow us to reveal further molecular events contributing to the hypervirulence of Beijing strains in the near future.

Evolution of the *M. tuberculosis* L4 Sublineage

M. tuberculosis strains of the phylogenetic lineage 4 are the cause for the majority of tuberculosis cases in the Americas, Europe, and large parts of Africa and are thus the most widespread of the *M. tuberculosis* sublineages on a global scale (93–99). The L4 lineage comprises *M. tuberculosis* strains that, according to molecular typing characteristics, belong to the Haarlem, the Latin American-Mediterranean (LAM), and the T-strain families, which are the predominant strains in Europe, Central and South America, and Africa, as well as the X family, which is highly prevalent in North and Central America (100). Within the relatively heterogenic L4 strains, some seem to have a higher outbreak potential as concluded from higher transmission and incidence rates. However, only few experimental data are available on the molecular events that might have driven the spread of L4 outbreak clones. One attempt to explain the spread of a dominant L4 clade comes from the so-called RD^Rio strains, which were associated with high rates of cavitary tuberculosis, higher bacillary load, and consequent higher transmission (101). These strains are part of the LAM family and are responsible for the majority of tuberculosis cases in Brazil (102). The fact that they were also identified in various regions around the world, including a predominant clone in Madrid, Spain (strain 5; ST20 or LAM1), predominant strains in South Africa (F9 and F10) and an emerging RD^Rio strain population in New York City, emphasizes their high transmissibility and thus global importance (101, 103, 104). The RD^Rio deletion is a 26-kb stretch of DNA including two PPE genes (PPE55 and PPE56), which belong to a family of mycobacterial-specific proteins with a Pro-Pro-Glu (PPE) motif with potential implications in virulence (105). Lazzarini et al. speculated that the deletion of the two PPE genes might have impacted the virulence of the RD^Rio strains through possible mechanisms of immune evasion, because PPE proteins together with the closely related PE (Pro-Glu) proteins were suggested to contribute to antigenic variation (102, 105). In addition, both PPE55 and PPE56 were earlier shown to be induced in murine and cellular models, further endorsing a potential function during infection (102). Yet, this hypothesis remains only speculative, because complementation studies on the effect of PPE55 and PPE56 in RD^Rio strains are missing.

Von Groll et al. further compared *in vitro* growth of LAM versus non-LAM strains as well as RD^{Rio} versus non-RD^{Rio} strains as a means to assess a potential fitness advantage of some strains over others. They found that, while LAM strains had a significantly faster growth rate than non-LAM strains (30.8 h versus 38.1 h), no growth advantage was detected between RD^{Rio} versus non-RD^{Rio} (106). Another dominant clade within the L4 strains is the Haarlem family, which was first described in 1999. It was named after Haarlem in the Netherlands, the city of residence of the patient infected by the first isolated strain of this family (107). Since then, several MDR tuberculosis outbreaks have been linked to Haarlem strains, as was seen by the so-called M strain in a hospital in Buenos Aires, Argentina, in the 1990s (108, 109), an outbreak in the Czech Republic in the late 1990s (110), or an outbreak in Tunisia in the beginning of the 2000s (111). The Haarlem family was also associated with drug resistance and found to be genetically more heterogeneous than the higher conserved Beijing strains (112). However, similarly to the Beijing family, missense mutations in the DNA repair genes *ogt* and *ung*, specific for the Haarlem family, could so far not be correlated to an increased emergence of multidrug resistance, suggesting other modes of resistance acquisition (113).

These examples emphasize the importance of evolutionary adaptation and selection of *M. tuberculosis*, in general, and certain lineages, in particular, which helps to understand the present epidemiological situation and to predict future trends. In particular, the question of the association of certain strains and strain families with drug resistance merits deeper investigations and discussions. Hence, in the following final paragraphs, we discuss some of the main principles and insights regarding drug resistance in *M. tuberculosis* and the MTBC obtained from different disciplines, including recent WGS approaches.

EVOLUTION OF DRUG-RESISTANT *M. TUBERCULOSIS* STRAINS

While drug resistance in other bacteria is mainly acquired through horizontal gene transfer (HGT) of antibiotic resistance cassettes, interstrain genetic resistance transfer has not been reported in the members of the MTBC, even though WGS of the early-branched *M. canettii* strains suggest an important impact of HGT on their evolution and the early evolution of MTBC strains (2, 114). *M. canettii* genomes display multiple putative recombination tracts, which show signatures very similar to recombination tracts acquired through a very particular mechanism of gene transfer, termed

distributive chromosomal transfer (DCT), found in the fast-growing nonpathogenic *Mycobacterium smegmatis* (114). DCT creates genetically blended progeny with alternating DNA sequences of the donor and the recipient with transferred segments of up to several hundred kilobase pairs, thus theoretically large enough to contain whole operons (115). Indeed, recent results from fluorescence-assisted mating assays and WGS have provided key experimental evidence of multiple chromosomal DNA transfer between selected donor and recipient *M. canettii* strains (116). However, no evidence of DNA exchange between MTBC strains was found, despite the use of the same experimental setup (116). These findings suggest that HGT may have played an important role during the evolution of tubercle bacilli and the emergence of MTBC from an *M. canettii*-like progenitor strain pool. However, the faculty of frequent DNA exchange seems to have been lost at some stage within the lineage of MTBC members, in agreement with the clonal population structure observed for the MTBC, with no apparent evidence of recent lateral gene transfer. These findings are supporting the concept of *de novo* acquisition of individual resistance mutations as the main mechanisms of antituberculosis drug resistance.

Ever since the discovery of the first antituberculosis compounds, streptomycin in 1943, isoniazid in 1952, and rifampin (rifampicin) in 1959, humanity has been confronted with the emergence of drug-resistant *M. tuberculosis* strains, which has made a combination of several drugs for successful treatment indispensable (117–120). The standard therapy used nowadays for drug-sensitive *M. tuberculosis* strains consists of a 2-month treatment with isoniazid, rifampin, pyrazinamide, and ethambutol, which is succeeded by a 4-month treatment with isoniazid and rifampin alone (121). The long duration of the therapy together with the severe side effects may cause noncompliance of the patient and interruption of the treatment, especially when patients are associated with unstable living conditions such as homelessness or substance abuse (9, 122–125). Insufficient or interrupted drug treatment provides the perfect breeding ground for development of drug-resistant and MDR strains, the latter defined as resistant to at least isoniazid and rifampin. The situation becomes particularly detrimental when already existing resistance mutations are not identified before treatment onset, because patients infected with MDR strains receiving the standard therapy bear a high risk of additionally developing resistances to the other drugs applied. Misuse and mismanagement of second-line drugs, which are less effective and have even more severe side effects, may lead to the emergence of XDR strains (126). XDR strains are MDR with additional resistance mechanisms against at least one of the three injectable drugs kanamycin, amikacin, and capreomycin, and to any fluoroquinolone used against *M. tuberculosis* (127). XDR-TB cases are practically untreatable, which makes an early diagnosis of MDR-TB and any additional resistance mutation together with a sufficiently well-organized drug management crucial for an appropriate treatment. A lot of work has thus been focused on determining the mutations that cause drug resistance to the major antituberculosis drugs.

Evolution of MDR-TB

Resistance to the first-line drug rifampin is caused by different mutations within an 81-bp rifampin resistance-determining region (RRDR, codons 428 to 456) in *rpoB*, the gene encoding the RNA polymerase subunit β (73, 128). Since rifampin, like many other drugs, targets an essential protein (RpoB), mutations in *rpoB*, in general, result in fitness defects and associated, potential lower transmissibility from one host to another (129). However, the negative effects of mycobacterial drug resistance can also be circumvented through introduction of compensatory mutations, explaining why some MDR-TB strains are better transmitted than others. The latter strains have the potential to cause outbreaks. Casali et al. found that 97% of Beijing MDR-TB cases in a Russian population that were caused by strains harboring the most common RpoB resistance mutation S450L (S531L in *Escherichia coli*), either had putative compensatory mutations in *rpoA* or *rpoC*, or several putative compensatory substitutions in RpoB itself (73) (Fig. 3). Meftahi et al. further studied Haarlem MDR-TB-causing strains that were responsible for an outbreak in Tunisia among HIV-negative, noninstitutionalized persons and found that, in addition to the frequently found RpoB S450L mutation, the isolates all had a mutation in RpoB V534M, which was restricted to the Tunisian outbreak. Phenotypic tests confirmed that V534M represents a secondary mutation that efficiently compensates the fitness cost caused by the RpoB S450L mutation and even further increases the level of rifampin resistance (130). Similarly, WGS of a collection of 252 clinical isolates belonging to the L4 M outbreak strain in Argentina revealed that those strains that showed putative phylogenetic transmission links harbored changes in either RpoB (V970A, 4 isolates), RpoC (D485H or A734T, 2 isolates each), or RpoA (T187N, 5 isolates) in addition to the RpoB S450L resistance mutation. However, while secondary RpoC mutations arose independently multiple times by convergent evolution, only the two above-mentioned were shared by pairs of related strains, thus questioning

the importance of *rpoC* secondary mutations for increased transmission (92). Hence, it was suggested that the decisive factors for a rifampin-resistant strain to be successful and transmissible were a low initial fitness cost, together with the ability to generate efficient compensatory mutations as well as a high rifampin minimal inhibitory concentration (MIC) (130, 131).

High-level resistance to isoniazid is conferred by mutations in the catalase-peroxidase KatG, which catalyzes the oxidation of the isoniazid prodrug to its active form (132–135). Low-level resistance, in turn, is associated with mutations in the NADH-dependent enoyl-acyl-carrier protein reductase InhA, involved in mycolic acid synthesis and the target of the drug (136). KatG is thought to protect *M. tuberculosis* from reactive oxygen radicals during infection (137), and its deletion or mutations in the catalase-peroxidase domain lead to an *in vivo* virulence attenuation (138–140). The most commonly found isoniazid resistance-conferring mutation is S315T of KatG (73, 129), which retains catalase-peroxidase activity, yet displays a decreased ability to activate isoniazid and is thus suggested to cause only low or no fitness cost for the bacilli (140). Other *katG* gene mutations as well as complete deletions were reported, which were associated, however, with high fitness costs. A compensation for the loss of KatG-peroxidase functions was suggested to be conferred by upregulation of the alkyl hydroperoxidase-encoding gene *ahpC* through mutations within the regulatory region (73, 129, 141). Furthermore, *M. tuberculosis* strains with mutations in the *inhA* promoter region in addition to *katG* mutations are resistant to even high levels of isoniazid (142) (Fig. 3). Another example of mutations that initially confer only low-level resistance to a particular drug, but result in high-level resistance in combination with other mutations, can be observed in the case of ethambutol resistance. Any nonsynonymous *ubiA* (Rv3806c) mutation, as well as mutations in some other genes (e.g., *nuoD*) in combination with the EmbB M306V mutation, were found to result in high-level ethambutol resistance. This finding is alarming, since standard phenotypic testing would fail to detect low-level resistant mutants due to low breakpoint concentrations to define drug resistance and thus subsequently potentially select for high-level resistance mutants (143).

Concerning the globally observed drug resistance patterns of *M. tuberculosis* strains, substantial variation can be observed. While the global estimates of rifampin resistance concern about 3.3% of all TB cases, individual rates are quite diverse. In the majority of western European countries the MDR-TB burden is low, but in some parts of the world, MDR *M. tuberculosis* strains

MDR-TB

RESISTANCE TO FIRST-LINE DRUGS

Isoniazide

katG

Resistance mutations	Resistance mutations + putative compensatory mutations
S315T	S315T + *inhA* prom-8;t-a/c
	S315T + ***inhA* prom-15;c-t**
	S315T + ***inhA* prom-17;g-t**
D63E, R104Q, A106V, W107R, H108Q, A109V, N138S/D, K143T, Y155C, G169S, D189X, W191R, Y229F, E261Q, A264T, K301aag..atag, G309V, S315I/N, Y337C, K345T, A350S, A379T, T394A, A409V, R463L, N493H, G495X, D573N, L587X, W728C, D735N, deletion	S315T + *inhA* prom-22;g-c
	S315T + *aphC* prom 0;t-c
	S315T + *aphC* prom-6;g-a
	S315T + *aphC* prom-54; t-tatgt
	D94G + *ahpC* prom-34;g-a
	L384R + *ahpC* prom-39;c-t
	S315N + *ahpC* prom-10;c-a
	A636E + *ahpC* prom-10;c-t
	L653P + *ahpC* prom-6;g-a
	T85P, G121C, Y155C, A162T, T251M, P280H, or E607K + *inhA* prom-15;c-t

inhA

Resistance mutations	Resistance mutations + putative compensatory mutations
prom-15; c-t	prom-15; c-t + *aphC* prom-30; c-t
prom-34	
prom-147; c-t	
I21T, S94A, I194T	
T241M,	

fabG1

Resistance mutations
prom-15; c-t
prom-8; t-c
prom-17; g-t

kasA

Resistance mutations
V142X, H253X

Rifampicin

rpoB

Resistance mutations	Putative compensatory mutations for *rpoB*-encoded S450L resistance mutation
S450L	V534M (Tunisian outbreak strain)
	L731P (Thai outbreak strain)†
S428R, L430P/R, S431G, Q432L/P/K, M434I/V, D435V/F/Y/G/A, H445Y/D/R/N/C/L/Q, S450W/F/P/L, L452P, G456S,	L42F, P45S, E82G, V170F/X, D259N, D265A, A286V, T399A, T400A, P479T, I480V, I487S, I488V, I491V/F, S493X, V496M/L, F503S, S540A, L554P, V555A, Y564H, D571A, V581M, H723Y, E761D, R824L, R827C, H835P/R, Q975H, **V970A**, H1028R, A1037S, Y1073S, I1106T

rpoA

Resistance mutations + putative compensatory mutations

P25L, G315/A, K177M, T181A, V183G, E184D, **T187N**/P/A, D190G, L304R, S307L

rpoC

L14R, G332S/R/C, N416T/S, S428A, V431M, G433S/C, P434R/T/Q, K445R, L449V, F452C/L, R459W, V483A/G, W484G, **D485H**/N/Y, **I491T**/V, L516P, V517L, E518A, G519D, A521D, H525Q/N, L527V, R572H, P678R, N698H/K/S, V709L, **A734T**/G/V, D747A, Q761R, R770H, N826K, I832V, S838C, L847R, Y849C, I885V, D943G, G945V, V1039A, P1040T/S/R, I4046M, V1252L, A1303V

Ethambutol

embA

Resistance mutations
prom-12

embB

Resistance mutations	Resistance mutations + resistance enhancing mutations	
C12T, **M306I/V/L**, Y319X, D354A, P404S, E405X, G406S/C/D/A, A409X, Q497P/R/K, H1002R, D1024N	M306I/V	
	D354A	
	G406C/S/D	+ any non-synonymous ***ubiA* mutation**
	Q497R	
	T1082A	
	M306V	+ *nuoD* A287S

ubiA

Resistance mutations
R237C, R240C

cadI

Resistance mutations
prom-39; c-t

Pyrazinamide

pncA

Resistance mutations
A3E, D8N, Q10P, D12E, C14R, H54X, W68X, H71X, T100P, Y103*, W119R, L120R, V128G, G132A, T135P, R140X, L151S, R154X, L159V
bp insertions (e.g. +c L172, +g A152)
bp deletions (e.g. g395_527del; Rv2042c_Rv2045cdel)
promoter mutations (e.g. prom-11)

† not confirmed by phenotypic test

XDR-TB (+MDR-TB mutations)

RESISTANCE TO SECOND-LINE DRUGS

Ofloxacin, Ciprofloxacin, Moxifloxacin

gyrA	gyrB
Resistance mutations	Resistance mutations
G88X, **A90V**, S91P, **D94G**/A/N/H/Y, R292G, N499D,	A504V+ gyrA A90V, A504V+ gyrA D94G, A504V+ gyrA L105R, D461V

Kanamycin, Capreomycin, Amikacin

rrs	eis (kanamycin, amikacin)	tlyA (capreomycin)
Resistance mutations	Resistance mutations	Resistance mutations
a1205g (capreomycin), a1400g, **a1401g**, c1483t	promoter mutations prom-10; c-g, prom-37	G196E, loss-of-function mutations (e.g. A217fs)

Ethionamide

ethR-fabG1	inhA	mshA
Resistance mutations	Resistance mutations	Resistance mutations
prom-15; c-t	S94X, prom-15;c-t, prom-8;t-c	L108fs

ethA	ndh
Resistance mutations	Resistance mutations
H22P, W69L, Q206L, S208P, Q215*, T232fs, S251fs, R259fs, F302S, V312G, A341E, E400fs, G437fs, R469P	A324fs, C98fs
prom-11;t-c	

Streptomycin

gidB	rrs	rpsL
Resistance mutations	Resistance mutations	Resistance mutations
L79S, V110fs, A134X, A138X, A141X	rrs a513c, rrs **a514c**, rrs 516, rrs **c517t**, rrs 904, rrs 905, rrs 906, rrs 907	**K43R**, K88R/M
130 bp deletion (L50-P93)		

D-cycloserine

ald	alr
Resistance mutations	Resistance mutations
bp deletions, bp insertions, Q153*	S22L, L89R, K319T, K133E, R373G, prom-8; g- t

Figure 3 Overview of a large number of potential drug resistance as well as compensatory mutations against first- and second-line drugs. Mutations shown in bold represent most commonly found mutations among resistant strains. Semibold secondary mutations in *rpoB*, *rpoC*, and *rpoB* were found to be shared by related strains, thus suggesting mutations favoring transmission. Any mutations leading to at least rifampin and isoniazid resistance confer an MDR phenotype, whereas MDR strains with additional mutations against at least one of the three injectable drugs, kanamycin, amikacin, and capreomycin, and to any fluoroquinolone used against *M. tuberculosis* are referred to as XDR strains. Table based on mutations found in the following publications (50, 58, 73, 89, 91, 92, 130, 133, 142, 143, 149, 151–154, 156, 163, 166).

cause up to 45.5% of all TB cases, as revealed by a study on the TB situation in Belarus (144). General estimates thus need to be interpreted with caution. Transmission of drug-resistant *M. tuberculosis* strains is enhanced in areas with high rates of human-to-human contacts among immunocompromised individuals, such as is the case in hospitals, for example, yet MDR-TB was also found to spread among immunocompetent hosts (108, 124, 145–148). Cohen et al. found that, in the majority of drug-resistant TB cases in KwaZulu-Natal, South Africa, resistance to isoniazid, conferred by the *katG* S315T mutation, developed first and was followed by resistance to rifampin and second-line drugs (149), which is in line with results obtained in other studies (66, 92, 150, 151). This finding is especially alarming since diagnosis of drug-resistant TB often primarily focuses on the detection of rifampin resistance and not resistance to isoniazid. Particular attention will be paid to this matter for future diagnostic TB tests to avoid selection of MDR-TB as response to inadequate drug treatment due to insufficient identification of prevailing resistance mutations.

Evolution of Resistance to Second-Line Drugs

While transmission of MDR *M. tuberculosis* strains seems to occur more regularly (see above), XDR *M. tuberculosis* strains, in general, appear to be a consequence of the stepwise acquisition of mutations in response to treatment with second-line drugs (73, 89, 91). Only a few XDR-TB outbreaks with confirmed patient-to-patient transmission have been identified so far. One example was the so-called Tugela Ferry outbreak in the province of KwaZulu Natal, South Africa, in 2005, where XDR-TB cases were caused by L4 LAM family *M. tuberculosis* strains that provoked a rapidly progressing form of TB with mainly fatal outcome in HIV coinfected patients (124). A study by Gandhi et al. came to the alarming result that more than half of the XDR-TB patients had never been treated with second-line drugs before, thus rather suggesting person-to-person transmission than *de novo* acquisition of resistance mutations (124). Later, WGS of a large collection of clinical strains from the KwaZulu-Natal region suggested that the progenitor of the Tugela Ferry XDR outbreak strain had acquired resistance mutations to the first-line drugs after their first introduction to the market about 50 years prior to the outbreak. Subsequently, resistance mutations to other drugs and emergence of XDR-TB followed in a stepwise manner over decades (149). Cohen et al. further found that the Tugela Ferry XDR clone was not re-

stricted to immunodeficient hosts, as initially thought, but was also isolated from HIV-negative patients, suggesting that this particular XDR-TB strain is fit enough for human-to-human transmission and disease progression even in immunocompetent patients (149). Furthermore, MDR and XDR-TB-causing strains other than the Tugela Ferry outbreak clone independently evolved 56 and 9 times, respectively, within the population of KwaZulu-Natal between 2008 and 2013, indicating frequent *de novo* evolution of drug resistance together with successful transmission of MDR and XDR clones (149). Most alarmingly, 13 LAM *M. tuberculosis* strains were identified within the specimen collection that were only one mutation away from reaching XDR-level resistance (149). The authors thus concluded that the emergence of drug-resistant strains in South Africa was a result of decades of poor TB control and that, due to incomplete knowledge of all resistance-conferring mutations, numerous drug-resistant TB infections might be diagnosed inadequately. These findings are in line with results obtained by other studies. Eldholm et al., for example, found that the M strain belonging to the L4 *M. tuberculosis* lineage, which was responsible for a large MDR-TB outbreak in a hospital in Buenos Aires in 1994 to 1995, gradually acquired additional resistance mutations over 4 decades and is now circulating as a pre-XDR strain in Argentina (92). Thus, a thorough understanding of the genes and mutations conferring drug resistance and a direct application for subsequent diagnosis is crucial for the prevention of XDR-TB emergence. WGS of resistant strains combined with phenotypic tests already helped identify a large number of putative resistance-conferring mutations in various genes for different first- and second-line drugs, even though phenotypic complementation is still lacking in many cases (Fig. 3) (73, 90–92, 129, 130, 149, 152–154). However, the big challenge we still face is the development of efficient, rapid, and affordable diagnostic tests that detect the vast majority of resistance mutations to the various antituberculosis drugs. In this respect, important efforts are currently being made to implement novel, accurate TB diagnostic procedures that can simultaneously identify the presence of *M. tuberculosis* and the most common *rpoB* drug resistance mutations (155). However, the extension of resistance mutations from first-line drugs to second-line drugs represents a significant technical challenge. In addition, despite growing knowledge of individual resistance-conferring mutations, several mechanisms of resistance are still incompletely understood. As one example of a recent study on the evolution of resistance mechanisms against second-line drugs, a study on D-cycloserine should be mentioned here. Desjardins et al. screened for new resistance-conferring mutations in a collection of 498 *M. tuberculosis* strains from South Africa and China, and found that loss-of-function mutations in a gene coding for the L-alanine dehydrogenase Ald (Rv2780) conferred resistance to D-cycloserine. They further observed that *ald* loss-of-function mutations evolved solely in MDR or XDR strains, suggesting that these mutations exclusively arise upon second-line drug treatment. By the integration of D-cycloserine resistance mechanisms in TB diagnostics, treatment with this drug that shows substantial toxicity could be reserved only for patients with susceptible TB disease (156).

Finally, it should be mentioned that analyses of large WGS-generated data sets from collections of clinical isolates and/or drug-resistant mutants also have the potential to identify and predict relevant drug-resistant mutations (157, 158). Indeed, independent comparative genomic analyses (90, 159) have identified a substantial number of new resistance-associated mutations not previously implicated in genetic drug resistance of *M. tuberculosis*, although the impact of these potentially novel resistance-associated mutations on mycobacterial pathogenesis remains currently unknown, and requires further investigations.

Microevolution During TB Infection as Driver of Genetic Heterogeneity

The recent availability of more and more affordable WGS tools led to their use in the track of inter- and intrapatient evolution during infection with *M. tuberculosis*. Subsequently, various studies came to the intrigu-ing conclusion that infections with single *M. tuberculosis* clones develop more genetic heterogeneity within infected patients than expected (150, 160–165). Genetic diversity of subpopulations within a single patient can be as high as that between different patients and can be found in extrapulmonary sites as well as within the lungs, where several variants can eventually be transmitted (160). Furthermore, it was shown that microevolution also plays a role in the emergence of multidrug resistance. A study by Eldholm and colleagues followed the emergence of an XDR-TB-causing strain from an initially susceptible clone in a single patient over 42 months. The authors found that a high genetic diversity of competing resistant subpopulations developed within the patient, and that antibiotic pressure subsequently drove clonal expansion of single resistant clones. Within the population, several resistance mutations developed independently for different drugs, of which only one, presumably with the least fitness cost, finally became fixed and consequently displaced others (162). Similar results were obtained by Black and colleagues, who found that during infection several heterogeneous variants may emerge in parallel. Upon drug treatment, those clones carrying low-cost resistance mutations to the respective drugs applied become dominant and consequently prevail over other variants. Finally, subsequent repeated genetic diversification results in genomic heterogeneity of the resistant population (163) (Fig. 4). In this light, it seems alarming that standard diagnostic sampling procedures mostly depend on specimen collection from single sputum samples and might not reflect the genetic diversity within the sites of infections, because it has been found that even collection of different sputum samples from the same patients contained different strain variants (161, 164).

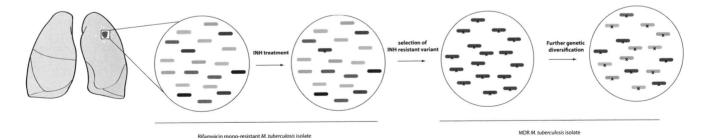

Figure 4 Suggested model for a selection bottleneck followed by random mutations on the population structure of *M. tuberculosis* clinical isolates. Genetic diversity of subpopulations is present in a rifampin monoresistant clinical *M. tuberculosis* isolate (each individual bacterium contains a rifampin resistance-conferring mutation). Upon isoniazid treatment clones carrying low-cost resistance mutations to the drug become dominant and prevail over other variants, resulting in the loss of numerous other genetic mutations. Subsequent repeated genetic diversification results in genomic heterogeneity of the MDR strain population. x represents an isoniazid resistance-causing mutation. Figure adapted from reference 163.

Furthermore, read frequency cutoff values used in standard variant filtering of WGS data are usually set at >70%, implying that low-frequency subpopulations are not identified (163). Thus, the importance of using low sequencing read frequency cutoffs, combined with techniques to accurately identify subpopulations carrying resistance mutations in sputum samples, is unequivocal. Hence, increasingly cost-effective WGS makes this technique an interesting option for diagnosis of drug resistance and drug susceptibility, even though a routine use, especially in low-income countries, might appear difficult in the near future (157).

CONCLUDING COMMENTS AND PERSPECTIVES

Our insights into the evolution of *M. tuberculosis* as a key pathogen are constantly increasing. With the identification and genomic characterization of the *M. canettii* strain pool, a plausible scenario of the early evolution of tuberculosis-causing mycobacteria can now be drawn, which contributes to the identification of molecular parameters that likely have contributed to the incursion, maintenance, and spread of selected MTBC members, in particular, mammalian hosts. This scenario is constantly refined with the accumulation of data on SNP diversity from different *M. tuberculosis* strains and other members of the MTBC. The insights we are continuing to gain from genome data are substantial, revealing long-hidden associations concerning global phylogeny, epidemiology, and evolution of drug resistance mechanisms that we have tried to summarize in this review, as a snapshot of current developments. Research into this important subject is ongoing and will hopefully help to facilitate rational decisions to positively impact the current situation of TB treatment and patient management.

Acknowledgments. The authors acknowledge support from a European Community grant (no. 260872), the EU-EFPIA Innovative Medicines Initiative (grant no. 115337), the Agence National de Recherche (ANR-14-JAMR-001-02), and the Fondation pour la Recherche Médicale FRM (DEQ2013 0326471). E.C.B. was supported by a stipend from the Pasteur–Paris University (PPU) International PhD program.

Citation. Boritsch EC, Brosch R. 2016. Evolution of *Mycobacterium tuberculosis*: new insights into pathogenicity and drug resistance. Microbiol Spectrum 4(5):TBTB2-0020-2016.

References

1. Koeck JL, Fabre M, Simon F, Daffé M, Garnotel E, Matan AB, Gérôme P, Bernatas JJ, Buisson Y, Pourcel C. 2011. Clinical characteristics of the smooth tubercle bacilli 'Mycobacterium canettii' infection suggest the existence of an environmental reservoir. *Clin Microbiol Infect* 17:1013–1019.

2. Supply P, Marceau M, Mangenot S, Roche D, Rouanet C, Khanna V, Majlessi L, Criscuolo A, Tap J, Pawlik A, Fiette L, Orgeur M, Fabre M, Parmentier C, Frigui W, Simeone R, Boritsch EC, Debrie AS, Willery E, Walker D, Quail MA, Ma L, Bouchier C, Salvignol G, Sayes F, Cascioferro A, Seemann T, Barbe V, Locht C, Gutierrez MC, Leclerc C, Bentley SD, Stinear TP, Brisse S, Médigue C, Parkhill J, Cruveiller S, Brosch R. 2013. Genomic analysis of smooth tubercle bacilli provides insights into ancestry and pathoadaptation of *Mycobacterium tuberculosis*. *Nat Genet* 45:172–179.

3. Springer B, Stockman L, Teschner K, Roberts GD, Böttger EC. 1996. Two-laboratory collaborative study on identification of mycobacteria: molecular versus phenotypic methods. *J Clin Microbiol* 34:296–303.

4. Veyrier F, Pletzer D, Turenne C, Behr MA. 2009. Phylogenetic detection of horizontal gene transfer during the step-wise genesis of *Mycobacterium tuberculosis*. *BMC Evol Biol* 9:196.

5. Tufariello JM, Kerantzas CA, Vilchèze C, Calder RB, Nordberg EK, Fischer JA, Hartman TE, Yang E, Driscoll T, Cole LE, Sebra R, Maqbool SB, Wattam AR, Jacobs WR Jr. 2015. The complete genome sequence of the emerging pathogen *Mycobacterium haemophilum* explains its unique culture requirements. *MBio* 6:e01313-15.

6. Le Chevalier F, Cascioferro A, Majlessi L, Herrmann JL, Brosch R. 2014. *Mycobacterium tuberculosis* evolutionary pathogenesis and its putative impact on drug development. *Future Microbiol* 9:969–985.

7. Cole ST, Brosch R, Parkhill J, Garnier T, Churcher C, Harris D, Gordon SV, Eiglmeier K, Gas S, Barry CE III, Tekaia F, Badcock K, Basham D, Brown D, Chillingworth T, Connor R, Davies R, Devlin K, Feltwell T, Gentles S, Hamlin N, Holroyd S, Hornsby T, Jagels K, Krogh A, McLean J, Moule S, Murphy L, Oliver K, Osborne J, Quail MA, Rajandream MA, Rogers J, Rutter S, Seeger K, Skelton J, Squares R, Squares S, Sulston JE, Taylor K, Whitehead S, Barrell BG. 1998. Deciphering the biology of *Mycobacterium tuberculosis* from the complete genome sequence. *Nature* 393:537–544.

8. Fleischmann RD, Alland D, Eisen JA, Carpenter L, White O, Peterson J, DeBoy R, Dodson R, Gwinn M, Haft D, Hickey E, Kolonay JF, Nelson WC, Umayam LA, Ermolaeva M, Salzberg SL, Delcher A, Utterback T, Weidman J, Khouri H, Gill J, Mikula A, Bishai W, Jacobs WR Jr, Venter JC, Fraser CM. 2002. Whole-genome comparison of *Mycobacterium tuberculosis* clinical and laboratory strains. *J Bacteriol* 184:5479–5490.

9. Roetzer A, Diel R, Kohl TA, Rückert C, Nübel U, Blom J, Wirth T, Jaenicke S, Schuback S, Rüsch-Gerdes S, Supply P, Kalinowski J, Niemann S. 2013. Whole genome sequencing versus traditional genotyping for investigation of a *Mycobacterium tuberculosis* outbreak: a longitudinal molecular epidemiological study. *PLoS Med* 10:e1001387.

10. Stinear TP, Seemann T, Harrison PF, Jenkin GA, Davies JK, Johnson PD, Abdellah Z, Arrowsmith C, Chillingworth

T, Churcher C, Clarke K, Cronin A, Davis P, Goodhead I, Holroyd N, Jagels K, Lord A, Moule S, Mungall K, Norbertczak H, Quail MA, Rabbinowitsch E, Walker D, White B, Whitehead S, Small PL, Brosch R, Ramakrishnan L, Fischbach MA, Parkhill J, Cole ST. 2008. Insights from the complete genome sequenceof *Mycobacterium marinum* on the evolution of Mycobacterium tuberculosis. *Genome Res* 18:729–741.

11. Wang J, McIntosh F, Radomski N, Dewar K, Simeone R, Enninga J, Brosch R, Rocha EP, Veyrier FJ, Behr MA. 2015. Insights on the emergence of *Mycobacterium tuberculosis* from the analysis of *Mycobacterium kansasii*. *Genome Biol Evol* 7:856–870.

12. Stinear TP, Seemann T, Pidot S, Frigui W, Reysset G, Garnier T, Meurice G, Simon D, Bouchier C, Ma L, Tichit M, Porter JL, Ryan J, Johnson PD, Davies JK, Jenkin GA, Small PL, Jones LM, Tekaia F, Laval F, Daffé M, Parkhill J, Cole ST. 2007. Reductive evolution and niche adaptation inferred from the genome of *Mycobacterium ulcerans*, the causative agent of Buruli ulcer. *Genome Res* 17:192–200.

13. Singh P, Benjak A, Schuenemann VJ, Herbig A, Avanzi C, Busso P, Nieselt K, Krause J, Vera-Cabrera L, Cole ST. 2015. Insight into the evolution and origin of leprosy bacilli from the genome sequence of *Mycobacterium lepromatosis*. *Proc Natl Acad Sci USA* 112:4459–4464.

14. Cole ST, Eiglmeier K, Parkhill J, James KD, Thomson NR, Wheeler PR, Honoré N, Garnier T, Churcher C, Harris D, Mungall K, Basham D, Brown D, Chillingworth T, Connor R, Davies RM, Devlin K, Duthoy S, Feltwell T, Fraser A, Hamlin N, Holroyd S, Hornsby T, Jagels K, Lacroix C, Maclean J, Moule S, Murphy L, Oliver K, Quail MA, Rajandream MA, Rutherford KM, Rutter S, Seeger K, Simon S, Simmonds M, Skelton J, Squares R, Squares S, Stevens K, Taylor K, Whitehead S, Woodward JR, Barrell BG. 2001. Massive gene decay in the leprosy bacillus. *Nature* 409:1007–1011.

15. Comas I, Chakravartti J, Small PM, Galagan J, Niemann S, Kremer K, Ernst JD, Gagneux S. 2010. Human T cell epitopes of *Mycobacterium tuberculosis* are evolutionarily hyperconserved. *Nat Genet* 42:498–503.

16. de Jong BC, Antonio M, Gagneux S. 2010. *Mycobacterium africanum*–review of an important cause of human tuberculosis in West Africa. *PLoS Negl Trop Dis* 4:e744

17. Gonzalo-Asensio J, Malaga W, Pawlik A, Astarie-Dequeker C, Passemar C, Moreau F, Laval F, Daffé M, Martin C, Brosch R, Guilhot C. 2014. Evolutionary history of tuberculosis shaped by conserved mutations in the PhoPR virulence regulator. *Proc Natl Acad Sci USA* 111:11491–11496.

18. Smith NH, Kremer K, Inwald J, Dale J, Driscoll JR, Gordon SV, van Soolingen D, Hewinson RG, Smith JM. 2006. Ecotypes of the *Mycobacterium tuberculosis* complex. *J Theor Biol* 239:220–225.

19. Garnier T, Eiglmeier K, Camus JC, Medina N, Mansoor H, Pryor M, Duthoy S, Grondin S, Lacroix C, Monsempe C, Simon S, Harris B, Atkin R, Doggett J, Mayes R, Keating L, Wheeler PR, Parkhill J, Barrell BG, Cole ST, Gordon SV, Hewinson RG. 2003. The complete genome sequence of *Mycobacterium bovis*. *Proc Natl Acad Sci USA* 100:7877–7882.

20. van Ingen J, Rahim Z, Mulder A, Boeree MJ, Simeone R, Brosch R, van Soolingen D. 2012. Characterization of *Mycobacterium orygis* as *M. tuberculosis* complex subspecies. *Emerg Infect Dis* 18:653–655.

21. Parsons SD, Drewe JA, Gey van Pittius NC, Warren RM, van Helden PD. 2013. Novel cause of tuberculosis in meerkats, South Africa. *Emerg Infect Dis* 19:2004–2007.

22. Cousins DV, Bastida R, Cataldi A, Quse V, Redrobe S, Dow S, Duignan P, Murray A, Dupont C, Ahmed N, Collins DM, Butler WR, Dawson D, Rodríguez D, Loureiro J, Romano MI, Alito A, Zumarraga M, Bernardelli A. 2003. Tuberculosis in seals caused by a novel member of the *Mycobacterium tuberculosis* complex: *Mycobacterium pinnipedii* sp. nov. *Int J Syst Evol Microbiol* 53:1305–1314.

23. Domogalla J, Prodinger WM, Blum H, Krebs S, Gellert S, Müller M, Neuendorf E, Sedlmaier F, Büttner M. 2013. Region of difference 4 in alpine *Mycobacterium caprae* isolates indicates three variants. *J Clin Microbiol* 51:1381–1388.

24. Coscolla M, Lewin A, Metzger S, Maetz-Rennsing K, Calvignac-Spencer S, Nitsche A, Dabrowski PW, Radonic A, Niemann S, Parkhill J, Couacy-Hymann E, Feldman J, Comas I, Boesch C, Gagneux S, Leendertz FH. 2013. Novel *Mycobacterium tuberculosis* complex isolate from a wild chimpanzee. *Emerg Infect Dis* 19:969–976.

25. Alexander KA, Sanderson CE, Larsen MH, Robbe-Austerman S, Williams MC, Palmer MV. 2016. Emerging tuberculosis pathogen hijacks social communication behavior in the group-living banded mongoose (*Mungos mungo*). *MBio* 7:e00281-16.

26. Stead WW. 1997. The origin and erratic global spread of tuberculosis. How the past explains the present and is the key to the future. *Clin Chest Med* 18:65–77.

27. Brosch R, Gordon SV, Marmiesse M, Brodin P, Buchrieser C, Eiglmeier K, Garnier T, Gutierrez C, Hewinson G, Kremer K, Parsons LM, Pym AS, Samper S, van Soolingen D, Cole ST. 2002. A new evolutionary scenario for the *Mycobacterium tuberculosis* complex. *Proc Natl Acad Sci USA* 99:3684–3689.

28. Mostowy S, Cousins D, Brinkman J, Aranaz A, Behr MA. 2002. Genomic deletions suggest a phylogeny for the *Mycobacterium tuberculosis* complex. *J Infect Dis* 186:74–80.

29. Smith NH, Hewinson RG, Kremer K, Brosch R, Gordon SV. 2009. Myths and misconceptions: the origin and evolution of *Mycobacterium tuberculosis*. *Nat Rev Microbiol* 7:537–544.

30. Gutierrez MC, Brisse S, Brosch R, Fabre M, Omaïs B, Marmiesse M, Supply P, Vincent V. 2005. Ancient origin and gene mosaicism of the progenitor of *Mycobacterium tuberculosis*. *PLoS Pathog* 1:e5

31. Blouin Y, Cazajous G, Dehan C, Soler C, Vong R, Hassan MO, Hauck Y, Boulais C, Andriamanantena D, Martinaud C, Martin É, Pourcel C, Vergnaud G. 2014. Progenitor "Mycobacterium canettii" clone responsible for lymph node tuberculosis epidemic, Djibouti. *Emerg Infect Dis* 20:21–28.

32. Canetti G. 1970. [Infection caused by atypical myco-bacteria and antituberculous immunity.] In French. *Lille Med* 15:280–282.

33. van Soolingen D, Hoogenboezem T, de Haas PE, Hermans PW, Koedam MA, Teppema KS, Brennan PJ, Besra GS, Portaels F, Top J, Schouls LM, van Embden JD. 1997. A novel pathogenic taxon of the *Mycobacterium tuberculosis* complex, Canetti: characterization of an exceptional isolate from Africa. *Int J Syst Bacteriol* 47:1236–1245.

34. Pfyffer GE, Auckenthaler R, van Embden JD, van Soolingen D. 1998. *Mycobacterium canettii*, the smooth variant of M. tuberculosis, isolated from a Swiss patient exposed in Africa. *Emerg Infect Dis* 4:631–634.

35. Koeck JL, Bernatas JJ, Gerome P, Fabre M, Houmed A, Herve V, Teyssou R. 2002. [Epidemiology of resistance to antituberculosis drugs in *Mycobacterium tuberculosis* complex strains isolated from adenopathies in Djibouti. Prospective study carried out in 1999.] In French. *Med Trop* 62:70–72.

36. Fabre M, Koeck JL, Le Flèche P, Simon F, Hervé V, Vergnaud G, Pourcel C. 2004. High genetic diversity revealed by variable-number tandem repeat genotyping and analysis of *hsp65* gene polymorphism in a large collection of "*Mycobacterium canettii*" strains indicates that the M. tuberculosis complex is a recently emerged clone of "*M. canettii*." *J Clin Microbiol* 42:3248–3255.

37. Fabre M, Hauck Y, Soler C, Koeck JL, van Ingen J, van Soolingen D, Vergnaud G, Pourcel C. 2010. Molecular characteristics of "*Mycobacterium canettii*" the smooth *Mycobacterium tuberculosis* bacilli. *Infect Genet Evol* 10:1165–1173.

38. Young JS, Gormley E, Wellington EM. 2005. Molecular detection of *Mycobacterium bovis* and *Mycobacterium bovis* BCG (Pasteur) in soil. *Appl Environ Microbiol* 71:1946–1952.

39. Mba Medie F, Ben Salah I, Henrissat B, Raoult D, Drancourt M. 2011. *Mycobacterium tuberculosis* complex mycobacteria as amoeba-resistant organisms. *PLoS One* 6:e20499.

40. Boritsch EC, Supply P, Honoré N, Seemann T, Stinear TP, Brosch R. 2014. A glimpse into the past and predictions for the future: the molecular evolution of the tuberculosis agent. *Mol Microbiol* 93:835–852.

41. Gopinath K, Moosa A, Mizrahi V, Warner DF. 2013. Vitamin B(12) metabolism in *Mycobacterium tuberculosis*. *Future Microbiol* 8:1405–1418.

42. Comas I, Coscolla M, Luo T, Borrell S, Holt KE, Kato-Maeda M, Parkhill J, Malla B, Berg S, Thwaites G, Yeboah-Manu D, Bothamley G, Mei J, Wei L, Bentley S, Harris SR, Niemann S, Diel R, Aseffa A, Gao Q, Young D, Gagneux S. 2013. Out-of-Africa migration and Neolithic coexpansion of *Mycobacterium tuberculosis* with modern humans. *Nat Genet* 45:1176–1182.

43. Young DB, Comas I, de Carvalho LP. 2015. Phylogenetic analysis of vitamin B12-related metabolism in *Mycobacterium tuberculosis*. *Front Mol Biosci* 2:6

44. Boritsch EC, Frigui W, Cascioferro A, Malaga W, Etienne G, Laval G, Pawlik A, Le Chevalier F, Orgeur M, Ma L, Bouchier C, Stinear TP, Supply P, Majlessi L, Daffé M, Guilhot C, Brosch R. 2016. *pks5*-recombination-mediated surface remodelling in *Mycobacterium tuberculosis* emergence. *Nat Microbiol* 1:15019

45. Bottai D, Brosch R. 2009. Mycobacterial PE, PPE and ESX clusters: novel insights into the secretion of these most unusual protein families. *Mol Microbiol* 73:325–328.

46. Zumbo A, Palucci I, Cascioferro A, Sali M, Ventura M, D'Alfonso P, Iantomasi R, Di Sante G, Ria F, Sanguinetti M, Fadda G, Manganelli R, Delogu G. 2013. Functional dissection of protein domains involved in the immunomodulatory properties of PE_PGRS33 of *Mycobacterium tuberculosis*. *Pathog Dis* 69:232–239.

47. Cascioferro A, Daleke MH, Ventura M, Donà V, Delogu G, Palù G, Bitter W, Manganelli R. 2011. Functional dissection of the PE domain responsible for translocation of PE_PGRS33 across the mycobacterial cell wall. *PLoS One* 6:e27713.

48. Talarico S, Cave MD, Foxman B, Marrs CF, Zhang L, Bates JH, Yang Z. 2007. Association of *Mycobacterium tuberculosis* PE PGRS33 polymorphism with clinical and epidemiological characteristics. *Tuberculosis (Edinb)* 87:338–346.

49. Danilchanka O, Sun J, Pavlenok M, Maueröder C, Speer A, Siroy A, Marrero J, Trujillo C, Mayhew DL, Doornbos KS, Muñoz LE, Herrmann M, Ehrt S, Berens C, Niederweis M. 2014. An outer membrane channel protein of Mycobacterium tuberculosis with exotoxin activity. *Proc Natl Acad Sci USA* 111:6750–6755.

50. Gagneux S, DeRiemer K, Van T, Kato-Maeda M, de Jong BC, Narayanan S, Nicol M, Niemann S, Kremer K, Gutierrez MC, Hilty M, Hopewell PC, Small PM. 2006. Variable host-pathogen compatibility in *Mycobacterium tuberculosis*. *Proc Natl Acad Sci USA* 103:2869–2873.

51. Filliol I, Motiwala AS, Cavatore M, Qi W, Hazbón MH, Bobadilla del Valle M, Fyfe J, García-García L, Rastogi N, Sola C, Zozio T, Guerrero MI, León CI, Crabtree J, Angiuoli S, Eisenach KD, Durmaz R, Joloba ML, Rendón A, Sifuentes-Osornio J, Ponce de León A, Cave MD, Fleischmann R, Whittam TS, Alland D. 2006. Global phylogeny of *Mycobacterium tuberculosis* based on single nucleotide polymorphism (SNP) analysis: insights into tuberculosis evolution, phylogenetic accuracy of other DNA fingerprinting systems, and recommendations for a minimal standard SNP set. *J Bacteriol* 188:759–772.

52. Baker L, Brown T, Maiden MC, Drobniewski F. 2004. Silent nucleotide polymorphisms and a phylogeny for *Mycobacterium tuberculosis*. *Emerg Infect Dis* 10:1568–1577.

53. Comas I, Hailu E, Kiros T, Bekele S, Mekonnen W, Gumi B, Tschopp R, Ameni G, Hewinson RG, Robertson BD, Goig GA, Stucki D, Gagneux S, Aseffa A, Young D, Berg S. 2015. Population genomics of *Mycobacterium tuberculosis* in Ethiopia contradicts the virgin soil hypothesis for human tuberculosis in Sub-Saharan Africa. *Curr Biol* 25:3260–3266.

54. Nebenzahl-Guimaraes H, Yimer SA, Holm-Hansen C, de Beer J, Brosch R, van Soolingen D. 2016. Genomic characterization of *Mycobacterium tuberculosis* lineage

7 and a proposed name: "Aethiops vetus." *Microb Genom* **2:**

55. Blouin Y, Hauck Y, Soler C, Fabre M, Vong R, Dehan C, Cazajous G, Massoure PL, Kraemer P, Jenkins A, Garnotel E, Pourcel C, Vergnaud G. 2012. Significance of the identification in the Horn of Africa of an exceptionally deep branching *Mycobacterium tuberculosis* clade. *PLoS One* **7:**e52841.

56. Firdessa R, Berg S, Hailu E, Schelling E, Gumi B, Erenso G, Gadisa E, Kiros T, Habtamu M, Hussein J, Zinsstag J, Robertson BD, Ameni G, Lohan AJ, Loftus B, Comas I, Gagneux S, Tschopp R, Yamuah L, Hewinson G, Gordon SV, Young DB, Aseffa A. 2013. Mycobacterial lineages causing pulmonary and extrapulmonary tuberculosis, Ethiopia. *Emerg Infect Dis* **19:** 460–463.

57. Reiling N, Homolka S, Walter K, Brandenburg J, Niwinski L, Ernst M, Herzmann C, Lange C, Diel R, Ehlers S, Niemann S. 2013. Clade-specific virulence patterns of *Mycobacterium tuberculosis* complex strains in human primary macrophages and aerogenically infected mice. *MBio* **4:**e00250-13.

58. Winglee K, Manson McGuire A, Maiga M, Abeel T, Shea T, Desjardins CA, Diarra B, Baya B, Sanogo M, Diallo S, Earl AM, Bishai WR. 2016. Whole genome sequencing of *Mycobacterium africanum* strains from Mali provides insights into the mechanisms of geographic restriction. *PLoS Negl Trop Dis* **10:**e0004332.

59. Coscolla M, Gagneux S. 2014. Consequences of genomic diversity in *Mycobacterium tuberculosis*. *Semin Immunol* **26:**431–444.

60. de Jong BC, Hill PC, Aiken A, Awine T, Antonio M, Adetifa IM, Jackson-Sillah DJ, Fox A, Deriemer K, Gagneux S, Borgdorff MW, McAdam KP, Corrah T, Small PM, Adegbola RA. 2008. Progression to active tuberculosis, but not transmission, varies by *Mycobacterium tuberculosis* lineage in The Gambia. *J Infect Dis* **198:**1037–1043.

61. Niobe-Eyangoh SN, Kuaban C, Sorlin P, Cunin P, Thonnon J, Sola C, Rastogi N, Vincent V, Gutierrez MC. 2003. Genetic biodiversity of *Mycobacterium tuberculosis* complex strains from patients with pulmonary tuberculosis in Cameroon. *J Clin Microbiol* **41:**2547–2553.

62. Godreuil S, Torrea G, Terru D, Chevenet F, Diagbouga S, Supply P, Van de Perre P, Carriere C, Bañuls AL. 2007. First molecular epidemiology study of *Mycobacterium tuberculosis* in Burkina Faso. *J Clin Microbiol* **45:**921–927.

63. Koro Koro F, Kamdem Simo Y, Piam FF, Noeske J, Gutierrez C, Kuaban C, Eyangoh SI. 2013. Population dynamics of tuberculous Bacilli in Cameroon as assessed by spoligotyping. *J Clin Microbiol* **51:**299–302.

64. Asante-Poku A, Yeboah-Manu D, Otchere ID, Aboagye SY, Stucki D, Hattendorf J, Borrell S, Feldmann J, Danso E, Gagneux S. 2015. *Mycobacterium africanum* is associated with patient ethnicity in Ghana. *PLoS Negl Trop Dis* **9:**e3370.

65. Brites D, Gagneux S. 2012. Old and new selective pressures on *Mycobacterium tuberculosis*. *Infect Genet Evol* **12:**678–685.

66. Merker M, et al. 2015. Evolutionary history and global spread of the *Mycobacterium tuberculosis* Beijing lineage. *Nat Genet* **47:**242–249.

67. van Soolingen D, Qian L, de Haas PE, Douglas JT, Traore H, Portaels F, Qing HZ, Enkhsaikan D, Nymadawa P, van Embden JD. 1995. Predominance of a single genotype of *Mycobacterium tuberculosis* in countries of east Asia. *J Clin Microbiol* **33:**3234–3238.

68. Luo T, Comas I, Luo D, Lu B, Wu J, Wei L, Yang C, Liu Q, Gan M, Sun G, Shen X, Liu F, Gagneux S, Mei J, Lan R, Wan K, Gao Q. 2015. Southern East Asian origin and coexpansion of *Mycobacterium tuberculosis* Beijing family with Han Chinese. *Proc Natl Acad Sci USA* **112:**8136–8141.

69. Mokrousov I. 2013. Insights into the origin, emergence, and current spread of a successful Russian clone of *Mycobacterium tuberculosis*. *Clin Microbiol Rev* **26:** 342–360.

70. Frieden TR, Sherman LF, Maw KL, Fujiwara PI, Crawford JT, Nivin B, Sharp V, Hewlett D Jr, Brudney K, Alland D, Kreisworth BN. 1996. A multi-institutional outbreak of highly drug-resistant tuberculosis: epidemiology and clinical outcomes. *JAMA* **276:**1229–1235.

71. Bifani PJ, Plikaytis BB, Kapur V, Stockbauer K, Pan X, Lutfey ML, Moghazeh SL, Eisner W, Daniel TM, Kaplan MH, Crawford JT, Musser JM, Kreiswirth BN. 1996. Origin and interstate spread of a New York City multidrug-resistant *Mycobacterium tuberculosis* clone family. *JAMA* **275:**452–457.

72. Almeida D, Rodrigues C, Ashavaid TF, Lalvani A, Udwadia ZF, Mehta A. 2005. High incidence of the Beijing genotype among multidrug-resistant isolates of *Mycobacterium tuberculosis* in a tertiary care center in Mumbai, India. *Clin Infect Dis* **40:**881–886.

73. Casali N, Nikolayevskyy V, Balabanova Y, Harris SR, Ignatyeva O, Kontsevaya I, Corander J, Bryant J, Parkhill J, Nejentsev S, Horstmann RD, Brown T, Drobniewski F. 2014. Evolution and transmission of drug-resistant tuberculosis in a Russian population. *Nat Genet* **46:**279–286.

74. Coscolla M, Barry PM, Oeltmann JE, Koshinsky H, Shaw T, Cilnis M, Posey J, Rose J, Weber T, Fofanov VY, Gagneux S, Kato-Maeda M, Metcalfe JZ. 2015. Genomic epidemiology of multidrug-resistant *Mycobacterium tuberculosis* during transcontinental spread. *J Infect Dis* **212:**302–310.

75. Pfyffer GE, Strässle A, van Gorkum T, Portaels F, Rigouts L, Mathieu C, Mirzoev F, Traore H, van Embden JD. 2001. Multidrug-resistant tuberculosis in prison inmates, Azerbaijan. *Emerg Infect Dis* **7:**855–861.

76. Johnson R, Warren RM, van der Spuy GD, Gey van Pittius NC, Theron D, Streicher EM, Bosman M, Coetzee GJ, van Helden PD, Victor TC. 2010. Drug-resistant tuberculosis epidemic in the Western Cape driven by a virulent Beijing genotype strain. *Int J Tuberc Lung Dis* **14:** 119–121.

77. López B, Aguilar D, Orozco H, Burger M, Espitia C, Ritacco V, Barrera L, Kremer K, Hernandez-Pando R, Huygen K, van Soolingen D. 2003. A marked difference in pathogenesis and immune response induced by differ-

ent *Mycobacterium tuberculosis* genotypes. *Clin Exp Immunol* 133:30–37.

78. Tsenova L, Harbacheuski R, Sung N, Ellison E, Fallows D, Kaplan G. 2007. BCG vaccination confers poor protection against *M. tuberculosis* HN878-induced central nervous system disease. *Vaccine* 25:5126–5132.

79. Parish T, Smith DA, Roberts G, Betts J, Stoker NG. 2003. The *senX3-regX3* two-component regulatory system of *Mycobacterium tuberculosis* is required for virulence. *Microbiology* 149:1423–1435.

80. Marmiesse M, Brodin P, Buchrieser C, Gutierrez C, Simoes N, Vincent V, Glaser P, Cole ST, Brosch R. 2004. Macro-array and bioinformatic analyses reveal mycobacterial 'core' genes, variation in the ESAT-6 gene family and new phylogenetic markers for the *Mycobacterium tuberculosis* complex. *Microbiology* 150: 483–496.

81. Huet G, Constant P, Malaga W, Lanéelle MA, Kremer K, van Soolingen D, Daffé M, Guilhot C. 2009. A lipid profile typifies the Beijing strains of *Mycobacterium tuberculosis*: identification of a mutation responsible for a modification of the structures of phthiocerol dimycocerosates and phenolic glycolipids. *J Biol Chem* 284:27101–27113.

82. Constant P, Perez E, Malaga W, Lanéelle MA, Saurel O, Daffé M, Guilhot C. 2002. Role of the *pks15/1* gene in the biosynthesis of phenolglycolipids in the *Mycobacterium tuberculosis* complex. Evidence that all strains synthesize glycosylated p-hydroxybenzoic methyl esters and that strains devoid of phenolglycolipids harbor a frameshift mutation in the *pks15/1* gene. *J Biol Chem* 277:38148–38158.

83. Reed MB, Domenech P, Manca C, Su H, Barczak AK, Kreiswirth BN, Kaplan G, Barry CE III. 2004. A glycolipid of hypervirulent tuberculosis strains that inhibits the innate immune response. *Nature* 431:84–87.

84. Sinsimer D, Huet G, Manca C, Tsenova L, Koo MS, Kurepina N, Kana B, Mathema B, Marras SA, Kreiswirth BN, Guilhot C, Kaplan G. 2008. The phenolic glycolipid of *Mycobacterium tuberculosis* differentially modulates the early host cytokine response but does not in itself confer hypervirulence. *Infect Immun* 76:3027–3036.

85. Reed MB, Gagneux S, Deriemer K, Small PM, Barry CE III. 2007. The W-Beijing lineage of *Mycobacterium tuberculosis* overproduces triglycerides and has the DosR dormancy regulon constitutively upregulated. *J Bacteriol* 189:2583–2589.

86. Fallow A, Domenech P, Reed MB. 2010. Strains of the East Asian (W/Beijing) lineage of *Mycobacterium tuberculosis* are DosS/DosT-DosR two-component regulatory system natural mutants. *J Bacteriol* 192:2228–2238.

87. Domenech P, Kolly GS, Leon-Solis L, Fallow A, Reed MB. 2010. Massive gene duplication event among clinical isolates of the *Mycobacterium tuberculosis* W/Beijing family. *J Bacteriol* 192:4562–4570.

88. Ebrahimi-Rad M, Bifani P, Martin C, Kremer K, Samper S, Rauzier J, Kreiswirth B, Blazquez J, Jouan M, van Soolingen D, Gicquel B. 2003. Mutations in

putative mutator genes of *Mycobacterium tuberculosis* strains of the W-Beijing family. *Emerg Infect Dis* 9: 838–845.

89. Merker M, Kohl TA, Roetzer A, Truebe L, Richter E, Rüsch-Gerdes S, Fattorini L, Oggioni MR, Cox H, Varaine F, Niemann S. 2013. Whole genome sequencing reveals complex evolution patterns of multidrug-resistant *Mycobacterium tuberculosis* Beijing strains in patients. *PLoS One* 8:e82551.

90. Zhang H, Li D, Zhao L, Fleming J, Lin N, Wang T, Liu Z, Li C, Galwey N, Deng J, Zhou Y, Zhu Y, Gao Y, Wang T, Wang S, Huang Y, Wang M, Zhong Q, Zhou L, Chen T, Zhou J, Yang R, Zhu G, Hang H, Zhang J, Li F, Wan K, Wang J, Zhang XE, Bi L. 2013. Genome sequencing of 161 *Mycobacterium tuberculosis* isolates from China identifies genes and intergenic regions associated with drug resistance. *Nat Genet* 45:1255–1260.

91. Ioerger TR, Feng Y, Chen X, Dobos KM, Victor TC, Streicher EM, Warren RM, Gey van Pittius NC, Van Helden PD, Sacchettini JC. 2010. The non-clonality of drug resistance in Beijing-genotype isolates of *Mycobacterium tuberculosis* from the Western Cape of South Africa. *BMC Genomics* 11:670.

92. Eldholm V, Monteserin J, Rieux A, Lopez B, Sobkowiak B, Ritacco V, Balloux F. 2015. Four decades of transmission of a multidrug-resistant Mycobacterium tuberculosis outbreak strain. *Nat Commun* 6:7119.

93. Click ES, Moonan PK, Winston CA, Cowan LS, Oeltmann JE. 2012. Relationship between *Mycobacterium tuberculosis* phylogenetic lineage and clinical site of tuberculosis. *Clin Infect Dis* 54:211–219.

94. Séraphin MN, Lauzardo M, Doggett RT, Zabala J, Morris JG Jr, Blackburn JK. 2016. Spatiotemporal clustering of *Mycobacterium tuberculosis* complex genotypes in Florida: genetic diversity segregated by country of birth. *PLoS One* 11:e0153575.

95. Anderson J, Jarlsberg LG, Grindsdale J, Osmond D, Kawamura M, Hopewell PC, Kato-Maeda M. 2013. Sublineages of lineage 4 (Euro-American) *Mycobacterium tuberculosis* differ in genotypic clustering. *Int J Tuberc Lung Dis* 17:885–891.

96. Lee RS, Radomski N, Proulx JF, Levade I, Shapiro BJ, McIntosh F, Soualhine H, Menzies D, Behr MA. 2015. Population genomics of *Mycobacterium tuberculosis* in the Inuit. *Proc Natl Acad Sci USA* 112:13609–13614.

97. Barletta F, Otero L, de Jong BC, Iwamoto T, Arikawa K, Van der Stuyft P, Niemann S, Merker M, Uwizeye C, Seas C, Rigouts L. 2015. Predominant *Mycobacterium tuberculosis* families and high rates of recent transmission among new cases are not associated with primary multidrug resistance in Lima, Peru. *J Clin Microbiol* 53: 1854–1863.

98. Guerra-Assunção JA, Crampin AC, Houben RM, Mzembe T, Mallard K, Coll F, Khan P, Banda L, Chiwaya A, Pereira RP, McNerney R, Fine PE, Parkhill J, Clark TG, Glynn JR. 2015. Large-scale whole genome sequencing of *M. tuberculosis* provides insights into transmission in a high prevalence area. *eLife* 4:e05166.

99. Homolka S, Post E, Oberhauser B, George AG, Westman L, Dafae F, Rüsch-Gerdes S, Niemann S. 2008. High ge-

netic diversity among *Mycobacterium tuberculosis* complex strains from Sierra Leone. *BMC Microbiol* 8:103.

100. Brudey K, et al. 2006. *Mycobacterium tuberculosis* complex genetic diversity: mining the fourth international spoligotyping database (SpolDB4) for classification, population genetics and epidemiology. *BMC Microbiol* 6:23.

101. Lazzarini LC, Spindola SM, Bang H, Gibson AL, Weisenberg S, da Silva Carvalho W, Augusto CJ, Huard RC, Kritski AL, Ho JL. 2008. RDRio *Mycobacterium tuberculosis* infection is associated with a higher frequency of cavitary pulmonary disease. *J Clin Microbiol* 46:2175–2183.

102. Lazzarini LC, Huard RC, Boechat NL, Gomes HM, Oelemann MC, Kurepina N, Shashkina E, Mello FC, Gibson AL, Virginio MJ, Marsico AG, Butler WR, Kreiswirth BN, Suffys PN, Lapa E Silva JR, Ho JL. 2007. Discovery of a novel *Mycobacterium tuberculosis* lineage that is a major cause of tuberculosis in Rio de Janeiro, Brazil. *J Clin Microbiol* 45:3891–3902.

103. Gibson AL, Huard RC, Gey van Pittius NC, Lazzarini LC, Driscoll J, Kurepina N, Zozio T, Sola C, Spindola SM, Kritski AL, Fitzgerald D, Kremer K, Mardassi H, Chitale P, Brinkworth J, Garcia de Viedma D, Gicquel B, Pape JW, van Soolingen D, Kreiswirth BN, Warren RM, van Helden PD, Rastogi N, Suffys PN, Lapa e Silva J, Ho JL. 2008. Application of sensitive and specific molecular methods to uncover global dissemination of the major RDRio Sublineage of the Latin American-Mediterranean *Mycobacterium tuberculosis* spoligotype family. *J Clin Microbiol* 46:1259–1267.

104. Weisenberg SA, Gibson AL, Huard RC, Kurepina N, Bang H, Lazzarini LC, Chiu Y, Li J, Ahuja S, Driscoll J, Kreiswirth BN, Ho JL. 2012. Distinct clinical and epidemiological features of tuberculosis in New York City caused by the RD(Rio) *Mycobacterium tuberculosis* sublineage. *Infect Genet Evol* 12:664–670.

105. Majlessi L, Prados-Rosales R, Casadevall A, Brosch R. 2015. Release of mycobacterial antigens. *Immunol Rev* 264:25–45.

106. Von Groll A, Martin A, Felix C, Prata PF, Honscha G, Portaels F, Vandame P, da Silva PE, Palomino JC. 2010. Fitness study of the RDRio lineage and Latin American-Mediterranean family of *Mycobacterium tuberculosis* in the city of Rio Grande, Brazil. *FEMS Immunol Med Microbiol* 58:119–127.

107. Kremer K, van Soolingen D, Frothingham R, Haas WH, Hermans PW, Martín C, Palittapongarnpim P, Plikaytis BB, Riley LW, Yakrus MA, Musser JM, van Embden JD. 1999. Comparison of methods based on different molecular epidemiological markers for typing of *Mycobacterium tuberculosis* complex strains: interlaboratory study of discriminatory power and reproducibility. *J Clin Microbiol* 37:2607–2618.

108. Ritacco V, Di Lonardo M, Reniero A, Ambroggi M, Barrera L, Dambrosi A, Lopez B, Isola N, de Kantor IN. 1997. Nosocomial spread of human immunodeficiency virus-related multidrug-resistant tuberculosis in Buenos Aires. *J Infect Dis* 176:637–642.

109. Palmero D, Ritacco V, Ambroggi M, Natiello M, Barrera L, Capone L, Dambrosi A, di Lonardo M, Isola

N, Poggi S, Vescovo M, Abbate E. 2003. Multidrug-resistant tuberculosis in HIV-negative patients, Buenos Aires, Argentina. *Emerg Infect Dis* 9:965–969.

110. Kubín M, Havelková M, Hyncicová I, Svecová Z, Kaustová J, Kremer K, van Soolingen D. 1999. A multidrug-resistant tuberculosis microepidemic caused by genetically closely related *Mycobacterium tuberculosis* strains. *J Clin Microbiol* 37:2715–2716.

111. Mardassi H, Namouchi A, Haltiti R, Zarrouk M, Mhenni B, Karboul A, Khabouchi N, Gey van Pittius NC, Streicher EM, Rauzier J, Gicquel B, Dellagi K. 2005. Tuberculosis due to resistant Haarlem strain, Tunisia. *Emerg Infect Dis* 11:957–961.

112. Ramazanzadeh R, Roshani D, Shakib P, Rouhi S. 2015. Prevalence and occurrence rate of *Mycobacterium tuberculosis* Haarlem family multi-drug resistant in the worldwide population: A systematic review and meta-analysis. *J Res Med Sci* 20:78–88.

113. Olano J, López B, Reyes A, Lemos MP, Correa N, Del Portillo P, Barrera L, Robledo J, Ritacco V, Zambrano MM. 2007. Mutations in DNA repair genes are associated with the Haarlem lineage of *Mycobacterium tuberculosis* independently of their antibiotic resistance. *Tuberculosis (Edinb)* 87:502–508. Edinb

114. Mortimer TD, Pepperell CS. 2014. Genomic signatures of distributive conjugal transfer among mycobacteria. *Genome Biol Evol* 6:2489–2500.

115. Gray TA, Krywy JA, Harold J, Palumbo MJ, Derbyshire KM. 2013. Distributive conjugal transfer in mycobacteria generates progeny with meiotic-like genome-wide mosaicism, allowing mapping of a mating identity locus. *PLoS Biol* 11:e1001602.

116. Boritsch EC, Khanna V, Pawlik A, Honoré N, Navas VH, Ma L, Bouchier L, Seemann T, Supply P, Stinear TP, Brosch R. Key experimental evidence of chromosomal DNA transfer among selected tuberculosis-causing mycobacteria. *Proc Natl Acad Sci USA* 113:9876–9881.

117. Schatz A, Waksman SA. 1944. Effect of streptomycin and other antibiotic substances upon *Mycobacterium tuberculosis* and related organisms. *Proc Soc Exp Biol Med* 57:244–248.

118. Medical Research Council. 1952. Treatment of pulmonary tuberculosis with isoniazid; an interim report to the Medical Research Council by their Tuberculosis Chemotherapy Trials Committee. *BMJ* 2:735–746.

119. Sensi P. 1983. History of the development of rifampin. *Rev Infect Dis* 5(Suppl 3):S402–S406.

120. Canetti G. 1965. Present aspects of bacterial resistance in tuberculosis. *Am Rev Respir Dis* 92:687–703.

121. Lienhardt C, Vernon A, Raviglione MC. 2010. New drugs and new regimens for the treatment of tuberculosis: review of the drug development pipeline and implications for national programmes. *Curr Opin Pulm Med* 16:186–193.

122. Gardy JL, Johnston JC, Ho Sui SJ, Cook VJ, Shah L, Brodkin E, Rempel S, Moore R, Zhao Y, Holt R, Varhol R, Birol I, Lem M, Sharma MK, Elwood K, Jones SJ, Brinkman FS, Brunham RC, Tang P. 2011. Whole-genome sequencing and social-network analysis of a tuberculosis outbreak. *N Engl J Med* 364:730–739.

123. Mitruka K, Oeltmann JE, Ijaz K, Haddad MB. 2011. Tuberculosis outbreak investigations in the United States, 2002–2008. *Emerg Infect Dis* **17:**425–431.

124. Gandhi NR, Moll A, Sturm AW, Pawinski R, Govender T, Lalloo U, Zeller K, Andrews J, Friedland G. 2006. Extensively drug-resistant tuberculosis as a cause of death in patients co-infected with tuberculosis and HIV in a rural area of South Africa. *Lancet* **368:**1575–1580.

125. Stucki D, Ballif M, Bodmer T, Coscolla M, Maurer AM, Droz S, Butz C, Borrell S, Längle C, Feldmann J, Furrer H, Mordasini C, Helbling P, Rieder HL, Egger M, Gagneux S, Fenner L. 2015. Tracking a tuberculosis outbreak over 21 years: strain-specific single-nucleotide polymorphism typing combined with targeted whole-genome sequencing. *J Infect Dis* **211:**1306–1316.

126. Centers for Disease Control and Prevention (CDC). 2006. Emergence of *Mycobacterium tuberculosis* with extensive resistance to second-line drugs–worldwide, 2000–2004. *MMWR Morb Mortal Wkly Rep* **55:**301–305.

127. WHO. 2015. *Global Tuberculosis Report 2015.* World Health Organization, Geneva, Switzerland.

128. Telenti A, Imboden P, Marchesi F, Matter L, Schopfer K, Bodmer T, Lowrie D, Colston MJ, Cole S. 1993. Detection of rifampicin-resistance mutations in *Mycobacterium tuberculosis. Lancet* **341:**647–651.

129. Gagneux S, Long CD, Small PM, Van T, Schoolnik GK, Bohannan BJ. 2006. The competitive cost of antibiotic resistance in *Mycobacterium tuberculosis. Science* **312:**1944–1946.

130. Meftahi N, Namouchi A, Mhenni B, Brandis G, Hughes D, Mardassi H. 2016. Evidence for the critical role of a secondary site *rpoB* mutation in the compensatory evolution and successful transmission of an MDR tuberculosis outbreak strain. *J Antimicrob Chemother* **71:**324–332.

131. Brandis G, Pietsch F, Alemayehu R, Hughes D. 2015. Comprehensive phenotypic characterization of rifampicin resistance mutations in *Salmonella* provides insight into the evolution of resistance in *Mycobacterium tuberculosis. J Antimicrob Chemother* **70:**680–685.

132. Zhang Y, Heym B, Allen B, Young D, Cole S. 1992. The catalase-peroxidase gene and isoniazid resistance of *Mycobacterium tuberculosis. Nature* **358:**591–593.

133. Cade CE, Dlouhy AC, Medzihradszky KF, Salas-Castillo SP, Ghiladi RA. 2010. Isoniazid-resistance conferring mutations in *Mycobacterium tuberculosis* KatG: catalase, peroxidase, and INH-NADH adduct formation activities. *Protein Sci* **19:**458–474.

134. Ghiladi RA, Medzihradszky KF, Rusnak FM, Ortiz de Montellano PR. 2005. Correlation between isoniazid resistance and superoxide reactivity in *mycobacterium tuberculosis* KatG. *J Am Chem Soc* **127:**13428–13442.

135. Shoeb HA, Bowman BU Jr, Ottolenghi AC, Merola AJ. 1985. Peroxidase-mediated oxidation of isoniazid. *Antimicrob Agents Chemother* **27:**399–403.

136. Banerjee A, Dubnau E, Quemard A, Balasubramanian V, Um KS, Wilson T, Collins D, de Lisle G, Jacobs WR Jr. 1994. *inhA,* a gene encoding a target for isoniazid and ethionamide in *Mycobacterium tuberculosis. Science* **263:**227–230.

137. Manca C, Paul S, Barry CE III, Freedman VH, Kaplan G. 1999. *Mycobacterium tuberculosis* catalase and peroxidase activities and resistance to oxidative killing in human monocytes in vitro. *Infect Immun* **67:**74–79.

138. Middlebrook G, Cohn ML. 1953. Some observations on the pathogenicity of isoniazid-resistant variants of tubercle bacilli. *Science* **118:**297–299.

139. Li Z, Kelley C, Collins F, Rouse D, Morris S. 1998. Expression of *katG* in *Mycobacterium tuberculosis* is associated with its growth and persistence in mice and guinea pigs. *J Infect Dis* **177:**1030–1035.

140. Pym AS, Saint-Joanis B, Cole ST. 2002. Effect of *katG* mutations on the virulence of *Mycobacterium tuberculosis* and the implication for transmission in humans. *Infect Immun* **70:**4955–4960.

141. Sherman DR, Mdluli K, Hickey MJ, Arain TM, Morris SL, Barry CE III, Stover CK. 1996. Compensatory *ahpC* gene expression in isoniazid-resistant *Mycobacterium tuberculosis. Science* **272:**1641–1643.

142. Guo H, Seet Q, Denkin S, Parsons L, Zhang Y. 2006. Molecular characterization of isoniazid-resistant clinical isolates of *Mycobacterium tuberculosis* from the USA. *J Med Microbiol* **55:**1527–1531.

143. Safi H, Lingaraju S, Amin A, Kim S, Jones M, Holmes M, McNeil M, Peterson SN, Chatterjee D, Fleischmann R, Alland D. 2013. Evolution of high-level ethambutol-resistant tuberculosis through interacting mutations in decaprenylphosphoryl-β-D-arabinose biosynthetic and utilization pathway genes. *Nat Genet* **45:**1190–1197.

144. Eldholm V, Balloux F. 2016. Antimicrobial resistance in *Mycobacterium tuberculosis*: the odd one out. *Trends Microbiol* **24:**637–648.

145. Frieden TR, Sterling T, Pablos-Mendez A, Kilburn JO, Cauthen GM, Dooley SW. 1993. The emergence of drug-resistant tuberculosis in New York City. *N Engl J Med* **328:**521–526.

146. Rullán JV, Herrera D, Cano R, Moreno V, Godoy P, Peiró EF, Castell J, Ibañez C, Ortega A, Agudo LS, Pozo F. 1996. Nosocomial transmission of multidrug-resistant *Mycobacterium tuberculosis* in Spain. *Emerg Infect Dis* **2:**125–129.

147. Hannan MM, Peres H, Maltez F, Hayward AC, Machado J, Morgado A, Proenca R, Nelson MR, Bico J, Young DB, Gazzard BS. 2001. Investigation and control of a large outbreak of multi-drug resistant tuberculosis at a central Lisbon hospital. *J Hosp Infect* **47:**91–97.

148. Harries AD, Kamenya A, Namarika D, Msolomba IW, Salaniponi FM, Nyangulu DS, Nunn P. 1997. Delays in diagnosis and treatment of smear-positive tuberculosis and the incidence of tuberculosis in hospital nurses in Blantyre, Malawi. *Trans R Soc Trop Med Hyg* **91:**15–17.

149. Cohen KA, Abeel T, Manson McGuire A, Desjardins CA, Munsamy V, Shea TP, Walker BJ, Bantubani N, Almeida DV, Alvarado L, Chapman SB, Mvelase NR, Duffy EY, Fitzgerald MG, Govender P, Gujja S, Hamilton S, Howarth C, Larimer JD, Maharaj K, Pearson MD, Priest ME, Zeng Q, Padayatchi N, Grosset J, Young SK, Wortman J, Mlisana KP, O'Donnell MR, Birren BW, Bishai WR, Pym AS, Earl AM. 2015. Evolu-

tion of extensively drug-resistant tuberculosis over four decades: whole genome sequencing and dating analysis of *Mycobacterium tuberculosis* isolates from KwaZulu-Natal. *PLoS Med* 12:e1001880.

150. Sun G, Luo T, Yang C, Dong X, Li J, Zhu Y, Zheng H, Tian W, Wang S, Barry CE III, Mei J, Gao Q. 2012. Dynamic population changes in *Mycobacterium tuberculosis* during acquisition and fixation of drug resistance in patients. *J Infect Dis* 206:1724–1733.

151. Casali N, Nikolayevskyy V, Balabanova Y, Ignatyeva O, Kontsevaya I, Harris SR, Bentley SD, Parkhill J, Nejentsev S, Hoffner SE, Horstmann RD, Brown T, Drobniewski F. 2012. Microevolution of extensively drug-resistant tuberculosis in Russia. *Genome Res* 22: 735–745.

152. Phelan J, Coll F, McNerney R, Ascher DB, Pires DE, Furnham N, Coeck N, Hill-Cawthorne GA, Nair MB, Mallard K, Ramsay A, Campino S, Hibberd ML, Pain A, Rigouts L, Clark TG. 2016. *Mycobacterium tuberculosis* whole genome sequencing and protein structure modelling provides insights into anti-tuberculosis drug resistance. *BMC Med* 14:31.

153. Comas I, Borrell S, Roetzer A, Rose G, Malla B, Kato-Maeda M, Galagan J, Niemann S, Gagneux S. 2011. Whole-genome sequencing of rifampicin-resistant *Mycobacterium tuberculosis* strains identifies compensatory mutations in RNA polymerase genes. *Nat Genet* 44:106–110.

154. Walker TM, Kohl TA, Omar SV, Hedge J, Del Ojo Elias C, Bradley P, Iqbal Z, Feuerriegel S, Niehaus KE, Wilson DJ, Clifton DA, Kapatai G, Ip CL, Bowden R, Drobniewski FA, Allix-Béguec C, Gaudin C, Parkhill J, Diel R, Supply P, Crook DW, Smith EG, Walker AS, Ismail N, Niemann S, Peto TE, Modernizing Medical Microbiology (MMM) Informatics Group. 2015. Whole-genome sequencing for prediction of *Mycobacterium tuberculosis* drug susceptibility and resistance: a retrospective cohort study. *Lancet Infect Dis* 15:1193–1202.

155. Shenai S, Amisano D, Ronacher K, Kriel M, Banada PP, Song T, Lee M, Joh JS, Winter J, Thayer R, Via LE, Kim S, Barry CE III, Walzl G, Alland D. 2013. Exploring alternative biomaterials for diagnosis of pulmonary tuberculosis in HIV-negative patients by use of the GeneXpert MTB/RIF assay. *J Clin Microbiol* 51: 4161–4166.

156. Desjardins CA, Cohen KA, Munsamy V, Abeel T, Maharaj K, Walker BJ, Shea TP, Almeida DV, Manson AL, Salazar A, Padayatchi N, O'Donnell MR, Mlisana KP, Wortman J, Birren BW, Grosset J, Earl AM, Pym AS. 2016. Genomic and functional analyses of *Mycobacterium tuberculosis* strains implicate *ald* in D-cycloserine resistance. *Nat Genet* 48:544–551.

157. Takiff HE, Feo O. 2015. Clinical value of whole-genome sequencing of *Mycobacterium tuberculosis*. *Lancet Infect Dis* 15:1077–1090.

158. Warner DF, Mizrahi V. 2013. Complex genetics of drug resistance in *Mycobacterium tuberculosis*. *Nat Genet* 45:1107–1108.

159. Farhat MR, Shapiro BJ, Kieser KJ, Sultana R, Jacobson KR, Victor TC, Warren RM, Streicher EM, Calver A, Sloutsky A, Kaur D, Posey JE, Plikaytis B, Oggioni MR, Gardy JL, Johnston JC, Rodrigues M, Tang PK, Kato-Maeda M, Borowsky ML, Muddukrishna B, Kreiswirth BN, Kurepina N, Galagan J, Gagneux S, Birren B, Rubin EJ, Lander ES, Sabeti PC, Murray M. 2013. Genomic analysis identifies targets of convergent positive selection in drug-resistant *Mycobacterium tuberculosis*. *Nat Genet* 45:1183–1189.

160. Pérez-Lago L, Comas I, Navarro Y, González-Candelas F, Herranz M, Bouza E, García-de-Viedma D. 2014. Whole genome sequencing analysis of intrapatient microevolution in *Mycobacterium tuberculosis*: potential impact on the inference of tuberculosis transmission. *J Infect Dis* 209:98–108.

161. Pérez-Lago L, Palacios JJ, Herranz M, Ruiz Serrano MJ, Bouza E, García-de-Viedma D. 2015. Revealing hidden clonal complexity in *Mycobacterium tuberculosis* infection by qualitative and quantitative improvement of sampling. *Clin Microbiol Infect* 21:147.e1–147.e7.

162. Eldholm V, Norheim G, von der Lippe B, Kinander W, Dahle UR, Caugant DA, Mannsåker T, Mengshoel AT, Dyrhol-Riise AM, Balloux F. 2014. Evolution of extensively drug-resistant *Mycobacterium tuberculosis* from a susceptible ancestor in a single patient. *Genome Biol* 15:490.

163. Black PA, de Vos M, Louw GE, van der Merwe RG, Dippenaar A, Streicher EM, Abdallah AM, Sampson SL, Victor TC, Dolby T, Simpson JA, van Helden PD, Warren RM, Pain A. 2015. Whole genome sequencing reveals genomic heterogeneity and antibiotic purification in *Mycobacterium tuberculosis* isolates. *BMC Genomics* 16:857.

164. Liu Q, Via LE, Luo T, Liang L, Liu X, Wu S, Shen Q, Wei W, Ruan X, Yuan X, Zhang G, Barry CE III, Gao Q. 2015. Within patient microevolution of *Mycobacterium tuberculosis* correlates with heterogeneous responses to treatment. *Sci Rep* 5:17507.

165. Niemann S, Köser CU, Gagneux S, Plinke C, Homolka S, Bignell H, Carter RJ, Cheetham RK, Cox A, Gormley NA, Kokko-Gonzales P, Murray LJ, Rigatti R, Smith VP, Arends FP, Cox HS, Smith G, Archer JA. 2009. Genomic diversity among drug sensitive and multidrug resistant isolates of *Mycobacterium tuberculosis* with identical DNA fingerprints. *PLoS One* 4:e7407.

166. Ioerger TR, Koo S, No EG, Chen X, Larsen MH, Jacobs WR Jr, Pillay M, Sturm AW, Sacchettini JC. 2009. Genome analysis of multi- and extensively-drug-resistant tuberculosis from KwaZulu-Natal, South Africa. *PLoS One* 4:e7778.

The Signature Problem of Tuberculosis Persistence

V

Tuberculosis and the Tubercle Bacillus, 2nd ed.
Edited by William R. Jacobs, Jr., Helen McShane, Valerie Mizrahi, and Ian M. Orme
© 2018 American Society for Microbiology, Washington, DC
doi:10.1128/microbiolspec.TBTB2-0003-2015

Acid-Fast Positive and Acid-Fast Negative *Mycobacterium tuberculosis*: The Koch Paradox

23

Catherine Vilchèze[1] and Laurent Kremer[2]

INTRODUCTION

Mycobacterium tuberculosis possesses a unique cell wall architecture that is distinct from both Gram-negative and Gram-positive bacteria. The cell wall consists of a thick, lipid-rich outer layer composed primarily of mycolic acids (1) (Fig. 1). This lipid layer lies on top of a layer of peptidoglycan and the polysaccharide arabinogalactan, which, in turn, are anchored to the inner lipid membrane common to all bacteria (2–4). The overall thick waxy coat renders acid-fast (AF) mycobacteria resistant to Gram staining. When stained with alternative dyes, the cell wall is resistant to decolorization with acid alcohol, thus giving these bacteria their sobriquet "acid-fast." This unique AF property has been the basis for the continuous development of staining procedures over the past century and remains the cornerstone for the diagnosis of tuberculosis (TB), especially in low-income and middle-income countries where more than 90% of TB cases occur (5). The Ziehl-Neelsen (ZN) stain, also known as the AF stain, which is used in microscopic detection of *M. tuberculosis*, was originally developed independently by Ziehl and Neelsen, who improved on the early work of Koch, Rindfleisch, and Ehrlich (see below).

Acid-fastness has been attributed to a number of mycobacterial cell wall components, including outer lipids, arabinogalactan-bound mycolic acids, and lipoglycans (6–8). The underlying theme in all of the proposed mechanisms is the presence of a lipid-rich, hydrophobic barrier that can be penetrated by phenol-based stains but is resistant to decolorization by acid-alcohol, although the precise molecular component(s) responsible for this unique staining property remains undetermined. Early studies of the effects of the first-line anti-TB drug isoniazid on staining characteristics of *M. tuberculosis* demonstrated a loss of acid-fastness after growth in the presence of isoniazid (9). Because isoniazid is known to inhibit the synthesis of mycolic acids (10), this observation suggested that these lipids may be the components responsible for AF staining and that mutants defective in mycolic acid production would be suitable candidates to study the phenomenon of acid-fastness. This stimulated more recent studies using defined *M. tuberculosis* mutants deleted in mycolic acid biosynthetic genes, culminating in the discovery that deletion of the β-ketoacyl acyl carrier protein (ACP) synthase encoded by *kasB* caused alterations in mycolic acid structure ultimately resulting in a loss of acid-fastness (11).

Nevertheless, it has been known for a long time that conversion of actively replicating AF-positive bacilli into dormant AF-negative bacteria can occur during infection in both human patients and in animal models (12). This loss of acid-fastness, also known as Koch's paradox, has recently been linked to physiological metabolic changes as well as modifications of the cell wall composition and/or architecture that must occur in the dormant bacilli. This may have important consequences for the diagnosis of TB as well as in clinical epidemiology.

This review article will mainly focus on Koch's paradox, highlighting recent contributions of new *in vitro* and cellular models to address the metabolic changes characterizing and linking persistence with loss of acid-fastness.

[1]Howard Hughes Medical Institute, Department of Microbiology and Immunology, Albert Einstein College of Medicine, Bronx, NY 10461;
[2]IRIM (ex-CPBS) UMR 9004, Infectious Disease Research Institute of Montpellier (IDRIM), Université de Montpellier, CNRS, 34293 Montpellier, France.

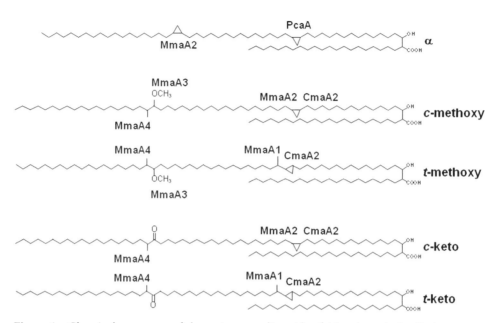

Figure 1 Chemical structures of the major mycolic acids of *M. tuberculosis*. Cyclopropane rings and methyl branches are shown and annotated with the *S*-adenosyl methionine-dependent methyl transferases responsible for their synthesis. *c*, *cis*; *t*, *trans*.

A BRIEF HISTORY OF AF STAINING

On 24 March 1882, Robert Koch gave his break-through lecture "Die Aetiologie der Tuberkulose" (13) on the discovery of the bacillus *M. tuberculosis*, in which he described the first successful attempt to stain *M. tuberculosis* by spreading mycobacteria-infected specimens on coverslips. After fixing the specimens, he dipped the coverslips into a hot, alkaline, ethanolic solution of methylene blue for 1 hour and then covered them with a solution of vesuvin (Bismarck brown) before rinsing with distilled water. This procedure allowed, for the first time, the visualization of *M. tuberculosis* as blue bacilli on a brown background. This important discovery in detecting the bacilli in infected human and animal specimens was quickly followed by several improvements on Koch's technique (14). On 1 May 1882, P. Ehrlich announced at the Association of Internal Medicine in Berlin that he had developed a staining protocol whereby Koch's methylene blue was replaced with an ethanolic solution of fuchsin or methylene violet dissolved in water saturated with aniline oil, followed by decolorization with 30% aqueous nitric acid solution and counterstaining with a yellow (Bismarck) or blue (methylene blue) dye (15). The bacilli appeared as a distinctive purple/blue on a yellow background or red on a blue background. Ehrlich's method was deemed a "great improvement" over Koch's staining protocol by none other than Koch himself.

On 12 August 1882, F. Ziehl published a modified version of Ehrlich's staining protocol in which carbolic acid (phenol) was used instead of aniline oil along with a weaker acid for decolorization. The bacilli appeared as strikingly colored as in Ehrlich's method but with the advantage that the carbol-fuchsin solution was more stable than Ehrlich's aniline-fuchsin solution. Rindfleisch then proposed in October 1882 to enhance Koch's protocol by heating the slides instead of dipping them in hot water, as reported by Koch. On 14 July 1883, F. Neelsen published a modified Ziehl's staining protocol that described the use of a 0.75% fuchsin solution in 5% carbolic acid followed by decolorization with a 25% sulfuric acid solution. It took only 16 months for this method of staining of the tubercle bacilli to be standardized and to become widely recognized a decade later as ZN staining, although the technique was based on the complementary work of five researchers: Koch, Ehrlich, Ziehl, Rindfleisch, and Neelsen. From then on, *M. tuberculosis* would be known as an AF bacillus for its ability to resist decolorization by an ethanolic acid wash (Fig. 2).

Despite the successful staining of *M. tuberculosis* with the ZN technique, numerous researchers continued modifying the ZN protocol. In 1887, H. S. Gabbett proposed shortening the protocol by combining the decolorization with sulfuric acid and the counterstaining with methylene blue (16), with the whole pro-

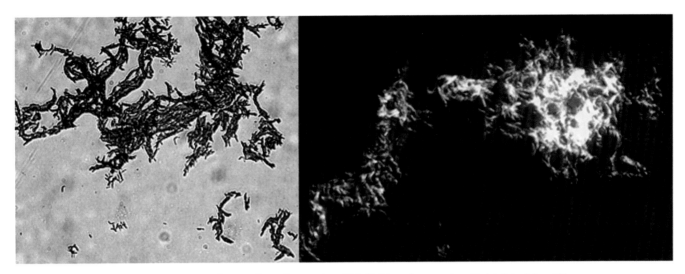

Figure 2 Staining of *M. tuberculosis* using ZN (left) and auramine O (right). Magnification, ×100.

cess taking no more than 6 minutes to complete. In 1915, J. Kinyoun published his procedure to examine sputum from TB-infected patients using a twist on the staining method that has become known as the "cold staining" technique (17). Kinyoun stated that Gabbett's decolorization solution did not work well on thick, unevenly spread slides and recommended the following protocol: (i) increased concentrations of fuchsin (3.1%) and phenol (6.25%) in the primary stain, which was done at room temperature, and (ii) decolorization with 3% hydrochloric acid instead of sulfuric acid (17). This protocol is the basis of the Kinyoun cold stain method, yet several modifications of this method can be found in the literature, which are described below.

V. Hallberg noticed that all the primary stain dyes used previously to stain *M. tuberculosis* were either water-soluble or formed semicolloidal solutions in water and decided to test the "Nachtblau" dye that forms colloidal solutions in water (18). Using a carbol-Nachtblau solution as the primary stain, followed by the ZN decolorization technique with carbol-fuchsin as the counterstain resulted in the bacilli being seen as dark blue on a red background. The new staining solution had the advantage of being stable for at least a year, and Hallberg and others reported higher sensitivity when compared to conventional ZN staining (19). However, F. Tison observed stability issues with Hallberg's Nachtblau staining solution and proposed a cold method in which the primary stain with the Nachtblau solution was performed for 24 hours at room temperature followed by decolorization with an ethanolic solution of 25% hydrochloric acid for 3 min-

utes and counterstaining with orange G (20). The bacilli appeared bright blue on an orange background, which gave color-blind people, who cannot distinguish between red and blue, the ability to read AF staining slides. In 1962, T. T. Hok proposed combining the Kinyoun primary stain with Gabbett's decolorization/counterstaining solution to produce a faster (4.5 minutes as opposed to 8 minutes for the traditional ZN staining protocol) and easier "cold staining" protocol (21). Experiencing problems with the decolorizing steps in the Hok's cold staining protocol, J. L. Allen devised a modified hot ZN staining protocol and compared it to the traditional hot ZN staining and Hok's cold staining methods. The modified hot ZN protocol consisted of combining the decolorizing and counterstaining steps (22). In her study of 122 pathology specimens, the majority (104) were smear-negative/culture-negative, 16 were smear-positive by the ZN method and culture-positive, and two were smear-positive by the modified ZN but culture-negative. Of the 18 smear-positive samples, the cold staining protocol detected only one. Both the ZN and the Kinyoun staining protocols are still currently used in clinical settings. The ZN primary stain consists of a 0.3% ethanolic fuchsin solution in 5% aqueous phenolic solution, whereas the Kinyoun primary stain is a 4% ethanolic fuchsin solution in 8% aqueous phenolic solution. Both methods use a 3% aqueous hydrochloric acid solution for decolorization and a 0.3% aqueous methylene blue solution for counterstaining.

The third staining technique for the detection of AF bacilli is auramine-rhodamine (AR) staining, which is a highly sensitive method but requires a fluorescence microscope. The use of the auramine dye to stain *M. tuberculosis* was introduced by Hagemann in 1938 (23) (Fig. 2). The auramine O staining method was more sensitive and faster in detecting tubercle bacilli than the ZN protocol, but the major drawback was the potential background fluorescence due to other bacteria/viruses or artifacts. J. Degommier recommended the use of two fluorochromes to easily distinguish *M. tuberculosis* from background artifacts, with auramine as the first stain, followed by decolorization and counterstaining with thiazine red, and resulting in *M. tuberculosis* bacilli appearing bright yellow while the artifacts or other microbes stained red (24). J. Augier instead proposed adding rhodamine to auramine to increase the contrast between tubercle bacilli and other microbes or artifacts (24). A counterstain with potassium permanganate that eliminated the fluorescence of all organisms/artifacts except for mycobacteria was later proposed (25). The authors also found that the AR combination was better at preventing the visualization of artifacts than auramine alone. The AR staining protocol, also called the Truant method, consists of staining with a solution of 1.2% auramine O, 0.6% rhodamine B, and 8% phenol in water/glycerol, followed by decolorization with 0.5% aqueous hydrochloric acid solution and counterstaining with 0.5% potassium permanganate.

Despite the apparent ease of use of these protocols, there are still numerous pitfalls to the staining of mycobacteria, which has encouraged researchers to continuously improve the staining techniques to make them faster, safer, and more reliable, especially since AF staining of sputum and sputum cultures is the primary tool for the diagnosis of active TB.

AF STAINING IN CLINICAL DIAGNOSIS OF TB

Considering the time required for sputum cultures to grow (6 to 8 weeks), analysis of sputum after AF staining is the quickest and easiest technique for diagnosing pulmonary TB. Nevertheless, AF staining faces numerous issues and, therefore, can lead to false-negative or false-positive results in clinical settings.

ZN staining is cost-effective, relatively simple, and fast to use. The processing of the samples, the thickness of the smears, the preparation and conservation of the reagents, the quality of the microscopes, the length of the primary and counterstaining, as well as the expertise of the technical staff play important roles in the sensitivity and specificity of AF staining (26–29). The sensitivity of the staining varies between 20 and 60%

(30, 31), and the concentrations of the primary stain (carbol-fuchsin) and counterstain (methylene blue) were shown to be important for the detection of *M. tuberculosis*. The World Health Organization recommends using 0.3% carbol-fuchsin and 0.3% methylene blue, but it was suggested that, in clinical settings, staining with 1% carbol-fuchsin for 10 minutes and counterstaining with 0.1% methylene blue for 1 minute gives better results (27). Others failed to observe significant differences in sensitivity with concentrations ranging between 0.3 and 1% carbol-fuchsin, but decreasing the concentration of carbol-fuchsin to 0.1% resulted in a significant decrease in sensitivity (32).

The sensitivity of ZN staining is also related to the bacillary counts in sputum. To obtain a positive AF diagnosis from a TB patient's sputum, around 5,000 to 10,000 bacilli per milliliter of sputum are required (33). Yet in extrapulmonary TB cases (34), TB patients coinfected with HIV (30, 35), or children infected with TB (36), the bacillary count might be lower than the minimum amount required for optimal ZN staining, resulting in poor sensitivity. To balance this issue, Shapiro and Hänscheid have shown that ZN-stained slides of unprocessed sputum, where *M. tuberculosis* was not easily detectable with bright-field microscopy, could be more readily observed by fluorescence microscopy (37). Other issues to consider are color blindness, given that the tubercle bacilli are seen as red on a blue background, as well as waste disposal. The ZN primary stain solution is phenol-based and is considered hazardous material requiring proper disposal.

The Kinyoun cold staining method has been found unreliable (22), giving more false-positive results than ZN staining (38, 39). The main advantage of this technique is that the duration of the different steps does not play such a critical role, although researchers have noted problems with the decolorization step and that far fewer bacilli are stained than when the samples are heated.

Staining of TB patients' sputa with auramine O is described as the most sensitive, reproducible, and specific method for detecting *M. tuberculosis* (40, 41). This increase in sensitivity has been attributed to mycolic acids in the mycobacterial cell wall that retain auramine O better than carbol-fuchsin (42), although others have reported that auramine O and fuchsin are bound to nucleic acids and not mycolic acids (43). The reading of auramine O-stained slides is conducted at a lower magnification, resulting in a larger field of view and rendering the process three times faster than ZN staining (44). In paucibacillary *M. tuberculosis* samples, such as from extrapulmonary TB cases, auramine O staining can detect *M. tuberculosis* even in culture-negative samples (45, 46). Staining with auramine O instead of the ZN staining protocol also generates a lower percentage of false-negative results (47). A combination of both protocols was tested using auramine and Kinyoun carbol fuchsin solutions as the primary stain, followed by acid wash and methylene blue counterstaining and scanning the slides on bright-field and fluorescence microscopes; although application of this dual staining solution was faster than staining two slides for both methods, the proposed protocol had specific issues such as decolorizing inefficiency and increased background fluorescence (48). Finally, color-blind personnel can easily identify the tubercle bacilli in auramine O-stained smears. The main drawbacks are false-positivity due to background staining, the requirement of a fluorescence microscope, and the classification of auramine O as a carcinogen (49, 50). However, the replacement of auramine O with acridine orange, a dye that stains nucleic acids in bacteria and eukaryotic cells, was shown to be as efficient as auramine O in detecting *M. tuberculosis* in specimen smears (51).

THE KOCH PARADOX

Non-AF tubercle bacilli were first reported a year after Koch published his technique for detecting and identifying *M. tuberculosis* from TB patients (52). Although these non-AF bacilli did not retain the primary stain upon acid wash, they were able to cause TB disease when used to infect animals, could be found in lesions of patients with caseous or miliary TB, and could be grown in laboratory cultures depending on the media and strains used (53). The non-AF bacilli were either fully virulent, were fully avirulent and behaving like saprophytic bacilli, or had lost some but not all of their virulence characteristics (54). Additionally, although initially non-AF, these bacteria could regain their acid-fastness upon passage in animals (52). The loss of acid-fastness was also observed in early studies of cultures treated with isoniazid. Rist et al. had noticed that, within 24 hours of isoniazid treatment, the bacilli appeared blue with ZN staining, whereas *M. tuberculosis* bacilli resistant to isoniazid were red (9). When it was later discovered that isoniazid inhibits mycolic acid biosynthesis (10), the field had the first indication that cell wall organization and specifically the mycolic acid composition were involved in the ability of mycobacteria to retain the primary stain and resist the acid wash.

The non-AF phenotype of *M. tuberculosis* had been attributed as early as 1910 to a specific stage in its life cycle: the "resting or latent form" (55), also termed the "L-form" (56), "mycococcus" (57), or "Much's granule"

form (58). Since then, *M. tuberculosis* has often been described as persisting in the host in a metabolically inactive, latent state as non-AF rods. In the next section, we will attempt to present how important cell envelope components can be linked to the AF property and how changes in the cell wall composition/structure may be altered in persistent bacilli.

ACID-FASTNESS, A UNIQUE ATTRIBUTE OF THE WAXY MYCOBACTERIAL CELL ENVELOPE

Current methods to visualize bacilli within infected tissue rely on (i) ZN and AR staining (41), (ii) detecting bacterial surface proteins by immunohistochemistry or immunofluorescence (12, 59), or (iii) detecting bacterial nucleic acid by *in situ* hybridization or intercalating dyes (60–62). Although AF stains have been around for decades, the exact cellular component(s) of *M. tuberculosis* recognized by the dyes is still being elucidated. Fuchsin, the main component of ZN and Kinyoun AF stains, has been shown to stain the vastly complex lipid portion of the mycobacterial cell wall (42, 63, 64). However, little is known regarding the specific target of the combined AR stain. Whereas auramine O is believed to bind to mycolic acid (42) and nucleic acids (43, 65), the exact target of rhodamine remains unknown. However, mycobacterial genetics has been particularly useful in recent years in searching for molecular target(s) responsible for the AF property of mycobacteria.

The Importance of Mycolic Acids

KasB represents one of the two β-ketoacyl-ACP synthases involved in the final elongation steps during biosynthesis of mycolic acids (66). Disruption of *kasB* in *Mycobacterium marinum* and *M. tuberculosis* resulted in the loss of cording and AF staining (11, 67, 68). Moreover, the *M. marinum kasB* mutant was found to be more sensitive to lysozyme and to human neutrophil defensin peptide, and during infection of macrophages, there was a partial loss of phagolysosomal fusion inhibition (67). The *M. tuberculosis kasB* mutant produced mycolic acid chains that were two to four carbons shorter than their wild-type counterparts and oxygenated mycolic acids that were defective in *trans*-cyclopropanation (11). Ultrastructural analyses by conventional transmission electron microscopy failed to reveal any detectable differences in the thickness of the cell envelope between the wild-type *M. tuberculosis* strain and the *kasB* deletion mutant. However, cryo-transmission electron microscopy indicated that the region between the inner and outer membranes of the mutant, mainly composed of cell wall-anchored mycolic acids, showed a notable decrease in electron density (68). It was therefore proposed that the *kasB* mutant cannot synthesize tight mycolic acid bundles, thus affecting the packing of the lipid-rich layer of the mycobacterial cell wall. The reduced bundle formation results in the loss of AF staining, whereas acid-fastness of the wild-type strain may be due to the rigid cell envelope structure provided by the densely packed mycolic acids. Importantly, the *M. tuberculosis kasB* deletion strain was strongly attenuated, did not cause disease in infected mice, and strikingly, was able to persist at constant low levels in the lungs and spleen of mice for 450 days post-aerosol infection (11).

The regulation of mycolic acid biosynthesis has only recently begun to be unraveled, and numerous studies have shown that most essential enzymes forming the central core of type II fatty acid synthase are phosphorylated by Ser/Thr protein kinases and that posttranslational phosphorylation inhibits the activity of these enzymes *in vitro* (69). These enzymes include the β-ketoacyl ACP synthases KasA and KasB, the β-ketoacyl-ACP reductase MabA, the β-hydroxyacyl-ACP dehydratases HadAB and HadBC, and the enoyl-ACP reductase InhA (70–74). Recent studies identified the phosphorylation sites of KasB as Thr334 and Thr336, and to investigate the *in vivo* role of KasB phosphorylation in regulating mycolic acid biosynthesis, a KasB phosphomimetic mutant of *M. tuberculosis* was constructed in which Thr334 and Thr336 were replaced by Asp residues (75). In this mutant, constitutive phosphorylation of KasB on both Thr334 and Thr336 negatively affected the condensing activity of KasB, resulting in an altered mycolic acid chain length and a defect in *trans*-cyclopropanation. Importantly, this mutant strain was found to be extremely attenuated in immunocompetent and immunocompromised mice and had lost AF staining (75) (Fig. 3).

These results provided new insights into the *in vivo* contribution and importance of Ser/Thr kinase-dependent phosphorylation in the control of (i) the clinically important feature of AF staining and (ii) the physiopathology of TB, suggesting that *M. tuberculosis* regulates these two related phenotypes through a signal transduction pathway. Interestingly, phosphorylation of KasB in *Mycobacterium bovis* BCG was more pronounced in stationary cultures than in replicating cultures, suggesting that phosphorylation is a mechanism by which mycobacteria might tightly control mycolic acid biosynthesis under nonreplicating conditions. It is tempting to speculate that the loss of acid-fastness

in persistent infections may be linked to signaling leading to increased phosphorylation of KasB. Further work is needed to elucidate the *in vivo* cues that activate the appropriate kinases under nonreplicating conditions. This knowledge may lead to a better understanding of the molecular signals that trigger reactivation and TB disease.

Whereas the above-mentioned results indicate that enzymatic and signaling pathways that control mycolic acid chain length are required to maintain the AF property, other enzymatic steps introducing additional structural elements to meromycolic acid are also essential to sustain both the integrity of the cell wall and acid-fastness. *M. tuberculosis* produces significant amounts of cyclopropanated mycolic acids: α-mycolic acids possess two *cis* cyclopropanes on the meromycolate chain, whereas oxygenated mycolates contain either a distal methoxy or ketone group and a proximal *cis* or *trans* cyclopropane (Fig. 1). The cyclopropane rings as well as the methyl branches of the lipids are synthesized by a family of S-adenosyl methionine-dependent methyl transferases (1) that are highly homologous in both primary sequence and three-dimensional structure (76). Despite their structural similarity, genetic deletion of each methyl transferase has revealed highly specific biosynthetic functions for each enzyme. To investigate the phenotypic consequences caused by the loss of meromycolic acid modification, a chemical inhibitory approach was applied in which dioctylamine was used to inhibit multiple mycolic acid methyltransferases in a dose-dependent fashion (77). Lipid analysis combined with extensive genetic characterization of mycolic acid modifications indicated that dioctylamine inhibited multiple sites of cyclopropanation and methylation catalyzed by MmaA2, MmaA3, MmaA4, CmaA2, and PcaA (Fig. 1). This inhibition resulted in decreased bacterial viability, pleiotropic alterations in the cell envelope structure, and loss of AF staining (77). *M. tuberculosis* mutant strains lacking any mycolic acid cyclopropanation were also found to exhibit less AF staining than the wild-type strain (7), confirming the results obtained with dioctylamine. A possible explanation of the phenotypes observed following either chemical or genetic inhibition of the mycolic acid methyl transferases involves dysregulation of membrane fluidity leading to impaired protein localization or cell division as well as altered cell wall permeability.

Non-Mycolic Acid-Containing Components

The PhoPR two-component system plays a crucial role in the physiology and pathogenicity of *M. tuberculosis* as well as in regulation of global gene expression (78).

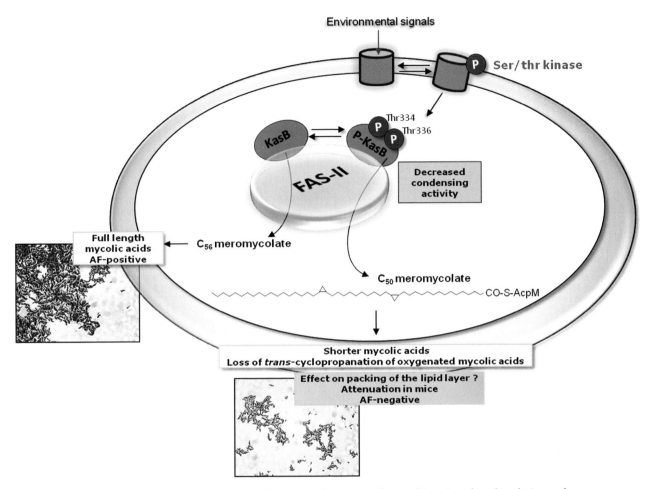

Figure 3 Ser/Thr kinase-dependent signaling cascade resulting in phosphorylation of KasB and loss of acid-fastness. Modification of the cell wall composition in response to exogenous cues is central for *M. tuberculosis* adaptation to different environmental conditions. In response to an external signal, mycobacterial Ser/Thr kinases phosphorylate the different FAS-II components, including the β-ketoacyl ACP synthase KasB involved in the addition of the last carbon atoms during the mycolic acid elongation step. Phosphorylation on Thr334 and Thr336 decreases the condensation activity of KasB, resulting in the production of shorter mycolic acids, which probably affects the packing of the lipid layer and also results in the loss of the AF property and severe attenuation in mice.

Disruption of *phoPR* caused a robust growth attenuation in human and mouse macrophages as well as in infected mice and prevented growth at low magnesium concentrations (6). Genes that were positively regulated by PhoPR include those found in the *pks2* and the *msl3* gene clusters that encode enzymes required for the biosynthesis of sulfolipids and diacyltrehalose/ pentaacyltrehalose, respectively. Consistent with these findings, lipid analysis revealed the absence of all three lipids in the *phoP* mutant (6, 79). Microscopic inspection of the *phoP* mutant not only revealed that the cells appeared smaller than the wild-type bacteria but that they had also lost AF staining, suggesting that sulfo-

lipids and/or diacyltrehalose/pentaacyltrehalose could explain the phenotypic traits of the *phoP* mutant (6).

Although acid-fastness has essentially been attributed to the waxy nature of the cell wall outer membrane, recent studies highlighted the important contribution of other components, especially lipomannan/lipoarabino-mannan (LM/LAM), which also participate in the immunomodulation of the host response. Ablation of the branch forming α-1,2-mannosyltransferase (*MSMEG_ 4247*) in *Mycobacterium smegmatis* leads to accumulation of branchless LAM and the complete absence of LM (80) and AF-negative bacteria (8). This strongly suggests that changes in the LM/LAM structures can affect the cell wall integrity and AF staining. However, an equivalent mutant in *M. tuberculosis* did not show a defect in AF staining, suggesting that the LM and LAM do not exert a significant impact on the AF staining of *M. tuberculosis* (8).

LIPID ACCUMULATION AND LOSS OF THE AF PROPERTY

Latent TB infection is characterized by the presence of *M. tuberculosis* bacilli that can persist in a nonreplicating state, known as the dormancy phase, inside lipid-rich foamy macrophages in granuloma (81, 82). Under these environmental conditions, persistence is favored by the storage of intracellular lipid inclusions (ILI) in the bacterial cytoplasm. These structures are essentially composed of triacylglycerols (TAG) resulting from the degradation of lipid bodies contained in foamy macrophages (83–85). ILI are thought to provide a source of carbon and energy prior to metabolic reactivation and replication, prerequisites ultimately leading to active TB (84). They are also found in bacilli derived from sputum of TB patients (86) and have been proposed as biomarkers for nonreplicating persistence, because a strong correlation between ILI and dormancy has been established (87). TAG degradation by *M. tuberculosis* involves a wide array of lipolytic enzymes, in the form of cell surface-associated/secreted enzymes for

lipid body degradation (88–90) or as intracellular enzymes for ILI degradation (91, 92). Although the origin of the lipid accumulation within ILI has begun to be elucidated (83), identification of the enzymes involved in the transfer of lipids from lipid bodies to ILI remains elusive (88). One possible enzyme is LipY (Rv3097c), a specific TAG hydrolase that plays a major role in the degradation of TAG-containing ILI under growth conditions mimicking dormancy (91, 92). It has been demonstrated that a *lipY* deletion mutation lost the capacity to utilize stored TAG and to escape dormancy (93).

Because most *in vitro* dormancy models use single stress factors and fail to generate a truly dormant population, a novel multi-stress model has recently been developed by applying the combined stresses of low oxygen (5%), high CO_2 (10%), low nutrients (10% Dubos medium), and acidic pH (5.0), thereby mimicking conditions encountered in the host (94). Under these conditions, *M. tuberculosis* stopped replicating, accumulated TAG and wax ester, acquired phenotypic antibiotic resistance, and lost acid-fastness. Dual staining of *M. tuberculosis* with the combination of auramine O and Nile red has been used to reveal AF staining properties and neutral lipid accumulation in the same cell (94) (Fig. 4A). When synchronous cultures of *M. tuberculosis* were subjected to the multi-stress conditions for increasing periods of time, a steady decrease in auramine

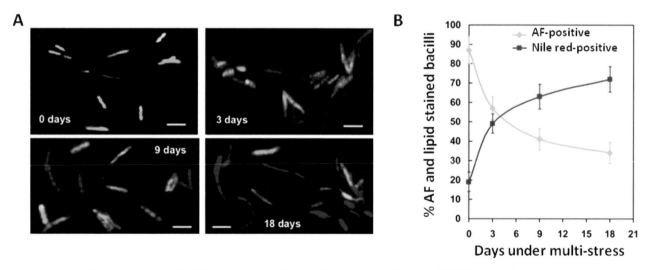

Figure 4   Loss of AF staining coincides with the accumulation of TAG-containing intracellular lipid inclusions. (**A**) Dual staining of *M. tuberculosis* grown under multiple stress conditions, using auramine O for AF-staining (green) and Nile red as a neutral lipid stain (red). Bacilli were observed by confocal laser scanning microscopy. Overlaid images of the dual-stained bacteria are shown. Bar = 4 μm. (**B**) Quantification of the number of AF-positive and lipid-stain-positive bacilli grown as in (A). Auramine O-stained and Nile red-stained positive cells were counted from multiple scans. (Adapted from Deb et al. *PLoS ONE* 4(6):e6077 with permission of the publisher.)

O-stained, green-fluorescent AF cells with a concomitant increase in Nile red-stained, red-fluorescent, ILI-containing cells was observed (Fig. 4B). After 18 days under multiple stresses, AF-positive cells decreased to about 30% of the population, while Nile red-stained cells with internal, red, spherical bodies (corresponding to ILI) increased from 10% to about 70% (94). This difference in dual-staining properties indicated the occurrence of at least three subpopulations under the multiple-stress condition: a subset of auramine O-positive cells (actively replicating), a second subset that stained with both auramine O and Nile red (presumably transitioning to a nonreplicating state), and a third subset that stained exclusively with Nile red (nonreplicating and dormant). Nile red-positive lipid droplets were found in *M. tuberculosis* cells from sputum samples, and these lipid-loaded bacteria from human patients were found to be dormant (86, 87).

The finding that TAG accumulation within ILI of Nile red-positive bacilli correlated with reduced acid-fastness was further confirmed through the use of a *tgs1* deletion mutant. The *tgs1* gene encodes a TAG synthase that is the dominant contributor to TAG storage when *M. tuberculosis* is exposed to various single stress factors (95, 96). The *tgs1* deletion mutant failed to accumulate TAG when subjected to the multi-stress treatment, and consistently lower proportions of Nile red-positive bacilli and higher percentages of AF-positive bacilli were observed than with the wild-type strain (94). Transcriptomic analyses of bacteria subjected to the multi-stress response revealed the achievement of a dormant state, the induction of stress-responsive genes, and the repression of energy generation, transcription, and translation machineries (94). Interestingly, among these genes, *kasB* was found to be downregulated, further substantiating the possible link between the loss of the AF property and the shutdown of mycolic acid biosynthesis.

Whether AF-negative bacilli and ILI accumulation occur as bacteria enter dormancy was subsequently addressed in granulomas using a biomimetic *in vitro* model of human TB granuloma (84). In a multi-stress model, granuloma sections and *M. tuberculosis* cells were subjected to the dual auramine O and Nile red staining. At day 0, *M. tuberculosis* exhibited few Nile red-stained but abundant auramine O-stained positive cells. In contrast, *M. tuberculosis*-infected granulomas contained a higher proportion of Nile red-positive cells at day 8 than at day 0. In addition, around 10% of the bacteria from the day 8 granuloma samples displayed tolerance to rifampicin compared to less than 1% at day 0. In this human TB granuloma model, *M. tuber-culosis* presents features of dormant mycobacteria as judged by the (i) loss of acid-fastness, (ii) accumulation of TAG-containing ILI, and (iii) induction of drug tolerance.

Neutralizing tumor necrosis factor alpha (TNFα) signaling results in the disruption of the granuloma structure *in vivo*, allowing the bacilli to escape the granuloma and ultimately leading to the induction of active TB. To investigate whether *M. tuberculosis* within granulomas can emerge from dormancy following anti-TNF treatment, resuscitation of the bacilli was monitored by comparing the characteristic dormancy phenotypes, including the auramine O/Nile red-staining profile and tolerance to rifampicin after treatment with anti-TNF antibodies. The vast majority of the cells from granulomas treated with anti-TNF were AF-positive and failed to accumulate large amounts of ILI and also exhibited significantly less rifampicin tolerance than mycobacteria from granulomas treated with a control antibody (84). Under these conditions, the *tgs1* mutant accumulated significantly fewer lipids in the form of ILI in the granulomas than did the control strain, and it was compromised in its ability to enter into a dormant state. Conversely, staining of the *lipY*-disrupted mutant from granulomas revealed a compromised ability to resuscitate and escape dormancy upon immunosuppression with anti-TNF treatment (84). Overall, these findings point to a critical role of the *tgs1/lipY* expression profile in influencing the lipid accumulation/consumption in *M. tuberculosis*, allowing the bacilli either to enter into dormancy with a loss of acid-fastness or promoting resuscitation and the escape from dormancy.

AF-NEGATIVE *M. TUBERCULOSIS* AND CELL WALL ALTERATIONS

The AF-negative phenotype of *M. tuberculosis* bacteria in established experimental animal infections (12) strongly suggests that cell wall changes are occurring. Consistent with these alterations, the cell wall of *M. tuberculosis* thickens when grown *in vitro* under hypoxic conditions, as revealed by transmission electron microscopy (97). These findings emphasize the need to understand the physical and spatial organization of the cell wall and the cell wall changes that occur during *in vivo* growth. Although the primary structure of the major cell wall components is fairly well established, details such as the degree of coverage of the peptidoglycan (PG) layer by covalently attached mycolic acids in the outer membrane, as well as the spatial organization of the components occurring in *in vivo*-grown bacilli, remain elusive. Thus, with the aim of addressing the spatial properties of the mycobacterial cell wall and to begin examining the differences between mycobacteria grown in cultures and in animals, the cell wall characteristics of *M. tuberculosis* grown *in vitro* were compared with those of *Mycobacterium leprae* grown in armadillos (98). The cell wall of *M. leprae* contained significantly more mycolic acids attached to PG than did the cell wall of *in vitro*-grown *M. tuberculosis* (mycolate:PG ratios of 21:10 versus 16:10, respectively). The greater coverage of *M. leprae* PG by mycolic acids may render this bacterium less permeable overall. However, whether similar changes may occur with *in vivo*-grown *M. tuberculosis* remains to be determined experimentally.

In light of these findings, there was the surprising observation that cortisone-forced reactivation of *M. tuberculosis* in infected guinea pigs, which had been previously treated with chemotherapy (rifampicin, pyrazinamide, and TMC207), revealed very weak AF staining despite the ability to cultivate very high numbers of bacilli from the lungs of the reactivating animals (99). Under these conditions, AF bacilli were sparse and difficult to see in the lung sections, further supporting the concept that despite drug treatment, the bacteria undergo physiological adaptation such as cell wall modification. By analogy with the *kasB* deletion mutant, which persisted indefinitely in mice and was characterized by shortened mycolic acids, loss of AF staining, and the inability to cause disease in mice (11), it appears reasonable to speculate that *M. tuberculosis* bacilli persisting in this model of chemotherapy may share similar properties with the *kasB* mutant, which could explain the basis for their poor AF staining *in vivo*.

LOSS OF ACID-FASTNESS AND PERSISTENCE

As already mentioned, ZN-negative cells correspond to *M. tuberculosis* bacilli in a dormant state displaying distinct cell wall alterations (12). In particular, it was demonstrated that the classical, cell wall composition-dependent staining with either ZN or AR was lost during persistent infection in mice. In contrast, detection of *M. tuberculosis* by cell wall composition-independent staining using a polyclonal, anti-*M. bovis* BCG serum was maintained during persistent infection (12). Because of its polyclonal nature, the antiserum recognizes multiple epitopes in the mycobacterial cell wall, and this recognition is independent of the spatial arrangement of cell wall components, thus explaining why the antiserum generated positive results at all times postinfection, even in tissue sections that were negative for

ZN staining. These observations were further corroborated by analyzing histopathological lung sections from patients with acute TB, reactivated TB, or persistent latent TB. Whereas *M. tuberculosis* in tissue sections from the patients with either acute or reactivated TB was positive for both ZN staining and for immunohistochemistry using the anti-*M. bovis* BCG serum, bacilli in tissue sections from the patients with latent TB were positive for staining with the antiserum but remained ZN-negative (12). Therefore, it can be inferred that in both latent, experimental TB and in patients with TB, loss of cell wall composition-dependent ZN staining represents a specific attribute of dormant bacilli that can best be explained by mycobacterial cell wall alterations abolishing ZN staining. Alternatively, reorganization of the cell wall may prevent entry of the ZN stain into the bacilli.

A similar dual-staining approach has also been successfully used to study and compare the multiple phenotypic subpopulations in *M. tuberculosis* cultures and in lung sections of *M. tuberculosis*-infected mice and guinea pigs (100). This experimental protocol included the combination of fluorescent AF staining and AR that targeted the mycolic acid-containing cell wall and an immunofluorescence assay that targeted bacterial proteins using an anti-*M. tuberculosis* whole cell lysate, polyclonal antisera. Two phenotypically different subpopulations were found in stationary cultures, whereas three subpopulations were observed in hypoxic cultures and in lung sections. Bacilli were either exclusively AF-positive, exclusively immunofluorescent, or AF-positive and immunofluorescent. The finding of a subpopulation of AF-negative bacilli, corresponding to dormant *M. tuberculosis*, is consistent with earlier work (12). By applying both staining methods simultaneously, it now becomes possible to detect AF-positive and AF-negative bacteria in the same microenvironments *in vitro* and *in vivo* (100). The discovery of heterogeneous phenotypes of *M. tuberculosis* in the same biological samples reveals new challenges, prompting future studies to investigate the metabolic changes of the bacilli in these microenvironments using genomic, proteomic, metabolomic, and lipidomic approaches.

CONCLUSION AND PERSPECTIVES

Because *in vivo* growth has been shown to induce dormancy in substantial subpopulations of *M. tuberculosis*, it is very likely that the ZN-negativity of dormant mycobacteria leads to an underestimation of bacterial burden, which has important consequences for diagnosis of TB as well as for clinical epidemiology. From the dual-staining approaches, combining both ZN and polyclonal serum staining, it seems reasonable to assert that a ZN-negative but antibody-positive specimen points toward a dormant infection rather than the absence of infection. Furthermore, ZN-negative granulomatous pathologies of unknown etiology may result from persistent mycobacteria. Therefore, the current AF-staining methods are not highly reliable for the diagnosis of TB, and further staining improvements are needed to better detect AF-negative cases. Furthermore, this article emphasizes the critical role of mycolic acids in the AF property of *M. tuberculosis*. If loss of acid-fastness correlates with a reduction in mycolic acid chain length, perhaps as a direct consequence of KasB phosphorylation in persistent bacteria, then a more reliable staining procedure that is not dependent on mycolic acid chain length may be warranted. Therefore, more precise knowledge of the dormant state of *M. tuberculosis* may not only help to improve the detection of the latent forms of the bacilli but would also have important implications for chemotherapy and vaccine developments. This may now be possible thanks to the recent development of multi-stress *in vitro* granuloma models that induce *M. tuberculosis* to enter a dormant-like state.

Acknowledgments. *The authors wish to thank Torin Weisbrod for the microscopy pictures, and Paras Jain, Tracy Kaiser, Lina Kaminski, Lawrence Leung, and Brian Weinrick for critical reading of the manuscript and helpful discussions.*

Citation. Vilchèze C, Kremer L. 2017. Acid-fast positive and acid-fast negative *Mycobacterium tuberculosis*: the Koch paradox. Microbiol Spectrum 5(2):TBTB2-0003-2015.

References

1. Pawełczyk J, Kremer L. 2014. The molecular genetics of mycolic acid biosynthesis. *Microbiol Spectr* 2:MGM2-0003-2013.

2. Brennan PJ, Nikaido H. 1995. The envelope of mycobacteria. *Annu Rev Biochem* 64:29–63.

3. Hoffmann C, Leis A, Niederweis M, Plitzko JM, Engelhardt H. 2008. Disclosure of the mycobacterial outer membrane: cryo-electron tomography and vitreous sections reveal the lipid bilayer structure. *Proc Natl Acad Sci USA* 105:3963–3967.

4. Zuber B, Chami M, Houssin C, Dubochet J, Griffiths G, Daffé M. 2008. Direct visualization of the outer membrane of mycobacteria and corynebacteria in their native state. *J Bacteriol* 190:5672–5680.

5. Foulds J, O'Brien R. 1998. New tools for the diagnosis of tuberculosis: the perspective of developing countries. *Int J Tuberc Lung Dis* 2:778–783.

6. Walters SB, Dubnau E, Kolesnikova I, Laval F, Daffe M, Smith I. 2006. The *Mycobacterium tuberculosis* PhoPR two-component system regulates genes essential for

virulence and complex lipid biosynthesis. *Mol Microbiol* 60:312–330.

7. Barkan D, Hedhli D, Yan HG, Huygen K, Glickman MS. 2012. *Mycobacterium tuberculosis* lacking all mycolic acid cyclopropanation is viable but highly attenuated and hyperinflammatory in mice. *Infect Immun* 80:1958–1968.

8. Fukuda T, Matsumura T, Ato M, Hamasaki M, Nishiuchi Y, Murakami Y, Maeda Y, Yoshimori T, Matsumoto S, Kobayashi K, Kinoshita T, Morita YS. 2013. Critical roles for lipomannan and lipoarabinomannan in cell wall integrity of mycobacteria and pathogenesis of tuberculosis. *MBio* 4:e00472-e12.

9. Rist N, Grumbach F, Cals S, Riebel J. 1952. Isonicotinic acid hydrazide (INH); antituberculous activity in mice; creation of resistant strains *in vitro*. [In French.] *Ann Inst Pasteur (Paris)* 82:757–760.

10. Takayama K, Wang L, David HL. 1972. Effect of isoniazid on the *in vivo* mycolic acid synthesis, cell growth, and viability of *Mycobacterium tuberculosis*. *Antimicrob Agents Chemother* 2:29–35.

11. Bhatt A, Fujiwara N, Bhatt K, Gurcha SS, Kremer L, Chen B, Chan J, Porcelli SA, Kobayashi K, Besra GS, Jacobs WR Jr. 2007. Deletion of *kasB* in *Mycobacterium tuberculosis* causes loss of acid-fastness and subclinical latent tuberculosis in immunocompetent mice. *Proc Natl Acad Sci USA* 104:5157–5162.

12. Seiler P, Ulrichs T, Bandermann S, Pradl L, Jörg S, Krenn V, Morawietz L, Kaufmann SHE, Aichele P. 2003. Cell-wall alterations as an attribute of *Mycobacterium tuberculosis* in latent infection. *J Infect Dis* 188:1326–1331.

13. Koch R. 1882. Die Atiologie der Tuberkulose. *Berl Klinischen Wochenschr* 15:221–230.

14. Bishop PJ, Neumann G. 1970. The history of the Ziehl-Neelsen stain. *Tubercle* 51:196–206.

15. Ehrlich P. 1882. A method for staining the tubercle bacillus. *Dtsch Med Wochenschr* 8:269–270.

16. Gabbett HS. 1887. Rapid staining of the tubercle bacillus. *Lancet* 129:757.

17. Kinyoun JJ. 1915. A note on Uhlenhuths method for sputum examination, for tubercle bacilli. *Am J Public Health (NY)* 5:867–870.

18. Hallberg V. 1946. Origin of the Nachtblau method for staining tubercle bacilli and its preliminary use. *Acta Med Scand Suppl* 180:6–8.

19. Hallberg V. 1946. Experiences with regard to the tubercle micro-organism obtained by the new staining method. *Acta Med Scand Suppl* 180:22–24.

20. Tison F. 1951. La coloration de Hallberg modifiée pour la mise en évidence du bacille tuberculeux. *Ann Inst Pasteur (Paris)* 80:207–210.

21. Hok TT. 1962. A simple and rapid cold-staining method for acid-fast bacteria. *Am Rev Respir Dis* 85:753–754.

22. Allen JL. 1992. A modified Ziehl-Neelsen stain for mycobacteria. *Med Lab Sci* 49:99–102.

23. Hagemann PKH. 1938. Fluoreszenzfarbung von Tuberkelbakterien mit Auramin. *Munch Med Wochenschr* 85:1066–1068.

24. Degommier J. 1957. Nouvelle technique de coloration des bacilles tuberculeux pour la recherche en fluorescence. *Ann Inst Pasteur (Paris)* **92**:692–694.

25. Truant JP, Brett WA, Thomas W Jr. 1962. Fluorescence microscopy of tubercle bacilli stained with auramine and rhodamine. *Henry Ford Hosp Med Bull* **10**:287–296.

26. Alausa KO, Osoba AO, Montefiore D, Sogbetun OA. 1977. Laboratory diagnosis of tuberculosis in a developing country 1968–1975. *Afr J Med Med Sci* **6**:103–108.

27. Angra P, Becx-Bleumink M, Gilpin C, Joloba M, Jost K, Kam KM, Kim SJ, Lumb R, Mitarai S, Ramsay A, Ridderhof J, Rieder HL, Selvakumar N, van Beers S, van Cleeff M, Van Deun A, Vincent V. 2007. Ziehl-Neelsen staining: strong red on weak blue, or weak red under strong blue? *Int J Tuberc Lung Dis* **11**:1160–1161.

28. Levy H, Feldman C, Sacho H, van der Meulen H, Kallenbach J, Koornhof H. 1989. A reevaluation of sputum microscopy and culture in the diagnosis of pulmonary tuberculosis. *Chest* **95**:1193–1197.

29. Petersen KF, Urbanczik R. 1982. Microscopic and cultural methods for the laboratory diagnosis of tuberculosis. A short historical review (author's transl). (In German.) *Zentralbl Bakteriol Mikrobiol Hyg [A]* **251**:308–325.

30. Siddiqi K, Lambert ML, Walley J. 2003. Clinical diagnosis of smear-negative pulmonary tuberculosis in low-income countries: the current evidence. *Lancet Infect Dis* **3**:288–296.

31. Aber VR, Allen BW, Mitchison DA, Ayuma P, Edwards EA, Keyes AB. 1980. Laboratory studies on isolated positive cultures and the efficiency of direct smear examination. *Tubercle* **61**:123–133.

32. Van Deun A, Hamid Salim A, Aung KJ, Hossain MA, Chambugonj N, Hye MA, Kawria A, Declercq E. 2005. Performance of variations of carbolfuchsin staining of sputum smears for AFB under field conditions. *Int J Tuberc Lung Dis* **9**:1127–1133.

33. Tuberculosis Division International Union Against Tuberculosis and Lung Disease. 2005. Tuberculosis bacteriology–priorities and indications in high prevalence countries: position of the technical staff of the Tuberculosis Division of the International Union Against Tuberculosis and Lung Disease. *Int J Tuberc Lung Dis* **9**:355–361.

34. Chakravorty S, Sen MK, Tyagi JS. 2005. Diagnosis of extrapulmonary tuberculosis by smear, culture, and PCR using universal sample processing technology. *J Clin Microbiol* **43**:4357–4362.

35. Karstaedt AS, Jones N, Khoosal M, Crewe-Brown HH. 1998. The bacteriology of pulmonary tuberculosis in a population with high human immunodeficiency virus seroprevalence. *Int J Tuberc Lung Dis* **2**:312–316.

36. Khan EA, Starke JR. 1995. Diagnosis of tuberculosis in children: increased need for better methods. *Emerg Infect Dis* **1**:115–123.

37. Shapiro HM, Hänscheid T. 2008. Fuchsin fluorescence in *Mycobacterium tuberculosis*: the Ziehl-Neelsen stain in a new light. *J Microbiol Methods* **74**:119–120.

38. Gruft H. 1978. Evaluation of mycobacteriology laboratories: the acid-fast smear. *Health Lab Sci* **15**:215–220.

39. Somoskövi A, Hotaling JE, Fitzgerald M, O'Donnell D, Parsons LM, Salfinger M. 2001. Lessons from a proficiency testing event for acid-fast microscopy. *Chest* **120**:250–257.

40. Ba F, Rieder HL. 1999. A comparison of fluorescence microscopy with the Ziehl-Neelsen technique in the examination of sputum for acid-fast bacilli. *Int J Tuberc Lung Dis* **3**:1101–1105.

41. Steingart KR, Ng V, Henry M, Hopewell PC, Ramsay A, Cunningham J, Urbanczik R, Perkins MD, Aziz MA, Pai M. 2006. Sputum processing methods to improve the sensitivity of smear microscopy for tuberculosis: a systematic review. *Lancet Infect Dis* **6**:664–674.

42. Richards OW. 1941. The staining of acid-fast tubercle bacteria. *Science* **93**:190.

43. Hänscheid T, Ribeiro CM, Shapiro HM, Perlmutter NG. 2007. Fluorescence microscopy for tuberculosis diagnosis. *Lancet Infect Dis* **7**:236–237.

44. Bhalla M, Sidiq Z, Sharma PP, Singhal R, Myneedu VP, Sarin R. 2013. Performance of light-emitting diode fluorescence microscope for diagnosis of tuberculosis. *Int J Mycobacteriol* **2**:174–178.

45. Kumar VA, Chandra PS. 2008. Auramine phenol staining of smears for screening acid fast bacilli in clinical specimens. *J Commun Dis* **40**:47–52.

46. Laifangbam S, Singh HL, Singh NB, Devi KM, Singh NT. 2009. A comparative study of fluorescent microscopy with Ziehl-Neelsen staining and culture for the diagnosis of pulmonary tuberculosis. *Kathmandu Univ Med J KUMJ* **7**:226–230. KUMJ.

47. Mutha A, Tiwari S, Khubnani H, Mall S. 2005. Application of bleach method to improve sputum smear microscopy for the diagnosis of pulmonary tuberculosis. *Indian J Pathol Microbiol* **48**:513–517.

48. Burdash NM, West ME, Bannister ER, Dyar C, Duncan RC. 1976. Evaluation of a dual-staining method for acid-fast bacilli. *J Clin Microbiol* **2**:149–150.

49. International Agency for Research on Cancer. 1979. Monographs on the evaluation of carcinogenic risk of chemicals to humans. Chemicals and industrial processes associated with cancer in humans. *IARC Monogr* **1**(Suppl.):24.

50. International Agency for Research on Cancer. 1982. Chemicals, industrial processes and industries associated with cancer in humans. an updating of Volumes 1 to 29. *IARC Monogr* **4**(Suppl.):14.

51. Katila ML, Mäntyjärvi RA. 1982. Acridine orange staining of smears for demonstration of *Mycobacterium tuberculosis*. *Eur J Clin Microbiol* **1**:351–353.

52. Mallassez L, Vignal W. 1883. Tuberculose zoologique. *Arch Physiol Norm Pathologique* **2**:369–412.

53. Miller FR. 1932. The induced development of non-acid-fast forms of bacillus tuberculosis and other mycobacteria. *J Exp Med* **56**:411–424.

54. Miller FR. 1931. Non-acid-fast tubercle bacilli. *Science* **74**:343–344.

55. Leonard WM. 1910. The paradox of the tubercle bacillus. *Boston Med Surg J* **162**:753–757.

56. Khomenko AG. 1987. The variability of *Mycobacterium tuberculosis* in patients with cavitary pulmonary

tuberculosis in the course of chemotherapy. *Tubercle* 68: 243–253.

57. Csillag A. 1964. The mycococcus form of mycobacteria. *Microbiology* 34:341–352.

58. Much DH. 1907. Über die granuläre, nach Ziehl nicht färbbare Form des Tuberkulosevirus. *Beitr Klin Tuberk* 8:85–99.

59. Ulrichs T, Lefmann M, Reich M, Morawietz L, Roth A, Brinkmann V, Kosmiadi GA, Seiler P, Aichele P, Hahn H, Krenn V, Göbel UB, Kaufmann SHE. 2005. Modified immunohistological staining allows detection of Ziehl-Neelsen-negative *Mycobacterium tuberculosis* organisms and their precise localization in human tissue. *J Pathol* 205:633–640.

60. Ryan GJ, Shapiro HM, Lenaerts AJ. 2014. Improving acid-fast fluorescent staining for the detection of myco-bacteria using a new nucleic acid staining approach. *Tuberculosis (Edinb)* 94:511–518.

61. St Amand AL, Frank DN, De Groote MA, Basaraba RJ, Orme IM, Pace NR. 2005. Use of specific rRNA oligo-nucleotide probes for microscopic detection of *Mycobacterium tuberculosis* in culture and tissue specimens. *J Clin Microbiol* 43:5369–5371.

62. Fenhalls G, Stevens L, Moses L, Bezuidenhout J, Betts JC, van Helden P, Lukey PT, Duncan K. 2002. *In situ* detection of *Mycobacterium tuberculosis* transcripts in human lung granulomas reveals differential gene expression in necrotic lesions. *Infect Immun* 70:6330–6338.

63. Harada K. 1976. The nature of mycobacterial acid-fastness. *Stain Technol* 51:255–260.

64. Goren MB, Cernich M, Brokl O. 1978. Some observations of mycobacterial acid-fastness. *Am Rev Respir Dis* 118:151–154.

65. Oster G. 1951. Fluorescence of auramine O in the presence of nucleic acid. *C R Hebd Seances Acad Sci* 232:1708–1710. (In French.)

66. Bhatt A, Molle V, Besra GS, Jacobs WR Jr, Kremer L. 2007. The *Mycobacterium tuberculosis* FAS-II condensing enzymes: their role in mycolic acid biosynthesis, acid-fastness, pathogenesis and in future drug development. *Mol Microbiol* 64:1442–1454.

67. Gao L-Y, Laval F, Lawson EH, Groger RK, Woodruff A, Morisaki JH, Cox JS, Daffe M, Brown EJ. 2003. Requirement for *kasB* in *Mycobacterium* mycolic acid biosynthesis, cell wall impermeability and intracellular survival: implications for therapy. *Mol Microbiol* 49:1547–1563.

68. Yamada H, Bhatt A, Danev R, Fujiwara N, Maeda S, Mitarai S, Chikamatsu K, Aono A, Nitta K, Jacobs WR Jr, Nagayama K. 2012. Non-acid-fastness in *Mycobacterium tuberculosis kasB* mutant correlates with the cell envelope electron density. *Tuberculosis (Edinb)* 92:351–357.

69. Molle V, Kremer L. 2010. Division and cell envelope regulation by Ser/Thr phosphorylation: *Mycobacterium* shows the way. *Mol Microbiol* 75:1064–1077.

70. Molle V, Brown AK, Besra GS, Cozzone AJ, Kremer L. 2006. The condensing activities of the *Mycobacterium*

tuberculosis type II fatty acid synthase are differentially regulated by phosphorylation. *J Biol Chem* 281:30094–30103.

71. Veyron-Churlet R, Zanella-Cléon I, Cohen-Gonsaud M, Molle V, Kremer L. 2010. Phosphorylation of the *Mycobacterium tuberculosis* beta-ketoacyl-acyl carrier protein reductase MabA regulates mycolic acid biosynthesis. *J Biol Chem* 285:12714–12725.

72. Molle V, Gulten G, Vilchèze C, Veyron-Churlet R, Zanella-Cléon I, Sacchettini JC, Jacobs WR Jr, Kremer L. 2010. Phosphorylation of InhA inhibits mycolic acid biosynthesis and growth of *Mycobacterium tuberculosis*. *Mol Microbiol* 78:1591–1605.

73. Slama N, Leiba J, Eynard N, Daffé M, Kremer L, Quémard A, Molle V. 2011. Negative regulation by Ser/Thr phosphorylation of HadAB and HadBC dehydratases from *Mycobacterium tuberculosis* type II fatty acid synthase system. *Biochem Biophys Res Commun* 412:401–406.

74. Khan S, Nagarajan SN, Parikh A, Samantaray S, Singh A, Kumar D, Roy RP, Bhatt A, Nandicoori VK. 2010. Phosphorylation of enoyl-acyl carrier protein reductase InhA impacts mycobacterial growth and survival. *J Biol Chem* 285:37860–37871.

75. Vilchèze C, Molle V, Carrère-Kremer S, Leiba J, Mourey L, Shenai S, Baronian G, Tufariello J, Hartman T, Veyron-Churlet R, Trivelli X, Tiwari S, Weinrick B, Alland D, Guérardel Y, Jacobs WR Jr, Kremer L. 2014. Phosphorylation of KasB regulates virulence and acid-fastness in *Mycobacterium tuberculosis*. *PLoS Pathog* 10:e1004115.

76. Huang CC, Smith CV, Glickman MS, Jacobs WR Jr, Sacchettini JC. 2002. Crystal structures of mycolic acid cyclopropane synthases from *Mycobacterium tuberculosis*. *J Biol Chem* 277:11559–11569.

77. Barkan D, Liu Z, Sacchettini JC, Glickman MS. 2009. Mycolic acid cyclopropanation is essential for viability, drug resistance, and cell wall integrity of *Mycobacterium tuberculosis*. *Chem Biol* 16:499–509.

78. Ryndak M, Wang S, Smith I. 2008. PhoP, a key player in *Mycobacterium tuberculosis* virulence. *Trends Microbiol* 16:528–534.

79. Gonzalo Asensio J, Maia C, Ferrer NL, Barilone N, Laval F, Soto CY, Winter N, Daffé M, Gicquel B, Martín C, Jackson M. 2006. The virulence-associated two-component PhoP-PhoR system controls the biosynthesis of polyketide-derived lipids in *Mycobacterium tuberculosis*. *J Biol Chem* 281:1313–1316.

80. Sena CBC, Fukuda T, Miyanagi K, Matsumoto S, Kobayashi K, Murakami Y, Maeda Y, Kinoshita T, Morita YS. 2010. Controlled expression of branch-forming mannosyltransferase is critical for mycobacterial lipoarabinomannan biosynthesis. *J Biol Chem* 285:13326–13336.

81. Peyron P, Vaubourgeix J, Poquet Y, Levillain F, Botanch C, Bardou F, Daffé M, Emile J-F, Marchou B, Cardona P-J, de Chastellier C, Altare F. 2008. Foamy macrophages from tuberculous patients' granulomas constitute a nutrient-rich reservoir for *M. tuberculosis* persistence. *PLoS Pathog* 4:e1000204.

82. Russell DG, Cardona P-J, Kim M-J, Allain S, Altare F. 2009. Foamy macrophages and the progression of the human tuberculosis granuloma. *Nat Immunol* 10:943–948.

83. Daniel J, Maamar H, Deb C, Sirakova TD, Kolattukudy PE. 2011. *Mycobacterium tuberculosis* uses host triacylglycerol to accumulate lipid droplets and acquires a dormancy-like phenotype in lipid-loaded macrophages. *PLoS Pathog* 7:e1002093.

84. Kapoor N, Pawar S, Sirakova TD, Deb C, Warren WL, Kolattukudy PE. 2013. Human granuloma *in vitro* model, for TB dormancy and resuscitation. *PLoS One* 8: e53657.

85. Caire-Brändli I, Papadopoulos A, Malaga W, Marais D, Canaan S, Thilo L, de Chastellier C, Flynn JL. 2014. Reversible lipid accumulation and associated division arrest of *Mycobacterium avium* in lipoprotein-induced foamy macrophages may resemble key events during latency and reactivation of tuberculosis. *Infect Immun* 82: 476–490.

86. Garton NJ, Christensen H, Minnikin DE, Adegbola RA, Barer MR. 2002. Intracellular lipophilic inclusions of mycobacteria *in vitro* and in sputum. *Microbiology* 148:2951–2958.

87. Garton NJ, Waddell SJ, Sherratt AL, Lee S-M, Smith RJ, Senner C, Hinds J, Rajakumar K, Adegbola RA, Besra GS, Butcher PD, Barer MR. 2008. Cytological and transcript analyses reveal fat and lazy persister-like bacilli in tuberculous sputum. *PLoS Med* 5:e75.

88. Dedieu L, Serveau-Avesque C, Kremer L, Canaan S. 2013. Mycobacterial lipolytic enzymes: a gold mine for tuberculosis research. *Biochimie* 95:66–73.

89. Daleke MH, Cascioferro A, de Punder K, Ummels R, Abdallah AM, van der Wel N, Peters PJ, Luirink J, Manganelli R, Bitter W. 2011. Conserved pro-Glu (PE) and Pro-Pro-Glu (PPE) protein domains target LipY lipases of pathogenic mycobacteria to the cell surface via the ESX-5 pathway. *J Biol Chem* 286:19024–19034.

90. Dhouib R, Laval F, Carrière F, Daffé M, Canaan S. 2010. A monoacylglycerol lipase from *Mycobacterium smegmatis* involved in bacterial cell interaction. *J Bacteriol* 192:4776–4785.

91. Deb C, Daniel J, Sirakova TD, Abomoelak B, Dubey VS, Kolattukudy PE. 2006. A novel lipase belonging to the hormone-sensitive lipase family induced under starvation to utilize stored triacylglycerol in *Mycobacterium tuberculosis*. *J Biol Chem* 281:3866–3875.

92. Mishra KC, de Chastellier C, Narayana Y, Bifani P, Brown AK, Besra GS, Katoch VM, Joshi B, Balaji KN, Kremer L. 2008. Functional role of the PE domain and immunogenicity of the *Mycobacterium tuberculosis* triacylglycerol hydrolase LipY. *Infect Immun* 76: 127–140.

93. Low KL, Rao PS, Shui G, Bendt AK, Pethe K, Dick T, Wenk MR. 2009. Triacylglycerol utilization is required for regrowth of *in vitro* hypoxic nonreplicating *Mycobacterium bovis* bacillus Calmette-Guerin. *J Bacteriol* 191:5037–5043.

94. Deb C, Lee C-M, Dubey VS, Daniel J, Abomoelak B, Sirakova TD, Pawar S, Rogers L, Kolattukudy PE. 2009. A novel *in vitro* multiple-stress dormancy model for *Mycobacterium tuberculosis* generates a lipid-loaded, drug-tolerant, dormant pathogen. *PLoS One* 4:e6077.

95. Daniel J, Deb C, Dubey VS, Sirakova TD, Abomoelak B, Morbidoni HR, Kolattukudy PE. 2004. Induction of a novel class of diacylglycerol acyltransferases and triacylglycerol accumulation in *Mycobacterium tuberculosis* as it goes into a dormancy-like state in culture. *J Bacteriol* 186:5017–5030.

96. Sirakova TD, Dubey VS, Deb C, Daniel J, Korotkova TA, Abomoelak B, Kolattukudy PE. 2006. Identification of a diacylglycerol acyltransferase gene involved in accumulation of triacylglycerol in *Mycobacterium tuberculosis* under stress. *Microbiology* 152:2717–2725.

97. Cunningham AF, Spreadbury CL. 1998. Mycobacterial stationary phase induced by low oxygen tension: cell wall thickening and localization of the 16-kilodalton alpha-crystallin homolog. *J Bacteriol* 180:801–808.

98. Bhamidi S, Scherman MS, Jones V, Crick DC, Belisle JT, Brennan PJ, McNeil MR. 2011. Detailed structural and quantitative analysis reveals the spatial organization of the cell walls of *in vivo* grown *Mycobacterium leprae* and *in vitro* grown *Mycobacterium tuberculosis*. *J Biol Chem* 286:23168–23177.

99. Obregon-Henao A, Shanley CA, Shang S, Caraway ML, Basaraba RJ, Duncan CG, Ordway DJ, Orme IM. 2012. Cortisone-forced reactivation of weakly acid fast positive *Mycobacterium tuberculosis* in guinea pigs previously treated with chemotherapy. *Mycobact Dis* 2:116.

100. Ryan GJ, Hoff DR, Driver ER, Voskuil MI, Gonzalez-Juarrero M, Basaraba RJ, Crick DC, Spencer JS, Lenaerts AJ. 2010. Multiple *M. tuberculosis* phenotypes in mouse and guinea pig lung tissue revealed by a dual-staining approach. *PLoS One* 5:e11108.

Tuberculosis and the Tubercle Bacillus, 2nd ed.
Edited by William R. Jacobs, Jr., Helen McShane, Valerie Mizrahi, and Ian M. Orme
© 2018 American Society for Microbiology, Washington, DC
doi:10.1128/microbiolspec.TBTB2-0024-2016

Mycobacterial Biofilms: Revisiting Tuberculosis Bacilli in Extracellular Necrotizing Lesions

24

Randall J. Basaraba[1] and Anil K. Ojha[2]

INTRODUCTION

The ongoing emergence of multidrug-resistant (MDR) and extensively drug-resistant (XDR) strains of *Mycobacterium tuberculosis* not only underscores the limitations of our current tuberculosis (TB) control strategies but is also escalating the TB epidemic to a new level. Realizing the imminent threats of MDR- and XDR-TB and the urgency for new TB control measures, the World Health Organization has maintained TB control as high priority and set an ambitious goal of eradicating the disease by 2030 (1). What remains an urgent need is the development of a shorter-duration combination of antimicrobial drug treatments that is more effective at eradicating drug-susceptible and drug-resistant strains of *M. tuberculosis*. However, progress toward this goal is hampered by a lack of understanding of factors that contribute to the expression of *in vivo* drug tolerance by *M. tuberculosis*, which contributes significantly to the need to treat patients from 6 to 9 months with antimicrobial drug combinations that have toxic side effects. In this review, we discuss the current state of our understanding of the host and pathogen factors that contribute to *M. tuberculosis* drug tolerance. Moreover, we highlight potential strategies that can be used to improve the efficacy of existing drugs against drug-tolerant *M. tuberculosis*. These strategies are based on our current knowledge of how and where drug-tolerant bacilli persist and on features of the complex host response that likely limit the penetration of antibiotics. A better understanding of the factors that contribute to the expression of drug tolerance reveals the potential value of adjunctive therapies

that can be used to potentiate the effectiveness of existing and future anti-TB drugs.

NECROTIZING LESIONS: THE CHARACTERISTIC PATHOLOGY OF ACTIVE PULMONARY TB

In general, the host response to *M. tuberculosis* infection is best characterized as mixed inflammation, composed primarily of macrophages and lymphocytes that accumulate at the site of primary infection in the lung or in extrapulmonary tissues. In humans and some animal model species, mixed inflammatory cells are organized into a nodular mass referred to as a granuloma. In other species, like most strains of mice, the inflammatory and immune cell types, although similar, fail to organize into discrete granulomas. The morphological features of TB granulomas are dynamic and variable, being influenced by combinations of host, pathogen, and environmental factors. Besides the aforementioned species-specific differences, granuloma composition and structure can also be influenced by the relative susceptibility of the host, stage of infection, virulence of the *M. tuberculosis* strain(s), presence/absence of comorbidities, and whether individuals are treated and responding appropriately to antimicrobial drug treatment. Despite the different granuloma morphotypes, the prototypical TB granuloma is composed of centrally located macrophages surrounded by an ill-defined rim of different lymphocyte subsets, fewer plasma cells, multinucleated giant cells, and granulocytes. In addition, granuloma morphology can be altered by the presence

[1]College of Veterinary Medicine and Biomedical Sciences, Colorado State University, Fort Collins, Co 80524; [2]Wadsworth Center, NY State Department of Health and University at Albany, Albany, NY 12208.

or absence of central necrosis, dystrophic calcification, and fibrous encapsulation. Calcification and fibrosis are indicative of wound or lesion healing that occurs concurrently with active inflammation, especially in patients with chronic TB. The development of granuloma necrosis and calcification is significant in that they represent, at the least, a localized loss of normal tissue structure and function and associated irreversible tissue damage that can persist for the life of the patient.

While the granuloma is recognized as the response to primary infection in humans and some animals, the clinical signs of active TB in humans are often the result of a post-primary manifestation that can occur years or decades following the initial exposure (2). The pathogenesis of postprimary tuberculosis is complex and poorly understood, and is not easily reproduced in animal models including non-human primates. An emerging hypothesis is that postprimary TB is associated with airway obstruction that alters the lung microenvironment to favor rapid *M. tuberculosis* proliferation, which stimulates an aggressive and destructive proinflammatory response that predisposes to cavitary disease and thus large numbers of extracellular bacilli (3, 4). Cavitary TB is the most severe manifestation of active TB disease, in which an unregulated immune response degrades and replaces normal lung parenchyma. The formation of an open cavity is determined in part by the location of the destructive inflammatory response and whether lesion necrosis develops adjacent to and communicates with conducting airways. The progression of TB disease to necrosis or lesion cavitation is not only detrimental to the host, but also represents an important transition from a predominantly intracellular infection to now include extracellular bacilli released from infected cells. In addition, the relatively normal oxygen concentration in lesions connected with airways supports the proliferation of high numbers of extracellular bacilli, which further contributes to inflammation and necrosis. This transition alone contributes to the complexity of the host microenvironment as well as the physiological state of different *M. tuberculosis* populations (5–7).

EXTRACELLULAR *M. TUBERCULOSIS* IN NECROTIZING LESIONS: A PROTECTED NICHE FOR THE PATHOGEN

It is generally accepted that granuloma formation in response to *M. tuberculosis* infection functions as a protective barrier that contains bacilli from spreading from the site of primary infection within a single host or between hosts. The accumulation of mixed immune cells that make up the granulomatous response acts not only

as a mechanical barrier, but also as a functional barrier given that cell-mediated immunity is critical to controlling *M. tuberculosis* infection. As mentioned above, the development of lesion necrosis and cavitation further contributes to the functional diversity of *M. tuberculosis* populations within individual lesions even within a single host. As infection of macrophages allows bacilli to evade innate and adaptive immune surveillance, extracellular bacilli also gain a survival advantage through physical separation from circulating immune cells and resistance to phagocytosis. By virtue of being associated with cellular and tissue necrosis, extracellular bacilli are sequestered within a microenvironment that has little or no blood supply that not only limits oxygen delivery, but also the ability of effector immune cells to circulate within lesions, and limits the penetration and accumulation of antimicrobial drugs (8–10). Moreover, even though *M. tuberculosis* requires oxygen to effectively replicate *in vitro* and *in vivo*, bacilli can survive or persist in a nonreplicative state for a long period of time under hypoxic or anoxic conditions (11–13). Studies have shown that, in humans and animal model species that typically form necrotic TB lesions and thus harbor viable, extracellular bacilli, lesions are measurably hypoxic (12) and drug penetration is limited or absent (10, 14). Besides host factors, the changing lesion microenvironment contributes to changes in bacilli physiology. *In vitro* studies have clearly demonstrated that hypoxia is among the most important inducers of the *dosRS*-dependent dormancy regulon in *M. tuberculosis* (15).

Since the discovery that *M. tuberculosis* infects and survives within macrophages *in vitro*, much has been learned about how *M. tuberculosis* circumvents intracellular killing (16, 17). However, very little is known about the importance of extracellular bacilli in the pathogenesis of active TB disease or the clinical manifestations of *in vivo* drug tolerance in humans and animals. Even in the pre-antibiotic era, investigators recognized the importance of extracellular *M. tuberculosis* in human TB lesions, especially those with central necrosis or cavitation (18–21). Typically, the distribution of both intracellular and extracellular bacilli in the context of naturally occurring TB in humans and experimental infections in animals has been studied through the use of acid-fast staining of histological sections postmortem or from surgical biopsies. Studies in both humans and animals using different staining techniques suggest that acid-fast positive bacilli represent a fraction of the organisms that make up the total bacterial burden in TB lesions (22). In humans, Nyka et al. demonstrated in multiple studies that acid-fast negative, extracellular bacilli in human TB lesions form large microbial communities morphologically resembling biofilms formed by other pathogenic bacteria that cause extracellular infection (23–26). Biofilms are defined as matrix-encapsulated microbial communities attached to biotic or abiotic surfaces that are self-assembled through a genetically programmed developmental process (27). The high cell density, cell-cell contacts, and different nutrient and oxygen gradients within the interiors of biofilms facilitate expression of several unique phenotypes, including antimicrobial tolerance, that are not expressed by the same organisms grown as unattached, free-living organisms referred to as planktonic growth (28, 29). The most striking and clinically significant feature of biofilm-forming bacteria is their extraordinary recalcitrance to antibiotics (30, 31). Several mycobacterial species including *M. tuberculosis* spontaneously form biofilms *in vitro* (32–36) (Fig. 1), although the architectural and functional properties of the extracellular *M. tuberculosis* aggregates in necrotizing lesions remain unknown.

Orme and, more recently, Wong et al. refer to these extracellular bacilli *in vivo* as necrosis-associated extracellular clusters or NECs (37, 38). As mentioned previously, a large proportion of these extracellular bacilli are acid-fast negative. In an effort to visualize heterogeneous populations of extracellular bacilli in animal models, Lenaerts et al. developed a fluorescent DNA-staining protocol that shows both acid-fast negative and positive bacilli. As a consequence, they confirmed that *M. tuberculosis* persists as large clusters of both intracellular and extracellular bacilli in the C3HFeJ strain of mice that develop necrotic lesions following aerosol exposure (22). These data show that the propensity of *M. tuberculosis* to form *in vivo* microbial communities is not limited to extracellular bacilli but can accumulate within an intracellular compartment as well. The concept of intracellular biofilm formation was first suggested in the study of uropathogenic *Escherichia coli* in the urinary bladder of patients with recurring urinary tract infections (39), and later shown

to persist against antibiotics within transitional epithelium (40–42). The possibility that intracellular and extracellular communities of *M. tuberculosis* contribute to the expression of drug tolerance *in vivo* is in need of further investigation.

EXTRACELLULAR *M. TUBERCULOSIS* PERSISTS AGAINST ANTIBIOTICS TREATMENT

Recent animal studies have found that extracellular bacilli are among the populations of *M. tuberculosis* that persist and express *in vivo* antimicrobial drug tolerance, especially in model species that develop necrotic granulomas (7, 43, 44). Using the guinea pig model, which develops well-organized TB granulomas similar to those in humans, Lenaerts et al. reported that the majority of the acid-fast *M. tuberculosis* bacilli that recovered from a truncated exposure of antibiotics were localized in acellular rims of necrotizing lesions (44). This was later verified by comparing the host response to *M. tuberculosis* infection in different strains of mice that do or do not form necrotic lung lesions (6). Drug treatment of *M. tuberculosis*-infected mice produced a more uniform decline in acid-fast bacilli across the lesions in strains that fail to develop lesion necrosis, whereas antimicrobial drug treatment of mice strains that do develop necrotic lesions, and of guinea pigs, resulted in disproportionately higher levels of extracellular, drug-tolerant bacilli (6). Although the visualization methods in these studies fail to clarify the live/dead status of the recovered acid-fast bacilli from drug-treated tissues, the findings nevertheless provide clues as to the host factors that contribute to the *in vivo* expression of antimicrobial drug by *M. tuberculosis*.

BIOFILMS: A NEW PERSPECTIVE OF EXTRACELLULAR *M. TUBERCULOSIS* IN NECROTIZING LESIONS

In the animal studies discussed above, the investigators made an intriguing observation of diffused rhodamine staining pattern around the acellular rims of necrotizing lesions. In light of the fact that rhodamine readily stains mycolic acids, the authors speculated that the diffused material could likely be *M. tuberculosis*-derived mycolic acids, either actively secreted by viable bacilli or accumulated after bacterial death and degradation (6). The former possibility assumes greater significance from the fact that mycolic acids are abundantly produced and secreted as free acids by *in vitro* cultures of mycobacteria in detergent-free medium, in which the bacilli

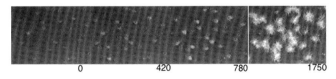

Figure 1 Visualization of *M. smegmatis* growth in a microfluidic device by time-lapse microscopy. The numbers at the bottom of the snapshots denote the time in minutes at which the snaps were taken. Note the distinct foci of multicellular communities from growth of individual cells. (Data collected by Jacob Richards in the laboratory of Anil Ojha).

typically grow as self-organized, surface-associated, multicellular communities, leading to development of pellicles on air-medium interface (33) or colonies on solid substratum (Fig. 1). Moreover, a direct role of free-mycolic acids (FM) in formation of pellicle is suggested by a *groEL1* mutant of *Mycobacterium smegmatis*, in which the defects of the mutant in forming pellicle are linked to instability of mycolic acid modulating enzyme KasA and KasB that results in lower abundance of FM (32, 45).

The phenotypic and functional characteristics of mycobacteria grown as pellicles *in vitro* adhere to the general definition of biofilms in a way that not only are the pellicles more resistant to antibiotics, but also that their development proceeds through genetically distinct stages (32, 33). Taken together, colocalization of diffused (secreted) mycolic acids and drug-tolerant persisters in the acellular rim of necrotizing lesions support the hypothesis that mycobacteria could likely grow as biofilms in such host niches. Interestingly, Wong and Jacobs suggested that the multicellular growth of mycobacteria inside the host could be an active process regulated by the pathogen (37). The authors found that *M. tuberculosis* actively produces signals through the ESX-1 pathway to induce lysis of macrophages. Subsequent release of host DNA in the extracellular compartment, also called extracellular traps, appears to facilitate aggregated growth of the pathogen (37). Given that DNA is a key component of extracellular matrix in biofilms produced by many pathogenic bacteria, it is reasonable to argue that host-derived DNA can also contribute significantly to the extracellular matrix of *M. tuberculosis* biofilms, especially in necrotic lesions (46).

Nick et al. showed that neutrophil-derived eDNA contributed significantly to biofilm formation by *Pseudomonas aeruginosa in vitro*, and that targeting DNA and the host cytoskeletal protein actin enzymatically dispersed microbial communities, which restored antimicrobial drug susceptibility (47, 48). Ackart et al. developed a similar *in vitro* assay in which lysed human neutrophils served as an attachment matrix for extracellular *M. tuberculosis*. They went on to show that *M. tuberculosis* formed complex microbial communities similar to those described for other known biofilm-forming bacterial species (49). Moreover, bacilli attached to host-derived macromolecules expressed a nonreplicating phenotype and extreme tolerance to first-line anti-TB drugs alone or in combination. This *in vitro* model system was used as a platform to screen a library of 2-aminoimidazole (2-AI)-based small molecules that have been shown to have biofilm-inhibiting and -dispersing

activity against a wide variety of Gram-positive and Gram-negative bacteria (50). These data showed that second-generation 2-AI small molecules were even more effective at restoring susceptibility of drug-tolerant bacilli to isoniazid and rifampin by directly targeting attached communities of *M. tuberculosis* (51). In more recent unpublished studies, these investigators have shown that 2-AI compounds are also effective at reversing the inherent resistance of *M. smegmatis* and *M. tuberculosis* to beta-lactam antibiotics. These data demonstrate the potential use of small molecules as adjunctive therapy to restore antimicrobial susceptibility of *M. tuberculosis* expressing drug tolerance through extracellular biofilm formation.

Besides an extraordinary recalcitrance to antibiotics, pathogenic bacterial biofilms also successfully subvert the host immunity to establish chronic infections. For example, biofilm formation by *Streptococcus pneumoniae* evades recognition by the immune system by inhibiting complement binding and phagocytosis (52). In an *in vitro* culture of *E. coli*, the phagocytosis of planktonic bacteria by macrophages was significantly more efficient than that of bacteria maintained as a biofilm (53). Biofilm formation can also impair antimicrobial killing by neutrophils. Neutrophils are often the first cells to encounter bacteria during the early stages of infection and have multiple antimicrobial strategies for killing both intracellular and extracellular bacteria. Recent studies have shown that microbial communities are not completely resistant to killing by neutrophils but the impairment of antimicrobial defenses is somewhat dependent on a combination of host and pathogen factors (54). In the case of *M. tuberculosis*, Lenaerts et al. showed that growth of bacilli under hypoxic conditions *in vitro* resulted in the secretion of extracellular DNA (22, 55), which may, in combination with host DNA and other macromolecules, impair phagocytosis and extracellular killing (56, 57). This raises a possible linkage between the characteristic chronic infection by *M. tuberculosis* and its ability to form aggregated community in extracellular niches.

SUMMARY AND OUTLOOK

Taken together, *in vivo* aggregates of extracellular *M. tuberculosis* represent an interesting and perhaps physiologically distinct entity that could influence the clinical characteristics of TB. For further investigation into the significance of these aggregates in *M. tuberculosis* persistence *in vivo*, *in vitro* studies on growth characteristics of the pathogen are crucial. Using *in vitro* growth models, addressing fundamental questions such as how do individual bacteria attach and aggregate to biotic and abiotic surfaces, what facilitates their adaptation to interior microenvironment of the aggregates, and how these processes impact their fitness against host defense and drug treatment stresses would provide molecular tools for characterization of *in vivo* aggregates. Mutational analysis is a powerful approach to address these questions. However, a straightforward genetic correlation between *in vitro* and *in vivo* phenotypes of a mutant is often difficult to infer because of multiple possible effects of a mutation on the pathogen. For example, *mmaA4*, a methyltransferase involved in synthesis of oxygenated mycolic acids, influences cell wall permeability of *M. tuberculosis* as well as host-pathogen interaction (58, 59). Because of such pleiotropic effects of *mmaA4*, its requirement in biofilm formation *in vitro* and growth *in vivo* offers limited correlation between the two phenotypes (60, 61). These limitations could be circumvented by an integrative approach that combines advanced microscopy with high-throughput genetics (Tn-seq), transcriptomics (RNAseq), and bioinformatics techniques to determine the specific biomarkers associated with *M. tuberculosis* biofilms *in vitro*. Such biomarkers could serve as valuable reagents for understanding the role of extracellular aggregate in *M. tuberculosis* persistence and pathogenesis.

Citation. Basaraba RJ, Ojha AK. 2017. Mycobacterial biofilms: revisiting tuberculosis bacilli in extracellular necrotizing lesions. Microbiol Spectrum 5(3):TBTB2-0024-2016.

References

1. WHO. 2015. *The WHO End TB Strategy*. http://www.who.int/tb/post2015_strategy/en/

2. Hunter RL, Actor JK, Hwang SA, Karev V, Jagannath C. 2014. Pathogenesis of post primary tuberculosis: immunity and hypersensitivity in the development of cavities. *Ann Clin Lab Sci* 44:365–387.

3. Hunter RL. 2011. Pathology of post primary tuberculosis of the lung: an illustrated critical review. *Tuberculosis (Edinb)* 91:497–509.

4. Hunter RL. 2016. Tuberculosis as a three-act play: a new paradigm for the pathogenesis of pulmonary tuberculosis. *Tuberculosis (Edinb)* 97:8–17.

5. Grosset J. 2003. *Mycobacterium tuberculosis* in the extracellular compartment: an underestimated adversary. *Antimicrob Agents Chemother* 47:833–836.

6. Hoff DR, Ryan GJ, Driver ER, Ssemakulu CC, De Groote MA, Basaraba RJ, Lenaerts AJ. 2011. Location of intra- and extracellular *M. tuberculosis* populations in lungs of mice and guinea pigs during disease progression and after drug treatment. *PLoS One* 6:e17550.

7. Lenaerts A, Barry CE III, Dartois V. 2015. Heterogeneity in tuberculosis pathology, microenvironments and therapeutic responses. *Immunol Rev* 264:288–307.

8. Barclay WR, Ebert RH, Manthei RW, Roth LJ. 1953. Distribution of C14 labeled isoniazid in sensitive and resistant tubercle bacilli and in infected and uninfected tissues in tuberculous patients. *Trans Annu Meet Natl Tuberc Assoc* 49:192–195.

9. Manthei RW, Roth LJ, Barclay WR, Ebert RH. 1954. The distribution of C14 labeled isoniazid in normal and infected guinea pigs. *Arch Int Pharmacodyn Ther* 98:183–192.

10. Prideaux B, ElNaggar MS, Zimmerman M, Wiseman JM, Li X, Dartois V. 2015. Mass spectrometry imaging of levofloxacin distribution in TB-infected pulmonary lesions by MALDI-MSI and continuous liquid micro-junction surface sampling. *Int J Mass Spectrom* 377:699–708.

11. Datta M, Via LE, Chen W, Baish JW, Xu L, Barry CE III, Jain RK. 2016. Mathematical model of oxygen transport in tuberculosis granulomas. *Ann Biomed Eng* 44:863–872.

12. Via LE, Lin PL, Ray SM, Carrillo J, Allen SS, Eum SY, Taylor K, Klein E, Manjunatha U, Gonzales J, Lee EG, Park SK, Raleigh JA, Cho SN, McMurray DN, Flynn JL, Barry CE III. 2008. Tuberculous granulomas are hypoxic in guinea pigs, rabbits, and nonhuman primates. *Infect Immun* 76:2333–2340.

13. Via LE, Schimel D, Weiner DM, Dartois V, Dayao E, Cai Y, Yoon YS, Dreher MR, Kastenmayer RJ, Laymon CM, Carny JE, Flynn JL, Herscovitch P, Barry CE III. 2012. Infection dynamics and response to chemotherapy in a rabbit model of tuberculosis using [18F]2-fluoro-deoxy-D-glucose positron emission tomography and computed tomography. *Antimicrob Agents Chemother* 56:4391–4402.

14. Prideaux B, Via LE, Zimmerman MD, Eum S, Sarathy J, O'Brien P, Chen C, Kaya F, Weiner DM, Chen PY, Song T, Lee M, Shim TS, Cho JS, Kim W, Cho SN, Olivier KN, Barry CE III, Dartois V. 2015. The association between sterilizing activity and drug distribution into tuberculosis lesions. *Nat Med* 21:1223–1227.

15. Karakousis PC, Yoshimatsu T, Lamichhane G, Woolwine SC, Nuermberger EL, Grosset J, Bishai WR. 2004. Dormancy phenotype displayed by extracellular *Mycobacterium tuberculosis* within artificial granulomas in mice. *J Exp Med* 200:647–657.

16. Goren MB, D'Arcy Hart P, Young MR, Armstrong JA. 1976. Prevention of phagosome-lysosome fusion in cultured macrophages by sulfatides of *Mycobacterium tuberculosis*. *Proc Natl Acad Sci USA* 73:2510–2514.

17. Weiss G, Schaible UE. 2015. Macrophage defense mechanisms against intracellular bacteria. *Immunol Rev* 264:182–203.

18. Canetti G. 1950. Exogenous reinfection and pulmonary tuberculosis a study of the pathology. *Tubercle* 31:224–233.

19. Canetti G. 1956. Dynamic aspects of the pathology and bacteriology of tuberculous lesions. *Am Rev Tuberc* 74:13–21, discussion, 22–27.

20. Canetti G, Israel R, Hertzog P, Daumet P, Toty L. 1954. [Koch's bacillus in resected tuberculous lesions after chemotherapy: 97 cases]. *Poumon Coeur* 10:465–485.

21. Canetti GJ. 1959. Changes in tuberculosis as seen by a pathologist. *Am Rev Tuberc* **79**:684–686.

22. Ryan GJ, Shapiro HM, Lenaerts AJ. 2014. Improving acid-fast fluorescent staining for the detection of mycobacteria using a new nucleic acid staining approach. *Tuberculosis (Edinb)* **94**:511–518.

23. Nyka W, O'Neill EF. 1970. A new approach to the study of non-acid-fast mycobacteria. *Ann N Y Acad Sci* **174** (2 Unusual Isola):862–871.

24. Nyka W. 1977. The chromophobic tubercle bacilli and the problem of endogenous reactivation of tuberculosis. *Mater Med Pol* **9**:175–185.

25. Nyka W. 1967. Method for staining both acid-fast and chromophobic tubercle bacilli with carbolfuschsin. *J Bacteriol* **93**:1458–1460.

26. Nyka W. 1963. Studies on *Mycobacterium tuberculosis* in lesions of the human lung. A new method of staining tubercle bacilli in tissue sections. *Am Rev Respir Dis* **88**:670–679.

27. Richards JP, Ojha AK. 2014. Mycobacterial biofilms. *Microbiol Spectr* **2**:

28. López D, Vlamakis H, Kolter R. 2010. Biofilms. *Cold Spring Harb Perspect Biol* **2**:a000398

29. Stoodley P, Sauer K, Davies DG, Costerton JW. 2002. Biofilms as complex differentiated communities. *Annu Rev Microbiol* **56**:187–209.

30. Mah TF, O'Toole GA. 2001. Mechanisms of biofilm resistance to antimicrobial agents. *Trends Microbiol* **9**:34–39.

31. Davies D. 2003. Understanding biofilm resistance to antibacterial agents. *Nat Rev Drug Discov* **2**:114–122.

32. Ojha A, Anand M, Bhatt A, Kremer L, Jacobs WR Jr, Hatfull GF. 2005. GroEL1: a dedicated chaperone involved in mycolic acid biosynthesis during biofilm formation in mycobacteria. *Cell* **123**:861–873.

33. Ojha AK, Baughn AD, Sambandan D, Hsu T, Trivelli X, Guerardel Y, Alahari A, Kremer L, Jacobs WR Jr, Hatfull GF. 2008. Growth of *Mycobacterium tuberculosis* biofilms containing free mycolic acids and harbouring drug-tolerant bacteria. *Mol Microbiol* **69**:164–174.

34. Recht J, Kolter R. 2001. Glycopeptidolipid acetylation affects sliding motility and biofilm formation in Mycobacterium smegmatis. *J Bacteriol* **183**:5718–5724.

35. Marsollier L, Brodin P, Jackson M, Korduláková J, Tafelmeyer P, Carbonnelle E, Aubry J, Milon G, Legras P, André JP, Leroy C, Cottin J, Guillou ML, Reysset G, Cole ST. 2007. Impact of *Mycobacterium ulcerans* biofilm on transmissibility to ecological niches and Buruli ulcer pathogenesis. *PLoS Pathog* **3**:e62.

36. Hall-Stoodley L, Brun OS, Polshyna G, Barker LP. 2006. *Mycobacterium marinum* biofilm formation reveals cording morphology. *FEMS Microbiol Lett* **257**:43–49.

37. Wong KW, Jacobs WR Jr. 2016. postprimary tuberculosis and macrophage necrosis: is there a big conNECtion? *MBio* **7**:e01589-15.

38. Orme IM. 2014. A new unifying theory of the pathogenesis of tuberculosis. *Tuberculosis (Edinb)* **94**:8–14.

39. Anderson GG, Dodson KW, Hooton TM, Hultgren SJ. 2004. Intracellular bacterial communities of uropathogenic *Escherichia coli* in urinary tract pathogenesis. *Trends Microbiol* **12**:424–430.

40. Berry RE, Klumpp DJ, Schaeffer AJ. 2009. Urothelial cultures support intracellular bacterial community formation by uropathogenic *Escherichia coli*. *Infect Immun* **77**:2762–2772.

41. Hunstad DA, Justice SS. 2010. Intracellular lifestyles and immune evasion strategies of uropathogenic *Escherichia coli*. *Annu Rev Microbiol* **64**:203–221.

42. Scott VC, Haake DA, Churchill BM, Justice SS, Kim JH. 2015. Intracellular bacterial communities: a potential etiology for chronic lower urinary tract symptoms. *Urology* **86**:425–431.

43. Lanoix JP, Lenaerts AJ, Nuermberger EL. 2015. Heterogeneous disease progression and treatment response in a C3HeB/FeJ mouse model of tuberculosis. *Dis Model Mech* **8**:603–610.

44. Lenaerts AJ, Hoff D, Aly S, Ehlers S, Andries K, Cantarero L, Orme IM, Basaraba RJ. 2007. Location of persisting mycobacteria in a Guinea pig model of tuberculosis revealed by r207910. *Antimicrob Agents Chemother* **51**: 3338–3345.

45. Ojha AK, Trivelli X, Guerardel Y, Kremer L, Hatfull GF. 2010. Enzymatic hydrolysis of trehalose dimycolate releases free mycolic acids during mycobacterial growth in biofilms. *J Biol Chem* **285**:17380–17389.

46. Basaraba RJ. 2008. Experimental tuberculosis: the role of comparative pathology in the discovery of improved tuberculosis treatment strategies. *Tuberculosis (Edinb)* **88** (Suppl 1):S35–S47.

47. Parks QM, Young RL, Poch KR, Malcolm KC, Vasil ML, Nick JA. 2009. Neutrophil enhancement of *Pseudomonas aeruginosa* biofilm development: human F-actin and DNA as targets for therapy. *J Med Microbiol* **58**:492–502.

48. Walker TS, Tomlin KL, Worthen GS, Poch KR, Lieber JG, Saavedra MT, Fessler MB, Malcolm KC, Vasil ML, Nick JA. 2005. Enhanced *Pseudomonas aeruginosa* biofilm development mediated by human neutrophils. *Infect Immun* **73**:3693–3701.

49. Ackart DF, Hascall-Dove L, Caceres SM, Kirk NM, Podell BK, Melander C, Orme IM, Leid JG, Nick JA, Basaraba RJ. 2014. Expression of antimicrobial drug tolerance by attached communities of *Mycobacterium tuberculosis*. *Pathog Dis* **70**:359–369.

50. Ackart DF, Lindsey EA, Podell BK, Melander RJ, Basaraba RJ, Melander C. 2014. Reversal of *Mycobacterium tuberculosis* phenotypic drug resistance by 2-aminoimidazole-based small molecules. *Pathog Dis* **70**: 370–378.

51. Furlani RE, Richardson MA, Podell BK, Ackart DF, Haugen JD, Melander RJ, Basaraba RJ, Melander C. 2015. Second generation 2-aminoimidazole based advanced glycation end product inhibitors and breakers. *Bioorg Med Chem Lett* **25**:4820–4823.

52. Domenech M, Ramos-Sevillano E, García E, Moscoso M, Yuste J. 2013. Biofilm formation avoids complement immunity and phagocytosis of *Streptococcus pneumoniae*. *Infect Immun* **81**:2606–2615.

53. Hernández-Jiménez E, Del Campo R, Toledano V, Vallejo-Cremades MT, Muñoz A, Largo C, Arnalich F, García-Rio F, Cubillos-Zapata C, López-Collazo E. 2013. Biofilm

vs. planktonic bacterial mode of growth: which do human macrophages prefer? *Biochem Biophys Res Commun* 441:947–952.

54. Hirschfeld J. 2014. Dynamic interactions of neutrophils and biofilms. *J Oral Microbiol* 6:26102.

55. Ryan GJ, Hoff DR, Driver ER, Voskuil MI, Gonzalez-Juarrero M, Basaraba RJ, Crick DC, Spencer JS, Lenaerts AJ. 2010. Multiple *M. tuberculosis* phenotypes in mouse and guinea pig lung tissue revealed by a dual-staining approach. *PLoS One* 5:e11108.

56. Arciola CR. 2010. Host defense against implant infection: the ambivalent role of phagocytosis. *Int J Artif Organs* 33:565–567.

57. Montanaro L, Poggi A, Visai L, Ravaioli S, Campoccia D, Speziale P, Arciola CR. 2011. Extracellular DNA in biofilms. *Int J Artif Organs* 34:824–831.

58. Yuan Y, Lee RE, Besra GS, Belisle JT, Barry CE III. 1995. Identification of a gene involved in the biosynthe-

sis of cyclopropanated mycolic acids in *Mycobacterium tuberculosis*. *Proc Natl Acad Sci USA* 92:6630–6634.

59. Dkhar HK, Nanduri R, Mahajan S, Dave S, Saini A, Somavarapu AK, Arora A, Parkesh R, Thakur KG, Mayilraj S, Gupta P. 2014. *Mycobacterium tuberculosis* keto-mycolic acid and macrophage nuclear receptor TR4 modulate foamy biogenesis in granulomas: a case of a heterologous and noncanonical ligand-receptor pair. *J Immunol* 193:295–305.

60. Sambandan D, Dao DN, Weinrick BC, Vilchèze C, Gurcha SS, Ojha A, Kremer L, Besra GS, Hatfull GF, Jacobs WR Jr. 2013. Keto-mycolic acid-dependent pellicle formation confers tolerance to drug-sensitive Mycobacterium tuberculosis. *MBio* 4:e00222-13.

61. Dubnau E, Chan J, Raynaud C, Mohan VP, Lanéelle MA, Yu K, Quémard A, Smith I, Daffé M. 2000. Oxygenated mycolic acids are necessary for virulence of *Mycobacterium tuberculosis* in mice. *Mol Microbiol* 36:630–637.

Tuberculosis and the Tubercle Bacillus, 2nd ed.
Edited by William R. Jacobs, Jr., Helen McShane, Valerie Mizrahi, and Ian M. Orme
© 2018 American Society for Microbiology, Washington, DC
doi:10.1128/microbiolspec.TBTB2-0028-2016

Killing *Mycobacterium tuberculosis* *In Vitro*: What Model Systems Can Teach Us

25

Tracy L. Keiser[1] and Georgiana E. Purdy[2]

INTRODUCTION

Mycobacterium tuberculosis is one of the oldest and most successful pathogens in human history due in large part to its coevolution with humans, resulting in an exquisite adaptation by the bacterium to its host. Detection of *M. tuberculosis* DNA in mummified human remains from both the Old and New World is evidence that tuberculosis (TB) has been part of our history for millennia (1). In addition, genomic analysis demonstrated that genetic expansion of the mycobacterial repertoire coincided with the geographical expansions of humans, solidifying the evidence that *M. tuberculosis* has evolved with its host (2). During this evolution, *M. tuberculosis* has developed numerous ways to subvert the human immune response (3–5). For instance, a hallmark of *M. tuberculosis* pathogenicity is its ability to establish a niche in macrophages, the host immune cells that should be the bacterium's ultimate undoing. Macrophages are a crucial cell subset of the innate immune system whose primary function is to patrol the host and seek out foreign particles. Bacteria and other pathogens are recognized via their pathogen-associated molecular patterns, which initiate a signaling cascade that results in phagocytosis of the pathogen and upregulation of a proinflammatory response. The most notable cytokines produced by macrophages associated with this proinflammatory state in TB are interleukin-1 (IL-1), IL-6, IL-8, IL-12, and tumor necrosis factor (TNF) (6). Ideally, bacteria are killed and degraded upon phagosome-lysosomal fusion, and as antigen-presenting cells (APCs), macrophages present *M. tuberculosis* peptides and lipid antigens, ultimately leading to a highly specific adaptive immune response. Therefore,

the primary encounter between *M. tuberculosis* and macrophages dictates the subsequent immune response. In TB, this immune response is focused on containment and eventual eradication of the bacterium in the granuloma.

TB is typically a pulmonary disease that is disseminated by aerosol from an actively infected person. When the bacterium enters the lung of a new host there are three possible outcomes: clearance of the infection by the immune system, the development of primary infection, and/or the establishment of latency. The majority (90%) of infections result in latent infections that may last for the lifetime of the host or possibly reactivate when the host becomes immunocompromised. Although *M. tuberculosis* is adept at subverting the host and establishing a long-lasting, latent infection, several lines of evidence highlight the relevance of innate defense mechanisms and macrophages in control of *M. tuberculosis* infection in its early stages. First, in people closely and repeatedly exposed to *M. tuberculosis*, only about 50% develop infection as evidenced by a positive tuberculin skin test (TST) reaction or interferon gamma response assay response (7). In the case of individuals who remain TST-negative, it is likely that at an early point of infection, the host was able to contain and clear the infection without implementing the adaptive immune response. Genetic studies of these individuals, so-called resisters, may reveal the underlying nature of this successful bactericidal response (8). Second, in individuals with evidence of infection (TST-positive), the precise location of *M. tuberculosis* is not known, and most do not have discernable granulomatous infection. In other words, these individuals were able to

[1]Department of Microbiology and Immunology, Albert Einstein College of Medicine, Bronx, NY 10461; [2]Department of Microbiology and Immunology, Oregon Health Sciences University, Portland OR, 97239.

contain and possibly clear the infection via a combined innate and adaptive immune response. Harnessing these early responses may lead to more effective vaccination strategies.

At the turn of the 20th century, scientists were armed with the knowledge that *M. tuberculosis* was the causative agent of TB, but there was still much to learn about its pathology and pathogenesis. In 1927, autopsy results of *M. tuberculosis*-infected tissue indicated that the bacilli could always be found within phagocytic cells (9). However, it should be noted that detailed postmortem analysis revealed that *M. tuberculosis* was infrequently cultured from the deceased tissue, and when it was cultured, there were equal odds of finding the bacterium in "normal" lung tissue versus a granuloma (10). Since alveolar macrophages are the first cells encountered by *M. tuberculosis*, *in vitro* work with macrophages is indispensable for understanding the basic biology of *M. tuberculosis*, its pathogenic mechanisms, and the mycobactericidal properties of the macrophage. In 1952, Suter published the first established *in vitro* model of infection using "peritoneal exudates" of normal guinea pigs (11). After 64 years, the general infection system has not changed much, but our knowledge and repertoire of available systems has become more refined as we strive toward a better molecular and immunological understanding of TB disease. The premise of this article was prompted by the question "Can a macrophage kill *M. tuberculosis*?" In an effort to answer that question, the first section of the article focuses on *in vitro* models of infection as well as the caveats of each system. The second section highlights the key findings obtained in these systems using cells obtained from mice, non-human primates (NHPs), and humans. Finally, coordinated innate and adaptive immune responses are important for containment and clearance of infection, and the third section discusses the *in vitro* model systems that address this complexity.

MODEL SYSTEMS OVERVIEW

It is generally accepted that for an infection to be established, *M. tuberculosis* is inhaled in small, aerosolized droplets that are then engulfed by alveolar macrophages in the lung. As a result, a multitude of studies aimed at understanding mechanisms underlying *M. tuberculosis* host pathogen interactions have been performed using macrophages or differentiated monocyte cell lines as well as primary macrophages. Although work has been done in a variety of animal systems, the majority of these studies have been performed on cells

obtained from mice, NHPs, and humans; the benefits and caveats of these systems are outlined below.

Mouse *In Vitro* Models

Cell lines

The RAW264.7 and J774 macrophage cell lines are the murine cell lines predominantly used for *M. tuberculosis in vitro* studies. RAW264.7 is a macrophage cell line derived from BALB/c mice and was immortalized via transformation with the Abelson murine leukemia virus (12). J774.1 macrophages also have a BALB/c mouse origin and were isolated from a sarcoma (13). These adherent cell lines have maintained phagocytic capacity and can be induced into an activated phenotype by cytokine or endotoxin (14, 15). The cytokine response to *M. tuberculosis* and *M. tuberculosis*-derived lipids is intact in RAW264.7 and J774 cells and is similar to that of bone marrow-derived macrophages (BMDMs). Cell lines produce TNF, IL-6, and IL-1β in response to intact bacteria as well as to purified trehalose dimycolate (TDM) (16–19). In addition, RAW264.7 macrophages produced nitric oxide (NO) species and TNF in response to lipoarabinomannan (20). However, direct comparison revealed differences in NO production by RAW264.7 and J774 cells. Similar to primary peritoneal macrophages, RAW264.7 produced NO in response to lipopolysaccharide (LPS), IFN-γ, heat-killed *Mycobacterium bovis* BCG, and purified protein derivative (PPD). Of these four potent inducers, J774 produced NO in response only to LPS, but not IFN-γ, heat-killed *M. bovis* BCG, or PPD (21).

Although the majority of cell lines available are in the BALB/c background, C57/B6 (C57Bl/6J) macrophages have been immortalized using the method of retroviral transduction of v-*raf* and v-*myc* oncogenes (22, 23). This approach can be used with wild-type BMDMs as well as those from knockout mice strains. Despite the potential of these cells of non-BALB/c origin, there are surprisingly few cases in which they have been used to study host-pathogen interactions between *M. tuberculosis* and the macrophage (24).

Even fewer studies have been attempted using cell lines of alveolar origin. The MH-S cell line was derived by transformation of BALB/c alveolar macrophages with the SV40 virus (25). MH-S cells were investigated as a potential cell line for studies with *M. tuberculosis* and were found to have similar phagocytic capacity to that of resident alveolar macrophages, although their capacity to control *M. tuberculosis* infection has not been reported (26). AMJ2-C11 are cloned, continuous, alveolar macrophage cell lines generated from C57Bl/6 mice by *in vitro* infection with the J2 retrovirus carrying the v-*raf* and v-*myc* oncogenes. These cells share many characteristics with the parental alveolar macrophages in that they are phagocytic and can be activated by cytokine and LPS. Activation with IFN-γ and LPS upregulates major histocompatibility complex-class II antigen presentation and the production of NO (27, 28). The potential for these cells as an *in vitro* model for *M. tuberculosis* appears underappreciated. One report used AMJ2-C11 cells to demonstrate that the *M. tuberculosis phoP* mutant was attenuated. This study also tested the survival of wild-type and mutant strains in the THP-1 human monocyte and J774 macrophage cell line, which allowed some comparison of the AMJ2-C11 ability to contain *M. tuberculosis*. It appears that the AMJ2-C11 cells were more similar to the J774 cells in preventing *M. tuberculosis* replication than the THP-1 cells, showing that wild-type *M. tuberculosis* replicated over 1 log during the course of a 6-day infection (29).

Primary cells

Primary cells isolated from mice, in particular BMDMs, are a popular choice for *in vitro* studies. These cells can be expanded to a certain extent and are responsive to cytokine stimulation and bacterial infection. Although alveolar macrophages are the more relevant cell type for *M. tuberculosis* infection, their dismal yield from mice discourages their use. As a result, peritoneal macrophages are sometimes used as representatives of resident macrophages.

Despite the spectrum of mice that have different susceptibilities to infection with *M. tuberculosis* and subsequent disease outcomes, most studies with primary murine macrophages use cells from either BALB/c or C57Bl/6 mice, which were recently characterized as "permissive-susceptible" and "permissive-resistant" mouse strains, respectively (30). During infection of BALB/c and C57Bl/6 mice, *M. tuberculosis* infects and initially replicates, but the C57Bl/6 mice are able to control the subsequent chronic, progressive infection via a Th1 immune response. In the BALB/c background in which a Th2 immune response predominates, lung lesions develop more rapidly with more apparent necrosis, which is reflected in the faster clinical deterioration of infected mice. These differences between *M. tuberculosis* infections of BALB/c and C57Bl/6 are most noticeable at later time points following infection (>60 days). The most common criticism of using BALB/c and C57Bl/6 mouse strains is that they do not develop the necrotizing granulomatous lesions that are the hallmark of human disease. An innately resistant mouse model for TB that more faithfully mimics human resis-

tance to disease has not been developed yet, and therefore it is not known how macrophages, other innate effector cells, and/or some other aspect of mucosal immunity contribute to control of *M. tuberculosis*.

The overwhelming advantage to using primary macrophages from C57Bl/6 mice is the availability of knockout mutants in this genetic background. While the fate of *M. tuberculosis* in a mouse infection can broadly define the role of specific host immune factors, *in vitro* studies with wild-type and knockout macrophages can further dissect the role of these proteins and pathways in the context of initial infection and innate immunity. For example, macrophages were obtained from mice that lack phagocyte oxidase (NOX2/gp91phox) and inducible NO synthase (iNOS), and they were invaluable in characterizing the role of these host defenses and the relevant resistance mechanisms of *M. tuberculosis* (31, 32) (discussed below in "Basic Principles of *M. tuberculosis* Macrophage Biology").

Benefits and caveats of murine *in vitro* models

The most obvious benefit to using cell lines or primary cells such as BMDMs from inbred mice is that these allow investigators to work with large or unlimited numbers of relatively homogenous cells with phenotypes that are consistent over time. In addition, the number of cells obtainable permits experiments that necessitate large numbers of cells. For instance, large-scale screens using libraries of more than 10,000 transposon mutants to analyze parameters of *M. tuberculosis*-macrophages have been facilitated through the use of resting and IFN-γ-activated C57Bl/6 macrophages (33). In some experimental systems, the numbers of cells needed to obtain sufficient material for analysis would be difficult to achieve without the use of cell lines or BMDMs. Dissecting the transcriptional response of *M. tuberculosis* and the host during initial stages of infection benefited greatly from the use of BMDMs (34, 35). Finally, the isolation and characterization of bioactive host molecules can also require large amounts of cellular material. Bactericidal peptides that were generated in the lysosome were isolated from C57Bl/6 BMDMs and RAW264.7 cells and identified via mass spectroscopy (36, 37).

As the predominant model system for infectious disease and immunology, a major advantage of using mice is the availability of reagents including recombinant cytokines and antibodies to facilitate experimentation *in vitro* and *in vivo*. Seminal work showed that activation of BMDMs with recombinant IFN-γ and/or TNF resulted in cells that were mycobacteriostatic, consistent with the prevailing model that activated macrophages contain infection (38). Cellular microbiology studies using recombinant cytokine enabled investigators to show that when mycobacteria are in activated macrophages, the block in phagosome maturation is no longer maintained and there is increased phagolysosomal fusion (39, 40). Although IFN-γ and TNF play a central role in the protective immune response, infection of macrophages also results in production of IL-1β via the NLRP3 inflammasome (41). A notable caveat to the applicability of cell lines to innate immune responses, and inflammasomes in particular, is that RAW264.7 cells do not express the protein ASC (apoptosis-associated speck-like protein containing a caspase activation and recruitment domain) and therefore cannot efficiently activate some inflammasome complexes (42).

Genetic manipulation of the host was an immediate advantage of using cell lines that remains relevant today. Early work demonstrating the potential role of reactive oxygen intermediates (ROIs) and reactive nitrogen intermediates (RNIs) was facilitated by work by Bloom and colleagues. An ROI-deficient strain of J774 cells was derived from a continuous ROI-positive clone using the mutagen N-methyl-N'nitro-N-nitrosoguanidine. ROI, but not RNI, production was impacted in the mutant cells. Survival of *M. tuberculosis* in ROI-deficient macrophages emphasized the importance of RNI (43, 44). Modern molecular approaches are now used to manipulate the host cell via gene knockdown and knockout. Cell lines and primary cells (to a certain extent) are amenable to genetic manipulation via small interfering RNA or expression of short hairpin RNA via lentivirus. Nonessential genes can be knocked out using CRISPR/Cas9 methodology. The applicability of such methods to studying host cell biology is readily appreciated. For example, a library of host-directed small interfering RNAs was used to identify host factors involved in *M. tuberculosis* survival in J774 cells. Those proteins were categorized into a range of functional classes from intracellular trafficking to immune signaling and host cell metabolic pathways (45). In the future, these host factors may provide additional targets for development of novel TB therapeutics.

NHP *in vitro* models

NHPs allow for the study of tuberculosis in a model that more faithfully recapitulates human tuberculosis disease progression, notably the development of latent tuberculosis and a spectrum of granulomas resembling those observed in human disease (46). NHPs are an excellent model to test new vaccines or therapeutic compounds. Since true latency can be achieved, reactivation

of disease upon HIV (simian immunodeficiency virus) coinfection or anti-TNF therapy can be assessed (47–49). There is also a benefit in using NHPs to tease apart host-pathogen interactions. Mycobacterial genes associated with virulence were identified by infecting NHPs with *M. tuberculosis* transposon mutants (50). When rhesus macaques were infected with a pool of 326 *M. tuberculosis* mutants, roughly 30% of the mutants were attenuated. When those attenuated mutants were tested in mice only 10% were attenuated, demonstrating the difference between the two infection models. These results suggest that the NHP environment is less permissive than the mouse to *M. tuberculosis* infection, reinforcing how exquisitely adapted *M. tuberculosis* is to its human host.

For *in vitro* studies using NHP cells, investigators are limited to primary cells. Alveolar macrophages can be readily purified from bronchoalveolar lavage fluid and used to answer questions regarding host innate immune control. The cytokine and gene responses of alveolar macrophages to infection by *M. tuberculosis* were examined in alveolar macrophages from macaques and mice. *M. tuberculosis* infection resulted in the upregulation of immune response-related genes, but only a small number of genes were similarly regulated in both macaque and murine cells (51). While these data suggest that investigators should not extrapolate upon mouse data too heavily, other studies have shown that certain aspects of immune control are conserved. We showed that autophagic killing of *M. tuberculosis* occurs in alveolar macrophages from rhesus macaques, recapitulating our previous experiments performed using murine BMDMs (36, 52). In addition, we used alveolar macrophages to ask whether this autophagic killing was impaired upon aging, since this pathway is thought to be diminished with age. We found no difference between control of *M. tuberculosis* by alveolar macrophages from young or old animals, suggesting that other aspects of immunosenescence contribute to the increased rate of TB in the elderly. BMDMs from rhesus macaques have also been used to investigate interactions of *M. tuberculosis* with the host *in vitro*, notably, to look at the gene response of macrophages infected with dormant versus actively replicating *M. tuberculosis* (53). These studies showed an induction of TNF gene expression and an increase in apoptosis in macrophages infected with the hypoxia-adapted bacteria compared to those infected with actively replicating *M. tuberculosis*. We predict that the combined use of the NHP model and primary cells will not only provide a more nuanced interpretation of the host immune response, but will likely elucidate novel *M. tuberculosis* pathways and effectors required for establishment and maintenance of infection.

Human *In Vitro* Models

Human cell lines

The two most utilized human cell lines are U937 and THP-1 cells. U937 is an immortalized monocyte cell line isolated from a histiocytic lymphoma patient. THP-1 cells were isolated from a young patient with acute monocytic leukemia. Standardized methods exist to generate macrophages from these immortalized monocyte precursors via stimulation with the phorbol esters phorbol 12-myristate 13-acetate (PMA) and 12-O-tetradecanoylphorbol-13 acetate (TPA), or with 1,25-dihydroxyvitamin D3 (VD3). Differentiated THP-1 cells become adherent, possess lysozyme activity, and demonstrate increased phagocytosis (54). However, maturation depends on the inducer used with PMA treatment, resulting in cells that are further differentiated than those obtained with vitamin D (55). Similar to primary monocyte-derived macrophages, PMA-differentiated THP-1 cells acquire macrophage surface markers and respond to LPS stimulation by producing TNF and IL-1β (56). A caveat concerning these cell lines is that they lack some of the key receptors and markers of mature macrophages, and one must proceed with caution when analyzing results. For instance, THP-1 cells lack the mannose receptor, which is a key marker for distinguishing macrophages from other lymphocytes. More importantly for cellular microbiology of *M. tuberculosis*, entry of *M. tuberculosis* via the mannose receptor contributes to the bacterium's ability to arrest phagosome maturation in primary human monocyte-derived macrophages (57, 58).

Human primary cells

Due to our inability to use a human *in vivo* model, human primary cells become the most appropriate system to study this human-specific pathogen. Whole blood from healthy human donors is processed to obtain peripheral blood monocyte cells (PBMCs). Monocyte-derived macrophages are then induced using either autologous serum or human recombinant cytokines, deriving these precursor monocytes into mature macrophages. Primary cells from multiple donors are needed to reflect the heterogeneous human population to accurately study *M. tuberculosis* infection and host-pathogen interactions. In addition to their use in *M. tuberculosis*-macrophage interaction studies, human primary cells have also been used to examine *M. tuberculosis* infection in macrophage-T cell coculture infection models and for establishing *in vitro* granulomas (discussed in

"Beyond the Macrophage," below). Such coculture infections require autologous T cells, which are more easily obtained in the mouse model and become a powerful tool for understanding basic principles of antigen recognition and immune control in the human system.

Induced pluripotent stem (iPS) cells

In an ideal world, nearly any cell type necessary for *in vitro* analysis of host-pathogen interactions could be generated from stem cells. The induction of a stem cell state in adult human cells brings the field closer to this goal (59). Cells obtained from a healthy human donor can be induced into a pluripotent stem cell state, rendering iPS cells by the expression of known transcription factors. These cells provide many positive possibilities in that they can be easily isolated from any donor, and methods are currently being developed to differentiate them into nearly any cell type. In 2008, the first methods using the cytokines M-CSF and IL-3 to elicit both monocytes and macrophages were published. These iPS-derived macrophages were tested for cell surface markers (e.g., PU-1, C/EBPα, EMR1, EMR2, MPEG1, CD1c, CD4, CD18, CD32, CD33, CD68), phagocytosis of foreign particles such as opsonized yeast and LPS, as well as the secretion of cytokines postperturbation and -activation by important cytokines such as IFN-γ and IL-4 (60, 61). The investigators concluded that the iPS-derived macrophages were not distinguishable from PBMCs. These cells have been used to elucidate the entry of HIV-1 in macrophages via CD4 containing lipid rafts (62), and it is likely that studies of the interactions between *M. tuberculosis* and host cells will also capitalize on these cells. Primary macrophages are notoriously difficult to manipulate genetically because they are programmed to recognize foreign DNA. The CRISPR-cas9 methods recently developed to generate null deletions combined with the limitless number of cells that can be generated in both type and volume make the iPS system an extremely powerful tool for the study of all diseases, both infectious and genetic.

Benefits and caveats of human *in vitro* models

The simplest benefit to using human cells to study TB is pathogen specificity. *M. tuberculosis* is an obligate intracellular human pathogen, and although the mouse model shares a great deal of similarity with humans, the overall disease progression is altered. The major drawback to using human *in vitro* cell culture systems is that they are typically limited both in cell number and to single or small cell systems, which do not always reflect how these cells work in a whole organism. Another drawback of using human cells is that there are vastly more reagents/tools developed and verified for mice. Unlike the strains of inbred mice normally used for *M. tuberculosis* studies, humans are an outbred population, and consistent and statistically significant results can be difficult to obtain. Lastly, the variables that affect a human over a lifetime are incalculable compared to an inbred mouse strain, where we control almost every variable in its lifetime.

A final point must be made about the applicability of the cell lines and primary cells described above to defining aspects of innate immune control and TB-macrophage biology. Even the use of primary human macrophages comes with the caveat that although these macrophages may restrict bacterial replication, they are not exceptionally bactericidal. Better understanding the differences observed between killing of *M. tuberculosis* among different research groups in these *in vitro* models will likely require genetic comparison of widely used cell lines and primary cells, in addition to thoughtful experiments utilizing *M. tuberculosis* mutants. Ultimately, effective killing mechanisms used by macrophages may be enhanced through pharmacological or therapeutic approaches. For instance, delivery of NO via inhalable microparticles to infected THP-1 macrophages resulted in a 2-log reduction in viable *M. tuberculosis* within 12 hours. Subsequent therapeutic use of these microparticles in infected mice resulted in a 2-log reduction in CFU in the lung, but not the spleen (63). In a host, it likely takes a coordinated effort of multiple cell types in both the innate and adaptive arms of immunity to control *M. tuberculosis*. *In vitro* models to address this complexity are discussed in "Beyond the Macrophage" below.

BASIC PRINCIPLES OF *M. TUBERCULOSIS*-MACROPHAGE BIOLOGY: LESSONS LEARNED FROM MICE AND HUMANS

The use of cultured macrophages revealed aspects of *M. tuberculosis* biology such as the alteration of host cell trafficking to promote phagosome maturation arrest, survival in the face of host antimycobacterial molecules, the modulation of cell death pathways, and the nature of subsequent signaling to promote *M. tuberculosis* survival and establishment of a granulomatous infection. As described above, a number of systems are used to assess these features, and it is a rare example where bacterial survival is compared between systems (64). One of the major concerns in using cell lines or the mouse model system is the possibility that a key molecule or activity with a dramatic impact on *M. tuberculosis* interactions differs between species or between

cell lines and primary cells from different sources. In this section we will outline some key findings on *M. tuberculosis* interactions with the macrophage and point out where *in vitro* systems reveal great conservation or major discrepancies.

Phagosome Maturation Arrest

A hallmark of *M. tuberculosis* cellular microbiology is its ability to arrest phagosome maturation and establish a niche in a vacuole that fails to acidify and retains characteristics of the early endosome (65–68). Studies *in vitro* using cultured macrophages have been key to defining the properties of the *M. tuberculosis*-containing vacuole and revealing the underlying mechanisms of phagosome maturation arrest. A multitude of studies contribute to our understanding of this complex phenotype and demonstrate that that the ability of *M. tuberculosis* to arrest phagosome maturation in resting macrophages depends on both cell wall lipids and protein effectors. TDM has long been appreciated for its immunomodulatory activity. The administration of purified TDM results in the production of high proinflammatory cytokines in mice and in macrophages *in vitro* (17). Trafficking of TDM-coated beads to the lysosome of J774 macrophages was reduced similarly to the trafficking of *M. tuberculosis*, indicating a role for cell wall lipids in mycobacterial phagosome maturation arrest (16). The roles of mannosylated lipid species lipoarabinomannan and phosphatidylinositol mannosides in phagosome maturation were also demonstrated in J774 cells (69, 70). *M. tuberculosis* transposon mutant screens performed in murine macrophages and cell lines identified other proteins that contribute to this aspect of *M. tuberculosis* biology (71, 72). Further characterization of *M. tuberculosis* in macrophages has defined metabolic changes in the bacterium and given clues to various nutrient sources used by the organism in its unique intracellular niche (73).

Survival in the Face of Host Antimycobacterial Molecules

Studies of murine macrophages are a powerful means for dissecting the mechanisms of bacterial resistance to the host innate and adaptive immune responses. Immune activation and the induction of autophagy shift the balance of *M. tuberculosis* infection to benefit the host by promoting production of mycobactericidal molecules and the enhanced maturation of the *M. tuberculosis*-containing phagosome. Of note, activated macrophages express NADPH phagocyte oxidase (gp91phox) and inducible NOS2. The study of *M. tuberculosis* mutants in primary macrophages isolated from gp91^{phox}- and/or NOS2-deficient mice was essential to establishing the role of several *M. tuberculosis* systems in detoxifying ROI and RNI. The *M. tuberculosis* detoxifying systems such as superoxide dismutase (SodA), catalase (KatG), and NADH-dependent peroxidase and peroxynitrite reductase (comprising the proteins AhpC, AhpD, DlaT, and Lpd) are important for survival in macrophages, and *M. tuberculosis* strains with mutation in the encoding genes showed altered growth or survival in mouse models of infection (74–77).

An often-cited difference between human and mouse macrophages is the intensity and effect of NOS2 induction, resulting in the free radical NO. In contrast to the effective production of NO via mouse macrophages upon immune activation, human macrophages have a less potent NOS2 response due to structural promoter elements and posttranscriptional modifications (31). Specifically, epigenetic silencing by CpG (5′-C-phosphate-G-3′) methylation, histone modification, and chromatin structure results in the lack of iNOS mRNA and protein in human alveolar macrophages (32). This is not to say that NOS2 does not contribute to the control of human *M. tuberculosis* infection, since NOS2 is constitutively expressed by human upper airway epithelial cells (78) and upregulated in airway epithelial cells in an IFN-γ-dependent manner (79, 80). Although RNI production by human macrophages and other immune cells is relatively low, it is likely balanced by higher ROI production than that found in comparable murine cells (81).

Activated and autophagic macrophages also promote bacterial killing by delivering the bacterium to the lysosome, an acidic and hydrolytic compartment that is enriched with bactericidal peptides including Ub- and Fau-derived peptides (36, 37, 82). *In vitro* studies indicate that *M. tuberculosis* possesses systems to maintain pH homeostasis although the contribution of the *M. tuberculosis* cell wall to the bacterium's intrinsic resistance to the macrophage environment cannot be dismissed (83, 84). *M. tuberculosis* also encounters antimicrobial peptides delivered to the *M. tuberculosis*-containing phagosome. In human-derived macrophages vitamin D and TLR2 stimulation induce cathelicidin, which colocalizes with *M. tuberculosis*, resulting in bacterial death (85, 86). Hepcidin also colocalizes with *M. tuberculosis* in IFN-γ-activated mouse macrophages, although this molecule is not highly bactericidal for mycobacteria *in vitro* (87).

While many antimicrobial peptides are conserved between species, recent work on the role of sulfolipid-1 (SL-1) in *M. tuberculosis* suggests that potential differences exist between human and mouse peptides. SL-1 is a tetra-acylated trehalose-based glycolipid unique to pathogenic mycobacteria and expressed on the bacterial cell surface. An *M. tuberculosis* mutant deficient in SL-1 biosynthesis displayed increased resistance to cathelicidin *in vitro* and replicated better than wild-type *M. tuberculosis* in THP-1 monocyte-derived macrophages (88). This phenotype was not recapitulated in murine macrophages, suggesting the presence of an antimicrobial mechanism specific to the human macrophage. In addition, the mutant did not have a phenotype that differed from the wild type in the mouse model of infection. This study might shed some light on the conflicting results investigators have obtained with regard to SL-1's role in virulence.

Modulation of Cell Death Pathways

The infection of macrophages by *M. tuberculosis* can lead to host cell death via either apoptosis or necrosis. In general, necrosis is thought to be detrimental to the host, whereas apoptosis is associated with host innate defenses and control of bacterial replication (89). More virulent species and strains of mycobacteria appear to inhibit apoptosis and promote necrosis in human alveolar macrophages (90, 91). These observations were replicated in the more utilized murine cell lines and primary macrophages (92–94). Further use of these cells allowed investigators to show that the *M. tuberculosis* protein ESAT6 and the CpnT toxin promote the necrotic death of infected macrophages (95, 96).

Innate Immune Sensing and Downstream Proinflammatory Signaling

The host cell recognizes a number of *M. tuberculosis* ligands via surface and intracellular pattern recognition receptors and initiates a proinflammatory cytokine response (97). TLR2, TLR9, NOD2, Mincle, and STING all contribute to innate immune signaling in response to *M. tuberculosis* infection. In many of these cases, investigators capitalized on the availability of BMDM from knockout mice to demonstrate reduced cytokine response to intact bacteria or bacterial products in the absence of the pattern recognition receptor (98–102). While the roles of TNF and IFN in immunity to *M. tuberculosis* are well appreciated, infection of macrophages with *M. tuberculosis* also stimulates production of IL-1β. Experiments performed using BMDM from wild-type and NALP3-/- knockout mice demonstrated that *M. tuberculosis* induces IL-1β via the NLRP3 inflammasome: subsequent work showed that *M. tuberculosis* actively reduces the activation of this system by inducing IFN-γ and inhibits the AIM2-inflammasome in an ESX-1-dependent manner (103, 104).

In addition to their role in innate control of pathogens, macrophages also function as APCs. A key difference between mouse and human macrophages is the absence of CD1 molecules. CD1 is a major histocompatibility complex-like presentation molecule on APC that presents self and microbial lipid antigens. Humans express CD1a-e, whereas mice only express the CD1d molecule (105). This difference is particularly important in the context of *M. tuberculosis* infection since human CD1-restricted T cells have been identified that recognize mycobacterial lipids and glycolipids presented via CD1a, CD1b, and CD1c molecules (106–108). Specific presentation of *M. tuberculosis* glycolipids by macrophages and other APCs to T cells and natural killer (NK) T cells is a critical component of recognition by the adaptive immune system.

BEYOND THE MACROPHAGE: DEVELOPMENT OF MORE NUANCED *IN VITRO* MODELS TO INVESTIGATE MTB INFECTION

Although the macrophage is the host niche and the most studied cell type in the context of *M. tuberculosis* infection, it takes multiple cell types to eliminate the organism and develop immunity against subsequent exposures to the pathogen. Other cell types are encountered during initial infection, including neutrophils, epithelial cells, innate T cells, and NK cells. In this section we will discuss these cells and the *in vitro* coculture systems, including granuloma models that are being used to look at the contribution of these cells to an appropriate innate and subsequently successful adaptive immune response.

Neutrophils

Neutrophils are rapidly recruited to sites of infection and can destroy pathogens by oxidative and nonoxidative mechanisms. Neutrophils can release granules into the phagosome that contain lysozyme, antimicrobial peptides, and myeloperoxidase. They can also kill bacteria via intracellular ROS and phagosome-lysosome fusion. Polymorphonuclear leukocytes also form neutrophil extracellular traps (NETs), which bind microbes and contribute to their killing. NET release is associated with a type of cell death termed NETosis, which requires elastase, ROI, and myeloperoxidase (109). Neutrophils are important innate immune responders to infection but also appear to have a role throughout *M. tuberculosis* infection. Neutrophils represent the main cell population in bronchoalveolar lavage and sputum of patients with active tuberculosis and are present in the granu-

loma caseum (110). Neutrophils are also present in lung granulomas in mice and guinea pigs, indicating a role during chronic TB infection of these small animal models (111).

In vitro culture models have examined the mycobactericidal capacity of neutrophils. Some studies showed that opsonized *M. tuberculosis* was not killed by neutrophils following engulfment (112, 113). However, other studies showed that neutrophils kill *M. tuberculosis* or inhibit *M. tuberculosis* replication (114). The mechanism by which this occurred was unclear since NETosis of polymorphonuclear leukocytes does not appear to be involved with control of *M. tuberculosis* (115). A recently developed *in vitro* model provided a more nuanced look at the *M. tuberculosis*-neutrophil interaction. Exposure of *M. tuberculosis* to alveolar lining fluid prior to infection of neutrophils resulted in a 10 to 30% reduction in bacterial CFU within 6 hours of infection. The mechanism appears to be via the delivery of *M. tuberculosis* to the lysosome rather than through the involvement of apoptosis, necrosis, or NETosis of the infected cell. In conclusion, neutrophils likely contribute to *M. tuberculosis* killing, but the experimental evidence from *in vitro* models is inconsistent, likely because of differences in the experimental setup and handling of the cells between research groups. It should be noted that there are inherent technical difficulties associated with working with nonadherent cells, and investigators working with polymorphonuclear leukocytes are also constrained by the cell's short *in vitro* half-life of only 6 to 12 hours (112, 113).

Coculture Systems with Innate and Conventional T Cells

Only ~50% of household contacts living among people with active TB develop infection as evidenced by a positive TST reaction or interferon gamma response assay, highlighting the relevance of the lung epithelium and mucosal defense mechanisms in control of *M. tuberculosis* infection. *M. tuberculosis* can infect and easily replicate in alveolar epithelial cells *in vitro* (116–118). It is likely that it infects human lung epithelial cells, since *M. tuberculosis* DNA can be isolated from nonphagocytic lung tissue in humans (119). The contribution of epithelial cells to TB infections is largely underappreciated, but there is increasing evidence that they contribute to early recognition of *M. tuberculosis* infection and subsequent immune control. Human lung epithelial cell lines (BEAS-2B and A549 cells) and primary human large airway epithelial cells infected with *M. tuberculosis* efficiently process and present bacterial antigens to both classically and nonclassically restricted T cells, including those restricted by MR1 (118, 120).

Mucosal-associated invariant T (MAIT) cells, which are CD8+ T cells that express a semi-invariant T cell receptor and that are restricted by the nonclassical molecule MR-1, can detect intracellular infection by a number of pathogens including *M. tuberculosis* (121). Detection is due in part to the nature of the MR-1 ligands, which include riboflavin and vitamin B metabolites. MAIT cells are enriched in the human respiratory tract, where they are ideally placed to recognize and respond to *M. tuberculosis* infection (120). MAIT cells produce IFN-γ *in vitro* upon coculture with *M. tuberculosis*-infected airway epithelial cells, macrophages, or dendritic cells (118, 120). Underscoring their innate properties, recognition of *M. tuberculosis* infection occurred with MAIT cells from both *M. tuberculosis*-naive and -infected individuals. The full effector repertoire of MAIT cells remains to be determined, but as innate responders, these cells can rapidly respond to and likely play a role in control of early *M. tuberculosis* infection. Studies in mice show that MR-1 was required for wild-type control of *M. bovis* BCG infection (122). Although the MR1 molecule is highly conserved, it is worth noting that the number of MAIT cells in humans is significantly higher than in mice. We have looked at potential bactericidal functions of human MAITs *in vitro* using a coculture model. Our data show that coculture of *M. tuberculosis*-infected THP-1 or BEAS-2B cells with MAIT cells reduced bacterial viability by 80% and 250%, respectively, over 4 days (G. E. Purdy, data not shown).

Innate-functioning T cells also include the NK T cells that express a semi-invariant T cell receptor and are restricted by CD1d, which binds to lipid antigens including mycolic acid-containing glycoconjugates. A role for NK T cells in control of *M. tuberculosis* was demonstrated using *M. tuberculosis*-infected mouse macrophages cocultured with splenocytes from a naive mouse. These studies showed that NK T cells not only contained replication of *M. tuberculosis* but also stimulated *M. tuberculosis* killing (123). In coculture with *M. tuberculosis*-infected macrophages, splenocytes secreted IFN-γ and subsequently upregulated production of NO by the infected macrophages, presumably providing the antibacterial mechanism. These results are consistent with an early innate role for NKT cells during *M. tuberculosis* infection. Consistent results were obtained *in vitro* using *M. tuberculosis*-infected human monocytes in coculture with NK cells (124). There was

a 63% and 70% decrease in intracellular H37Rv using cells from PPD-positive and PPD-negative donors, respectively. Apoptosis of the infected monocytes was implicated as the bactericidal mechanism.

In addition to innate-functioning T cells, *in vitro* coculture systems also suggest the potential of CD4+ and CD8+ T cells to control *M. tuberculosis* in infected monocytes or macrophages. A 75% and 85% reduction in viable *M. tuberculosis* was observed upon coculture of *M. tuberculosis*-infected human monocyte-derived macrophages with autologous CD4+ and CD8+ T cells, respectively (125). In a separate household contact study, addition of autologous CD8+ T cells, but not CD4+ T cells, to *M. tuberculosis*-infected alveolar macrophages significantly reduced bacterial replication but was not bactericidal (126). The mechanism underlying the mycobactericidal activity observed for CD8+ T cells is their ability to recognize *M. tuberculosis*-infected cells and respond by secreting proinflammatory cytokines, exocytosing granules that induce apoptosis of the target cells and deliver antimicrobial peptides such as granulysin (127–129).

In Vitro Granuloma Models

Granulomas are the hallmark of TB infection, where the aforementioned cell types act in a coordinated fashion to wall off the bacteria. Granulomas can be considered a second line of defense by the immune system. There is some debate as to whether granuloma formation is the last best chance of the host to control infection or whether this is elicited by the bacteria as a safe place to replicate outside a macrophage (130). In the best-case scenario, this barricade is tightly formed and able to control microbial growth. However, examination of human and NHP TB infections reveals that the nature of granulomas is heterogeneous. The inner part of some granulomas is sterile, whereas others possess a large bacterial burden in the caseus or necrotic center (46). Although we have uncovered the cellular makeup of these granulomas from NHP, rabbit, and guinea pig models along with postautopsy clinical analysis, the initiation and progression of granuloma development during the course of TB infection remain unclear.

Until recently, granuloma formation had to be studied *in vivo* because this formation requires the coordination of both innate and adaptive immune cells. Several approaches have been taken to model granuloma formation *in vitro* using PBMCs. In the context of mycobacteria or mycobacterial antigens, the aggregation of cells occurs within days and can recapitulate the generation of mulitnucleated cells and epithelioid macrophages that associate with surrounding macrophages and lymphocytes (131). *In vitro* granuloma models using human PBMCs from TST-positive and TST-negative subjects showed that granuloma formation is faster, tighter, and more able to control the microbial burden in TST-positive donors compared to their TST-negative counterparts (132). Granuloma formation in humans is also associated with the presence of nonreplicating, persistent bacteria. This aspect of granuloma formation was achieved by embedding PBMCs and *M. tuberculosis* in a collagen matrix with dormancy confirmed by the loss of acid-fastness, accumulation of lipid droplets, and transcriptional profiling (133).

While not strictly an *in vitro* model, another system that has some merit is the use of *Mycobacterium marinum* in the zebra fish. While this model allows for live, real-time imaging of granuloma formation, a major caveat is the use of the surrogate organism *M. marinum* in a system that inherently lacks lymphocytes. That issue notwithstanding, these studies suggest that the initiation and progression of the granuloma is largely dictated by macrophages. Macrophage death induced via the *M. tuberculosis* Esx-1 secretion system forms the basis for the necrotic core of the newly forming granuloma. The number and type of macrophages that are recruited are both too low and skewed in their ability to effectively counter *M. tuberculosis* infection (134). The development of a three-dimensional computational model based on these data assessed how variables such as oxygen availability within the granuloma modified disease progression (135). Although these model systems do not mirror the exact nature of granulomas *in vivo*, they can provide insight into TB progression that is not limited by the expense of the NHP.

CONCLUSIONS

What have these *in vitro* models told us about *M. tuberculosis*, and how can we capitalize on this information to eradicate or prevent TB disease? They tell us that macrophages, even activated macrophages, are largely permissive to *M. tuberculosis* replication. Obviously *M. tuberculosis* has a number of mechanisms to resist killing by the host as illustrated by the number of *M. tuberculosis* mutants that have reduced survival in macrophages. Those *M. tuberculosis* mutants that show the greatest attenuation give some indication of which host-mediated pressures are the strongest. As discussed above, *M. tuberculosis* mutants that fail to arrest phagosome maturation or lack detoxifying enzymes are less able to survive or replicate in the macrophage. In addition, auxotrophic mutants have reduced

survival in macrophages, indicating that the bacterium is sensitive to nutrient restriction in the host. The severe attenuation of the methionine auxotroph in the mouse model relative to others suggests that, in the complex environment of the host, certain nutrients are more critical for the bacteria to survive (136). Macrophages do not act alone in the context of human disease, and coculture of *M. tuberculosis*-infected macrophages with T cells can achieve up to 1 log killing of the bacteria. Even exposure of the bacterium to human alveolar lining fluid increased killing of *M. tuberculosis* by monocyte-derived macrophages (137). With the use of increasingly sophisticated coculture models, we can tease apart the important variables for control of *M. tuberculosis*. Some of these, such as the methionine biosynthetic pathway, may be appealing targets for novel therapeutics, whereas others, such as the innate functioning T cell classes, may be modulated to provide more effective control via improved vaccination strategies.

The human immune system can successfully clear *M. tuberculosis*, but the trick is to establish effective mycobactericidal activity early in infection. Correlating with what is observed in the clinic, studies in the NHP model show that *M. tuberculosis* infection has variable outcomes. In-depth analysis of infected macaques revealed that granulomas exhibiting a range of histopathological features exist within an individual animal. After four weeks of infection, sterilization occurs in some lesions, while significant bacterial replication is apparent in others (138). Even animals with active disease possess sterilized granulomas. Further data from this model suggest that clearance of *M. tuberculosis* within the granuloma is maximally achieved with a coordinated innate and adaptive immune system (139). There is also heterogeneity within the bacterial population during infection. For this reason, *in vitro* infection of macrophages results in a percentage of *M. tuberculosis* delivered to the lysosome while the remainder of the bacterial cells arrest phagosome maturation and replicate. In the context of antibiotic treatment, a subpopulation of "persisters" remains in both the test tube and the human host. *In vitro* models that accurately mimic latency and the variety of granulomas encountered during human infection would facilitate our understanding of the signals *M. tuberculosis* senses to enter into a dormant state, the changes in its metabolism and physiology that permit it to resist host insults, and ultimately how and if it emerges from this quiescent state.

A better understanding of the early events in infection—before the establishment of granulomas and the emergence of nonreplicating persistent bacteria—

will greatly aid development of interventions. *In vitro* models in conjunction with small animal and NHP models of infection will continue to move the field forward and to find a way to kill *M. tuberculosis*. To finally address the question "Can a macrophage kill *M. tuberculosis*?" the short answer is yes. It has become more evident that the capacity of an individual to clear this pathogen requires a well-coordinated innate and adaptive immune system, and increasingly more complex *in vitro* studies will help us understand this disease one piece at a time.

Citation. Keiser TL, Purdy GE. 2017. Killing *Mycobacterium tuberculosis in vitro*: what model systems can teach us. Microbiol Spectrum 5(3):TBTB2-0028-2016.

References

1. **Anastasiou E, Mitchell PD.** 2013. Palaeopathology and genes: investigating the genetics of infectious diseases in excavated human skeletal remains and mummies from past populations. *Gene* 528:33–40.

2. **Comas I, Coscolla M, Luo T, Borrell S, Holt KE, Kato-Maeda M, Parkhill J, Malla B, Berg S, Thwaites G, Yeboah-Manu D, Bothamley G, Mei J, Wei L, Bentley S, Harris SR, Niemann S, Diel R, Aseffa A, Gao Q, Young D, Gagneux S.** 2013. Out-of-Africa migration and Neolithic coexpansion of *Mycobacterium tuberculosis* with modern humans. *Nat Genet* 45:1176–1182.

3. **Hmama Z, Peña-Díaz S, Joseph S, Av-Gay Y.** 2015. Immunoevasion and immunosuppression of the macrophage by *Mycobacterium tuberculosis*. *Immunol Rev* 264:220–232.

4. **Murray PJ, Wynn TA.** 2011. Protective and pathogenic functions of macrophage subsets. *Nat Rev Immunol* 11:723–737.

5. **Khan N, Vidyarthi A, Javed S, Agrewala JN.** 2016. Innate immunity holding the flanks until reinforced by adaptive immunity against *Mycobacterium tuberculosis* infection. *Front Microbiol* 7:328.

6. **Arango Duque G, Descoteaux A.** 2014. Macrophage cytokines: involvement in immunity and infectious diseases. *Front Immunol* 5:491.

7. **Rieder HL.** 1999. *Epidemiologic Basis of Tuberculosis Control*, p 17–43. International Union against Tuberculosis and Lung Disease, Paris, France.

8. **Sobota RS, Stein CM, Kodaman N, Scheinfeldt LB, Maro I, Wieland-Alter W, Igo RP Jr, Magohe A, Malone LL, Chervenak K, Hall NB, Modongo C, Zetola N, Matee M, Joloba M, Froment A, Nyambo TB, Moore JH, Scott WK, Lahey T, Boom WH, von Reyn CF, Tishkoff SA, Sirugo G, Williams SM.** 2016. A locus at 5q33.3 confers resistance to tuberculosis in highly susceptible individuals. *Am J Hum Genet* 98:514–524.

9. **Opie EL, Aronson JD.** 1927. Tubercle bacilli in latent tuberculous lesions in lung tissue without tuberculous lesions. *Arch Pathol Lab Med* 4:1–21.

10. **Canetti G.** 1946. *Le Bacille de Koch dans la Lésion Tuberculeuse du Poumon.* Éditions Médicales Flammarion, Paris, France.

11. **Suter E.** 1952. The multiplication of tubercle bacilli within normal phagocytes in tissue culture. *J Exp Med* 96:137–150.

12. **Raschke WC, Baird S, Ralph P, Nakoinz I.** 1978. Functional macrophage cell lines transformed by Abelson leukemia virus. *Cell* 15:261–267.

13. **Ralph P, Nakoinz I.** 1975. Phagocytosis and cytolysis by a macrophage tumour and its cloned cell line. *Nature* 257:393–394.

14. **Ralph P, Nakoinz I.** 1977. Antibody-dependent killing of erythrocyte and tumor targets by macrophage-related cell lines: enhancement by PPD and LPS. *J Immunol* 119:950–954.

15. **Ralph P, Nakoinz I.** 1981. Differences in antibody-dependent cellular cytotoxicity and activated killing of tumor cells by macrophage cell lines. *Cancer Res* 41:3546–3550.

16. **Indrigo J, Hunter RL Jr, Actor JK.** 2003. Cord factor trehalose 6,6′-dimycolate (TDM) mediates trafficking events during mycobacterial infection of murine macrophages. *Microbiology* 149:2049–2059.

17. **Perez RL, Roman J, Roser S, Little C, Olsen M, Indrigo J, Hunter RL, Actor JK.** 2000. Cytokine message and protein expression during lung granuloma formation and resolution induced by the mycobacterial cord factor trehalose-6,6′-dimycolate. *J Interferon Cytokine Res* 20:795–804.

18. **Rao V, Fujiwara N, Porcelli SA, Glickman MS.** 2005. Mycobacterium tuberculosis controls host innate immune activation through cyclopropane modification of a glycolipid effector molecule. *J Exp Med* 201:535–543.

19. **Rao V, Gao F, Chen B, Jacobs WR Jr, Glickman MS.** 2006. Trans-cyclopropanation of mycolic acids on trehalose dimycolate suppresses *Mycobacterium tuberculosis*-induced inflammation and virulence. *J Clin Invest* 116:1660–1667.

20. **Adams LB, Fukutomi Y, Krahenbuhl JL.** 1993. Regulation of murine macrophage effector functions by lipoarabinomannan from mycobacterial strains with different degrees of virulence. *Infect Immun* 61:4173–4181.

21. **Stuehr DJ, Marletta MA.** 1987. Synthesis of nitrite and nitrate in murine macrophage cell lines. *Cancer Res* 47:5590–5594.

22. **Radzioch D, Hudson T, Boulé M, Barrera L, Urbance JW, Varesio L, Skamene E.** 1991. Genetic resistance/susceptibility to mycobacteria: phenotypic expression in bone marrow derived macrophage lines. *J Leukoc Biol* 50:263–272.

23. **Blasi E, Mathieson BJ, Varesio L, Cleveland JL, Borchert PA, Rapp UR.** 1985. Selective immortalization of murine macrophages from fresh bone marrow by a raf/myc recombinant murine retrovirus. *Nature* 318:667–670.

24. **Manzanillo PS, Shiloh MU, Portnoy DA, Cox JS.** 2012. *Mycobacterium tuberculosis* activates the DNA-dependent cytosolic surveillance pathway within macrophages. *Cell Host Microbe* 11:469–480.

25. Mbawuike IN, Herscowitz HB. 1989. MH-S, a murine alveolar macrophage cell line: morphological, cytochemical, and functional characteristics. *J Leukoc Biol* **46**:119–127.

26. Melo MD, Stokes RW. 2000. Interaction of *Mycobacterium tuberculosis* with MH-S, an immortalized murine alveolar macrophage cell line: a comparison with primary murine macrophages. *Tuber Lung Dis* **80**:35–46.

27. Palleroni AV, Hajos S, Wright RB, Palleroni NJ. 1998. Nitric oxide synthase induction in lines of macrophages from different anatomical sites. *Cell Mol Biol* **44**:527–535.

28. Palleroni AV, Varesio L, Wright RB, Brunda MJ. 1991. Tumoricidal alveolar macrophage and tumor infiltrating macrophage cell lines. *Int J Cancer* **49**:296–302.

29. Walters SB, Dubnau E, Kolesnikova I, Laval F, Daffe M, Smith I. 2006. The *Mycobacterium tuberculosis* PhoPR two-component system regulates genes essential for virulence and complex lipid biosynthesis. *Mol Microbiol* **60**:312–330.

30. Kramnik I, Beamer G. 2016. Mouse models of human TB pathology: roles in the analysis of necrosis and the development of host-directed therapies. *Semin Immunopathol* **38**:221–237.

31. Bogdan C. 2015. Nitric oxide synthase in innate and adaptive immunity: an update. *Trends Immunol* **36**:161–178.

32. Gross TJ, Kremens K, Powers LS, Brink B, Knutson T, Domann FE, Philibert RA, Milhem MM, Monick MM. 2014. Epigenetic silencing of the human NOS2 gene: rethinking the role of nitric oxide in human macrophage inflammatory responses. *J Immunol* **192**:2326–2338.

33. Rengarajan J, Bloom BR, Rubin EJ. 2005. Genome-wide requirements for *Mycobacterium tuberculosis* adaptation and survival in macrophages. *Proc Natl Acad Sci USA* **102**:8327–8332.

34. Ehrt S, Schnappinger D, Bekiranov S, Drenkow J, Shi S, Gingeras TR, Gaasterland T, Schoolnik G, Nathan C. 2001. Reprogramming of the macrophage transcriptome in response to interferon-gamma and *Mycobacterium tuberculosis*: signaling roles of nitric oxide synthase-2 and phagocyte oxidase. *J Exp Med* **194**:1123–1140.

35. Homolka S, Niemann S, Russell DG, Rohde KH. 2010. Functional genetic diversity among *Mycobacterium tuberculosis* complex clinical isolates: delineation of conserved core and lineage-specific transcriptomes during intracellular survival. *PLoS Pathog* **6**:e1000988.

36. Alonso S, Pethe K, Russell DG, Purdy GE. 2007. Lysosomal killing of *Mycobacterium* mediated by ubiquitin-derived peptides is enhanced by autophagy. *Proc Natl Acad Sci USA* **104**:6031–6036.

37. Ponpuak M, Davis AS, Roberts EA, Delgado MA, Dinkins C, Zhao Z, Virgin HW IV, Kyei GB, Johansen T, Vergne I, Deretic V. 2010. Delivery of cytosolic components by autophagic adaptor protein p62 endows autophagosomes with unique antimicrobial properties. *Immunity* **32**:329–341.

38. Flesch IE, Kaufmann SH. 1990. Activation of tuberculostatic macrophage functions by gamma interferon,

interleukin-4, and tumor necrosis factor. *Infect Immun* **58**:2675–2677.

39. Via LE, Fratti RA, McFalone M, Pagan-Ramos E, Deretic D, Deretic V. 1998. Effects of cytokines on mycobacterial phagosome maturation. *J Cell Sci* **111**:897–905.

40. Schaible UE, Sturgill-Koszycki S, Schlesinger PH, Russell DG. 1998. Cytokine activation leads to acidification and increases maturation of *Mycobacterium avium*-containing phagosomes in murine macrophages. *J Immunol* **160**:1290–1296.

41. Briken V, Ahlbrand SE, Shah S. 2013. *Mycobacterium tuberculosis* and the host cell inflammasome: a complex relationship. *Front Cell Infect Microbiol* **3**:62

42. Pelegrin P, Surprenant A. 2009. The P2X(7) receptor-pannexin connection to dye uptake and IL-1beta release. *Purinergic Signal* **5**:129–137.

43. Damiani G, Kiyotaki C, Soeller W, Sasada M, Peisach J, Bloom BR. 1980. Macrophage variants in oxygen metabolism. *J Exp Med* **152**:808–822.

44. Chan J, Xing Y, Magliozzo RS, Bloom BR. 1992. Killing of virulent *Mycobacterium tuberculosis* by reactive nitrogen intermediates produced by activated murine macrophages. *J Exp Med* **175**:1111–1122.

45. Jayaswal S, Kamal MA, Dua R, Gupta S, Majumdar T, Das G, Kumar D, Rao KV. 2010. Identification of host-dependent survival factors for intracellular *Mycobacterium tuberculosis* through an siRNA screen. *PLoS Pathog* **6**:e1000839.

46. Flynn JL, Gideon HP, Mattila JT, Lin PL. 2015. Immunology studies in non-human primate models of tuberculosis. *Immunol Rev* **264**:60–73.

47. Lin PL, Myers A, Smith L, Bigbee C, Bigbee M, Fuhrman C, Grieser H, Chiosea I, Voitenek NN, Capuano SV, Klein E, Flynn JL. 2010. Tumor necrosis factor neutralization results in disseminated disease in acute and latent *Mycobacterium tuberculosis* infection with normal granuloma structure in a cynomolgus macaque model. *Arthritis Rheum* **62**:340–350.

48. Diedrich CR, Mattila JT, Klein E, Janssen C, Phuah J, Sturgeon TJ, Montelaro RC, Lin PL, Flynn JL. 2010. Reactivation of latent tuberculosis in cynomolgus macaques infected with SIV is associated with early peripheral T cell depletion and not virus load. *PLoS One* **5**:e9611.

49. Mehra S, Golden NA, Dutta NK, Midkiff CC, Alvarez X, Doyle LA, Asher M, Russell-Lodrigue K, Monjure C, Roy CJ, Blanchard JL, Didier PJ, Veazey RS, Lackner AA, Kaushal D. 2011. Reactivation of latent tuberculosis in rhesus macaques by coinfection with simian immunodeficiency virus. *J Med Primatol* **40**:233–243.

50. Dutta NK, Karakousis PC. 2014. Latent tuberculosis infection: myths, models, and molecular mechanisms. *Microbiol Mol Biol Rev* **78**:343–371.

51. Zinman G, Brower-Sinning R, Emeche CH, Ernst J, Huang GT, Mahony S, Myers AJ, O'Dee DM, Flynn JL, Nau GJ, Ross TM, Salter RD, Benos PV, Bar Joseph Z, Morel PA. 2011. Large scale comparison of innate responses to viral and bacterial pathogens in mouse and macaque. *PLoS One* **6**:e22401.

52. Pacheco SA, Powers KM, Engelmann F, Messaoudi I, Purdy GE. 2013. Autophagic killing effects against *Mycobacterium tuberculosis* by alveolar macrophages from young and aged rhesus macaques. *PLoS One* 8: e66985.

53. Gautam US, Mehra S, Ahsan MH, Alvarez X, Niu T, Kaushal D. 2014. Role of TNF in the altered interaction of dormant *Mycobacterium tuberculosis* with host macrophages. *PLoS One* 9:e95220.

54. Tsuchiya S, Kobayashi Y, Goto Y, Okumura H, Nakae S, Konno T, Tada K. 1982. Induction of maturation in cultured human monocytic leukemia cells by a phorbol diester. *Cancer Res* 42:1530–1536.

55. Schwende H, Fitzke E, Ambs P, Dieter P. 1996. Differences in the state of differentiation of THP-1 cells induced by phorbol ester and 1,25-dihydroxyvitamin D3. *J Leukoc Biol* 59:555–561.

56. Daigneault M, Preston JA, Marriott HM, Whyte MK, Dockrell DH. 2010. The identification of markers of macrophage differentiation in PMA-stimulated THP-1 cells and monocyte-derived macrophages. *PLoS One* 5:e8668.

57. Schlesinger LS. 1993. Macrophage phagocytosis of virulent but not attenuated strains of *Mycobacterium tuberculosis* is mediated by mannose receptors in addition to complement receptors. *J Immunol* 150:2920–2930.

58. Schlesinger LS. 1996. Role of mononuclear phagocytes in *M tuberculosis* pathogenesis. *J Investig Med* 44: 312–323.

59. Takahashi K, Okita K, Nakagawa M, Yamanaka S. 2007. Induction of pluripotent stem cells from fibroblast cultures. *Nat Protoc* 2:3081–3089.

60. Karlsson KR, Cowley S, Martinez FO, Shaw M, Minger SL, James W. 2008. Homogeneous monocytes and macrophages from human embryonic stem cells following coculture-free differentiation in M-CSF and IL-3. *Exp Hematol* 36:1167–1175.

61. van Wilgenburg B, Browne C, Vowles J, Cowley SA. 2013. Efficient, long term production of monocyte-derived macrophages from human pluripotent stem cells under partly-defined and fully-defined conditions. *PLoS One* 8:e71098.

62. van Wilgenburg B, Moore MD, James WS, Cowley SA. 2014. The productive entry pathway of HIV-1 in macrophages is dependent on endocytosis through lipid rafts containing CD4. *PLoS One* 9:e86071.

63. Verma RK, Agrawal AK, Singh AK, Mohan M, Gupta A, Gupta P, Gupta UD, Misra A. 2013. Inhalable microparticles of nitric oxide donors induce phagosome maturation and kill *Mycobacterium tuberculosis*. *Tuberculosis (Edinb)* 93:412–417.

64. Jordao L, Bleck CK, Mayorga L, Griffiths G, Anes E. 2008. On the killing of mycobacteria by macrophages. *Cell Microbiol* 10:529–548 10.1111/j.1462-5822.2007. 01067.x.

65. Sturgill-Koszycki S, Schlesinger PH, Chakraborty P, Haddix PL, Collins HL, Fok AK, Allen RD, Gluck SL, Heuser J, Russell DG. 1994. Lack of acidification in *Mycobacterium* phagosomes produced by exclusion of the vesicular proton-ATPase. *Science* 263:678–681.

66. Clemens DL, Lee BY, Horwitz MA. 2000. Deviant expression of Rab5 on phagosomes containing the intracellular pathogens *Mycobacterium tuberculosis* and *Legionella pneumophila* is associated with altered phagosomal fate. *Infect Immun* 68:2671–2684.

67. Via LE, Deretic D, Ulmer RJ, Hibler NS, Huber LA, Deretic V. 1997. Arrest of mycobacterial phagosome maturation is caused by a block in vesicle fusion between stages controlled by rab5 and rab7. *J Biol Chem* 272:13326–13331.

68. d'Arcy Hart P. 1975. Response of macrophages to bacterial infection with special reference to their lysosomes. *Pathol Biol (Paris)* 23:451–452.

69. Vergne I, Chua J, Deretic V. 2003. Tuberculosis toxin blocking phagosome maturation inhibits a novel Ca2+/calmodulin-PI3K hVPS34 cascade. *J Exp Med* 198:653–659.

70. Vergne I, Fratti RA, Hill PJ, Chua J, Belisle J, Deretic V. 2004. *Mycobacterium tuberculosis* phagosome maturation arrest: mycobacterial phosphatidylinositol analog phosphatidylinositol mannoside stimulates early endosomal fusion. *Mol Biol Cell* 15:751–760.

71. Pethe K, Swenson DL, Alonso S, Anderson J, Wang C, Russell DG. 2004. Isolation of *Mycobacterium tuberculosis* mutants defective in the arrest of phagosome maturation. *Proc Natl Acad Sci USA* 101:13642–13647.

72. MacGurn JA, Cox JS. 2007. A genetic screen for *Mycobacterium tuberculosis* mutants defective for phagosome maturation arrest identifies components of the ESX-1 secretion system. *Infect Immun* 75:2668–2678.

73. Baker JJ, Johnson BK, Abramovitch RB. 2014. Slow growth of *Mycobacterium tuberculosis* at acidic pH is regulated by phoPR and host-associated carbon sources. *Mol Microbiol* 94:56–69.

74. Ng VH, Cox JS, Sousa AO, MacMicking JD, McKinney JD. 2004. Role of KatG catalase-peroxidase in mycobacterial pathogenesis: countering the phagocyte oxidative burst. *Mol Microbiol* 52:1291–1302.

75. Edwards KM, Cynamon MH, Voladri RK, Hager CC, DeStefano MS, Tham KT, Lakey DL, Bochan MR, Kernodle DS. 2001. Iron-cofactored superoxide dismutase inhibits host responses to *Mycobacterium tuberculosis*. *Am J Respir Crit Care Med* 164:2213–2219.

76. Dussurget O, Stewart G, Neyrolles O, Pescher P, Young D, Marchal G. 2001. Role of *Mycobacterium tuberculosis* copper-zinc superoxide dismutase. *Infect Immun* 69:529–533.

77. Shi S, Ehrt S. 2006. Dihydrolipoamide acyltransferase is critical for *Mycobacterium tuberculosis* pathogenesis. *Infect Immun* 74:56–63.

78. Guo FH, De Raeve HR, Rice TW, Stuehr DJ, Thunnissen FB, Erzurum SC. 1995. Continuous nitric oxide synthesis by inducible nitric oxide synthase in normal human airway epithelium *in vivo*. *Proc Natl Acad Sci USA* 92: 7809–7813.

79. Asano K, Chee CB, Gaston B, Lilly CM, Gerard C, Drazen JM, Stamler JS. 1994. Constitutive and inducible nitric oxide synthase gene expression, regulation, and activity in human lung epithelial cells. *Proc Natl Acad Sci USA* 91:10089–10093.

80. Guo FH, Uetani K, Haque SJ, Williams BR, Dweik RA, Thunnissen FB, Calhoun W, Erzurum SC. 1997. Interferon gamma and interleukin 4 stimulate prolonged expression of inducible nitric oxide synthase in human airway epithelium through synthesis of soluble mediators. *J Clin Invest* **100**:829–838.

81. Wink DA, Hines HB, Cheng RY, Switzer CH, Flores-Santana W, Vitek MP, Ridnour LA, Colton CA. 2011. Nitric oxide and redox mechanisms in the immune response. *J Leukoc Biol* **89**:873–891.

82. Gutierrez MG, Master SS, Singh SB, Taylor GA, Colombo MI, Deretic V. 2004. Autophagy is a defense mechanism inhibiting BCG and *Mycobacterium tuberculosis* survival in infected macrophages. *Cell* **119**: 753–766.

83. Vandal OH, Pierini LM, Schnappinger D, Nathan CF, Ehrt S. 2008. A membrane protein preserves intrabacterial pH in intraphagosomal *Mycobacterium tuberculosis*. *Nat Med* **14**:849–854.

84. Purdy GE, Niederweis M, Russell DG. 2009. Decreased outer membrane permeability protects mycobacteria from killing by ubiquitin-derived peptides. *Mol Microbiol* **73**:844–857.

85. Liu PT, Stenger S, Li H, Wenzel L, Tan BH, Krutzik SR, Ochoa MT, Schauber J, Wu K, Meinken C, Kamen DL, Wagner M, Bals R, Steinmeyer A, Zügel U, Gallo RL, Eisenberg D, Hewison M, Hollis BW, Adams JS, Bloom BR, Modlin RL. 2006. Toll-like receptor triggering of a vitamin D-mediated human antimicrobial response. *Science* **311**:1770–1773.

86. Liu PT, Stenger S, Tang DH, Modlin RL. 2007. Cutting edge: vitamin D-mediated human antimicrobial activity against *Mycobacterium tuberculosis* is dependent on the induction of cathelicidin. *J Immunol* **179**: 2060–2063.

87. Sow FB, Florence WC, Satoskar AR, Schlesinger LS, Zwilling BS, Lafuse WP. 2007. Expression and localization of hepcidin in macrophages: a role in host defense against tuberculosis. *J Leukoc Biol* **82**:934–945.

88. Gilmore SA, Schelle MW, Holsclaw CM, Leigh CD, Jain M, Cox JS, Leary JA, Bertozzi CR. 2012. Sulfolipid-1 biosynthesis restricts *Mycobacterium tuberculosis* growth in human macrophages. *ACS Chem Biol* **7**:863–870.

89. Behar SM, Martin CJ, Booty MG, Nishimura T, Zhao X, Gan HX, Divangahi M, Remold HG. 2011. Apoptosis is an innate defense function of macrophages against *Mycobacterium tuberculosis*. *Mucosal Immunol* **4**:279–287.

90. Keane J, Balcewicz-Sablinska MK, Remold HG, Chupp GL, Meek BB, Fenton MJ, Kornfeld H. 1997. Infection by *Mycobacterium tuberculosis* promotes human alveolar macrophage apoptosis. *Infect Immun* **65**:298–304.

91. Keane J, Remold HG, Kornfeld H. 2000. Virulent *Mycobacterium tuberculosis* strains evade apoptosis of infected alveolar macrophages. *J Immunol* **164**:2016–2020.

92. Gan H, Lee J, Ren F, Chen M, Kornfeld H, Remold HG. 2008. *Mycobacterium tuberculosis* blocks cross linking of annexin-1 and apoptotic envelope formation on infected macrophages to maintain virulence. *Nat Immunol* **9**:1189–1197.

93. Divangahi M, Chen M, Gan H, Desjardins D, Hickman TT, Lee DM, Fortune S, Behar SM, Remold HG. 2009. *Mycobacterium tuberculosis* evades macrophage defenses by inhibiting plasma membrane repair. *Nat Immunol* **10**:899–906.

94. Keane J, Shurtleff B, Kornfeld H. 2002. TNF-dependent BALB/c murine macrophage apoptosis following *Mycobacterium tuberculosis* infection inhibits bacillary growth in an IFN-gamma independent manner. *Tuberculosis (Edinb)* **82**:55–61.

95. Wong KW, Jacobs WR Jr. 2011. Critical role for NLRP3 in necrotic death triggered by *Mycobacterium tuberculosis*. *Cell Microbiol* **13**:1371–1384.

96. Sun J, Siroy A, Lokareddy RK, Speer A, Doornbos KS, Cingolani G, Niederweis M. 2015. The tuberculosis necrotizing toxin kills macrophages by hydrolyzing NAD. *Nat Struct Mol Biol* **22**:672–678.

97. Cooper AM, Mayer-Barber KD, Sher A. 2011. Role of innate cytokines in mycobacterial infection. *Mucosal Immunol* **4**:252–260.

98. Underhill DM, Ozinsky A, Smith KD, Aderem A. 1999. Toll-like receptor-2 mediates mycobacteria-induced proinflammatory signaling in macrophages. *Proc Natl Acad Sci USA* **96**:14459–14463.

99. Bafica A, Scanga CA, Feng CG, Leifer C, Cheever A, Sher A. 2005. TLR9 regulates Th1 responses and cooperates with TLR2 in mediating optimal resistance to *Mycobacterium tuberculosis*. *J Exp Med* **202**: 1715–1724.

100. Schoenen H, Bodendorfer B, Hitchens K, Manzanero S, Werninghaus K, Nimmerjahn F, Agger EM, Stenger S, Andersen P, Ruland J, Brown GD, Wells C, Lang R. 2010. Cutting edge: mincle is essential for recognition and adjuvanticity of the mycobacterial cord factor and its synthetic analog trehalose-dibehenate. *J Immunol* **184**:2756–2760.

101. Watson RO, Bell SL, MacDuff DA, Kimmey JM, Diner EJ, Olivas J, Vance RE, Stallings CL, Virgin HW, Cox JS. 2015. The cytosolic sensor cGAS detects *Mycobacterium tuberculosis* DNA to induce type I interferons and activate autophagy. *Cell Host Microbe* **17**:811–819.

102. Pandey AK, Yang Y, Jiang Z, Fortune SM, Coulombe F, Behr MA, Fitzgerald KA, Sassetti CM, Kelliher MA. 2009. NOD2, RIP2 and IRF5 play a critical role in the type I interferon response to *Mycobacterium tuberculosis*. *PLoS Pathog* **5**:e1000500.

103. Shah S, Bohsali A, Ahlbrand SE, Srinivasan L, Rathinam VA, Vogel SN, Fitzgerald KA, Sutterwala FS, Briken V. 2013. Cutting edge: mycobacterium tuberculosis but not nonvirulent mycobacteria inhibits IFN-β and AIM2 inflammasome-dependent IL-1β production via its ESX-1 secretion system. *J Immunol* **191**:3514–3518.

104. Stanley SA, Johndrow JE, Manzanillo P, Cox JS. 2007. The Type I IFN response to infection with *Mycobacterium tuberculosis* requires ESX-1-mediated secretion and contributes to pathogenesis. *J Immunol* **178**: 3143–3152.

105. Dutronc Y, Porcelli SA. 2002. The CD1 family and T cell recognition of lipid antigens. *Tissue Antigens* 60: 337–353.

106. Moody DB, Reinhold BB, Guy MR, Beckman EM, Frederique DE, Furlong ST, Ye S, Reinhold VN, Sieling PA, Modlin RL, Besra GS, Porcelli SA. 1997. Structural requirements for glycolipid antigen recognition by CD1b-restricted T cells. *Science* 278:283–286.

107. Van Rhijn I, Ly D, Moody DB. 2013. CD1a, CD1b, and CD1c in immunity against mycobacteria. *Adv Exp Med Biol* 783:181–197.

108. Moody DB, Ulrichs T, Mühlecker W, Young DC, Gurcha SS, Grant E, Rosat JP, Brenner MB, Costello CE, Besra GS, Porcelli SA. 2000. CD1c-mediated T-cell recognition of isoprenoid glycolipids in *Mycobacterium tuberculosis* infection. *Nature* 404:884–888.

109. Brinkmann V, Zychlinsky A. 2007. Beneficial suicide: why neutrophils die to make NETs. *Nat Rev Microbiol* 5:577–582.

110. Eum SY, Kong JH, Hong MS, Lee YJ, Kim JH, Hwang SH, Cho S-N, Via LE, Barry CE III. 2010. Neutrophils are the predominant infected phagocytic cells in the airways of patients with active pulmonary TB. *Chest* 137:122–128.

111. Orme IM. 2014. A new unifying theory of the pathogenesis of tuberculosis. *Tuberculosis (Edinb)* 94:8–14.

112. Denis M. 1991. Human neutrophils, activated with cytokines or not, do not kill virulent *Mycobacterium tuberculosis*. *J Infect Dis* 163:919–920.

113. Corleis B, Korbel D, Wilson R, Bylund J, Chee R, Schaible UE. 2012. Escape of *Mycobacterium tuberculosis* from oxidative killing by neutrophils. *Cell Microbiol* 14:1109–1121.

114. Martineau AR, Newton SM, Wilkinson KA, Kampmann B, Hall BM, Nawroly N, Packe GE, Davidson RN, Griffiths CJ, Wilkinson RJ. 2007. Neutrophil-mediated innate immune resistance to mycobacteria. *J Clin Invest* 117:1988–1994.

115. Ramos-Kichik V, Mondragón-Flores R, Mondragón-Castelán M, Gonzalez-Pozos S, Muñiz-Hernandez S, Rojas-Espinosa O, Chacón-Salinas R, Estrada-Parra S, Estrada-García I. 2009. Neutrophil extracellular traps are induced by *Mycobacterium tuberculosis*. *Tuberculosis (Edinb)* 89:29–37.

116. McDonough KA, Kress Y. 1995. Cytotoxicity for lung epithelial cells is a virulence-associated phenotype of *Mycobacterium tuberculosis*. *Infect Immun* 63: 4802–4811.

117. Bermudez LE, Goodman J. 1996. *Mycobacterium tuberculosis* invades and replicates within type II alveolar cells. *Infect Immun* 64:1400–1406.

118. Harriff MJ, Cansler ME, Toren KG, Canfield ET, Kwak S, Gold MC, Lewinsohn DM. 2014. Human lung epithelial cells contain Mycobacterium tuberculosis in a late endosomal vacuole and are efficiently recognized by CD8+ T cells. *PLoS One* 9:e97515.

119. Hernández-Pando R, Jeyanathan M, Mengistu G, Aguilar D, Orozco H, Harboe M, Rook GA, Bjune G. 2000. Persistence of DNA from *Mycobacterium tuber-culosis* in superficially normal lung tissue during latent infection. *Lancet* 356:2133–2138.

120. Gold MC, Cerri S, Smyk-Pearson S, Cansler ME, Vogt TM, Delepine J, Winata E, Swarbrick GM, Chua WJ, Yu YY, Lantz O, Cook MS, Null MD, Jacoby DB, Harriff MJ, Lewinsohn DA, Hansen TH, Lewinsohn DM. 2010. Human mucosal associated invariant T cells detect bacterially infected cells. *PLoS Biol* 8: e1000407.

121. Gold MC, Napier RJ, Lewinsohn DM. 2015. MR1-restricted mucosal associated invariant T (MAIT) cells in the immune response to *Mycobacterium tuberculosis*. *Immunol Rev* 264:154–166.

122. Chua WJ, Truscott SM, Eickhoff CS, Blazevic A, Hoft DF, Hansen TH. 2012. Polyclonal mucosa-associated invariant T cells have unique innate functions in bacterial infection. *Infect Immun* 80:3256–3267.

123. Sada-Ovalle I, Chiba A, Gonzales A, Brenner MB, Behar SM. 2008. Innate invariant NKT cells recognize *Mycobacterium tuberculosis*-infected macrophages, produce interferon-gamma, and kill intracellular bacteria. *PLoS Pathog* 4:e1000239.

124. Brill KJ, Li Q, Larkin R, Canaday DH, Kaplan DR, Boom WH, Silver RF. 2001. Human natural killer cells mediate killing of intracellular *Mycobacterium tuberculosis* H37Rv via granule-independent mechanisms. *Infect Immun* 69:1755–1765.

125. Canaday DH, Wilkinson RJ, Li Q, Harding CV, Silver RF, Boom WH. 2001. CD4(+) and CD8(+) T cells kill intracellular *Mycobacterium tuberculosis* by a perforin and Fas/Fas ligand-independent mechanism. *J Immunol* 167:2734–2742.

126. Carranza C, Juárez E, Torres M, Ellner JJ, Sada E, Schwander SK. 2006. *Mycobacterium tuberculosis* growth control by lung macrophages and CD8 cells from patient contacts. *Am J Respir Crit Care Med* 173: 238–245.

127. Stenger S, Hanson DA, Teitelbaum R, Dewan P, Niazi KR, Froelich CJ, Ganz T, Thoma-Uszynski S, Melián A, Bogdan C, Porcelli SA, Bloom BR, Krensky AM, Modlin RL. 1998. An antimicrobial activity of cytolytic T cells mediated by granulysin. *Science* 282:121–125.

128. Stenger S, Mazzaccaro RJ, Uyemura K, Cho S, Barnes PF, Rosat JP, Sette A, Brenner MB, Porcelli SA, Bloom BR, Modlin RL. 1997. Differential effects of cytolytic T cell subsets on intracellular infection. *Science* 276:1684–1687.

129. Tan BH, Meinken C, Bastian M, Bruns H, Legaspi A, Ochoa MT, Krutzik SR, Bloom BR, Ganz T, Modlin RL, Stenger S. 2006. Macrophages acquire neutrophil granules for antimicrobial activity against intracellular pathogens. *J Immunol* 177:1864–1871.

130. Paige C, Bishai WR. 2010. Penitentiary or penthouse condo: the tuberculous granuloma from the microbe's point of view. *Cell Microbiol* 12:301–309.

131. Puissegur MP, Botanch C, Duteyrat JL, Delsol G, Caratero C, Altare F. 2004. An *in vitro* dual model of mycobacterial granulomas to investigate the molecular interactions between mycobacteria and human host cells. *Cell Microbiol* 6:423–433.

132. Guirado E, Mbawuike U, Keiser TL, Arcos J, Azad AK, Wang SH, Schlesinger LS. 2015. Characterization of host and microbial determinants in individuals with latent tuberculosis infection using a human granuloma model. *MBio* **6:**e02537–e14.

133. Kapoor N, Pawar S, Sirakova TD, Deb C, Warren WL, Kolattukudy PE. 2013. Human granuloma *in vitro* model, for TB dormancy and resuscitation. *PLoS One* **8:**e53657.

134. Pagán AJ, Ramakrishnan L. 2014. Immunity and immunopathology in the tuberculous granuloma. *Cold Spring Harb Perspect Med* **5:**a018499.

135. Sershen CL, Plimpton SJ, May EE. 2016. Oxygen modulates the effectiveness of granuloma mediated host response to *Mycobacterium tuberculosis*: a multiscale computational biology approach. *Front Cell Infect Microbiol* **6:**6.

136. Berney M, Berney-Meyer L, Wong KW, Chen B, Chen M, Kim J, Wang J, Harris D, Parkhill J, Chan J, Wang F, Jacobs WR Jr. 2015. Essential roles of methio-

nine and S-adenosylmethionine in the autarkic lifestyle of *Mycobacterium tuberculosis*. *Proc Natl Acad Sci USA* **112:**10008–10013.

137. Arcos J, Sasindran SJ, Fujiwara N, Turner J, Schlesinger LS, Torrelles JB. 2011. Human lung hydrolases delineate *Mycobacterium tuberculosis*-macrophage interactions and the capacity to control infection. *J Immunol* **187:**372–381.

138. Lin PL, Ford CB, Coleman MT, Myers AJ, Gawande R, Ioerger T, Sacchettini J, Fortune SM, Flynn JL. 2014. Sterilization of granulomas is common in active and latent tuberculosis despite within-host variability in bacterial killing. *Nat Med* **20:**75–79.

139. Gideon HP, Phuah J, Myers AJ, Bryson BD, Rodgers MA, Coleman MT, Maiello P, Rutledge T, Marino S, Fortune SM, Kirschner DE, Lin PL, Flynn JL. 2015. Variability in tuberculosis granuloma T cell responses exists, but a balance of pro- and anti-inflammatory cytokines is associated with sterilization. *PLoS Pathog* **11:**e1004603.

Tuberculosis and the Tubercle Bacillus, 2nd ed.
Edited by William R. Jacobs, Jr., Helen McShane, Valerie Mizrahi, and Ian M. Orme
© 2018 American Society for Microbiology, Washington, DC
doi:10.1128/microbiolspec.TBTB2-0005-2015

Epigenetic Phosphorylation Control of *Mycobacterium tuberculosis* Infection and Persistence

26

Melissa Richard-Greenblatt and Yossef Av-Gay

PROTEIN PHOSPHORYLATION IN *MYCOBACTERIUM TUBERCULOSIS*

Protein phosphorylation is known to occur across all three kingdoms of life; however, the study of posttranslational modification in bacteria was neglected for a considerable amount of time. Early attempts to detect its presence were unsuccessful, generating the dogma that protein phosphorylation was a regulatory mechanism that emerged late in evolution to meet the needs of organisms composed of multiple and differentiated cells. The pioneering work of several groups in the 1970s identified protein kinase activity in both *Escherichia coli* and *Salmonella typhimurium* (1–3), which soon led to the discovery of the histidine/aspartate kinases of the two-component systems (4, 5). The first aspect of this system involves the stimulation of a histidine kinase by a particular environmental or intracellular signal resulting in autophosphorylation on a key histidine residue. The phospho-histidine can then be used as a substrate by the cognate response regulator for its own autophosphorylation on an aspartate residue. The majority of response regulators are DNA binding proteins that trigger expression from target promoters. Unlike the cross-reactivity observed with serine/threonine/tyrosine (Ser/Thr/Tyr) kinases in eukaryotic cell signaling cascades, two-component systems work in isolation, where a given pairing of histidine kinase and response regulator is highly selective for each other via protein-protein interaction.

During the initial phase of the two-component system discovery, these systems were regarded as the major signal transduction pathway in bacteria, which led to the hypothesis that Ser/Thr/Tyr phosphorylation was a eukaryotic trait, whereas His/Asp phosphorylation was exclusive to prokaryotes. Since this time, our knowledge of protein phosphorylation has been revised. Hundreds of two-component systems have been discovered in eukaryotic cells (6), and recent genomic data indicate that "eukaryotic-like" Ser/Thr protein kinases (STPKs) are as prevalent in prokaryotes as in their histidine kinase counterparts (7). However, two-component systems remain the main signaling mechanism in all phyla of bacteria, with STPKs most abundant among *Acidobacteria*, *Actinobacteria* (including the genus *Mycobacterium*), various groups of *Cyanobacteria*, as well as bacteria belonging to the order of *Myxococcales*.

The pathogenic success of *M. tuberculosis* is largely dependent on its ability to sense and adapt to the dynamic environment of the host. As a result, *M. tuberculosis* has evolved an extensive intracellular signaling network consisting of 12 paired two-component regulatory systems (also including 4 orphan regulators), 11 STPKs, a single tyrosine kinase, and 3 phosphatases, which have been extensively reviewed in the past 2 decades (8–10). The presence of Ser/Thr and Tyr protein kinases, and two-component systems that phosphorylate substrates on Asp, enables the cell to generate phosphorylated residues with far greater stability. Generally, the hydrolytic half-time of phosphoryl-asp is only a couple of hours, whereas Ser/Thr/Tyr phosphoresters, or *O*-phosphorylation, can produce signals that remain stable for weeks and require a phosphatase to be reversed (11). Consequently, *M. tuberculosis* uses phosphoryl-asp for rapid, short-term signal transduction and Ser/Thr/Tyr phosphorylation for long-term,

Division of Infectious Diseases, Department of Medicine, University of British Columbia, Vancouver, BC V6H 3Z6, Canada.

Table 1 Biochemically verified substrates of *M. tuberculosis* serine/threonine protein kinases[a]

Kinase	Substrate function	Substrate
PknA (Rv0015c)	Cell division	FipA (179), FtsZ (85), ParB (180), Wag31 (66)
	Arabinan biosynthesis	EmbR (181)
	MA biosynthesis	KasA (101), KasB (101), FabD (101), FabH (102), HadAB/BC (99), InhA (97,98), MabA (96)
	PG biosynthesis	MurD (74)
	TCA cycle	Mdh (172)
	Methionine cycle	SahH (182)
	Signaling	PstP (183), PtkA (22)
	Protein chaperone	GroEL1 (184)
	Proteasome	PrcA (56)
	Hypothetical	Rv1422/CuvA (66)
PknB (Rv0014c)	Cell division	HupB (185), ParB (180)
	Arabinan biosynthesis	EmbR (181)
	MA biosynthesis	KasA (101), KasB (101), FabD (101), HadAB/BC (99), InhA (97, 98), MabA (96)
	PG biosynthesis	FhaA (186, 187), GlmU (67), MviN (68), PbpA (87), PonA1 (79)
	α-Glucan biosynthesis	GlgE (143)
	PDIM biosynthesis	PapA5 (115, 116)
	Erothioneine biosynthesis	EgtD (132)
	TCA cycle	GarA (40, 167, 188)
	Methionine cycle	SahH (182, 189)
	Signaling	PstP (183), PtpA (51)
	Protein chaperone	GroEL1 (184)
	Protein synthesis	EF-Tu (190)
	Proteasome	PrcA (56)
	Stress response	RshA (55), SigH (55)
	Hypothetical	Rv1422/CuvA (66), Rv0516c (30), Rv1747 (186)
PknD (Rv0931c)	Cell division	ParB (180)
	MA biosynthesis	FabD (101), FabH (102), HadAB/BC (99), KasA (101), KasB (101), MabA (96), PcaA (191)
	Ergothioneine biosynthesis	EgtD (132)
	TCA cycle	GarA (188), Mdh (172)
	Signaling	PtkA (22), PtpA (51)
	Protein chaperone	GroEL1 (184)
	Transport	MmpL7 (114), Rv1747 (186)
	Osmotic stress	OprA (30)
	Anti-antisigma factor?	Rv0516c (30)
PknE (Rv1743)	Cell division	HupB (185)
	Arabinan biosynthesis	EmbR (192), EmbR2 (192)
	MA biosynthesis	FabD (101), FabH (96), KasA (101), KasB (101), HadAB/BC (99), PcaA (191)
	PDIM biosynthesis	PapA5 (115)
	TCA cycle	GarA (188), Mdh (172)
	Methionine cycle	SahH (182)
	Signaling	PtpA (51)
	Protein chaperone	GroEL1 (184)
	Transport	Rv1747 (186)
	Stress response	RshA (30)
	Anti-antisigma factor	RsfA (30), Rv0516c (30), Rv1904 (30)
PknF (Rv1746)	Cell division	HupB (185), ParB (180)
	Arabinan biosynthesis	EmbR (192), EmbR2 (192)
	MA biosynthesis	FabD (101), FabH (96), KasA (101), KasB (101), HadAB/BC (99), InhA (98), PcaA (191)
	PG biosynthesis	FhaA (186)

(Continued)

Table 1 *(Continued)*

Kinase	Substrate function	Substrate
	TCA cycle	GarA (188)
	Methionine cycle	SahH (182)
	Signaling	PtkA (22)
	Protein chaperone	GroE1 (184)
	Transport	Rv1747 (164)
PknG (Rv0410c)	TCA cycle	GarA (40, 167), Mdh (172)
	Oxidative stress/biofilm growth	L13 (193)
PknH (Rv1266c)	Arabinan biosynthesis	EmbR (25, 194)
	MA biosynthesis	FadD (101), FabH (102), HadAB/BC (99), InhA (98), KasA (101), KasB (101), PcaA (191)
	PG biosynthesis	DacB1 (78)
	TCA cycle	Mdh (172)
	Methionine cycle	SahH (182)
	Signaling	PtpA (51)
	Protein chaperone	GroEL1 (184)
	Dormancy	DosR (27)
	Transcription	Rv0681 (78)
PknI (Rv2914c)	MA biosynthesis	FadD (101)
PknJ (Rv2088)	Arabinan biosynthesis	EmbR (195)
	MA biosynthesis	MmaA4 (195)
	TCA cycle	Mdh (172)
	Glycolysis	PykA (162, 165)
	Dipeptidase	PepE (195)
PknK (Rv3080c)	MA biosynthesis	FabD (196), VirS (14)
	Ergothioneine biosynthesis	EgtD (132)
	Signaling	PtkA (22)
PknL (Rv2176)	MA biosynthesis	FadD (101), InhA (97), KasA (101), KasB (101), MabA (96)
	Protein chaperone	GroEL1 (184)
	Methionine cycle	SahH (182)
	Signaling	PtpA (51)
	DNA binding?	Rv2175c (197)

*a*Abbreviations: MA, mycolic acid; PG, peptidoglycan biosynthesis; TCA, tricarboxylic acid.

global responses, giving cells the advantage to adapt and survive in complex environments.

The discovery of *M. tuberculosis* STPKs originated from the identification of 11 genes encoding for the subdomains of the Hank's superfamily of kinases, resulting in their annotation as "eukaryotic-like" STPKs (12). Yet it is possible that not all STPKs involved in O-phosphorylation have been identified due to our use of a eukaryotic-like biased paradigm. Of the 11 STPKs (PknA to PknL, with the exception of PknC), the sequences of 9 contain a transmembrane region that connects the intracellular N-terminal kinase domain to a C-terminal sensory component located extracellularly. Current structural data indicate that these transmembrane receptor kinases are activated by dimerization of their kinase domains, resulting in the phosphorylation of the activation loop and ultimately leading to kinase activation (13). The remaining two

kinases, PknK and PknG, lack a transmembrane domain. Yet subcellular fractions of *M. tuberculosis* lysates showed PknK to be present in the cell wall/membrane fraction rather than the cytosol through an unknown anchoring mechanism (14). Therefore, PknG is described as the sole soluble STPK in *M. tuberculosis*.

Due to the lack of Tyr kinases in the *M. tuberculosis* genome, Tyr phosphorylation was believed to be absent from *M. tuberculosis* despite the presence of two protein Tyr phosphatases: PtpA and PtpB (15). As a result, these protein phosphatases were originally hypothesized to be solely involved in the interference of host signaling pathways, which was shown by the ability of PtpA to inhibit host vesicular trafficking and phagosome acidification (16, 17). However, preliminary immunoblot evidence suggesting the existence of an *M. tuberculosis* protein phosphorylated on Tyr (18) led us to identify the first *M. tuberculosis* protein tyrosine kinase, PtkA, located within the same operon as its cognate substrate PtpA (19). Recent phosphoproteomic data have indeed found *M. tuberculosis* to support extensive Tyr phosphorylation (63 sites on 49 proteins) (20). Yet bioinformatic analysis has been unsuccessful in identifying any of the traditional bacterial tyrosine kinases (known as BY-kinases), suggesting that Tyr phosphorylation might be carried out strictly by a novel and "odd" family of Tyr kinases in *M. tuberculosis* (21). However, recent investigation by Kusebauch et al. (20) found that *M. tuberculosis* STPKs undergo Tyr phosphorylation in their activation segment, suggesting their action as dual-specificity (Ser/Thr/Tyr) kinases. Although plausible, this hypothesis has to be proven experimentally because none of the STPKs have been shown to phosphorylate their substrates on Tyr. On the other hand, the tyrosine kinase PtkA was shown to be Ser/Thr phosphorylated by and interact with several STPKs (22), strengthening the idea of cross-phosphorylation between STPKs and Tyr kinases in *M. tuberculosis*.

Similar to other prokaryotes, the overall extent of O-phosphorylation in *M. tuberculosis* is limited, amounting to 7.5% of all proteins being phosphorylated (23), compared to the 40 to 45% of eukaryotes (24). As expected, the number of Ser/Thr phosphorylation sites in *M. tuberculosis* is significantly greater than that of Tyr, with over 500 sites identified (23). These findings indicate that each STPK can act on multiple substrates (Table 1). However, little is known regarding STPK signaling cascades and kinase hierarchy in *M. tuberculosis*. In contrast to His-kinases, which typically phosphorylate a single response regulator, the cross-reactivity observed with Ser/Thr/Tyr kinases results in complex signaling cascades. Rarely does the direct output of *M. tuberculosis* Ser/Thr phosphorylation involve the direct regulation of expression of target genes; however, some evidence exists of signaling organization typical of two-component systems (14, 25–27).

Recently, *in vitro* analysis of the interactions between all STPKs has added a novel layer of signaling in *M. tuberculosis* (28). Mapping of STPK phosphorylation suggests a three-layered architecture that includes master regulator (PknB and PknH), signal transducer (PknE and PknJ), and terminal substrate kinases (PknA, PknD, PknF, PknK, and PknL) as shown in Fig. 1. Master regulator kinases exclusively undergo autophosphorylation to achieve activation, which can in turn cross-phosphorylate downstream kinases. Signal transducing kinases can also autophosphorylate as well as cross-phosphorylate downstream kinases, which is likely to act as a mode to propagate signals to intracel-

lular substrates. The remaining substrate kinases were unable to transfer phosphates to other STPKs, indicating that their molecular targets are limited to other protein substrates. Furthermore, four of these kinases (PknA, PknF, PknK, PknL) are thought to lack the machinery to detect extracellular signals and therefore rely on cross-phosphorylation by the upstream kinases for activation (28). Recent evidence showed PknA to autophosphorylate its own activation loop independent of PknB; however, the extracytoplasmic domain appears to be dispensable for PknA function (29). Unlike the other substrate kinases, PknD contains an extracellular β-propeller used by *M. tuberculosis* to sense osmotic stress and is also strategically positioned in the intracellular signaling network to regulate the "stressosome" in response to upstream STPKs (30–32). However, little is known about which ligands bind to these sensor domains or about what environmental stimuli they respond to (Table 2). Furthermore, it is evident that transcriptional data offer limited information about the environmental cues that are sensed by *M. tuberculosis* STPKs. Conditions have been reported where the transcriptional levels of STPKs have increased and meanwhile their protein levels remained unchanged (33). Furthermore, STPKs require activation through auto- or cross-phosphorylation prior to initiating any downstream signaling events. Therefore, it is recommended that caution be used when inferring relationships between environmental conditions and STPK function.

Our understanding of bacterial signal transduction has become very significant due to its role in *M. tuberculosis* pathogenicity. In recent years, STPKs have been shown to play a crucial role in the growth and survival of *M. tuberculosis* during infection. The intracellular cascades induced by STPKs culminate in alterations in gene transcription, enzymatic activity, cellular localization, and protein-protein interactions which translate into the rapid metabolic adaptation of the bacterium. Through our knowledge of their corresponding environmental stimuli and substrates, along with the bacilli's physiological responses, we dedicate this article to describing the role of STPKs in the growth and/or survival of *M. tuberculosis* to establish a persistent infection.

ESTABLISHING INFECTION THROUGH SUBVERSION OF INNATE IMMUNE RESPONSE BY STPKs

Following internalization by host macrophages, *M. tuberculosis* resides and replicates in intracellular membrane-bound vacuoles. Bacterial compartmentalization

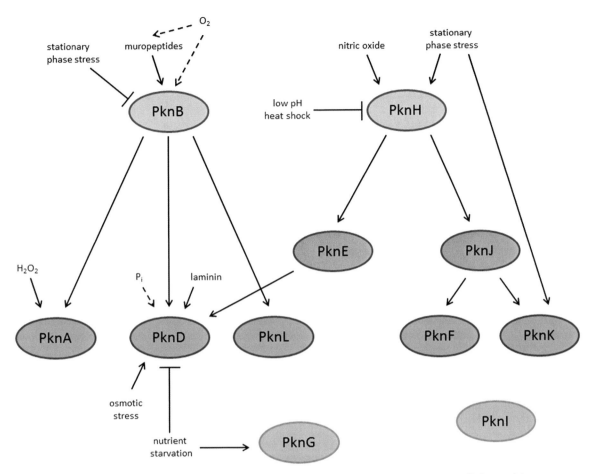

Figure 1 Hierarchy of *M. tuberculosis* STPK activation in response to extracellular and intracellular signals. Master STPKs (blue) sense environmental signals and further cross-phosphorylate the kinase domains of signal transducing (purple) and substrate (red) STPKs to propagate signals and regulate specific downstream proteins. (Figure modified from reference 28).

provides an enclosed space for the host cell to localize high concentrations of reactive oxygen species, reactive nitrogen intermediates, and enzymes that eliminate invading pathogens. Typically during infection, the phagosome fuses with endosomes and lysosomes, resulting in lumen acidification and the acquisition of proteolytic enzymes for lysosome-mediated degradation of invading microorganisms. The classical mechanism *M. tuberculosis* uses to evade the innate immune response is through inhibition of these cellular pathways, namely, phagosomal acidification and blockage of the fusion of phagosomes with lysosomes (34, 35). Therefore, sensing the intracellular environment of the macrophage, adapting its physiology, and responding to host defense mechanisms are an integral part of *M. tuberculosis* pathophysiology.

One of the fascinating strategies used by *M. tuberculosis* is its recently discovered ability to directly in-

terfere with host signaling pathways. The best and first studied example of such interference is the utilization of the mycobacterial secreted Tyr phosphatase PtpA. PtpA was shown to possess phosphatase activity against the host vacuolar protein sorting 33B and glycogen synthase kinase-α, resulting in the arrest of phagosome maturation and prevention of macrophage apoptosis, respectively (16, 36). In addition, PtpA binds subunit H of the macrophage ATPase pump, resulting in blockage of phagosomal acidification and leading to subversion of one of the key characteristics of innate immunity (37, 38).

Inhibition of Phagosome-Lysosome Fusion

M. tuberculosis STPKs are mainly localized to the mycobacterial membrane, and as such possess a limited role in the direct interaction with the host immune system. The only exception described has been that of PknG,

Table 2 Growth and persistence phenotypes of *M. tuberculosis* serine/threoneine protein kinase mutants[a]

STPK	In vitro[b]	Other in vitro conditions[c]	Ex vivo survival	In vivo survival
PknA[d]	Essential (29)			Negligible histopathology, no bacilli recovered from lung or spleen of mice (88)
PknB[d]	Essential (88)			Negligible histopathology, no bacilli recovered from lung or spleen of mice (88)
PknD	N.D. (198)	↓P_i poor conditions following 24 h starvation (199)	N.D. murine macrophages (173)	Required for invasion of brain endothelia (173) N.D. lungs for mouse or guinea pig (198)
PknE	N.D. (43)	↓DTT, glutathione, zinc, cadmium, ↑SNP, GSNO, acidified nitrite (43)	↓120 h THP-1 cells (43)	↑Guinea pigs (200)[e] N.D. BALB/c mice (44)
PknF[f]	Faster growth, shortened cells (163)			
PknG	↓Exponential, more pronounced stationary (41)	↓Nutrient depleted (41)		↓Lung, spleen, and liver in BALB/c and CD-1 mice (41)
PknH	N.D. (44)	↑Acidified nitrite stress ↓H_2O_2, O_2^- (44)	↓120 h THP-1 cells (44)	↑Lung and spleen in BALB/c mice (44)
PknI	↓Exponential (135)	↑Acidic pH and hypoxia ↓Acidic pH and oxygenated (135)	↑120 h THP-1 cells (135)	Hypervirulent SCID mice (135)
PknK	N.D. exponential ↑Stationary phase Shortened cells (133)	↑Acidic pH, hypoxia, H_2O_2 (133)	–	↓Acute phase lung, ↑persistent phase lung and spleen in C57BL/6 (133)

[a]Abbreviations: DTT, dithiothreitol; SNP, sodium nitroprusside; GSNO, S-nitrosoglutathione; THP-1, human monocytic cell line derived from an acute monocytic leukemia patient; ND, no observed difference in phenotype.

[b]In vitro growth under nutrient-rich, oxygenated conditions based on optical density or CFU data.

[c]In vitro growth conditions showing STPK mutant phenotypes varying from wild type. Based on optical density or CFU data.

[d]In vivo work performed with conditional depletion mutant of PknA or PknB.

[e]Polar effect was not ruled out due to lack of complemented strain.

[f]Results represent work performed with a *pknF* antisense mutant.

which was shown to be secreted and suggested to directly phosphorylate host proteins (39). Although a direct host substrate was not yet identified, PknG was suggested to control phagosome-lysosome fusion of *Mycobacterium bovis* Bacille Calmette-Guérin (BCG)-containing phagosomes within macrophages (39), in contrast to *Mycobacterium smegmatis*, which was directly transferred to lysosomal compartments upon infection. However, PknG was shown to have a direct role in *M. tuberculosis* physiology (40). Since no host substrates or mechanism for PknG blockage of phagosome-lysosome fusion has been described, the effect on host response might be indirect and can be explained by the growth deficiency of the PknG mutant in macrophages and animal models (41).

Apoptosis

Consistent with *M. tuberculosis*'s ability to evade immune-mediated destruction, blockage of macrophage apoptosis upon infection enables bacterial persistence (42). PknE was shown to have a role in *M. tuberculosis* pathogenicity because the mutant demonstrated decreased survival due to increased host-apoptosis in both macrophage and murine models of infection (43, 44). In line with the role of nitric oxide (NO) in regulating the intrinsic apoptotic events of the cell (45), apoptosis occurred following treatment of the Δ*pknE* mutant with NO (43). Furthermore, *pknE* expression was shown to be upregulated in the presence of nitrate stress in *M. smegmatis*, although a polar effect of the mutation was not ruled out. Despite the study lacking a complement, these findings suggest that PknE senses NO inside the host and possibly interacts with other mycobacterial and/or host cell components, leading to inhibition of apoptosis.

The exact mechanism underlying the inhibition of apoptosis by PknE remains unknown; however, a role for PknE in modulating the expression of apoptotic proteins was suggested (46, 47). The *pknE* gene was shown to modulate the expression of Toll-like receptors (TLRs), in agreement with their previously identified role in *M. tuberculosis* infections, by regulating apoptosis and inflammatory responses (48, 49). In addition, a number of PknE substrates are involved in regulating mycolic acid synthesis (Table 1). The uptake of mycolic acids has been previously shown to prolong the survival and increase Bcl-2 expression of the macrophage (50). Furthermore, mycolic acid extracted from *M. tuberculosis* was also shown to reduce the macrophage response to TLR2 agonists, which could prevent the induction of apoptosis (48). Therefore, PknE may prevent apoptosis of the infected macrophage by altering

its cell wall to avoid triggering activation of TLRs associated with cell death.

Another potential mechanism by which PknE may be involved in blocking apoptosis is through regulation of PtpA, which has been shown to be a substrate of PknE (51). Several studies have described substrates of PtpA in the host and its ability to directly interfere with host cell signaling pathways (16, 36–38). Dephosphorylation of one of the PtpA substrates, GSK3α, was indeed shown to decrease apoptosis of the host cell early in infection (36). Furthermore, a kinome analysis identified additional substrates for PtpA, including other apoptotic proteins (36). Therefore, it would be of interest to determine if PknE is able to suppress apoptosis through the regulation of PtpA.

Defense Against Host-Generated Reactive Oxygen and Nitrogen Species

Although *M. tuberculosis* is able to avoid immune recognition, the bacterium is still required to overcome the hostile environment of the phagosome. Upon phagocytosis, *M. tuberculosis* is immediately exposed to a considerable amount of reactive oxygen species, while reactive nitrogen species levels only increase after 72 h (52).

The alternate sigma factor, SigH, is a central regulator of mycobacterial adaptation to redox, heat, and acid stress and is induced upon phagocytosis of the macrophage (53). In addition to undergoing autoregulation of its promoter, SigH interacts posttranslationally with its cognate antisigma factor, RshA (54). Under oxidizing conditions the interaction between RshA and SigH is disrupted, leading to a strong induction of the SigH regulon. However, if the regulation of SigH was employed by this mechanism alone, by the time the intracellular environment became significantly oxidized and RshA dissociated from SigH, damage to *M. tuberculosis* biomolecules would have already occurred. Therefore, the binding of RshA to SigH undergoes further kinase-mediated regulation by PknB, allowing *M. tuberculosis* to generate a more rapid response to an oxidative environment (55). To overcome challenge by oxidative stress, phosphorylation of RshA decreases its interaction with SigH *in vitro*, leading to increased SigH activity *in vivo*. In addition, phosphorylation of SigH was also demonstrated by PknB *in vitro*, but this modification had no effect on the SigH-RshA interaction. It is hypothesized that phosphorylation of SigH may alter binding or transcriptional activation at individual promoters under conditions of increased *pknB* expression; however, this remains to be determined.

In addition to PknB, PknA has also been shown to be involved in responding to oxidative stress. In the presence of H_2O_2, PknA increases its autophosphorylation levels (56). The implication of the observed enhancement of PknA activation was specifically observed to hinder proteasome assembly. The α-subunit (PrcA) and β-subunit (pre-PrcB) of the *M. tuberculosis* proteasome core complex are phosphorylated by both PknB and PknA, with PknB phosphorylation leading to enhanced degradation of the proteasomal substrate, Ino1 (56, 57). In contrast, phosphorylation of PrcA by PknA did not affect the proteasomal degradation *in vitro*. Rather, phosphorylation of both pre-PrcB and PrcA by H_2O_2-induced PknA activation inhibited the assembly of the holo-proteasome complex. Depletion of the proteasomal system was originally found to impair *M. tuberculosis* growth in the presence of NO but provided 2- to 3-fold greater resistance to H_2O_2 (58, 59). Thus, under conditions of oxidative stress, PknA inhibition of proteasome assembly is able to enhance *M. tuberculosis* resistance to H_2O_2 (56).

M. tuberculosis resistance to nitrosative stress has also been linked to the activity of STPKs. The production of NO in response to cytokines or pathogen-derived molecules is an important host defense mechanism against intracellular pathogens and has been shown to be essential in controlling *M. tuberculosis* infection (60, 61). Although *M. tuberculosis* is able to inhibit the colocalization of inducible nitric oxide synthase (iNOS) to the phagosomal membrane (62), it is unlikely that the bacilli can maintain this inhibition throughout the course of infection. Thus, it would be advantageous for the bacterium to possess additional protective mechanisms to ensure its survival. Deletion of either the *pknE* or *pknH* genes resulted in increased resistance to NO donors (43, 44, 46). However, the increased resistance to nitrosative stress of either mutant coincided with increased sensitivity to the oxidants tested. These findings implicate both PknE and PknH in sensing the host's redox environment and orchestrating a physiological response to enhance the survival of *M. tuberculosis*.

STPKs REGULATE *M. TUBERCULOSIS* MORPHOLOGY TO ENSURE COLONIZATION OF THE HOST

Bacterial proliferation can be thought of in two steps: elongation of the mother cell and division into two daughter cells. In the case of the tubercule bacillus, elongation is characterized by polar growth which requires the synthesis and incorporation of new materials into the cell wall. During the initial stages of infection, *M. tuberculosis* actively replicates inside the macrophage to ensure colonization of the host. The extensive regulation of the mycobacterial cell envelope biogenesis and division results in size and cell wall composition heterogeneity of daughter cells (63, 64). This physicochemical diversity is suggested to increase the survival odds for *M. tuberculosis* by enabling reservoirs within subpopulations that are able withstand diverse dynamic stressors encountered by the bacilli (65).

Cell Size

PknA and PknB have been shown to regulate the growth and morphology of the mycobacterial cell through a number of cell elongation and division proteins (29, 66). PknB is largely involved in regulating cell size through peptidoglycan biosynthesis (Table 1). PknB was shown to inhibit the acetyltransferase activity of GlmU, a protein involved in the synthesis of the peptidoglycan precursor UDP-N-acetylglucosamine (67). At the same time, the insertion of lipid II, the final intermediate in peptidoglycan biosynthesis, into the extracellular space is also regulated by PknB. In this situation, the membrane protein MviN responsible for the physical inversion of lipid II is negatively regulated by phosphorylation, ultimately impeding peptidoglycan biosynthesis (68). Furthermore, prior to insertion into the mycobacterial cell wall, lipid II undergoes extensive modification by a family of Mur synthases (69). These synthases are responsible for catalyzing the addition of acetyl, glycosyl, and amino groups to the peptide side chain of lipid II. Modification to peptidoglycan has been described to provide bacteria with resistance to hydrolysis by lysozymes, thereby limiting their detection by host pattern recognition receptors (70) as well as to regulate immunogenicity through the nucleotide-binding oligomerization domain-containing 2 immune receptor (71, 72). Both PknA and PknB have been shown to interact with MurC-F, suggesting that they regulate the modification of muropeptides in response to the environment of *M. tuberculosis* (73, 74).

The final stages of peptidoglycan biosynthesis involve a family of penicillin binding proteins (PBPs) that are responsible for catalyzing cross-linking between peptidoglycan, a modification which also influences cell expansion. Traditionally, peptidoglycan precursors inserted into the cell wall are linked by transpeptidases to produce 4-3 cross-links. In contrast, up to 80% of *M. tuberculosis* peptidoglycan contains 3-3 peptide cross-links (75, 76), and this modification is crucial for persistence *in vivo* (77). Remodeling of peptidoglycan by the PBP DacB1 is believed to be responsible for maintaining 3-3 cross-links. Although the effect of phosphorylation on DacB1 activity is unknown, the PBP is a substrate of PknH *in vitro* (78). It is plausible that PknH regulates peptidoglycan cross-linking to increases during infection to promote cell wall rigidity and bacterial survival under stress. In addition, the PBP PonA1 is a substrate of PknB. Phosphorylation of PonA1 by PknB inhibits its transglycosylation activity and slows polar elongation, resulting in shorter cells (79). Lastly, PknA also coordinates peptidoglycan biosynthesis through the elongation complex, a macromolecular machine composed of peptidoglycan synthases and hydrolases that drive peptidoglycan remodeling during elongation. To localize elongation to the poles, Wag31 acts as an anchor at this site and provides a basis for the recruitment of the remaining complex components (80). Localization of Wag31 to cell poles is dependent on its phosphorylation by PknA, and growth of the *M. smegmatis* Wag31 phosphomimicking mutant resulted in shorter and wider cells (66).

In contrast to other bacterial species, mycobacterial septa are placed over a wide zone within the cell body (81, 82), further contributing to differences in daughter cell size as well as the distribution of proteins and small molecules between daughter cells (83). FtsZ, a homolog of eukaryotic tubulin, is the principal driving force of cytokinesis in mycobacteria. Through its self-activating GTPase activity, FtsZ undergoes polymerization to form a ring-like structure, known as the Z-ring (84), that was shown to be regulated by PknA among other mechanisms (85). This structure acts as a cytoskeletal scaffold for the recruitment and assembly of the divisome and provides energy for membrane constriction during cell division (86). Phosphorylated FtsZ showed a reduction in GTP hydrolysis and polymerization activity *in vitro*. Overexpression of PknA in *E. coli* resulted in phosphorylation of *E. coli* FtsZ and the production of elongated cells, indicating dysregulation in septum formation (85). In addition, the localization of PbpA, a peptidoglycan synthase part of the divisome, to the septum is thought to be mediated via phosphorylation by PknB (87). PbpA is a substrate of PknB *in vitro*, and the absence of phosphorylated PbpA prevents PbpA localization to the septa and causes the elongated growth of *M. smegmatis in vitro* (87).

As outlined earlier, PknA and PknB play a crucial role in polar elongation and septal localization. Therefore, these two kinases are likely responsible, in part, for differences in the size of daughter cells observed *in vivo*. This notion is supported by the fact that overexpression of these kinases results in short bulging cells, while their depletion causes narrow and elongated bacilli (66). Not only are PknA and PknB essential for *M. tuberculosis* growth *in vitro*, but they also are indispensible in the survival and pathogenesis

of *M. tuberculosis* during murine infection (29, 88) (Table 2). Thus, PknB senses host environmental factors that enable its orchestration of downstream signaling to tightly regulate growth and generate a heterogeneous population that enables *M. tuberculosis* to persist in the presence of host innate and acquired immunity.

Cell Wall Composition

Transcriptional analysis of *M. tuberculosis* isolated from tuberculosis patients identified substantial changes in the expression of cell wall biosynthetic genes, including the upregulation of lipid synthesis genes (89). Thickening of the cell wall restricts the transit of toxic molecules including antibiotics. Lipids can also act as a sink for toxic by-products generated by β-oxidation during *in vivo* growth (90), absorb oxidative radicals (91), and manipulate the host immune response (92). Of these lipids, mycolic acids, phthiocerol dimycocerosate (PDIM), and sulfolipid 1 (SL-1) were all found to increase in abundance and/or alter their composition during *M. tuberculosis* growth *in vivo* (89, 93, 94).

The outer layer of the *M. tuberculosis* cell wall is composed of long-carbon-chain mycolic acids that give rise to the observed thick waxy coat and the remarkable impermeability of mycobacteria (95). The biosynthetic pathway of mycolic acids begins with the *de novo* synthesis of fatty acids from acetyl-CoA. The mycobacterial fatty acid synthase (FAS) II is composed of four sets of enzymes that are essential in catalyzing each cycle of elongation: β-ketoacyl-ACP reductase (MabA), β-hydroxylacyl-ACP dehydratases (HadAB/HadBC), NADH-dependent *trans*-2-enoyl-ACP reductase (InhA), and β-ketoacyl-ACP synthases (KasA or KasB). Interestingly, each FAS-II enzyme is phosphorylated by multiple STPKs (Table 1), enabling regulation of mycolic acid biosynthesis in response to variable growth environments (96–101). STPKs are also involved in reducing the production of the FAS-II system precursors by phosphorylating malonyl-CoA-ACP (FabD) (101) and the β-ketoacyl-ACP synthase (FabH) (102). Being the target of multiple STPKs and the fact that phosphorylation of individual enzymes results in only the partial reduction of its activity enable fine-tuning of the FAS-II system (Table 3). Furthermore, the observation that PknA and PknB negatively regulate these enzymes indicates that even under conditions of growth, mycolic acid biosynthesis is being constrained. Mycolic acid biosynthesis is an expensive process, and in addition, *M. tuberculosis* resides in nutrient-limited phagosomes. Thus, it would be beneficial to carefully balance mycolic acid biosynthesis with cell expansion.

Table 3 Effect of phosphorylation on *M. tuberculosis* serine/threonine protein kinase substrates[a]

Substrate	Function	Effect of phosphorylation	Kinase	References[b]
DosR	Dormancy	Enhances its binding activity to dosR regulon promoter	PknH	27
EF-Tu	Cell division	Reduces interaction with GTP	PknB	190
EgtD	EGT biosynthesis	Inhibits methylation activity	PknD	132
EmbR	Arabinan biosynthesis	Enhances EmbR binding to *embCAB* promoter	PknH	25
FabD	MA biosynthesis	Decreases its condensing activity	PknF	96
FipA	Cell division	Enhances interaction with FtsZ	PknA	179
FtsZ	Cell division	Impairs GTP hydrolysis and polymerization	PknA	85
GarA	TCA cycle	Inhibits binding to KDH, GDH, and GltS	PknB	40, 167
			PknG	40
GlgE	α-glucan biosynthesis	Decreases maltosyltransferase activity	PknB	143
GlmU	PG biosynthesis	Decreases acetyltransferase activity	PknB	67
HupB	Cell division	Inhibits its DNA binding activity	PknE	185
InhA	MA biosynthesis	Decreases enoyl reductase activity	PknA	98
			PknB	98
			PknE	98
			PknL	98
KasB	MA biosynthesis	Decreases its condensing activity	PknF	100
L13	Oxidative stress	Promotes its association with RenU and enhances RenU hydrolysis of NADH	PknG	193
MabA	MA biosynthesis	Decreases β-ketoacyl-ACP reductase activity	PknB	96
Mdh	TCA cycle	Inhibits dehydrogenase activity	PknD	172
MviN	PG biosynthesis	Induces dimerization with FhaA	PknB	68
OprA	Osmotic stress	Enables SigF binding to RNA polymerase	PknD	31
ParB	Cell division	Inhibits DNA binding to *parS* and interaction with ParA	PknA	180
			PknB	180
			PknD	180
			PknF	180
PonA1	PG biosynthesis	Inhibits transglycosylation activity	PknB	79
PrcA	Proteasome	Inhibits proteasome assembly	PknA	56
		Enhances degradation of Ino1	PknB	56
PstP	Signaling	Decreases phosphatase activity	PknA	183
PtpA	Signaling	Enhances phosphatase activity	PknA	51
RshA	Stress response	Inhibits its interaction with SigH	PknB	55
Rv0516c	Anti-antisigma factor?	Inhibits association with Rv268	PknD	30
Rv1747	ABC transporter	Enhances enzymatic activity	PknF	201
Rv2175c	DNA binding?	Inhibits its DNA binding	PknL	26, 197
SahH	Methionine cycle	Decreases hydrolase activity	PknA	182
		Decreases hydrolase activity and its affinity to NAD$^+$	PknB	182, 189
			PknD	182
			PknE	182
			PknF	182
			PknL	182
VirS	MA biosynthesis?	Enhances binding to *mym* promoter under physiological conditions	PknK	14
Wag31	Cell division	Localizes it to the cell poles and enhances oligomerization of the elongation complex	PknA	202

[a]Abbreviations: EGT, ergothioneine; GDH, glutamate dehydrogenase; KDH, α-ketoglutarate dehydrogenase complex; MA, mycolic acid; TCA, tricarboxylic acid; PG, peptidoglycan.
[b]Reference of the effect of phosphorylation on the target substrate identified *in vitro* and/or *in vivo*. Only cases where the effect of phosphorylation by the specific STPK tested and/or phosphorylation sites are mentioned in the table. We do not assume that the STPKs phosphorylate their substrates on the same residues and have the same effect. Table only includes analysis of *M. tuberculosis* proteins.

Differentially regulating FAS-II enzymes may also provide opportunity for the full extension of mycolic acids. The importance of extending these chains has been observed in the *M. tuberculosis kasB* mutant. Production of shorter mycolates in this strain resulted in impaired growth, increased cell wall permeability, and severe defects in resisting host defenses and antibiotic action (103, 104). Lastly, it has also been proposed that mycolic acids are recycled under conditions that damage the cell envelope (105, 106). Consistent with this notion, gene expression profiling of *M. bovis* BCG suggests that "new" mycolic acids are synthesized via the remodeling of older chains during infection (107).

The *mymA* operon (*rv3803-rv3809*) is predicted to encode for the gene products involved in an alternative approach for the condensation of long fatty acids for the synthesis of mycolic acids (108). *M. tuberculosis* disrupted in the *mymA* genes has impaired survival in both activated macrophages and guinea pigs as well as increased cell wall permeability (109). The *mymA* operon has considerable basal activity, which is further enhanced 2- to 3-fold by the transcriptional regulator, VirS, under acidic conditions (14, 109, 110). Interestingly, VirS undergoes posttranslational modification by PknK, enhancing its DNA binding affinity for the *mymA* promoter; however, PknK was only found to stimulate VirS-mediated transcription of the *mym* promoter under physiological conditions (14). Therefore, in the absence of acid stress, PknK may enhance VirS activity, modulating mycolic acid biosynthesis through a FAS-II-independent pathway during infection.

In the past decade, evidence of STPK involvement in PDIM biosynthesis and export has slowly been accumulating. PDIM is implicated in protecting *M. tuberculosis* from reactive nitrogen species generated by the host (111), and thus it is not surprising that PknH, activated by nitrate stress (44, 112), has been found to positively regulate PDIM biosynthesis (113). The exact mechanism behind PknH regulation of PDIM biosynthesis is unknown, but it could be speculated that nitrate stress leads to the downstream activation of PknD and PknE, which have targets in PDIM transport (114) and biosynthesis (115), respectively. In addition to PknE, PknB was also found to phosphorylate PapA5, an acyltransferase that catalyzes the dual esterification of mycocerosate onto phthiocerol to complete the biosynthesis of PDIM (115, 116). Although identified as substrates of *M. tuberculosis* STPKs, it remains unknown what effect phosphorylation has on the activity of PapA5 or the PDIM transporter, MmpL7. Since PknE is also implicated in sensing nitrate stress (43), it

is suspected that phosphorylation of PapA5 may positively regulate its enzymatic activity.

PDIM and sulfolipid-1 (SL-1) production are coupled via the metabolic flux of methylmalonyl-coenzyme A (MMCoA) (93), and as a result STPK downregulation of PDIM biosynthesis would lead to an increase in SL-1 production. SL-1 has been found to negatively regulate *M. tuberculosis* growth in human macrophages as well as provide protection against human cationic antimicrobial peptides *in vitro* (117). Enhancing PDIM production via STPK would reduce the quantity of SL-1 (93) while increasing *M. tuberculosis* resistance to reactive nitrogen species (111). The early immune response to *M. tuberculosis* is also subdued by the presence of PDIM, which is shown to inhibit the secretion of tumor necrosis factor-α and interleukin-6 from resting macrophages and dendritic cells (111). Therefore, STPK regulation of PDIM production and export may contribute to the intracellular growth and survival of *M. tuberculosis* during the initial stage of infection.

STPKs COORDINATE *M. TUBERCULOSIS* PHYSIOLOGY TO ACHIEVE NONREPLICATING PERSISTENCE

As the disease progresses, *M. tuberculosis* can further diversify in response to pressure from anatomical location, the host immune response, and drug treatment. These adaptations lead to differences in gene expression profiles, metabolism, growth rate, and other functional characteristics, resulting in a heterogeneous population of bacteria (118). Often, conditions in the host give rise to a subpopulation of dormant-like bacteria characterized as nonreplicating with low metabolic activity. It is these dormant-like bacteria that are the reservoir for *M. tuberculosis* persistence and reactivation of the disease. To successfully enter a dormant-like state, *M. tuberculosis* senses a number of unfavorable growth conditions resulting in growth arrest, cell wall remodeling, and downregulation of metabolism (Fig. 2).

Growth Arrest

M. tuberculosis infection is primarily characterized by the formation of granulomas, organized structures of immune cells that act to control and prevent the dissemination of infection. Despite the heightened immune response that is usually associated with granulomas, *M. tuberculosis* is still able to persist long-term within this structure. Survival under these conditions is likely due to arrested growth and cellular respiration of *M. tuberculosis* in response to NO generated from acti-

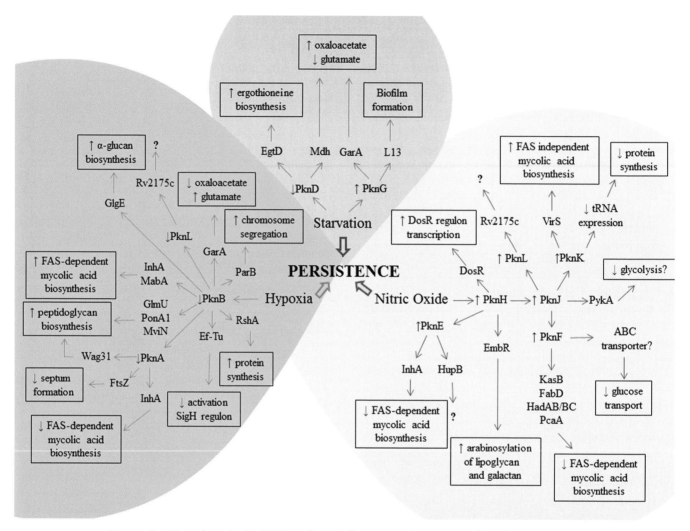

Figure 2 *M. tuberculosis* STPK cell signaling network associated with persistence. STPKs sense specific environmental cues (starvation, hypoxia, and nitric oxide) and coordinate a physiological response that triggers *M. tuberculosis* to enter a state of nonreplicating persistence.

vated macrophages and the hypoxic environment of the granuloma (119, 120). The *M. tuberculosis* state of quiescence, termed nonreplicating persistence (NRP), is entered upon the activation of the DosR regulon, a set of 48 genes that downregulate cellular respiration. DosR is regulated by two cognate sensor kinases, DosS and DosT (121, 122), which activate the DosR regulon under conditions of hypoxia (123–125), NO (120), and carbon monoxide (126, 127). Interestingly, PknH was shown to sense host NO and trigger the induction of the DosR regulon (27, 44, 112, 128). Further evidence describes *pknH* transcription to be upregulated during stationary phase growth *in vitro* (129), and the *pknH* deletion mutant showed higher bacillary loads in mouse organs than did wild type (44). Taken together, these

findings implicate PknH in slowing the growth of *M. tuberculosis* to achieve a state of NRP during infection, and perhaps specifically in response to the granuloma's environment (Fig. 2).

The induction of NRP is not limited to the redox environment of *M. tuberculosis*. The other well-known contributing factor leading to NRP is nutrient deprivation (Fig. 2). Both the phagosome and granuloma are sites of nutrient deprivation for pathogens, and *M. tuberculosis* isolated from lung lesions demonstrated an altered morphology and staining properties that were similar to cultures starved in distilled water for 2 years (130). Furthermore, Loebel et al. (131) and Betts et al. (128) identified that starvation of *M. tuberculosis* in phosphate-buffered saline resulted in the gradual shutdown of respiration to minimal levels, and the bacteria remained viable but nonreplicating. Among the 323 genes involved in adaptation in this model of persistence, *pknB* and *pknD* were both found to be significantly downregulated (128). As a result, it is tempting to speculate that PknB senses the extracellular signal of starvation terminating downstream STPK signaling pathways involved in cell proliferation via posttranslational modification. However, regulation of bacteriostasis by PknB was shown to be specific to oxygen levels, rather than nutrient starvation (33).

PknD also has a functional extracellular domain (32), and its kinase activity is regulated under a variety of processes (Fig. 1), suggesting broad use of this kinase by *M. tuberculosis*. However, the relevance of the downregulation of PknD during nutrient deprivation (128) became apparent when we discovered that PknD negatively regulates ergothioneine biosynthesis in *M. tuberculosis* (132). Ergothioneine is a sulfur-containing amino acid derived from histidine, and very little is known about its physiological role in microorganisms. However, ergothioneine is required for *M. tuberculosis* survival under long-term starvation (132), suggesting that the downregulation of PknD is essential for persistence. In contrast, nutrient starvation (128) and hypoxia (33) show no influence on the transcript levels and activity of PknH *in vitro*.

PknK and PknI have also been implicated in slowing the growth of mycobacteria *in vitro*, which was further shown to be relevant because the *M. tuberculosis* ΔpknK and ΔpknI mutants both demonstrate enhanced growth during macrophage and/or mouse infection (133–135). PknH indirectly regulates the activity of PknK through the signal transduction kinase PknJ (28) (Fig. 1); however, PknK is also positively regulated at a transcriptional level during stationary phase (133). The slowing of *M. tuberculosis* growth is thought to be the consequence of PknK regulating the expression of a variety of genes, including those involved in cell wall processes and lipid metabolism. Perhaps the most notable observation from this study was the inhibitory effect on transcription and translation processes of tRNAs resulting in the repression of protein synthesis in *M. tuberculosis* (134). The exact mechanism of how PknK regulates the expression of a variety of genes is unknown; however, it is plausible that PknK targets a variety of transcriptional regulatory proteins, as observed in the case of VirS (14), to ultimately slow *M. tuberculosis* growth.

PknI is not part of the *M. tuberculosis* STPK interaction network described by Baer et al. (28), and little is known about its activation (Fig. 1). The ΔpknI mutant showed enhanced growth under acidic pH and limited oxygen availability (Table 2), suggesting that PknI is involved in slowing *M. tuberculosis* growth in response to the macrophage environment (135). However, two independent groups have shown that *pknI* expression is not induced upon infection of the macrophage (133, 136), again suggesting that expression data must be interpreted with caution for STPKs. However, it remains possible that PknI expression is not detected during infection because the signaling cascade is only induced at very early stages of infection (<18 h), an event similar to what is observed with PknK (133). Alternatively, the initial expression levels of PknI may be sufficient for its activity within macrophages (135). Currently, there is a single known *in vitro* substrate for PknI: FabD (Table 1); however, the effect of phosphorylation remains to be investigated. In addition, due to its positioning in the *M. tuberculosis* genome, PknI has been proposed to play a role in cell wall synthesis and division (12).

Cell Wall Remodeling

M. tuberculosis halts cell division and undergoes extensive cell wall remodeling while transitioning into a state of NRP (137). Cunningham and Spreadbury (138) reported a very prominent thickening of the cell wall outer layer in *M. tuberculosis*, which was later attributed to the gradual accumulation of loosely bound extracellular material around the bacilli in the form of a capsule (129). This matrix is primarily composed of proteins and polysaccharides (139), with only a small proportion (2 to 3%) containing lipids (140). The major carbohydrates making up 80% of the extracellular capsule are α-glucans, and *M. tuberculosis* strains defective in the production of capsular α-glucans showed attenuated survival in mice during the persistence phase of infection (141).

The biosynthesis of α-glucan in *M. tuberculosis* occurs through three known pathways. Of these, the GlgE pathway has been described as a nonclassical type responsible for the conversion of trehalose into branched α-glucan through maltose 1-phosphate (142). In this pathway the linear backbone of α-glucans is directly synthesized from maltose 1-phosphate by the essential maltosyltransferase, GlgE. To ensure the appropriate channeling of trehalose in the formation of the cell wall, it is expected that the GlgE pathway would be negatively regulated during cell growth. Consistent with this idea, Molle and colleagues (143) identified PknB to negatively regulate GlgE activity and ultimately α-glucan biosynthesis.

Another mechanism employed by *M. tuberculosis* to adapt to a state of NRP is to increase the abundance of free mycolates in the cell wall lipids (129). Free mycolates have been shown to play a key role in the formation of mycobacterial pellicle biofilms (144), and *M. tuberculosis* biofilms have been observed within the caseum of human granulomas (119). The production of free mycolates occurs as the result of the direct cleavage of trehalose dimycolate (145), and free trehalose is then transported back to the cytoplasm (146). Since *pknB* transcripts are downregulated in the absence of *M. tuberculosis* growth (66, 128), it is plausible that α-glucan biosynthesis via GlgE would thereby increase, contributing to the observed thickening of the *M. tuberculosis* capsule during NRP.

Remodeling of the mycobacterial cell wall during NRP was also found to include increased arabinosylation and abundance of lipoglycans in response to *in vitro* nutrient starvation (129). In mycobacteria, the lipoglycans, lipomannan and lipoarabinomannan (LAM), are associated with the cell wall and are exposed on the outer surface of the bacterium (147). Both of these lipoglycans are ligands of the TLR2; however, lipomannan is a stronger inducer of this receptor's response relative to LAM (148). EmbC is an arabinofuranosyltransferase which serves to elongate the arabinan domain of LAM (149). Transcriptome analyses identified *embC* to be upregulated during stationary phase (129, 149), which most likely contributes to the corresponding increase in LAM arabinosylation observed during NRP (129). The enhanced expression of *embC* is indirectly regulated by PknH through the phosphorylation of the response regulator EmbR (25). Additionally, *pknH* is also upregulated during stationary phase (129). These results implicate PknH in sensing a growth-limiting factor, resulting in a signaling cascade to increase *embC* expression and ultimately the arabinose content of LAM.

In vitro environmental conditions, such as anoxic and nutrient starvation, responsible for directing *M. tuberculosis* into a state of NRP are also found to produce cultures that lose their acid-fastness (130, 150–152). The involvement of mycolic acids in acid-fast staining arose when Jacobs and colleagues (103) observed that the deletion of *kasB* resulted in a loss of acid-fastness. Furthermore, this *M. tuberculosis kasB* mutant displayed significant *in vivo* growth attenuation that led to a long-term persistent infection reminiscent of latent tuberculosis. Prior to these findings, the condensing activities of KasB were found to be under the regulation of STPKs (101), implicating these kinases as major players in the progression of the disease to a latent state. Interestingly, the original study identifying KasB as a substrate of multiple STPKs identified PknA to positively regulate KasB; however, more recent work by the same group showed that phosphorylation of KasB by PknF resulted in shortened mycolic acids that lacked *trans*-cyclopropanation (100). The relevance of the *in vitro* observation of KasB phosphorylation by PknA remains questionable. Nonetheless, further analysis of the KasB phosphomimetic mutant showed a complete loss of acid-fast staining as well as the incapacity to grow yet establish a long-term persistent infection in mice (100).

The core structure of mycolic acids is conserved across mycobacteria; however, pathogenic mycobacteria produce significant quantities of cyclopropanated mycolic acids. Following elongation, the meromycolic chain produced by the FAS-II system can undergo cyclopropanation by a number of *M. tuberculosis* methyltransferases (MmaA 1 to 4, PcaA, and CmaA2). PcaA and MmaA2 have been analyzed for their ability to act as substrates for *M. tuberculosis* STPKs, with only PcaA acting as a substrate for PknF and PknH (153). PcaA methyltransferase activity was decreased upon phosphorylation by PknF. Since *M. tuberculosis* PcaA is implicated in persistence (154) and attenuated immunopathology (155), these findings suggest that mycolic acid modifications have an immunomodulatory function, and specifically, cyclopropanation acts to suppress the immune response to *M. tuberculosis*. However, in the presence of NO, PknH and its downstream signaling effectors, including PknF, are activated, leading to the negative regulation of mycolic acid elongation and cyclopropanation (27, 28). This regulatory mechanism may function to simply act as part of the observed shutdown of mycolic acid biosynthesis when *M. tuberculosis* enters a dormant state (128, 156) and/or may be used to modulate the immune response later in infection (157, 158).

Slowing Central Metabolism

Based on early observations by Bloch and Segal (159), it is accepted that *M. tuberculosis* preferentially utilizes fatty acids as a carbon source during infection. Although the *M. tuberculosis* genome encodes for transporters and enzymes known to metabolize sugars (160), the conditions in which carbohydrates can be utilized for *in vivo* growth still need to be determined. Interestingly, a double mutant of *M. tuberculosis* glucokinases, the enzymes responsible for generating glucose-6-P in the first step of glycolysis, was unable to persist during the chronic phase of infection (161). From these findings, it remains plausible that *M. tuberculosis* has access to glucose during infection; however, the production of glucose-6-P may, rather, be the consequence of gluconeogenesis. The regulatory mechanisms of glucose metabolism further support the notion that glucose availability is limited inside the host. The activity of the glycolytic enzyme pyruvate kinase A (PykA) has been shown to be a substrate of PknJ in *M. tuberculosis* (162). Although the effect of phosphorylation was not studied in depth, a phosphomutant of PykA suggests negative regulation. As PknJ is activated by PknH, decreasing PykA activity during NRP would impede the production of pyruvate, enabling gluconeogenesis to proceed. Furthermore, glucose transport has also been shown to be mediated by STPKs. *M. tuberculosis* expressing antisense *pknF* demonstrated an increase in [¹⁴C]glucose uptake *in vitro* (163). Molle et al. (164) identified Rv1747 to be a substrate of PknF, suggesting that other ABC transporters could be regulated by this mechanism and mediate glucose transport. PknJ (165) and PknF (163) have been shown to decrease the growth rate of *M. bovis* BCG and *M. tuberculosis*, respectively. Perhaps, together PknJ and PknF coordinate the shutdown of carbohydrate catabolism during the *M. tuberculosis* life cycle in the host to slow bacterial growth and prepare the cell for entering a quiescent state.

The observed shutdown of the glycolytic pathway during infection and the inability of carbohydrate transporters to promote the survival of *M. tuberculosis in vivo* suggest that glucose is primarily generated via gluconeogenesis (161). This thought is consistent with the dramatic loss of virulence in a mutant strain that lacks the gluconeogenic enzyme, phosphoenolpyruvate kinase (166). During stationary phase and when grown in nutrient-depleted media, an *M. tuberculosis* mutant deficient in PknG displays reduced growth, and upon further analysis was found to accumulate both glutamate and glutamine (41). Glutamate is one of the major gluconeogenic precursors for cells. The amino acid is broken down by glutamate dehydrogenase to produce α-ketoglutarate and ammonium. A small forkhead associated domain protein known as GarA regulates α-ketoglutarate entry into the tricarboxylic acid (TCA) cycle. GarA binds and inhibits both the α-ketoglutarate dehydrogenase complex and glutamate dehydrogenase (40). In the meantime, GarA also promotes glutamate synthesis by activating glutamine oxoglutarate aminotransferase, an enzyme which assimilates glutamine together with α-ketoglutarate to produce glutamate (167). PknG was shown to phosphorylate GarA and prevent binding to its enzyme partners. Therefore, GarA phosphorylation impedes glutamate synthesis and relieves TCA cycle inhibition in *M. tuberculosis* (40).

PknG has been shown to be upregulated during infection (133) and contribute to the survival of a number of mycobacterial species both in macrophages (39, 168–170) and in mice (41, 168). The macrophage phagosome is presumed to be nutrient-poor, which likely results in the activation of PknG-mediated signaling to upregulate gluconeogenic pathways (Fig. 2). It should be considered that during *in vivo* growth, gluconeogenesis may be acting to support the anabolism of cell wall components, such as mannosylated LAM (171), or other pathways, which in turn results in the blockage of phagosome-lysosome fusion, a phenotype noted earlier to be associated with PknG. A second enzyme involved in gluconeogenesis and the TCA cycle, malate dehydrogenase, is also a substrate of a number of STPKs, including PknD (172). Phosphorylation by PknD has a negative effect on malate dehydrogenase activity. Thus, in conditions resulting in nutrient starvation where *pknD* transcripts are reduced, one would expect an increase in oxaloacetate. In addition, PknD is not required for growth in macrophages (173), indicating that this kinase may also contribute to the regulation of gluconeogenesis during infection.

THE SWITCH: SENSING WHEN TO EXIT NRP

Little is known about the environmental conditions that are associated with the transition between latency and reactivation. Previous work has shown that growth of hypoxia-arrested *M. tuberculosis* occurs upon reaeration of *in vitro* cultures (33, 174). These findings are consistent with anatomically related reactivation, which commonly occurs in the upper lobes, the area of the lungs that have the highest oxygen tension (175), while bacterial dormancy is associated with the oxygen-limited granuloma (176, 177). The regulation of oxygen-dependent replication is mediated in part by PknB (33). PknB protein levels were found to be upregulated in response to oxygen, where PknB decreased during hypoxia. Regulation of bacteriostasis was found to be limited to oxygen, because other conditions known to inhibit growth such as nitric oxide, low pH, and nutrient starvation had no effect on the growth and survival of a *pknB* over-expression strain (33).

The exact mechanism by which PknB senses changes in oxygen tension still needs to be defined, because its extracellular PMP and Ser/Thr Kinase Associated (PASTA) domains are not believed to be involved in oxygen sensing (178). It is thought that *M. tuberculosis* uses resuscitation-promoting factors(Rpfs) to initiate regrowth following dormancy (118). *Micrococcus luteus* Rpf orthologs possess a conserved domain predicted to have lysozyme activity and may therefore cleave peptidoglycan and in turn activate PknB during reaeration.

Alternatively, PknB activation was suggested to go through cross-phosphorylation by another STPK or two-component signaling system in response to oxygen levels (33) as previously exemplified (27).

From the above findings, it is clear that PknB is critical in transducing growth and replication signals in response to oxygen levels. Careful regulation of its activity is required at every stage of the life cycle of *M. tuberculosis*. As suggested, PknB may therefore represent a highly vulnerable drug target for *M. tuberculosis* during both active and latent disease.

CONCLUSION

To establish persistence, *M. tuberculosis* STPKs regulate mycobacterial proteins to adapt the bacilli's physiology. Furthermore, to ensure survival inside the phagosome, *M. tuberculosis* interferes with the host intracellular signaling of the infected macrophage through the secreted phosphatases PtpA and SapM. Currently, little evidence exists that demonstrates secretion and direct association of *M. tuberculosis* STPKs with host effector proteins. Rather, the role STPKs play in evading the host immune response is mainly through the regulation of cell growth, cell wall remodeling, and the activation of specific stress responses during infection.

Generally, as shown in Table 1, multiple STPKs can act on a defined single substrate and have a similar effect, suggesting that *M. tuberculosis* carefully fine-tunes its physiological response to match the associated conditions of the bacterium. In addition, multiple enzymes that belong to the same pathway or cell process are also regulated by multiple STPKs. Such regulatory flexibility can lead to a population differing in cell size, growth rate, and cell wall composition. As a result, the heterogeneity of this population may improve the fitness of *M. tuberculosis* by providing bacteria with the physiological diversity to successfully grow in a range of host microenvironments or persist in a quiescent state.

Currently, our knowledge of the conditions that activate STPKs during infection is limited. Therefore, it is difficult to link the physiological adaptation of *M. tuberculosis* with the host response. We can predict that *M. tuberculosis* replicates during the initial stage of infection as well as during disease reactivation, a process which is regulated for the most part by PknA and PknB. However, under conditions of limited oxygen and nutrients as well as in the presence of NO, *M. tuberculosis* enters a state of NRP to ensure its long-term survival in the host. Although these conditions can be encountered at any point during the life cycle of the bacilli, *M. tuberculosis* primarily exists in a state of NRP in the granuloma. As summarized in Fig. 2, the hypoxic environment of the granuloma likely shuts down PknB and its downstream signaling pathway to arrest growth and increase peptidoglycan and α-glucan biosynthesis to enhance rigidity and thickness, respectively, of the cell wall. In parallel, *de novo* biosynthesis of mycolic acids is downregulated by both the activation of PknH and the inhibition of PknB signaling cascades to potentially reduce *M. tuberculosis* immunogenicity. The activation of PknH by NO generated from activated macrophages additionally enhances the induction of the DosR regulon to further prevent bacterial replication and inhibit aerobic respiration. In addition to DosR, PknH coordinates slowing of *M. tuberculosis* growth through PknJ and its downstream targets PknF and PknK to inhibit glucose catabolism and protein synthesis. Despite reduced metabolic activity during NRP, *M. tuberculosis* relies on gluconeogenesis for biomass production and survival throughout infection. It is likely that PknG plays a crucial role in this process through its regulation of GarA. Furthermore, the downregulation of PknD is potentially crucial for the survival of *M. tuberculosis* during NRP due to its role in gluconeogenesis and ergothioneine biosynthesis.

Understanding the mechanisms behind host signaling pathways targeted by *M. tuberculosis*, as well as how the bacilli physiologically adapt to persist within the host, is crucial for effective management of chronic infection. In the past two decades, the field of oncology has been dedicated to developing libraries of compounds that block protein kinase activity due to their role in uncontrolled cell division. Therefore, it may be possible to use our knowledge of how *M. tuberculosis* interferes with host signaling pathways and enhance the immune response with an appropriate compound. Alternatively, screening these libraries for antimicrobial activity against *M. tuberculosis* may also prove beneficial. Because *M. tuberculosis* STPKs play a crucial role in regulating a wide variety of cell processes involved in bacterial growth and persistence, altering the activity of these kinases may represent a promising approach for novel drug discovery.

Acknowledgments. *Funding for this work was provided by the British Columbia Lung Association and the University of British Columbia's Four Year Doctoral Fellowship and Friedman Scholars Program. We would additionally like to thank Xingji Zheng for his insightful comments and Joseph Chao for his careful editing of the manuscript.*

Citation. Richard-Greenblatt M, Av-Gay Y. 2017. Epigenetic phosphorylation control of *Mycobacterium tuberculosis* infection and persistence. Microbiol Spectrum 5(2):TBTB2-0005-2015.

References

1. Wang JY, Koshland DE Jr. 1978. Evidence for protein kinase activities in the prokaryote *Salmonella typhimurium*. *J Biol Chem* **253**:7605–7608.

2. Garnak M, Reeves HC. 1979. Phosphorylation of isocitrate dehydrogenase of *Escherichia coli*. *Science* **203**:1111–1112.

3. Manai M, Cozzone AJ. 1979. Analysis of the protein-kinase activity of *Escherichia coli* cells. *Biochem Biophys Res Commun* **91**:819–826.

4. Mizuno T, Wurtzel ET, Inouye M. 1982. Osmoregulation of gene expression. II. DNA sequence of the envZ gene of the ompB operon of *Escherichia coli* and characterization of its gene product. *J Biol Chem* **257**:13692–13698.

5. Tommassen J, de Geus P, Lugtenberg B, Hackett J, Reeves P. 1982. Regulation of the pho regulon of *Escherichia coli* K-12: cloning of the regulatory genes phoB and phoR and identification of their gene products. *J Mol Biol* **157**:265–274.

6. Grebe TW, Stock JB. 1999. The histidine protein kinase superfamily. *Adv Microb Physiol* **41**:139–227.

7. Kannan N, Taylor SS, Zhai Y, Venter JC, Manning G. 2007. Structural and functional diversity of the microbial kinome. *PLoS Biol* **5**:e17.

8. Chao J, Wong D, Zheng X, Poirier V, Bach H, Hmama Z, Av-Gay Y. 2010. Protein kinase and phosphatase signaling in *Mycobacterium tuberculosis* physiology and pathogenesis. *Biochim Biophys Acta* **1804**:620–627.

9. Wong D, Chao JD, Av-Gay Y. 2013. *Mycobacterium tuberculosis*-secreted phosphatases: from pathogenesis to targets for TB drug development. *Trends Microbiol* **21**:100–109.

10. Prisic S, Husson RN. 2014. Mycobacterium tuberculosis serine/threonine protein kinases. *Microbiol Spectr* **2**:2.

11. Sickmann A, Meyer HE. 2001. Phosphoamino acid analysis. *Proteomics* **1**:200–206.

12. Av-Gay Y, Everett M. 2000. The eukaryotic-like Ser/Thr protein kinases of *Mycobacterium tuberculosis*. *Trends Microbiol* **8**:238–244.

13. Alber T. 2009. Signaling mechanisms of the *Mycobacterium tuberculosis* receptor Ser/Thr protein kinases. *Curr Opin Struct Biol* **19**:650–657.

14. Kumar P, Kumar D, Parikh A, Rananaware D, Gupta M, Singh Y, Nandicoori VK. 2009. The *Mycobacterium tuberculosis* protein kinase K modulates activation of transcription from the promoter of mycobacterial monooxygenase operon through phosphorylation of the transcriptional regulator VirS. *J Biol Chem* **284**:11090–11099.

15. Koul A, Choidas A, Treder M, Tyagi AK, Drlica K, Singh Y, Ullrich A. 2000. Cloning and characterization of secretory tyrosine phosphatases of *Mycobacterium tuberculosis*. *J Bacteriol* **182**:5425–5432.

16. Bach H, Papavinasasundaram KG, Wong D, Hmama Z, Av-Gay Y. 2008. *Mycobacterium tuberculosis* virulence is mediated by PtpA dephosphorylation of human vacuolar protein sorting 33B. *Cell Host Microbe* **3**:316–322.

17. Bach H, Ko HH, Raizman EA, Attarian R, Cho B, Biet F, Enns R, Bressler B. 2011. Immunogenicity of *Mycobacterium avium* subsp. *paratuberculosis* proteins in Crohn's disease patients. *Scand J Gastroenterol* **46**:30–39.

18. Chow K, Ng D, Stokes R, Johnson P. 1994. Protein tyrosine phosphorylation in *Mycobacterium tuberculosis*. *FEMS Microbiol Lett* **124**:203–207.

19. Bach H, Wong D, Av-Gay Y. 2009. *Mycobacterium tuberculosis* PtkA is a novel protein tyrosine kinase whose substrate is PtpA. *Biochem J* **420**:155–162.

20. Kusebauch U, Ortega C, Ollodart A, Rogers RS, Sherman DR, Moritz RL, Grundner C. 2014. *Mycobacterium tuberculosis* supports protein tyrosine phosphorylation. *Proc Natl Acad Sci USA* **111**:9265–9270.

21. Chao KL, Gorlatova NV, Eisenstein E, Herzberg O. 2014. Structural basis for the binding specificity of human Recepteur d'Origine Nantais (RON) receptor tyrosine kinase to macrophage-stimulating protein. *J Biol Chem* **289**:29948–29960.

22. Zhou P, Wong D, Li W, Xie J, Av-Gay Y. 2015. Phosphorylation of *Mycobacterium tuberculosis* protein tyrosine kinase A PtkA by Ser/Thr protein kinases. *Biochem Biophys Res Commun* **467**:421–426.

23. Prisic S, Dankwa S, Schwartz D, Chou MF, Locasale JW, Kang CM, Bemis G, Church GM, Steen H, Husson RN. 2010. Extensive phosphorylation with overlapping specificity by *Mycobacterium tuberculosis* serine/threonine protein kinases. *Proc Natl Acad Sci USA* **107**:7521–7526.

24. Jünger MA, Aebersold R. 2014. Mass spectrometry-driven phosphoproteomics: patterning the systems biology mosaic. *Wiley Interdiscip Rev Dev Biol* **3**:83–112.

25. Sharma K, Gupta M, Pathak M, Gupta N, Koul A, Sarangi S, Baweja R, Singh Y. 2006. Transcriptional control of the mycobacterial embCAB operon by PknH through a regulatory protein, EmbR, *in vivo*. *J Bacteriol* **188**:2936–2944.

26. Cohen-Gonsaud M, Barthe P, Canova MJ, Stagier-Simon C, Kremer L, Roumestand C, Molle V. 2009. The *Mycobacterium tuberculosis* Ser/Thr kinase substrate Rv2175c is a DNA-binding protein regulated by phosphorylation. *J Biol Chem* **284**:19290–19300.

27. Chao JD, Papavinasasundaram KG, Zheng X, Chávez-Steenbock A, Wang X, Lee GQ, Av-Gay Y. 2010. Convergence of Ser/Thr and two-component signaling to coordinate expression of the dormancy regulon in *Mycobacterium tuberculosis*. *J Biol Chem* **285**:29239–29246.

28. Baer CE, Iavarone AT, Alber T, Sassetti CM. 2014. Biochemical and spatial coincidence in the provisional Ser/Thr protein kinase interaction network of *Mycobacterium tuberculosis*. *J Biol Chem* **289**:20422–20433.

29. Nagarajan SN, Upadhyay S, Chawla Y, Khan S, Naz S, Subramanian J, Gandotra S, Nandicoori VK. 2015. Protein kinase A (PknA) of *Mycobacterium tuberculosis* is independently activated and is critical for growth *in vitro* and survival of the pathogen in the host. *J Biol Chem* **290**:9626–9645.

30. Greenstein AE, MacGurn JA, Baer CE, Falick AM, Cox JS, Alber T. 2007. *M. tuberculosis* Ser/Thr protein kinase D phosphorylates an anti-anti-sigma factor homolog. *PLoS Pathog* 3:e49.

31. Hatzios SK, Baer CE, Rustad TR, Siegrist MS, Pang JM, Ortega C, Alber T, Grundner C, Sherman DR, Bertozzi CR. 2013. Osmosensory signaling in *Mycobacterium tuberculosis* mediated by a eukaryotic-like Ser/Thr protein kinase. *Proc Natl Acad Sci USA* 110: E5069–E5077.

32. Good MC, Greenstein AE, Young TA, Ng HL, Alber T. 2004. Sensor domain of the *Mycobacterium tuberculosis* receptor Ser/Thr protein kinase, PknD, forms a highly symmetric beta propeller. *J Mol Biol* 339:459–469.

33. Ortega C, Liao R, Anderson LN, Rustad T, Ollodart AR, Wright AT, Sherman DR, Grundner C. 2014. *Mycobacterium tuberculosis* Ser/Thr protein kinase B mediates an oxygen-dependent replication switch. *PLoS Biol* 12: e1001746.

34. Armstrong JA, Hart PD. 1971. Response of cultured macrophages to *Mycobacterium tuberculosis*, with observations on fusion of lysosomes with phagosomes. *J Exp Med* 134:713–740.

35. Sturgill-Koszycki S, Schlesinger PH, Chakraborty P, Haddix PL, Collins HL, Fok AK, Allen RD, Gluck SL, Heuser J, Russell DG. 1994. Lack of acidification in *Mycobacterium* phagosomes produced by exclusion of the vesicular proton-ATPase. *Science* 263:678–681.

36. Poirier V, Bach H, Av-Gay Y. 2014. *Mycobacterium tuberculosis* promotes anti-apoptotic activity of the macrophage by PtpA protein-dependent dephosphorylation of host GSK3α. *J Biol Chem* 289:29376–29385.

37. Wong D, Bach H, Sun J, Hmama Z, Av-Gay Y. 2011. *Mycobacterium tuberculosis* protein tyrosine phosphatase (PtpA) excludes host vacuolar-H+-ATPase to inhibit phagosome acidification. *Proc Natl Acad Sci USA* 108: 19371–19376.

38. Wang J, Li BX, Ge PP, Li J, Wang Q, Gao GF, Qiu XB, Liu CH. 2015. *Mycobacterium tuberculosis* suppresses innate immunity by coopting the host ubiquitin system. *Nat Immunol* 16:237–245.

39. Walburger A, Koul A, Ferrari G, Nguyen L, Prescianotto-Baschong C, Huygen K, Klebl B, Thompson C, Bacher G, Pieters J. 2004. Protein kinase G from pathogenic mycobacteria promotes survival within macrophages. *Science* 304:1800–1804.

40. O'Hare HM, Durán R, Cerveñansky C, Bellinzoni M, Wehenkel AM, Pritsch O, Obal G, Baumgartner J, Vialaret J, Johnsson K, Alzari PM. 2008. Regulation of glutamate metabolism by protein kinases in mycobacteria. *Mol Microbiol* 70:1408–1423.

41. Cowley S, Ko M, Pick N, Chow R, Downing KJ, Gordhan BG, Betts JC, Mizrahi V, Smith DA, Stokes RW, Av-Gay Y. 2004. The *Mycobacterium tuberculosis* protein serine/threonine kinase PknG is linked to cellular glutamate/glutamine levels and is important for growth *in vivo*. *Mol Microbiol* 52:1691–1702.

42. Keane J, Remold HG, Kornfeld H. 2000. Virulent *Mycobacterium tuberculosis* strains evade apoptosis of infected alveolar macrophages. *J Immunol* 164:2016–2020.

43. Jayakumar D, Jacobs WR Jr, Narayanan S. 2008. Protein kinase E of *Mycobacterium tuberculosis* has a role in the nitric oxide stress response and apoptosis in a human macrophage model of infection. *Cell Microbiol* 10:365–374.

44. Papavinasasundaram KG, Chan B, Chung JH, Colston MJ, Davis EO, Av-Gay Y. 2005. Deletion of the *Mycobacterium tuberculosis* pknH gene confers a higher bacillary load during the chronic phase of infection in BALB/c mice. *J Bacteriol* 187:5751–5760.

45. Li CQ, Wogan GN. 2005. Nitric oxide as a modulator of apoptosis. *Cancer Lett* 226:1–15.

46. Kumar D, Narayanan S. 2012. pknE, a serine/threonine kinase of *Mycobacterium tuberculosis* modulates multiple apoptotic paradigms. *Infect Genet Evol* 12: 737–747.

47. Parandhaman DK, Hanna LE, Narayanan S. 2014. PknE, a serine/threonine protein kinase of *Mycobacterium tuberculosis* initiates survival crosstalk that also impacts HIV coinfection. *PLoS One* 9:e83541.

48. Sequeira PC, Senaratne RH, Riley LW. 2014. Inhibition of toll-like receptor 2 (TLR-2)-mediated response in human alveolar epithelial cells by mycolic acids and *Mycobacterium tuberculosis* mce1 operon mutant. *Pathog Dis* 70:132–140.

49. Sánchez D, Rojas M, Hernández I, Radzioch D, García LF, Barrera LF. 2010. Role of TLR2- and TLR4-mediated signaling in *Mycobacterium tuberculosis*-induced macrophage death. *Cell Immunol* 260:128–136.

50. Nuzzo I, Galdiero M, Bentivoglio C, Galdiero R, Romano Carratelli C. 2002. Apoptosis modulation by mycolic acid, tuberculostearic acid and trehalose 6,6′-dimycolate. *J Infect* 44:229–235.

51. Zhou P, Li W, Wong D, Xie J, Av-Gay Y. 2015. Phosphorylation control of protein tyrosine phosphatase A activity in *Mycobacterium tuberculosis*. *FEBS Lett* 589: 326–331.

52. Vishwanath V, Meera R, Narayanan PR, Puvanakrishnan R. 1997. Fate of *Mycobacterium tuberculosis* inside rat peritoneal macrophages *in vitro*. *Mol Cell Biochem* 175: 169–175.

53. Sachdeva P, Misra R, Tyagi AK, Singh Y. 2010. The sigma factors of *Mycobacterium tuberculosis*: regulation of the regulators. *FEBS J* 277:605–626.

54. Song T, Dove SL, Lee KH, Husson RN. 2003. RshA, an anti-sigma factor that regulates the activity of the mycobacterial stress response sigma factor SigH. *Mol Microbiol* 50:949–959.

55. Park ST, Kang CM, Husson RN. 2008. Regulation of the SigH stress response regulon by an essential protein kinase in *Mycobacterium tuberculosis*. *Proc Natl Acad Sci USA* 105:13105–13110.

56. Anandan T, Han J, Baun H, Nyayapathy S, Brown JT, Dial RL, Moltalvo JA, Kim MS, Yang SH, Ronning DR, Husson RN, Suh J, Kang CM. 2014. Phosphorylation regulates mycobacterial proteasome. *J Microbiol* 52: 743–754.

57. Festa RA, McAllister F, Pearce MJ, Mintseris J, Burns KE, Gygi SP, Darwin KH. 2010. Prokaryotic ubiquitin-

like protein (Pup) proteome of *Mycobacterium tuberculosis*. *PLoS One* 5:e8589.

58. Darwin KH, Ehrt S, Gutierrez-Ramos JC, Weich N, Nathan CF. 2003. The proteasome of *Mycobacterium tuberculosis* is required for resistance to nitric oxide. *Science* 302:1963–1966.

59. Gandotra S, Schnappinger D, Monteleone M, Hillen W, Ehrt S. 2007. *In vivo* gene silencing identifies the *Mycobacterium tuberculosis* proteasome as essential for the bacteria to persist in mice. *Nat Med* 13:1515–1520.

60. MacMicking JD, North RJ, LaCourse R, Mudgett JS, Shah SK, Nathan CF. 1997. Identification of nitric oxide synthase as a protective locus against tuberculosis. *Proc Natl Acad Sci USA* 94:5243–5248.

61. Miller CC, Rawat M, Johnson T, Av-Gay Y. 2007. Innate protection of *Mycobacterium smegmatis* against the antimicrobial activity of nitric oxide is provided by mycothiol. *Antimicrob Agents Chemother* 51:3364–3366.

62. Davis AS, Vergne I, Master SS, Kyei GB, Chua J, Deretic V. 2007. Mechanism of inducible nitric oxide synthase exclusion from mycobacterial phagosomes. *PLoS Pathog* 3:e186.

63. Aldridge BB, Fernandez-Suarez M, Heller D, Ambravaneswaran V, Irimia D, Toner M, Fortune SM. 2012. Asymmetry and aging of mycobacterial cells lead to variable growth and antibiotic susceptibility. *Science* 335:100–104.

64. Santi I, Dhar N, Bousbaine D, Wakamoto Y, McKinney JD. 2013. Single-cell dynamics of the chromosome replication and cell division cycles in mycobacteria. *Nat Commun* 4:2470.

65. Kieser KJ, Rubin EJ. 2014. How sisters grow apart: mycobacterial growth and division. *Nat Rev Microbiol* 12:550–562.

66. Kang CM, Abbott DW, Park ST, Dascher CC, Cantley LC, Husson RN. 2005. The *Mycobacterium tuberculosis* serine/threonine kinases PknA and PknB: substrate identification and regulation of cell shape. *Genes Dev* 19:1692–1704.

67. Parikh A, Verma SK, Khan S, Prakash B, Nandicoori VK. 2009. PknB-mediated phosphorylation of a novel substrate, N-acetylglucosamine-1-phosphate uridyltransferase, modulates its acetyltransferase activity. *J Mol Biol* 386:451–464.

68. Gee CL, Papavinasasundaram KG, Blair SR, Baer CE, Falick AM, King DS, Griffin JE, Venghatakrishnan H, Zukauskas A, Wei JR, Dhiman RK, Crick DC, Rubin EJ, Sassetti CM, Alber T. 2012. A phosphorylated pseudokinase complex controls cell wall synthesis in mycobacteria. *Sci Signal* 5:ra7.

69. Mahapatra S, Yagi T, Belisle JT, Espinosa BJ, Hill PJ, McNeil MR, Brennan PJ, Crick DC. 2005. Mycobacterial lipid II is composed of a complex mixture of modified muramyl and peptide moieties linked to decaprenyl phosphate. *J Bacteriol* 187:2747–2757.

70. Davis KM, Weiser JN. 2011. Modifications to the peptidoglycan backbone help bacteria to establish infection. *Infect Immun* 79:562–570.

71. Hansen JM, Golchin SA, Veyrier FJ, Domenech P, Boneca IG, Azad AK, Rajaram MV, Schlesinger LS, Divangahi M, Reed MB, Behr MA. 2014. N-glycolylated peptidoglycan contributes to the immunogenicity but not pathogenicity of *Mycobacterium tuberculosis*. *J Infect Dis* 209:1045–1054.

72. Coulombe F, Divangahi M, Veyrier F, de Léséleuc L, Gleason JL, Yang Y, Kelliher MA, Pandey AK, Sassetti CM, Reed MB, Behr MA. 2009. Increased NOD2-mediated recognition of N-glycolyl muramyl dipeptide. *J Exp Med* 206:1709–1716.

73. Munshi T, Gupta A, Evangelopoulos D, Guzman JD, Gibbons S, Keep NH, Bhakta S. 2013. Characterisation of ATP-dependent Mur ligases involved in the biogenesis of cell wall peptidoglycan in *Mycobacterium tuberculosis*. *PLoS One* 8:e60143.

74. Thakur M, Chakraborti PK. 2008. Ability of PknA, a mycobacterial eukaryotic-type serine/threonine kinase, to transphosphorylate MurD, a ligase involved in the process of peptidoglycan biosynthesis. *Biochem J* 415:27–33.

75. Kumar P, Arora K, Lloyd JR, Lee IY, Nair V, Fischer E, Boshoff HI, Barry CE III. 2012. Meropenem inhibits D,D-carboxypeptidase activity in *Mycobacterium tuberculosis*. *Mol Microbiol* 86:367–381.

76. Lavollay M, Arthur M, Fourgeaud M, Dubost L, Marie A, Veziris N, Blanot D, Gutmann L, Mainardi JL. 2008. The peptidoglycan of stationary-phase *Mycobacterium tuberculosis* predominantly contains cross-links generated by L,D-transpeptidation. *J Bacteriol* 190:4360–4366.

77. Gupta R, Lavollay M, Mainardi JL, Arthur M, Bishai WR, Lamichhane G. 2010. The *Mycobacterium tuberculosis* protein LdtMt2 is a nonclassical transpeptidase required for virulence and resistance to amoxicillin. *Nat Med* 16:466–469.

78. Zheng X, Papavinasasundaram KG, Av-Gay Y. 2007. Novel substrates of *Mycobacterium tuberculosis* PknH Ser/Thr kinase. *Biochem Biophys Res Commun* 355:162–168.

79. Kieser KJ, Boutte CC, Kester JC, Baer CE, Barczak AK, Meniche X, Chao MC, Rego EH, Sassetti CM, Fortune SM, Rubin EJ. 2015. Phosphorylation of the peptidoglycan synthase PonA1 governs the rate of polar elongation in mycobacteria. *PLoS Pathog* 11:e1005010.

80. Meniche X, Otten R, Siegrist MS, Baer CE, Murphy KC, Bertozzi CR, Sassetti CM. 2014. Subpolar addition of new cell wall is directed by DivIVA in mycobacteria. *Proc Natl Acad Sci USA* 111:E3243–E3251.

81. Joyce G, Williams KJ, Robb M, Noens E, Tizzano B, Shahrezaei V, Robertson BD. 2012. Cell division site placement and asymmetric growth in mycobacteria. *PLoS One* 7:e44582.

82. Singh B, Nitharwal RG, Ramesh M, Pettersson BM, Kirsebom LA, Dasgupta S. 2013. Asymmetric growth and division in *Mycobacterium* spp.: compensatory mechanisms for non-medial septa. *Mol Microbiol* 88:64–76.

83. Kysela DT, Brown PJ, Huang KC, Brun YV. 2013. Biological consequences and advantages of asymmetric bacterial growth. *Annu Rev Microbiol* 67:417–435.

84. Adams DW, Errington J. 2009. Bacterial cell division: assembly, maintenance and disassembly of the Z ring. *Nat Rev Microbiol* **7:**642–653.

85. Thakur M, Chakraborti PK. 2006. GTPase activity of mycobacterial FtsZ is impaired due to its transphosphorylation by the eukaryotic-type Ser/Thr kinase, PknA. *J Biol Chem* **281:**40107–40113.

86. Typas A, Banzhaf M, Gross CA, Vollmer W. 2011. From the regulation of peptidoglycan synthesis to bacterial growth and morphology. *Nat Rev Microbiol* **10:** 123–136.

87. Dasgupta A, Datta P, Kundu M, Basu J. 2006. The serine/threonine kinase PknB of *Mycobacterium tuberculosis* phosphorylates PBPA, a penicillin-binding protein required for cell division. *Microbiology* **152:**493–504. [Retraction.]

88. Chawla Y, Upadhyay S, Khan S, Nagarajan SN, Forti F, Nandicoori VK. 2014. Protein kinase B (PknB) of *Mycobacterium tuberculosis* is essential for growth of the pathogen *in vitro* as well as for survival within the host. *J Biol Chem* **289:**13858–13875.

89. Rachman H, Strong M, Ulrichs T, Grode L, Schuchhardt J, Mollenkopf H, Kosmiadi GA, Eisenberg D, Kaufmann SH. 2006. Unique transcriptome signature of *Mycobacterium tuberculosis* in pulmonary tuberculosis. *Infect Immun* **74:**1233–1242.

90. Griffin JE, Pandey AK, Gilmore SA, Mizrahi V, McKinney JD, Bertozzi CR, Sassetti CM. 2012. Cholesterol catabolism by *Mycobacterium tuberculosis* requires transcriptional and metabolic adaptations. *Chem Biol* **19:**218–227.

91. Dubnau E, Chan J, Raynaud C, Mohan VP, Lanéelle MA, Yu K, Quémard A, Smith I, Daffé M. 2000. Oxygenated mycolic acids are necessary for virulence of *Mycobacterium tuberculosis* in mice. *Mol Microbiol* **36:** 630–637.

92. Vander Beken S, Al Dulayymi JR, Naessens T, Koza G, Maza-Iglesias M, Rowles R, Theunissen C, De Medts J, Lanckacker E, Baird MS, Grooten J. 2011. Molecular structure of the *Mycobacterium tuberculosis* virulence factor, mycolic acid, determines the elicited inflammatory pattern. *Eur J Immunol* **41:**450–460.

93. Jain M, Petzold CJ, Schelle MW, Leavell MD, Mougous JD, Bertozzi CR, Leary JA, Cox JS. 2007. Lipidomics reveals control of *Mycobacterium tuberculosis* virulence lipids via metabolic coupling. *Proc Natl Acad Sci USA* **104:**5133–5138.

94. Bhamidi S, Shi L, Chatterjee D, Belisle JT, Crick DC, McNeil MR. 2012. A bioanalytical method to determine the cell wall composition of *Mycobacterium tuberculosis* grown *in vivo*. *Anal Biochem* **421:**240–249.

95. Barry CE III, Lee RE, Mdluli K, Sampson AE, Schroeder BG, Slayden RA, Yuan Y. 1998. Mycolic acids: structure, biosynthesis and physiological functions. *Prog Lipid Res* **37:**143–179.

96. Veyron-Churlet R, Zanella-Cléon I, Cohen-Gonsaud M, Molle V, Kremer L. 2010. Phosphorylation of the *Mycobacterium tuberculosis* beta-ketoacyl-acyl carrier protein reductase MabA regulates mycolic acid biosynthesis. *J Biol Chem* **285:**12714–12725.

97. Molle V, Gulten G, Vilchèze C, Veyron-Churlet R, Zanella-Cléon I, Sacchettini JC, Jacobs WR Jr, Kremer L. 2010. Phosphorylation of InhA inhibits mycolic acid biosynthesis and growth of *Mycobacterium tuberculosis*. *Mol Microbiol* **78:**1591–1605.

98. Khan S, Nagarajan SN, Parikh A, Samantaray S, Singh A, Kumar D, Roy RP, Bhatt A, Nandicoori VK. 2010. Phosphorylation of enoyl-acyl carrier protein reductase InhA impacts mycobacterial growth and survival. *J Biol Chem* **285:**37860–37871.

99. Slama N, Leiba J, Eynard N, Daffé M, Kremer L, Quémard A, Molle V. 2011. Negative regulation by Ser/Thr phosphorylation of HadAB and HadBC dehydratases from *Mycobacterium tuberculosis* type II fatty acid synthase system. *Biochem Biophys Res Commun* **412:**401–406.

100. Vilchèze C, Molle V, Carrère-Kremer S, Leiba J, Mourey L, Shenai S, Baronian G, Tufariello J, Hartman T, Veyron-Churlet R, Trivelli X, Tiwari S, Weinrick B, Alland D, Guérardel Y, Jacobs WR Jr, Kremer L. 2014. Phosphorylation of KasB regulates virulence and acid-fastness in *Mycobacterium tuberculosis*. *PLoS Pathog* **10:**e1004115.

101. Molle V, Brown AK, Besra GS, Cozzone AJ, Kremer L. 2006. The condensing activities of the *Mycobacterium tuberculosis* type II fatty acid synthase are differentially regulated by phosphorylation. *J Biol Chem* **281:**30094–30103.

102. Veyron-Churlet R, Molle V, Taylor RC, Brown AK, Besra GS, Zanella-Cléon I, Fütterer K, Kremer L. 2009. The *Mycobacterium tuberculosis* beta-ketoacyl-acyl carrier protein synthase III activity is inhibited by phosphorylation on a single threonine residue. *J Biol Chem* **284:** 6414–6424.

103. Bhatt A, Fujiwara N, Bhatt K, Gurcha SS, Kremer L, Chen B, Chan J, Porcelli SA, Kobayashi K, Besra GS, Jacobs WR Jr. 2007. Deletion of kasB in *Mycobacterium tuberculosis* causes loss of acid-fastness and subclinical latent tuberculosis in immunocompetent mice. *Proc Natl Acad Sci USA* **104:**5157–5162.

104. Gao LY, Laval F, Lawson EH, Groger RK, Woodruff A, Morisaki JH, Cox JS, Daffé M, Brown EJ. 2003. Requirement for kasB in i mycolic acid biosynthesis, cell wall impermeability and intracellular survival: implications for therapy. *Mol Microbiol* **49:**1547–1563.

105. Wilson M, DeRisi J, Kristensen HH, Imboden P, Rane S, Brown PO, Schoolnik GK. 1999. Exploring drug-induced alterations in gene expression in *Mycobacterium tuberculosis* by microarray hybridization. *Proc Natl Acad Sci USA* **96:**12833–12838.

106. Voskuil MI. 2013. *Mycobacterium tuberculosis* cholesterol catabolism requires a new class of acyl coenzyme A dehydrogenase. *J Bacteriol* **195:**4319–4321.

107. Rienksma RA, Suarez-Diez M, Mollenkopf HJ, Dolganov GM, Dorhoi A, Schoolnik GK, Martins Dos Santos VA, Kaufmann SH, Schaap PJ, Gengenbacher M. 2015. Comprehensive insights into transcriptional adaptation of intracellular mycobacteria by microbe-enriched dual RNA sequencing. *BMC Genomics* **16:**34.

108. Asselineau C, Asselineau J, Lanéelle G, Lanéelle MA. 2002. The biosynthesis of mycolic acids by mycobac-

teria: current and alternative hypotheses. *Prog Lipid Res* 41:501–523.

109. Singh A, Gupta R, Vishwakarma RA, Narayanan PR, Paramasivan CN, Ramanathan VD, Tyagi AK. 2005. Requirement of the mymA operon for appropriate cell wall ultrastructure and persistence of *Mycobacterium tuberculosis* in the spleens of guinea pigs. *J Bacteriol* 187:4173–4186.

110. Singh A, Jain S, Gupta S, Das T, Tyagi AK. 2003. mymA operon of *Mycobacterium tuberculosis*: its regulation and importance in the cell envelope. *FEMS Microbiol Lett* 227:53–63.

111. Rousseau C, Winter N, Pivert E, Bordat Y, Neyrolles O, Avé P, Huerre M, Gicquel B, Jackson M. 2004. Production of phthiocerol dimycocerosates protects *Mycobacterium tuberculosis* from the cidal activity of reactive nitrogen intermediates produced by macrophages and modulates the early immune response to infection. *Cell Microbiol* 6:277–287.

112. Sharma K, Chandra H, Gupta PK, Pathak M, Narayan A, Meena LS, D'Souza RC, Chopra P, Ramachandran S, Singh Y. 2004. PknH, a transmembrane Hank's type serine/threonine kinase from *Mycobacterium tuberculosis* is differentially expressed under stress conditions. *FEMS Microbiol Lett* 233:107–113.

113. Gómez-Velasco A, Bach H, Rana AK, Cox LR, Bhatt A, Besra GS, Av-Gay Y. 2013. Disruption of the serine/threonine protein kinase H affects phthiocerol dimycocerosates synthesis in *Mycobacterium tuberculosis*. *Microbiology* 159:726–736.

114. Pérez J, Garcia R, Bach H, de Waard JH, Jacobs WR Jr, Av-Gay Y, Bubis J, Takiff HE. 2006. *Mycobacterium tuberculosis* transporter MmpL7 is a potential substrate for kinase PknD. *Biochem Biophys Res Commun* 348:6–12.

115. Touchette MH, Bommineni GR, Delle Bovi RJ, Gadbery JE, Nicora CD, Shukla AK, Kyle JE, Metz TO, Martin DW, Sampson NS, Miller WT, Tonge PJ, Seeliger JC. 2015. Diacyltransferase activity and chain length specificity of *Mycobacterium tuberculosis* PapA5 in the synthesis of alkyl β-diol lipids. *Biochemistry* 54:5457–5468.

116. Gupta M, Sajid A, Arora G, Tandon V, Singh Y. 2009. Forkhead-associated domain-containing protein Rv0019c and polyketide-associated protein PapA5, from substrates of serine/threonine protein kinase PknB to interacting proteins of *Mycobacterium tuberculosis*. *J Biol Chem* 284:34723–34734.

117. Gilmore SA, Schelle MW, Holsclaw CM, Leigh CD, Jain M, Cox JS, Leary JA, Bertozzi CR. 2012. Sulfolipid-1 biosynthesis restricts *Mycobacterium tuberculosis* growth in human macrophages. *ACS Chem Biol* 7:863–870.

118. Gengenbacher M, Kaufmann SH. 2012. *Mycobacterium tuberculosis*: success through dormancy. *FEMS Microbiol Rev* 36:514–532.

119. Canetti G. 1955. The tubercle bacillus in the pulmonary lesion of man, p 111–126. *In* Dubos RJ, McDermott W (ed), *Growth of the Tubercle Bacillus in the Tuberculosis Lesion*. Springer, New York, NY.

120. Voskuil MI, Schnappinger D, Visconti KC, Harrell MI, Dolganov GM, Sherman DR, Schoolnik GK. 2003. Inhibition of respiration by nitric oxide induces a *Mycobacterium tuberculosis* dormancy program. *J Exp Med* 198:705–713.

121. Saini DK, Malhotra V, Tyagi JS. 2004. Cross talk between DevS sensor kinase homologue, Rv2027c, and DevR response regulator of *Mycobacterium tuberculosis*. *FEBS Lett* 565:75–80.

122. Kumar A, Toledo JC, Patel RP, Lancaster JR Jr, Steyn AJ. 2007. *Mycobacterium tuberculosis* DosS is a redox sensor and DosT is a hypoxia sensor. *Proc Natl Acad Sci USA* 104:11568–11573.

123. Sherman DR, Voskuil M, Schnappinger D, Liao R, Harrell MI, Schoolnik GK. 2001. Regulation of the *Mycobacterium tuberculosis* hypoxic response gene encoding alpha-crystallin. *Proc Natl Acad Sci USA* 98:7534–7539. [Erratum,]

124. Park HD, Guinn KM, Harrell MI, Liao R, Voskuil MI, Tompa M, Schoolnik GK, Sherman DR. 2003. Rv3133c/dosR is a transcription factor that mediates the hypoxic response of *Mycobacterium tuberculosis*. *Mol Microbiol* 48:833–843.

125. Rosenkrands I, Slayden RA, Crawford J, Aagaard C, Barry CE III, Andersen P. 2002. Hypoxic response of *Mycobacterium tuberculosis* studied by metabolic labeling and proteome analysis of cellular and extracellular proteins. *J Bacteriol* 184:3485–3491.

126. Kumar A, Deshane JS, Crossman DK, Bolisetty S, Yan BS, Kramnik I, Agarwal A, Steyn AJ. 2008. Heme oxygenase-1-derived carbon monoxide induces the *Mycobacterium tuberculosis* dormancy regulon. *J Biol Chem* 283:18032–18039.

127. Shiloh MU, Manzanillo P, Cox JS. 2008. *Mycobacterium tuberculosis* senses host-derived carbon monoxide during macrophage infection. *Cell Host Microbe* 3:323–330.

128. Betts JC, Lukey PT, Robb LC, McAdam RA, Duncan K. 2002. Evaluation of a nutrient starvation model of *Mycobacterium tuberculosis* persistence by gene and protein expression profiling. *Mol Microbiol* 43:717–731.

129. Bacon J, Alderwick LJ, Allnutt JA, Gabasova E, Watson R, Hatch KA, Clark SO, Jeeves RE, Marriott A, Rayner E, Tolley H, Pearson G, Hall G, Besra GS, Wernisch L, Williams A, Marsh PD. 2014. Non-replicating *Mycobacterium tuberculosis* elicits a reduced infectivity profile with corresponding modifications to the cell wall and extracellular matrix. *PLoS One* 9:e87329.

130. Nyka W. 1974. Studies on the effect of starvation on mycobacteria. *Infect Immun* 9:843–850.

131. Loebel RO, Shorr E, Richardson HB. 1933. The influence of adverse conditions upon the respiratory metabolism and growth of human tubercle bacilli. *J Bacteriol* 26:167–200.

132. Richard-Greenblatt M, Bach H, Adamson J, Peña-Diaz S, Li W, Steyn AJ, Av-Gay Y. 2015. Regulation of ergothioneine biosynthesis and its effect on *Mycobacterium tuberculosis* growth and infectivity. *J Biol Chem* 290:23064–23076.

133. Malhotra V, Arteaga-Cortés LT, Clay G, Clark-Curtiss JE. 2010. *Mycobacterium tuberculosis* protein kinase K confers survival advantage during early infection in mice and regulates growth in culture and during persistent infection: implications for immune modulation. *Microbiology* 156:2829–2841.

134. Malhotra V, Okon BP, Clark-Curtiss JE. 2012. *Mycobacterium tuberculosis* protein kinase K enables growth adaptation through translation control. *J Bacteriol* 194:4184–4196.

135. Gopalaswamy R, Narayanan S, Chen B, Jacobs WR, Av-Gay Y. 2009. The serine/threonine protein kinase PknI controls the growth of *Mycobacterium tuberculosis* upon infection. *FEMS Microbiol Lett* 295:23–29.

136. Singh A, Singh Y, Pine R, Shi L, Chandra R, Drlica K. 2006. Protein kinase I of *Mycobacterium tuberculosis*: cellular localization and expression during infection of macrophage-like cells. *Tuberculosis (Edinb)* 86:28–33.

137. Rittershaus ES, Baek SH, Sassetti CM. 2013. The normalcy of dormancy: common themes in microbial quiescence. *Cell Host Microbe* 13:643–651.

138. Cunningham AF, Spreadbury CL. 1998. Mycobacterial stationary phase induced by low oxygen tension: cell wall thickening and localization of the 16-kilodalton alpha-crystallin homolog. *J Bacteriol* 180:801–808.

139. Ortalo-Magné A, Dupont MA, Lemassu A, Andersen AB, Gounon P, Daffé M. 1995. Molecular composition of the outermost capsular material of the tubercle bacillus. *Microbiology* 141:1609–1620.

140. Ortalo-Magné A, Lemassu A, Lanéelle MA, Bardou F, Silve G, Gounon P, Marchal G, Daffé M. 1996. Identification of the surface-exposed lipids on the cell envelopes of *Mycobacterium tuberculosis* and other mycobacterial species. *J Bacteriol* 178:456–461.

141. Sambou T, Dinadayala P, Stadthagen G, Barilone N, Bordat Y, Constant P, Levillain F, Neyrolles O, Gicquel B, Lemassu A, Daffé M, Jackson M. 2008. Capsular glucan and intracellular glycogen of *Mycobacterium tuberculosis*: biosynthesis and impact on the persistence in mice. *Mol Microbiol* 70:762–774.

142. Chandra G, Chater KF, Bornemann S. 2011. Unexpected and widespread connections between bacterial glycogen and trehalose metabolism. *Microbiology* 157:1565–1572.

143. Leiba J, Syson K, Baronian G, Zanella-Cléon I, Kalscheuer R, Kremer L, Bornemann S, Molle V. 2013. *Mycobacterium tuberculosis* maltosyltransferase GlgE, a genetically validated antituberculosis target, is negatively regulated by Ser/Thr phosphorylation. *J Biol Chem* 288:16546–16556.

144. Ojha AK, Baughn AD, Sambandan D, Hsu T, Trivelli X, Guerardel Y, Alahari A, Kremer L, Jacobs WR Jr, Hatfull GF. 2008. Growth of *Mycobacterium tuberculosis* biofilms containing free mycolic acids and harbouring drug-tolerant bacteria. *Mol Microbiol* 69:164–174.

145. Ojha AK, Trivelli X, Guerardel Y, Kremer L, Hatfull GF. 2010. Enzymatic hydrolysis of trehalose dimycolate releases free mycolic acids during mycobacterial growth in biofilms. *J Biol Chem* 285:17380–17389.

146. Kalscheuer R, Weinrick B, Veeraraghavan U, Besra GS, Jacobs WR Jr. 2010. Trehalose-recycling ABC transporter LpqY-SugA-SugB-SugC is essential for virulence of *Mycobacterium tuberculosis*. *Proc Natl Acad Sci USA* 107:21761–21766.

147. Pitarque S, Larrouy-Maumus G, Payré B, Jackson M, Puzo G, Nigou J. 2008. The immunomodulatory lipoglycans, lipoarabinomannan and lipomannan, are exposed at the mycobacterial cell surface. *Tuberculosis (Edinb)* 88:560–565.

148. Vignal C, Guérardel Y, Kremer L, Masson M, Legrand D, Mazurier J, Elass E. 2003. Lipomannans, but not lipoarabinomannans, purified from *Mycobacterium chelonae* and *Mycobacterium kansasii* induce TNF-alpha and IL-8 secretion by a CD14-toll-like receptor 2-dependent mechanism. *J Immunol* 171:2014–2023.

149. Goude R, Amin AG, Chatterjee D, Parish T. 2008. The critical role of embC in *Mycobacterium tuberculosis*. *J Bacteriol* 190:4335–4341.

150. Deb C, Lee CM, Dubey VS, Daniel J, Abomoelak B, Sirakova TD, Pawar S, Rogers L, Kolattukudy PE. 2009. A novel *in vitro* multiple-stress dormancy model for *Mycobacterium tuberculosis* generates a lipid-loaded, drug-tolerant, dormant pathogen. *PLoS One* 4:e6077.

151. Gillespie J, Barton LL, Rypka EW. 1986. Phenotypic changes in mycobacteria grown in oxygen-limited conditions. *J Med Microbiol* 21:251–255.

152. Daniel J, Maamar H, Deb C, Sirakova TD, Kolattukudy PE. 2011. *Mycobacterium tuberculosis* uses host triacylglycerol to accumulate lipid droplets and acquires a dormancy-like phenotype in lipid-loaded macrophages. *PLoS Pathog* 7:e1002093.

153. Corrales RM, Molle V, Leiba J, Mourey L, de Chastellier C, Kremer L. 2012. Phosphorylation of mycobacterial PcaA inhibits mycolic acid cyclopropanation: consequences for intracellular survival and for phagosome maturation block. *J Biol Chem* 287:26187–26199.

154. Rao V, Fujiwara N, Porcelli SA, Glickman MS. 2005. *Mycobacterium tuberculosis* controls host innate immune activation through cyclopropane modification of a glycolipid effector molecule. *J Exp Med* 201:535–543.

155. Glickman MS, Cox JS, Jacobs WR Jr. 2000. A novel mycolic acid cyclopropane synthetase is required for cording, persistence, and virulence of *Mycobacterium tuberculosis*. *Mol Cell* 5:717–727.

156. Galagan JE, Minch K, Peterson M, Lyubetskaya A, Azizi E, Sweet L, Gomes A, Rustad T, Dolganov G, Glotova I, Abeel T, Mahwinney C, Kennedy AD, Allard R, Brabant W, Krueger A, Jaini S, Honda B, Yu WH, Hickey MJ, Zucker J, Garay C, Weiner B, Sisk P, Stolte C, Winkler JK, Van de Peer Y, Iazzetti P, Camacho D, Dreyfuss J, Liu Y, Dorhoi A, Mollenkopf HJ, Drogaris P, Lamontagne J, Zhou Y, Piquenot J, Park ST, Raman S, Kaufmann SH, Mohney RP, Chelsky D, Moody DB, Sherman DR, Schoolnik GK. 2013. The *Mycobacterium tuberculosis* regulatory network and hypoxia. *Nature* 499:178–183.

157. Barkan D, Hedhli D, Yan HG, Huygen K, Glickman MS. 2012. *Mycobacterium tuberculosis* lacking all

mycolic acid cyclopropanation is viable but highly attenuated and hyperinflammatory in mice. *Infect Immun* 80:1958–1968.

158. Barkan D, Liu Z, Sacchettini JC, Glickman MS. 2009. Mycolic acid cyclopropanation is essential for viability, drug resistance, and cell wall integrity of *Mycobacterium tuberculosis*. *Chem Biol* 16:499–509.

159. Bloch H, Segal W. 1956. Biochemical differentiation of *Mycobacterium tuberculosis* grown *in vivo* and *in vitro*. *J Bacteriol* 72:132–141.

160. Cole ST, Brosch R, Parkhill J, Garnier T, Churcher C, Harris D, Gordon SV, Eiglmeier K, Gas S, Barry CE III, Tekaia F, Badcock K, Basham D, Brown D, Chillingworth T, Connor R, Davies R, Devlin K, Feltwell T, Gentles S, Hamlin N, Holroyd S, Hornsby T, Jagels K, Krogh A, McLean J, Moule S, Murphy L, Oliver K, Osborne J, Quail MA, Rajandream MA, Rogers J, Rutter S, Seeger K, Skelton J, Squares R, Squares S, Sulston JE, Taylor K, Whitehead S, Barrell BG. 1998. Deciphering the biology of *Mycobacterium tuberculosis* from the complete genome sequence. *Nature* 393:537–544.

161. Marrero J, Trujillo C, Rhee KY, Ehrt S. 2013. Glucose phosphorylation is required for *Mycobacterium tuberculosis* persistence in mice. *PLoS Pathog* 9:e1003116.

162. Arora G, Sajid A, Gupta M, Bhaduri A, Kumar P, Basu-Modak S, Singh Y. 2010. Understanding the role of PknJ in *Mycobacterium tuberculosis*: biochemical characterization and identification of novel substrate pyruvate kinase A. *PLoS One* 5:e10772.

163. Deol P, Vohra R, Saini AK, Singh A, Chandra H, Chopra P, Das TK, Tyagi AK, Singh Y. 2005. Role of *Mycobacterium tuberculosis* Ser/Thr kinase PknF: implications in glucose transport and cell division. *J Bacteriol* 187:3415–3420.

164. Molle V, Soulat D, Jault JM, Grangeasse C, Cozzone AJ, Prost JF. 2004. Two FHA domains on an ABC transporter, Rv1747, mediate its phosphorylation by PknF, a Ser/Thr protein kinase from *Mycobacterium tuberculosis*. *FEMS Microbiol Lett* 234:215–223.

165. Singh DK, Singh PK, Tiwari S, Singh SK, Kumari R, Tripathi DK, Srivastava KK. 2014. Phosphorylation of pyruvate kinase A by protein kinase J leads to the altered growth and differential rate of intracellular survival of mycobacteria. *Appl Microbiol Biotechnol* 98:10065–10076.

166. Marrero J, Rhee KY, Schnappinger D, Pethe K, Ehrt S. 2010. Gluconeogenic carbon flow of tricarboxylic acid cycle intermediates is critical for *Mycobacterium tuberculosis* to establish and maintain infection. *Proc Natl Acad Sci USA* 107:9819–9824.

167. Nott TJ, Kelly G, Stach L, Li J, Westcott S, Patel D, Hunt DM, Howell S, Buxton RS, O'Hare HM, Smerdon SJ. 2009. An intramolecular switch regulates phosphoindependent FHA domain interactions in *Mycobacterium tuberculosis*. *Sci Signal* 2:ra12.

168. Tiwari D, Singh RK, Goswami K, Verma SK, Prakash B, Nandicoori VK. 2009. Key residues in *Mycobacterium tuberculosis* protein kinase G play a role in regulating kinase activity and survival in the host. *J Biol Chem* 284:27467–27479.

169. Chaurasiya SK, Srivastava KK. 2009. Downregulation of protein kinase C-alpha enhances intracellular survival of mycobacteria: role of PknG. *BMC Microbiol* 9:271.

170. Scherr N, Müller P, Perisa D, Combaluzier B, Jenö P, Pieters J. 2009. Survival of pathogenic mycobacteria in macrophages is mediated through autophosphorylation of protein kinase G. *J Bacteriol* 191:4546–4554.

171. Kang PB, Azad AK, Torrelles JB, Kaufman TM, Beharka A, Tibesar E, DesJardin LE, Schlesinger LS. 2005. The human macrophage mannose receptor directs *Mycobacterium tuberculosis* lipoarabinomannan-mediated phagosome biogenesis. *J Exp Med* 202:987–999.

172. Wang XM, Soetaert K, Peirs P, Kalai M, Fontaine V, Dehaye JP, Lefèvre P. 2015. Biochemical analysis of the NAD+-dependent malate dehydrogenase, a substrate of several serine/threonine protein kinases of *Mycobacterium tuberculosis*. *PLoS One* 10:e0123327.

173. Be NA, Bishai WR, Jain SK. 2012. Role of *Mycobacterium tuberculosis* pknD in the pathogenesis of central nervous system tuberculosis. *BMC Microbiol* 12:7.

174. Wayne LG. 1977. Synchronized replication of *Mycobacterium tuberculosis*. *Infect Immun* 17:528–530.

175. Schmitt SK, Longworth DL. 2014. Pulmonary infections, 505–524. *In* Kacmarek RM, Stoller JK, Heuer A (ed), *Egan's Fundamentals of Respiratory Care*, 10th ed. Elsevier Health Sciences, St. Louis, MO.

176. Tsai MC, Chakravarty S, Zhu G, Xu J, Tanaka K, Koch C, Tufariello J, Flynn J, Chan J. 2006. Characterization of the tuberculous granuloma in murine and human lungs: cellular composition and relative tissue oxygen tension. *Cell Microbiol* 8:218–232.

177. Via LE, Lin PL, Ray SM, Carrillo J, Allen SS, Eum SY, Taylor K, Klein E, Manjunatha U, Gonzales J, Lee EG, Park SK, Raleigh JA, Cho SN, McMurray DN, Flynn JL, Barry CE III. 2008. Tuberculous granulomas are hypoxic in guinea pigs, rabbits, and nonhuman primates. *Infect Immun* 76:2333–2340.

178. Barthe P, Mukamolova GV, Roumestand C, Cohen-Gonsaud M. 2010. The structure of PknB extracellular PASTA domain from *Mycobacterium tuberculosis* suggests a ligand-dependent kinase activation. *Structure* 18:606–615.

179. Sureka K, Hossain T, Mukherjee P, Chatterjee P, Datta P, Kundu M, Basu J. 2010. Novel role of phosphorylation-dependent interaction between FtsZ and FipA in mycobacterial cell division. *PLoS One* 5:e8590.

180. Baronian G, Ginda K, Berry L, Cohen-Gonsaud M, Zakrzewska-Czerwińska J, Jakimowicz D, Molle V. 2015. Phosphorylation of *Mycobacterium tuberculosis* ParB participates in regulating the ParABS chromosome segregation system. *PLoS One* 10:e0119907.

181. Sharma K, Gupta M, Krupa A, Srinivasan N, Singh Y. 2006. EmbR, a regulatory protein with ATPase activity, is a substrate of multiple serine/threonine kinases and phosphatase in *Mycobacterium tuberculosis*. *FEBS J* 273:2711–2721.

182. Corrales RM, Leiba J, Cohen-Gonsaud M, Molle V, Kremer L. 2013. *Mycobacterium tuberculosis* S-adenosyl-l-homocysteine hydrolase is negatively regulated by Ser/

Thr phosphorylation. *Biochem Biophys Res Commun* 430:858–864.

183. Sajid A, Arora G, Gupta M, Upadhyay S, Nandicoori VK, Singh Y. 2011. Phosphorylation of *Mycobacterium tuberculosis* Ser/Thr phosphatase by PknA and PknB. *PLoS One* 6:e17871.

184. Canova MJ, Kremer L, Molle V. 2009. The *Mycobacterium tuberculosis* GroEL1 chaperone is a substrate of Ser/Thr protein kinases. *J Bacteriol* 191:2876–2883.

185. Gupta M, Sajid A, Sharma K, Ghosh S, Arora G, Singh R, Nagaraja V, Tandon V, Singh Y. 2014. HupB, a nucleoid-associated protein of *Mycobacterium tuberculosis*, is modified by serine/threonine protein kinases *in vivo*. *J Bacteriol* 196:2646–2657.

186. Grundner C, Gay LM, Alber T. 2005. *Mycobacterium tuberculosis* serine/threonine kinases PknB, PknD, PknE, and PknF phosphorylate multiple FHA domains. *Protein Sci* 14:1918–1921.

187. Roumestand C, Leiba J, Galophe N, Margeat E, Padilla A, Bessin Y, Barthe P, Molle V, Cohen-Gonsaud M. 2011. Structural insight into the *Mycobacterium tuberculosis* Rv0020c protein and its interaction with the PknB kinase. *Structure* 19:1525–1534.

188. Villarino A, Duran R, Wehenkel A, Fernandez P, England P, Brodin P, Cole ST, Zimny-Arndt U, Jungblut PR, Cerveñansky C, Alzari PM. 2005. Proteomic identification of *M. tuberculosis* protein kinase substrates: PknB recruits GarA, a FHA domain-containing protein, through activation loop-mediated interactions. *J Mol Biol* 350:953–963.

189. Singhal A, Arora G, Sajid A, Maji A, Bhat A, Virmani R, Upadhyay S, Nandicoori VK, Sengupta S, Singh Y. 2013. Regulation of homocysteine metabolism by *Mycobacterium tuberculosis* S-adenosylhomocysteine hydrolase. *Sci Rep* 3:2264.

190. Sajid A, Arora G, Gupta M, Singhal A, Chakraborty K, Nandicoori VK, Singh Y. 2011. Interaction of *Mycobacterium tuberculosis* elongation factor Tu with GTP is regulated by phosphorylation. *J Bacteriol* 193:5347–5358.

191. Corrales RM, Molle V, Leiba J, Mourey L, de Chastellier C, Kremer L. 2012. Phosphorylation of mycobacterial PcaA inhibits mycolic acid cyclopropanation: consequences for intracellular survival and for phagosome maturation block. *J Biol Chem* 287:26187–26199.

192. Molle V, Reynolds RC, Alderwick LJ, Besra GS, Cozzone AJ, Fütterer K, Kremer L. 2008. EmbR2, a structural homologue of EmbR, inhibits the *Mycobacterium tuberculosis* kinase/substrate pair PknH/EmbR. *Biochem J* 410:309–317.

193. Wolff KA, de la Peña AH, Nguyen HT, Pham TH, Amzel LM, Gabelli SB, Nguyen L. 2015. A redox regulatory system critical for mycobacterial survival in macrophages and biofilm development. *PLoS Pathog* 11:e1004839.

194. Molle V, Kremer L, Girard-Blanc C, Besra GS, Cozzone AJ, Prost JF. 2003. An FHA phosphoprotein recognition domain mediates protein EmbR phosphorylation by PknH, a Ser/Thr protein kinase from *Mycobacterium tuberculosis*. *Biochemistry* 42:15300–15309.

195. Jang J, Stella A, Boudou F, Levillain F, Darthuy E, Vaubourgeix J, Wang C, Bardou F, Puzo G, Gilleron M, Burlet-Schiltz O, Monsarrat B, Brodin P, Gicquel B, Neyrolles O. 2010. Functional characterization of the *Mycobacterium tuberculosis* serine/threonine kinase PknJ. *Microbiology* 156:1619–1631.

196. Kumari R, Saxena R, Tiwari S, Tripathi DK, Srivastava KK. 2013. Rv3080c regulates the rate of inhibition of mycobacteria by isoniazid through FabD. *Mol Cell Biochem* 374:149–155.

197. Canova MJ, Veyron-Churlet R, Zanella-Cleon I, Cohen-Gonsaud M, Cozzone AJ, Becchi M, Kremer L, Molle V. 2008. The *Mycobacterium tuberculosis* serine/threonine kinase PknL phosphorylates Rv2175c: mass spectrometric profiling of the activation loop phosphorylation sites and their role in the recruitment of Rv2175c. *Proteomics* 8:521–533.

198. Rifat D, Bishai WR, Karakousis PC. 2009. Phosphate depletion: a novel trigger for *Mycobacterium tuberculosis* persistence. *J Infect Dis* 200:1126–1135.

199. Vanzembergh F, Peirs P, Lefevre P, Celio N, Mathys V, Content J, Kalai M. 2010. Effect of PstS sub-units or PknD deficiency on the survival of *Mycobacterium tuberculosis*. *Tuberculosis (Edinb)* 90:338–345.

200. Kumar D, Palaniyandi K, Challu VK, Kumar P, Narayanan S. 2013. PknE, a serine/threonine protein kinase from *Mycobacterium tuberculosis* has a role in adaptive responses. *Arch Microbiol* 195:75–80.

201. Spivey VL, Molle V, Whalan RH, Rodgers A, Leiba J, Stach L, Walker KB, Smerdon SJ, Buxton RS. 2011. Forkhead-associated (FHA) domain containing ABC transporter Rv1747 is positively regulated by Ser/Thr phosphorylation in *Mycobacterium tuberculosis*. *J Biol Chem* 286:26198–26209.

202. Jani C, Eoh H, Lee JJ, Hamasha K, Sahana MB, Han JS, Nyayapathy S, Lee JY, Suh JW, Lee SH, Rehse SJ, Crick DC, Kang CM. 2010. Regulation of polar peptidoglycan biosynthesis by Wag31 phosphorylation in mycobacteria. *BMC Microbiol* 10:327.

Tuberculosis and the Tubercle Bacillus, 2nd ed.
Edited by William R. Jacobs, Jr., Helen McShane, Valerie Mizrahi, and Ian M. Orme
© 2018 American Society for Microbiology, Washington, DC
doi:10.1128/microbiolspec.TBTB2-0027-2016

DNA Replication in *Mycobacterium tuberculosis*

27

Zanele Ditse[1], Meindert H. Lamers[2], and Digby F. Warner[3,4]

INTRODUCTION

The transfer of genetic material through successive generations is essential to the survival and evolution of all living organisms, including bacteria. As causative agent of tuberculosis (TB), *Mycobacterium tuberculosis* must complete successive cycles of transmission, infection, and disease in order to maintain a viable presence in the human population. And, like other pathogens (1), *M. tuberculosis* is faced with the extra problem of regulating DNA replication, chromosomal segregation, and cell division while residing in diverse anatomical and cellular loci within its human host—including extra- and intracellular compartments (2, 3). Therefore, in addition to the metabolic challenges faced during infection of dynamic and often hostile environments (4, 5), *M. tuberculosis* is likely to encounter multiple stresses that are directly or indirectly genotoxic (6–8). In patients with active TB disease, these stresses might arise from host-derived antimicrobial immune effectors, generation of toxic by-products from host and/or mycobacterial metabolism, changes in intracellular redox potential as a function of shifts in metabolic activity, pH, or oxygen availability, or even exposure to anti-TB drugs. However, given that the number of active TB cases (although devastatingly high in absolute terms) is small relative to the total number of estimated infections (9), an additional feature of *M. tuberculosis* is the ability of infecting bacilli to persist for decades in a poorly understood subclinical state (10, 11), in some cases reactivating decades later to cause postprimary TB (12, 13). Under these conditions, DNA replication and repair pathways are predicted to be essential for preserving the genetic content and viability of bacilli located in lesions characterized by different states of immune activation at various stages throughout the disease cycle (14).

Of course, the evolutionary imperative to survive while adapting to the stresses and fluctuating environments encountered during long-term infection requires that there must be an intrinsic capacity for error even in the processes that function to maintain genomic integrity (15). This reinforces the importance of understanding DNA metabolism in *M. tuberculosis* as a key component of both mycobacterial virulence and mycobacterial evolution (including the development of drug resistance) and, in turn, identifies the mycobacterial DNA metabolic machinery as a potential source of new targets for novel anti-TB chemotherapies designed to inhibit growth while limiting emergence of drug resistance. Unlike many other bacterial pathogens, drug resistance in *M. tuberculosis* arises exclusively from mutations in chromosomal genes that are associated with drug action: there is no evidence of horizontal gene transfer in the modern evolution of *M. tuberculosis* strains (16–18). So, chromosomal mutagenesis drives the microevolution of this obligate pathogen within its human host, in which case the interplay between high-fidelity DNA replication and repair, on the one hand, and low-fidelity damage tolerance pathways, on the other, might be critical to the ability of *M. tuberculosis* to maintain viability under otherwise lethal antibiotic exposure, and to adapt under changing selection pressures (19).

In this review, we summarize recent progress in our understanding of the machinery responsible for DNA

[1]Centre for HIV and STIs, National Institute for Communicable Diseases of the National Health Laboratory Service, Johannesburg, 2131, South Africa; [2]Medical Research Council Laboratory of Molecular Biology, Cambridge, CB2 0QH United Kingdom; [3]South African Medical Research Council (SAMRC)/National Health Laboratory Services (NHLS)/University of Cape Town (UCT) Molecular Mycobacteriology Research Unit, Department of Science and Technology (DST)/National Research Foundation (NRF) Centre of Excellence for Biomedical TB Research, Department of Pathology, Faculty of Health Sciences, University of Cape Town, Rondebosch 7700, South Africa; [4]Institute of Infectious Disease and Molecular Medicine, Faculty of Health Sciences, University of Cape Town, Rondebosch 7700, South Africa.

replication in *M. tuberculosis*, with a specific focus on the different mycobacterial DNA polymerases and their potential roles as specialists in different aspects of DNA replication and repair. In addition, we highlight key results suggesting the utility of targeting DNA replication for anti-TB drug development. Finally, given that the regulation of DNA replication and its coordination with cell division are critical to cell cycle progression, we consider the impact of transient interruptions of DNA replication on mycobacterial drug susceptibility as well as the emergence and fixation of genetic mutations in a pathogen increasingly associated with multidrug resistance. As applies to all specialist review articles, the treatment in this case of DNA replication in *M. tuberculosis* and its potential role in pathogenesis is neither exhaustive nor definitive: the reader is encouraged to consult the large number of related articles on this subject, some of which are cited here as well (8, 20–24).

BACTERIAL DNA REPLICATION

Bacterial DNA replication is performed by a large, multiprotein replisome that synthesizes leading and lagging strands in a highly coordinated fashion. Together, the replisome proteins catalyze a large number of events such as DNA unwinding, RNA primer synthesis, clamp loading, and DNA synthesis (Fig. 1). From comparative genomic analyses, it is evident that most of the replisome components are conserved across bacteria (25). This observation remains valid for a small panel of mycobacteria including *Mycobacterium leprae* (Tables 1 and 2), an obligate pathogen whose genome displays evidence of extensive decay (26), as well as the nonpathogenic environmental mycobacterium *Mycobacterium smegmatis*, which has served as tractable model in the majority of live-cell investigations of mycobacterial DNA replication and cell division (27–33).

As noted elsewhere (22, 34, 35), replisome function has been most thoroughly studied in *Escherichia coli* (36) and *Bacillus subtilis* (37), from which models of the bacterial replisome have been constructed (Fig. 1). The replisome can be divided into three catalytic centers (Fig. 2): the helicase-primase complex (25), the core complex, and the clamp loader complex (35, 38). Together with the β clamp, the core complex and clamp-loader complex form the DNA polymerase III holoenzyme (PolIII HE) (39, 40). The helicase-primase

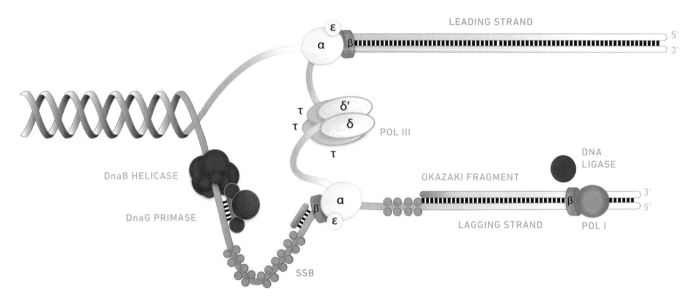

Figure 1   A working model of the mycobacterial replisome. Schematic representation of the model replisome consisting of the PolIII core polymerase, the homodimeric β_2-sliding clamp, the $\tau_3\delta\delta'$ clamp-loader complex, DnaB helicase (red hexamer), DnaG primase (blue), PolI (pink) DNA ligase (purple), and SSB (orange). Recent biochemical evidence suggests that, in *M. tuberculosis*, the ε proofreader forms part of the core replicase together with the β_2 and α subunits (42). As noted in the main text, the precise stoichiometry and architecture of the mycobacterial replisome remain to be established; similarly, it is not known whether the mycobacterial replisome functions as a di- or tripolymerase system, nor whether DnaE2 is able to access the replisome under non-DNA-damaging conditions in the absence of ImuB and ImuA' accessory factors.

complex contains a DnaB helicase that unwinds the two DNA strands, and a DnaG primase that synthesizes the short RNA primers on the lagging strand that form the initiation site for the replicative DNA polymerase, PolIIIα. Two core complexes—comprising PolIIIα, the exonuclease ε, and the small subunit θ—synthesize the new DNA strand on both the leading and lagging strands. To ensure processivity, the core complex binds to the β clamp, a torroidal protein that encircles the DNA. Together, the core-clamp complex synthesizes DNA fragments with lengths of up 100,000 base pairs (41). The $\tau_3\delta_1\delta'_1\chi_1\psi_1$ clamp-loader complex loads β clamps onto newly synthesized RNA primers. The τ subunits furthermore bind to the PolIIIα subunits, thus coupling leading- and lagging-strand synthesis. Finally, the χ/ψ subunits guide SSB molecules onto the single-stranded DNA lagging strand.

The genes predicted to be involved in DNA replication in *M. tuberculosis* are shown in Tables 1 and 2. The mycobacterial replisome lacks obvious homologs of several components that perform key functions in the model organism; for example, there are no obvious homologs of the initiation proteins, DnaC, DnaT, PriB, and PriC; the *holE*-encoded θ subunit; or the *holC*- and *holD*-encoded χ and ψ clamp-loader subunits (22). However, comparative genomics has established that this reduced gene complement is typical of many bacteria. In fact, the *M. tuberculosis* genome was included among the set that contributed to the definition of a basic bacterial replication module comprising the replication initiator protein, DnaA, the DnaB helicase, DnaG primase, PolIIIα, the β2-sliding clamp, ε proofreading subunit, τ, δ, and δ', SSB, DNA ligase, and PolI (25, 35). Key recent studies have provided additional insights into the composition of the mycobacterial replisome and its functional organization (42, 43) (detailed below). Nevertheless, it remains relatively poorly characterized, and the working model of the full *M. tuberculosis* replisome is therefore inferred largely through comparison with model organisms (39, 40), and from the limited number of genetic and biochemical studies that have focused on specific mycobacterial replication proteins (Tables 1 and 2). As a result, there are a number of important gaps that need to be addressed. For example, the stoichiometry and architecture of the mycobacterial replisome are unknown; what is the complement of replisome components present at the replication fork during active replication? And how does this alter under conditions of slow growth, metabolic quiescence, or stress? What are the factors that determine the rates of chromosomal replication and cell division in *M. tuberculosis* during host infection?

In addition, the potential for other cellular factors to affect (or modify) both function and composition of the replisome—such as the relative levels of deoxyribonucleotide triphosphates (dNTPs) and ribonucleotide triphosphates (rNTPs), the building blocks of DNA and RNA, respectively, or the presence of specialist DNA polymerases and other repair enzymes—remains unresolved. Some of these questions are explored further below.

The Mycobacterial Replication Machinery

Despite significant genetic differences across bacterial phyla, there appears to be strong functional conservation in the mechanics of chromosomal replication (25, 34). For simplicity, it is useful to reference the *E. coli* model when considering the overall process of DNA replication in *M. tuberculosis*, although a number of recent observations have suggested that the mycobacterial system is likely to differ in some key respects.

The DnaA-ATP interaction is critical for replication initiation, since it results in the opening of the DNA duplex to allow loading of DnaB, and the *dnaA* promoter remains active during replication to ensure progression through the cell cycle (44). *M. tuberculosis oriC* is located in the 527-bp intergenic region between *dnaA* and *dnaN*, and contains multiple predicted and confirmed DnaA-binding sites. Interestingly, this region also serves as a common locus for the insertion of IS*6110* transposable elements. To date, however, there is no evidence to suggest the insertions have any effect on the replication process, including the timing of replication initiation. Instead, these sites have been exploited as useful markers for restriction fragment length polymorphism (RFLP) fingerprinting of clinical *M. tuberculosis* isolates (45). In *E. coli*, DnaA recruits the hexameric DnaB replicative helicase to the origin to initiate strand separation. Recent work has confirmed the physical interaction of *M. tuberculosis* DnaA and DnaB, and has further implicated DnaB in controlling DnaA complex formation and the interaction with *oriC* (46). In contrast, *M. tuberculosis* does not possess a homolog of the DnaC helicase loader, which is required for loading DnaB helicase onto the DNA in *E. coli* (Table 1). This suggests that the DnaC function must be performed by another protein, or that DnaA alone might be sufficient for DnaB loading, as has been suggested for other organisms that lack a DnaC helicase loader (47). Similarly, and as noted above, *M. tuberculosis* does not possess either θ, χ, or ψ subunits; moreover, the mycobacterial *dnaX* gene does not contain the alternative STOP codon that, in *E. coli*,

Table 1 Components of the bacterial replisome

E. coli protein	E. coli gene	M. tuberculosis / M. smegmatis / M. leprae	Function	Catalytic activity	Essentiality in M. tuberculosis in vitro[a]/comments	Reference(s)
Primosome (loading of replicative helicase DnaB)						
DnaA	dnaA	Rv0001 MSMEG_6947 ML0001	Replication initiator	ATPase, DNA unwinding	Essential; required for regulation of DNA replication	46, 190
DnaC	dnaC	Absent Absent Absent	Helicase loader, replication restart	ATPase		
DnaT	dnaT	Absent Absent Absent	Helicase loader, replication restart			
PriA	priA	Rv1402 MSMEG_3061 ML0548	Helicase loader, replication restart	ATPase, helicase	Essential	
PriB	priB	Absent Absent Absent	Helicase loader, replication restart			
PriC	priC	Absent Absent Absent	Helicase loader, replication restart			
Helicase-primase (DNA unwinding, RNA primer synthesis, lagging-strand protection)						
DnaB helicase	dnaB	Rv0058 MSMEG_6892 ML2680	Replicative helicase	ATPase, helicase	Essential; controls DnaA complex formation and interaction with oriC	46
DnaG primase	dnaG	Rv2343c MSMEG_4482 ML0833	RNA primase	RNA primase	Essential; required for regulation of DNA replication	191
SSB	ssb	Rv0054 MSMEG_6896 ML2684	Single-stranded DNA binding protein		Essential[b]	32
Core-clamp (leading- and lagging-strand DNA synthesis)						
PolIIIα	dnaE	Rv1547 MSMEG_3178 ML1207	α subunit, polymerase activity	DNA polymerase	Essential; high-fidelity replicative polymerase	42, 43, 69
ε-Exonuclease	dnaQ	Rv3711c MSMEG_6275 Absent	ε subunit, proofreading activity	Exonuclease	Nonessential; component of M. tuberculosis $\alpha\beta_2\varepsilon$ core replicase, interacts with β but not DnaE1; deletion does not result in increased mutation rate phenotype in vitro	42, 43, 77
θ	holE	Absent Absent Absent	ε stabilizer			

Protein	Gene	Identifier	Function	Activity	Notes	Ref
β clamp	*dnaN*	Rv0002, MSMEG_0001, ML0002	β$_2$-sliding clamp		Essential; processivity factor, component of *M. tuberculosis* αβ$_2$ε core replicase, interacting separately with α and ε subunits	42, 43
Clamp loader (clamp loading, SSB loading, polymerase connection)						
τ/γ	*dnaX*	Rv3721c, MSMEG_6285, ML2335	Clamp loading, connects leading- and lagging-strand polymerase	ATPase	Essential; the alternative gene product γ has not been observed in mycobacteria	
δ	*holA*	Rv2413c, MSMEG_4572, ML0603	Clamp loading	Inactive ATPase	Essential	
δ′	*holB*	Rv3644c, MSMEG_6153, ML0202	Clamp loading	ATPase	Essential	
χ	*holC*	Absent, Absent, Absent	SSB loading			
ψ	*holD*	Absent, Absent, Absent	SSB loading			
Okazaki maturation: removal of RNA primer, synthesis and ligation of single-stranded gap						
Pol I	*polA*	Rv1629, MSMEG_3839, ML1381	Removal of RNA primer, Closing of ssDNA gap	DNA polymerase	Essential; lacks a proofreading 3′-5′ exonuclease activity, *polA* mutant displayed a DNA damage phenotype following UV irradiation and hydrogen peroxide treatment	94, 95
DNA ligase I	*ligA*	Rv3014c, MSMEG_2362, ML1705	Closing of nicks on lagging strand	NAD-dependent DNA ligase	Essential	192
Topoisomerases, gyrases						
Topoisomerase I	*topA*	Rv3646c, MSMEG_6157, ML0200	DNA topoisomerase I	Relax supercoiling	Essential; role in DNA repair	193
GyrA	*gyrA*	Rv0006, MSMEG_0006, ML0006	DNA gyrase, subunit A (DNA topoisomerase II)	Negative supercoiling, ATPase	Essential	194
GyrB	*gyrB*	Rv0005, MSMEG_0005, ML0005	DNA gyrase, subunit B (DNA topoisomerase II)	Negative supercoiling, ATPase	Essential	194
Translesion polymerases and associated proteins						
Pol II	*polB*	Absent, Absent, Absent	Translesion DNA polymerase	DNA polymerase		

(Continued)

Table 1 Components of the bacterial replisome *(Continued)*

E. coli protein	E. coli gene	M. tuberculosis / M. smegmatis / M. leprae	Catalytic activity	Function	Essentiality in M. tuberculosis in vitro[a]/comments	Reference(s)
Pol IV	dinB	Rv1537 / MSMEG_3172 / Absent	DNA polymerase	Translesion DNA polymerase	Nonessential; capacity for ribonucleotide discrimination during DNA synthesis	99, 105, 106
Pol IV	dinB	Rv3056 / MSMEG_2294 / Absent	DNA polymerase	Translesion DNA polymerase	Nonessential; dispensable for DNA damage tolerance; capacity for ribonucleotide incorporation	99, 105, 106
Pol V (UmuC)	umuC	Absent / Absent / Absent	DNA polymerase	Translesion DNA polymerase		
Pol V (UmuD)	umuD	Absent / Absent / Absent		Translesion DNA polymerase subunit		

[a]*In vitro* essentiality, as determined by transposon site hybridization (TraSH) (201, 202).
[b]*Rv0054* did not satisfy the strict criterion for essentiality in the study by Griffin et al. (201); however, no transposon (Tn) insertions were identified in any of the five possible TA dinucleotides in the open reading frame, suggesting that the gene is likely to be essential.

creates the γ protein through ribosomal slippage (48). All four proteins are, however, not generally conserved in bacterial replisomes and, in some cases, may even be unique to the *E. coli* replisome. The θ subunit is nonessential and found only in a small group of *Enterobacteriaceae* (49, 50). The clamp-loader subunits, χ and ψ, connect to SSB on the lagging DNA strand (51, 52), and their deletion in *E. coli* leads to a reduction in viability (53). Yet, in several organisms, χ and ψ appear to be absent (54). In *E. coli*, the γ protein is a shorter version of the τ protein, containing only the first ~430 residues that oligomerize into the pentameric clamp-loader complex, but lacking the C-terminal ~210 residues that bind the DNA polymerase. Deletion of γ has no effect on *E. coli* viability (55), and the subunit is absent in several bacteria (56–58), supporting the notion that it is nonessential for replication.

Leading-strand synthesis is highly processive and involves the continuous extension of DNA; this is in contrast to lagging-strand synthesis, which requires discontinuous replication via the extension and ligation of Okazaki fragments (Fig. 1). DnaG primase fulfills the essential function of producing the short RNA primers for extension by PolIII, and has been identified as a potential target for novel TB drugs (59).

THE MYCOBACTERIAL C-FAMILY DNA POLYMERASES

As detailed above, the core complex in the well-studied bacterium, *E. coli*, contains three subunits: the PolIIIα subunit that functions as active DNA polymerase, the *dnaQ*-encoded ε subunit possessing 3′-5′ exonuclease proofreading activity, and the *holE*-encoded θ subunit, that stabilizes the ε subunit. PolIIIα subunits are C-family DNA polymerases (60), restricted exclusively to the bacterial kingdom and a few bacteriophages (61) and classified into two major groups: PolC-type (62) and DnaE-type (63, 64), the last of which is further subdivided into the DnaE1, DnaE2, and DnaE3 groups. PolC is present in low-GC Gram-positive bacteria such as *B. subtilis*, whereas DnaE1 serves as PolIIIα in the widely studied Gram-negative model organism, *E. coli*, and also in *M. tuberculosis*.

C-family DNA polymerases possess a set of four highly conserved and ordered domains within a single polypeptide that folds broadly into the shape of a cupped right hand (Fig. 3). These are the Polymerase and Histidinol Phosphatase (PHP) domain, which is limited to the C-family polymerases as well as some PolX members and, in some organisms, possesses proofreading activity; the Palm domain, which contains the catalytic residues

TABLE 2 Unique components of the mycobacterial replisome/repair—not present in *E. coli*

M. tuberculosis protein	M. tuberculosis gene	M. tuberculosis / M. smegmatis / M. leprae	Function	Catalytic activity	Essentiality in M. tuberculosis in vitro[a]/Comments	References
DnaE2	*dnaE2*	*Rv3370c* MSMEG_1633 pseudogene	Translesion DNA polymerase	DNA polymerase	Nonessential; required for DNA damage-induced mutagenesis; implicated in the emergence of drug resistance *in vivo*	67, 69
ImuA'	*imuA'*	*Rv3395c* MSMEG_1620 Absent	Not known	Not determined	Nonessential; required for DNA damage-induced mutagenesis	67
ImuB	*imuB*	*Rv3394c* MSMEG_1622 Absent	Predicted translesion DNA polymerase	Not determined	Nonessential; required for DNA damage-induced mutagenesis	67
PolX	*polX*	*Rv3856c* MSMEG_6445 Absent	DNA PolX	Unknown[b]	Nonessential	
LigB	*ligB*	*Rv3062* MSMEG_2277 Absent	DNA ligase	ATP-dependent DNA ligase	Nonessential; role in DNA repair	195
LigC	*ligC*	*Rv3731* MSMEG_6304 Absent	DNA ligase	ATP-dependent DNA ligase	Nonessential; role in Ku-dependent nonhomologous end-joining (NHEJ) DSB repair pathway	195
RnhB	*rnhB*	*Rv2902c* MSMEG_2442 ML1611	RNase HII	RNase	Nonessential	196
LigD	*ligD*	*Rv0938* MSMEG_5570 Absent	DNA ligase, DSB repair	ATP-dependent DNA ligase	Nonessential; plays a central role in the mutagenic NHEJ pathway of DSB repair	197, 198
RnhA-CobC		*Rv2228c* MSMEG 4305ML1637	Chimeric protein; N-terminal RNase HI domain, C-terminal CobC-like α-ribazole phosphatase domain	RNase/α-ribazole phosphatase	Essential; deletion of *rnhB* in *M. smegmatis* does not alter genome stability	199
DnaQ-UvrC		*Rv2191* MSMEG_4259 Absent	Fusion protein; N-terminal 3'-5' exonuclease domain, C-terminal UvrC-like endonuclease domain	Exonuclease/Endonuclease	Nonessential; RecA-independent induction of expression in response to mitomycin C treatment; expressed during chronic infection in rabbits *in vivo*	43, 81, 200

[a]In vitro essentiality, as determined by transposon site hybridization (TraSH) (201, 202).
[b]A natural truncation in the polymerase domain of Rv3856c is predicted to eliminate catalytic activity, suggesting that Rv3856c does not function as *de facto* PolX.

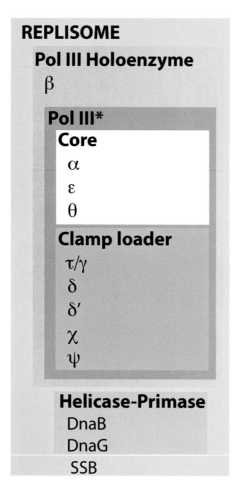

Figure 2 Subcomplex division in the bacterial replisome. The replisome contains three catalytic centers: core, clamp loader, and helicase-primase. The core complex and clamp-loader complex assemble into a larger, stable complex termed Pol III*. Together with the β clamp, they form the Pol III holoenzyme. The DnaB helicase and DnaG primase form a transient complex to synthesize primers on the lagging strand. Modified with permission from the *Annual Review of Biochemistry*, Volume 74 © 2005 by Annual Reviews, http://www.annualreviews.org

required for template elongation; the Thumb domain, which binds the DNA backbone and inserts a loop into the major groove; and the Fingers domain, which, together with the palm domain, forms a preinsertion nucleotide-binding pocket that positions the incoming dNTP for transfer to the catalytic binding site (35). The arrangement of additional domains, such as the oligonucleotide/oligosaccharide binding (OB) domain that binds single-stranded DNA (35, 65, 66), distinguishes DnaE and PolC subfamilies: in the DnaE family, the OB domain is located C-terminal from the polymerase, whereas in the PolC family it is located at the N-terminal end (Fig. 3B). DnaE2 polymerases differ from both

DnaE1 and DnaE3 types in that no DnaE2 appears to possess the C-terminal domain, which includes both OB-fold and τ-binding domains. In contrast, the DnaE3 polymerases are characterized by a domain organization that is similar to the DnaE1 group, albeit with a smaller (degraded), disordered PHP domain (61). DnaE2 also lacks the C-terminal τ-binding domain that is critical for connecting DNA to the rest of the replisome during DNA replication, and is instead characterized by a C-terminal pentapeptide motif, SRDF[H/R], which is conserved among most DnaE2 homologs (61). It has been hypothesized that this motif is required for mediating protein-protein interactions, including during function of the mycobacterial mutasome (67); however, this remains to be demonstrated.

The majority of bacterial genomes sequenced to date contain two, three, or even four putative C-family polymerases (61). Most encode a single replicative polymerase of the DnaE1 type, which functions as the sole high-fidelity replicative C-family DNA polymerase in the cell (61, 68); this is the case for *M. tuberculosis*, which encodes a single DnaE1 subunit, Rv1547 (Tables 1 and 2). Based on distributions across bacterial genomes, DnaE1 appears to be the only C-family polymerase that is able to exist alone or in combination with DnaE2 and PolC (68); in contrast, the other C-family members (PolC, DnaE2 or DnaE3) always occur in combination with representatives from at least one of the other groups. Only DnaE2 subunits—which are common among aerobic bacteria with large, GC-rich genomes—do not conform to phylogenetic boundaries, and can coexist with DnaE1 or PolC (61). Consistent with this observation, in addition to the DnaE1 replicative subunit, *M. tuberculosis* possesses a second, DnaE2-type polymerase, which has been implicated in DNA damage-induced mutagenesis as part of the mycobacterial DNA damage (or SOS) response (61, 69).

DnaE1 PHP Domain Proofreading Activity in Maintaining Replication Fidelity

The *in vitro* mutation rate in *M. tuberculosis* has been calculated at ~2.9 × 10^{-10} per base pair per round of replication (70), a figure comparable to that determined for *E. coli* (71). However, whereas *E. coli* has a well-characterized pathway for postreplicative mismatch repair (MMR), like all actinomycetes, *M. tuberculosis* does not possess an identifiable MMR system (21). Loss of MMR function in *E. coli* results in a mutator phenotype, with MMR-deficient cells exhibiting mutation rates more than 100-fold higher than wild-type, MMR-proficient cells (71). This is not surprising: the overall error rate of 10^{-10} is a function of the in-

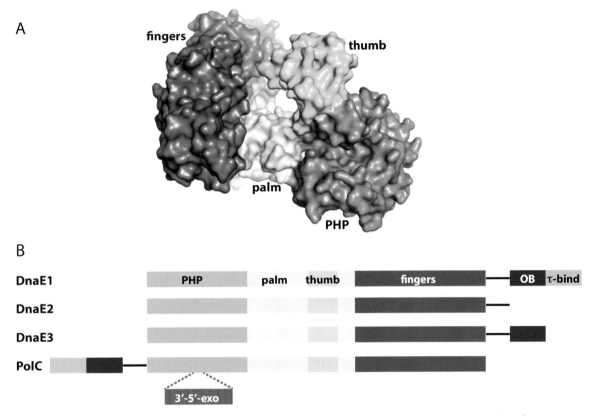

Figure 3 Structure of the C-family polymerases. (**A**) Computational model of *M. tuberculosis* DnaE1 based on the crystal structure of *T. aquaticus* PolIII. Different domains indicated in separate colors (C-terminal domains not shown). (**B**) Domain organization in the different polymerase families. The DnaE families are defined by the presence of the C-terminal domains, whereas PolC forms a distinct class where an ε-like exonuclease domain is inserted into the PHP domain.

trinsic replication fidelity of the replicative polymerase (which contributes an error rate of ~10^{-5}), the 3′-5′ exonuclease activity of the replicative polymerase itself or its interacting proofreading subunit, DnaQ (contributing an error rate ~10^{-2}), and MMR (for which the escape rate is estimated at ~10^{-3}); therefore, the loss of this critical fidelity mechanism can be expected to impact mutation rates (72). What is surprising, however, is that *M. tuberculosis* is not a mutator despite the natural absence of MMR (20), which suggests that intrinsic polymerase fidelity and/or proofreading are able to preserve the mycobacterial error rate. It is possible that an alternative, nonorthologous system catalyzes MMR in mycobacteria (20, 21), or that a recently identified archaeal mismatch-specific endonuclease (73) is functional in *M. tuberculosis*, but this remains to be tested.

A key recent study by Rock and colleagues has highlighted the hazards of investigating all bacterial systems in the context of the well-established *E. coli* model in which proofreading is predominantly the function of the exonuclease subunit. Using a combination of biochemical, microbiological, and bioinformatics approaches, the authors located intrinsic exonuclease function in the PHP domain of the essential PolIIIα subunit, DnaE1 (43). Critically, this study established that, although *M. tuberculosis* encodes two putative homologs of the *E. coli* ε subunit (74), Rv3711c (*dnaQ*) and Rv2191 (comprising a putative N-terminal 3′-5′ exonuclease domain fused to a C-terminal UvrC-like endonuclease domain) (Table 2), neither appears essential to the maintenance of replication fidelity during normal growth *in vitro*: deletion of *Rv3711c* had no impact on the *M. tuberculosis* mutation rate in fluctuation assays, an observation reinforced in the faster-growing *M. smegmatis* in which knockouts lacking either one or both DnaQ homologs retained wild-type mutation rates. In contrast, *M. smegmatis* mutants carrying targeted substitutions of amino acids essential for PHP exonuclease function (owing to their roles in metal cofactor coordination) exhibited severe growth defects that were coupled with massively elevated mutation rates in excess of 2,300-fold greater than the wild-type parental strain. Moreover, whole-genome sequence (WGS) analyses of the PHP domain mutants revealed an accumulation of insertion and deletion events, confirming the requirement for a functional PHP domain in maintaining genomic integrity.

In *E. coli*, the replicase maintains a weak interaction between the ε proofreading subunit and the β clamp in the polymerization mode of DNA synthesis, which is disrupted to enable the transition to alternative conformational states which allow transient access of other polymerases and clamp-binding proteins, for example, during proofreading or translesion synthesis (75). In their study of mycobacterial replication fidelity, Rock and colleagues raised important questions about the applicability of this *E. coli* paradigm to *M. tuberculosis*: in particular, they observed that, while *M. tuberculosis* DnaQ possessed exonuclease activity in biochemical assays *in vitro*, the putative proofreading subunit did not interact stably with the *dnaE1*-encoded α subunit (43). This result was confirmed subsequently in another key study by Lijun Bi and colleagues (42), who reconstituted a functional *M. tuberculosis* DNA PolIII HE comprising recombinant α (DnaE1), ε (DnaQ), β (DnaN), τ (DnaZX), δ (HolA), δ′ (HolB), and SSB (Ssb) subunits *in vitro*. From a series of biochemical assays, the authors concluded that the core mycobacterial replicase consists of αβ₂ε, with β₂ functioning as bridge protein to compensate for the lack of interaction between the α and ε proteins. Consistent with the *E. coli* model, however, *M. tuberculosis* DNA PolIII replicase was shown to transition between polymerization and proofreading modes, with these results implicating the β₂ clamp (which maintains the αβ₂ε replicase in polymerization mode) and dNTP availability in mediating this switch.

Although largely in agreement, these studies did highlight a potential disconnect between the phenotypes observed in whole-cell (microbiological) assays (43) and the enzymatic properties characterized *in vitro* (42): that is, no increase in mutation rate was detected in any of the *dnaQ*-deficient deletion mutants (43) despite the apparently integral role of DnaQ in the mycobacterial replicase that was inferred from biochemical assays. This suggests that there may be additional factors that determine the relative contributions of PHP and DnaQ to proofreading in live *M. tuberculosis* cells, including during host infection. While this remains to be resolved, it is worth noting that comparative genomics of clinical strains has identified *dnaQ* as highly poly-

morphic (76) and possibly linked to the emergence of *M. tuberculosis* drug resistance (77). Both observations suggest that *dnaQ* is under strong selective pressure; however, further work is required to verify this inference.

Specialist Function: DnaE1 Versus DnaE2

M. tuberculosis is unusual in that it contains both SOS-dependent (78) and SOS-independent (79, 80) DNA damage responses, with some repair components induced by both mechanisms (81). Of the complement of DNA polymerases encoded in the *M. tuberculosis* genome, only *dnaE1* and *dnaE2* are upregulated in the mycobacterial DNA damage response (67, 69) (discussed further below). Given the essentiality of the DnaE1 subunit for chromosomal replication (and hence bacillary survival), it is challenging to determine the specific reason for increased *dnaE1* expression under damage conditions. In contrast, the nonessential nature of *dnaE2* has enabled the elucidation of a DnaE2-dependent mutagenic pathway that might be considered the functional analog of the PolV mutasome in *E. coli* (67).

Loss of DnaE2 activity rendered *M. tuberculosis* hypersensitive to DNA damage and eliminated induced mutagenesis *in vitro* (67, 69). Moreover, a *dnaE2* deletion mutant was associated with attenuated virulence and reduced frequency of drug resistance in a mouse model (69). Coupled with the induction of *dnaE2* during stationary infection, these observations implicated a DnaE2-mediated mutagenic mechanism in both pathogenesis and the evolution of drug resistance during therapy. Subsequent studies demonstrated that DnaE2 operates in a novel mutagenic pathway comprising two additional accessory proteins, ImuA′ and ImuB. ImuB is one of three putative Y-family polymerase homologs in the *M. tuberculosis* genome, but it appears from sequence analysis to be catalytically inactive (67). Although this prediction requires formal demonstration, the current model for the mycobacterial "mutasome" holds that DnaE2 functions as the translesion synthesis (TLS) polymerase with ImuB acting as hub protein that interacts with both ImuA′ and DnaE2 via the C-terminal domain, and with the β₂ clamp via a clamp-binding motif (67). The basis for the functional specialization of C-family replicative and TLS polymerases in *M. tuberculosis* and other Gram-positive bacteria remains unclear (82, 83). Unlike Y-family polymerases whose structures are adapted to specialist lesion bypass (84), sequence analysis reveals few clues about DnaE2 function. DnaE1 and DnaE2 are similar in terms of amino acid identity, yet perform different functions (69). Moreover, although DnaE2 appears to be a central player in the DNA damage response in *M. tuberculosis*, its role as an error-prone TLS polymerase is not generally conserved across bacterial phyla. For example, *Pseudomonas putida* DnaE2 has been shown to have antimutator properties (85), while the homologous protein in *Pseudomonas aeruginosa* appears dispensable for damage tolerance (86) but not for induced mutagenesis (87). In addition, in *Streptomyces coelicolor*, DnaE2 is SOS inducible, but dispensable for DNA replication, linear chromosome end patching, ultraviolet resistance, and mutagenesis (88). This suggests that, in addition to intrinsic structural determinants such as active-site architecture, differential interactions with other DNA metabolic proteins might modulate polymerase function and fidelity.

Most major DNA PolIIIα structural features are readily identifiable in both DnaE1 and DnaE2, except for the C-terminal τ-interacting domain that is absent in DnaE2 (Fig. 3B) (61, 67). The α-τ interaction enables dimerization of leading- and lagging-strand polymerases in *E. coli* (35), which suggests that the absence of this region might account (at least partially) for the inability of DnaE2 and other nonessential polymerases to substitute essential replicative function (69, 82, 83). DnaE2 also lacks a consensus β$_2$-clamp-binding motif, QL[S/D]LF, which suggests that it must bind another β$_2$-clamp-binding protein(s) for access to the DNA (89) and, in addition, does not possess the complete set of metal coordinating residues required for PHP domain proofreading function (90, 91). As noted above, the interaction between PolIIIα and the *dnaQ*-encoded ε subunit is essential for fidelity in *E. coli*; moreover, disruptions to proofreading activity enable PolIII-mediated TLS in the absence of specialist DNA repair pols IV and V (92, 93), while in organisms such as *Streptococcus pyogenes*, the essential DnaE subunit that catalyzes error-prone TLS does not bind DnaQ (83). In combination, these observations raise the possibility that differential interactions with DnaQ (Rv3711c) or Rv2191 might impact DnaE2 function in *M. tuberculosis*, but this remains to be determined.

OTHER DNA POLYMERASES AT THE REPLICATION FORK?

In addition to the C-family DNA polymerases, DnaE1 (42, 43) and DnaE2 (67, 69), the *M. tuberculosis* genome encodes six other DNA polymerases (Tables 1 and 2): the A-family polymerase, PolI (*polA*; Rv1629) (94, 95); three polymerases of the archaeo-eukaryotic primase (AEP) superfamily, LigD-POL (Rv0938) (96), PolD1 (Rv3730c), and PolD2 (Rv0269c) (97, 98); and

two Y-family polymerases, DinB1 (Rv1537) and DinB2 (Rv3056) (99–101). Homologs of *E. coli* PolII (*polA*) or PolV (*umuD*, *umuC*) are not found in *M. tuberculosis*. As discussed previously (22), dynamic polymerase exchange is critical to chromosomal replication and repair in bacteria (72). For example, both PolI (*polA*) and PolII (*polB*) contribute directly to the fidelity of normal chromosomal replication in *E. coli*, (35, 72), as well as functioning with the Y-family polymerases, PolIV (*dinB*) and PolV (*umuD*$_2$C), as specialist TLS polymerases in the DNA damage response (72). Owing to their roles in response to stress, many specialist polymerases—especially Y-family TLS polymerases—have been implicated in induced mutagenesis (102). In turn, this suggests that the different DNA polymerases in *M. tuberculosis* are likely also to encode specialist functions, and so highlights the importance of elucidating the conditions under which each (or a combination thereof) is preferentially active.

M. tuberculosis does not encode a PolII enzyme, but possesses two PolIV homologs, DinB1 and DinB2 (99), which are Y-family TLS polymerases. The *E. coli* genome contains three TLS polymerases, all of which are upregulated in the DNA damage or SOS response: the B-family polymerase PolII, and the Y-family polymerases PolIV and PolV that are encoded by *dinB* and *umuDC*, respectively (103). Since *M. tuberculosis* does not encode a B-family DNA polymerase, it was assumed that all specialist bypass function in *M. tuberculosis* depended on the two PolIV homologs, originally annotated as DinP (DinB2) and DinX (DinB1) (21). However, numerous studies have confirmed that, in contrast to most bacterial systems, neither *dinB1*- nor *dinB2*-encoded PolIV homolog is upregulated in the mycobacterial damage response (67, 69, 81, 104); instead, both genes are expressed constitutively during logarithmic growth and stationary phase (99). Notably, *M. tuberculosis* deletion mutants lacking one or both of *dinB1* and *dinB2* were not hypersensitive to multiple DNA-damaging agents *in vitro*, and showed no phenotype in a mouse model of TB; furthermore, overexpression of either *M. tuberculosis dinB1* or *dinB2* gene in *M. smegmatis* did not increase the spontaneous mutation rate (99).

These observations, which supported the dispensability of the mycobacterial Y-family polymerases for damage tolerance and induced mutagenesis, presented a genuine puzzle until recently. Then, two elegant biochemical studies by Stewart Shuman and colleagues elucidated potential specialist function differentiating DinB1 as a *bona fide* DNA-dependent DNA polymerase, whereas DinB2 was shown to possess the additional capacity to catalyze the incorporation of ribonucleotides (105, 106). As the authors demonstrated, an aromatic steric gate side chain in DinB1 and most other DNA polymerases enables rNTP discrimination; this is notably absent in DinB2, which carries a leucine residue in the corresponding position and so lacks the ability to differentiate between dNTPs and rNTPs during template-directed synthesis. In addition to a surprising capacity to synthesize long stretches of RNA from a DNA template (106), these studies also revealed that *M. smegmatis* DinB2 is a low-fidelity enzyme, displaying characteristic signatures of misincorporation opposite undamaged DNA during both DNA and RNA synthesis *in vitro* (105). Moreover, DinB2 is promiscuous in its incorporation of both 8-oxo-dGMP and oxo-rGTP, as well as misincorporation of rNTPs opposite 8-oxo-dG lesions. It seems likely, therefore, that DinB2 might function as "ribo patch" DNA repair polymerase during dNTP starvation or under conditions of oxidative stress (105); however, this prediction needs to be tested.

THE MYCOBACTERIAL REPLICATION RATE

The term "replication rate" is often applied to mycobacteria to denote the rate at which an individual bacillus divides; that is, the time taken for one (parent) cell to generate two (daughter) cells. Although convenient, this is not strictly accurate, for two principal reasons. In the first place, the stem "replica" demands that the products of the reproduction process are near-identical. For chromosomes, this mostly holds true: replication of the genome is accomplished with high fidelity by a replisome complex with a very low error rate. In contrast, for whole organisms, the products of cell division—the daughter cells—will generally fail to satisfy this criterion owing to unequal cellular division and/or distribution of cellular constituents including macromolecules, metabolites, and cofactors. Accumulating evidence reinforces this interpretation and its implications for understanding *M. tuberculosis* population dynamics in the infected host: mycobacteria divide asymmetrically, producing daughter cells that are morphologically similar but vary in length (one cell is often longer), composition (the distribution of the "old" and "new" cell poles means that some cells are much older than others), and cellular content (macromolecules are not evenly distributed during division) (107, 108). A number of single-cell analyses have shown that all these factors can have significant physiological and survival consequences, most notably in the form of differential susceptibility to antibiotics (28, 30, 107, 109) (discussed below).

The second reason for caution is that the chromosomal replication rate is not strictly concordant with cell division: although mycobacteria complete only one round of chromosomal replication per cell division cycle (29, 31), there are instances in which these processes appear to be uncoupled. For example, mycobacteria in hypoxia-induced nonreplicating persistence are reported to be diploid, and initiate RNA synthesis, cell division, and then DNA replication in an ordered sequence following reexposure to oxygen (110). Similarly, although it has not been directly investigated, it is tempting to speculate that the filamentous mycobacteria that develop during infection of macrophages (111, 112) might also be polyploid. It is worth noting, too, that separating concepts of cell division from chromosomal replication appears consistent with the idea that it may be simplistic to assume that mycobacterial metabolism (including DNA metabolism) has been selected to generate maximal bacillary numbers within a given microenvironment during host infection (23). As discussed previously, bacillary numbers determined from individual pulmonary lesions in a non-human primate model of TB suggest that the infecting population maintains a fairly consistent bacterial load throughout active disease (14), and that maximal growth may even be detrimental to the immediate fate of the infecting bacillus (individual host outcome) or to its long-term survival (evolutionary persistence within the human population). In turn, this reinforces the likelihood that *M. tuberculosis* infection is characterized by a spectrum of disease that extends from nonreplicating persisting organisms, to replicating but asymptomatic infections, to low-level disease with higher numbers of actively replicating bacteria, to full-blown disease pathology and transmission (14, 113, 114). It seems inevitable, therefore, that both the replication and cell division rates will vary within specific lesions, and over time, as a function of metabolic and environmental pressures. The growing appreciation that low metabolic activity and limited to no growth represent the dominant states of most bacteria in their natural environments (115) further underscores the need to move away from the more experimentally tractable laboratory-based studies that are predicated on maximal growth rates in nutrient-replete conditions.

M. tuberculosis divides every ~18 to 24 hours during optimal growth *in vitro*, a period in which the bacillus undergoes a single round of chromosomal replication (29) with an accompanying mutation rate of $\sim 10^{-10}$ errors per base pair per round of replication (70). As discussed previously (20), there are limited to no data on the rates of chromosomal replication, cell division, and mutagenesis in *M. tuberculosis* bacilli during host infection, especially through periods of clinical latency. What is now known, however, is that the replication rate achieved by the recombinant DnaE1 polymerase in biochemical assays is at least as fast as (if not faster than) *E. coli* PolIIIα (43), which contradicts any notion that intrinsic replicative (in)capacity necessarily limits the mycobacterial growth rate. This observation must be contrasted with evidence from single-cell analyses of mycobacterial growth and division by time-lapse fluorescence microscopy which indicate that chromosomal replication in *M. smegmatis* accounts for approximately 70% of the bacterial cell cycle (that is, approximately 140 min of the standard 180- to 200-min period between successive division events) (29, 31). As noted by Trojanowski and colleagues (29), this corresponds to a DNA synthesis rate of ~400 bases (b)/s, which is approximately 8 times faster than that estimated for *M. tuberculosis* (44, 116), but 1.5 to 2.5 times slower than the fast-growing *E. coli*, which is capable of multifork replication at rates approaching 600 to 1,000 bp/s. The disconnect between the rate of DNA synthesis estimated from the activity of recombinant replicase proteins *in vitro* and that inferred from whole bacterial cells implicates other factors in determining the *in vivo* replication rate. These are likely to include the supply of dNTPs for incorporation into DNA, as well as the need to coordinate chromosomal replication with cell division; in addition, it must be remembered that, where DNA replication occurs in the context of a living cell, numerous other DNA transactions (including DNA repair, RNA transcription, dsDNA folding and packaging, and binding and unbinding of transcriptional regulators) are taking place at the same time. It seems certain that intracellular dNTP concentrations must also play a critical role in determining the rate and fidelity of DNA replication in *M. tuberculosis*. However, while numerous studies have investigated the ribonucleotide reductase and thymidylate synthase enzymes responsible for the provision of dATP/dCTP/dGTP and dTTP, respectively (117–130), the measurement of dNTP pool sizes remains an elusive (23), but high-priority, research focus.

The Evidence from *In Vivo* Infection Models and Clinical *M. tuberculosis* Strains

Molecular epidemiological studies have established the capacity for endogenous reactivation of *M. tuberculosis* after three decades of latent infection (12) and this risk increases 10% per year in HIV-infected patients relative to immune-competent individuals (131). Previous models of latent TB infection (LTBI) suggested that,

during the latent phase, *M. tuberculosis* enters a very slowly replicating or nonreplicating (but probably metabolically active) state in which bacilli are insensitive to killing by host immune effector molecules and anti-TB drugs (110). In contrast, alternative models by Sherman and colleagues, which are based on the use of a "clock" plasmid that is lost from daughter cells during division, instead propose a stable balance *in vivo* between bacillary replication and death, probably as a consequence of active immune surveillance (132).

To gain insight into the mutational capacity of *M. tuberculosis* during different stages of infection, Ford and colleagues used WGS to measure the mutation rate of *M. tuberculosis* isolates from cynomolgus macaques with active, latent, and reactivated disease (70). Given that the *in vivo* generation time of *M. tuberculosis* in this model is unknown, the mutation rate was calculated allowing for a broad range of generation times (between 18 and 240 h). Interestingly, the authors observed similar replication and mutation rates in *M. tuberculosis* isolates from latent, reactivated, and actively infected macaques. In addition, they demonstrated that bacilli isolated from macaques with clinically latent infection had acquired mutations at rates similar to those of rapidly replicating bacteria *in vitro* (70)—an intriguing observation since these would be expected to differ on the basis that mutation rates determined *in vitro* often involve large mycobacterial populations either at exponential or stationary phases of growth (133) that do not represent *in vivo* conditions. Instead, the findings from this study suggest that *M. tuberculosis* continues to divide actively during the entire course of prolonged clinical latency, and that active replication is balanced by robust killing. The authors further concluded that the mutation rates observed during latency are likely attributable to oxidative DNA damage rather than replicative errors. In summary, these observations were interpreted as suggesting that the mutational capacity of *M. tuberculosis* during latent infection might be determined primarily by the length of time the organism spends in the host environment rather than the replicative capacity and replicative errors of the organism during infection (70).

In contrast, findings from clinical *M. tuberculosis* samples suggest that the non-human primate model might not appropriately recapitulate latent TB in humans (134). Again using WGS, Alland and colleagues calculated the replication and mutation rates of latent *M. tuberculosis* by comparing the genome sequence of a single strain that had been transmitted from a single, incident TB case that subsequently resulted in TB disease in close contacts over a period of 20 years. Unlike the findings in macaques, these analyses yielded lower mutation rates during latency, for any given generation time, even after adjusting for the predicted higher mutation rate that was considered likely to occur during the final stage of infection as the individual progressed to active TB (134). Moreover, the mutation spectrum in the human LTBI model did not reveal a higher proportion of mutations associated with oxidative damage (GC>AT or GC>TA mutations) as observed in macaques; instead, there were fewer mutations associated with oxidative damage, suggesting that, during latent infection in humans, mutations are driven by replicative error rather than oxidative stress. By analyzing four strains derived from the same index case, two of which were classified as latent for more than 20 years, these authors further showed that the mutation rate was likely to be 10 times lower during latency than active disease, possibly indicating less selective pressure on the organism during latency, and therefore, a reduced likelihood that adaptive mutations would become fixed in the infecting population.

A very recent study has tested this notion by applying WGS to matched pairs of clinical *M. tuberculosis* isolates obtained from individuals thought to have harbored latent TB infection for prolonged periods of as much as 3 decades (13). The estimated mutation rate from these analyses was 0.2 to 0.3 single nucleotide polymorphisms (SNPs) per genome per year over 33 years, which again places the rate at which *M. tuberculosis* accumulates mutations during clinical latency in a range that is very similar to those calculated for active TB disease in infection models (70) and from outbreak studies (135–137). In summary, therefore, it appears that further analyses of this nature are required, but will require the careful selection of clinical *M. tuberculosis* isolates that have been obtained and archived sequentially during disease progression.

COORDINATING CHROMOSOMAL REPLICATION AND CELL DIVISION

In eukaryotic cells, the genetic material is encapsulated within a defined intracellular organelle, the nucleus. For bacteria, however, chromosomal DNA is located in an undefined region of the cytoplasm called the nucleoid that often consumes a major portion of the total cell volume (138, 139). Therefore, to avoid damaging the genetic material, DNA replication and repair must be coordinated with mycobacterial cell division. In turn, this implies that these pathways are tightly regulated to ensure successful completion of the growth and division cycle: once initiated, sustained interruptions to

cell division, or chromosomal replication and segregation, are likely to be lethal. The mechanisms governing these processes in mycobacteria have been the subject of intense recent research, enabled largely through the increasing availability of advanced single-cell imaging techniques. A series of comprehensive reviews has documented the significant progress made (107, 108); therefore, in the context of this review, it is considered sufficient to provide a brief overview, highlighting those aspects of special relevance to chromosomal replication.

All bacteria, including *M. tuberculosis*, have evolved rigorous control mechanisms to regulate the initiation of DNA replication, and to ensure that it does not occur at random sequences throughout the chromosome (140). In some bacteria, including *E. coli*, replication is initiated at a single site (the origin, *ori*) in the mid-cell region, with sister replisomes proceeding bidirectionally around the chromosome until the two replication forks meet in the replication terminus (*ter*), a region located approximately opposite *ori*. For organisms such as *Caulobacter crescentus* and *Helicobacter pylori*, the *ori* is located at the old cell pole, with the replisomes moving toward the mid-cell before terminating. In contrast, in *B. subtilis* and *P. aeruginosa*, the chromosome is spooled through a "replication factory" comprising sister replisomes colocalized at the mid-cell (141, 142). Largely irrespective of the location of the replisomes, chromosomal replication requires that the two strands of the template DNA are separated at the origin, yielding two fork structures. Replicative DNA polymerases and accessory proteins are assembled onto each of these forks, and synthesize new DNA bidirectionally around the circular chromosome until the two replication forks meet in the *ter*, yielding two copies of the bacterial chromosome, each containing one strand from the parental chromosome and one nascent strand. Moreover, since this must occur only once during the cell cycle, a diverse array of regulatory mechanisms ensures that the assembly of the replication machinery is triggered at the appropriate stage (22, 25).

As noted elsewhere (107), the application of advanced live-cell imaging techniques has facilitated key insights into mycobacterial growth and division. However, the results have not always been consistent across different groups, especially on the question of the (a) symmetry of mycobacterial cell division: this has necessitated an attempt to rationalize the different experimental observations (107). It seems that further work is required in order to establish definitely the timing and location of cell division in *M. tuberculosis*, particularly under conditions that prevail during host infection. Recent observations (29, 32), however, appear to a support a general model which holds that, in *M. smegmatis*, the replisome is positioned near mid-cell, with the two replication forks remaining colocalized (or, at least, in very close proximity to each other) (29) throughout the DNA replication cycle, broadly consistent with the "replication factory" model of *B. subtilis* and *P. aeruginosa* (32). These studies also agree on the critical role played by ParB in chromosome segregation and positioning of the *oriC* region, as well as in the localization of newly assembled replisomes.

Bacterial chromosomes are folded and functionally organized according to a hierarchy of organizational units of different nucleobase lengths so that individual chromosomal loci occupy specific subcellular locations within the cell (139, 141, 142). Together with the structural maintenance of chromosome (SMC) protein, ParB functions as part of the ParABS chromosome partitioning system to ensure that the spatial arrangement of the chromosome is restored in the daughter cells after completion of chromosome replication and segregation. In recent years, advanced methods for determining chromosomal architecture and topography have been developed that have been profitably applied in some bacteria (143). This suggests the need to obtain equivalent insight into the *M. tuberculosis* chromosome to understand the physical/structural properties of the genome that affect (or are affected by) fundamental processes such as DNA replication and RNA transcription (144) and, in turn, that might impact the propensity for mutagenesis.

MUTAGENESIS IN *M. TUBERCULOSIS*

As noted above, *M. tuberculosis* is not a natural mutator (70). However, since evolution in this organism (including the emergence of drug resistance) occurs exclusively through chromosomal rearrangements and point mutations, determining the rate and cause of these mutagenic events is critical to understand evolutionary dynamics during host infection. Numerous studies have provided both experimental and clinical evidence demonstrating that *M. tuberculosis* strains from different lineages vary in their capacity to cause disease (145–148) and to acquire drug resistance (149–152). However, the evidence for an association between specific *M. tuberculosis* strains and an elevated mutation rate is mixed. Gicquel and colleagues demonstrated that *M. tuberculosis* strains from the Beijing family contain mutations in genes whose disruption in other bacteria confers a mutator phenotype (153). Moreover, strains from this lineage have also been

shown to have polymorphisms in DNA replication, recombination, and repair genes, raising the possibility that they have higher mutation rates (154). Also consistent with these observations, Fortune and colleagues used WGS to demonstrate strain-based differences in mutation rates between lineage 2 (East Asian) and lineage 4 (Euro-American) strains (155). Specifically, the authors reported that *M. tuberculosis* lineage 2 strains acquire drug resistance *in vitro* more rapidly than lineage 4 strains and, further, that the observed differences were not due to the enhanced ability of lineage 2 strains to adapt to antibiotic pressure but rather due to a higher basal mutation rate in the presence of the drug. Nevertheless, the mechanism underlying the inferred difference in mutation rates between the selected lineages remains to be determined (155).

In contrast to these studies, previous *in vitro* analyses observed no differences between the mutation rates of the Beijing versus non-Beijing strains (156), consistent with the idea that multiple factors other than the mutation rate contribute to the apparent success of the Beijing clade (157). It is possible that the apparent discrepancies reflect the representative Beijing versus non-Beijing strains that were used in each case. Therefore, while these findings offer compelling evidence of strain-based differences in mutation rates, it is worth noting that the CDC155 strain employed as an exemplar lineage 4 strain in the Fortune study is a minor branch within this lineage, with its own mode of evolution (158); similarly, HN878, which was used as representative lineage 2 strain, has also separated from other Beijing family members in constructed phylogenies (158). Whether these are genuine caveats is not clear; however, it does appear that further studies are required to address this important question adequately.

TARGETING THE REPLISOME FOR NEW TB DRUG DEVELOPMENT

The essential role of DNA replication in survival and pathogenesis suggests the possibility of targeting the mycobacterial replication and repair machinery with novel chemotherapeutic agents (25). Until recently, however, the replisome has largely failed to yield candidate drugs—with the exception of DNA gyrase inhibitors, for which several antibiotic classes exist (15, 22, 25). There are some encouraging results, however: for example, 6-anilinouracils and their derivatives have been shown to inhibit DNA PolIII and have antibacterial activity against low GC Gram-positive bacteria (159, 160). Moreover, a recent study identified a panel of novel imidazoline compounds that disrupt replication by displacing the replisome from the nucleoid, and are bactericidal against both replicating and nonreplicating *M. tuberculosis* and Gram-positive cocci (161). The bacterial β$_2$-sliding clamp has also emerged as a potentially vulnerable target owing to its central role in DNA replication as a protein-protein interaction hub (162, 163): small molecule inhibitors (163) and tetrahydrocarbazole derivatives have been shown to inhibit DNA replication in both Gram-positive and Gram-negative organisms (162), suggesting the need to test these compounds in *M. tuberculosis*.

New technologies, including structure-based drug design and fragment-based lead generation, might be usefully applied to identify replication components suitable for chemical inhibition (164), but these are dependent on the availability of high-quality structural data that currently do not exist for the majority of *M. tuberculosis* replisome components. In the meantime, natural products seem likeliest to provide the best leads based on very recent evidence: specifically, the exciting identification of two unrelated natural product classes targeting the bacterial replisome. The first of these is nargenicin, a macrolide produced by *Nocardia argentinensis*, which has recently been shown by researchers at Merck Research Laboratories to target the DnaE subunit in both Gram-positive and Gram-negative bacteria (165). A related patent application from the same group claims that nargenicin is bactericidal against *M. tuberculosis* (International Patent Number WO2016/061772A1), but there are no additional reports describing its antimycobacterial activity. In addition, even though resistance in *Staphylococcus aureus* mapped to a single SNP in *dnaE*, that mutation was distal to the DnaE active site, suggesting that further work is required to elucidate the exact mechanism of action (and resistance) against different bacterial pathogens.

The second natural product targeting the replisome, the griselimycins, are cyclic peptides isolated from *Streptomyces griseus* (166). Although described over 50 years ago, the key pharmacological liabilities of these compounds were considered insurmountable until recently, when a revived program generated a series of fully synthetic griselimycin analogs with superior pharmacokinetic properties (167). Griselimycins are potently active against *M. tuberculosis*, binding to the *dnaN*-encoded β-sliding clamp with high affinity and so disrupting DNA replication. Spontaneous resistance to griselimycin results from amplification of the *dnaN* gene—a novel mechanism that, although it incurs a severe fitness cost (167), simultaneously highlights the daunting number of routes to drug resistance that are seemingly available to bacterial mutants (168).

Consistent with their inferred importance for mycobacterial pathogenesis, DNA damage tolerance pathways might offer an additional option for novel antibacterial therapies. There has been considerable discussion of the possibility of inhibiting tolerance mechanisms, particularly inducible mutagenesis pathways, in order to protect current drugs by targeting the mechanisms that underlie the evolution of resistance (169). In some respects, this approach can be considered analogous to inhibiting efflux pathways (170): on its own, a specific efflux pump(s) is not an attractive target but, in combination with the appropriate frontline drug, its inhibition might be critical to efficacy by ensuring that the active compound is maintained at an elevated intracellular concentration (170–172). *M. tuberculosis* DnaE2 represents a good candidate for this approach since it is not essential for normal growth *in vitro*, yet loss of DnaE2 activity attenuates virulence *in vivo* and reduces the frequency of drug-resistance mutations during chronic infection (69). Furthermore, DnaE2 has been demonstrated to function in association with other DNA damage response proteins as a split "mutagenic cassette" (67), suggesting an alternative strategy of targeting the other pathway components, for example, by disrupting the protein-protein interactions that are essential to mutasome function (162, 163).

Recent evidence implicating the lethal incorporation of oxidized guanine into DNA as a major cause of antibiotic-induced bacterial cell death (173) suggests that DNA replication and repair pathways might contribute significantly to intrinsic drug resistance and, for that reason, further supports the call for DNA metabolic pathways to be targeted aggressively as potentially novel antimicrobial therapies.

DNA REPLICATION AND MYCOBACTERIAL PERSISTENCE

The fixation of chromosomal mutations through spontaneous replicative error, or via the operation of error-prone DNA repair or damage tolerance pathways, provides a clear route to the generation of drug-resistant isolates. Less certain, however, are the roles that DNA replication and repair might play in the ability of a genetically susceptible mycobacterial population to exhibit phenotypic tolerance of an applied drug. The terminology relating to "antibiotic tolerance" (a phrase often used interchangeably with "persistence") can be confusing (174, 175), and a thorough discussion of the various functional definitions is beyond the scope of this review. However, it does seem intuitive that, by altering the replicative status of all bacilli exposed to a genotoxic stress, a general, regulated response—such as the LexA/RecA-dependent DNA damage (or SOS) response—might impact the susceptibility of the *entire* population to an applied antibiotic. In contrast, spontaneous blocks to replication—whether mediated by errors in cellular function, or temporary halts to the replication cycle to enable repair of endogenous DNA damage—will occur in individual cells (or even a very small subpopulation of cells) within a population, where the effect will not be generalized; this effect is captured in the Persistence as Stuff Happens (or PaSH) model of Johnson and Levin (176).

The framework developed recently by Balaban and colleagues (177) for classifying the drug response of bacteria according to specific definitions of "resistance," "tolerance," and "persistence" is instructive in this context. Using the combined parameters of antibiotic susceptibility (minimum inhibitory concentration, MIC), and kill dynamics (minimum duration for killing, MDK), the authors proposed a practical algorithm to distinguish tolerance and persistence phenotypes. Critically, the Balaban framework defines tolerance as a population effect—whether by slow growth, or by extended lag phase—whereas persistence is a property of a subpopulation of cells. So, for a tolerant population, the MDK$_{99}$ value (minimum duration for killing 99% of the population) will be greater than for a susceptible population; in contrast, a persistence phenotype (often manifest as a biphasic kill curve) is revealed only in the MDK$_{99.99}$ value (denoting the MDK for 99.99% of the population) which will be much greater for the minority persister subpopulation than for the remainder of the (susceptible) population.

In the context of mycobacterial replication, this suggests that a general, population-wide effect on replication (e.g., slow growth as a result of dNTP starvation, or SOS-induced replication arrest) will give rise to a tolerant state (Fig. 4). On the other hand, where replication is arrested in only a small fraction (or subpopulation) of mycobacterial cells owing to transient disruptions to cell function (as proposed in the PaSH model [176]), the effect will be of persistence. This is key, since it in turn implies a general framework (Fig. 4) in which the capacity for population heterogeneity is minimized at theoretical extremes: where there is limited (or no) stress—such as under logarithmic growth in nutrient-rich medium or under minimal host immune pressure—or under high stress, in which every cell in the population responds similarly—such as by triggering expression of a regulatory program like the SOS response. It is perhaps worth noting that the bulk of the mycobacterial phenotypes modeled *in vitro* (including in TB drug discovery) are located in either

of these extremes (logarithmic growth, or under a generalized stress such as low pH or hypoxia)—largely for practical reasons. Yet, it seems intuitive to predict that the majority of environments encountered in the host during natural infection are more likely to impose conditions that occur somewhere between those experimentally tractable extremes (depicted inside the theoretical dotted lines in Fig. 4), thereby increasing the propensity for phenotypic heterogeneity (a mixture of tolerant and persistent phenotypes). In turn, this suggests that the true impact of population heterogeneity on drug susceptibility (and other relevant pathogenic phenotypes) remains largely unknown.

Is There a Link Between Persistence and Resistance?

It has been argued that the quiescent metabolic state of tolerant (or persistent) cells necessarily precludes the *de novo* generation and fixation of resistance mutations (a process that requires active replication); that is, (nongenetic) tolerance/persistence and (genetic) resistance cannot be linked since growth and replication are halted. However, recent evidence indicating that persister cells *can* replicate in the presence of a lethal antibiotic (109, 178) does suggest the possibility for tolerant (or persister) cells to be implicated in the emergence of genetic drug resistance. Consistent with the predictions of the PaSH model (176), spontaneous DNA damage and breakage events occur at detectable frequencies in *E. coli* cells during normal growth *in vitro* (179, 180) and induce the bacterial SOS response (181), which regulates the coordinated expression of multiple genes and operons to minimize the effects of genotoxic stress (182). Since the SOS regulon includes elements involved in transiently halting the progression of cellular division (78–80, 183) to enable DNA repair and, as described above (Fig. 4), can be induced by endogenous (metabolic) (179–181) and exogenous (host immune-mediated) damage, as well as applied (antibiotic-mediated) (184–186) stress, activation of the SOS response in bacteria including *M. tuberculosis* might invoke a physiological state analogous to persistence in a single organism or subpopulation of bacilli, or tolerance at a population level (187). That is, the elements necessary for both phenotypic heterogeneity (through growth arrest, damage repair, and detoxification) and genetic heterogeneity (through mutagenesis) are united in a single regulon.

Some support for this possibility is provided in a set of studies by Robert Austin and colleagues describing the accelerated emergence of drug resistance in *E. coli* cells exposed to the genotoxic antibiotic, ciprofloxacin

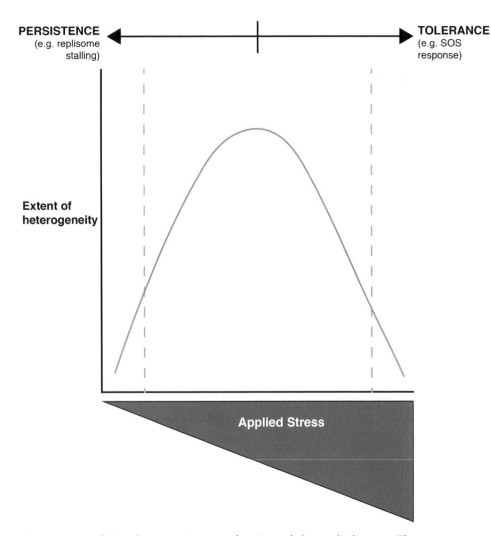

Figure 4 Population heterogeneity as a function of the applied stress. The cartoon summarizes the notion that the degree (or strength) of applied stress might determine the extent of phenotypic heterogeneity within a specific (myco)bacterial population. So, as the applied stress (e.g., genotoxin, antibiotic, nutrient deprivation, pH, oxygen starvation) increases toward a critical point or concentration (which will differ for each stress), the degree of heterogeneity within the population increases. Beyond that critical point (the vertex of the parabola), the result is more likely to be manifest as a general, regulated response at the population level; this has the effect of reducing the extent of heterogeneity within the population. At each extreme (low/absent stress versus high/severe stress), the degree of heterogeneity approaches a minimum. Importantly, for conditions under which both the applied stress and the degree of heterogeneity are low, a small subpopulation of persister cells might enable survival, consistent with the framework proposed by Balaban and colleagues (177). At the other extreme—high/severe stress, low heterogeneity—any observed tolerance will exist at the population level, and will be mediated by a dominant regulatory mechanism(s), such as the LexA/RecA-dependent SOS response.

(188, 189). Using microfluidics and time-lapse imaging, the authors first demonstrated that resistant mutants could emerge in a fully susceptible population, provided the bacteria were located in connected microenvironments that created an antibiotic concentration gradient (188). Importantly, these studies established

that, for a resistant population to emerge, the total bacterial numbers in the antibiotic-treated population need not be especially high: resistant mutants were obtained from a starting (antibiotic-treated) population of as few as ~100 bacteria. However, essential to the emergence of resistance under treatment was the SOS-dependent induction of a filamentation phenotype, in which cells exposed to sublethal antibiotic concentrations elongated without division. The resulting polyploid filaments occasionally generated a viable "bud," which possessed a chromosome containing a drug-resistance mutation that consequently enabled resumption of normal cell division. Although the precise mutagenic mechanism was not determined (it seems intuitive that any of the SOS-inducible TLS polymerases in *E. coli* might be involved, for example), these studies nevertheless hinted at the potential for a tolerance phenotype (SOS-induced division arrest and bacterial filamentation) to create the transient opportunity for the generation (and fixation) of a resistance mutation(s) under strong selective pressure. Additional research will be required to test this notion, which seems to be of special relevance to *M. tuberculosis*, an obligate human pathogen that is increasingly associated with genetic diversity and microvariation, including the development of drug resistance under chemotherapy (19).

Acknowledgments. A portion of the review presented here was submitted by Z.D. in partial fulfilment of the requirements for a Doctor of Philosophy in Medical Microbiology at the University of Cape Town. We thank Valerie Mizrahi and members of the MMRU for many helpful discussions and critical review of this manuscript. Work in the MMRU on mycobacterial DNA replication and repair is funded by grants from the US National Institute of Child Health and Human Development (NICHD) U01HD085531-02 (to D.F.W.); the Department of Science and Technology (DST) of South Africa; the South African Medical Research Council; and the National Research Foundation of South Africa (to D.F.W.). We gratefully acknowledge the support of the Carnegie Corporation of New York (to Z.D.); the National Research Foundation of South Africa (to Z.D.); and the German Academic Exchange Service (DAAD), in partnership with the National Research Foundation of South Africa (to Z.D.). We thank Herman de Klerk and Anastasia Koch for technical assistance with the preparation of the figures.

Citation. Ditse Z, Lamers MH, Warner DF. 2017. DNA replication in *Mycobacterium tuberculosis*. Microbiol Spectrum 5(2):TBTB2-0027-2016.

References

1. **Ambur OH, Davidsen T, Frye SA, Balasingham SV, Lagesen K, Rognes T, Tønjum T.** 2009. Genome dynamics in major bacterial pathogens. *FEMS Microbiol Rev* **33:**453–470.
2. **Russell DG.** 2016. The ins and outs of the *Mycobacterium tuberculosis*-containing vacuole. *Cell Microbiol* **18:**1065–1069.
3. **Dartois V.** 2014. The path of anti-tuberculosis drugs: from blood to lesions to mycobacterial cells. *Nat Rev Microbiol* **12:**159–167.
4. **Olive AJ, Sassetti CM.** 2016. Metabolic crosstalk between host and pathogen: sensing, adapting and competing. *Nat Rev Microbiol* **14:**221–234.
5. **Warner DF.** 2014. *Mycobacterium tuberculosis* metabolism. *Cold Spring Harb Perspect Med* **5:**5.
6. **Darwin KH, Nathan CF.** 2005. Role for nucleotide excision repair in virulence of *Mycobacterium tuberculosis*. *Infect Immun* **73:**4581–4587.
7. **Dutta NK, Mehra S, Didier PJ, Roy CJ, Doyle LA, Alvarez X, Ratterree M, Be NA, Lamichhane G, Jain SK, Lacey MR, Lackner AA, Kaushal D.** 2010. Genetic requirements for the survival of tubercle bacilli in primates. *J Infect Dis* **201:**1743–1752.
8. **Gorna AE, Bowater RP, Dziadek J.** 2010. DNA repair systems and the pathogenesis of *Mycobacterium tuberculosis*: varying activities at different stages of infection. *Clin Sci (Lond)* **119:**187–202.
9. **WHO.** 2015. *Global Tuberculosis Report 2015.* World Health Organization, Geneva, Switzerland.
10. **Chao MC, Rubin EJ.** 2010. Letting sleeping dogs lie: does dormancy play a role in tuberculosis? *Annu Rev Microbiol* **64:**293–311.
11. **Lipworth S, Hammond RJ, Baron VO, Hu Y, Coates A, Gillespie SH.** 2016. Defining dormancy in mycobacterial disease. *Tuberculosis (Edinb)* **99:**131–142.
12. **Lillebaek T, Dirksen A, Baess I, Strunge B, Thomsen VO, Andersen AB.** 2002. Molecular evidence of endogenous reactivation of *Mycobacterium tuberculosis* after 33 years of latent infection. *J Infect Dis* **185:**401–404.
13. **Lillebaek T, Norman A, Rasmussen EM, Marvig RL, Folkvardsen DB, Andersen AB, Jelsbak L.** 2016. Substantial molecular evolution and mutation rates in prolonged latent *Mycobacterium tuberculosis* infection in humans. *Int J Med Microbiol* **306:**580–585.
14. **Lin PL, Ford CB, Coleman MT, Myers AJ, Gawande R, Ioerger T, Sacchettini J, Fortune SM, Flynn JL.** 2014. Sterilization of granulomas is common in active and latent tuberculosis despite within-host variability in bacterial killing. *Nat Med* **20:**75–79.
15. **Warner DF.** 2010. The role of DNA repair in *M. tuberculosis* pathogenesis. *Drug Discov Today Dis Mech* **7:**e5–e11.
16. **Almeida Da Silva PE, Palomino JC.** 2011. Molecular basis and mechanisms of drug resistance in *Mycobacterium tuberculosis*: classical and new drugs. *J Antimicrob Chemother* **66:**1417–1430.
17. **Sandgren A, Strong M, Muthukrishnan P, Weiner BK, Church GM, Murray MB.** 2009. Tuberculosis drug resistance mutation database. *PLoS Med* **6:**e1000002.
18. **Boritsch EC, Khanna V, Pawlik A, Honoré N, Navas VH, Ma L, Bouchier C, Seemann T, Supply P, Stinear TP, Brosch R.** 2016. Key experimental evidence of chromosomal DNA transfer among selected tuberculosis-causing mycobacteria. *Proc Natl Acad Sci USA* **113:**9876–9881.
19. **Warner DF, Koch A, Mizrahi V.** 2015. Diversity and disease pathogenesis in *Mycobacterium tuberculosis*. *Trends Microbiol* **23:**14–21.
20. **McGrath M, Gey van Pittius NC, van Helden PD, Warren RM, Warner DF.** 2014. Mutation rate and the emergence of drug resistance in *Mycobacterium tuberculosis*. *J Antimicrob Chemother* **69:**292–302.

21. Mizrahi V, Andersen SJ. 1998. DNA repair in *Mycobacterium tuberculosis*. What have we learnt from the genome sequence? *Mol Microbiol* 29:1331–1339.

22. Warner DF, Evans JC, Mizrahi V. 2014. Nucleotide metabolism and DNA replication. *Microbiol Spectr* 2:MGM2-0001-2013.

23. Warner DF, Tønjum T, Mizrahi V. 2013. DNA metabolism in mycobacterial pathogenesis. *Curr Top Microbiol Immunol* 374:27–51.

24. Davis EO, Forse LN. 2009. DNA repair: key to survival, p 79–117. *In* Parish T, Brown A (ed), *Mycobacterium Genomics and Molecular Biology*. Caister Academic Press, Norfolk, UK.

25. Robinson A, Causer RJ, Dixon NE. 2012. Architecture and conservation of the bacterial DNA replication machinery, an underexploited drug target. *Curr Drug Targets* 13:352–372.

26. Cole ST, Eiglmeier K, Parkhill J, James KD, Thomson NR, Wheeler PR, Honoré N, Garnier T, Churcher C, Harris D, Mungall K, Basham D, Brown D, Chillingworth T, Connor R, Davies RM, Devlin K, Duthoy S, Feltwell T, Fraser A, Hamlin N, Holroyd S, Hornsby T, Jagels K, Lacroix C, Maclean J, Moule S, Murphy L, Oliver K, Quail MA, Rajandream MA, Rutherford KM, Rutter S, Seeger K, Simon S, Simmonds M, Skelton J, Squares R, Squares S, Stevens K, Taylor K, Whitehead S, Woodward JR, Barrell BG. 2001. Massive gene decay in the leprosy bacillus. *Nature* 409:1007–1011.

27. Ginda K, Bezulska M, Ziółkiewicz M, Dziadek J, Zakrzewska-Czerwińska J, Jakimowicz D. 2013. ParA of *Mycobacterium smegmatis* co-ordinates chromosome segregation with the cell cycle and interacts with the polar growth determinant DivIVA. *Mol Microbiol* 87:998–1012.

28. Richardson K, Bennion OT, Tan S, Hoang AN, Cokol M, Aldridge BB. 2016. Temporal and intrinsic factors of rifampicin tolerance in mycobacteria. *Proc Natl Acad Sci USA* 113:8302–8307.

29. Trojanowski D, Ginda K, Pióro M, Hołówka J, Skut P, Jakimowicz D, Zakrzewska-Czerwińska J. 2015. Choreography of the Mycobacterium replication machinery during the cell cycle. *MBio* 6:e02125-14.

30. Aldridge BB, Fernandez-Suarez M, Heller D, Ambravaneswaran V, Irimia D, Toner M, Fortune SM. 2012. Asymmetry and aging of mycobacterial cells lead to variable growth and antibiotic susceptibility. *Science* 335:100–104.

31. Santi I, Dhar N, Bousbaine D, Wakamoto Y, McKinney JD. 2013. Single-cell dynamics of the chromosome replication and cell division cycles in mycobacteria. *Nat Commun* 4:2470.

32. Santi I, McKinney JD. 2015. Chromosome organization and replisome dynamics in *Mycobacterium smegmatis*. *MBio* 6:e01999-14.

33. Joyce G, Williams KJ, Robb M, Noens E, Tizzano B, Shahrezaei V, Robertson BD. 2012. Cell division site placement and asymmetric growth in mycobacteria. *PLoS One* 7:e44582.

34. Beattie TR, Reyes-Lamothe R. 2015. A replisome's journey through the bacterial chromosome. *Front Microbiol* 6:562.

35. McHenry CS. 2011. DNA replicases from a bacterial perspective. *Annu Rev Biochem* 80:403–436.

36. Reyes-Lamothe R, Sherratt DJ, Leake MC. 2010. Stoichiometry and architecture of active DNA replication machinery in *Escherichia coli*. *Science* 328:498–501.

37. Sanders GM, Dallmann HG, McHenry CS. 2010. Reconstitution of the *B. subtilis* replisome with 13 proteins including two distinct replicases. *Mol Cell* 37:273–281.

38. Johnson A, O'Donnell M. 2005. Cellular DNA replicases: components and dynamics at the replication fork. *Annu Rev Biochem* 74:283–315.

39. Johnson A, O'Donnell M. 2005. Cellular DNA replicases: components and dynamics at the replication fork. *Annu Rev Biochem* 74:283–315.

40. O'Donnell M. 2006. Replisome architecture and dynamics in *Escherichia coli*. *J Biol Chem* 281:10653–10656.

41. Yao NY, Georgescu RE, Finkelstein J, O'Donnell ME. 2009. Single-molecule analysis reveals that the lagging strand increases replisome processivity but slows replication fork progression. *Proc Natl Acad Sci USA* 106:13236–13241.

42. Gu S, Li W, Zhang H, Fleming J, Yang W, Wang S, Wei W, Zhou J, Zhu G, Deng J, Hou J, Zhou Y, Lin S, Zhang XE, Bi L. 2016. The β2 clamp in the *Mycobacterium tuberculosis* DNA polymerase III αβ2ε replicase promotes polymerization and reduces exonuclease activity. *Sci Rep* 6:18418.

43. Rock JM, Lang UF, Chase MR, Ford CB, Gerrick ER, Gawande R, Coscolla M, Gagneux S, Fortune SM, Lamers MH. 2015. DNA replication fidelity in *Mycobacterium tuberculosis* is mediated by an ancestral prokaryotic proofreader. *Nat Genet* 47:677–681.

44. Nair N, Dziedzic R, Greendyke R, Muniruzzaman S, Rajagopalan M, Madiraju MV. 2009. Synchronous replication initiation in novel *Mycobacterium tuberculosis* dnaA cold-sensitive mutants. *Mol Microbiol* 71:291–304.

45. Turcios L, Casart Y, Florez I, de Waard J, Salazar L. 2009. Characterization of IS6110 insertions in the dnaA-dnaN intergenic region of *Mycobacterium tuberculosis* clinical isolates. *Clin Microbiol Infect* 15:200–203.

46. Xie Y, He ZG. 2009. Characterization of physical interaction between replication initiator protein DnaA and replicative helicase from *Mycobacterium tuberculosis* H37Rv. *Biochemistry (Mosc)* 74:1320–1327.

47. Stelter M, Gutsche I, Kapp U, Bazin A, Bajic G, Goret G, Jamin M, Timmins J, Terradot L. 2012. Architecture of a dodecameric bacterial replicative helicase. *Structure* 20:554–564.

48. Flower AM, McHenry CS. 1990. The γ subunit of DNA polymerase III holoenzyme of *Escherichia coli* is produced by ribosomal frameshifting. *Proc Natl Acad Sci USA* 87:3713–3717.

49. Slater SC, Lifsics MR, O'Donnell M, Maurer R. 1994. *holE*, the gene coding for the theta subunit of DNA

polymerase III of *Escherichia coli*: characterization of a *holE* mutant and comparison with a *dnaQ* (epsilon-subunit) mutant. *J Bacteriol* **176**:815–821.

50. Taft-Benz SA, Schaaper RM. 2004. The theta subunit of *Escherichia coli* DNA polymerase III: a role in stabilizing the epsilon proofreading subunit. *J Bacteriol* **186**:2774–2780.

51. Kelman Z, Yuzhakov A, Andjelkovic J, O'Donnell M. 1998. Devoted to the lagging strand-the subunit of DNA polymerase III holoenzyme contacts SSB to promote processive elongation and sliding clamp assembly. *EMBO J* **17**:2436–2449.

52. Witte G, Urbanke C, Curth U. 2003. DNA polymerase III chi subunit ties single-stranded DNA binding protein to the bacterial replication machinery. *Nucleic Acids Res* **31**:4434–4440.

53. Viguera E, Petranovic M, Zahradka D, Germain K, Ehrlich DS, Michel B. 2003. Lethality of bypass polymerases in *Escherichia coli* cells with a defective clamp loader complex of DNA polymerase III. *Mol Microbiol* **50**:193–204.

54. Gulbis JM, Kazmirski SL, Finkelstein J, Kelman Z, O'Donnell M, Kuriyan J. 2004. Crystal structure of the chi:psi sub-assembly of the *Escherichia coli* DNA polymerase clamp-loader complex. *Eur J Biochem* **271**:439–449.

55. Blinkova A, Hervas C, Stukenberg PT, Onrust R, O'Donnell ME, Walker JR. 1993. The *Escherichia coli* DNA polymerase III holoenzyme contains both products of the dnaX gene, tau and gamma, but only tau is essential. *J Bacteriol* **175**:6018–6027.

56. Bruck I, Georgescu RE, O'Donnell M. 2005. Conserved interactions in the *Staphylococcus aureus* DNA PolC chromosome replication machine. *J Biol Chem* **280**:18152–18162.

57. Jarvis TC, Beaudry AA, Bullard JM, Janjic N, McHenry CS. 2005. Reconstitution of a minimal DNA replicase from *Pseudomonas aeruginosa* and stimulation by non-cognate auxiliary factors. *J Biol Chem* **280**:7890–7900.

58. Sanders GM, Dallmann HG, McHenry CS. 2010. Reconstitution of the *B. subtilis* replisome with 13 proteins including two distinct replicases. *Mol Cell* **37**:273–281.

59. Biswas T, Resto-Roldán E, Sawyer SK, Artsimovitch I, Tsodikov OV. 2013. A novel non-radioactive primase-pyrophosphatase activity assay and its application to the discovery of inhibitors of *Mycobacterium tuberculosis* primase DnaG. *Nucleic Acids Res* **41**:e56.

60. Ito J, Braithwaite DK. 1991. Compilation and alignment of DNA polymerase sequences. *Nucleic Acids Res* **19**:4045–4057.

61. Timinskas K, Balvočiūtė M, Timinskas A, Venclovas Č. 2014. Comprehensive analysis of DNA polymerase III α subunits and their homologs in bacterial genomes. *Nucleic Acids Res* **42**:1393–1413.

62. Evans RJ, Davies DR, Bullard JM, Christensen J, Green LS, Guiles JW, Pata JD, Ribble WK, Janjic N, Jarvis TC. 2008. Structure of PolC reveals unique DNA binding and fidelity determinants. *Proc Natl Acad Sci USA* **105**:20695–20700.

63. Bailey S, Wing RA, Steitz TA. 2006. The structure of *T. aquaticus* DNA polymerase III is distinct from eukaryotic replicative DNA polymerases. *Cell* **126**:893–904.

64. Lamers MH, Georgescu RE, Lee S-G, O'Donnell M, Kuriyan J. 2006. Crystal structure of the catalytic alpha subunit of *E. coli* replicative DNA polymerase III. *Cell* **126**:881–892.

65. Huang YP, Ito J. 1999. DNA polymerase C of the thermophilic bacterium *Thermus aquaticus*: classification and phylogenetic analysis of the family C DNA polymerases. *J Mol Evol* **48**:756–769.

66. Lamers MH, O'Donnell M. 2008. A consensus view of DNA binding by the C family of replicative DNA polymerases. *Proc Natl Acad Sci USA* **105**:20565–20566.

67. Warner DF, Ndwandwe DE, Abrahams GL, Kana BD, Machowski EE, Venclovas C, Mizrahi V. 2010. Essential roles for *imuA′*- and *imuB*-encoded accessory factors in DnaE2-dependent mutagenesis in *Mycobacterium tuberculosis*. *Proc Natl Acad Sci USA* **107**:13093–13098.

68. Zhao XQ, Hu JF, Yu J. 2006. Comparative analysis of eubacterial DNA polymerase III alpha subunits. *Genomics Proteomics Bioinformatics* **4**:203–211.

69. Boshoff HI, Reed MB, Barry CE III, Mizrahi V. 2003. DnaE2 polymerase contributes to *in vivo* survival and the emergence of drug resistance in *Mycobacterium tuberculosis*. *Cell* **113**:183–193.

70. Ford CB, Lin PL, Chase MR, Shah RR, Iartchouk O, Galagan J, Mohaideen N, Ioerger TR, Sacchettini JC, Lipsitch M, Flynn JL, Fortune SM. 2011. Use of whole genome sequencing to estimate the mutation rate of *Mycobacterium tuberculosis* during latent infection. *Nat Genet* **43**:482–486.

71. Lee H, Popodi E, Tang H, Foster PL. 2012. Rate and molecular spectrum of spontaneous mutations in the bacterium *Escherichia coli* as determined by whole-genome sequencing. *Proc Natl Acad Sci USA* **109**:E2774–E2783.

72. Fijalkowska IJ, Schaaper RM, Jonczyk P. 2012. DNA replication fidelity in *Escherichia coli*: a multi-DNA polymerase affair. *FEMS Microbiol Rev* **36**:1105–1121.

73. Ishino S, Nishi Y, Oda S, Uemori T, Sagara T, Takatsu N, Yamagami T, Shirai T, Ishino Y. 2016. Identification of a mismatch-specific endonuclease in hyperthermophilic Archaea. *Nucleic Acids Res* **44**:2977–2986.

74. Barros T, Guenther J, Kelch B, Anaya J, Prabhakar A, O'Donnell M, Kuriyan J, Lamers MH. 2013. A structural role for the PHP domain in *E. coli* DNA polymerase III. *BMC Struct Biol* **13**:8.

75. Jergic S, Horan NP, Elshenawy MM, Mason CE, Urathamakul T, Ozawa K, Robinson A, Goudsmits JM, Wang Y, Pan X, Beck JL, van Oijen AM, Huber T, Hamdan SM, Dixon NE. 2013. A direct proofreader-clamp interaction stabilizes the Pol III replicase in the polymerization mode. *EMBO J* **32**:1322–1333.

76. Dos Vultos T, Mestre O, Rauzier J, Golec M, Rastogi N, Rasolofo V, Tonjum T, Sola C, Matic I, Gicquel B. 2008. Evolution and diversity of clonal bacteria: the paradigm of Mycobacterium tuberculosis. *PLoS One* **3**:e1538.

77. Farhat MR, Shapiro BJ, Kieser KJ, Sultana R, Jacobson KR, Victor TC, Warren RM, Streicher EM, Calver A, Sloutsky A, Kaur D, Posey JE, Plikaytis B, Oggioni MR, Gardy JL, Johnston JC, Rodrigues M, Tang PK, Kato-Maeda M, Borowsky ML, Muddukrishna B, Kreiswirth BN, Kurepina N, Galagan J, Gagneux S, Birren B, Rubin EJ, Lander ES, Sabeti PC, Murray M. 2013. Genomic analysis identifies targets of convergent positive selection in drug-resistant *Mycobacterium tuberculosis*. *Nat Genet* 45:1183–1189.

78. Smollett KL, Smith KM, Kahramanoglou C, Arnvig KB, Buxton RS, Davis EO. 2012. Global analysis of the regulon of the transcriptional repressor LexA, a key component of SOS response in *Mycobacterium tuberculosis*. *J Biol Chem* 287:22004–22014.

79. Gamulin V, Cetkovic H, Ahel I. 2004. Identification of a promoter motif regulating the major DNA damage response mechanism of *Mycobacterium tuberculosis*. *FEMS Microbiol Lett* 238:57–63.

80. Wang Y, Huang Y, Xue C, He Y, He ZG. 2011. ClpR protein-like regulator specifically recognizes RecA protein-independent promoter motif and broadly regulates expression of DNA damage-inducible genes in mycobacteria. *J Biol Chem* 286:31159–31167.

81. Rand L, Hinds J, Springer B, Sander P, Buxton RS, Davis EO. 2003. The majority of inducible DNA repair genes in *Mycobacterium tuberculosis* are induced independently of RecA. *Mol Microbiol* 50:1031–1042.

82. Le Chatelier E, Bécherel OJ, d'Alençon E, Canceill D, Ehrlich SD, Fuchs RP, Jannière L. 2004. Involvement of DnaE, the second replicative DNA polymerase from *Bacillus subtilis*, in DNA mutagenesis. *J Biol Chem* 279:1757–1767.

83. Bruck I, Goodman MF, O'Donnell M. 2003. The essential C family DnaE polymerase is error-prone and efficient at lesion bypass. *J Biol Chem* 278:44361–44368.

84. Yang W, Woodgate R. 2007. What a difference a decade makes: insights into translesion DNA synthesis. *Proc Natl Acad Sci USA* 104:15591–15598.

85. Koorits L, Tegova R, Tark M, Tarassova K, Tover A, Kivisaar M. 2007. Study of involvement of ImuB and DnaE2 in stationary-phase mutagenesis in *Pseudomonas putida*. *DNA Repair (Amst)* 6:863–868.

86. Cirz RT, O'Neill BM, Hammond JA, Head SR, Romesberg FE. 2006. Defining the *Pseudomonas aeruginosa* SOS response and its role in the global response to the antibiotic ciprofloxacin. *J Bacteriol* 188:7101–7110.

87. Sanders LH, Rockel A, Lu H, Wozniak DJ, Sutton MD. 2006. Role of *Pseudomonas aeruginosa* dinB-encoded DNA polymerase IV in mutagenesis. *J Bacteriol* 188:8573–8585.

88. Tsai HH, Shu HW, Yang CC, Chen CW. 2012. Translesion-synthesis DNA polymerases participate in replication of the telomeres in *Streptomyces*. *Nucleic Acids Res* 40:1118–1130.

89. Dalrymple BP, Kongsuwan K, Wijffels G, Dixon NE, Jennings PA. 2001. A universal protein-protein interaction motif in the eubacterial DNA replication and repair systems. *Proc Natl Acad Sci USA* 98:11627–11632.

90. Baños B, Lázaro JM, Villar L, Salas M, de Vega M. 2008. Editing of misaligned 3′-termini by an intrinsic 3′-5′ exonuclease activity residing in the PHP domain of a family X DNA polymerase. *Nucleic Acids Res* 36:5736–5749.

91. Stano NM, Chen J, McHenry CS. 2006. A coproofreading Zn(2+)-dependent exonuclease within a bacterial replicase. *Nat Struct Mol Biol* 13:458–459.

92. Borden A, O'Grady PI, Vandewiele D, Fernández de Henestrosa AR, Lawrence CW, Woodgate R. 2002. *Escherichia coli* DNA polymerase III can replicate efficiently past a T-T cis-syn cyclobutane dimer if DNA polymerase V and the 3′ to 5′ exonuclease proofreading function encoded by *dnaQ* are inactivated. *J Bacteriol* 184:2674–2681.

93. Vandewiele D, Borden A, O'Grady PI, Woodgate R, Lawrence CW. 1998. Efficient translesion replication in the absence of *Escherichia coli* Umu proteins and 3′-5′ exonuclease proofreading function. *Proc Natl Acad Sci USA* 95:15519–15524.

94. Gordhan BG, Andersen SJ, De Meyer AR, Mizrahi V. 1996. Construction by homologous recombination and phenotypic characterization of a DNA polymerase domain *polA* mutant of *Mycobacterium smegmatis*. *Gene* 178:125–130.

95. Mizrahi V, Huberts P. 1996. Deoxy- and dideoxynucleotide discrimination and identification of critical 5′ nuclease domain residues of the DNA polymerase I from *Mycobacterium tuberculosis*. *Nucleic Acids Res* 24:4845–4852.

96. Zhu H, Nandakumar J, Aniukwu J, Wang LK, Glickman MS, Lima CD, Shuman S. 2006. Atomic structure and nonhomologous end-joining function of the polymerase component of bacterial DNA ligase D. *Proc Natl Acad Sci USA* 103:1711–1716.

97. Brissett NC, Pitcher RS, Juarez R, Picher AJ, Green AJ, Dafforn TR, Fox GC, Blanco L, Doherty AJ. 2007. Structure of a NHEJ polymerase-mediated DNA synaptic complex. *Science* 318:456–459.

98. Zhu H, Bhattarai H, Yan HG, Shuman S, Glickman MS. 2012. Characterization of *Mycobacterium smegmatis* PolD2 and PolD1 as RNA/DNA polymerases homologous to the POL domain of bacterial DNA ligase D. *Biochemistry* 51:10147–10158.

99. Kana BD, Abrahams GL, Sung N, Warner DF, Gordhan BG, Machowski EE, Tsenova L, Sacchettini JC, Stoker NG, Kaplan G, Mizrahi V. 2010. Role of the DinB homologs Rv1537 and Rv3056 in *Mycobacterium tuberculosis*. *J Bacteriol* 192:2220–2227.

100. Ghosh S, Samaddar S, Kirtania P, Das Gupta SK. 2015. A DinB ortholog enables mycobacterial growth under dTTP-limiting conditions induced by the expression of a mycobacteriophage-derived ribonucleotide reductase gene. *J Bacteriol* 198:352–362.

101. Sharma A, Nair DT. 2012. MsDpo4—a DinB homolog from *Mycobacterium smegmatis*—is an error-prone DNA polymerase that can promote G:T and T:G mismatches. *J Nucleic Acids* 2012:285481.

102. Andersson DI, Koskiniemi S, Hughes D. 2010. Biological roles of translesion synthesis DNA polymerases in eubacteria. *Mol Microbiol* 77:540–548.

103. Goodman MF. 2002. Error-prone repair DNA polymerases in prokaryotes and eukaryotes. *Annu Rev Biochem* **71:**17–50.

104. Davis EO, Springer B, Gopaul KK, Papavinasasundaram KG, Sander P, Böttger EC. 2002. DNA damage induction of recA in *Mycobacterium tuberculosis* independently of RecA and LexA. *Mol Microbiol* **46:**791–800.

105. Ordonez H, Shuman S. 2014. *Mycobacterium smegmatis* DinB2 misincorporates deoxyribonucleotides and ribonucleotides during templated synthesis and lesion bypass. *Nucleic Acids Res* **42:**12722–12734.

106. Ordonez H, Uson ML, Shuman S. 2014. Characterization of three mycobacterial DinB (DNA polymerase IV) paralogs highlights DinB2 as naturally adept at ribonucleotide incorporation. *Nucleic Acids Res* **42:** 11056–11070.

107. Uhía I, Williams KJ, Shahrezaei V, Robertson BD. 2015. Mycobacterial growth. *Cold Spring Harb Perspect Med* **5:**a021097.

108. Hett EC, Rubin EJ. 2008. Bacterial growth and cell division: a mycobacterial perspective. *Microbiol Mol Biol Rev* **72:**126–156.

109. Wakamoto Y, Dhar N, Chait R, Schneider K, Signorino-Gelo F, Leibler S, McKinney JD. 2013. Dynamic persistence of antibiotic-stressed mycobacteria. *Science* **339:** 91–95.

110. Wayne LG. 1977. Synchronized replication of *Mycobacterium tuberculosis*. *Infect Immun* **17:**528–530.

111. Caire-Brändli I, Papadopoulos A, Malaga W, Marais D, Canaan S, Thilo L, de Chastellier C, Flynn JL. 2014. Reversible lipid accumulation and associated division arrest of *Mycobacterium avium* in lipoprotein-induced foamy macrophages may resemble key events during latency and reactivation of tuberculosis. *Infect Immun* **82:**476–490.

112. Chauhan A, Madiraju MV, Fol M, Lofton H, Maloney E, Reynolds R, Rajagopalan M. 2006. *Mycobacterium tuberculosis* cells growing in macrophages are filamentous and deficient in FtsZ rings. *J Bacteriol* **188:**1856–1865.

113. Ernst JD. 2012. The immunological life cycle of tuberculosis. *Nat Rev Immunol* **12:**581–591.

114. Gupta A, Kaul A, Tsolaki AG, Kishore U, Bhakta S. 2012. *Mycobacterium tuberculosis*: immune evasion, latency and reactivation. *Immunobiology* **217:**363–374.

115. Bergkessel M, Basta DW, Newman DK. 2016. The physiology of growth arrest: uniting molecular and environmental microbiology. *Nat Rev Microbiol* **14:**549–562.

116. Hiriyanna KT, Ramakrishnan T. 1986. Deoxyribonucleic acid replication time in *Mycobacterium tuberculosis* H37 Rv. *Arch Microbiol* **144:**105–109.

117. Liu AM, Barra AL, Rubin H, Lu GZ, Graslund A. 2000. Heterogeneity of the local electrostatic environment of the tyrosyl radical in *Mycobacterium tuberculosis* ribonucleotide reductase observed by high-field electron paramagnetic resonance. *J Am Chem Soc* **122:** 1974–1978.

118. Elleingand E, Gerez C, Un S, Knüpling M, Lu G, Salem J, Rubin H, Sauge-Merle S, Laulhère JP, Fontecave M. 1998. Reactivity studies of the tyrosyl radical in ribonucleotide reductase from *Mycobacterium tuberculosis* and *Arabidopsis thaliana*–comparison with *Escherichia coli* and mouse. *Eur J Biochem* **258:**485–490.

119. Hammerstad M, Røhr AK, Andersen NH, Gräslund A, Högbom M, Andersson KK. 2014. The class Ib ribonucleotide reductase from *Mycobacterium tuberculosis* has two active R2F subunits. *J Biol Inorg Chem* **19:** 893–902.

120. Georgieva ER, Narvaez AJ, Hedin N, Gräslund A. 2008. Secondary structure conversions of *Mycobacterium tuberculosis* ribonucleotide reductase protein R2 under varying pH and temperature conditions. *Biophys Chem* **137:**43–48.

121. Uppsten M, Davis J, Rubin H, Uhlin U. 2004. Crystal structure of the biologically active form of class Ib ribonucleotide reductase small subunit from *Mycobacterium tuberculosis*. *FEBS Lett* **569:**117–122.

122. Basta T, Boum Y, Briffotaux J, Becker HF, Lamarre-Jouenne I, Lambry JC, Skouloubris S, Liebl U, Graille M, van Tilbeurgh H, Myllykallio H. 2012. Mechanistic and structural basis for inhibition of thymidylate synthase ThyX. *Open Biol* **2:**120120.

123. Hunter JH, Gujjar R, Pang CK, Rathod PK. 2008. Kinetics and ligand-binding preferences of *Mycobacterium tuberculosis* thymidylate synthases, ThyA and ThyX. *PLoS One* **3:**e2237.

124. Liu A, Pötsch S, Davydov A, Barra AL, Rubin H, Gräslund A. 1998. The tyrosyl free radical of recombinant ribonucleotide reductase from *Mycobacterium tuberculosis* is located in a rigid hydrophobic pocket. *Biochemistry* **37:**16369–16377.

125. Yang F, Lu G, Rubin H. 1994. Isolation of ribonucleotide reductase from *Mycobacterium tuberculosis* and cloning, expression, and purification of the large subunit. *J Bacteriol* **176:**6738–6743.

126. Mowa MB, Warner DF, Kaplan G, Kana BD, Mizrahi V. 2009. Function and regulation of class I ribonucleotide reductase-encoding genes in mycobacteria. *J Bacteriol* **191:**985–995.

127. Singh V, Brecik M, Mukherjee R, Evans JC, Svetlíková Z, Blaško J, Surade S, Blackburn J, Warner DF, Mikušová K, Mizrahi V. 2015. The complex mechanism of antimycobacterial action of 5-fluorouracil. *Chem Biol* **22:** 63–75.

128. Fivian-Hughes AS, Houghton J, Davis EO. 2012. *Mycobacterium tuberculosis* thymidylate synthase gene thyX is essential and potentially bifunctional, while thyA deletion confers resistance to p-aminosalicylic acid. *Microbiology* **158:**308–318.

129. Dawes SS, Warner DF, Tsenova L, Timm J, McKinney JD, Kaplan G, Rubin H, Mizrahi V. 2003. Ribonucleotide reduction in *Mycobacterium tuberculosis*: function and expression of genes encoding class Ib and class II ribonucleotide reductases. *Infect Immun* **71:**6124–6131.

130. Yang F, Curran SC, Li LS, Avarbock D, Graf JD, Chua MM, Lu G, Salem J, Rubin H. 1997. Characterization of two genes encoding the *Mycobacterium tuberculosis* ribonucleotide reductase small subunit. *J Bacteriol* **179:** 6408–6415.

131. Nahid P, Daley CL. 2006. Prevention of tuberculosis in HIV-infected patients. *Curr Opin Infect Dis* **19:** 189–193.

132. Gill WP, Harik NS, Whiddon MR, Liao RP, Mittler JE, Sherman DR. 2009. A replication clock for *Mycobacterium tuberculosis*. *Nat Med* **15:**211–214.

133. Gillespie SH. 2002. Evolution of drug resistance in *Mycobacterium tuberculosis*: clinical and molecular perspective. *Antimicrob Agents Chemother* **46:**267–274.

134. Colangeli R, Arcus VL, Cursons RT, Ruthe A, Karalus N, Coley K, Manning SD, Kim S, Marchiano E, Alland D. 2014. Whole genome sequencing of *Mycobacterium tuberculosis* reveals slow growth and low mutation rates during latent infections in humans. *PLoS One* **9:** e91024.

135. Eldholm V, Monteserin J, Rieux A, Lopez B, Sobkowiak B, Ritacco V, Balloux F. 2015. Four decades of transmission of a multidrug-resistant *Mycobacterium tuberculosis* outbreak strain. *Nat Commun* **6:**7119.

136. Guerra-Assunção JA, Crampin AC, Houben RM, Mzembe T, Mallard K, Coll F, Khan P, Banda L, Chiwaya A, Pereira RP, McNerney R, Fine PE, Parkhill J, Clark TG, Glynn JR. 2015. Large-scale whole genome sequencing of *M. tuberculosis* provides insights into transmission in a high prevalence area. *eLife* **4:** e05166.

137. Walker TM, Ip CL, Harrell RH, Evans JT, Kapatai G, Dedicoat MJ, Eyre DW, Wilson DJ, Hawkey PM, Crook DW, Parkhill J, Harris D, Walker AS, Bowden R, Monk P, Smith EG, Peto TE. 2013. Whole-genome sequencing to delineate *Mycobacterium tuberculosis* outbreaks: a retrospective observational study. *Lancet Infect Dis* **13:**137–146.

138. Adams DW, Wu LJ, Errington J. 2014. Cell cycle regulation by the bacterial nucleoid. *Curr Opin Microbiol* **22:**94–101.

139. Dame RT, Tark-Dame M. 2016. Bacterial chromatin: converging views at different scales. *Curr Opin Cell Biol* **40:**60–65.

140. Reyes-Lamothe R, Nicolas E, Sherratt DJ. 2012. Chromosome replication and segregation in bacteria. *Annu Rev Genet* **46:**121–143.

141. Badrinarayanan A, Le TB, Laub MT. 2015. Bacterial chromosome organization and segregation. *Annu Rev Cell Dev Biol* **31:**171–199.

142. Wang X, Montero Llopis P, Rudner DZ. 2013. Organization and segregation of bacterial chromosomes. *Nat Rev Genet* **14:**191–203.

143. Marbouty M, Le Gall A, Cattoni DI, Cournac A, Koh A, Fiche JB, Mozziconacci J, Murray H, Koszul R, Nollmann M. 2015. Condensin- and replication-mediated bacterial chromosome folding and origin condensation revealed by Hi-C and super-resolution imaging. *Mol Cell* **59:**588–602.

144. Le TB, Laub MT. 2016. Transcription rate and transcript length drive formation of chromosomal interaction domain boundaries. *EMBO J* **35:**1582–1595.

145. de Jong BC, Hill PC, Aiken A, Awine T, Antonio M, Adetifa IM, Jackson-Sillah DJ, Fox A, Deriemer K, Gagneux S, Borgdorff MW, McAdam KP, Corrah T, Small PM, Adegbola RA. 2008. Progression to active tuberculosis, but not transmission, varies by *Mycobacterium tuberculosis* lineage in The Gambia. *J Infect Dis* **198:**1037–1043.

146. Coscolla M, Gagneux S. 2010. Does *M. tuberculosis* genomic diversity explain disease diversity? *Drug Discov Today Dis Mech* **7:**e43–e59.

147. Kato-Maeda M, Shanley CA, Ackart D, Jarlsberg LG, Shang S, Obregon-Henao A, Harton M, Basaraba RJ, Henao-Tamayo M, Barrozo JC, Rose J, Kawamura LM, Coscolla M, Fofanov VY, Koshinsky H, Gagneux S, Hopewell PC, Ordway DJ, Orme IM. 2012. Beijing sublineages of *Mycobacterium tuberculosis* differ in pathogenicity in the guinea pig. *Clin Vaccine Immunol* **19:**1227–1237.

148. Glynn JR, Whiteley J, Bifani PJ, Kremer K, van Soolingen D. 2002. Worldwide occurrence of Beijing/W strains of *Mycobacterium tuberculosis*: a systematic review. *Emerg Infect Dis* **8:**843–849.

149. Anh DD, Borgdorff MW, Van LN, Lan NT, van Gorkom T, Kremer K, van Soolingen D. 2000. *Mycobacterium tuberculosis* Beijing genotype emerging in Vietnam. *Emerg Infect Dis* **6:**302–305.

150. Huang HY, Tsai YS, Lee JJ, Chiang MC, Chen YH, Chiang CY, Lin NT, Tsai PJ. 2010. Mixed infection with Beijing and non-Beijing strains and drug resistance pattern of *Mycobacterium tuberculosis*. *J Clin Microbiol* **48:**4474–4480.

151. Sun G, Luo T, Yang C, Dong X, Li J, Zhu Y, Zheng H, Tian W, Wang S, Barry CE III, Mei J, Gao Q. 2012. Dynamic population changes in *Mycobacterium tuberculosis* during acquisition and fixation of drug resistance in patients. *J Infect Dis* **206:**1724–1733.

152. Johnson R, Warren RM, van der Spuy GD, Gey van Pittius NC, Theron D, Streicher EM, Bosman M, Coetzee GJ, van Helden PD, Victor TC. 2010. Drug-resistant tuberculosis epidemic in the Western Cape driven by a virulent Beijing genotype strain. *Int J Tuberc Lung Dis* **14:**119–121.

153. Ebrahimi-Rad M, Bifani P, Martin C, Kremer K, Samper S, Rauzier J, Kreiswirth B, Blazquez J, Jouan M, van Soolingen D, Gicquel B. 2003. Mutations in putative mutator genes of *Mycobacterium tuberculosis* strains of the W-Beijing family. *Emerg Infect Dis* **9:**838–845.

154. Mestre O, Luo T, Dos Vultos T, Kremer K, Murray A, Namouchi A, Jackson C, Rauzier J, Bifani P, Warren R, Rasolofo V, Mei J, Gao Q, Gicquel B. 2011. Phylogeny of *Mycobacterium tuberculosis* Beijing strains constructed from polymorphisms in genes involved in DNA replication, recombination and repair. *PLoS One* **6:** e16020.

155. Ford CB, Shah RR, Maeda MK, Gagneux S, Murray MB, Cohen T, Johnston JC, Gardy J, Lipsitch M, Fortune SM. 2013. *Mycobacterium tuberculosis* mutation rate estimates from different lineages predict substantial differences in the emergence of drug-resistant tuberculosis. *Nat Genet* **45:**784–790.

156. Werngren J, Hoffner SE. 2003. Drug-susceptible *Mycobacterium tuberculosis* Beijing genotype does not

develop mutation-conferred resistance to rifampin at an elevated rate. *J Clin Microbiol* **41:**1520–1524.

157. Parwati I, van Crevel R, van Soolingen D. 2010. Possible underlying mechanisms for successful emergence of the *Mycobacterium tuberculosis* Beijing genotype strains. *Lancet Infect Dis* **10:**103–111.

158. Mokrousov I. 2014. Widely-used laboratory and clinical *Mycobacterium tuberculosis* strains: to what extent they are representative of their phylogenetic lineages? *Tuberculosis (Edinb)* **94:**355–356.

159. Xu WC, Wright GE, Brown NC, Long ZY, Zhi CX, Dvoskin S, Gambino JJ, Barnes MH, Butler MM. 2011. 7-Alkyl-N²-substituted-3-deazaguanines. Synthesis, DNA polymerase III inhibition and antibacterial activity. *Bioorg Med Chem Lett* **21:**4197–4202.

160. Zhi C, Long ZY, Gambino J, Xu WC, Brown NC, Barnes M, Butler M, LaMarr W, Wright GE. 2003. Synthesis of substituted 6-anilinouracils and their inhibition of DNA polymerase IIIC and Gram-positive bacterial growth. *J Med Chem* **46:**2731–2739.

161. Harris KK, Fay A, Yan HG, Kunwar P, Socci ND, Pottabathini N, Juventhala RR, Djaballah H, Glickman MS. 2014. Novel imidazoline antimicrobial scaffold that inhibits DNA replication with activity against mycobacteria and drug resistant Gram-positive cocci. *ACS Chem Biol* **9:**2572–2583.

162. Yin Z, Whittell LR, Wang Y, Jergic S, Liu M, Harry EJ, Dixon NE, Beck JL, Kelso MJ, Oakley AJ. 2014. Discovery of lead compounds targeting the bacterial sliding clamp using a fragment-based approach. *J Med Chem* **57:**2799–2806.

163. Georgescu RE, Yurieva O, Kim SS, Kuriyan J, Kong XP, O'Donnell M. 2008. Structure of a small-molecule inhibitor of a DNA polymerase sliding clamp. *Proc Natl Acad Sci USA* **105:**11116–11121.

164. Sanyal G, Doig P. 2012. Bacterial DNA replication enzymes as targets for antibacterial drug discovery. *Expert Opin Drug Discov* **7:**327–339.

165. Painter RE, Adam GC, Arocho M, DiNunzio E, Donald RG, Dorso K, Genilloud O, Gill C, Goetz M, Hairston NN, Murgolo N, Nare B, Olsen DB, Powles M, Racine F, Su J, Vicente F, Wisniewski D, Xiao L, Hammond M, Young K. 2015. Elucidation of DnaE as the antibacterial target of the natural product, nargenicin. *Chem Biol* **22:**1362–1373.

166. Hoagland DT, Liu J, Lee RB, Lee RE. 2016. New agents for the treatment of drug-resistant *Mycobacterium tuberculosis*. *Adv Drug Deliv Rev* **102:**55–72.

167. Kling A, Lukat P, Almeida DV, Bauer A, Fontaine E, Sordello S, Zaburannyi N, Herrmann J, Wenzel SC, König C, Ammerman NC, Barrio MB, Borchers K, Bordon-Pallier F, Brönstrup M, Courtemanche G, Gerlitz M, Geslin M, Hammann P, Heinz DW, Hoffmann H, Klieber S, Kohlmann M, Kurz M, Lair C, Matter H, Nuermberger E, Tyagi S, Fraisse L, Grosset JH, Lagrange S, Müller R. 2015. Targeting DnaN for tuberculosis therapy using novel griselimycins. *Science* **348:**1106–1112.

168. Warrier T, Kapilashrami K, Argyrou A, Ioerger TR, Little D, Murphy KC, Nandakumar M, Park S, Gold B, Mi J, Zhang T, Meiler E, Rees M, Somersan-Karakaya S, Porras-De Francisco E, Martinez-Hoyos M, Burns-Huang K, Roberts J, Ling Y, Rhee KY, Mendoza-Losana A, Luo M, Nathan CF. 2016. N-methylation of a bactericidal compound as a resistance mechanism in *Mycobacterium tuberculosis*. *Proc Natl Acad Sci USA* **113:**E4523–E4530.

169. Smith PA, Romesberg FE. 2007. Combating bacteria and drug resistance by inhibiting mechanisms of persistence and adaptation. *Nat Chem Biol* **3:**549–556.

170. Adams KN, Takaki K, Connolly LE, Wiedenhoft H, Winglee K, Humbert O, Edelstein PH, Cosma CL, Ramakrishnan L. 2011. Drug tolerance in replicating mycobacteria mediated by a macrophage-induced efflux mechanism. *Cell* **145:**39–53.

171. Adams KN, Szumowski JD, Ramakrishnan L. 2014. Verapamil, and its metabolite norverapamil, inhibit macrophage-induced, bacterial efflux pump-mediated tolerance to multiple anti-tubercular drugs. *J Infect Dis* **210:**456–466.

172. Gupta S, Tyagi S, Bishai WR. 2015. Verapamil increases the bactericidal activity of bedaquiline against *Mycobacterium tuberculosis* in a mouse model. *Antimicrob Agents Chemother* **59:**673–676.

173. Foti JJ, Devadoss B, Winkler JA, Collins JJ, Walker GC. 2012. Oxidation of the guanine nucleotide pool underlies cell death by bactericidal antibiotics. *Science* **336:**315–319.

174. Balaban NQ, Gerdes K, Lewis K, McKinney JD. 2013. A problem of persistence: still more questions than answers? *Nat Rev Microbiol* **11:**587–591.

175. Lewis K. 2010. Persister cells. *Annu Rev Microbiol* **64:**357–372.

176. Johnson PJ, Levin BR. 2013. Pharmacodynamics, population dynamics, and the evolution of persistence in *Staphylococcus aureus*. *PLoS Genet* **9:**e1003123.

177. Brauner A, Fridman O, Gefen O, Balaban NQ. 2016. Distinguishing between resistance, tolerance and persistence to antibiotic treatment. *Nat Rev Microbiol* **14:** 320–330.

178. Cohen NR, Lobritz MA, Collins JJ. 2013. Microbial persistence and the road to drug resistance. *Cell Host Microbe* **13:**632–642.

179. Elez M, Murray AW, Bi LJ, Zhang XE, Matic I, Radman M. 2010. Seeing mutations in living cells. *Curr Biol* **20:**1432–1437.

180. Shee C, Cox BD, Gu F, Luengas EM, Joshi MC, Chiu LY, Magnan D, Halliday JA, Frisch RL, Gibson JL, Nehring RB, Do HG, Hernandez M, Li L, Herman C, Hastings PJ, Bates D, Harris RS, Miller KM, Rosenberg SM. 2013. Engineered proteins detect spontaneous DNA breakage in human and bacterial cells. *eLife* **2:** e01222.

181. Pennington JM, Rosenberg SM. 2007. Spontaneous DNA breakage in single living *Escherichia coli* cells. *Nat Genet* **39:**797–802.

182. Durbach SI, Andersen SJ, Mizrahi V. 1997. SOS induction in mycobacteria: analysis of the DNA-binding activity of a LexA-like repressor and its role in DNA damage induction of the *recA* gene from *Mycobacterium smegmatis*. *Mol Microbiol* **26:**643–653.

183. Chauhan A, Lofton H, Maloney E, Moore J, Fol M, Madiraju MV, Rajagopalan M. 2006. Interference of *Mycobacterium tuberculosis* cell division by Rv2719c, a cell wall hydrolase. *Mol Microbiol* 62:132–147.

184. Malik M, Chavda K, Zhao X, Shah N, Hussain S, Kurepina N, Kreiswirth BN, Kerns RJ, Drlica K. 2012. Induction of mycobacterial resistance to quinolone class antimicrobials. *Antimicrob Agents Chemother* 56: 3879–3887.

185. Miller C, Thomsen LE, Gaggero C, Mosseri R, Ingmer H, Cohen SN. 2004. SOS response induction by β-lactams and bacterial defense against antibiotic lethality. *Science* 305:1629–1631.

186. O'Sullivan DM, Hinds J, Butcher PD, Gillespie SH, McHugh TD. 2008. *Mycobacterium tuberculosis* DNA repair in response to subinhibitory concentrations of ciprofloxacin. *J Antimicrob Chemother* 62:1199–1202.

187. Debbia EA, Roveta S, Schito AM, Gualco L, Marchese A. 2001. Antibiotic persistence: the role of spontaneous DNA repair response. *Microb Drug Resist* 7:335–342.

188. Zhang Q, Lambert G, Liao D, Kim H, Robin K, Tung CK, Pourmand N, Austin RH. 2011. Acceleration of emergence of bacterial antibiotic resistance in connected microenvironments. *Science* 333:1764–1767.

189. Bos J, Zhang Q, Vyawahare S, Rogers E, Rosenberg SM, Austin RH. 2015. Emergence of antibiotic resistance from multinucleated bacterial filaments. *Proc Natl Acad Sci USA* 112:178–183.

190. Leonard AC, Grimwade JE. 2011. Regulation of DnaA assembly and activity: taking directions from the genome. *Annu Rev Microbiol* 65:19–35.

191. Klann AG, Belanger AE, Abanes-De Mello A, Lee JY, Hatfull GF. 1998. Characterization of the *dnaG* locus in *Mycobacterium smegmatis* reveals linkage of DNA replication and cell division. *J Bacteriol* 180:65–72.

192. Srivastava SK, Dube D, Kukshal V, Jha AK, Hajela K, Ramachandran R. 2007. NAD+-dependent DNA ligase (Rv3014c) from *Mycobacterium tuberculosis*: novel structure-function relationship and identification of a specific inhibitor. *Proteins* 69:97–111.

193. Yang Q, Huang F, Hu L, He ZG. 2012. Physical and functional interactions between 3-methyladenine DNA glycosylase and topoisomerase I in mycobacteria. *Biochemistry (Mosc)* 77:378–387.

194. Mérens A, Matrat S, Aubry A, Lascols C, Jarlier V, Soussy CJ, Cavallo JD, Cambau E. 2009. The penta-peptide repeat proteins MfpAMt and QnrB4 exhibit opposite effects on DNA gyrase catalytic reactions and on the ternary gyrase-DNA-quinolone complex. *J Bacteriol* 191:1587–1594.

195. Gong C, Bongiorno P, Martins A, Stephanou NC, Zhu H, Shuman S, Glickman MS. 2005. Mechanism of non-homologous end-joining in mycobacteria: a low-fidelity repair system driven by Ku, ligase D and ligase C. *Nat Struct Mol Biol* 12:304–312.

196. Minias AE, Brzostek AM, Minias P, Dziadek J. 2015. The deletion of *rnhB* in *Mycobacterium smegmatis* does not affect the level of RNase HII substrates or influence genome stability. *PLoS One* 10:e0115521.

197. Gong C, Martins A, Bongiorno P, Glickman M, Shuman S. 2004. Biochemical and genetic analysis of the four DNA ligases of mycobacteria. *J Biol Chem* 279:20594–20606.

198. Heaton BE, Barkan D, Bongiorno P, Karakousis PC, Glickman MS. 2014. Deficiency of double-strand DNA break repair does not impair *Mycobacterium tuberculosis* virulence in multiple animal models of infection. *Infect Immun* 82:3177–3185.

199. Watkins HA, Baker EN. 2010. Structural and functional characterization of an RNase HI domain from the bifunctional protein Rv2228c from *Mycobacterium tuberculosis*. *J Bacteriol* 192:2878–2886.

200. Kesavan AK, Brooks M, Tufariello J, Chan J, Manabe YC. 2009. Tuberculosis genes expressed during persistence and reactivation in the resistant rabbit model. *Tuberculosis (Edinb)* 89:17–21.

201. Griffin JE, Gawronski JD, Dejesus MA, Ioerger TR, Akerley BJ, Sassetti CM. 2011. High-resolution phenotypic profiling defines genes essential for mycobacterial growth and cholesterol catabolism. *PLoS Pathog* 7: e1002251.

202. Sassetti CM, Boyd DH, Rubin EJ. 2003. Genes required for mycobacterial growth defined by high density mutagenesis. *Mol Microbiol* 48:77–84.

Tuberculosis and the Tubercle Bacillus, 2nd ed.
Edited by William R. Jacobs, Jr., Helen McShane, Valerie Mizrahi, and Ian M. Orme
© 2018 American Society for Microbiology, Washington, DC
doi:10.1128/microbiolspec.TBTB2-0013-2016

The Sec Pathways and Exportomes of *Mycobacterium tuberculosis*

28

Brittany K. Miller, Katelyn E. Zulauf, and Miriam Braunstein

INTRODUCTION

Approximately 20% of bacterial proteins have functions outside the cytoplasm (1). Consequently, all bacteria possess protein export pathways that transport proteins made in the cytoplasm beyond the cytoplasmic membrane. These exported proteins may remain in the bacterial cell envelope or be further secreted to the extracellular environment. Many exported proteins function in essential physiological processes. Additionally, in bacterial pathogens, many exported proteins have functions in virulence. Consequently, the pathways that export proteins are commonly essential and/or are important for pathogenesis. Across bacteria, including mycobacteria, there are conserved protein export pathways: the general secretion (Sec) and the twin-arginine translocation (Tat) pathways. Both Sec and Tat pathways are essential to the viability of *Mycobacterium tuberculosis* and both also contribute to virulence (L. Rank and M. Braunstein, unpublished; 2–4). In addition to these conserved pathways, bacterial pathogens commonly have specialized protein export systems that are important for pathogenesis due to their role in exporting virulence factors. Mycobacteria also have specialized protein export systems: the SecA2 export pathway and five ESX (type VII) pathways. In this article, we focus on the conserved Sec pathway and the specialized SecA2 pathway, review what is known about their respective exportomes, and discuss their importance during *M. tuberculosis* replication and persistence within the host.

THE CONSERVED Sec (SecA1) PATHWAY

Most protein export in bacteria is carried out by the Sec pathway, which is highly conserved and essential in all bacteria (5). The Sec pathway transports proteins from the cytoplasm across the cytoplasmic membrane. Sec-exported proteins can then remain in the cell envelope or be fully secreted into the extracellular space. Sec-exported proteins are transported in an unfolded state through the SecYEG membrane channel (Fig. 1). SecY is an essential integral membrane protein which forms the central core of the channel (6). SecE is an essential integral membrane protein that is suggested to stabilize the open SecY conformation before and during translocation (7). SecG is not essential but improves the efficiency of translocation (8). Additional membrane-bound components of the Sec pathway also serve to improve export efficiency: SecD, SecF, and YajC (9). In addition to fully exporting proteins across the cytoplasmic membrane, the Sec pathway is involved in the delivery and insertion of integral membrane proteins into the cytoplasmic membrane. Complete export across the membrane by the Sec pathway is a posttranslational process, whereas the role of the Sec pathway in integral membrane protein localization is a cotranslational process that involves the conserved, essential, ribonucleoprotein signal recognition particle (SRP) (10). SRP is composed of the Ffh protein bound to SRP RNA (11). SRP recognizes the transmembrane domain on a nascent integral membrane protein and then delivers it as a ribosome-mRNA-nascent protein complex to the SRP receptor FtsY (12). In turn, FtsY delivers the integral membrane protein to SecYEG, where a lateral gate in SecY allows passage of transmembrane domains into the cytoplasmic membrane (13). The discussion of the Sec pathway mechanism below focuses on posttranslational export of fully synthesized proteins across the cytoplasmic membrane.

In addition to the Sec proteins discussed above, Sec export requires the essential SecA ATPase that is peripherally associated with SecYEG. SecA is a multifunc-

Department of Microbiology and Immunology, University of North Carolina – Chapel Hill, Chapel Hill, NC 27599.

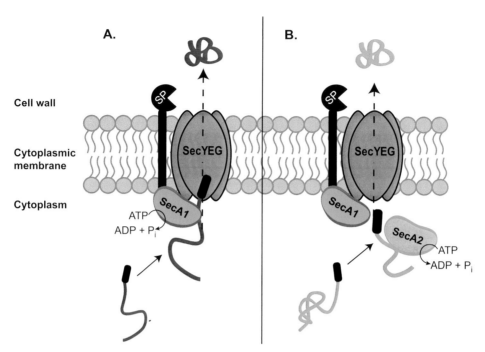

Figure 1 Models of SecA1 and SecA2 export in *M. tuberculosis*. **(A)** SecA1 uses ATP hydrolysis to export preproteins through the SecYEG channel in an unfolded, export-competent state. Sec signal peptides (black rectangle) target preproteins (blue ribbon) for export through SecYEG and are then cleaved by a signal peptidase (SP). **(B)** SecA2 also uses the SecYEG channel and possibly SecA1 to export its own subset of preproteins (green ribbon). The signal peptide (black rectangle) is indistinguishable from canonical Sec signal peptides. Instead, the mature domain's propensity for cytoplasmic folding is predicted to confer specificity for SecA2.

tional protein that binds to Sec-exported proteins in the cytoplasm, targets them to SecYEG, and harnesses energy from repeated rounds of ATP binding and hydrolysis to drive stepwise export of proteins through the SecYEG channel (14). An unusual feature of mycobacteria is that two SecA paralogs (SecA1 and SecA2) exist (15). These two SecAs have unique functions, with SecA1 being the essential SecA that functions in the conserved Sec pathway of mycobacteria to transport the majority of exported proteins.

Proteins exported by the Sec pathway have specific characteristics. Sec-exported proteins are synthesized as preproteins with N-terminal signal peptides. The signal peptide has a positively charged N-terminus, a hydrophobic central domain, and an uncharged polar C-terminus containing a cleavage site (16). Additionally, lipoproteins exported by the Sec pathway contain a lipobox motif at the C-terminal end of the signal peptide with an invariant cysteine that is the site of lipid attachment (17). The signal peptide and portions of the mature domain are recognized by SecA. After export, the signal peptide is removed by one of two signal peptidases (the type I signal peptidase LepB or the type

II signal peptidase LspA) on the extracytoplasmic side of the membrane to release the protein, which then folds into its mature conformation (18).

Another feature of Sec-exported preproteins is that they must be in an unfolded conformation to be exported through SecY (19). Cytosolic chaperones, such as SecB in Gram-negative bacteria, can help preproteins maintain an unfolded and translocation-competent state compatible with transport through SecYEG (20). SecB also has a role in delivering preproteins to SecA (21). However, not all preproteins require a SecB chaperone, and Gram-positive bacteria lack a SecB ortholog. While there is a SecB-like protein (Rv1957) in *M. tuberculosis*, the available data indicate that it is a chaperone for the HigBA toxin-antitoxin system and not a chaperone for Sec export (22).

THE CONSERVED SecA1 EXPORTOME

Due to the large bulk of protein export carried out by the conserved Sec pathway and the importance of exported proteins to physiological processes and host interactions in bacterial pathogens, the Sec pathway is important to both bacterial homeostasis and virulence. The essentiality of SecA1 and other components of the pathway makes it impossible to study the roles of the Sec pathway in virulence using deletion mutants, due to the lethality of these mutations. Instead, studies involving partial or conditional loss-of-function mutants can be used to address this issue, such as a conditional *secA1* mutant of *M. tuberculosis* (Rank and Braunstein, unpublished). In other pathogens, these approaches have been used to confirm the role of the Sec pathway in virulence. In pathogenic *Listeria monocytogenes* and *Staphylococcus aureus*, ∆*secDF* mutants (nonessential components of the Sec machinery) exhibit reduced export of virulence factors and are defective for growth in macrophages and animals (23, 24). In *Chlamydia trachomatis* and *Francisella tularensis*, the Sec export pathway is also shown to export virulence factors as demonstrated using ∆*secB* mutants (nonessential chaperone of the Sec pathway in Gram-negative bacteria) (25, 26).

Of the 4,024 open reading frames in the *M. tuberculosis* genome, 997 are predicted to be exported out of the cytoplasm due to the presence of an N-terminal Sec signal peptide and/or transmembrane domain (27, 28). In support of these bioinformatics predictions, our lab recently identified 593 of these proteins as being exported during *M. tuberculosis* infection of mice, using an *in vivo* selection strategy to identify exported fusion proteins (Perkowski and Braunstein, unpublished). While the specific pathway responsible for the export of most of these proteins has not been directly investigated, the majority of them are likely exported by the Sec pathway since they possess conserved Sec export signals and only a small subset are exported in a SecA2-dependent manner (see below). This presumed SecA1 exportome consists of 213 proteins in *M. tuberculosis* that are predicted to be essential for bacterial viability using saturating transposon mutagenesis screens such as transposon site hybridization or Tnseq (2, 29). Additionally, 239 proteins of this exportome are predicted to be important in virulence based on screens of transposon mutant libraries in mice, macrophages, and macaques (30–33). Below, we highlight a few members of the presumed SecA1 exportome with roles in essential processes, virulence, and entrance/reactivation from dormancy.

Cell Wall Synthesis and Remodeling Factors

All bacteria must maintain a structurally sound cell wall and coordinate the synthesis and breakdown of cell wall components during and after cell division. The proteins that perform these functions are typically exported to the cell wall and often are essential. There are many examples of cell wall synthesis and remodeling factors among the predicted SecA1 exportome (34). One of the more thoroughly studied cell wall remodeling enzymes is RipA. In *M. tuberculosis*, RipA is an essential protein with a Sec signal peptide that is exported to the cell wall (35). RipA is a peptidoglycan-hydrolyzing endopeptidase that localizes to the septa of dividing bacteria, where it is thought to degrade the layer of peptidoglycan connecting the two daughter cells (35). Depletion of *ripA* in *Mycobacterium smegmatis* results in a significant decrease in growth, formation of long, branched chains, and increased sensitivity to cell wall-targeting antibiotics (36).

A prominent category of cell wall synthesis/remodeling factors is the penicillin binding proteins (PBPs), which carry out the final stages of peptidoglycan synthesis and are involved in processes such as cell wall expansion, cell shape maintenance, and division (37). *M. tuberculosis* has eight annotated PBPs, all of which have predicted Sec export signals (34). Two of these PBPs (PBPB and Rv3627c) are suggested to be essential in *M. tuberculosis* by transposon site hybridization and Tnseq studies (2, 29). Alternatively, PonA1, PonA2, DacB2, and PBPA are not essential *in vitro* but are required for virulence, according to screens of transposon libraries in macrophages and animals, suggesting that some cell wall modifications are important in the host environment and that the enzymes responsible for these modifications are crucial for pathogenesis (31–33). Both PonA1 and PonA2 are predicted to be exported; PonA1 has a predicted transmembrane domain and PonA2 has a Sec signal peptide (38, 39). PonA1 and PonA2 are bifunctional PBPs that can both polymerize glycan strands and cross-link peptides in peptidoglycan (40). Single *M. tuberculosis* mutants lacking either *ponA1* or *ponA2* are defective for growth in mice (41, 42).

Lipoproteins

Sec-exported lipoproteins contribute to *M. tuberculosis* virulence as shown by virulence defects of an ∆*lspA* mutant. LspA, the type II signal peptidase that cleaves Sec signal peptides from lipoproteins following export via the Sec pathway, is not essential, but an *M. tuberculosis* ∆*lspA* mutant is attenuated in macrophages and in mouse models of infection (43). This suggests that at least some lipoproteins exported by the Sec pathway are important for virulence. Furthermore, 20 Sec signal peptide-containing lipoproteins have been identified by transposon site hybridization or Tnseq as being required for virulence in macrophages and animals (30–33).

LprG is a Sec signal peptide-containing lipoprotein that is exported to the cell wall and required for virulence of *M. tuberculosis* in macrophages and mice (44). It is suggested to have dual functions in *M. tuberculosis*. LprG binds to lipoarabinomannan and transfers it from the plasma membrane, where it is synthesized to the mycobacterial outer membrane, where one of its functions is to inhibit phagosome-lysosome fusion (44). Additionally, *lprG* forms an operon with *rv1410c*, which encodes a putative integral membrane transporter for export of triacylglyceride to the cell wall (45).

LpqH (19-kDa lipoprotein) is another Sec signal peptide-containing lipoprotein exported to the cell wall of *M. tuberculosis* with a role in virulence (38). It is an adhesin that binds mannose receptor and promotes phagocytosis of mycobacteria (46). LpqH is also immunomodulatory; it can limit major histocompatibility complex (MHC)-II antigen processing and presentation in *M. tuberculosis*-infected macrophages by inhibiting gamma interferon-induced upregulation of MHC-II (47). An *M. tuberculosis* Δ*lpqH* mutant is severely attenuated for replication in mice (48).

Exported Virulence Factors with Unknown Functions

Of the mycobacterial proteins with Sec export signals, 60% are not assigned a predicted function (compared to 49% of proteins without export signals that have unassigned functions) (49). Further studies of these exported proteins with unknown functions may reveal additional Sec substrates with novel roles in pathogenesis. For example, Erp (exported, repetitive protein) is a mycobacteria-specific, Sec signal peptide-containing, cell wall protein that was the first mycobacterial virulence protein to be characterized by targeted deletion (50). The contribution of Erp to virulence is well demonstrated; mutants lacking *erp* in *M. tuberculosis* and *Mycobacterium marinum* are attenuated for growth in macrophages and in animals (mice and zebra fish) (50, 51). Erp-deficient mutants have a defect early during infection, particularly in intracellular growth and survival in macrophages; however, the function of Erp remains unknown (51). *M. smegmatis* Δ*erp* mutants are more sensitive to detergents and lipophilic antibiotics and have altered colony morphology, suggesting that the function of Erp may be in cell wall synthesis or modulation; however, this possibility requires further study (51, 52).

More recently, Rv0888 was identified as an exported protein with a Sec signal peptide that contributes to virulence (53, 54). Using a biotin probe, Rv0888 was shown to be surface-exposed on the outer membrane of *M. tuberculosis* (53). Additionally, Rv0888 activity was detected in the supernatants of *M. tuberculosis* cultures, suggesting that some Rv0888 is also secreted (53). A Δ*rv0888* mutant of *M. tuberculosis* has replication defects in THP-1 cells and BALB/c mice, but not C57BL/6 mice (53, 54). Recent studies suggest that Rv0888 may function as an extracellular nuclease and/ or a sphingomyelinase (53, 54).

Entering Dormancy

Following initial *M. tuberculosis* infection, most individuals mount a cell-mediated immune response and control the bacilli within multicellular granulomas. These individuals are considered to have latent tuberculosis because *M. tuberculosis* can persist in granulomas in a dormant state and later reactivate. Dormant bacteria are viable, but they exhibit reduced metabolic activity and are in a state of low- to nonreplicating persistence. *In vitro* models of dormancy have been developed to study nonreplicating persistence of *M. tuberculosis*, the most common being oxygen deprivation or nutrient starvation (55). The essential type I signal peptidase LepB that cleaves Sec signal peptides following export via the Sec pathway is required for *M. tuberculosis* viability *in vitro* during replicating as well as nonreplicating persistence conditions, suggesting that the essentiality of the Sec export machinery is not diminished during dormancy (56).

Environmental stresses such as hypoxia, nutrient deprivation, and iron restriction induce dormancy. The transition from active growth to dormancy depends on specific changes to the cell, including modifications to the peptidoglycan that increase cell wall thickness. The dormancy-related cell wall modifications in *M. tuberculosis* include increasing the number of 3→3 diaminopimelic acid (DAP-DAP) cross-links in the peptidoglycan (up to 80% of cross-linkages in dormant bacteria) (57). Increased DAP-DAP cross-linking also signifies the transition from active growth to a nonreplicating state in other bacteria, such as *Escherichia coli* and *Enterococcus faecalis* (58, 59). Exported L,D-transpeptidases are responsible for the 3-3 cross-linking between DAP. *M. tuberculosis* has three L,D-transpeptidases with predicted Sec signal peptides: LdtMt2, PBPA, and Rv1433. All of these proteins were predicted to function in virulence by screening transposon mutants in animals and macrophages, although none have been directly tested for a role in dormancy (32, 33). The PBP PonA2 may also be important for dormancy. In a model of nonreplicating persistence utilizing anaerobic *M. smegmatis* cultures, a Δ*ponA2* mutant exhibits reduced survival and altered cell morphology (39).

Reactivation/Resuscitation from Dormancy

Reactivation of dormant *M. tuberculosis*, which is defined by the re-establishment of metabolic and replicative activity, is initiated by resuscitation (60). The environmental signals that trigger the transition from dormancy to replication during infection are not clear. However, secreted resuscitation-promoting factors (Rpfs) appear to be involved in this transition in mycobacteria as well as in other actinomycetes that undergo some form of dormancy. Rpfs, which restore culturability when added to dormant bacteria, were first identified in *Micrococcus luteus* (61). *M. tuberculosis* has five Rpf homologs (RpfA-E), all with predicted Sec signal peptides. Several studies confirm that single or multi-*rpf* deletion mutants of *M. tuberculosis* have defects in reactivation. A Δ*rpfB* mutant of *M. tuberculosis* has delayed kinetics of reactivation in a mouse model of dormancy (62). Different combinations of double or triple *rpf* mutants in *M. tuberculosis* are impaired *in vitro* for resuscitation out of a state of nonreplicating persistence and for the ability to resume replication in mice from a state of persistence (63, 64). Finally, an Δ*rpfA-E* quintuple mutant is attenuated for growth and persistence in mice (65).

The specific mechanisms of action by which Rpf proteins induce reactivation remain unknown. Rpf proteins are predicted to be transglycolases involved in remodeling peptidoglycan. Interestingly, RpfB and RpfE interact with the peptidoglycan-hydrolyzing endopeptidase RipA and localize to the septa (35). Peptidoglycan remodeling could cause restructuring of the bacterial cell wall, allowing resumption of cell division, or could create specific breakdown products of peptidoglycan that function as second messengers to signal the cell to reactivate (66).

Summary

In all likelihood, the SecA1 exportome is important for both the viability and virulence of *M. tuberculosis*. However, to date, the majority of proteins with Sec signal peptides lack experimental evidence for being specifically exported by the SecA1 pathway versus other pathways. While the essentiality of components of the SecA1 export machinery presents challenges to comprehensively identifying members of the SecA1 exportome of *M. tuberculosis*, a dedicated effort to conduct such an analysis is warranted, particularly for understanding the contribution of the SecA1 export pathway to virulence and dormancy. The role of peptidoglycan modifications for entering dormancy and reactivation, as well as the requirement of Rpfs for resuscitation following dormancy, makes it highly likely that members of the SecA1 exportome are also important for latency.

THE SecA2 PROTEIN EXPORT PATHWAY

Identification

The first report of a second SecA paralog in bacteria was in mycobacteria (15). However, two SecA proteins also exist in other actinomycetes and in a small set of Gram-positive bacteria including *Listeria*, *Staphylococcus*, and some *Streptococci*. In bacteria with two SecA proteins, SecA1 is the name given to the SecA with higher sequence similarity to the well-studied SecA protein of *E. coli*, and SecA2 refers to the second paralog of SecA. In mycobacteria, the two SecAs are demonstrated to have unique functions. Even when SecA2 is overexpressed, *secA1* cannot be deleted, indicating that SecA2 cannot substitute for SecA1 (15). Similarly, overexpression of SecA1 does not rescue the phenotypes of a Δ*secA2* deletion mutant. As mentioned above, the mycobacterial SecA1 is essential and functions in the conserved Sec pathway. In contrast to SecA1, the mycobacterial SecA2 is not essential for growth *in vitro* and exports a smaller subset of proteins. However, SecA2 contributes to the virulence of the pathogenic mycobacteria *M. tuberculosis* and *M. marinum* in macrophage and animal models of infection (67–71). In other bacterial pathogens with SecA2 proteins, such as *L. monocytogenes*, *S. aureus*, *Streptococcus gordonii*, and *Streptococcus parasanguinis*, SecA2 is also nonessential but has a role in virulence (72–75).

SecA2 systems can be divided into two groups: those that only possess a single copy of *secY* and those that also include an accessory copy of *secY*. Systems with an accessory SecY (SecY2) are referred to as SecA2/Y2 systems. The best-studied SecA2/Y2 systems are those of *S. gordonii* and *S. parasanguinis*. In SecA2/Y2 systems, a single, large, glycosylated substrate is secreted, presumably through the SecY2 channel. The genes encoding SecA2, SecY2, and the substrate are arranged in a conserved locus along with the glycosylation factors that modify the substrate (74). However, there is only a single copy of *secY* in mycobacteria. Furthermore, the mycobacterial SecA2 pathway exports multiple, diverse substrates and is referred to as a SecA2-only or multisubstrate SecA2 system (76, 77). In contrast to the SecA2/Y2 systems, studies suggest that the SecA2 proteins of the SecA2-only systems of mycobacteria, *L. monocytogenes*, and *Clostridium difficile* likely work with the canonical SecYEG channel for the export of their specific subsets of SecA2-dependent proteins (78–80).

Mechanism

Studies of the mechanism of SecA2-dependent export in mycobacteria have been conducted in *M. tuberculosis* and *M. marinum* as well as in the nonpathogenic model organism *M. smegmatis*. Complementation experiments show that the *secA2* of *M. tuberculosis* and *M. smegmatis* can substitute for one another to complement Δ*secA2* deletion mutant phenotypes, indicating that SecA2 is functionally conserved between *M. smegmatis* and *M. tuberculosis* (81).

Although it is understood that *M. tuberculosis* SecA1 and SecA2 are functionally distinct, it is not clear what structural differences contribute to their individual roles. SecA2 shares only 38% amino acid sequence identity with SecA1 and is approximately 20 kDa smaller. However, crystal structures of *M. tuberculosis* SecA1 and SecA2 reveal a high level of structural similarity, with most functional domains identified in conserved SecAs being present in both SecA1 and SecA2 (82, 83), including several residues that are critical for interacting with SecYEG. The most notable difference revealed by the structures is that SecA2 lacks the helical wing domain (HWD) present in SecA1 and other conserved SecAs (83). The function of the HWD is unknown, but it undergoes conformational changes in response to substrate binding and may be involved in signal peptide recognition and binding (84, 85). SecA2 homologs in other actinomycetes and Gram-positive bacteria also have absent or truncated HWDs (83). Future studies exploring the consequences of a deleted HWD are warranted.

In vitro experiments demonstrate that, like SecA1, SecA2 has ATPase activity (86). Further, ATP binding is necessary for SecA2 function in *M. tuberculosis* and *M. smegmatis* as shown with a SecA2 variant harboring an amino acid substitution in the ATP-binding site of *M. smegmatis* SecA2 (K129R), which corresponds to *M. tuberculosis* SecA2 (K115R) (81, 86). SecA2 K129R cannot bind ATP and is defective in protein export, and in *M. tuberculosis* SecA2 K115R fails to carry out the SecA2 role in promoting growth in macrophages (81, 86). In *M. smegmatis*, SecA2 K129R is dominant negative and is associated with phenotypes that are more severe than those exhibited by a *secA2* null mutant. These results are indicative of SecA2 K129R being locked in a nonfunctional complex with SecA2-interacting proteins. Expression of *secA2 K129R* also results in reduced levels of the sole SecY of mycobacteria, and increased SecY levels can suppress the severe phenotypes of the *M. smegmatis secA2 K129R* mutant (78). This suggests that SecA2 K129R is locked in a nonproductive interaction with SecYEG and that increased

SecY levels overcome the effect of this dominant negative interaction. In the SecA2-only system of *L. monocytogenes*, suppressor mutations of a *secA2* mutant also map to *secY*, which is consistent with SecA2 working with SecY in other SecA2-only systems as well (79). Additionally, intragenic suppressor mutants of *secA2 K129R* in *M. smegmatis* map to residues where similar mutations disrupt *E. coli* SecA binding to SecYEG, further supporting a model where SecA2 uses the canonical SecY channel to export its own set of substrates (Fig. 1) (83).

SecA1, along with SecY, may also be important for SecA2-dependent export. Numerous reports establish the ability of SecA proteins to dimerize, and a recent study demonstrates heterodimer formation (as well as homodimer formation) *in vitro* of recombinant *M. tuberculosis* SecA1 and SecA2 purified out of *E. coli* (87, 88). However, it remains to be demonstrated if SecA1-SecA2 heterodimers exist and are biologically relevant in mycobacteria. Further, the oligomeric state of SecA during protein export is controversial. SecA is suggested to function either as a monomer or as a dimer during translocation (87). However, another finding in support of a role of SecA1 in the SecA2 pathway is that export of SecA2-dependent substrates in *M. smegmatis* is compromised when SecA1 is depleted, although it is also possible that this result could reflect a role for SecA1 in assembling the SecYEG channel (81).

Current data support a model where SecA2 works with the conserved SecYEG channel, and possibly SecA1 as well, to export its specific subset of preproteins. One outstanding question is how SecA2 recognizes and exports its unique set of substrates and not the larger population of SecA1 preproteins. Recent observations suggest that ADP binding induces conformational changes of *M. tuberculosis* SecA2 that are not observed in *M. tuberculosis* SecA1 or *E. coli* SecA (89). While the biological outcomes of these structural changes are unknown, it is hypothesized that the conformational changes result in the closure of a clamp in SecA2 that is thought to bind the mature domain of the preprotein (89). It is possible that closure of the clamp prevents recognition of SecA1 substrates by ADP-bound SecA2. In this scenario, SecA2 binding to an unknown factor or a SecA2-dependent substrate could promote ADP release and open the clamp to enable SecA2 activity. Additionally, the absence of the HWD in SecA2 leaves the signal peptide binding cleft more open and solvent-exposed (83). This structural difference could help SecA2 recognize its unique substrates and exclude SecA1 substrates. Further studies of how SecA1 and SecA2 cooperate for export through the SecYEG channel are necessary to understand the complexities of the relationship between SecA2 and the conserved SecA1 pathway.

Features of SecA2-Dependent Substrates

Studies of *M. tuberculosis*, *M. marinum*, and *M. smegmatis* have identified proteins that are exported in a SecA2-dependent manner (the composition of the SecA2 exportome is described in more detail below) (38, 70, 90). The list of SecA2-dependent proteins includes examples with N-terminal Sec signal peptides as well as proteins lacking recognizable signal peptides (e.g., SodA and PknG). Interestingly, the SecA2-only systems of other pathogens such as *L. monocytogenes* are also associated with export of proteins with or without signal peptides (91).

The best-studied SecA2-dependent substrates are the *M. smegmatis* lipoproteins Msmeg1704 and Msmeg1712 (90). These are both solute binding proteins (SBPs) that are synthesized as preproteins with Sec signal peptides containing lipobox motifs. SBP lipoproteins are also identified in *M. tuberculosis* and *M. marinum* as a category of protein exported by the SecA2 pathway (38, 70). However, the lipidated nature of these proteins does not confer their SecA2-dependency for export; an amino acid substitution of the invariant cysteine in the lipoboxes of Msmeg1704 and Msmeg1712, which prevents lipid attachment, does not eliminate the requirement for SecA2 in export (92). Although Msmeg1704 and Msmeg1712 require signal peptides to be exported, their signal peptides do not contain any distinguishing features targeting them to SecA2 for export (92). If their signal peptides are swapped for the signal peptide of a SecA1-dependent substrate, Msmeg1704 and Msmeg1712 retain their SecA2-dependency. Thus, the mature domains of these proteins, not signal peptides, impart the requirement for SecA2 in their export.

One possible defining feature of the mature domains of SecA2-dependent substrates is a propensity to fold in the cytoplasm prior to export. In support of this idea, when the Sec signal peptide of Msmeg1704 is exchanged for a signal peptide that directs preproteins for export through the Tat pathway, Msmeg1704 is exported by the Tat pathway (92). The Tat pathway differs from the Sec system in that it requires preproteins to be folded prior to export. Thus, the fact that the mature domain of a SecA2 substrate is compatible with export by the Tat pathway suggests that SecA2-dependent substrates can fold in the cytoplasm prior to export. Furthermore, it suggests that the role of SecA2 may be to facilitate export of these problematic substrates through the SecYEG channel, which requires proteins to be unfolded. It remains unclear how SecA2 may assist in the export of these substrates. Two nonexclusive possibilities for how SecA2 could influence export are that SecA2 serves a chaperone-like role of keeping preproteins unfolded prior to export or that it cooperates with SecA1 to provide additional energy to translocate challenging substrates through SecYEG.

SecA2-dependent features of the mature domain may also help to explain the SecA2-dependence of *M. tuberculosis* proteins lacking signal peptides (e.g., SodA and PknG). SodA proteins lacking signal peptides are reported to be exported by the canonical Sec pathway in *Rhizobium leguminosarum* and by the SecA2-only pathway in *L. monocytogenes* (93, 94). Further studies are needed for these unconventional exported proteins lacking signal peptides, because it also remains possible that the effect of SecA2 on exported proteins such as SodA is indirect. There may be unidentified signal peptide-containing proteins exported by SecA2 that are themselves components of a different specialized export machinery responsible for secreting unconventional proteins such as SodA.

THE SecA2 EXPORTOME

As indicated by the virulence defects of Δ*secA2* mutants of *M. tuberculosis* and *M. marinum*, the SecA2-dependent pathway exports proteins with roles in pathogenesis (67–71). Early studies identified a small number of SecA2-exported proteins using comparative two-dimensional gel electrophoresis of cell wall or secreted proteins of *M. smegmatis* and *M. tuberculosis* (15, 90). More recent quantitative mass spectrometry analyses of cell wall and cell envelope fractions of Δ*secA2* mutants of *M. tuberculosis* and *M. marinum* identified additional SecA2 substrates (38, 70). While the mass spectrometry studies dramatically increase our knowledge of the SecA2 exportome, further studies are required to validate the SecA2-dependency of many of the more recently identified proteins. Below, we highlight validated examples of SecA2 substrates along with common themes among proteins in the SecA2 exportome.

SBPs

Msmeg1704 and Msmeg1712 lipoproteins of *M. smegmatis* represent one class of SecA2-dependent substrates, SBPs. SBPs are cell wall localized proteins that deliver solutes to permease components of ATP-binding cassette transporters for import using energy from ATP hydrolysis (Fig. 2).

Although *M. tuberculosis* does not have a direct homolog of Msmeg1704 or Msmeg1712, quantitative mass spectrometry reveals numerous SBPs that are also

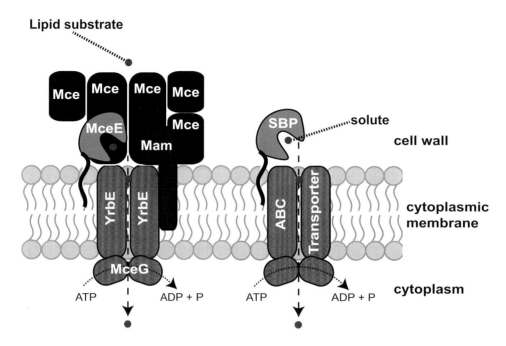

Figure 2 Solute-binding proteins and Mce proteins are exported by the SecA2 pathway. Two classes of SecA2-dependent substrates are SBPs and Mce proteins. Both SBPs and Mce proteins are involved in solute acquisition. In the case of SBPs this involves import of a solute through an ABC transporter permease using energy provided by ATP hydrolysis. Mce transporters are thought to function in a similar manner as ABC transporters to import a lipid substrate through a YrbE permease in an ATP-dependent manner. Although the diagram of an Mce transporter is speculative, the similarities between these two systems are compelling.

SecA2-dependent in *M. tuberculosis* and *M. marinum* (38, 70). In *M. tuberculosis*, nearly all of the SBPs identified in the cell wall fraction (13 out of 15) are present at lower levels in the Δ*secA2* mutant cell wall (38). All of the *M. tuberculosis* SecA2-dependent SBPs are lipoproteins with predicted signal peptides. Three SBPs with predicted Sec signal peptides were also identified as SecA2-dependent in *M. marinum* (70). Given the possibility of SecA2 substrates having a tendency to fold prior to export, it is notable that 4 of the 13 SBPs reduced in the Δ*secA2* mutant of *M. tuberculosis* have predicted or proven signal peptides for the Tat export pathway, which exports folded proteins (4, 38). There are also examples of SBPs with Tat signal peptides in other bacteria, suggesting that cytoplasmic folding is a common property of the SBP family (95, 96). The trend of SBPs being SecA2-dependent may extend to other SecA2-only systems, because there is some evidence that SecA2 may also export SBPs in *Listeria* (72).

Although most SBPs in *M. tuberculosis* have not been directly studied and their substrates remain unknown, SBPs can import a wide range of solutes (97). Thus, the role of SecA2 in exporting SBPs could be im-

portant for nutrient acquisition and affect the ability of *M. tuberculosis* to thrive in the host.

Mce Transporters

Another class of proteins exported by SecA2 is Mce transporter components. Mce transporters are importer complexes that are thought to function similarly to ATP-binding cassette transporters in that they recognize an extracytoplasmic substrate (in this case a lipid) and import it into the cytoplasm using ATP hydrolysis (98). Mce transporters are composed of two YrbE membrane proteins forming a putative permease, five exported Mce proteins, one exported Mce lipoprotein, and in some cases, one or more Mam transmembrane proteins (Fig. 2). All of these components are exported proteins that possess either a transmembrane domain or a signal peptide. The five Mce proteins and the Mce lipoprotein are proposed to recognize the lipid substrate and deliver it to the permease and, therefore, are functionally similar to SBPs of ATP-binding cassette transporters (98). Supporting this speculated similarity, there are presumed lipid-importing SBPs of Gram-negative bacteria that possess Mce-like domains (99).

M. tuberculosis has four Mce transporters. The best-studied Mce transporter is Mce4, which imports cholesterol (100). Because cholesterol catabolism is critical to *M. tuberculosis* pathogenesis, Mce4 has an important role in virulence (100, 101). Furthermore, studies in mice suggest that Mce4 is required for *M. tuberculosis* persistence during chronic infection (100). Mce1 is proposed to be a mycolic acid re-importer (102, 103). Mce1 is required for optimal growth in mice and in macrophages; however, there are also conflicting reports concerning these phenotypes (31, 102, 104–107).

Multiple exported components of Mce1 and Mce4 transporters are identified by quantitative mass spectrometry as being SecA2-dependent in *M. tuberculosis*. Six components of Mce1 and six components of Mce4 are significantly reduced in the Δ*secA2* mutant cell wall (38). Although Mce2 and Mce3 transporter components were not detected in the *M. tuberculosis* mass spectrometry dataset, Mce3E, along with Mce4D, was identified as reduced in the Δ*secA2* mutant of *M. marinum* (Fig. 3) (38, 70). This suggests that SecA2 may also export Mce2 and Mce3 system components, in addition to Mce1 and Mce4. Levels of MceG, the presumed ATPase for Mce transporters, are also reduced in the Δ*secA2* mutant of *M. tuberculosis* (38). While MceG is predicted to be cytoplasmic, MceG levels are shown to depend on the presence of other Mce transporter components (104). Therefore, the

reduction in MceG may be a consequence of reduced export of Mce transporter components in the Δ*secA2* mutant. Collectively, these data suggest a link between SecA2 and lipid transport in mycobacteria.

It is striking that SecA2 impacts multiple components of Mce transporters. This result presents two possibilities. First, SecA2 may export multiple components of Mce transporters. Second, SecA2 may export only one or a small number of proteins that make up the Mce transporter complex, but when that protein(s) is not exported (i.e., in a Δ*secA2* mutant) the entire Mce complex may fail to assemble and/or be destabilized. Because of the proposed similarity with SBPs, our identification of Mce proteins and Mce lipoproteins as SecA2-dependent is intriguing in terms of common features of proteins in the SecA2 exportome (Fig. 2). Because Mce systems are important for virulence, the role of SecA2 in the export of Mce transporters may also contribute to the pathogenesis of *M. tuberculosis*. More specifically, because of the impact on the Mce4 transporter, SecA2 may be required for cholesterol catabolism during infection, which could translate to a role for SecA2 in persistence.

SodA and KatG

The Fe-superoxide dismutase SodA is another protein identified as being exported in a SecA2-dependent manner (67). The Δ*secA2* mutant of *M. tuberculosis* secretes less SodA protein and exhibits less secreted

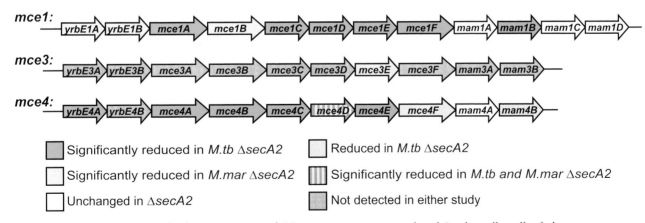

Figure 3 Multiple components of Mce transporters are reduced in the cell wall of the Δ*secA2* mutant. The *M. tuberculosis* genome contains four *mce* loci encoding putative lipid transporters. The genomic regions encoding Mce1, Mce3, and Mce4 transporters are shown with open reading frames colored for Mce proteins that are reduced in quantitative mass spectrometry studies of the *M. tuberculosis* (*M.tb*) and *M. marinum* (*M.mar*) Δ*secA2* mutant cell wall or cell envelope fractions (38, 70). In dark blue and/or green are *mce* genes for proteins that are significantly reduced (*P* < 0.01 for *M. tuberculosis* and *P* < 0.05 for *M. marinum*) in the Δ*secA2* mutant; in light blue are genes for Mce proteins that are reduced in the *M. tuberculosis* Δ*secA2* mutant but did not reach statistical significance.

superoxide dismutase activity than wild-type or complemented strains (67, 108). As an antioxidant that converts superoxide to hydrogen peroxide and oxygen, secreted SodA could be important for counteracting the macrophage antimicrobial oxidative burst (109). SodA can be found in the mycobacterial cytoplasm in addition to being secreted (67). SodA is an example of a SecA2-dependent protein lacking a signal peptide. In *L. monocytogenes* a Mn-superoxide dismutase that lacks a signal peptide is also SecA2-dependent, which provides another example of similarities between SecA2-only systems (94).

The catalase-peroxidase KatG is another antioxidant reported to be SecA2-dependent for secretion (67). KatG works with SodA to detoxify oxygen radicals by converting damaging hydrogen peroxide to oxygen and water (110). KatG is also able to detoxify the reaction product of superoxide and nitric oxide: peroxynitrite (111). Like SodA, KatG lacks a signal peptide and can be found in the mycobacterial cytoplasm (67). The role of SecA2 in the export of SodA and KatG could translate to a function of the SecA2 pathway in protecting *M. tuberculosis* from the oxidative burst of macrophages.

PknG

The eukaryotic-like serine-threonine kinase PknG is also dependent on SecA2 for export (38, 70). Recent studies of *M. tuberculosis* and *M. marinum* identified reduced levels of PknG in the cell wall of the Δ*secA2* mutant compared to wild-type or complemented strains (38, 70). Like SodA and KatG, PknG lacks a signal peptide. Additionally, like SodA and KatG, PknG can be found in both the mycobacterial cytoplasm and its exported location (112, 113). Intriguingly, *pknG* is transcribed in a proposed operon downstream of the gene for the SecA2-dependent SBP *glnH*. The connection, if any, between these two SecA2 substrates remains to be investigated.

PknG functions in both mycobacterial metabolism and pathogenesis, and an *M. tuberculosis* Δ*pknG* mutant has an *in vitro* growth defect and is attenuated in mice (112). In addition to regulating glutamate metabolism and redox homeostasis in the mycobacterial cytoplasm, during *M. tuberculosis* infection of macrophages, exported PknG is detected in the host cell cytosol and is considered a virulence effector (112, 114, 115). A hallmark of macrophage infections with *M. tuberculosis* is that the bacterium arrests the normal process of phagosome maturation (116, 117). Consequently, *M. tuberculosis* avoids delivery to a mature, fully acidified phagolysosome (116, 117). Although the

mechanistic details remain unclear, PknG plays a role in phagosome maturation arrest. A Δ*pknG* mutant of *Mycobacterium bovis* bacilli Calmette-Guérin (BCG) localizes to mature phagosomes, and a strain of *M. smegmatis* expressing the BCG *pknG* prevents phagosome-lysosome fusion unlike wild-type *M. smegmatis* (114). This specific role of PknG in phagosome maturation is intriguing because studies of Δ*secA2* mutants of *M. tuberculosis* and *M. marinum* demonstrate a role of the SecA2 pathway in phagosome maturation arrest (69, 70). As discussed below, experiments with the Δ*secA2* mutant of *M. marinum* suggest that SecA2-dependent export of PknG can partly explain the role of the SecA2 pathway in promoting phagosome maturation arrest (70).

Summary

SecA2 exports a variety of proteins with a wide range of functions. Despite the recent expansion of our knowledge of SecA2 substrates, the list of known SecA2-exported proteins likely remains incomplete. Commonly, SecA2 substrates are only partially dependent on SecA2 for export; residual export of these substrates occurs in Δ*secA2* mutants through yet unidentified mechanisms (38, 67, 70, 90). Interestingly, Δ*secA2* mutants of other SecA2-only systems also exhibit incomplete export defects (72, 91, 94, 118). The partial dependency of SecA2 substrates creates a unique challenge in identifying substrates and understanding how SecA2 export contributes to *M. tuberculosis* pathogenesis.

SecA2 AND THE DosR REGULON

An unexpected discovery of quantitative mass spectrometry studies of the *M. tuberculosis* Δ*secA2* mutant is the identification of multiple DosR-regulated cytoplasmic proteins as being more abundant in the Δ*secA2* mutant (38). The DosR regulon consists of 49 genes that are under the control of the DosR/S/T two-component system (119). DosR-regulated proteins are induced by a number of stresses associated with infection, including hypoxia and nitric oxide stress, and the regulon is strongly induced during *M. tuberculosis* infection of macrophages, mice, guinea pigs, and humans (119). DosR-regulated proteins are important for *M. tuberculosis* dormancy. A Δ*dosR* mutant is attenuated during hypoxia and other nonreplicating conditions associated with dormancy (119). Moreover, while a Δ*dosR* mutant is able to grow comparably to wild-type *M. tuberculosis* in the initial stages of infection in macaques, it is unable to persist in the host (120).

A transcriptional effect can account for the increase in DosR-regulated proteins in the Δ*secA2* mutant. Transcript levels of the DosR-regulated gene, *hspX*, and the response regulator, *dosR*, are both higher in the mutant (38). Further, under conditions that induce the DosR regulon, the Δ*secA2* mutant responds quicker and to a much higher degree than wild type, leading to transiently higher levels of DosR-regulated proteins (38). The earlier induction of the DosR regulon may be due to an increased sensitivity of the Δ*secA2* mutant to DosR-inducing stimuli or due to a basal level of stress in the Δ*secA2* mutant that primes the mutant to respond more quickly to stimuli. Since DosR is known to be induced in macrophages, this increased induction of the DosR regulon in the Δ*secA2* mutant is likely to occur *in vivo* (121). Furthermore, macrophages infected with the Δ*secA2* mutant produce higher levels of reactive nitrogen intermediates (discussed below), which is a stimulus for induction of the DosR regulon, so this DosR upregulation may be even more pronounced during infection (68, 121, 122). It is possible that increased induction of DosR-regulated proteins contributes to the phenotypes of the Δ*secA2* mutant *in vivo*. For example, one DosR-regulated protein increased in the Δ*secA2* mutant, Rv0079, induces macrophage production of proinflammatory cytokines, including tumor necrosis factor alpha, which is a phenotype elicited by the Δ*secA2* mutant in macrophages (discussed below) (123).

SecA2 AND VIRULENCE

In *M. tuberculosis*, SecA2 is not required for growth *in vitro*, but it is required for virulence (67). A Δ*secA2* mutant of *M. tuberculosis* is attenuated in the mouse model of infection. Mice infected with the Δ*secA2* mutant (either by intravenous injection or aerosol) have reduced bacterial burden throughout the course of infection (67, 68). Mice infected with the Δ*secA2* mutant also survive significantly longer than mice infected with wild-type *M. tuberculosis* (67, 68). The SecA2 pathway is also required for virulence in *M. marinum*, a mycobacterial pathogen of fish and frogs. In both embryonic and adult zebra fish, infection with a Δ*secA2* mutant of *M. marinum* results in reduced bacterial burden, increased fish survival time, and a reduction in granuloma number compared to wild-type-infected animals (70, 71). The *M. marinum* Δ*secA2* mutant also has a phenotype in the murine tail vein infection model (fewer tail lesions) (71).

Growth in macrophages is vital for *M. tuberculosis* pathogenesis, and a Δ*secA2* mutant of *M. tuberculosis* has a significant growth defect in macrophages (68). While our understanding of how *M. tuberculosis* survives in macrophages and elicits disease remains incomplete, *M. tuberculosis* is known to limit many antimicrobial activities of macrophages (e.g., phagosome-lysosome fusion, attack by reactive oxygen and nitrogen intermediates [ROIs, RNIs], apoptosis, inflammatory responses, and antigen presentation) (116). Studies of the *M. tuberculosis* Δ*secA2* mutant in macrophages reveal roles for the SecA2 pathway in these processes (Fig. 4).

The SecA2 Pathway and Phagosome Maturation Arrest

Following phagocytosis by a macrophage, *M. tuberculosis* replicates intracellularly. Typically, once phagocytosed, microbes are delivered to phagosomes that subsequently mature, acidify, and fuse with a lysosome, resulting in destruction of the microbe. In contrast, *M. tuberculosis* arrests this process at an early stage, and *M. tuberculosis* avoids delivery to acidified phagolysosomes (116). One of the most striking phenotypes exhibited by *M. tuberculosis* and *M. marinum* Δ*secA2* mutants in macrophages is that a Δ*secA2* mutant fails to arrest phagosome maturation, which results in the mutant residing in a more mature, acidic phagosome (69, 70). When phagosome acidification is chemically inhibited, the *M. tuberculosis* Δ*secA2* mutant grows comparably to wild type, indicating that SecA2 inhibition of phagosome maturation is required for intracellular growth in macrophages (69).

PknG is a SecA2 substrate with a function in phagosome maturation arrest, which makes it a leading candidate for being a SecA2-dependent effector of this process (114). To determine if PknG export accounts for the role of the SecA2 pathway in phagosome maturation arrest, a Δ*secA2* mutant of *M. marinum* was engineered to overexpress *pknG* with the goal of restoring PknG export in the Δ*secA2* mutant (70). Increased PknG export partially restores the ability of the Δ*secA2* mutant to arrest phagosome maturation and also partially rescues growth of the Δ*secA2* mutant in zebra fish (70). These data indicate that SecA2 export of PknG is important for *M. tuberculosis* to arrest phagosome maturation and, more broadly, is required for virulence. However, the partial nature of these phenotypes suggests that additional SecA2-dependent proteins also contribute to these processes. Phagosome maturation arrest is a complex process involving multiple, sometimes redundant, virulence factors; thus, it is not surprising that more than one SecA2 substrate is required (116).

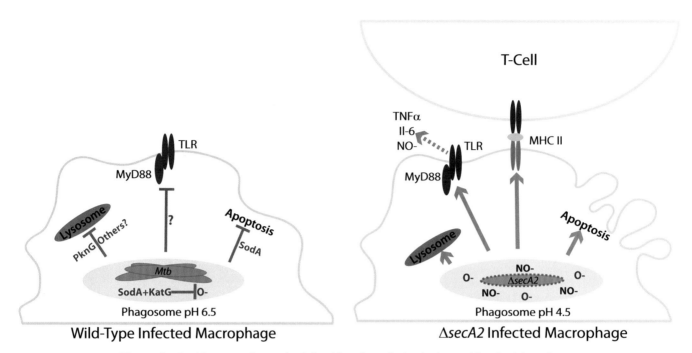

Figure 4 SecA2 export is required for *M. tuberculosis* virulence. The SecA2 pathway combats multiple host immune mechanisms of macrophages. SecA2 export of PknG in addition to other unknown effectors prevents phagosome acidification and fusion with degradative lysosomes. Export of SodA and KatG by SecA2 combats harmful reactive oxygen radicals and limits apoptosis. SecA2 also inhibits signaling through MyD88 by unknown mechanisms, resulting in lower levels of the proinflammatory cytokines interleukin-6 and tumor necrosis factor alpha along with nitric oxide. Additionally, SecA2 reduces gamma interferon-induced MHC II levels, which could impact antigen presentation to CD4+ T cells.

The SecA2 Pathway and Inhibition of Apoptosis

Another phenotype exhibited by macrophages infected with the Δ*secA2* mutant is increased apoptosis, which indicates a role for the *M. tuberculosis* SecA2 pathway in blocking macrophage apoptosis (108). Macrophage apoptosis is detrimental to *M. tuberculosis* because subsequent efferocytosis of *M. tuberculosis*-infected, apoptotic macrophages will kill the bacteria (124). Apoptosis can also drive establishment of a protective immune response, which is detrimental to the pathogen, by promoting antigen presentation to T cells (108, 125). Interestingly, superoxide can be a signal for apoptosis, and the proapoptotic phenotype of the Δ*secA2* mutant is attributed to the defect in SodA export (108, 109). When secretion of SodA is restored in a Δ*secA2* mutant, by overexpressing a version of SodA with a Sec signal peptide fused at its N terminus (α–SodA), secreted superoxide dismutase activity and antiapoptotic activity are restored (69, 108). However, when tested in macrophages and mice, virulence of the Δ*secA2* mutant expressing α-SodA remains attenuated

(69). Thus, on its own, inhibition of apoptosis is insufficient to explain the role of the SecA2 pathway in pathogenesis. However, it is common for bacterial pathogens to have overlapping virulence mechanisms, and the role of SecA2 in limiting macrophage apoptosis may still contribute to *M. tuberculosis* survival in macrophages and limiting of antigen presentation to the immune system.

The SecA2 Pathway and Immunomodulation

In response to infection with the Δ*secA2* mutant, macrophages produce increased levels of MyD88-dependent RNI and proinflammatory cytokines such as tumor necrosis factor alpha and interleukin-6 in comparison to macrophages infected with wild-type *M. tuberculosis* (68). This altered cytokine profile suggests that the SecA2 pathway has an immunomodulatory effect of inhibiting the innate immune responses of macrophages to *M. tuberculosis* infection. On its own, the altered immune response to the Δ*secA2* mutant is insufficient to explain the attenuated phenotype of the Δ*secA2* mutant in macrophages because the Δ*secA2* mutant remains attenuated in *myd88–/–* macrophages and mice (69). While these results indicate that immunomodulation by the SecA2 pathway is not the sole function of this export pathway, it may still be important for pathogenesis. SecA2 substrates may also function in suppressing the adaptive immune response, because the SecA2 pathway additionally impacts the level of gamma interferon-induced MHC II levels during *M. tuberculosis* infection (68). The SecA2 exported proteins that produce immunomodulatory effects are currently unknown.

The SecA2 Pathway and Reactive Radicals

Because SodA and KatG, enzymes important for detoxifying oxygen radicals, are secreted in a SecA2-dependent manner, an additional function of the SecA2 pathway could be to protect against the damaging reactive oxygen radicals produced by infected macrophages (67). The SecA2 pathway also limits production of RNI produced by macrophages (mentioned above) (68). Both ROI and RNI are important for controlling microbial growth in macrophages (126). However, when *phox–/–* macrophages, which fail to undergo an oxidative burst, or *NOS2–/–* macrophages, which fail to produce RNI, are infected with the Δ*secA2* mutant, the mutant remains attenuated for intracellular growth (68). While these results indicate that protection from reactive radicals is not the sole function of the SecA2 pathway in pathogenesis, this role for SecA2 may still contribute to virulence.

Summary

SecA2 affects several diverse host immune pathways, highlighting the importance of the SecA2 pathway and its exported proteins in mycobacterial infection. While the role of the SecA2 pathway in phagosome maturation arrest is proven to be critical for *M. tuberculosis* virulence, additional effects of SecA2 export on macrophages may also be significant (69). The significance of these other SecA2 effects may be masked by redundant virulence mechanisms because *M. tuberculosis* has additional, and likely SecA2-independent, apoptotic inhibitory factors, ROI resistance mechanisms, and immunomodulatory factors (116). More research is needed to understand all of the distinct roles SecA2 substrates play in promoting pathogenesis.

SecA2 AND DORMANCY

As discussed above, the SecA2 pathway is required in the initial stages of infection (i.e., promoting growth in macrophages), but SecA2 may also be involved in later stages of persistent infection. The increased and earlier induction of the DosR regulon in the Δ*secA2* mutant suggests that the SecA2 pathway has the potential to affect the timing of *M. tuberculosis* entry into dormancy (38). Although it has not been studied, it is possible that the correct timing of induction of the DosR regulon is important for *M. tuberculosis* survival in the host. Additionally, SecA2 export of Mce4 transporter proteins may be important for *M. tuberculosis* persistence in the host because the Mce4 transporter is required for persistence in mice (38, 100, 101).

Studies of the SecA2 pathway in *M. marinum* also support a possible role in dormancy. A Δ*secA2* mutant of *M. marinum* elicits significantly reduced granuloma formation in zebra fish when compared to a wild-type strain (70). In another study utilizing a mouse tail vein lesion model, granulomas formed from an infection with a Δ*secA2* mutant of *M. marinum* were found to be less stable (lesions resolved significantly faster), suggesting that SecA2 is involved in granuloma stability (71). The SecA2 substrates important for granuloma formation and stability remain unknown. A possible connection between SecA2 and dormancy is an aspect of the SecA2 pathway that has not been directly studied to date and deserves attention.

THE *SecA2* MUTANT AS A VACCINE CANDIDATE

The only licensed vaccine for tuberculosis is the live attenuated *M. bovis* strain BCG. The BCG vaccine induces potent cellular immune responses in infants and protects against disseminated tuberculosis in early childhood (127). However, the duration of protection is inconsistent and the vaccine shows, at best, variable protection in adults (128). Additionally, BCG can cause severe, disseminated infection in HIV-positive infants, with high mortality rates (129). Animal models of tuberculosis demonstrate that BCG vaccination does not give complete control or clearance of infection. This has been attributed to a lack of appropriate T cell responses, particularly a failure of BCG to induce a CD8+ T cell response (130). Consequently, new tuberculosis vaccines that are safer and more efficacious than BCG are urgently needed.

Several features of the virulence and export defects of the Δ*secA2* mutant make it an appealing candidate for a live vaccine for tuberculosis. The Δ*secA2* mutant induces higher levels of proinflammatory cytokines and apoptosis than wild-type *M. tuberculosis* in infected macrophages and higher levels of antigen-specific CD8+ T cells *in vivo* (108). The Δ*secA2* mutant is also defective in arresting phagosome maturation and, therefore, resides in a hydrolytic, degradative phagosome, which may be advantageous for antigen presentation and immunogenicity of vaccines (69, 125). When tested as a vaccine candidate in mice and guinea pig models, the attenuated Δ*secA2* mutant of *M. tuberculosis* and double or triple deletion strains (Δ*lysA*Δ*secA2*, Δ*panCD*Δ*leuCD*Δ*secA2*) exhibit superior protection against *M. tuberculosis* challenge as well as superior safety compared to the BCG vaccine, including a more robust CD8+ T cell response (108, 131–133). Furthermore, results of testing a Δ*panCD*Δ*leuCD*Δ*secA2* vaccine candidate in simian immunodeficiency virus-positive infant macaques suggest that a Δ*secA2* mutant derivative vaccine may be a safe alternative for HIV-positive infants (133). The increased expression of latency-associated, DosR-regulated proteins in the Δ*secA2* mutant could also be beneficial to a Δ*secA2* mutant vaccine in that it may be better able to elicit immune responses to latency antigens and, thereby, be better equipped to prevent latent *M. tuberculosis* infections (134). An alternative to a live-attenuated *M. tuberculosis* vaccine could be to improve the immunogenicity of the current BCG vaccine. Vaccination with BCGΔ*secA2*Δ*sigH* induced more cytokine-producing CD8+ T cells, a greater CD4+ lymphocyte response during memory phase, and greater clearance of challenge bacilli than the conventional BCG vaccine (135).

The live-attenuated Δ*secA2* mutant and its derivatives represent a promising avenue of vaccine candidates. Improved understanding of the SecA2 export system and its substrates will lead not only to a better understanding of *M. tuberculosis* pathogenesis but will also benefit development of a viable vaccine based on the Δ*secA2* mutant.

CONCLUSIONS

The exportomes of the SecA1 and SecA2 pathways of *M. tuberculosis* contain proteins with diverse functions that work together to coordinate successful pathogenicity. Despite progress in understanding these pathways in recent years, we still do not have a full picture of the complete list of SecA1 and SecA2 substrates. In part, this gap in understanding is due to the intrinsic difficulty of studying an essential pathway (SecA1) where deletion mutants are not viable, as well as the challenges associated with studying a pathway (SecA2) that when absent has some residual export of its substrates.

In this article, we highlighted examples of better-understood exported proteins. However, the largest category of exported proteins is proteins with unknown function. Characterizing the functions of these under-studied proteins will not only improve our understanding of the roles played by the protein export systems of *M. tuberculosis* but will serve to increase our overall knowledge of *M. tuberculosis* pathogenesis. In particular, the roles of protein export pathways and specific exported proteins in the context of dormancy deserve research attention to fully understand how *M. tuberculosis* uses protein export during infection.

Citation. Miller BK, Zulauf KE, Braunstein M. 2017. The Sec pathways and exportomes of *Mycobacterium tuberculosis*. *Microbiol Spectrum* 5(2):TBTB2-0013-2016.

References

1. Schneider G. 1999. How many potentially secreted proteins are contained in a bacterial genome? *Gene* 237:113–121.

2. Sassetti CM, Boyd DH, Rubin EJ. 2003. Genes required for mycobacterial growth defined by high density mutagenesis. *Mol Microbiol* 48:77–84.

3. Saint-Joanis B, Demangel C, Jackson M, Brodin P, Marsollier L, Boshoff H, Cole ST. 2006. Inactivation of Rv2525c, a substrate of the twin arginine translocation (Tat) system of *Mycobacterium tuberculosis*, increases β-lactam susceptibility and virulence. *J Bacteriol* 188:6669–6679.

4. McDonough JA, Hacker KE, Flores AR, Pavelka MS Jr, Braunstein M. 2005. The twin-arginine translocation pathway of *Mycobacterium smegmatis* is functional and required for the export of mycobacterial β-lactamases. *J Bacteriol* 187:7667–7679.

5. Vrontou E, Economou A. 2004. Structure and function of SecA, the preprotein translocase nanomotor. *Biochim Biophys Acta* 1694:67–80.

6. Meyer TH, Ménétret J-F, Breitling R, Miller KR, Akey CW, Rapoport TA. 1999. The bacterial SecY/E translocation complex forms channel-like structures similar to those of the eukaryotic Sec61p complex. *J Mol Biol* 285:1789–1800.

7. Kihara A, Akiyama Y, Ito K. 1995. FtsH is required for proteolytic elimination of uncomplexed forms of SecY, an essential protein translocase subunit. *Proc Natl Acad Sci USA* 92:4532–4536.

8. Nishiyama K, Suzuki T, Tokuda H. 1996. Inversion of the membrane topology of SecG coupled with SecA-dependent preprotein translocation. *Cell* 85:71–81.

9. Duong F, Wickner W. 1997. Distinct catalytic roles of the SecYE, SecG and SecDFyajC subunits of preprotein translocase holoenzyme. *EMBO J* 16:2756–2768.

10. Luirink J, Sinning I. 2004. SRP-mediated protein targeting: structure and function revisited. *Biochim Biophys Acta* 1694:17–35.

11. Wild K, Rosendal KR, Sinning I. 2004. A structural step into the SRP cycle. *Mol Microbiol* 53:357–363.

12. Valent QA, de Gier J-WL, von Heijne G, Kendall DA, ten Hagen-Jongman CM, Oudega B, Luirink J. 1997.

Nascent membrane and presecretory proteins synthesized in *Escherichia coli* associate with signal recognition particle and trigger factor. *Mol Microbiol* 25:53–64.

13. Egea PF, Stroud RM. 2010. Lateral opening of a translocon upon entry of protein suggests the mechanism of insertion into membranes. *Proc Natl Acad Sci USA* 107:17182–17187.

14. Economou A, Wickner W. 1994. SecA promotes preprotein translocation by undergoing ATP-driven cycles of membrane insertion and deinsertion. *Cell* 78:835–843.

15. Braunstein M, Brown AM, Kurtz S, Jacobs WR Jr. 2001. Two nonredundant SecA homologues function in mycobacteria. *J Bacteriol* 183:6979–6990.

16. von Heijne G. 1990. The signal peptide. *J Membr Biol* 115:195–201.

17. Nakayama H, Kurokawa K, Lee BL. 2012. Lipoproteins in bacteria: structures and biosynthetic pathways. *FEBS J* 279:4247–4268.

18. Paetzel M, Karla A, Strynadka NCJ, Dalbey RE. 2002. Signal peptidases. *Chem Rev* 102:4549–4580.

19. Bassford PJ Jr, Silhavy TJ, Beckwith JR. 1979. Use of gene fusion to study secretion of maltose-binding protein into *Escherichia coli* periplasm. *J Bacteriol* 139:19–31.

20. Sala A, Bordes P, Genevaux P. 2014. Multitasking SecB chaperones in bacteria. *Front Microbiol* 5:666.

21. Fisher AC, DeLisa MP. 2004. A little help from my friends: quality control of presecretory proteins in bacteria. *J Bacteriol* 186:7467–7473.

22. Bordes P, Cirinesi A-M, Ummels R, Sala A, Sakr S, Bitter W, Genevaux P. 2011. SecB-like chaperone controls a toxin-antitoxin stress-responsive system in *Mycobacterium tuberculosis*. *Proc Natl Acad Sci USA* 108:8438–8443.

23. Burg-Golani T, Pozniak Y, Rabinovich L, Sigal N, Nir Paz R, Herskovits AA. 2013. Membrane chaperone SecDF plays a role in the secretion of *Listeria monocytogenes* major virulence factors. *J Bacteriol* 195:5262–5272.

24. Quiblier C, Zinkernagel AS, Schuepbach RA, Berger-Bächi B, Senn MM. 2011. Contribution of SecDF to *Staphylococcus aureus* resistance and expression of virulence factors. *BMC Microbiol* 11:72.

25. Margolis JJ, El-Etr S, Joubert L-M, Moore E, Robison R, Rasley A, Spormann AM, Monack DM. 2010. Contributions of *Francisella tularensis* subsp. *novicida* chitinases and Sec secretion system to biofilm formation on chitin. *Appl Environ Microbiol* 76:596–608.

26. Chen D, Lei L, Lu C, Flores R, DeLisa MP, Roberts TC, Romesberg FE, Zhong G. 2010. Secretion of the chlamydial virulence factor CPAF requires the Sec-dependent pathway. *Microbiology* 156:3031–3040.

27. Petersen TN, Brunak S, von Heijne G, Nielsen H. 2011. SignalP 4.0: discriminating signal peptides from transmembrane regions. *Nat Methods* 8:785–786.

28. Möller S, Croning MDR, Apweiler R. 2001. Evaluation of methods for the prediction of membrane spanning regions. *Bioinformatics* 17:646–653.

29. Griffin JE, Gawronski JD, Dejesus MA, Ioerger TR, Akerley BJ, Sassetti CM. 2011. High-resolution phenotypic profiling defines genes essential for mycobacterial growth and cholesterol catabolism. *PLoS Pathog* 7:e1002251.

30. Sassetti CM, Rubin EJ. 2003. Genetic requirements for mycobacterial survival during infection. *Proc Natl Acad Sci USA* 100:12989–12994.

31. Rengarajan J, Bloom BR, Rubin EJ. 2005. Genome-wide requirements for *Mycobacterium tuberculosis* adaptation and survival in macrophages. *Proc Natl Acad Sci USA* 102:8327–8332.

32. Dutta NK, Mehra S, Didier PJ, Roy CJ, Doyle LA, Alvarez X, Ratterree M, Be NA, Lamichhane G, Jain SK, Lacey MR, Lackner AA, Kaushal D. 2010. Genetic requirements for the survival of tubercle bacilli in primates. *J Infect Dis* 201:1743–1752.

33. Zhang YJ, Reddy MC, Ioerger TR, Rothchild AC, Dartois V, Schuster BM, Trauner A, Wallis D, Galaviz S, Huttenhower C, Sacchettini JC, Behar SM, Rubin EJ. 2013. Tryptophan biosynthesis protects mycobacteria from CD4 T-cell-mediated killing. *Cell* 155:1296–1308.

34. Machowski EE, Senzani S, Ealand C, Kana BD. 2014. Comparative genomics for mycobacterial peptidoglycan remodelling enzymes reveals extensive genetic multiplicity. *BMC Microbiol* 14:75.

35. Hett EC, Chao MC, Steyn AJ, Fortune SM, Deng LL, Rubin EJ. 2007. A partner for the resuscitation-promoting factors of *Mycobacterium tuberculosis*. *Mol Microbiol* 66:658–668.

36. Hett EC, Chao MC, Deng LL, Rubin EJ. 2008. A mycobacterial enzyme essential for cell division synergizes with resuscitation-promoting factor. *PLoS Pathog* 4:e1000001.

37. Goffin C, Ghuysen J-M. 1998. Multimodular penicillin-binding proteins: an enigmatic family of orthologs and paralogs. *Microbiol Mol Biol Rev* 62:1079–1093.

38. Feltcher ME, Gunawardena HP, Zulauf KE, Malik S, Griffin JE, Sassetti CM, Chen X, Braunstein M. 2015. Label-free quantitative proteomics reveals a role for the *Mycobacterium tuberculosis* SecA2 pathway in exporting solute binding proteins and Mce transporters to the cell wall. *Mol Cell Proteomics* 14:1501–1516.

39. Patru M-M, Pavelka MS Jr. 2010. A role for the class A penicillin-binding protein PonA2 in the survival of *Mycobacterium smegmatis* under conditions of nonreplication. *J Bacteriol* 192:3043–3054.

40. Kieser KJ, Baranowski C, Chao MC, Long JE, Sassetti CM, Waldor MK, Sacchettini JC, Ioerger TR, Rubin EJ. 2015. Peptidoglycan synthesis in *Mycobacterium tuberculosis* is organized into networks with varying drug susceptibility. *Proc Natl Acad Sci USA* 112:13087–13092.

41. Kieser KJ, Boutte CC, Kester JC, Baer CE, Barczak AK, Meniche X, Chao MC, Rego EH, Sassetti CM, Fortune SM, Rubin EJ. 2015. Phosphorylation of the peptidoglycan synthase PonA1 governs the rate of polar elongation in mycobacteria. *PLoS Pathog* 11:e1005010.

42. Vandal OH, Roberts JA, Odaira T, Schnappinger D, Nathan CF, Ehrt S. 2009. Acid-susceptible mutants

of *Mycobacterium tuberculosis* share hypersusceptibility to cell wall and oxidative stress and to the host environment. *J Bacteriol* **191**:625–631.

43. Sander P, Rezwan M, Walker B, Rampini SK, Kroppenstedt RM, Ehlers S, Keller C, Keeble JR, Hagemeier M, Colston MJ, Springer B, Böttger EC. 2004. Lipoprotein processing is required for virulence of *Mycobacterium tuberculosis*. *Mol Microbiol* **52**:1543–1552.

44. Gaur RL, Ren K, Blumenthal A, Bhamidi S, Gibbs S, Jackson M, Zare RN, Ehrt S, Ernst JD, Banaei N. 2014. LprG-mediated surface expression of lipoarabinomannan is essential for virulence of Mycobacterium tuberculosis. *PLoS Pathog* **10**:e1004376. (Erratum, **11**:e1005336.)

45. Martinot AJ, Farrow M, Bai L, Layre E, Cheng T-Y, Tsai JH, Iqbal J, Annand JW, Sullivan ZA, Hussain MM, Sacchettini J, Moody DB, Seeliger JC, Rubin EJ. 2016. Mycobacterial metabolic syndrome: LprG and Rv1410 regulate triacylglyceride levels, growth rate and virulence in *Mycobacterium tuberculosis*. *PLoS Pathog* **12**:e1005351.

46. Diaz-Silvestre H, Espinosa-Cueto P, Sanchez-Gonzalez A, Esparza-Ceron MA, Pereira-Suarez AL, Bernal-Fernandez G, Espitia C, Mancilla R. 2005. The 19-kDa antigen of *Mycobacterium tuberculosis* is a major adhesin that binds the mannose receptor of THP-1 monocytic cells and promotes phagocytosis of mycobacteria. *Microb Pathog* **39**:97–107.

47. Fulton SA, Reba SM, Pai RK, Pennini M, Torres M, Harding CV, Boom WH. 2004. Inhibition of major histocompatibility complex II expression and antigen processing in murine alveolar macrophages by *Mycobacterium bovis* BCG and the 19-kilodalton mycobacterial lipoprotein. *Infect Immun* **72**:2101–2110.

48. Henao-Tamayo M, Junqueira-Kipnis AP, Ordway D, Gonzales-Juarrero M, Stewart GR, Young DB, Wilkinson RJ, Basaraba RJ, Orme IM. 2007. A mutant of *Mycobacterium tuberculosis* lacking the 19-kDa lipoprotein Rv3763 is highly attenuated *in vivo* but retains potent vaccinogenic properties. *Vaccine* **25**:7153–7159.

49. Lew JM, Kapopoulou A, Jones LM, Cole ST. 2011. TubercuList: 10 years after. *Tuberculosis (Edinb)* **91**:1–7.

50. Berthet F-X, Lagranderie M, Gounon P, Laurent-Winter C, Ensergueix D, Chavarot P, Thouron F, Maranghi E, Pelicic V, Portnoï D, Marchal G, Gicquel B. 1998. Attenuation of virulence by disruption of the *Mycobacterium tuberculosis erp* gene. *Science* **282**:759–762.

51. Cosma CL, Klein K, Kim R, Beery D, Ramakrishnan L. 2006. *Mycobacterium marinum* Erp is a virulence determinant required for cell wall integrity and intracellular survival. *Infect Immun* **74**:3125–3133.

52. Kocíncová D, Sondén B, de Mendonça-Lima L, Gicquel B, Reyrat J-M. 2004. The Erp protein is anchored at the surface by a carboxy-terminal hydrophobic domain and is important for cell-wall structure in *Mycobacterium smegmatis*. *FEMS Microbiol Lett* **231**:191–196.

53. Speer A, Sun J, Danilchanka O, Meikle V, Rowland JL, Walter K, Buck BR, Pavlenok M, Hölscher C, Ehrt S, Niederweis M. 2015. Surface hydrolysis of sphingo-

myelin by the outer membrane protein Rv0888 supports replication of *Mycobacterium tuberculosis* in macrophages. *Mol Microbiol* **97**:881–897.

54. Dang G, Cao J, Cui Y, Song N, Chen L, Pang H, Liu S. 2016. Characterization of Rv0888, a novel extracellular nuclease from *Mycobacterium tuberculosis*. *Sci Rep* **6**:19033.

55. Dutta NK, Karakousis PC. 2014. Latent tuberculosis infection: myths, models, and molecular mechanisms. *Microbiol Mol Biol Rev* **78**:343–371.

56. Ollinger J, O'Malley T, Ahn J, Odingo J, Parish T. 2012. Inhibition of the sole type I signal peptidase of *Mycobacterium tuberculosis* is bactericidal under replicating and nonreplicating conditions. *J Bacteriol* **194**:2614–2619.

57. Lavollay M, Arthur M, Fourgeaud M, Dubost L, Marie A, Veziris N, Blanot D, Gutmann L, Mainardi J-L. 2008. The peptidoglycan of stationary-phase *Mycobacterium tuberculosis* predominantly contains cross-links generated by L,D-transpeptidation. *J Bacteriol* **190**:4360–4366.

58. Pisabarro AG, de Pedro MA, Vázquez D. 1985. Structural modifications in the peptidoglycan of *Escherichia coli* associated with changes in the state of growth of the culture. *J Bacteriol* **161**:238–242.

59. Signoretto C, del Mar Lleò M, Tafi MC, Canepari P. 2000. Cell wall chemical composition of *Enterococcus faecalis* in the viable but nonculturable state. *Appl Environ Microbiol* **66**:1953–1959.

60. Gopinath V, Raghunandanan S, Gomez RL, Jose L, Surendran A, Ramachandran R, Pushparajan AR, Mundayoor S, Jaleel A, Kumar RA. 2015. Profiling the proteome of *Mycobacterium tuberculosis* during dormancy and reactivation. *Mol Cell Proteomics* **14**:2160–2176.

61. Mukamolova GV, Turapov OA, Kazarian K, Telkov M, Kaprelyants AS, Kell DB, Young M. 2002. The *rpf* gene of *Micrococcus luteus* encodes an essential secreted growth factor. *Mol Microbiol* **46**:611–621.

62. Tufariello JM, Mi K, Xu J, Manabe YC, Kesavan AK, Drumm J, Tanaka K, Jacobs WR Jr, Chan J. 2006. Deletion of the *Mycobacterium tuberculosis* resuscitation-promoting factor Rv1009 gene results in delayed reactivation from chronic tuberculosis. *Infect Immun* **74**:2985–2995.

63. Downing KJ, Mischenko VV, Shleeva MO, Young DI, Young M, Kaprelyants AS, Apt AS, Mizrahi V. 2005. Mutants of *Mycobacterium tuberculosis* lacking three of the five *rpf*-like genes are defective for growth *in vivo* and for resuscitation *in vitro*. *Infect Immun* **73**:3038–3043.

64. Biketov S, Potapov V, Ganina E, Downing K, Kana BD, Kaprelyants A. 2007. The role of resuscitation promoting factors in pathogenesis and reactivation of *Mycobacterium tuberculosis* during intra-peritoneal infection in mice. *BMC Infect Dis* **7**:146.

65. Kana BD, Gordhan BG, Downing KJ, Sung N, Vostroktunova G, Machowski EE, Tsenova L, Young M, Kaprelyants A, Kaplan G, Mizrahi V. 2008. The resuscitation-promoting factors of *Mycobacterium tu-*

berculosis are required for virulence and resuscitation from dormancy but are collectively dispensable for growth *in vitro*. *Mol Microbiol* 67:672–684.

66. **Mukamolova GV, Murzin AG, Salina EG, Demina GR, Kell DB, Kaprelyants AS, Young M.** 2006. Muralytic activity of *Micrococcus luteus* Rpf and its relationship to physiological activity in promoting bacterial growth and resuscitation. *Mol Microbiol* 59:84–98.

67. **Braunstein M, Espinosa BJ, Chan J, Belisle JTR, Jacobs WR Jr.** 2003. SecA2 functions in the secretion of superoxide dismutase A and in the virulence of *Mycobacterium tuberculosis*. *Mol Microbiol* 48:453–464.

68. **Kurtz S, McKinnon KP, Runge MS, Ting JPY, Braunstein M.** 2006. The SecA2 secretion factor of Mycobacterium tuberculosis promotes growth in macrophages and inhibits the host immune response. *Infect Immun* 74:6855–6864.

69. **Sullivan JT, Young EF, McCann JR, Braunstein M.** 2012. The *Mycobacterium tuberculosis* SecA2 system subverts phagosome maturation to promote growth in macrophages. *Infect Immun* 80:996–1006.

70. **van der Woude AD, Stoop EJM, Stiess M, Wang S, Ummels R, van Stempvoort G, Piersma SR, Cascioferro A, Jiménez CR, Houben ENG, Luirink J, Pieters J, van der Sar AM, Bitter W.** 2014. Analysis of SecA2-dependent substrates in *Mycobacterium marinum* identifies protein kinase G (PknG) as a virulence effector. *Cell Microbiol* 16:280–295.

71. **Watkins BY, Joshi SA, Ball DA, Leggett H, Park S, Kim J, Austin CD, Paler-Martinez A, Xu M, Downing KH, Brown EJ.** 2012. *Mycobacterium marinum* SecA2 promotes stable granulomas and induces tumor necrosis factor alpha *in vivo*. *Infect Immun* 80:3512–3520.

72. **Lenz LL, Mohammadi S, Geissler A, Portnoy DA.** 2003. SecA2-dependent secretion of autolytic enzymes promotes *Listeria monocytogenes* pathogenesis. *Proc Natl Acad Sci USA* 100:12432–12437.

73. **Siboo IR, Chambers HF, Sullam PM.** 2005. Role of SraP, a serine-rich surface protein of *Staphylococcus aureus*, in binding to human platelets. *Infect Immun* 73:2273–2280.

74. **Bensing BA, Sullam PM.** 2002. An accessory sec locus of *Streptococcus gordonii* is required for export of the surface protein GspB and for normal levels of binding to human platelets. *Mol Microbiol* 44:1081–1094.

75. **Chen Q, Wu H, Fives-Taylor PM.** 2004. Investigating the role of *secA2* in secretion and glycosylation of a fimbrial adhesin in *Streptococcus parasanguis* FW213. *Mol Microbiol* 53:843–856.

76. **Rigel NW, Braunstein M.** 2008. A new twist on an old pathway: accessory secretion systems. *Mol Microbiol* 69:291–302.

77. **Bensing BA, Seepersaud R, Yen YT, Sullam PM.** 2014. Selective transport by SecA2: an expanding family of customized motor proteins. *Biochim Biophys Acta* 1843:1674–1686.

78. **Ligon LS, Rigel NW, Romanchuk A, Jones CD, Braunstein M.** 2013. Suppressor analysis reveals a role for SecY in the SecA2-dependent protein export pathway of *Mycobacteria*. *J Bacteriol* 195:4456–4465.

79. **Durack J, Burke TP, Portnoy DA.** 2015. A *prl* mutation in SecY suppresses secretion and virulence defects of *Listeria monocytogenes secA2* mutants. *J Bacteriol* 197:932–942.

80. **Fagan RP, Fairweather NF.** 2011. *Clostridium difficile* has two parallel and essential Sec secretion systems. *J Biol Chem* 286:27483–27493.

81. **Rigel NW, Gibbons HS, McCann JR, McDonough JA, Kurtz S, Braunstein M.** 2009. The accessory SecA2 system of *Mycobacteria* requires ATP binding and the canonical SecA1. *J Biol Chem* 284:9927–9936.

82. **Sharma V, Arockiasamy A, Ronning DR, Savva CG, Holzenburg A, Braunstein M, Jacobs WR Jr, Sacchettini JC.** 2003. Crystal structure of *Mycobacterium tuberculosis* SecA, a preprotein translocating ATPase. *Proc Natl Acad Sci USA* 100:2243–2248.

83. **Swanson S, Ioerger TR, Rigel NW, Miller BK, Braunstein M, Sacchettini JC.** 2015. Structural similarities and differences between two functionally distinct SecA proteins: the *Mycobacterium tuberculosis* SecA1 and SecA2. *J Bacteriol* 198:720–730.

84. **Bhanu MK, Zhao P, Kendall DA.** 2013. Mapping of the SecA signal peptide binding site and dimeric interface by using the substituted cysteine accessibility method. *J Bacteriol* 195:4709–4715.

85. **Auclair SM, Oliver DB, Mukerji I.** 2013. Defining the solution state dimer structure of *Escherichia coli* SecA using Förster resonance energy transfer. *Biochemistry* 52:2388–2401.

86. **Hou JM, D'Lima NG, Rigel NW, Gibbons HS, McCann JR, Braunstein M, Teschke CM.** 2008. ATPase activity of *Mycobacterium tuberculosis* SecA1 and SecA2 proteins and its importance for SecA2 function in macrophages. *J Bacteriol* 190:4880–4887.

87. **Sardis MF, Economou A.** 2010. SecA: a tale of two protomers. *Mol Microbiol* 76:1070–1081.

88. **Prabudiansyah I, Kusters I, Driessen AJM.** 2015. *In vitro* interaction of the housekeeping SecA1 with the accessory SecA2 protein of *Mycobacterium tuberculosis*. *PLoS One* 10:e0128788.

89. **D'Lima NG, Teschke CM.** 2014. ADP-dependent conformational changes distinguish *Mycobacterium tuberculosis* SecA2 from SecA1. *J Biol Chem* 289:2307–2317.

90. **Gibbons HS, Wolschendorf F, Abshire M, Niederweis M, Braunstein M.** 2007. Identification of two *Mycobacterium smegmatis* lipoproteins exported by a SecA2-dependent pathway. *J Bacteriol* 189:5090–5100.

91. **Renier S, Chambon C, Viala D, Chagnot C, Hébraud M, Desvaux M.** 2013. Exoproteomic analysis of the SecA2-dependent secretion in *Listeria monocytogenes* EGD-e. *J Proteomics* 80:183–195.

92. **Feltcher ME, Gibbons HS, Ligon LS, Braunstein M.** 2013. Protein export by the mycobacterial SecA2 system is determined by the preprotein mature domain. *J Bacteriol* 195:672–681.

93. **Krehenbrink M, Edwards A, Downie JA.** 2011. The superoxide dismutase SodA is targeted to the periplasm in a SecA-dependent manner by a novel mechanism. *Mol Microbiol* 82:164–179.

94. Archambaud C, Nahori M-A, Pizarro-Cerda J, Cossart P, Dussurget O. 2006. Control of *Listeria* superoxide dismutase by phosphorylation. *J Biol Chem* **281:** 31812–31822.

95. Chater KF, Biró S, Lee KJ, Palmer T, Schrempf H. 2010. The complex extracellular biology of *Streptomyces. FEMS Microbiol Rev* **34:**171–198.

96. Shruthi H, Madan Babu M, Sankaran K. 2010. TAT-pathway-dependent lipoproteins as a niche-based adaptation in prokaryotes. *J Mol Evol* **70:**359–370.

97. Braibant M, Gilot P, Content J. 2000. The ATP binding cassette (ABC) transport systems of *Mycobacterium tuberculosis. FEMS Microbiol Rev* **24:**449–467.

98. Casali N, Riley LW. 2007. A phylogenomic analysis of the *Actinomycetalesmce* operons. *BMC Genomics* **8:**60.

99. Malinverni JC, Silhavy TJ. 2009. An ABC transport system that maintains lipid asymmetry in the Gram-negative outer membrane. *Proc Natl Acad Sci USA* **106:** 8009–8014.

100. Pandey AK, Sassetti CM. 2008. Mycobacterial persistence requires the utilization of host cholesterol. *Proc Natl Acad Sci USA* **105:**4376–4380. (Erratum, doi: 10.1073/pnas.0804298105.)

101. Senaratne RH, Sidders B, Sequeira P, Saunders G, Dunphy K, Marjanovic O, Reader JR, Lima P, Chan S, Kendall S, McFadden J, Riley LW. 2008. *Mycobacterium tuberculosis* strains disrupted in *mce3* and *mce4* operons are attenuated in mice. *J Med Microbiol* **57:** 164–170.

102. Forrellad MA, McNeil M, Santangelo ML, Blanco FC, García E, Klepp LI, Huff J, Niederweis M, Jackson M, Bigi F. 2014. Role of the Mce1 transporter in the lipid homeostasis of *Mycobacterium tuberculosis. Tuberculosis (Edinb)* **94:**170–177.

103. Cantrell SA, Leavell MD, Marjanovic O, Iavarone AT, Leary JA, Riley LW. 2013. Free mycolic acid accumulation in the cell wall of the *mce1* operon mutant strain of *Mycobacterium tuberculosis. J Microbiol* **51:**619–626.

104. Joshi SM, Pandey AK, Capite N, Fortune SM, Rubin EJ, Sassetti CM. 2006. Characterization of mycobacterial virulence genes through genetic interaction mapping. *Proc Natl Acad Sci USA* **103:**11760–11765.

105. Gioffré A, Infante E, Aguilar D, Santangelo MP, Klepp L, Amadio A, Meikle V, Etchechoury I, Romano MI, Cataldi A, Hernández RP, Bigi F. 2005. Mutation in mce operons attenuates *Mycobacterium tuberculosis* virulence. *Microbes Infect* **7:**325–334.

106. Shimono N, Morici L, Casali N, Cantrell S, Sidders B, Ehrt S, Riley LW. 2003. Hypervirulent mutant of *Mycobacterium tuberculosis* resulting from disruption of the mce1 operon. *Proc Natl Acad Sci USA* **100:**15918–15923.

107. McCann JR, McDonough JA, Sullivan JT, Feltcher ME, Braunstein M. 2011. Genome-wide identification of *Mycobacterium tuberculosis* exported proteins with roles in intracellular growth. *J Bacteriol* **193:**854–861.

108. Hinchey J, Lee S, Jeon BY, Basaraba RJ, Venkataswamy MM, Chen B, Chan J, Braunstein M, Orme IM, Derrick SC, Morris SL, Jacobs WR Jr, Porcelli SA. 2007. Enhanced priming of adaptive immunity by a pro-apoptotic mutant of *Mycobacterium tuberculosis. J Clin Invest* **117:**2279–2288.

109. De Groote MA, Ochsner UA, Shiloh MU, Nathan C, McCord JM, Dinauer MC, Libby SJ, Vazquez-Torres A, Xu Y, Fang FC. 1997. Periplasmic superoxide dismutase protects *Salmonella* from products of phagocyte NADPH-oxidase and nitric oxide synthase. *Proc Natl Acad Sci USA* **94:**13997–14001.

110. Heym B, Zhang Y, Poulet S, Young D, Cole ST. 1993. Characterization of the *katG* gene encoding a catalase-peroxidase required for the isoniazid susceptibility of *Mycobacterium tuberculosis. J Bacteriol* **175:** 4255–4259.

111. Wengenack NL, Jensen MP, Rusnak F, Stern MK. 1999. *Mycobacterium tuberculosis* KatG is a peroxynitritase. *Biochem Biophys Res Commun* **256:**485–487.

112. Cowley S, Ko M, Pick N, Chow R, Downing KJ, Gordhan BG, Betts JC, Mizrahi V, Smith DA, Stokes RW, Av-Gay Y. 2004. The *Mycobacterium tuberculosis* protein serine/threonine kinase PknG is linked to cellular glutamate/glutamine levels and is important for growth *in vivo. Mol Microbiol* **52:**1691–1702.

113. O'Hare HM, Durán R, Cerveñansky C, Bellinzoni M, Wehenkel AM, Pritsch O, Obal G, Baumgartner J, Vialaret J, Johnsson K, Alzari PM. 2008. Regulation of glutamate metabolism by protein kinases in mycobacteria. *Mol Microbiol* **70:**1408–1423.

114. Walburger A, Koul A, Ferrari G, Nguyen L, Prescianotto-Baschong C, Huygen K, Klebl B, Thompson C, Bacher G, Pieters J. 2004. Protein kinase G from pathogenic mycobacteria promotes survival within macrophages. *Science* **304:**1800–1804.

115. Wolff KA, de la Peña AH, Nguyen HT, Pham TH, Amzel LM, Gabelli SB, Nguyen L. 2015. A redox regulatory system critical for mycobacterial survival in macrophages and biofilm development. *PLoS Pathog* **11:** e1004839.

116. Hussain Bhat K, Mukhopadhyay S. 2015. Macrophage takeover and the host-bacilli interplay during tuberculosis. *Future Microbiol* **10:**853–872.

117. Armstrong JA, Hart PDA. 1971. Response of cultured macrophages to *Mycobacterium tuberculosis*, with observations on fusion of lysosomes with phagosomes. *J Exp Med* **134:**713–740.

118. Nguyen-Mau S-M, Oh S-Y, Kern VJ, Missiakas DM, Schneewind O. 2012. Secretion genes as determinants of *Bacillus anthracis* chain length. *J Bacteriol* **194:** 3841–3850.

119. Boon C, Dick T. 2012. How *Mycobacterium tuberculosis* goes to sleep: the dormancy survival regulator DosR a decade later. *Future Microbiol* **7:**513–518.

120. Mehra S, Foreman TW, Didier PJ, Ahsan MH, Hudock TA, Kissee R, Golden NA, Gautam US, Johnson A-M, Alvarez X, Russell-Lodrigue KE, Doyle LA, Roy CJ, Niu T, Blanchard JL, Khader SA, Lackner AA, Sherman DR, Kaushal D. 2015. The DosR regulon modulates adaptive immunity and is essential for *Mycobacterium tuberculosis* persistence. *Am J Respir Crit Care Med* **191:**1185–1196.

121. Schnappinger D, Ehrt S, Voskuil MI, Liu Y, Mangan JA, Monahan IM, Dolganov G, Efron B, Butcher PD, Nathan C, Schoolnik GK. 2003. Transcriptional adaptation of *Mycobacterium tuberculosis* within macrophages: insights into the phagosomal environment. *J Exp Med* 198:693–704.

122. Voskuil MI, Schnappinger D, Visconti KC, Harrell MI, Dolganov GM, Sherman DR, Schoolnik GK. 2003. Inhibition of respiration by nitric oxide induces a *Mycobacterium tuberculosis* dormancy program. *J Exp Med* 198:705–713.

123. Kumar A, Lewin A, Rani PS, Qureshi IA, Devi S, Majid M, Kamal E, Marek S, Hasnain SE, Ahmed N. 2013. Dormancy associated translation inhibitor (DATIN/Rv0079) of *Mycobacterium tuberculosis* interacts with TLR2 and induces proinflammatory cytokine expression. *Cytokine* 64:258–264.

124. Martin CJ, Booty MG, Rosebrock TR, Nunes-Alves C, Desjardins DM, Keren I, Fortune SM, Remold HG, Behar SM. 2012. Efferocytosis is an innate antibacterial mechanism. *Cell Host Microbe* 12:289–300.

125. Schaible UE, Winau F, Sieling PA, Fischer K, Collins HL, Hagens K, Modlin RL, Brinkmann V, Kaufmann SHE. 2003. Apoptosis facilitates antigen presentation to T lymphocytes through MHC-I and CD1 in tuberculosis. *Nat Med* 9:1039–1046.

126. Nathan C, Shiloh MU. 2000. Reactive oxygen and nitrogen intermediates in the relationship between mammalian hosts and microbial pathogens. *Proc Natl Acad Sci USA* 97:8841–8848.

127. Murray RA, Mansoor N, Harbacheuski R, Soler J, Davids V, Soares A, Hawkridge A, Hussey GD, Maecker H, Kaplan G, Hanekom WA. 2006. Bacillus Calmette Guerin vaccination of human newborns induces a specific, functional CD8+ T cell response. *J Immunol* 177:5647–5651.

128. Andersen P, Doherty TM. 2005. The success and failure of BCG: implications for a novel tuberculosis vaccine. *Nat Rev Microbiol* 3:656–662.

129. Hesseling AC, Marais BJ, Gie RP, Schaaf HS, Fine PEM, Godfrey-Faussett P, Beyers N. 2007. The risk of disseminated bacille Calmette-Guerin (BCG) disease in HIV-infected children. *Vaccine* 25:14–18.

130. Panas MW, Sixsmith JD, White K, Korioth-Schmitz B, Shields ST, Moy BT, Lee S, Schmitz JE, Jacobs WR Jr, Porcelli SA, Haynes BF, Letvin NL, Gillard GO. 2014. Gene deletions in *Mycobacterium bovis* BCG stimulate increased CD8+ T cell responses. *Infect Immun* 82:5317–5326.

131. Hinchey J, Jeon BY, Alley H, Chen B, Goldberg M, Derrick S, Morris S, Jacobs WR Jr, Porcelli SA, Lee S. 2011. Lysine auxotrophy combined with deletion of the SecA2 gene results in a safe and highly immunogenic candidate live attenuated vaccine for tuberculosis. *PLoS One* 6:e15857.

132. Ranganathan UDK, Larsen MH, Kim J, Porcelli SA, Jacobs WR Jr, Fennelly GJ. 2009. Recombinant pro-apoptotic *Mycobacterium tuberculosis* generates CD8+ T cell responses against human immunodeficiency virus type 1 Env and *M. tuberculosis* in neonatal mice. *Vaccine* 28:152–161.

133. Jensen K, Ranganathan UDK, Van Rompay KKA, Canfield DR, Khan I, Ravindran R, Luciw PA, Jacobs WR Jr, Fennelly G, Larsen MH, Abel K. 2012. A recombinant attenuated *Mycobacterium tuberculosis* vaccine strain is safe in immunosuppressed simian immunodeficiency virus-infected infant macaques. *Clin Vaccine Immunol* 19:1170–1181.

134. Geluk A, van Meijgaarden KE, Joosten SA, Commandeur S, Ottenhoff THM. 2014. Innovative strategies to identify *M. tuberculosis* antigens and epitopes using genome-wide analyses. *Front Immunol* 5:256.

135. Sadagopal S, Braunstein M, Hager CC, Wei J, Daniel AK, Bochan MR, Crozier I, Smith NE, Gates HO, Barnett L, Van Kaer L, Price JO, Blackwell TS, Kalams SA, Kernodle DS. 2009. Reducing the activity and secretion of microbial antioxidants enhances the immunogenicity of BCG. *PLoS One* 4:e5531.

Tuberculosis and the Tubercle Bacillus, 2nd ed.
Edited by William R. Jacobs, Jr., Helen McShane, Valerie Mizrahi, and Ian M. Orme
© 2018 American Society for Microbiology, Washington, DC
doi:10.1128/microbiolspec.TBTB2-0001-2015

The Role of ESX-1 in *Mycobacterium tuberculosis* Pathogenesis

29

Ka-Wing Wong

BACKGROUND

The identification of ESAT-6 secretion system-1 (ESX-1) as a virulence determinant of *Mycobacterium tuberculosis* is a major discovery in the history of tuberculosis research. ESX-1 is encoded by a genetic locus known as RD1, which stands for "region of difference" and is one of the deleted regions in the vaccine strain *Mycobacterium bovis* bacille Calmette-Guérin (BCG) for humans (1). The first evidence emerges from the finding that the absence of RD1 is responsible for the attenuation of BCG's virulence (2–4). Introduction of RD1 into BCG is sufficient to induce BCG growth in lung and spleen, granuloma formation in lung, splenomegaly, and inflammation and abscesses in liver and kidney in mice (4). Conversely, deletion of RD1 in the virulent H37Rv *M. tuberculosis* strain inactivates the ability of H37Rv to enable rapid bacterial replication in lung and spleen, to cause lung histopathology and death in mice (2, 3). Lung sections from infected mice show evidence of macrophage lysis, which is a RD1-dependent process (2). Consistent with this observation, Lewis et al. describe the requirement of RD1 for H37Rv to grow within and kill human macrophages (3).

Macrophage is the primary cell harboring *M. tuberculosis* during tuberculosis infection in humans (5). Accordingly, the discovery that RD1 mediates the induction of macrophage death by *M. tuberculosis* suggests that the outcome of the interaction between RD1 and macrophage host cell will be a key determinant of the virulence of *M. tuberculosis* pathogenesis. Significant progress toward understanding how ESX-1/RD1 facilitates tuberculosis pathogenesis has been made recently. In this article, we aim to provide an updated overview about the progress and put forward emerging concepts for improving our understanding of the nature of ESX-1-induced pathogenesis. In doing so, we also highlight some recent developments in designing intervention strategies based on targeting the RD1-encoded proteins.

ESX-1 SECRETION SYSTEM

The RD1 locus encodes a type VII secretion system known as ESAT-6 secretion system-1 (ESX-1) in *Mycobacterium* species (6). RD1 comprises nine genes, two of which are the secreted protein ESAT-6 (early secreted antigenic target of 6 kDa) and CFP-10 (culture filtrate protein of 10 kDa). Both of these proteins are immunodominant antigens and major virulence factors of *M. tuberculosis*. ESAT-6 and CFP-10 are cosecreted as a heterodimeric complex and are also essential components of the ESX-1 secretion system. Other RD1 genes encode the ATPase Rv3871, the transmembrane protein Rv3870, and the channel protein Rv3877. The ESAT-6-CFP-10 complex is recognized by the ATPase Rv3871, which is localized to the inner membrane through its interaction with Rv3870. The complex is then translocated across the inner membrane, most likely through the channel protein Rv3877. Other RD-1 genes might facilitate the biogenesis of the secretion system. Non-RD-1 genes are also required for proper functioning of ESX-1. EspR is a transcriptional regulator of ESX-1. EspA is an ESX-1-secreted substrate, and its secretion is required for the secretion of ESAT-6 and CFP-10. Additional detail about how the ESX-1 secretion system works is beyond the scope of this article. Interested readers should consult the comprehensive review by Abdallah et al. (6).

Shanghai Public Health Clinical Center, Key Laboratory of Medical Molecular Virology, School of Basic Medical Sciences, Shanghai Medical College of Fudan University, Shanghai 200032, People's Republic of China.

KEY OBSERVATIONS LEADING TO RECENT EVIDENCE OF PHAGOSOME DISRUPTION BY ESX-1

M. tuberculosis is phagocytized by alveolar macrophage after it is inhaled into the lungs of an individual. The internalized bacteria then reside within a membrane-bound compartment called phagosome. Armstrong and Hart used electron microscopy to examine these compartments in detail (7). Phagosomes containing non-pathogenic BCG normally undergo maturation, which is then followed by fusion with multiple lysosomes. The fusion events bring lysosomal digestive enzymes into the lumen of the phagosome for degradation. Indeed, damaged BCG is frequently observed. Using a sophisticated electron microscopy technique, Peters' group revisited the pioneer work of Armstrong and Hart (8). To their surprise, they found evidence of phagosome maturation and lysosome fusion in phagosomes containing H37Rv that contain ESX-1 (8). These are transient events and are only observed during early infections. In contrast, phagosome maturation and lysosome fusion are uninterrupted and occur continuously in macrophages infected with BCG. The authors show that, after the early engagement with lysosome, *M. tuberculosis* translocates from phagosome into cytosol and this process requires ESX-1 (8). This translocation has been proposed as a virulence mechanism (9). Similar observations were made earlier by McDonough et al. (10).

How does *M. tuberculosis* impair phagosome-lysosome fusion? The fusion requires membrane localizations of lysosome-associated proteins (LAMP)-1 and LAMP-2 on phagosomes (11). Membrane disruption should therefore affect phagosome-lysosome fusion. Importantly, membrane disruption by *M. tuberculosis* was first observed in 1984 by Leake et al. and Myrvik et al. using electron microscopy (12, 13). The disruption is observed only in macrophages infected with virulent *M. tuberculosis* H37Rv but not with attenuated BCG or H37Ra, consistent with the results of Armstrong and Hart. This finding has recently been confirmed by other methods. Damaged phagosomes can be marked by galectin-3 and are indeed observed in *M. tuberculosis*-infected macrophages in an-ESX-1-dependent fashion (14, 15). Simeone et al. have developed a single-cell fluorescence resonance energy transfer assay to monitor phagosome disruption (16). Using this assay, the authors demonstrate phagosome disruption in mouse spleen and lungs as revealed by the assay based on fluorescence resonance energy transfer (17). *In vitro*, the assay reveals evidence of phagosome disruption within 24 h of macrophage infections (17). Interestingly, most

of the cytosolic translocation event for *M. tuberculosis* requires 2 or 3 days to occur (9).

It is possible that the appearance of cytosolic localization of *M. tuberculosis* arises from collapse of phagosomal membrane as a result of continuous disruption of the phagosomal membrane. According to this scenario, cytosolic translocation of *M. tuberculosis* and impairment of phagosome-lysosome fusion can be seen as downstream effects of phagosome disruption. This has an important implication in *M. tuberculosis* pathogenesis. Phagosome disruption is a proposed mechanism of "patterns of pathogenesis." This concept was proposed by Vance, Isberg, and Portnoy to help in understanding pathogenic host responses to virulent microorganisms (18). In the next section, we will present new evidence that fits the idea that phagosome disruption is responsible for all major pathogenic responses as a result of tuberculosis infections. Therapeutic implication of this idea will then be discussed.

DAMAGE OF THE *M. TUBERCULOSIS*-CONTAINING PHAGOSOME: CONSEQUENCES OF CYTOSOLIC ACCESS BY *M. TUBERCULOSIS*

Phagosome disruption compromises the integrity of the phagosomal membrane and can lead to cytosolic access of the lumen content within the phagosome compartments. There are at least four major cellular responses as a result of such cytosolic access of *M. tuberculosis*-derived materials. And for each of the responses, the element of pathogenesis can be readily identified. First, phagosome disruption can lead to activation of the cytosolic inflammasome receptor NLRP3 (15). NLRP3 is activated by *M. tuberculosis* ESX-1 and the activation triggers downstream activation of caspase-1, which then facilitates secretion of cytokines interleukin 1 beta (IL-1beta) and interleukin 18 (IL-18) (19). These cytokine productions are protective against *M. tuberculosis* infections (20, 21). NLRP3 activation can also lead to the induction of a programmed necrotic death in *M. tuberculosis*-infected macrophages (15). *M. tuberculosis* mutants carrying a defective ESAT-6 that are unable to disrupt the phagosome cannot activate NLRP3 (as measured by IL-18 production) and cannot induce necrosis (15). This programmed cell death is not known to have any negative impact on the viability of *M. tuberculosis*. This kind of death is necrotic and highly inflammatory, which contributes to significant tissue damage. Indeed, macrophage necrosis is suggested to play a key role in all major stages of tuberculosis (22). It is presently unclear how NLRP3 senses phagosome disruption. NLRP3 is known to sense cell swelling and hyperosmotic stress (23, 24). It remains to be shown whether ESAT-6 promotes cell swelling and alters cellular osmolarity through its phagosome-disrupting activity. This scenario is possible since it has been shown that ESX-1 can cause residual effects on plasma membrane upon contact with macrophages (25).

Second, cytosolic access can activate a cytosolic surveillance pathway that triggers induction of type I interferon production. This induction by *M. tuberculosis* is dependent on ESX-1 (26). The phagosome-disrupting effect of ESX-1 provides cytosolic access of *M. tuberculosis* materials such as extracellular DNA, which acts as a specific activating ligand for the STING-TBK1-IRF3 signaling axis for type I interferon production (27). The cytosolic DNA sensor that is responsible for direct recognition of *M. tuberculosis* DNA and for activating STING has recently been identified by three independent groups to be cyclic GMP-AMP synthase (28–30). Interestingly, mice deficient in IRF3 are resistant to long-term *M. tuberculosis* infection (27). This observation is consistent with the idea that phagosome disruption is a pattern of pathogenesis. According to the pattern of pathogenesis model, phagosome disruption is sensed by a host mechanism that initiates a pathogenic response. In our case of *M. tuberculosis* infection in macrophage, cytosolic localization of *M. tuberculosis* DNA as a result of phagosome disruption triggers the STING-IRF3-type I interferon pathway responsible for pathogenesis. Indeed, prolonged induction of type I interferon by intranasal poly-L-lysine and carboxymethyl cellulose exacerbates tuberculosis in mice (31). Limiting excessive type I induction by IL-1beta confers host resistance against tuberculosis in mice (32). But *M. tuberculosis* has an ability to inhibit IL-1beta production, through a yet-to-be-defined ESX-1-dependent mechanism to suppress the AIM2 inflammasome that normally activates caspase-1 and triggers IL-1beta production upon recognizing cytosolic DNA (33). Consistent with these observations, excessive induction of type I interferon and reduced IL-1beta responses in tuberculosis patients are associated with tuberculosis exacerbation (32). Furthermore, transcriptional signature dominated by type I interferon signaling correlates strongly with the radiological extent of disease in patients with active tuberculosis and the signature reverts back to the levels seen in healthy controls after anti-*M. tuberculosis* treatment (34). Taken together, phagosome disruption as a result of ESX-1 is responsible for the pathogenesis of tuberculosis, at least in part through induction of type I interferon production by cytosolic *M. tuberculosis* DNA.

Third, cytosolic access enables peptidoglycan recognition by the cytosolic receptor NOD2 (35). *M. tuberculosis* induces the NOD2 pathway in an ESX-1-dependent fashion (36). This induction triggers type I interferon expression (36). Additionally, the NOD2 pathway also plays an important role in apoptosis (35). A role for NOD2 in apoptosis is consistent with the demonstration of a key role for ESX-1 in apoptosis induction by Aguilo et al. (37). Although the authors do not show that the ESAT-6-induced apoptosis is mediated by the NOD2 pathway, they do show that induction of apoptosis requires p38 MAPK activity, which is known to mediate signaling from the NOD2 pathway (38).

The fourth consequence of ESX-1-induced phagosome disruption is impairment of autophagic flux and fusions with lysosome. Autophagy is a cellular mechanism for degradation of intracellular protein aggregate. A selective form of autophagy known as xenophagy targets damaged organelles or intracellular pathogens. Indeed, autophagy has been shown to target *M. tuberculosis* for degradation in mouse macrophages (39). The initial step of autophagy involves the processing of microtubule-associated protein 1 light chain 3 (LC3) into the smaller isoform 2 (LC3-II). The processed LC3-II is then associated physically with the so-called isolation membrane, which is used eventually to engulf its targeting intracellular materials to create a closed membrane compartment known as autophagosome. Processed LC3-II recognizes polyubiquitin chains that mark intracellular contents destined for autophagy. In the case of damaged mitochondria or *M. tuberculosis*-disrupted phagosomes, the polyubiquitin chain is produced by the ubiquitin ligase parkin and then is recognized by the autophagy receptors NDP52 and p62 for LC3-II binding (40, 41). ESX-1 is necessary for polyubiquitin chain labeling and recruitments of NDP52, p62, and LC3-II on *M. tuberculosis*-containing phagosomes (42). It has been further shown that recognition of cytosolic DNA by the STING-dependent pathway is required for the polyubiquitination of *M. tuberculosis*-containing phagosome for autophagy (42). To complete the autophagy process, the autophagosome must fuse with lysosome for degradation of the phagosomal content. It is this step where autophagy is interrupted by ESX-1 (43). Indeed, ESX-1 genes are found to be critical for blocking phagosome maturation (44, 45). It remains unclear whether ESX-1 can directly permeabilize the outer autophagosomal double membrane to block fusion with lysosomes. *M. tuberculosis*-secreted effectors previously shown to block phagosome acidification and fusions with endosome or lysosome include

PtpA, SapM, and EsxH (46–48). It is probable that ESX-1 could provide access of these effectors into the cytosol and impair the autophagosome-lysosome fusion through its membrane-permeabilizing effect.

IS *M. TUBERCULOSIS* AN AMYLOID DISEASE MEDIATED BY ESX-1?

In their investigation about the role for ESX-1 in tuberculosis pathogenesis, Hsu et al. study how an ESX-1-secreted product mediates the lysis of macrophage. The authors first notice an earlier report from Ralph Isberg's group, which shows that host cell lysis caused by *Legionella pneumophila* is mediated by lethal ion fluxes as a result of the pore-forming ability of a protein secretion system and that exogenous glycine can prevent such ion fluxes as well as host lysis (49). To test whether *M. tuberculosis* may process similar pore-forming ability, Hsu et al. find that pretreatment of glycine prevents the *M. tuberculosis*-promoted macrophage lysis (2). Hsu et al. then show further that purified ESAT-6 induces ion fluxes across artificial bilayer membrane and eventual total destruction of the artificial membrane (2). Therefore, their results strongly indicate that ESAT-6 can form pores on membrane.

To further understand how ESAT-6 forms pores, Hsu et al. also observed that ESAT-6 forms structures similarly observed in amyloidogenic intermediate soluble protein (2). This intermediate structure is believed to be the precursor of insoluble amyloid fibril. In humans, amyloid aggregate is associated with several pathological conditions, including Alzheimer's disease, Parkinson diseases, and type 2 diabetes mellitus. Current consensus on amyloid diseases suggests that amyloidogenic prefibril intermediate is the most toxic entity and that aggregation of the amyloidogenic intermediate into insoluble form is a detoxification mechanism (50). The toxic species in amyloid diseases are small oligomers with pore-forming activity composed by the amyloidogenic intermediate (51). By analogy, it is possible that the amyloidogenic nature of ESAT-6 can similarly form small oligomer with pore-forming capability. According to this possibility, *M. tuberculosis* expressing an ESAT-6 mutant defective for amyloid aggregate should not possess pore-forming activity and, as a result, should not produce phenotypes associated with phagosome disruption. Such ESAT-6 mutants that are defective for forming amyloid aggregate have been described biochemically by the laboratory of David Eisenberg (52). When introduced in *M. tuberculosis*, these ESAT-6 mutants can no longer induce macrophage lysis, induce NLRP3 inflammasome, and damage phagosome (15). These observations are therefore consistent with the idea that the amyloidogenic nature of ESAT-6 is critical for disrupting the phagosomal membrane during macrophage infections. Nevertheless, this idea must be confirmed further by a demonstration of the existence of amyloid-like ESAT-6 aggregate, as well as by identification of ESAT-6 amyloid-forming inhibitors that block ESAT-6's cellular effects. In addition, ESAT-6 will not be able to form amyloid within macrophages if it cannot be present without binding to CFP-10. Thus, the amyloid hypothesis is critically dependent on showing that ESAT-6 exists in macrophages without CFP-10, which remains to be shown.

There has been some new exciting progress in Alzheimer's disease research using the approach of targeting amyloid in treating Alzheimer's disease (53). If ESAT-6 does indeed form toxic amyloid-like intermediate, the opportunity to disrupt such behavior may represent new opportunities for therapeutic intervention.

REGULATIONS OF ESX-1

ESX-1 secretion is regulated by at least two two-component sensing regulatory systems. The first one is PhoPR. A point mutation in PhoP causes drastic reduction of ESAT-6 secretion (54, 55). ESAT-6 secretion is dependent on EspA secretion (56). Expression of *espA* in turn is regulated positively by PhoPR as well as the PhoPR-regulated transcriptional factor EspR (57). Accordingly, ESAT-6 secretion can be triggered by PhoPR, since it induces *espR* and *espA* expressions. Interestingly, the transcriptional factor EspR is also a substrate of ESX-1 and is secreted by ESX-1. Raghavan et al. suggest that the secretion of the positive regulator EspR represents a negative feedback loop for the ESX-1 secretion (58). EspR is exported when ESX-1 secretion is activated. If its intracellular level falls below a threshold necessary to drive *espA* expression to replace the secreted EspA, there will not be enough EspA and ESX-1 secretion will shut down (58). However, ESX-1 secretion can resume when EspA accumulates as a result of signaling from PhoPR.

Tan et al. identify acidic pH and increase in chloride concentration as two synergistic cues sensed by PhoPR (59). These two cues correlate with phagosome maturation and immune activation. In response to these immune stresses PhoPR signals *M. tuberculosis* to turn on ESX-1 secretion. Phagosome maturation is promoted by interferon gamma (IFN-γ) (60). In mice macrophages, immune activation by IFN-γ induces effective *M. tuberculosis*-killing activities (61, 62). But IFN-γ fails to do so in human macrophages infected with *M. tuberculosis*.

Instead, it promotes necrosis in *M. tuberculosis*-infected human macrophages without harming *M. tuberculosis* (63). We have recently reported that IFN-γ promotes necrosis in *M. tuberculosis*-infected human macrophages and this process is dependent on the ESX-1 system (64). It seems plausible, although not demonstrated, that the necrosis promoted by IFN-γ is mediated by the ability of IFN-γ to promote phagosome maturation, which then activates PhoPR to promote ESX-1 secretion and ultimately cause necrosis.

Another two-component system that regulates ESX-1 is MprAB, which senses envelope stress such as protein misfolding in extracytoplasmic space. The absence of MprAB blocks secretions of ESAT-6 and EspA, but not secretion of CFP-10 (57). In the *mprAB* mutant, protein levels of EspA and ESAT-6 are unchanged although transcription of *espA* increases (57). It has been proposed that the absence of MprAB causes increased degradation resulting in defective secretion (57).

ESX-1 secretion is also regulated by ATP levels in *M. tuberculosis*. Zhang et al. show that low ATP levels shut down ESX-1 secretion system (65). Bedquiline inhibits ATP production in *Mycobacterium* species and completely blocks ESX-1 secretion (65). Sensing of low ATP levels is mediated by EspI, which is encoded by a gene within the RD1/ESX-1 locus. Mutations within the ATP-binding motif in EspI prevent turning off ESX-1 secretion, even in the presence of bedquiline (65).

ESPB: AN ESX-1 SUBSTRATE THAT TARGETS INNATE IMMUNE MECHANISMS

ESX-1 also secretes other proteins in addition to ESAT-6. One example is the 60-kDa protein EspB encoded by a gene within the RD1 locus. Chen et al. report that the *espB* mutant of *M. tuberculosis* is defective for cytotoxicity against the human macrophage cell line THP-1 (66). Interestingly, purified EspB is capable of binding to phosphatidic acid and phosphatidylserine (66). Phosphatidylserine is an "eat me" signal on the cell surface of apoptotic cells for clearance by macrophages through a mechanism known as efferocytosis. This mechanism is very effective in killing *M. tuberculosis* that resides within apoptotic cells (67). EspB could therefore block efferocytosis through disrupting phosphatidylserine signaling, although this idea awaits confirmation (66). In addition, EspB can inhibit autophagosome formation induced by INF-γ in murine macrophages (68). This result is consistent with the phosphatidic acid binding ability of EspB, because phosphatidic acid is an important intracellular signal for autophagy (69). Taken together, EspB can affect membrane-mediated innate immune mechanisms through binding of phosphatidic acid and phosphatidylserine. Two recent structural studies suggest that exported EspB forms an oligomeric structure with a central pore (70, 71). Since EspB can interact with membrane, it is very possible that the oligomeric EspB can form a membrane pore that facilitates phagosome permeabilization within infected macrophages.

INTERVENTIONS BY TARGET ESX-1 SECRETION

Since *M. tuberculosis* mutants carrying a defect in ESX-1 lose the ability to cause diseases in multiple animal models, drugs that target ESX-1 may lead to potential antituberculosis drugs. Several groups have performed compound library screens and have succeeded in identifying several ESX-1 inhibitors (72). Using a *M. tuberculosis* strain carrying a fluorescence reporter under an acid-inducible PhoPR promoter, Johnson et al. screen for inhibitors that block the PhoPR regulation (73). They identify ethozolamide as an ESX-1 inhibitor. Interestingly, the compound inhibits *M. tuberculosis* carbonic anhydrase activity, which has not previously been linked to PhoPR signaling (73).

Rybniker et al. screen for inhibitors that prevent fibroblast killing by *M. tuberculosis* (72). Their identified inhibitors were able to block ESAT-6 secretion, avert the block in phagosome maturation, reduce bacterial loads, and prevent *M. tuberculosis*-induced lysis. All these effects are consistent with the known roles for ESX-1 during macrophage interactions. Additionally, the screen identifies an inhibitor that targets the histidine kinase MprB and another one that affects *M. tuberculosis* metal-ion homeostasis. This observation has led the authors to uncover zinc stress as a previously unrecognized activating signal for ESX-1 (72). Just as in the previous study, Rybniker's study identifies inhibitors that target bacterial activities that have not previously been linked to regulating ESX-1.

SUMMARY

In this article, we have described several cellular pathological effects caused by the *M. tuberculosis* ESX-1. The effects include induction of necrosis, NOD2 signaling, type I interferon production, and autophagy. We then attempted to suggest that these pathological effects are mediated by the cytosolic access of *M. tuberculosis*-derived materials as a result of the phagosome-disrupting activity of the major ESX-1 substrate ESAT-6. Such activity of ESAT-6 is most likely due to its pore-forming activity at the membrane. The amyloidogenic characteristic of ESAT-6, first observed by Hsu et al., is reviewed here as a potential mechanism of membrane pore formation. In addition to ESAT-6, the ESX-1 substrate EspB interferes with membrane-mediated innate immune mechanisms such as efferocytosis and autophagy, most likely through its ability to bind phospholipids. Overall, the *M. tuberculosis* ESX-1 secretion system appears to be a specialized system for the deployment of host membrane-target proteins, whose primary function is to interrupt key steps in innate immune mechanisms against pathogens. Inhibitors that block the ESX-1 system or block host factors critical for ESX-1 toxicity have been identified and should represent attractive potential new antituberculosis drugs.

Citation. Wong K-W. 2017. The Role of ESX-1 in *Mycobacterium tuberculosis* Pathogenesis. Microbiol Spectrum 5(3): TBTB2-0001-2015.

References

1. **Behr MA, Wilson MA, Gill WP, Salamon H, Schoolnik GK, Rane S, Small PM.** 1999. Comparative genomics of BCG vaccines by whole-genome DNA microarray. *Science* **284:**1520–1523.

2. **Hsu T, Hingley-Wilson SM, Chen B, Chen M, Dai AZ, Morin PM, Marks CB, Padiyar J, Goulding C, Gingery M, Eisenberg D, Russell RG, Derrick SC, Collins FM, Morris SL, King CH, Jacobs WR Jr.** 2003. The primary mechanism of attenuation of bacillus Calmette-Guerin is a loss of secreted lytic function required for invasion of lung interstitial tissue. *Proc Natl Acad Sci USA* **100:** 12420–12425.

3. **Lewis KN, Liao R, Guinn KM, Hickey MJ, Smith S, Behr MA, Sherman DR.** 2003. Deletion of RD1 from *Mycobacterium tuberculosis* mimics bacille Calmette-Guérin attenuation. *J Infect Dis* **187:**117–123.

4. **Pym AS, Brodin P, Brosch R, Huerre M, Cole ST.** 2002. Loss of RD1 contributed to the attenuation of the live tuberculosis vaccines *Mycobacterium bovis* BCG and *Mycobacterium microti*. *Mol Microbiol* **46:**709–717.

5. **Russell DG, Cardona PJ, Kim MJ, Allain S, Altare F.** 2009. Foamy macrophages and the progression of the human tuberculosis granuloma. *Nat Immunol* **10:** 943–948.

6. **Abdallah AM, Gey van Pittius NC, Champion PA, Cox J, Luirink J, Vandenbroucke-Grauls CM, Appelmelk BJ, Bitter W.** 2007. Type VII secretion–mycobacteria show the way. *Nat Rev Microbiol* **5:**883–891.

7. **Armstrong JA, Hart PD.** 1971. Response of cultured macrophages to *Mycobacterium tuberculosis*, with observations on fusion of lysosomes with phagosomes. *J Exp Med* **134:**713–740.

8. **van der Wel N, Hava D, Houben D, Fluitsma D, van Zon M, Pierson J, Brenner M, Peters PJ.** 2007. M. tuberculo-

sis and *M. leprae* translocate from the phagolysosome to the cytosol in myeloid cells. *Cell* **129:**1287–1298.

9. **Houben D, Demangel C, van Ingen J, Perez J, Baldeón L, Abdallah AM, Caleechurn L, Bottai D, van Zon M, de Punder K, van der Laan T, Kant A, Bossers-de Vries R, Willemsen P, Bitter W, van Soolingen D, Brosch R, van der Wel N, Peters PJ.** 2012. ESX-1-mediated translocation to the cytosol controls virulence of mycobacteria. *Cell Microbiol* **14:**1287–1298.

10. **McDonough KA, Kress Y, Bloom BR.** 1993. Pathogenesis of tuberculosis: interaction of *Mycobacterium tuberculosis* with macrophages. *Infect Immun* **61:**2763–2773.

11. **Huynh KK, Eskelinen EL, Scott CC, Malevanets A, Saftig P, Grinstein S.** 2007. LAMP proteins are required for fusion of lysosomes with phagosomes. *EMBO J* **26:**313–324.

12. **Leake ES, Myrvik QN, Wright MJ.** 1984. Phagosomal membranes of *Mycobacterium bovis* BCG-immune alveolar macrophages are resistant to disruption by *Mycobacterium tuberculosis* H37Rv. *Infect Immun* **45:**443–446.

13. **Myrvik QN, Leake ES, Wright MJ.** 1984. Disruption of phagosomal membranes of normal alveolar macrophages by the H37Rv strain of *Mycobacterium tuberculosis*. A correlate of virulence. *Am Rev Respir Dis* **129:**322–328.

14. **Paz I, Sachse M, Dupont N, Mounier J, Cederfur C, Enninga J, Leffler H, Poirier F, Prevost MC, Lafont F, Sansonetti P.** 2010. Galectin-3, a marker for vacuole lysis by invasive pathogens. *Cell Microbiol* **12:**530–544.

15. **Wong KW, Jacobs WR Jr.** 2011. Critical role for NLRP3 in necrotic death triggered by *Mycobacterium tuberculosis*. *Cell Microbiol* **13:**1371–1384.

16. **Simeone R, Bobard A, Lippmann J, Bitter W, Majlessi L, Brosch R, Enninga J.** 2012. Phagosomal rupture by *Mycobacterium tuberculosis* results in toxicity and host cell death. *PLoS Pathog* **8:**e1002507.

17. **Simeone R, Sayes F, Song O, Gröschel MI, Brodin P, Brosch R, Majlessi L.** 2015. Cytosolic access of *Mycobacterium tuberculosis*: critical impact of phagosomal acidification control and demonstration of occurrence in vivo. *PLoS Pathog* **11:**e1004650.

18. **Vance RE, Isberg RR, Portnoy DA.** 2009. Patterns of pathogenesis: discrimination of pathogenic and non-pathogenic microbes by the innate immune system. *Cell Host Microbe* **6:**10–21.

19. **Mishra BB, Moura-Alves P, Sonawane A, Hacohen N, Griffiths G, Moita LF, Anes E.** 2010. *Mycobacterium tuberculosis* protein ESAT-6 is a potent activator of the NLRP3/ASC inflammasome. *Cell Microbiol* **12:**1046–1063.

20. **Schneider BE, Korbel D, Hagens K, Koch M, Raupach B, Enders J, Kaufmann SH, Mittrücker HW, Schaible UE.** 2010. A role for IL-18 in protective immunity against *Mycobacterium tuberculosis*. *Eur J Immunol* **40:**396–405.

21. **Mayer-Barber KD, Barber DL, Shenderov K, White SD, Wilson MS, Cheever A, Kugler D, Hieny S, Caspar P, Núñez G, Schlueter D, Flavell RA, Sutterwala FS, Sher A.** 2010. Caspase-1 independent IL-1beta production is critical for host resistance to *Mycobacterium tuberculosis* and does not require TLR signaling in vivo. *J Immunol* **184:**3326–3330.

22. Orme IM. 2014. A new unifying theory of the pathogenesis of tuberculosis. *Tuberculosis (Edinb)* 94:8–14.

23. Compan V, Baroja-Mazo A, López-Castejón G, Gomez AI, Martínez CM, Angosto D, Montero MT, Herranz AS, Bazán E, Reimers D, Mulero V, Pelegrín P. 2012. Cell volume regulation modulates NLRP3 inflammasome activation. *Immunity* 37:487–500.

24. Ip WK, Medzhitov R. 2015. Macrophages monitor tissue osmolarity and induce inflammatory response through NLRP3 and NLRC4 inflammasome activation. *Nat Commun* 6:6931.

25. King CH, Mundayoor S, Crawford JT, Shinnick TM. 1993. Expression of contact-dependent cytolytic activity by *Mycobacterium tuberculosis* and isolation of the genomic locus that encodes the activity. *Infect Immun* 61:2708–2712.

26. Stanley SA, Johndrow JE, Manzanillo P, Cox JS. 2007. The Type I IFN response to infection with *Mycobacterium tuberculosis* requires ESX-1-mediated secretion and contributes to pathogenesis. *J Immunol* 178:3143–3152.

27. Manzanillo PS, Shiloh MU, Portnoy DA, Cox JS. 2012. *Mycobacterium tuberculosis* activates the DNA-dependent cytosolic surveillance pathway within macrophages. *Cell Host Microbe* 11:469–480.

28. Collins AC, Cai H, Li T, Franco LH, Li XD, Nair VR, Scharn CR, Stamm CE, Levine B, Chen ZJ, Shiloh MU. 2015. Cyclic GMP-AMP synthase is an innate immune DNA sensor for *Mycobacterium tuberculosis*. *Cell Host Microbe* 17:820–828.

29. Wassermann R, Gulen MF, Sala C, Perin SG, Lou Y, Rybniker J, Schmid-Burgk JL, Schmidt T, Hornung V, Cole ST, Ablasser A. 2015. *Mycobacterium tuberculosis* differentially activates cGAS- and inflammasome-dependent intracellular immune responses through ESX-1. *Cell Host Microbe* 17:799–810.

30. Watson RO, Bell SL, MacDuff DA, Kimmey JM, Diner EJ, Olivas J, Vance RE, Stallings CL, Virgin HW, Cox JS. 2015. The cytosolic sensor cGAS detects *Mycobacterium tuberculosis* DNA to induce type I interferons and activate autophagy. *Cell Host Microbe* 17:811–819.

31. Antonelli LR, Gigliotti Rothfuchs A, Gonçalves R, Roffê E, Cheever AW, Bafica A, Salazar AM, Feng CG, Sher A. 2010. Intranasal poly-IC treatment exacerbates tuberculosis in mice through the pulmonary recruitment of a pathogen-permissive monocyte/macrophage population. *J Clin Invest* 120:1674–1682.

32. Mayer-Barber KD, Andrade BB, Oland SD, Amaral EP, Barber DL, Gonzales J, Derrick SC, Shi R, Kumar NP, Wei W, Yuan X, Zhang G, Cai Y, Babu S, Catalfamo M, Salazar AM, Via LE, Barry CE III, Sher A. 2014. Host-directed therapy of tuberculosis based on interleukin-1 and type I interferon crosstalk. *Nature* 511:99–103.

33. Shah S, Bohsali A, Ahlbrand SE, Srinivasan L, Rathinam VA, Vogel SN, Fitzgerald KA, Sutterwala FS, Briken V. 2013. Cutting edge: mycobacterium tuberculosis but not nonvirulent mycobacteria inhibits IFN-β and AIM2 inflammasome-dependent IL-1β production via its ESX-1 secretion system. *J Immunol* 191:3514–3518.

34. Berry MP, Graham CM, McNab FW, Xu Z, Bloch SA, Oni T, Wilkinson KA, Banchereau R, Skinner J, Wilkinson RJ, Quinn C, Blankenship D, Dhawan R, Cush JJ, Mejias A, Ramilo O, Kon OM, Pascual V, Banchereau J, Chaussabel D, O'Garra A. 2010. An interferon-inducible neutrophil-driven blood transcriptional signature in human tuberculosis. *Nature* 466:973–977.

35. Inohara N, Nuñez G. 2003. NODs: intracellular proteins involved in inflammation and apoptosis. *Nat Rev Immunol* 3:371–382.

36. Pandey AK, Yang Y, Jiang Z, Fortune SM, Coulombe F, Behr MA, Fitzgerald KA, Sassetti CM, Kelliher MA. 2009. NOD2, RIP2 and IRF5 play a critical role in the type I interferon response to *Mycobacterium tuberculosis*. *PLoS Pathog* 5:e1000500.

37. Aguilo JI, Alonso H, Uranga S, Marinova D, Arbués A, de Martino A, Anel A, Monzon M, Badiola J, Pardo J, Brosch R, Martin C. 2013. ESX-1-induced apoptosis is involved in cell-to-cell spread of *Mycobacterium tuberculosis*. *Cell Microbiol* 15:1994–2005.

38. Yao Q. 2013. Nucleotide-binding oligomerization domain containing 2: structure, function, and diseases. *Semin Arthritis Rheum* 43:125–130.

39. Gutierrez MG, Master SS, Singh SB, Taylor GA, Colombo MI, Deretic V. 2004. Autophagy is a defense mechanism inhibiting BCG and *Mycobacterium tuberculosis* survival in infected macrophages. *Cell* 119:753–766.

40. Manzanillo PS, Ayres JS, Watson RO, Collins AC, Souza G, Rae CS, Schneider DS, Nakamura K, Shiloh MU, Cox JS. 2013. The ubiquitin ligase parkin mediates resistance to intracellular pathogens. *Nature* 501:512–516.

41. Geisler S, Holmström KM, Skujat D, Fiesel FC, Rothfuss OC, Kahle PJ, Springer W. 2010. PINK1/Parkin-mediated mitophagy is dependent on VDAC1 and p62/SQSTM1. *Nat Cell Biol* 12:119–131.

42. Watson RO, Manzanillo PS, Cox JS. 2012. Extracellular M. tuberculosis DNA targets bacteria for autophagy by activating the host DNA-sensing pathway. *Cell* 150:803–815.

43. Romagnoli A, Etna MP, Giacomini E, Pardini M, Remoli ME, Corazzari M, Falasca L, Goletti D, Gafa V, Simeone R, Delogu G, Piacentini M, Brosch R, Fimia GM, Coccia EM. 2012. ESX-1 dependent impairment of autophagic flux by *Mycobacterium tuberculosis* in human dendritic cells. *Autophagy* 8:1357–1370.

44. Brodin P, Poquet Y, Levillain F, Peguillet I, Larrouy-Maumus G, Gilleron M, Ewann F, Christophe T, Fenistein D, Jang J, Jang MS, Park SJ, Rauzier J, Carralot JP, Shrimpton R, Genovesio A, Gonzalo-Asensio JA, Puzo G, Martin C, Brosch R, Stewart GR, Gicquel B, Neyrolles O. 2010. High content phenotypic cell-based visual screen identifies *Mycobacterium tuberculosis* acyltrehalose-containing glycolipids involved in phagosome remodeling. *PLoS Pathog* 6:e1001100.

45. MacGurn JA, Cox JS. 2007. A genetic screen for *Mycobacterium tuberculosis* mutants defective for phagosome maturation arrest identifies components of the ESX-1 secretion system. *Infect Immun* 75:2668–2678.

46. Mehra A, Zahra A, Thompson V, Sirisaengtaksin N, Wells A, Porto M, Köster S, Penberthy K, Kubota Y, Dricot A, Rogan D, Vidal M, Hill DE, Bean AJ, Philips

JA. 2013. *Mycobacterium tuberculosis* type VII secreted effector EsxH targets host ESCRT to impair trafficking. *PLoS Pathog* 9:e1003734.

47. Wong D, Bach H, Sun J, Hmama Z, Av-Gay Y. 2011. *Mycobacterium tuberculosis* protein tyrosine phosphatase (PtpA) excludes host vacuolar-H+-ATPase to inhibit phagosome acidification. *Proc Natl Acad Sci USA* 108:19371–19376.

48. Vergne I, Chua J, Lee HH, Lucas M, Belisle J, Deretic V. 2005. Mechanism of phagolysosome biogenesis block by viable *Mycobacterium tuberculosis*. *Proc Natl Acad Sci USA* 102:4033–4038.

49. Kirby JE, Vogel JP, Andrews HL, Isberg RR. 1998. Evidence for pore-forming ability by *Legionella pneumophila*. *Mol Microbiol* 27:323–336.

50. Lansbury PT Jr. 1999. Evolution of amyloid: what normal protein folding may tell us about fibrillogenesis and disease. *Proc Natl Acad Sci USA* 96:3342–3344.

51. Demuro A, Mina E, Kayed R, Milton SC, Parker I, Glabe CG. 2005. Calcium dysregulation and membrane disruption as a ubiquitous neurotoxic mechanism of soluble amyloid oligomers. *J Biol Chem* 280:17294–17300.

52. Wang L, Maji SK, Sawaya MR, Eisenberg D, Riek R. 2008. Bacterial inclusion bodies contain amyloid-like structure. *PLoS Biol* 6:e195.

53. Reardon S. 2015. Antibody drugs for Alzheimer's show glimmers of promise. *Nature* 523:509–510.

54. Frigui W, Bottai D, Majlessi L, Monot M, Josselin E, Brodin P, Garnier T, Gicquel B, Martin C, Leclerc C, Cole ST, Brosch R. 2008. Control of *M. tuberculosis* ESAT-6 secretion and specific T cell recognition by PhoP. *PLoS Pathog* 4:e33.

55. Lee JS, Krause R, Schreiber J, Mollenkopf HJ, Kowall J, Stein R, Jeon BY, Kwak JY, Song MK, Patron JP, Jorg S, Roh K, Cho SN, Kaufmann SH. 2008. Mutation in the transcriptional regulator PhoP contributes to avirulence of *Mycobacterium tuberculosis* H37Ra strain. *Cell Host Microbe* 3:97–103.

56. Fortune SM, Jaeger A, Sarracino DA, Chase MR, Sassetti CM, Sherman DR, Bloom BR, Rubin EJ. 2005. Mutually dependent secretion of proteins required for mycobacterial virulence. *Proc Natl Acad Sci USA* 102:10676–10681.

57. Cao G, Howard ST, Zhang P, Wang X, Chen XL, Samten B, Pang X. 2015. EspR, a regulator of the ESX-1 secretion system in *Mycobacterium tuberculosis*, is directly regulated by the two-component systems MprAB and PhoPR. *Microbiology* 161:477–489.

58. Raghavan S, Manzanillo P, Chan K, Dovey C, Cox JS. 2008. Secreted transcription factor controls *Mycobacterium tuberculosis* virulence. *Nature* 454:717–721.

59. Tan S, Sukumar N, Abramovitch RB, Parish T, Russell DG. 2013. *Mycobacterium tuberculosis* responds to chloride and pH as synergistic cues to the immune status of its host cell. *PLoS Pathog* 9:e1003282.

60. Via LE, Fratti RA, McFalone M, Pagan-Ramos E, Deretic D, Deretic V. 1998. Effects of cytokines on mycobacterial phagosome maturation. *J Cell Sci* 111:897–905.

61. Denis M. 1991. Interferon-gamma-treated murine macrophages inhibit growth of tubercle bacilli via the generation of reactive nitrogen intermediates. *Cell Immunol* 132:150–157.

62. Herbst S, Schaible UE, Schneider BE. 2011. Interferon gamma activated macrophages kill mycobacteria by nitric oxide induced apoptosis. *PLoS One* 6:e19105.

63. Warwick-Davies J, Dhillon J, O'Brien L, Andrew PW, Lowrie DB. 1994. Apparent killing of *Mycobacterium tuberculosis* by cytokine-activated human monocytes can be an artefact of a cytotoxic effect on the monocytes. *Clin Exp Immunol* 96:214–217.

64. Wong KW, Jacobs WR Jr. 2013. *Mycobacterium tuberculosis* exploits human interferon γ to stimulate macrophage extracellular trap formation and necrosis. *J Infect Dis* 208:109–119.

65. Zhang M, Chen JM, Sala C, Rybniker J, Dhar N, Cole ST. 2014. EspI regulates the ESX-1 secretion system in response to ATP levels in *Mycobacterium tuberculosis*. *Mol Microbiol* 93:1057–1065.

66. Chen JM, Zhang M, Rybniker J, Boy-Röttger S, Dhar N, Pojer F, Cole ST. 2013. *Mycobacterium tuberculosis* EspB binds phospholipids and mediates EsxA-independent virulence. *Mol Microbiol* 89:1154–1166.

67. Martin CJ, Booty MG, Rosebrock TR, Nunes-Alves C, Desjardins DM, Keren I, Fortune SM, Remold HG, Behar SM. 2012. Efferocytosis is an innate antibacterial mechanism. *Cell Host Microbe* 12:289–300.

68. Huang D, Bao L. 2016. *Mycobacterium tuberculosis* EspB protein suppresses interferon-γ-induced autophagy in murine macrophages. *J Microbiol Immunol Infect* 49:859–865. 10.1016/j.jmii.2014.11.008.

69. Bruntz RC, Lindsley CW, Brown HA. 2014. Phospholipase D signaling pathways and phosphatidic acid as therapeutic targets in cancer. *Pharmacol Rev* 66:1033–1079.

70. Korotkova N, Piton J, Wagner JM, Boy-Röttger S, Japaridze A, Evans TJ, Cole ST, Pojer F, Korotkov KV. 2015. Structure of EspB, a secreted substrate of the ESX-1 secretion system of *Mycobacterium tuberculosis*. *J Struct Biol* 191:236–244.

71. Solomonson M, Setiaputra D, Makepeace KA, Lameignere E, Petrotchenko EV, Conrady DG, Bergeron JR, Vuckovic M, DiMaio F, Borchers CH, Yip CK, Strynadka NC. 2015. Structure of EspB from the ESX-1 type VII secretion system and insights into its export mechanism. *Structure* 23:571–583.

72. Rybniker J, Chen JM, Sala C, Hartkoorn RC, Vocat A, Benjak A, Boy-Röttger S, Zhang M, Székely R, Greff Z, Orfi L, Szabadkai I, Pató J, Kéri G, Cole ST. 2014. Anticytolytic screen identifies inhibitors of mycobacterial virulence protein secretion. *Cell Host Microbe* 16:538–548.

73. Johnson BK, Colvin CJ, Needle DB, Mba Medie F, Champion PA, Abramovitch RB. 2015. The carbonic anhydrase inhibitor ethoxzolamide inhibits the *Mycobacterium tuberculosis* PhoPR regulon and Esx-1 secretion and attenuates virulence. *Antimicrob Agents Chemother* 59:4436–4445.

Tuberculosis and the Tubercle Bacillus, 2nd ed.
Edited by William R. Jacobs, Jr., Helen McShane, Valerie Mizrahi, and Ian M. Orme
© 2018 American Society for Microbiology, Washington, DC
doi:10.1128/microbiolspec.TBTB2-0025-2016

The Minimal Unit of Infection: *Mycobacterium tuberculosis* in the Macrophage

30

Brian C. VanderVen,[1] Lu Huang,[1]
Kyle H. Rohde,[2] and David G. Russell[1]

INTRODUCTION

Mycobacterium tuberculosis is the causative agent of human tuberculosis. The bacterium has the capacity to persist in its human host for decades prior to progressing to active disease. In fact, on balance, humans deal with *M. tuberculosis* infection quite effectively with only an estimated 5 to 10% of those infected actually ending up with clinical disease. However, because of the extraordinary penetrance of this infectious agent across the global population, this accounts for in excess of 1 million deaths due to tuberculosis every year. The combination with HIV in sub-Saharan Africa is catastrophic, and *M. tuberculosis* is now the leading cause of mortality among individuals living with HIV.

The success of *M. tuberculosis* as an infectious agent is due in large part to its ability to persist in its host, and this is due to the extraordinarily intimate association that is formed between the bacterium and its host cell. We believe firmly that, in considering tuberculosis, one should consider the infected macrophage as the "minimal unit of infection." Much of our research interests over the past 2 decades has centered on understanding how the physiology and metabolism of both bacterium and host cell are influenced and shaped by this enduring association.

Our understanding of the early events following infection is restricted predominantly to data from murine infections, and the phagocyte populations in the lung during early *M. tuberculosis* infection of mice are extremely plastic. Ernst and colleagues conducted detailed analysis of the different phagocytes infected with

green fluorescent protein (GFP)-expressing *M. tuberculosis* at different times postinfection (1). They showed that *M. tuberculosis* was differentially distributed in alveolar macrophages, recruited interstitial macrophages, monocytes, dendritic cells, and neutrophils. The potential significance of this phagocyte heterogeneity was illustrated by Leeman and colleagues who demonstrated that bulk depletion of macrophages prior to infection with a lethal challenge dose of *M. tuberculosis* improved survival of the mice; however, in contrast, specific depletion of activated macrophages was detrimental to the mice (2, 3). One interpretation of these data is that certain macrophages are required to provide a permissive niche for bacterial growth, but that depletion of classically activated macrophages reduces control of the infection. The idea that disease progression can be influenced both positively and negatively by the relative expansion of distinct subsets of phagocytes was shown elegantly by the work of Antonelli and colleagues (4). They treated mice intranasally with the type 1 interferon (IFN) inducer poly(I:C) prior to infection with *M. tuberculosis* and found that this induced a marked increase in bacterial load in the lungs. More recently, Dorhoi and colleagues showed that type 1 IFN receptor-deficient mice were partially protected from *M. tuberculosis* challenge and exhibited depressed recruitment of inflammatory monocytes to the lung (5). The data all reinforce the perception that the identity and characteristics of the host phagocyte populations present and recruited to the site of infection have a fundamental impact on bacterial survival and growth.

[1]Microbiology and Immunology, College of Veterinary Medicine, Cornell University, Ithaca, NY 14853; [2]Burnett School of Biomedical Sciences, College of Medicine, University of Central Florida, Orlando, FL 32827.

These studies all focused on the initial stages of infection prior to and during development of the acquired immune response. However, phagocyte heterogeneity is also observed in established granulomas in non-human primates (NHPs). Flynn and colleagues demonstrated that TB granulomas in macaques contain many diverse types of phagocytes that express different surface markers and activation proteins such as Arg1, Arg2, inducible nitric oxide synthase (iNOS), and endothelial nitric oxide synthase (eNOS) (6). These data were the basis for a model for granuloma progression driven by macrophage polarization developed by Kirschner and Flynn (7). They argue that macrophage polarization ratios are predictive of granuloma outcome and that stable, necrotic granulomas with low bacterial burden and limited inflammation are characterized by transient intervals of NF-κB activation. The heterogeneity in phagocyte phenotype is also reflected in the heterogeneous balance of lymphocyte subsets in different granulomas in *M. tuberculosis*-infected macaques (8).

Clearly, the dynamics of the *M. tuberculosis*-phagocyte interaction *in vivo* are extremely complex. How does one start to unravel the potential significance of this *in vivo* heterogeneity in phagocyte populations on bacteria fitness and growth, and the progression of disease? In this review, we explore how the understanding of experimental *M. tuberculosis* infections of murine bone marrow-derived macrophage in tissue culture, as a defined, manipulable model system, can be used to develop and validate tools to probe the extraordinary heterogeneity of the *in vivo* infection. Finally, and more significantly, the incorporation of the host phagocyte into drug discovery programs allows identification of metabolic targets unique to the intracellular environment exploited by *M. tuberculosis*.

PHAGOCYTOSIS AND BEYOND

M. tuberculosis is internalized by classic phagocytosis. Normally, particles phagocytosed by macrophages are delivered to the acidic, hydrolytic environment of the lysosome, but *M. tuberculosis* has evolved strategies to arrest phagosome maturation (9). The compartment in which *M. tuberculosis* resides has a slightly acidified pH (pH 6.4), remains accessible to the endosomal network, and exhibits minimal acquisition of lysosomal hydrolases. Classic activation of the macrophage with gamma interferon (IFN-γ) prior to infection enables the macrophage to overcome this blockade and deliver the bacterium to a more acidic compartment (10, 11). The ultimate killing of *M. tuberculosis* by activated

macrophages is dependent on multiple factors, most significantly, the production of nitric oxide (NO), the low pH of the lysosome, and the delivery of antimicrobial peptides through the process of autophagy (12–14).

Several publications document the ability of *M. tuberculosis* to escape the phagosome and access the cytosol of its host cell (15–18). However, this event appears to precipitate the necrotic death of the infected macrophage; therefore, we feel it is a transient event that may have significance with respect to the pathology observed in late-stage disease, but is of less importance to the long-term survival of the pathogen across the phagocyte populations of its host. We believe that, temporally and spatially, the intravacuolar population of *M. tuberculosis* represents a more significant target for therapeutics (19).

RESPONSE OF *M. TUBERCULOSIS* TO THE INTRACELLULAR ENVIRONMENT

Schnappinger and colleagues published the first transcriptional profiling analysis of *M. tuberculosis* in macrophages under differing levels of immune activation (20). These data indicate that *M. tuberculosis* perceived the environment within the macrophage as a hostile environment and exhibited upregulation of the expression of genes associated with both DNA damage and cell wall attack. The bacterium also showed upregulation of genes linked to fatty acid metabolism as opposed to glucose metabolism.

More recently, we have probed the response of *M. tuberculosis* to the phagosomal environment by transcriptional profiling with two goals in mind (21, 22). The first goal was to link transcriptional responses to specific environmental cues encountered within the phagosome of the macrophage, and the second was to exploit that information to build fluorescent reporter bacterial strains that could be used to inform us of the functionally significant heterogeneity of the bacterial populations in different infection models (23). Transcriptional profiling is an extremely powerful approach, but the data generated are always going to represent an average across the bacterial population; because heterogeneity exists in both the host phagocytes and the bacterial population, it is critical that we develop effective means of assessing bacterial fitness and growth across the spectrum of phagocyte populations that the bacterium infects *in vivo*.

Rohde and colleagues developed a long-term culture infection model that allowed us to maintain *M. tuberculosis* in macrophage culture for 14 days (Fig. 1) (24).

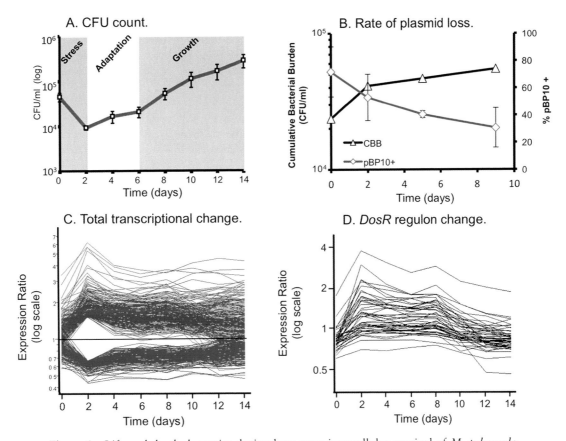

Figure 1 Life and death dynamics during long-term intracellular survival of *M. tuberculosis*. (**A**) Survival assays. Resting murine bone marrow-derived macrophages were infected at low multiplicity of infection (~1:1) with *M. tuberculosis* CDC1551. Viable CFU were quantified at day 0 and at 2-day intervals postinfection (p.i.) over a 14-day time course by lysis of monolayers, serial dilution, and plating on 7H10 medium. Error bars indicate standard error of the mean. (**B**) Replication clock plasmid. The percentage of bacteria containing the pBP10 plasmid during growth in resting macrophages was determined by comparing CFU (mean ± standard deviation) recovered on kanamycin versus nonselective media (red). The cumulative bacterial burden (CBB) (black) was determined by mathematical modeling based on total viable CFU and plasmid frequency data. Data shown represent two independent experiments. (**C**) The "bottleneck" response. Temporal expression profiles of genes differentially regulated at day 2 p.i., including genes from A that were upregulated (red) or downregulated (blue) >1.5-fold (shown as ratio of signal intensity relative to control). Note the maximal change in transcript levels at day 2 p.i. followed by majority trending back toward control levels. (**D**) "Guilt by association" analysis. Genes regulated in sync with known virulence regulons. i.e., the DosR regulon, were identified by using a highly regulated member of this regulon, *hspX*, in place of synthetic profiles. This figure is reproduced from Rohde et al. (24).

Interestingly, the most marked transcriptional response was at 2 days postinfection, with the profile trending toward the mean over the rest of the infection period. Determination of the CFU counts indicated that there was an initial drop in bacterial viability over the first 2 days, confirming that the transition was stressful for *M. tuberculosis*. Interestingly, analysis of bacterial replication rates utilizing a clock plasmid developed by Gill and coworkers (25) demonstrated that bacterial

replication was rapid during early infection, slowed considerably from day 2 to 4, and then recommenced from day 4 to 6 onward. These data indicate that rapid bacterial growth appears to be inconsistent with survival within the phagosomal environment of the macrophage. If one maps the temporal changes in transcriptional profile of genes of known association, such as those in the DosR stress regulon, one observes increased expression from day 0 to 2, a relatively sustained level of expression from day 2 to 6, and then decreasing abundance of transcripts from day 6 onward, as the bacterial population reenters growth phase.

Homolka and colleagues extended these analyses in a comparison between two laboratory strains (CDC1551 and H37Rv) and 15 clinical isolates that represented the genetic diversity of the *M. tuberculosis* complex that currently circulate within humans across the globe (26). The goal of this study was to identify the "core" or a common transcriptome expressed by *M. tuberculosis* inside macrophages. Once again, the induced expression of genes associated with hypoxia, oxidative and nitrosative stress, cell wall and DNA repair, and fatty acid metabolism across the panel of clinical isolates confirmed the previous single-strain data (20, 21).

LINKING ENVIRONMENTAL CUES AND RESPONSES

The next step in our analysis was to link the transcriptional responses to specific environmental cues. Phagosome maturation is a continuum, and it would be logical for *M. tuberculosis* to have evolved the capacity to sense and respond to gradients linked to the maturation status of its vacuole. In initial studies, we blocked phagosomal acidification with the V-ATPase inhibitor concanamycin A and compared the transcriptional profile with bacteria in unperturbed phagosomes (23, 27). In control macrophages, *M. tuberculosis* upregulated the expression of 68 genes 2 h postinternalization, whereas, in the nonacidified phagosomal environment, only 38 of these genes were upregulated. Much of this pH-dependent response was regulated by the two-component regulator *phoPR*, which included a locus, *aprABC*, that regulates the expression of genes linked to the synthesis of triacylglycerol (TAG) and phthiocerol-dimycocerosate (PDIM). In fact, *M. tuberculosis* exposed to reduced pH exhibits enhanced production of PDIMs such as phthiodiolone and phthiocerol A, which are virulence-associated lipids that are also linked to the utilization of 3-carbon intermediates like propionyl coenzyme A (propionyl-CoA) generated from the breakdown of cholesterol (28). This is discussed in greater depth later in this review.

Chloride is one of the counterions that balance the activity of the proton-ATPase responsible for phagosome acidification, and analysis of phagosome maturation using fluorogenic chemical readouts shows that the concentration of Cl⁻ increases in proportion to the reduction of pH, reaching a maximal concentration of approximately 100 mM. We have found that *M. tuber-*

culosis senses and responds to Cl⁻ over this physiological concentration range and that the expression of several genes is upregulated synergistically by exposure to a combination of lowered pH and increased Cl⁻ concentration (29).

These types of complex multigenic responses to relatively simple environmental cues are excellent examples of how bacterial regulons are molded by evolutionary pressure to facilitate pathogens, such as *M. tuberculosis*, to rapidly realign their physiology to exploit the different environmental niches to which they are exposed within their host.

CONSTRUCTION OF REPORTER STRAINS

We utilized our transcriptional profiling data to select genes that were specifically and markedly upregulated in response to environmental cues of interest. We cloned putative promoter regions from these open reading frames into a plasmid upstream of *M. tuberculosis* codon-optimized *gfp* and tested for enhanced expression of GFP under appropriate environmental conditions (23, 29). For reasons we did not pursue, many constructs did not work! Nonetheless, we currently have a panel of reporter *M. tuberculosis* strains that respond to environmental stimuli. In addition to the inducible GFP expression, these reporter plasmids also contain the mCherry gene downstream of the constitutive promoter from *smyc* (30).

We next developed a murine model of vaccination to probe the phenotype(s) of our reporter strains in the context of both naive and vaccinated hosts (31). Mice were vaccinated with heat-killed Erdman *M. tuberculosis* and challenged with three different reporter strains of Erdman *M. tuberculosis*. The bacterial strains we used responded to pH and chloride ions (*rv2390c´*::GFP, *smyc´*::mCherry), NO radicals (*hspX´*::GFP, *smyc´*::mCherry), and a replication reporter strain that contained a translational fusion between the single-strand binding protein (SSB) with the GFP protein (SSB-GFP, *smyc´*::mCherry). This latter construct had been used previously in *Escherichia coli*, where replicating bacteria form green fluorescent puncta that are associated with chromosomal replication (32). In *M. tuberculosis*, we found that this SSB-GFP positive complex persists for 70 to 80% of the replication cycle of the bacterium. We euthanized mice at 14 and 28 days postchallenge to quantify and determine the bacterial responses through imaging of thick sections from formaldehyde-fixed tissue.

The response of the *rv2390c´*::GFP, *smyc´*::mCherry reporter construct was theorized to correspond to vacuolar maturation. Interestingly, we found that the levels of induction of GFP in this reporter strain were lower in vaccinated versus naive mice at early time points, which appears counterintuitive. The data suggest that, in mock-treated mice, *M. tuberculosis* initially encounters a high [Cl⁻]/low pH environment consistent with increased phagosomal maturation, which trends toward a lower [Cl⁻]/higher pH environment at later time points. This indication of early stress during the establishment of infection is consistent with published studies in both macrophage and murine infections, which implies that bacteria coming from broth culture have to realign their physiology to be compatible with intracellular survival (22, 27). During this adjustment period, rapidly growing organisms survive poorly. The reduced expression of *rv2390c´*::GFP in the presence of an acquired immune response, observed in the current study, could be explained by either of two mechanistically divergent scenarios. First, while the adjustment in bacterial physiology required to support intracellular survival may come at a cost with respect to bacterial numbers, the realignment of bacterial physiology in the surviving bacteria may be accelerated by the presence of a preexisting immune response to *M. tuberculosis*. Or, second, bacilli expressing higher levels of *rv2390c´*::GFP may be the very bacteria that are killed most effectively by the preexisting immune response. Although the underlying mechanisms may differ, the outcome is the same: the accelerated generation of a bacterial population better equipped to survive in its host.

The presence of a preexisting immune response against *M. tuberculosis* should lead to immune activation of infected macrophages and the induction of expression of the inducible nitric oxide synthase (NOS2). Our second reporter strain, *hspX´*::GFP, *smyc´*::mCherry, was selected because of the robustness of the response of *hspX* expression to NO in culture. In this bacterium the level of expression of GFP was markedly enhanced in the vaccinated mice at day 14 postinfection but equivalent at day 28 postinfection, suggesting that expression closely mirrored development of an acquired immune response (Fig. 2). Furthermore, the levels of expression of GFP in IFN-γ-deficient and NOS2-deficient mice were considerably lower than those of wild-type mice. In addition, colabeling of the tissue with antibodies against the NOS2 demonstrated that the regions of tissue positive for NOS2 enzyme corresponded to those regions containing GFP-positive bacilli.

Our final reporter strain used in these studies contained the plasmid SSB-GFP, *smyc´*::mCherry, which reports on bacterial replication. At 14 days postchallenge, there was considerable diversity in the percentage of actively replicating *M. tuberculosis* within the various treatment groups, and no statistically significant differences between *M. tuberculosis* in vaccinated and naive mice were observed. In contrast, there were distinct differences in the relative replication status of *M. tuberculosis* between experimental groups at 28 days postchallenge. Confocal microscopy of infected tissue showed that fewer *M. tuberculosis* exhibiting SSB-GFP foci were observed in vaccinated mice as opposed to naive mice. Furthermore, consistent with the increased growth of *M. tuberculosis* in IFN-γ-deficient mice at 28 days postchallenge, we observed a greater number of bacteria positive for SSB-GFP foci in these mice. These data are consistent with the conventional view that vaccination will lead to a reduction in the number of actively replicating *M. tuberculosis* in the host.

MOVING TO THE SINGLE-CELL SUSPENSION

In these early studies, performed primarily to validate the reporter strains, we relied on histological approaches to visualize and quantify the bacterium's response to the host immune environment. Moving forward, we wanted to exploit these reporters to probe phenotypes of *M. tuberculosis* within the context of the different host phagocyte populations, utilizing methods similar to those developed by Ernst and colleagues (1, 33).

In our first study probing bacterial phenotypes in the context of phagocyte subsets during the course of infection, we investigated the impact of the immune status of the host cell on the susceptibility of the intracellular *M. tuberculosis* in response to different front-line drugs (Fig. 3) (34). Mice were infected with *M. tuberculosis* expressing mCherry for 21 days prior to euthanasia, and we generated single-cell suspensions from the infected lung tissue. We identified infected phagocytes by gating on cells that were CD11b-positive and contained mCherry-expressing *M. tuberculosis*. We then sorted infected myeloid cells into CD80-high and CD80-low populations to segregate activated versus resting *M. tuberculosis*-infected cells. Further flow cytometric analysis of these sorted populations showed that the CD80-high cells also expressed high levels of major histocompatibility complex class II and NOS2, confirming their immune-activated state. These cells were then established in culture and incubated with isoniazid (INH) or rifampin (RIF) for 24 h. Bacterial survival was then scored by counting CFUs from these isolated cells. Normalizing the bacterial burden from the drug-treated cell populations to the appropriate control

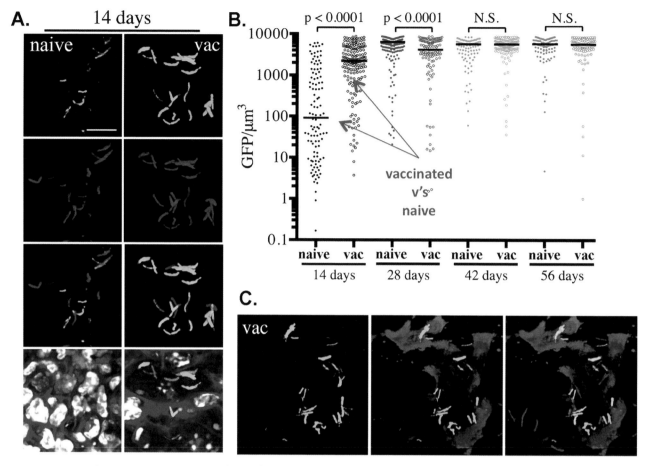

Figure 2 Demonstrating the usefulness of the *hspX´::GFP* reporter strain in assessing and reporting on the localized induction of iNOS at the site of infection. Phosphate-buffered saline-immunized (naive) mice and mice vaccinated with heat-killed *M. tuberculosis* (vac) were infected with the *hspX´*::GFP, *smyc´*::mCherry Erdman *M. tuberculosis* reporter strain. Fluorescence induction of the *hspX* promoter-dependent GFP is higher at 14 days in the vaccinated animals, as assessed by confocal microscopy of thick tissue sections (**A**) that were scored subsequently by Volocity (**B**). (**C**) The thick tissue sections were probed with antibodies against murine NOS2 (magenta), demonstrating the colocalization between GFP induction and NOS2 expression at the site(s) of infection. N.S., not significant. Data shown are detailed in Sukumar et al. (31).

populations revealed that *M. tuberculosis* in activated myeloid cells exhibited markedly decreased sensitivity to both INH and RIF. We subsequently determined that immune activation of macrophages in tissue culture induced drug tolerance to INH, RIF, pyrazinamide (PZA), and ethambutol (EMB) in the intracellular *M. tuberculosis*. We went on to demonstrate, with NOS2-deficient mice, that the expression of NO was a dominant driver of this drug-tolerant phenotype. However, the stress response induced in drug-tolerant *M. tuberculosis* is multigenic and involved upregulation of four major regulons, *dosR*, *mprA*, *phoP*, and *sigK*. The expression of the genes in these regulons is upregulated in response to exposure to NO, low pH, oxidative stress, hypoxia, membrane damage, and nutrient starvation, implying that the acquisition of a drug-tolerant phenotype could result from exposure to different host-derived stresses. These data are consistent with the previous report by Manina and colleagues documenting the phenotypic heterogeneity that the immune response to infection induces in *M. tuberculosis* and how this links to metabolic activity and drug tolerance (35).

We are currently probing the phagocyte subsets with greater resolution to determine the bacterial fitness in the different host cell populations. Similarly to the reported findings of Srivastava and colleagues

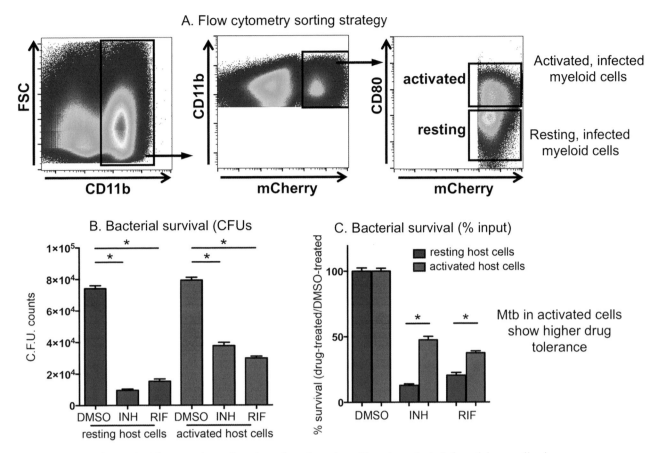

Figure 3 Flow sorting of activated and resting *M. tuberculosis*-infected host cells demonstrates that the drug sensitivity of *M. tuberculosis* recovered from *in vivo* infection correlates inversely with the immune activation status of the host phagocyte. (**A to C**) *M. tuberculosis* recovered from activated host cells *in vivo* were more tolerant to both INH and RIF than those recovered from resting host cells. C57BL/6J mice were infected with mCherry-expressing *M. tuberculosis* Erdman for 21 days, and *M. tuberculosis*-containing myeloid cells with different immune activation status isolated from lung tissue by using flow cytometry. (**A**) CD11b+ mCherry+ CD80^high cells (activated population) and CD11b+ mCherry+ CD80^low cells (resting population) were sorted according to the depicted gating strategies. (**B and C**) Isolated cells were established in culture and subjected to treatment with 1 μg/ml INH or RIF or an equivalent volume of dimethyl sulfoxide (DMSO). Following 24 h of drug treatment, bacterial survival was determined by CFU enumeration (**B**), and the percentage of *M. tuberculosis* surviving drug treatment was quantified by normalizing bacterial load in drug-treated samples against that in DMSO-treated samples (**C**). This figure is modified from the work of Liu et al. (34).

(1, 33), we detect *M. tuberculosis* in alveolar macrophages, neutrophils, recruited interstitial macrophages, and monocyte-derived dendritic cells. The relative number of bacteria in the different phagocyte subsets is extremely dynamic during the first 4 weeks of infection as the mouse transitions from a naive host to one with an acquired immune response. Some preliminary analysis of the dynamic nature of this interaction is illustrated in Fig. 4 (Huang and Russell, unpublished data). We show analysis of the single-cell suspensions isolated

from infected mouse lung tissue. The flow cytometric analysis involves the identification of live cells that are infected with reporter strains of *M. tuberculosis*, in this case the *hspX´*::GFP, *smyc´*::mCherry strain. Gating on the mCherry-positive cells, these can be subjected to preliminary assignment as alveolar macrophages, monocyte-derived dendritic cells, and recruited interstitial macrophages on the basis of the levels of surface expression of SiglecF and CD11c. The cells are fixed for further analysis to correlate the bacteria's stress

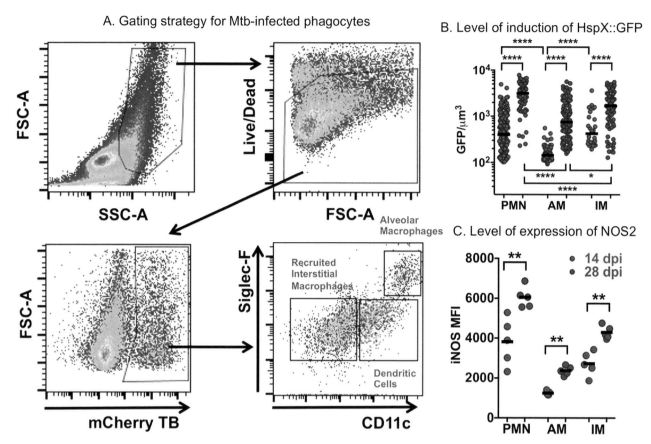

Figure 4 Examination of the bacterial stress reporter *M. tuberculosis* strain *hspX´*::GFP, *smyc´*::mCherry Erdman at the level of different host phagocyte populations in murine lung infection model. (**A**) The flow cytometry gating strategy for the identification of *M. tuberculosis*-infected phagocyte subsets from infected mouse lung, showing preliminary identification of alveolar macrophages, recruited interstitial macrophages, and monocyte-derived dendritic cell populations. (**B**) The level of expression of NO-driven GFP under regulation of the *hspX* promoter, identifying those phagocytes that induce the highest level of bacterial stress, and how the stress intensifies from 14 to 28 days postinfection. The levels of induction of expression of GFP indicate that the most stressful host cells appear to be neutrophils and the least stressful appear to be alveolar macrophages. C. Labeling of the host cells with antibody against NOS2 demonstrates the direct correlation between expression levels of the host nitric oxide synthase, NOS2, and levels of expression of the bacterial stress response reporter *hspX* ´::GFP, shown in panel B. MFI, mean fluorescence intensity; PMN, polymorphonuclear leukocytes; IM, recruited interstitial macrophages; AM, alveolar macrophages.

response status (*hspX´*::GFP) with the level of expression of the host nitric oxide synthase (NOS2). The level of induction of GFP expression in *M. tuberculosis* increases between the 14- and 28-day time points, which is consistent with the increased expression of NOS2 in the different cell subsets. The level of expression of NOS2 is lowest in the alveolar macrophages, as is the level of induction of GFP in those *M. tuberculosis*. These data suggest that the alveolar macrophage population represents a less stressful host cell environment than the other phagocyte populations shown here, but a more extensive analysis of the hypothesis that

these different phagocyte populations present differing degrees of permissiveness or control of bacterial growth is in progress. This figure is intended to show the experimental approaches behind this rationale, and not to provide a definitive answer.

Nonetheless, what these reporter strain studies have shown us is that the environment(s) within the host phagocytes is heterogeneous, both spatially and temporally, and that this heterogeneity has fundamental consequences on bacterial fitness and growth and ultimately on the progression of the infection to active disease.

CHEMICAL GENETICS OF
M. TUBERCULOSIS INFECTION
IN MACROPHAGES

Intracellular pathogens such as *M. tuberculosis* have evolved to specifically survive within their respective host cells, and these pathogens are inextricably linked to the unique constraints of the various cells they infect. With this in mind, we conducted an unbiased chemical screen designed to identify small molecules that specifically target pathways required for *M. tuberculosis* replication in macrophages. In collaboration with Vertex Pharmaceuticals, we screened a collection of ~340,000 small molecules and identified 1,359 compounds that inhibit *M. tuberculosis* replication in macrophages. Characterization of these hits revealed that only ~50% of the 300 most potent compounds (IC_{50} values < 5.0 μM in the macrophage assay) displayed equivalent inhibitory activity when *M. tuberculosis* was grown in standard Middlebrook 7H9 OADC medium. Unfortunately, the majority of these "universally active" compounds have previously been described in the literature. These compounds were likely discovered because of their ability to inhibit *M. tuberculosis* growth in standard media formulations. This class of compounds represents the classic type of antibiotics that inhibit *M. tuberculosis* growth and target essential bacterial pathways regardless of the growth conditions.

The remaining ~50% of the most potent compounds from the macrophage assay displayed no inhibitory activity against *M. tuberculosis* in 7H9 OADC media, indicating that this "macrophage active" group of compounds likely targets some aspect of *M. tuberculosis* physiology that is required for replication in macrophages (36). To begin to understand the mechanism of action for these "macrophage active" compounds, we evaluated the compounds against *M. tuberculosis* cultured in conditions thought to mimic the intraphagosomal environment. We tested these compounds when *M. tuberculosis* was exposed to *in vitro* pH and NO stresses or during growth in media that contained either fatty acids or cholesterol as carbon sources. To our surprise, we found that ~50% of the ~150 "macrophage active" compounds are cholesterol dependent and inhibit *M. tuberculosis* when the bacteria are grown in cholesterol media. On the basis of this observation, we hypothesized that some of these compounds directly target aspects of cholesterol metabolism or propionyl-CoA assimilation. To identify compounds involved in these pathways, we counterscreened all of the 1,359 hits to discover specific inhibitors of enzymes involved in propionyl-CoA assimilation through the methylcitrate cycle (MCC) or required for cholesterol breakdown. To do this, we focused on compounds that rescue *M. tuberculosis* growth from a cholesterol-dependent intoxication in an *M. tuberculosis* ΔIcl1 mutant. In this assay, compounds that inhibit key bottleneck enzymes involved in cholesterol breakdown or propionyl-CoA assimilation reversed toxicity in the *M. tuberculosis* ΔIcl1 mutant and allowed the bacteria to grow in the presence of cholesterol (36). Using this method, we have now discovered ~20 inhibitors that specifically block these metabolic pathways in *M. tuberculosis*, and these compounds have IC_{50} values between 5 and 20 μM in macrophages.

The rescue approach using the *M. tuberculosis* ΔIcl1 mutant did not reveal any putative targets for our most potent cholesterol-dependent, "macrophage active" compounds. To understand the mechanism of action for these compounds, we used transcriptional profiling to characterize the response of *M. tuberculosis* to these compounds in cholesterol media. By this approach, we discovered seven structurally unrelated compounds that prevent *M. tuberculosis* from metabolizing cholesterol as indicated by the strong downregulation of the KstR regulon (36). To further understand these compounds, we next screened an *M. tuberculosis* transposon library and isolated mutants resistant to these compounds, and we found that inactivating Rv1625c/cya conferred resistance to all seven of these compounds. The protein Rv1625c/cya is a well-characterized adenylyl cyclase that forms cAMP from ATP (37, 38). We have now confirmed that this group of compounds directly stimulates Rv1625c/cya to overproduce cAMP. These compounds are unusual in that they inhibit cholesterol utilization and induce very high levels of cAMP in *M. tuberculosis*, which can potentially perturb multiple different pathways (39–45). In addition, the high levels of cAMP produced by the *M. tuberculosis* in response to these compounds may modulate tumor necrosis factor alpha production in the infected cell by activating cytosolic sensors of cAMP in the infected macrophage (46).

Together, these data are consistent with previous observations (47–51) indicating that cholesterol is an important nutrient for *M. tuberculosis* and that pathways associated with the utilization of this molecule are required for growth in macrophages (52–55). This work further demonstrates that the cholesterol utilization pathways are "druggable" and tractable as targets for drug discovery. However, these observations do raise some new and puzzling questions such as (i) why do other nutrients, such as fatty acids, not substitute for cholesterol in supporting *M. tuberculosis* growth in macrophages; (ii) what is the link between cAMP and cholesterol metabolism; and (iii) is there an equivalent to carbon catabolite repression in *M. tuberculosis* that is activated in macrophages to govern the utilization by *M. tuberculosis* of host-derived nutrients? In recent years, our field has gained new insight into these aspects of *M. tuberculosis* physiology and pathogenesis, and here we incorporate these findings with our own observations and current understanding of *M. tuberculosis* metabolism in macrophages.

LIPID UTILIZATION BY *M. TUBERCULOSIS* IN MACROPHAGES

Although *M. tuberculosis* likely utilizes many different nutrients *in vivo* and during infection in macrophages, the bacterium appears to preferentially utilize host-derived lipids (fatty acids and cholesterol) as carbon sources to produce energy and fuel biosynthetic pathways. The notion that *M. tuberculosis* preferentially metabolizes host lipids during infection began with classic experiments reported by Segal and Bloch in 1954. These studies demonstrated that *ex vivo* respiration rates of *M. tuberculosis* isolated from mouse lung tissues were stimulated by fatty acid substrates, but not by carbohydrates (56). Consistent with the idea that lipids are important nutrients, the early genome annotation efforts revealed that *M. tuberculosis* has an expanded repertoire of genes associated with lipid metabolism and β-oxidation, which exceeded 250 genes (57). Although several of the *M. tuberculosis* genes originally annotated as having a β-oxidation function are now known to have anabolic activities (58, 59) or to act in multimeric complexes to oxidize lipids (60, 61), the *M. tuberculosis* genome still encodes more genes involved in lipid metabolism and β-oxidation relative to other bacteria. Another critical pathway that is required when bacteria metabolize lipids is the anaplerotic glyoxylate cycle, and a key enzyme in this pathway is isocitrate lyase (Icl). Early gene expression studies demonstrated that Icl1 is strongly induced by *M. tuberculosis* during infection in macrophages (62–64) and that the Icl1 gene is required for *M. tuberculosis* pathogenesis *in vivo* (53). A series of elegant experiments from John McKinney's laboratory established that *M. tuberculosis* expresses two Icl homologs (Icl1/Icl2) and that these enzymes play critical roles in lipid metabolism in the glyoxylate cycle and the methyl citrate cycle (MCC) (55, 65, 66). Early transcriptional profiling experiments of *M. tuberculosis* during infection in macrophages, reported by Schnappinger et al., found that numerous genes associated with lipid metabolism were induced in *M. tuberculosis* (20). Importantly, over one-half of the genes associated with

metabolic adaptations in this report are now known to be involved in cholesterol metabolism (FadD19, FadE27, EchA19, FadA5, FadD3, FadE28, FadE29, FadE31, and FadA6) and/or propionyl-CoA assimilation through the MCC (Icl1 and PrpC) in *M. tuberculosis* (67–69). More recent transcriptional studies on *M. tuberculosis* in macrophages demonstrated that genes involved in propionyl-CoA assimilation, lipid breakdown, and cholesterol metabolic genes are induced in *M. tuberculosis* across a 14-day infection period in macrophages (24). Last, the growth of *M. tuberculosis* on lipid-based substrates during infection in macrophages would also necessitate that *M. tuberculosis* synthesizes carbohydrates *de novo* through gluconeogenesis. Recent studies have confirmed that PckA, a key bottleneck enzyme in gluconeogenesis, is required for optimal *M. tuberculosis* growth in macrophages (70). In total, these observations continue to support the idea that *M. tuberculosis* relies heavily on lipids (fatty acids and cholesterol) as carbon sources and that the flux of propionyl-CoA through the MCC represents a critical axis in *M. tuberculosis* central metabolism during infection in macrophages.

FATTY ACIDS

M. tuberculosis can utilize exogenously acquired fatty acids as substrates for β-oxidation to produce energy and as acyl primers for polyketide lipid synthesis, or can assimilate them into phospholipids and/or TAG (59, 71). The fatty acid oxidation pathways in *M. tuberculosis* still remain largely uncharacterized, and the lipid substrates for the various β-oxidation enzymes are poorly defined. In addition to catabolism, fatty acids can be used as acyl-AMP primers for the biosynthesis of polyketide lipids (PDIM), polyacylated trehaloses (PATS), and sulfolipid (SL) (72). Interestingly, the fate of fatty acids in *M. tuberculosis* can be impacted when the bacteria metabolizes cholesterol. *M. tuberculosis* produces more PDIM and SL when the bacterium metabolizes cholesterol, and this is also observed during infection in mouse tissues (52, 73, 74). During growth on cholesterol, *M. tuberculosis* also synthesizes a modified form of PDIM and SL lipids that contain additional methyl branching, which is consistent with the assimilation of more methylmalonyl-CoA (derived from propionyl-CoA) into these lipids (52, 73, 74). Thus, metabolizing cholesterol induces the production of methyl-branched polyketide lipids, which requires a pool of available fatty acids as acyl primers. Metabolic labeling experiments with infected macrophages were used to track exogenously added ^{14}C-labeled fatty acids into PDIM and TAG (28), and we demonstrated that the growth defect of *M. tuberculosis* ΔIcl1 mutant in macrophages can be overcome by stimulating foam cell formation through the provision of excess fatty acid to the host macrophages (28). This is consistent with the idea that, during infection, fatty acids can be shunted into the anabolism of methyl-branched lipids and TAG to act as a sink for the assimilation of excess propionyl-CoA during infection (75). Fatty acids can also be assimilated directly into cell membrane phospholipids or converted into TAG. Phospholipids are required to maintain cytoplasmic membrane integrity, while TAG is classically thought to function as a carbon storage molecule that can be turned over when nutrients are limiting (71, 76). Cytosolic accumulation of TAG also negatively regulates *M. tuberculosis* growth, and exporting TAG from the bacterial cytosol appears to be required for optimal growth of *M. tuberculosis* in macrophages (77, 78). In addition to fueling biosynthesis and energy production, lipid metabolic pathways can influence the physiology of *M. tuberculosis* during infection. For example, TAG synthesis can also reduce *M. tuberculosis* growth rate and antibiotic sensitivity by reducing acetyl-CoA availability (79). The balance of fatty acid catabolism and anabolism can also influence cytosolic redox homeostasis during infection in macrophages (75).

CHOLESTEROL

Cholesterol has been repeatedly shown to be required for optimal growth and persistence of *M. tuberculosis* during infection (36, 47–49, 51, 80). Mechanisms involved in cholesterol import, side chain degradation, and early ring cleavage events have been partially characterized in *M. tuberculosis* (49, 52, 80–94). The current model is that, when cholesterol is broken down by *M. tuberculosis*, the 2- and 3-carbon intermediates acetyl-CoA, propionyl-CoA, and pyruvate are generated. The 3-carbon intermediate, propionyl-CoA, plays an important role in *M. tuberculosis* physiology, and recent studies have indicated that cholesterol is the major source of propionyl-CoA during infection in macrophages. The MCC genes (*prpC* and *prpD*) are induced by propionate and cholesterol, indicating that the transcriptional induction of *prpC* and *prpD* is activated by propionate or propionyl-CoA (52, 95). Griffin et al. demonstrated deleting the Mce4 cholesterol transporter in *M. tuberculosis* could reverse propionyl-CoA toxicity induced by the Icl1 inhibitor 3-nitropropionate (3-NP) during infection in macrophages (52). It is now understood that 3-NP not only inhibits *M. tuberculosis*

Icl1 enzyme (55), but also inhibits the *M. tuberculosis* succinate dehydrogenase in intact cells (96). Since the *prpD* promoter is responsive to cholesterol-derived propionate or propionyl-CoA, we fused the promoter region of *prpD* to GFP and made a cholesterol reporter strain in *M. tuberculosis*, *prpD´*::GFP, *smyc´*::mCherry. This reporter strain responds to cholesterol and stoichiometric amounts of propionate (Fig. 5). Importantly, the GFP signal in this reporter strain is strongly induced during infection in macrophages, and an inhibitor of *M. tuberculosis* cholesterol metabolism completely abolishes the GFP signal (Fig. 5). Together these observations support the idea that cholesterol is the major source of propionyl-CoA for *M. tuberculosis* during infection. In addition, it is likely that other sources of propionyl-CoA, such as branched-chain amino acids or odd-chain fatty acids, are minor contributors to the bacterial pools of propionyl-CoA during infection in macrophages. Whether the requirement for cholesterol for optimal growth in macrophages reflects the abundance or availability of the molecule, or a preference for the catabolic intermediates released from the molecule, remains unclear. Given that *M. tuberculosis* has the capacity to simultaneously metabolize simple substrates (97), it is puzzling why other nutrients such as fatty acids do not fully substitute for cholesterol during infection. Since the cholesterol catabolism produces only 2- and 3-carbon intermediates, this molecule may fulfill a dedicated role in *M. tuberculosis* metabolism. Fatty acids are more versatile substrates in metabolism and can be β-oxidized, stored, or used for biosynthesis. Perhaps *M. tuberculosis* uses cholesterol to fuel central metabolism and signals the bacterium to shunt fatty acids away from oxidation pathways during infection. This might explain why genetically and chemically inactivating cholesterol metabolism negatively impacts bacterial growth in macrophages despite the presence of other nutrients such as fatty acids. Clearly, this is a poorly understood area of *M. tuberculosis* physiology, and perhaps a potential therapeutic intervention could be developed that disrupts these complex pathways.

THE ROLE OF Icl AND THE MCC

It has been repeatedly demonstrated that the *M. tuberculosis* Icl enzymes are required for optimal bacterial growth in macrophages. Our understanding of this growth phenotype is complicated by the fact that *M. tuberculosis* expresses two Icl enzymes, termed Icl1 and Icl2 (65). These enzymes are also bifunctional and catalyze the isocitrate lyase reaction in the glyoxylate cycle and the methyl-isocitrate lyase reaction in

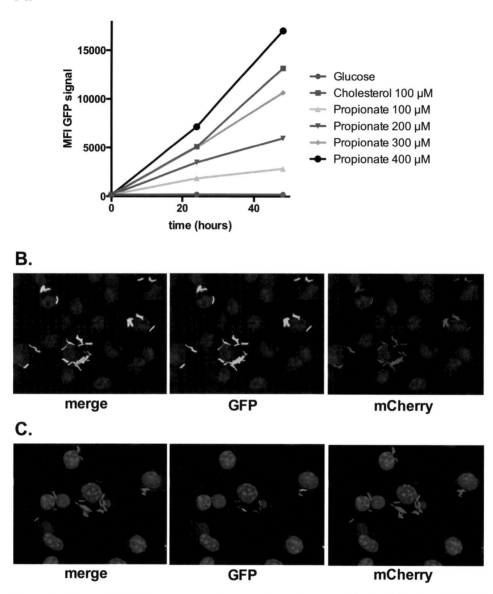

Figure 5 The *prpD´*::GFP reporter strain responds to cholesterol during infection. (**A**) GFP expression is induced with propionate and cholesterol. The GFP mean fluorescence intensity (MFI) was determined from 10,000 bacteria by flow cytometery. (**B**) Resting bone marrow-derived macrophages were infected with the *M. tuberculosis prpD´*::GFP reporter strain for 24 h. Within macrophages the *prpD´*::GFP reporter is active. (**C**) Treating macrophages infected with the *M. tuberculosis prpD´*::GFP reporter strain with one of the inhibitors of cholesterol breakdown, identified in a recent drug screen (36), abolishes induction of the reporter signal. Nuclei are stained with DAPI, and the images are courtesy of Kaley Wilburn. DAPI, 4´,6-diamidino-2-phenylindole.

the MCC, which are required for the assimilation of acetyl-CoA and propionyl-CoA, respectively. Recently, Eoh and Rhee reported a metabolomic-based characterization of the effects of blocking propionyl-CoA and acetyl-CoA assimilation in an *M. tuberculosis* Icl1/

Icl2 mutant. This work demonstrated that, when the *M. tuberculosis* Icl1/Icl2 mutant is provided, acetate or propionate inactivation of the methyl-isocitrate lyase activity is primarily responsible for bactericidal effect of the Icl1/Icl2 mutation, which depletes central metabolic intermediates, blocks gluconeogenesis, and perturbs multiple downstream aspects of cellular homeostasis (98). These studies required defined growth conditions and carbon sources to carefully quantify the isotopically labeled substrates that would make these experiments difficult to conduct with intracellular bacteria. That said, our studies with intracellular *M. tuberculosis* also indicate that the methyl-isocitrate lyase activity is principally responsible for the growth defect of the *M. tuberculosis* ΔIcl1 mutant. It is established that vitamin B$_{12}$ activates the methylmalonyl pathway and can reroute propionyl-CoA into central metabolism, bypassing the MCC (99). Adding vitamin B$_{12}$ to macrophages infected with *M. tuberculosis* ΔIcl1 mutant restores growth of the mutant to wild-type levels (28). This vitamin B$_{12}$-dependent growth restoration could be interpreted as simply opening an additional anaplerotic pathway that fuels central metabolism, but we do not think this is the case, because chemically or genetically inactivating *prpC* in an *M. tuberculosis* ΔIcl1 background also rescues growth of the bacteria to wild-type levels in 7H9 OADC containing cholesterol and in macrophages (36). Because this chemical and genetic rescue occurs without seemingly opening any anaplerotic route for propionyl-CoA, it is likely that the "dead-ended" MCC pathway in the *M. tuberculosis* ΔIcl1 mutant allows the accumulation of a toxic intermediate metabolite of the MCC and is responsible for the growth defect of this mutant.

LIPID ACQUISITION FROM THE HOST CELL

The mechanisms required for the bacterial acquisition of host-derived lipids are another poorly understood aspect of *M. tuberculosis* pathogenesis and physiology. Microscopy-based studies indicate that phagosomes containing *M. tuberculosis* can interact with lipid-loaded droplets in foamy macrophages (100, 101), and exogenously added radiolabeled fatty acids can be incorporated by *M. tuberculosis* during intracellular growth (28, 71). However, it remains unclear whether the fatty acids were acquired from host lipid droplets, membrane bilayers, or other sources. One possibility is that *M. tuberculosis* acquires cholesterol and fatty acids from serum-derived lipoproteins that traffic within the macrophage endocytic network (102). Serum lipoproteins can be internalized by macrophages using the same scavenger receptor as the *M. tuberculosis* bacillus (103).

On the bacterial side, the mycobacterial Mce4 cholesterol transporter complex is involved in the assimilation of host cholesterol during infection (50). Interestingly, a mutant lacking the permease subunit of

the Mce4 transporter can grow on cholesterol as a sole carbon source after a lag period, and the mutant can partially metabolize the substrate (50). This suggests that cholesterol transport is redundant, or a compensatory pathway exists in *M. tuberculosis* to assimilate either the intact sterol or some form of the molecule. In preliminary studies we have observed a ~50% reduction in GFP expression using our *prpD'*::GFP, *smyc'*::mCherry reporter in an *M. tuberculosis* ΔMce4 mutant during infection in macrophages (data not shown). Together, these observations indicate that Mce4 is clearly involved in cholesterol assimilation, but, during infection, some form of the sterol may still be metabolized to propionyl-CoA in the Mce4 mutant. Despite the important role fatty acids play in *M. tuberculosis* physiology, our understanding of how fatty acids are transported across the *M. tuberculosis* cell envelope remains incomplete.

MANIPULATING THE HOST CELL FOR NUTRITIONAL PURPOSES

The immune response mounted against *M. tuberculosis* also perturbs the host cell metabolism to seemingly favor *M. tuberculosis* survival. For example, chronic inflammation observed in human tuberculosis leads to the accumulation of lipid-loaded foamy macrophages that are infected with *M. tuberculosis*, and the development of these cells is associated with transcriptional and metabolic reprogramming of cells within the granuloma (100, 104). One mechanism involved in remodeling the macrophage is reliant on *M. tuberculosis* activation of peroxisome proliferator-activated receptors (PPARs) (105). PPARs are a family of transcription factors that respond to fatty acid metabolites and that, during *M. tuberculosis* infection, increase PPARγ expression in a Toll-like receptor 2-dependent manner, leading to foam cell formation (105–107). Conversely, antagonists of PPARγ downregulate the lipid content of infected macrophages, which has a negative effect on intracellular growth of *M. tuberculosis* (106–108). Many of the mechanisms involved in foam cell formation remain uncharacterized, but a recent report suggested that *M. tuberculosis* infection may stimulate PPARγ to increase the expression of CD36 through testicular receptor 4 (109). CD36 is a low-density lipoprotein receptor that is involved in uptake of serum-derived lipoproteins, and this may increase the lipid concentration and drive foam cell formation. Another mechanism, recently described by Singh et al., demonstrates that *M. tuberculosis* infection induces glycolysis in infected macrophages, which can drive foam cell formation (110). Specifically, *M. tuberculosis*-directed dysregulation of the antilipolytic G-protein-coupled receptor GPR109A in infected cells leads to increased lipid droplet accumulation and a permissive bacterial growth environment.

CONCLUSION

The interaction between *M. tuberculosis* and its host cell is highly complex and extremely intimate. Were it not for the disease, one might regard this interaction at the cellular level as an almost symbiotic one. The metabolic activity and physiology of both cells are shaped by this coexistence. We believe that where this appreciation has greatest significance is in the field of drug discovery. Evolution rewards efficiency, and recent data from many groups discussed in this review indicate that *M. tuberculosis* has evolved to utilize the environmental cues within its host to control large genetic responses or regulons. However, these regulons may represent chinks in the bacterium's armor because they can constrain the metabolic plasticity of *M. tuberculosis*. The prime example is how the presence of cholesterol within the host cell appears to limit the ability of *M. tuberculosis* to utilize or assimilate other carbon sources (36). And that is the reason for this title of this review. We believe firmly that to understand the physiology of *M. tuberculosis*, and to identify new drug targets, it is imperative that the bacterium be interrogated within the context of its host cell. The *M. tuberculosis*-infected macrophage truly is the "minimal unit of infection."

Acknowledgments. The authors would like to acknowledge the support of the U.S. Public Health Services through the National Institutes of Health awards AI118582, AI067027, and HL055936 (to D.G.R.) and AI099569 and AI119122 (to B.C.V.). D.G.R. is also grateful for the support of the Bill & Melinda Gates Foundation.

Citation. VanderVen BC, Huang L, Rohde KH, Russell DG. 2016. The minimal unit of infection: *Mycobacterium tuberculosis* in the macrophage. Microbiol Spectrum 4(6):TBTB2-0025-2016.

References

1. Srivastava S, Ernst JD, Desvignes L. 2014. Beyond macrophages: the diversity of mononuclear cells in tuberculosis. *Immunol Rev* 262:179–192.
2. Leemans JC, Juffermans NP, Florquin S, van Rooijen N, Vervoordeldonk MJ, Verbon A, van Deventer SJ, van der Poll T. 2001. Depletion of alveolar macrophages exerts protective effects in pulmonary tuberculosis in mice. *J Immunol* 166:4604–4611.
3. Leemans JC, Thepen T, Weijer S, Florquin S, van Rooijen N, van de Winkel JG, van der Poll T. 2005. Macrophages play a dual role during pulmonary tuberculosis in mice. *J Infect Dis* 191:65–74.
4. Antonelli LR, Gigliotti Rothfuchs A, Gonçalves R, Roffê E, Cheever AW, Bafica A, Salazar AM, Feng CG, Sher A. 2010. Intranasal Poly-IC treatment exacerbates tuberculosis in mice through the pulmonary recruitment of a pathogen-permissive monocyte/macrophage population. *J Clin Invest* 120:1674–1682.
5. Dorhoi A, Yeremeev V, Nouailles G, Weiner J III, Jörg S, Heinemann E, Oberbeck-Müller D, Knaul JK, Vogelzang A, Reece ST, Hahnke K, Mollenkopf HJ, Brinkmann V, Kaufmann SH. 2014. Type I IFN signaling triggers immunopathology in tuberculosis-susceptible mice by modulating lung phagocyte dynamics. *Eur J Immunol* 44:2380–2393.
6. Mattila JT, Ojo OO, Kepka-Lenhart D, Marino S, Kim JH, Eum SY, Via LE, Barry CE III, Klein E, Kirschner DE, Morris SM Jr, Lin PL, Flynn JL. 2013. Microenvironments in tuberculous granulomas are delineated by distinct populations of macrophage subsets and expression of nitric oxide synthase and arginase isoforms. *J Immunol* 191:773–784.
7. Marino S, Cilfone NA, Mattila JT, Linderman JJ, Flynn JL, Kirschner DE. 2015. Macrophage polarization drives granuloma outcome during *Mycobacterium tuberculosis* infection. *Infect Immun* 83:324–338.
8. Gideon HP, Phuah J, Myers AJ, Bryson BD, Rodgers MA, Coleman MT, Maiello P, Rutledge T, Marino S, Fortune SM, Kirschner DE, Lin PL, Flynn JL. 2015. Variability in tuberculosis granuloma T cell responses exists, but a balance of pro- and anti-inflammatory cytokines is associated with sterilization. *PLoS Pathog* 11: e1004603.
9. Tan S, Russell DG. 2015. Trans-species communication in the *Mycobacterium tuberculosis*-infected macrophage. *Immunol Rev* 264:233–248.
10. Schaible UE, Sturgill-Koszycki S, Schlesinger PH, Russell DG. 1998. Cytokine activation leads to acidification and increases maturation of *Mycobacterium avium*-containing phagosomes in murine macrophages. *J Immunol* 160:1290–1296.
11. Via LE, Fratti RA, McFalone M, Pagan-Ramos E, Deretic D, Deretic V. 1998. Effects of cytokines on mycobacterial phagosome maturation. *J Cell Sci* 111:897–905.
12. Alonso S, Pethe K, Russell DG, Purdy GE. 2007. Lysosomal killing of *Mycobacterium* mediated by ubiquitin-derived peptides is enhanced by autophagy. *Proc Natl Acad Sci USA* 104:6031–6036.
13. Gutierrez MG, Master SS, Singh SB, Taylor GA, Colombo MI, Deretic V. 2004. Autophagy is a defense mechanism inhibiting BCG and *Mycobacterium tuberculosis* survival in infected macrophages. *Cell* 119:753–766.
14. MacMicking JD, North RJ, LaCourse R, Mudgett JS, Shah SK, Nathan CF. 1997. Identification of nitric oxide synthase as a protective locus against tuberculosis. *Proc Natl Acad Sci USA* 94:5243–5248.
15. McDonough KA, Kress Y, Bloom BR. 1993. Pathogenesis of tuberculosis: interaction of *Mycobacterium tuberculosis* with macrophages. *Infect Immun* 61:2763–2773.

16. **Myrvik QN, Leake ES, Wright MJ.** 1984. Disruption of phagosomal membranes of normal alveolar macrophages by the H37Rv strain of *Mycobacterium tuberculosis*. A correlate of virulence. *Am Rev Respir Dis* **129**: 322–328.

17. **Simeone R, Bobard A, Lippmann J, Bitter W, Majlessi L, Brosch R, Enninga J.** 2012. Phagosomal rupture by *Mycobacterium tuberculosis* results in toxicity and host cell death. *PLoS Pathog* **8**:e1002507.

18. **van der Wel N, Hava D, Houben D, Fluitsma D, van Zon M, Pierson J, Brenner M, Peters PJ.** 2007. *M. tuberculosis* and *M. leprae* translocate from the phagolysosome to the cytosol in myeloid cells. *Cell* **129**: 1287–1298.

19. **Russell DG.** 2016. The ins and outs of the *Mycobacterium tuberculosis*-containing vacuole. *Cell Microbiol* **18**:1065–1069.

20. **Schnappinger D, Ehrt S, Voskuil MI, Liu Y, Mangan JA, Monahan IM, Dolganov G, Efron B, Butcher PD, Nathan C, Schoolnik GK.** 2003. Transcriptional adaptation of *Mycobacterium tuberculosis* within macrophages: insights into the phagosomal environment. *J Exp Med* **198**:693–704.

21. **Rohde KH, Abramovitch RB, Russell DG.** 2007. *Mycobacterium tuberculosis* invasion of macrophages: linking bacterial gene expression to environmental cues. *Cell Host Microbe* **2**:352–364.

22. **Rohde KH, Veiga DF, Caldwell S, Balázsi G, Russell DG.** 2012. Linking the transcriptional profiles and the physiological states of *Mycobacterium tuberculosis* during an extended intracellular infection. *PLoS Pathog* **8**: e1002769.

23. **Abramovitch RB, Rohde KH, Hsu FF, Russell DG.** 2011. aprABC: a *Mycobacterium tuberculosis* complex-specific locus that modulates pH-driven adaptation to the macrophage phagosome. *Mol Microbiol* **80**:678–694.

24. **Rohde KH, Veiga DF, Caldwell S, Balázsi G, Russell DG.** 2012. Linking the transcriptional profiles and the physiological states of *Mycobacterium tuberculosis* during an extended intracellular infection. *PLoS Pathog* **8**: e1002769.

25. **Gill WP, Harik NS, Whiddon MR, Liao RP, Mittler JE, Sherman DR.** 2009. A replication clock for *Mycobacterium tuberculosis*. *Nat Med* **15**:211–214.

26. **Homolka S, Niemann S, Russell DG, Rohde KH.** 2010. Functional genetic diversity among *Mycobacterium tuberculosis* complex clinical isolates: delineation of conserved core and lineage-specific transcriptomes during intracellular survival. *PLoS Pathog* **6**:e1000988.

27. **Rohde K, Yates RM, Purdy GE, Russell DG.** 2007. *Mycobacterium tuberculosis* and the environment within the phagosome. *Immunol Rev* **219**:37–54.

28. **Lee W, VanderVen BC, Fahey RJ, Russell DG.** 2013. Intracellular *Mycobacterium tuberculosis* exploits host-derived fatty acids to limit metabolic stress. *J Biol Chem* **288**:6788–6800.

29. **Tan S, Sukumar N, Abramovitch RB, Parish T, Russell DG.** 2013. *Mycobacterium tuberculosis* responds to chloride and pH as synergistic cues to the immune status of its host cell. *PLoS Pathog* **9**:e1003282

30. **Ehrt S, Guo XV, Hickey CM, Ryou M, Monteleone M, Riley LW, Schnappinger D.** 2005. Controlling gene expression in mycobacteria with anhydrotetracycline and Tet repressor. *Nucleic Acids Res* **33**:e21.

31. **Sukumar N, Tan S, Aldridge BB, Russell DG.** 2014. Exploitation of *Mycobacterium tuberculosis* reporter strains to probe the impact of vaccination at sites of infection. *PLoS Pathog* **10**:e1004394.

32. **Reyes-Lamothe R, Possoz C, Danilova O, Sherratt DJ.** 2008. Independent positioning and action of *Escherichia coli* replisomes in live cells. *Cell* **133**:90–102.

33. **Wolf AJ, Linas B, Trevejo-Nuñez GJ, Kincaid E, Tamura T, Takatsu K, Ernst JD.** 2007. *Mycobacterium tuberculosis* infects dendritic cells with high frequency and impairs their function in vivo. *J Immunol* **179**:2509–2519.

34. **Liu Y, Tan S, Huang L, Abramovitch RB, Rohde KH, Zimmerman MD, Chen C, Dartois V, VanderVen BC, Russell DG.** 2016. Immune activation of the host cell induces drug tolerance in *Mycobacterium tuberculosis* both in vitro and in vivo. *J Exp Med* **213**:809–825.

35. **Manina G, Dhar N, McKinney JD.** 2015. Stress and host immunity amplify *Mycobacterium tuberculosis* phenotypic heterogeneity and induce nongrowing metabolically active forms. *Cell Host Microbe* **17**:32–46.

36. **VanderVen BC, Fahey RJ, Lee W, Liu Y, Abramovitch RB, Memmott C, Crowe AM, Eltis LD, Perola E, Deininger DD, Wang T, Locher CP, Russell DG.** 2015. Novel inhibitors of cholesterol degradation in *Mycobacterium tuberculosis* reveal how the bacterium's metabolism is constrained by the intracellular environment. *PLoS Pathog* **11**:e1004679.

37. **Guo YL, Seebacher T, Kurz U, Linder JU, Schultz JE.** 2001. Adenylyl cyclase Rv1625c of *Mycobacterium tuberculosis*: a progenitor of mammalian adenylyl cyclases. *EMBO J* **20**:3667–3675.

38. **Ketkar AD, Shenoy AR, Ramagopal UA, Visweswariah SS, Suguna K.** 2006. A structural basis for the role of nucleotide specifying residues in regulating the oligomerization of the Rv1625c adenylyl cyclase from *M. tuberculosis*. *J Mol Biol* **356**:904–916.

39. **Agarwal N, Lamichhane G, Gupta R, Nolan S, Bishai WR.** 2009. Cyclic AMP intoxication of macrophages by a *Mycobacterium tuberculosis* adenylate cyclase. *Nature* **460**:98–102.

40. **Choudhary E, Bishai W, Agarwal N.** 2014. Expression of a subset of heat stress induced genes of *Mycobacterium tuberculosis* is regulated by 3′,5′-cyclic AMP. *PLoS One* **9**:e89759.

41. **Kahramanoglou C, Cortes T, Matange N, Hunt DM, Visweswariah SS, Young DB, Buxton RS.** 2014. Genomic mapping of cAMP receptor protein (CRP Mt) in *Mycobacterium tuberculosis*: relation to transcriptional start sites and the role of CRPMt as a transcription factor. *Nucleic Acids Res* **42**:8320–8329.

42. **Knapp GS, Lyubetskaya A, Peterson MW, Gomes AL, Ma Z, Galagan JE, McDonough KA.** 2015. Role of intragenic binding of cAMP responsive protein (CRP) in regulation of the succinate dehydrogenase genes Rv0249c-Rv0247c in TB complex mycobacteria. *Nucleic Acids Res* **43**:5377–5393.

43. Lee HJ, Lang PT, Fortune SM, Sassetti CM, Alber T. 2012. Cyclic AMP regulation of protein lysine acetylation in *Mycobacterium tuberculosis*. *Nat Struct Mol Biol* 19:811–818.

44. Shleeva M, Goncharenko A, Kudykina Y, Young D, Young M, Kaprelyants A. 2013. Cyclic AMP-dependent resuscitation of dormant Mycobacteria by exogenous free fatty acids. *PLoS One* 8:e82914. (Erratum, 9:e97206.)

45. Xu H, Hegde SS, Blanchard JS. 2011. Reversible acetylation and inactivation of *Mycobacterium tuberculosis* acetyl-CoA synthetase is dependent on cAMP. *Biochemistry* 50:5883–5892.

46. Aronoff DM, Canetti C, Serezani CH, Luo M, Peters-Golden M. 2005. Cutting edge: macrophage inhibition by cyclic AMP (cAMP): differential roles of protein kinase A and exchange protein directly activated by cAMP-1. *J Immunol* 174:595–599.

47. Chang JC, Harik NS, Liao RP, Sherman DR. 2007. Identification of mycobacterial genes that alter growth and pathology in macrophages and in mice. *J Infect Dis* 196:788–795.

48. Hu Y, van der Geize R, Besra GS, Gurcha SS, Liu A, Rohde M, Singh M, Coates A. 2010. 3-Ketosteroid 9-alpha-hydroxylase is an essential factor in the pathogenesis of *Mycobacterium tuberculosis*. *Mol Microbiol* 75:107–121.

49. Nesbitt NM, Yang X, Fontán P, Kolesnikova I, Smith I, Sampson NS, Dubnau E. 2010. A thiolase of *Mycobacterium tuberculosis* is required for virulence and production of androstenedione and androstadienedione from cholesterol. *Infect Immun* 78:275–282.

50. Pandey AK, Sassetti CM. 2008. Mycobacterial persistence requires the utilization of host cholesterol. *Proc Natl Acad Sci USA* 105:4376–4380 (Erratum, 105:9130.)

51. Van der Geize R, Yam K, Heuser T, Wilbrink MH, Hara H, Anderton MC, Sim E, Dijkhuizen L, Davies JE, Mohn WW, Eltis LD. 2007. A gene cluster encoding cholesterol catabolism in a soil actinomycete provides insight into *Mycobacterium tuberculosis* survival in macrophages. *Proc Natl Acad Sci USA* 104:1947–1952.

52. Griffin JE, Pandey AK, Gilmore SA, Mizrahi V, McKinney JD, Bertozzi CR, Sassetti CM. 2012. Cholesterol catabolism by *Mycobacterium tuberculosis* requires transcriptional and metabolic adaptations. *Chem Biol* 19:218–227.

53. McKinney JD, Höner zu Bentrup K, Muñoz-Elías EJ, Miczak A, Chen B, Chan WT, Swenson D, Sacchettini JC, Jacobs WR Jr, Russell DG. 2000. Persistence of *Mycobacterium tuberculosis* in macrophages and mice requires the glyoxylate shunt enzyme isocitrate lyase. *Nature* 406:735–738.

54. McKinney JD, Höner zu Bentrup K, Muñoz-Elías EJ, Miczak A, Chen B, Chan W-T, Swenson D, Sacchettini JC, Jacobs WR Jr, Russell DG. 2000. Persistence of *Mycobacterium tuberculosis* in macrophages and mice requires the glyoxylate shunt enzyme isocitrate lyase. *Nature* 406:735–738.

55. Muñoz-Elías EJ, McKinney JD. 2005. Mycobacterium tuberculosis isocitrate lyases 1 and 2 are jointly required for in vivo growth and virulence. *Nat Med* 11:638–644.

56. Bloch H, Segal W. 1956. Biochemical differentiation of *Mycobacterium tuberculosis* grown in vivo and in vitro. *J Bacteriol* 72:132–141.

57. Cole ST, Brosch R, Parkhill J, Garnier T, Churcher C, Harris D, Gordon SV, Eiglmeier K, Gas S, Barry CE III, Tekaia F, Badcock K, Basham D, Brown D, Chillingworth T, Connor R, Davies R, Devlin K, Feltwell T, Gentles S, Hamlin N, Holroyd S, Hornsby T, Jagels K, Krogh A, McLean J, Moule S, Murphy L, Oliver K, Osborne J, Quail MA, Rajandream MA, Rogers J, Rutter S, Seeger K, Skelton J, Squares R, Squares S, Sulston JE, Taylor K, Whitehead S, Barrell BG. 1998. Deciphering the biology of *Mycobacterium tuberculosis* from the complete genome sequence. *Nature* 393:537–544.

58. Krithika R, Marathe U, Saxena P, Ansari MZ, Mohanty D, Gokhale RS. 2006. A genetic locus required for iron acquisition in *Mycobacterium tuberculosis*. *Proc Natl Acad Sci USA* 103:2069–2074.

59. Trivedi OA, Arora P, Sridharan V, Tickoo R, Mohanty D, Gokhale RS. 2004. Enzymic activation and transfer of fatty acids as acyl-adenylates in mycobacteria. *Nature* 428:441–445.

60. Yang M, Guja KE, Thomas ST, Garcia-Diaz M, Sampson NS. 2014. A distinct MaoC-like enoyl-CoA hydratase architecture mediates cholesterol catabolism in *Mycobacterium tuberculosis*. *ACS Chem Biol* 9:2632–2645.

61. Yang M, Lu R, Guja KE, Wipperman MF, St Clair JR, Bonds AC, Garcia-Diaz M, Sampson NS. 2015. Unraveling cholesterol catabolism in *Mycobacterium tuberculosis*: ChsE4-ChsE5 α2β2 acyl-CoA dehydrogenase initiates β-oxidation of 3-oxo-cholest-4-en-26-oyl CoA. *ACS Infect Dis* 1:110–125.

62. Graham JE, Clark-Curtiss JE. 1999. Identification of *Mycobacterium tuberculosis* RNAs synthesized in response to phagocytosis by human macrophages by selective capture of transcribed sequences (SCOTS). *Proc Natl Acad Sci USA* 96:11554–11559.

63. Höner Zu Bentrup K, Miczak A, Swenson DL, Russell DG. 1999. Characterization of activity and expression of isocitrate lyase in *Mycobacterium avium* and *Mycobacterium tuberculosis*. *J Bacteriol* 181:7161–7167.

64. Sturgill-Koszycki S, Haddix PL, Russell DG. 1997. The interaction between *Mycobacterium* and the macrophage analyzed by two-dimensional polyacrylamide gel electrophoresis. *Electrophoresis* 18:2558–2565.

65. Gould TA, van de Langemheen H, Muñoz-Elías EJ, McKinney JD, Sacchettini JC. 2006. Dual role of isocitrate lyase 1 in the glyoxylate and methylcitrate cycles in *Mycobacterium tuberculosis*. *Mol Microbiol* 61:940–947.

66. Muñoz-Elías EJ, Upton AM, Cherian J, McKinney JD. 2006. Role of the methylcitrate cycle in *Mycobacterium tuberculosis* metabolism, intracellular growth, and virulence. *Mol Microbiol* 60:1109–1122.

67. Ouellet H, Johnston JB, de Montellano PR. 2011. Cholesterol catabolism as a therapeutic target in *Mycobacterium tuberculosis*. *Trends Microbiol* 19:530–539.

68. Wipperman MF, Sampson NS, Thomas ST. 2014. Pathogen roid rage: cholesterol utilization by *Mycobacterium tuberculosis*. *Crit Rev Biochem Mol Biol* 49:269–293.

69. Yam KC, Okamoto S, Roberts JN, Eltis LD. 2011. Adventures in *Rhodococcus* — from steroids to explosives. *Can J Microbiol* 57:155–168.

70. Marrero J, Rhee KY, Schnappinger D, Pethe K, Ehrt S. 2010. Gluconeogenic carbon flow of tricarboxylic acid cycle intermediates is critical for *Mycobacterium tuberculosis* to establish and maintain infection. *Proc Natl Acad Sci USA* 107:9819–9824.

71. Daniel J, Maamar H, Deb C, Sirakova TD, Kolattukudy PE. 2011. *Mycobacterium tuberculosis* uses host triacylglycerol to accumulate lipid droplets and acquires a dormancy-like phenotype in lipid-loaded macrophages. *PLoS Pathog* 7:e1002093.

72. Quadri LE. 2014. Biosynthesis of mycobacterial lipids by polyketide synthases and beyond. *Crit Rev Biochem Mol Biol* 49:179–211.

73. Jain M, Petzold CJ, Schelle MW, Leavell MD, Mougous JD, Bertozzi CR, Leary JA, Cox JS. 2007. Lipidomics reveals control of *Mycobacterium tuberculosis* virulence lipids via metabolic coupling. *Proc Natl Acad Sci USA* 104:5133–5138.

74. Yang X, Nesbitt NM, Dubnau E, Smith I, Sampson NS. 2009. Cholesterol metabolism increases the metabolic pool of propionate in *Mycobacterium tuberculosis*. *Biochemistry* 48:3819–3821.

75. Singh A, Crossman DK, Mai D, Guidry L, Voskuil MI, Renfrow MB, Steyn AJ. 2009. *Mycobacterium tuberculosis* WhiB3 maintains redox homeostasis by regulating virulence lipid anabolism to modulate macrophage response. *PLoS Pathog* 5:e1000545.

76. Daniel J, Deb C, Dubey VS, Sirakova TD, Abomoelak B, Morbidoni HR, Kolattukudy PE. 2004. Induction of a novel class of diacylglycerol acyltransferases and triacylglycerol accumulation in *Mycobacterium tuberculosis* as it goes into a dormancy-like state in culture. *J Bacteriol* 186:5017–5030.

77. Gaur RL, Ren K, Blumenthal A, Bhamidi S, Gibbs S, Jackson M, Zare RN, Ehrt S, Ernst JD, Banaei N. 2014. LprG-mediated surface expression of lipoarabinomannan is essential for virulence of *Mycobacterium tuberculosis*. *PLoS Pathog* 10:e1004376 (Erratum, 10:e1004489, e1004494.)

78. Martinot AJ, Farrow M, Bai L, Layre E, Cheng TY, Tsai JH, Iqbal J, Annand JW, Sullivan ZA, Hussain MM, Sacchettini J, Moody DB, Seeliger JC, Rubin EJ. 2016. Mycobacterial metabolic syndrome: LprG and Rv1410 regulate triacylglyceride levels, growth rate and virulence in *Mycobacterium tuberculosis*. *PLoS Pathog* 12:e1005351.

79. Baek SH, Li AH, Sassetti CM. 2011. Metabolic regulation of mycobacterial growth and antibiotic sensitivity. *PLoS Biol* 9:e1001065.

80. Yam KC, D'Angelo I, Kalscheuer R, Zhu H, Wang JX, Snieckus V, Ly LH, Converse PJ, Jacobs WR Jr, Strynadka N, Eltis LD. 2009. Studies of a ring-cleaving dioxygenase illuminate the role of cholesterol metabolism in the pathogenesis of *Mycobacterium tuberculosis*. *PLoS Pathog* 5:e1000344.

81. Capyk JK, Casabon I, Gruninger R, Strynadka NC, Eltis LD. 2011. Activity of 3-ketosteroid 9α-hydroxylase

82. Capyk JK, D'Angelo I, Strynadka NC, Eltis LD. 2009. Characterization of 3-ketosteroid 9alpha-hydroxylase, a Rieske oxygenase in the cholesterol degradation pathway of *Mycobacterium tuberculosis*. *J Biol Chem* 284:9937–9946.

83. Capyk JK, Kalscheuer R, Stewart GR, Liu J, Kwon H, Zhao R, Okamoto S, Jacobs WR Jr, Eltis LD, Mohn WW. 2009. Mycobacterial cytochrome p450 125 (cyp125) catalyzes the terminal hydroxylation of c27 steroids. *J Biol Chem* 284:35534–35542.

84. Casabon I, Crowe AM, Liu J, Eltis LD. 2013. FadD3 is an acyl-CoA synthetase that initiates catabolism of cholesterol rings C and D in actinobacteria. *Mol Microbiol* 87:269–283.

85. Casabon I, Swain K, Crowe AM, Eltis LD, Mohn WW. 2014. Actinobacterial acyl coenzyme A synthetases involved in steroid side-chain catabolism. *J Bacteriol* 196:579–587.

86. Casabon I, Zhu SH, Otani H, Liu J, Mohn WW, Eltis LD. 2013. Regulation of the KstR2 regulon of *Mycobacterium tuberculosis* by a cholesterol catabolite. *Mol Microbiol* 89:1201–1212.

87. Dresen C, Lin LY, D'Angelo I, Tocheva EI, Strynadka N, Eltis LD. 2010. A flavin-dependent monooxygenase from *Mycobacterium tuberculosis* involved in cholesterol catabolism. *J Biol Chem* 285:22264–22275.

88. Driscoll MD, McLean KJ, Levy C, Mast N, Pikuleva IA, Lafite P, Rigby SE, Leys D, Munro AW. 2010. Structural and biochemical characterization of *Mycobacterium tuberculosis* CYP142: evidence for multiple cholesterol 27-hydroxylase activities in a human pathogen. *J Biol Chem* 285:38270–38282.

89. Frank DJ, Madrona Y, Ortiz de Montellano PR. 2014. Cholesterol ester oxidation by mycobacterial cytochrome P450. *J Biol Chem* 289:30417–30425.

90. Griffin JE, Gawronski JD, DeJesus MA, Ioerger TR, Akerley BJ, Sassetti CM. 2011. High-resolution phenotypic profiling defines genes essential for mycobacterial growth and cholesterol catabolism. *PLoS Pathog* 7:e1002251.

91. Lack NA, Yam KC, Lowe ED, Horsman GP, Owen RL, Sim E, Eltis LD. 2010. Characterization of a carbon-carbon hydrolase from *Mycobacterium tuberculosis* involved in cholesterol metabolism. *J Biol Chem* 285:434–443.

92. Ouellet H, Guan S, Johnston JB, Chow ED, Kells PM, Burlingame AL, Cox JS, Podust LM, de Montellano PRO. 2010. *Mycobacterium tuberculosis* CYP125A1, a steroid C27 monooxygenase that detoxifies intracellularly generated cholest-4-en-3-one. *Mol Microbiol* 77:730–742.

93. Thomas ST, VanderVen BC, Sherman DR, Russell DG, Sampson NS. 2011. Pathway profiling in *Mycobacterium tuberculosis*: elucidation of cholesterol-derived catabolite and enzymes that catalyze its metabolism. *J Biol Chem* 286:43668–43678.

94. Yang X, Nesbitt NM, Dubnau E, Smith I, Sampson NS. 2009. Cholesterol metabolism increases the metabolic pool of propionate in *Mycobacterium tuberculosis*. *Biochemistry* 48:3819–3821.

95. Masiewicz P, Brzostek A, Wolański M, Dziadek J, Zakrzewska-Czerwińska J. 2012. A novel role of the PrpR as a transcription factor involved in the regulation of methylcitrate pathway in *Mycobacterium tuberculosis*. *PLoS One* 7:e43651 (Erratum, 9:e113015.)

96. Eoh H, Rhee KY. 2013. Multifunctional essentiality of succinate metabolism in adaptation to hypoxia in *Mycobacterium tuberculosis*. *Proc Natl Acad Sci USA* 110:6554–6559.

97. de Carvalho LP, Fischer SM, Marrero J, Nathan C, Ehrt S, Rhee KY. 2010. Metabolomics of *Mycobacterium tuberculosis* reveals compartmentalized co-catabolism of carbon substrates. *Chem Biol* 17:1122–1131.

98. Eoh H, Rhee KY. 2014. Methylcitrate cycle defines the bactericidal essentiality of isocitrate lyase for survival of *Mycobacterium tuberculosis* on fatty acids. *Proc Natl Acad Sci USA* 111:4976–4981.

99. Savvi S, Warner DF, Kana BD, McKinney JD, Mizrahi V, Dawes SS. 2008. Functional characterization of a vitamin B12-dependent methylmalonyl pathway in *Mycobacterium tuberculosis*: implications for propionate metabolism during growth on fatty acids. *J Bacteriol* 190:3886–3895.

100. Kim MJ, Wainwright HC, Locketz M, Bekker LG, Walther GB, Dittrich C, Visser A, Wang W, Hsu FF, Wiehart U, Tsenova L, Kaplan G, Russell DG. 2010. Caseation of human tuberculosis granulomas correlates with elevated host lipid metabolism. *EMBO Mol Med* 2:258–274.

101. Peyron P, Vaubourgeix J, Poquet Y, Levillain F, Botanch C, Bardou F, Daffé M, Emile JF, Marchou B, Cardona PJ, de Chastellier C, Altare F. 2008. Foamy macrophages from tuberculous patients' granulomas constitute a nutrient-rich reservoir for *M. tuberculosis* persistence. *PLoS Pathog* 4:e1000204

102. Graham A, Allen AM. 2015. Mitochondrial function and regulation of macrophage sterol metabolism and inflammatory responses. *World J Cardiol* 7:277–286.

103. Philips JA, Rubin EJ, Perrimon N. 2005. Drosophila RNAi screen reveals CD36 family member required for mycobacterial infection. *Science* 309:1251–1253.

104. Russell DG, Cardona P-J, Kim M-J, Allain S, Altare F. 2009. Foamy macrophages and the progression of the human tuberculosis granuloma. *Nat Immunol* 10:943–948.

105. Almeida PE, Silva AR, Maya-Monteiro CM, Töröcsik D, D'Avila H, Dezsö B, Magalhães KG, Castro-Faria-Neto HC, Nagy L, Bozza PT. 2009. *Mycobacterium bovis* bacillus Calmette-Guérin infection induces TLR2-dependent peroxisome proliferator-activated receptor gamma expression and activation: functions in inflammation, lipid metabolism, and pathogenesis. *J Immunol* 183:1337–1345.

106. Almeida PE, Carneiro AB, Silva AR, Bozza PT. 2012. PPARγ expression and function in mycobacterial infection: roles in lipid metabolism, immunity, and bacterial killing. *PPAR Res* 2012:383829.

107. Rajaram MV, Brooks MN, Morris JD, Torrelles JB, Azad AK, Schlesinger LS. 2010. *Mycobacterium tuberculosis* activates human macrophage peroxisome proliferator-activated receptor gamma linking mannose receptor recognition to regulation of immune responses. *J Immunol* 185:929–942.

108. Salamon H, Bruiners N, Lakehal K, Shi L, Ravi J, Yamaguchi KD, Pine R, Gennaro ML. 2014. Cutting edge: vitamin D regulates lipid metabolism in *Mycobacterium tuberculosis* infection. *J Immunol* 193:30–34.

109. Mahajan S, Dkhar HK, Chandra V, Dave S, Nanduri R, Janmeja AK, Agrewala JN, Gupta P. 2012. *Mycobacterium tuberculosis* modulates macrophage lipid-sensing nuclear receptors PPARγ and TR4 for survival. *J Immunol* 188:5593–5603.

110. Singh V, Jamwal S, Jain R, Verma P, Gokhale R, Rao KV. 2012. *Mycobacterium tuberculosis*-driven targeted recalibration of macrophage lipid homeostasis promotes the foamy phenotype. *Cell Host Microbe* 12:669–681.

Tuberculosis and the Tubercle Bacillus, 2nd ed.
Edited by William R. Jacobs, Jr., Helen McShane, Valerie Mizrahi, and Ian M. Orme
© 2018 American Society for Microbiology, Washington, DC
doi:10.1128/microbiolspec.TBTB2-0026-2016

Metabolic Perspectives on Persistence

31

Travis E. Hartman,[1] Zhe Wang,[1] Robert S. Jansen,[1]
Susana Gardete,[1] and Kyu Y. Rhee[1,2]

INTRODUCTION

DNA evidence indicates that *Mycobacterium tuberculosis* and humans have cohabited with one another since the emergence of *Homo sapiens* as a species (1). In humans, *M. tuberculosis* resides chiefly within and amidst cells of the immune system. *M. tuberculosis* has thus evolved in close physical and functional proximity to host immunity.

In most hosts, *M. tuberculosis* occupies the majority of its natural life cycle in a clinically asymptomatic state of slowed or arrested replication. However, *M. tuberculosis* is widely recognized for its ability to cause clinical disease in immunocompetent hosts years, if not decades, after successful containment of primary infection and successfully transmit itself to new hosts. This suggests that *M. tuberculosis* has evolved specific mechanisms to sense, withstand, and recover from prolonged periods of immune-imposed suppression, a trait that became evident with the discovery of increased rates of disease and mortality in immunosuppressed and/or immunodeficient populations (2).

In addition to host immunity, *M. tuberculosis* is equally well recognized for its ability to persist in the face of even effective chemotherapy, a trait often referred to as nonheritable antibiotic resistance or phenotypic tolerance. Phenotypic tolerance is widely believed to explain the need for treatment durations longer than for virtually any other bacterial infection, which in turn have inadvertently promoted the emergence of drug resistance itself (3).

Persistence has thus emerged as a central feature of both the physiology and pathogenicity of *M. tuberculosis*. However, like most phenotypic traits, persistence has come to encompass an increasingly diverse and het-erogeneous array of physiologic states and mechanisms. For *M. tuberculosis*, persistence has been linked to both deterministically and stochastically encoded programs in majority and minority subpopulations, respectively (4). The number and nature of states and/or mechanisms mediating persistence in latent infection, clinical disease, drug tolerance, treatment relapse, and heritable drug resistance, however, remain undefined.

Here, we provide a focused review of metabolic characteristics associated with *M. tuberculosis* persistence. We focus on metabolism because it is the biochemical foundation of all physiologic processes and a distinguishing hallmark of *M. tuberculosis* physiology and pathogenicity (5). In addition, it serves as the chemical interface between host and pathogen. However, existing knowledge of metabolism derives largely from physiologic contexts in which replication is the primary biochemical objective. The goal of this chapter is to review existing knowledge of mechanism- and/or model-specific and -independent metabolic features of *M. tuberculosis* persistence in which replicative quiescence often features as a key distinguishing characteristic. Such a perspective may help guide ongoing efforts to develop more efficient cures and inform on novel strategies to break the cycle of transmission sustaining the pandemic.

TERMS OF DISCOURSE

Medical evidence of clinically latent infection by *M. tuberculosis* predates current terminology by centuries. However, the terms used to describe the microbiologic features of this state have been used somewhat ambiguously. For the purposes of clarity, we have adapted the

[1]Department of Medicine and [2]Department of Microbiology & Immunology, Division of Infectious Diseases, Weill Cornell Medical College, New York, NY 10065.

definitions offered by Gomez and McKinney (6) as follows:

- **Persistence.** The ability of an organism to maintain infection in the face of either antibiotic treatment or host immunity. Its adjective form, "persistent," describes the subpopulation of organisms that display this property regardless of its size or location.
- **Latency.** The presence of infectious organisms despite asymptomatic lesions in the host.
- **Dormancy.** The property of slowly dividing or nondividing bacteria *in* or *ex vivo*.
- **Drug tolerance.** A form of phenotypic drug resistance that is demonstrably independent of specific mutations or alleles that confer that resistance. This phenotype is reversible (not genetically encoded) and can occur independently of dormancy.

These definitions emphasize the potential diversity of contexts and mechanisms in or by which persistence can arise. For the purposes of the current discussion, we take a clinical perspective in which persistence arises in two distinct contexts: host immunity and chemotherapy. Both share the ability to slow or arrest *M. tuberculosis* replication but act through a diverse and heterogeneous set of selective pressures whose overlap (or lack thereof) with one another remains unresolved and are thus considered as two functionally distinct classes.

In discussing persistence, it is equally important to highlight a commonly overlooked distinction between metabolism and nutrition. Though often used interchangeably, metabolism describes the entirety of chemical reactions used to maintain the living state of cells and organisms, while nutrition refers to the subset of processes used to fuel metabolism. In the context of persistence, this distinction is important because it recognizes a broader range of specific physiologic roles for metabolism beyond that of a central warehouse of precursors and energy, or conduit to the extracellular environment. Indeed, recent work has identified a growing number of cell-intrinsic metabolic functions that are dissociated from uptake of nutrients in the extracellular environment (7–10). Metabolism thus serves cellular physiology in ways that are as qualitatively as quantitatively specific.

MODELS

Experimental evidence of persistence in *M. tuberculosis* infection was first reported by McDermott, who showed that mice infected with *M. tuberculosis* and effectively cured with chemotherapy (as measured by

recovery of colony-forming units from the entire carcass of infected animals) harbored viable bacilli that could be unmasked (or reactivated) only upon immunosuppression (11). Numerous studies had previously reported the presence of visible bacteria in tuberculous lesions of humans after months of chemotherapy. However, few, if any, had recovered viable organisms. McDermott and colleagues further demonstrated that the recovered bacilli remained susceptible to the same antibiotics used to achieve cure and had not arisen from the acquisition of resistance alleles (11). Indeed, Ford and colleagues subsequently showed that heritable drug resistance was linked to basal mutation rates, rather than to pre-exposure to antibiotics (12). McDermott's work thus not only demonstrated that persistence could be mediated by a subpopulation of dormant organisms but that this subpopulation could also survive the joint pressure of host immunity and antibiotic selection. In support of this view, work by Gill et al., using a plasmid-based reporter of growth rate, recently showed that organisms recovered from the chronic (or persistent) phase of infection in mice exhibited slowed, but measurable, rates of growth despite steady titers (13).

The issue of persistence in human disease was first raised by W. W. Stead, who questioned whether new disease occurred because of reactivation of a clinically latent (or contained) infection or due to a new infectious event (14). If reactivation was simply the result of a secondary infection acquired by proximity with an infectious host, there was no reason to believe that persisters were anything more than dying *M. tuberculosis*, incapable of causing disease. However, population-based epidemiologic studies, combined with molecular strain typing methods, showed that disease relapse in countries with low burden was largely due to the same strain causing the initial episode of disease, suggestive of reactivation (15–18), while relapse in high-burden areas was associated with different strains, suggestive of reinfection (19, 20). Work by Vandiviere, comparing bacilli recovered from resected lesions of patients receiving chemotherapy that were either in communication with (open) or closed off from (closed) the airways, showed that bacteria recovered from closed lesions were uniformly drug susceptible, while those from open lesions were drug resistant despite similar levels of drug penetration (21). Clinical studies conducted by the British Medical Research Council subsequently showed that the duration of tuberculosis (TB) chemotherapy could be shortened by the inclusion of drugs such as rifampin and pyrazinamide that exhibited activity against non- or slowly replicating *M. tuber-*

culosis cultures *in vitro* (22, 23). These findings thus demonstrated that persistence was not only a feature of human TB but was also mediated by a subpopulation of *M. tuberculosis* refractory to sterilization by host immunity and conventional chemotherapy.

Prior to recognition of persistence in latent infection or chemotherapy, *M. tuberculosis* was long noted for its *in vitro* resilience to a broad range of environmental stresses. Indeed, seminal work by Corper and Cohn showed that clinical *M. tuberculosis* isolates could not only survive in a sealed culture vessel for 12 years at 37°C but could also retain their virulence (24). *M. tuberculosis* exposed to host- or chemotherapy-derived stresses has since served as useful *in vitro* models of persistence. In humans, *M. tuberculosis* occupies a dynamic and heterogeneous range of intra- and extracellular microenvironments, each of which includes multiple biochemical conditions capable of restricting its replication *in vitro*. Known stringencies include nutritional and micronutritional (vitamin and cofactor) deficiencies and oxidative, nitrosative, acidic, hypoxic, and membrane-perturbing stresses (25). In addition, sublethal exposure to antibiotics has been reported to slow *M. tuberculosis*'s replication and induce persistence to the same and other antibiotics (26). *In vitro* models have thus enabled detailed mechanistic studies of persistence. However, fundamental uncertainties concerning the location of host- and drug-induced persistent *M. tuberculosis*, and heterogeneity of conditions encountered therein, have hindered efforts to establish physiologic relevance.

In a practical illustration of the potential dissociation between *in vitro* and *in vivo* studies, Pethe et al. reported the results of a drug screen that focused on a class of pyrimidine imidazoles with strong *in vitro* efficacy but no antitubercular activity in the murine model (27). Investigating the cause of this dissociation, the authors discovered that the *in vitro* activity of these compounds required the inclusion of glycerol in the culture medium. Studies of *M. tuberculosis* mutants unable to metabolize glycerol (due to deletion of the activating enzyme, glycerol kinase) in mice, however, failed to reveal a survival defect. This finding thus highlighted an important, but previously unrecognized, limitation of commonly used culture conditions that had been selected for their ability to promote maximal *in vitro*, but not *in vivo*, growth (28).

Recognizing the physiologic complexity of the host niche, studies of persistence have also used cell culture-based models. Macrophages are the primary cell type infected by *M. tuberculosis* and constitute the largest cellular reservoir of *M. tuberculosis* during the estab-

lishment and maintenance of chronic infection (29). Within macrophages, *M. tuberculosis* resides chiefly within the phagosomal compartment, where it is often able to persist for days *in vitro* and years *in vivo* (30, 31). At the same time, *M. tuberculosis*-containing phagosomes have long been noted for their heterogeneity with respect to their biochemical composition and ability to restrict *M. tuberculosis*. For example, nascent phagosomes, while hypoxic and nutrient poor, are capable of slowing but not suppressing *M. tuberculosis* replication, while fusion with endomembrane compartments and immune activation by cytokines enables the host to suppress, and sometimes even kill, *M. tuberculosis* by altering its chemistry to include acidic pH, lytic (or cell wall-perturbing) enzymes, and/or antimicrobial peptides, oxygenated lipids, and reactive oxygen and nitrogen species (32, 33). Recent studies have suggested that *M. tuberculosis* can even escape the phagosome to reside in cytosol (34). Given this potential range of heterogeneity, it is not surprising that the utility of these models has been defined by the type, differentiation program, and immune activation status of the cells used, each of which can influence the nature and degree of *M. tuberculosis* persistence.

The largest and most complex model of *M. tuberculosis* persistence, short of humans, is the experimentally infected animal. Inbred mice are the historically oldest and most extensively studied model of TB. While murine models of TB fail to fully recapitulate the pathology of both latent and active human TB, the availability of various inbred strains, reagents, and genetically altered mutants and the ease with which mice can be infected and analyzed have allowed for the clear identification of genes associated with *M. tuberculosis* pathogenicity (35). In addition, experimental infections of other animal models with genetically altered *M. tuberculosis* mutants have been performed only rarely. In the most commonly used aerosol model of pulmonary TB in C57/Bl6 mice, *M. tuberculosis* persists at a stable bacterial burden, following the onset of adaptive immunity, that was found to represent a state of balanced growth and death in which the replication rate of growing organisms was approximately 20% of that observed during the initial establishment of infection and unrestricted *in vitro* growth (13). As with cell culture models, the availability of genetic mutants and biochemical and immunological reagents has made it possible to identify host and bacterial determinants of persistence. In a recent application of this approach, Liu et al. identified specific determinants of host immunity associated with drug-induced persistence (36). Nonetheless, the growing use of other animal models such as the guinea pig, rabbit, and non-human primates has begun to yield important insight into those aspects of TB pathogenesis not modeled by the mouse.

METHODS

Despite over 50 years of research, studies of persistence have been hindered, in part, by fundamental uncertainties regarding the heterogeneity, size, and location of clinically relevant persister organisms and their relationship to the multiplicity of potential mechanisms described above. Indeed, while bacterial numbers during latent infection and following chemotherapy often reach undetectable levels, clinico-pathologic studies have demonstrated large bacterial burdens at the center or acellular rim of necrotic or cavitary lesions that are often hypoxic and rank among the strongest known risk factors for treatment relapse (37). As a result, studies of persistence have been heavily influenced by the technical bias of available experimental methods and their compatibility with existing models. This bias initially favored the study of deterministic factors associated with persistence of majority subpopulations of *M. tuberculosis*. However, recent advances in single-cell technologies in combination with molecular genetic approaches have expanded this scope to enable the discovery of stochastic factors and minority subpopulations (38–40).

Agar-based culture methods have long served as the "gold standard" measure of persistence. Predating the recognition of persistence as a pathophysiologic trait, these methods provided the first evidence of *M. tuberculosis*'s unusually robust tolerance to a wide range of *ex vivo* stresses. Agar-based methods subsequently enabled the foundational discovery of persistence as a microbiologic trait and have since served as the chief modality for its detection and enumeration. Interestingly, recent work has suggested that, despite their historical significance, these methods may fail to detect a significant proportion of viable organisms. Such organisms have been found to be selectively recoverable from liquid- but not agar-based media, suggesting the existence of additional persistent subpopulations (41). From a broader perspective, however, the inherent requirement for growth under artificial conditions has restricted the utility of all culture-based methods outside of detection and enumeration to *in vitro* settings.

The advent of nucleic acid-based technologies subsequently enabled systems-level studies of *M. tuberculosis* incubated under conditions thought to represent the persister niche *in vitro* and *ex vivo*, as well as *M. tuberculosis* recovered from its native milieu in the lungs of

infected animals and humans. These technologies initially provided descriptive transcriptional profiles but were soon followed by functional methods that enabled the identification of specific genes required for persistence. The latter methods specifically entailed competitive negative selection assays comparing an input pool of transposon mutants to the pool recovered after some stress (42) and found applications in *in vitro* and animal models of host- or drug-induced persistence where bacterial biomass at physiological loads is limiting (43–48). The impact of these methods, however, was somewhat tempered by their general dependence on the accuracy and completeness of their accompanying bioinformatic annotations and limited coverage of genes also required for optimal *in vitro* growth. Limitations notwithstanding, these approaches have provided broad qualitative insights into *M. tuberculosis* persistence as manifest *in vitro* and in macrophages, animal models, and humans.

Advances in analytical chemistry, mass spectrometry, and nuclear magnetic resonance have recently enabled conceptually analogous systems-level biochemical studies. These technologies have thus far contributed specific insight into the *in vitro* proteome, *in situ* metabolome, and *in vivo* metabolome of persistent *M. tuberculosis* recovered from or resident in *in vitro* culture systems, macrophages, and the lungs of infected animals (49–55). Owing chiefly to limitations in sensitivity, however, these approaches have been primarily restricted to models in which persistence is manifest as a deterministic property of the majority population of *M. tuberculosis* present.

While direct studies of persistence mediated by minority subpopulations and/or stochastic mechanisms were once refractory to traditional experimental technologies, this hurdle has also been recently overcome by advances in robotic high-throughput screening and single-cell imaging technologies. These technologies have specifically enabled the discovery of a form of chemotherapeutically induced persistence in which *M. tuberculosis* is able to withstand sterilization by the frontline drug isoniazid through the temporally stochastic extinction of transcription of its activating enzyme, catalase (38). High-throughput robotics have similarly enabled the screening of vast chemical libraries for compounds active against non- or slowly replicating *M. tuberculosis* populations (56–58).

MEASUREMENTS

Focusing on metabolism, existing knowledge of persistence derives from a mosaic of experimental models and methods of varying physiologic relevance. Such uncertainties have made it difficult to relate the findings from one experimental setting to another as well as to the physiologically distinct forms of persistence observed *in vivo*. In the case of metabolism, this challenge has been further complicated by the fact that metabolic enzymes serve pathways that are often organism- and/or condition-specific and thus functionally unannotated.

Host-Induced Persistence

Limitations notwithstanding, evidence of a number of model-specific and -independent characteristics has slowly begun to emerge. Chief among this evidence is that pertaining to respiration. Though classified as a strict aerobe, *M. tuberculosis* is able to survive within intra- and extracellular niches that are either directly or functionally limiting for oxygen. Indeed, direct biochemical measurements have reported oxygen concentrations within mouse and human macrophage phagosomes as low as 1%, while those of *M. tuberculosis*-containing lesions in mice, rabbits, and non-human primates were generally less than 5% (59–62). Oxygen concentrations aside, *M. tuberculosis* also encounters nitric oxide (NO) as an inflammatory product of immune activated macrophages, resulting in a functional poisoning of its respiratory chain. At the same time, auto-oxidation of NO also gives rise to nitrate, which can serve as an alternative terminal electron acceptor, second only to molecular oxygen. Interestingly, *M. tuberculosis*'s ability to respire nitrate has been found to accompany a transcriptionally mediated program that is activated upon gradual oxygen depletion to levels below 1% and to facilitate survival in response to mild acid stress (pH = 5.5) similar to that achieved upon immune activation (60). *In vitro* studies have further shown that reductions in oxygen concentration below 1 to 2% and availability of nitrate are also linked to marked decreases in drug susceptibility. Respiration has thus attracted specific interest as a metabolic feature of persistence in the setting of both natural infection and chemotherapy.

Microbiologic studies first demonstrated that while *M. tuberculosis* is unable to survive abrupt transfer from vigorous aeration to anaerobic conditions *in vitro*, it is able to survive for extended periods of time at oxygen tensions as low as 0.28 mm Hg (0.03%) if allowed to adapt to gradual oxygen depletion (63). As oxygen depletes, *M. tuberculosis* first reduces its respiratory rate at a dissolved oxygen concentration of ~6%, though growth continues unabated (64). At oxygen concentrations of ~1 to 2% (nonreplicating persistence, or

NRP-1), growth slows with an arrest of DNA synthesis and a decrease in ATP levels and with an increase in levels of a glycine dehydrogenase-like activity (63). Consistent with these changes, transcriptional profiling studies of *M. tuberculosis* subjected to hypoxia or NO, or recovered from infected macrophages and mice, have shown increased expression of a type II (non-proton translocating) NADH dehydrogenase and less energy-efficient, but higher oxygen affinity cytochrome *bd* oxidase, and decreased expression of ATP synthase (65–67). Genetic deletion of the cytochrome *bd* oxidase has been further shown to impair survival of *M. tuberculosis* during transition to the chronic (or persistent) phase of infection (65). As oxygen depletes further (typically below 0.06%, or NRP-2), both DNA and RNA synthesis arrests and glycine dehydrogenase activity decreases, while *M. tuberculosis* resides in a physiologically quiescent state as shown by the synchronized resumption of RNA synthesis immediately upon re-aeration and delayed re-initiation of DNA replication until after completion of the first division (68).

Interestingly, adaptation to 1% oxygen, sublethal concentrations of NO, and residence within macrophage cell cultures and mice are all accompanied by a transcriptional increase in expression of the nitrate transporter, *narK2* (69). This increase in expression has been further shown to be accompanied by a biochemical increase in nitrate respiration. These findings thus support the physiologic relevance of nitrate as a prevalent feature of the hypoxic niches occupied by *M. tuberculosis*, independent of its specific production as an auto-oxidation product of NOS2, which requires oxygen as a substrate and loses 80 to 90% of its activity at 1% oxygen (70). Moreover, recent work has shown that respiration of nitrate gives rise to nitrite that alters *M. tuberculosis* physiology through mechanisms independent of its potential dismutation back into NO and nitrate. These mechanisms include inhibition of ATP consumption, oxidation of iron from the ferrous to ferric state, disrupting iron sulfur clusters and perhaps contributing to resistance to the frontline drug isoniazid (by potentially suppressing its activation by the heme-containing catalase), and inhibition of growth upon aeration (60).

From a metabolic perspective, ^{13}C tracing studies conducted in two independent studies have shown that the foregoing changes in respiration are linked to accompanying alterations in the structure of its tricarboxylic acid (TCA) cycle (71, 72). As oxygen is depleted to ~1%, *M. tuberculosis* increases expression of the glyoxylate shunt enzyme isocitrate lyase (ICL) to produce a large amount of succinate. This increased production of succinate is hypothesized to enable *M. tuberculosis* to flexibly sustain membrane potential, ATP synthesis, and anaplerosis at a rate proportional to its respiratory capacity, such that some of the unused excess can be secreted to maintain membrane potential while the remainder is stored to facilitate immediate resumption of carbon flow and ATP synthesis upon re-aeration. Accordingly, provision of nitrate at 1% oxygen abolished succinate secretion and restored TCA cycle activity, ATP levels, and NADH/NAD ratios to near aerobic levels (72). As oxygen levels are depleted further, *M. tuberculosis* has been shown to upregulate expression of genes of the reductive arm of its TCA cycle with an accompanying increase in reductive half-cycle activity which also produces succinate as an end product (71, 72). In this setting, the near neutral midpoint potential of the succinate/fumarate redox couple ($\varepsilon^0 = +0.03$ V) makes it suitable to accumulate as a fermentation product of fumarate reductase and facilitate redox balance. Generation of succinate thus appears to serve as a type of multifunctional "metabolic battery" capable of flexibly sustaining membrane potential, ATP synthesis, and TCA cycle precursors and functioning as a biochemical bridge between oxidative and fermentative metabolic states.

In a more functionally oriented approach, Hartman and colleagues characterized the impact of genetically deleting the membrane anchor subunit of *M. tuberculosis* succinate dehydrogenase (*sdh1*; *rv0249c*) (64). *sdh1* has dual roles in the TCA cycle and respiratory chain, where it oxidizes succinate to fumarate and delivers two electrons to the membrane electron carrier menaquinone. Accordingly, isotope-labeling studies of *M. tuberculosis* strains harboring clean deletions of *sdh1* confirmed that succinate oxidation was diminished during aerobic growth but continued uncontrolled when shifted into an anaerobic environment. This mismatch between succinate metabolism and respiration resulted in a 10-fold decrease in bacterial titers in the lungs of mice that developed severely hypoxic lesions.

Arguably, the most compelling line of evidence in support of hypoxic respiration as a critical feature of host-induced persistence is the clinical efficacy of bedaquiline (BDQ) and pretomanid (PA-824) (and its related nitroimidazo-oxazole, Delamanid [OPC-67683]) in human studies (73–75). BDQ is a potent inhibitor of *M. tuberculosis* ATP synthase that binds to the membrane-embedded rotor (c ring) and prevents the shuttling of Na^+ and/or H^+ ions needed to power ATP synthesis (76). Moreover, microbiologic and animal studies indicate that BDQ is capable of killing both replicating and nonreplicating *M. tuberculosis* as modeled

in vitro by hypoxia and nutrient starvation, and *in vivo* in an established model of chronic infection, wherein activity manifests as an accelerated bactericidal activity (77–81). PA-824, in contrast, is a bicyclic nitroimidazole compound whose activity against hypoxic *M. tuberculosis* is mediated by intrabacterial release of NO by a deazaflavin-dependent nitroreductase (Ddn; Rv3547) (82, 83). However, like BDQ, PA-824 was also found to exhibit activity during the continuation phase of chemotherapy in a high-dose aerosol challenge model of TB thought to model persistent *M. tuberculosis in vivo* (84, 85), as well as in patients with smear-positive disease (86, 87). Taken together, these findings unequivocally establish hypoxic respiration as a clinically relevant feature of *M. tuberculosis* persistence.

Respiration aside, knowledge of metabolic adaptations specific to host-induced persistence remains considerably more model-specific and dependent on bioinformatically derived inferences. These inferences derive chiefly from gene expression and mutant analysis studies of *M. tuberculosis* (i) incubated under host-relevant *in vitro* conditions thought to model persistence or (ii) recovered from the chronic phase of infection in animals and humans.

Studies of the former category have specifically examined nutrient starvation (modeled by incubation in phosphate-buffered saline), acid pH (approximating that of resting and immune activated macrophage phagosomes), bacteriostatic concentrations of NO (as described above), and a multistress model consisting of 5% oxygen, 10% CO_2, pH = 5, and 10% Dubos medium. Interestingly, exposure to both types of nutrient starvation identified a generalized downregulation of genes associated with aerobic respiration suggestive of metabolic changes similar to those associated with hypoxia (described above) (88). These included downregulation of subunits of its type I NADH dehydrogenase and ATP synthase and upregulation of its fumarate reductase and ICL, while expression of annotated genes of central carbon metabolism was generally reduced and oxygen consumption rates were significantly reduced.

Exposure to acid pH identified a surprisingly small number of annotated genes of metabolic function, of which only upregulation components of the ESX-1 secretion system were observed in an independent study (89, 90). Nonetheless, a comparison of *in vitro* acid stress (pH = 7 versus 6.5 versus 5.5) to infection of bone marrow-derived murine macrophages treated (or not) with concanamycin A, a specific inhibitor of the vacuolar ATPase mediating phagosomal acidification, identified an increase in expression of acid-specific genes involved in lipid metabolism (*lipF*-Rv3487c, *whiB3*-Rv3416) and polyketide biosynthesis (*papA1*-Rv3824c, *pks2*-Rv3825c, *pks3*-Rv1180) (89), though none of the latter set of genes was found to be essential for chronic phase survival in the murine lung (91).

Exposure to the complex stress described above identified related alterations in expression of genes associated with nutrient starvation, hypoxic adaptation, and lipid metabolism (*nuoB, ctaD, qcrC, atpA, atpD*), similar to those observed in bacteria recovered from sputa from patients prior to treatment (92, 93). Other microarray-based transcriptional profiling studies in mice and humans during the chronic (or persistent) phase of infection have similarly reported alterations in expression of genes involved in central carbon metabolism and/or respiration (*aceA, narK2, nuo, nadC, menA, lld2, ppdK*) and lipid metabolism (*aceA, echA15*), similar to those observed in *in vitro* models. However, the overlap of specific genes identified in all models has been small and primarily limited to those involved in respiration (67, 94, 95).

Studies of the latter category have primarily emerged from the use of genetically inbred mice. Such studies were initially restricted to the identification of metabolic genes dispensable for *in vitro* growth and/or survival but have since been expanded to include genes required for *in vitro* growth thanks to the advent of conditionally regulated gene expression systems (96). Together, these approaches have enabled a systematic inventorying of metabolically annotated genes required for persistence.

The first such gene to be identified was *icl1*, one of *M. tuberculosis*'s two annotated ICLs (97). ICL is a canonical enzyme of the glyoxylate shunt, a pathway required for assimilation of even-chain fatty acids. Deletion of *icl1* was specifically found to attenuate *M. tuberculosis* survival during the chronic, but not acute, phase of infection in mice and during infection of interferon gamma-activated, but not resting, bone marrow-derived macrophages. Based on these findings, ICL was interpreted to be essential for persistence due to its role in metabolism of even-chain fatty acids. However, subsequent work showed that *icl1* also encoded activity as a methylisocitrate lyase, an enzyme involved in metabolism of the odd-chain fatty acid propionate through the parallel methylcitrate cycle (98, 99). Moreover, studies of *M. tuberculosis* strains lacking both ICLs revealed a bactericidal vulnerability to both even- and odd-chain fatty acids that could be genetically complemented by *icl1* alone. This vulnerability was ultimately shown to be due to loss of methylisocitrate lyase, rather than ICL activity (99, 100). These studies thus raised the possibility that the persistence defect of ICL-deficient *M. tuberculosis* observed in mice might reflect an inability to metabolize propionate instead of, or in addition to, acetate. Efforts to resolve this ambiguity, however, were complicated by the discovery of two additional physiologic roles for ICL unrelated to fatty acid metabolism altogether: adaptation to hypoxia (discussed above) and antibiotic tolerance (discussed below) (9, 101).

A second example that emerged with the use of conditionally regulated mutants was the discovery of *pckA*, a gene annotated to encode the enzyme phosphoenol-pyruvate carboxykinase, which catalyzes the first committed step in gluconeogenesis. Transcriptional silencing of *pckA* during the chronic (or persistent) phase of an aerosol infection in mice led to its clearance (102). In conjunction with evidence for the importance of fatty acid metabolism, these data implicated an essential role for gluconeogenesis in mediating persistence. However, this survival defect could not be recapitulated when culturing *pckA*-deficient *M. tuberculosis* on fatty acids or in resting or immune activated bone marrow-derived macrophages. Thus, like the case for ICL, these studies identified *pckA* as a clear determinant of persistence but failed to reveal its specific metabolic role, owing to limitations in the accuracy and completeness of bioinformatic annotations and *in vitro* biochemical studies. Indeed, follow-up biochemical studies demonstrated that *M. tuberculosis* PckA could catalyze the reverse reaction in an anaplerotic, rather than gluconeogenic, direction under reducing conditions such as those associated with hypoxia (103). Experimentally based computational models of metabolic flux have similarly suggested that *M. tuberculosis* PckA may operate in an anaplerotic direction during intracellular growth within a THP-1 macrophage-like cell line (55).

Studies of additional gene deletion mutants in central carbon metabolism have similarly identified essential, but incompletely defined, roles for two glucokinases (*ppgK, glkA*), fructose bisphosphate aldolase (*fba*), lipoamide dehydrogenase (*lpd*), and 2-hydroxy-3-oxoadipate synthase (*hoas/kgd*) (8, 104–106). However, like the case for *icl1/2* and *pckA*, interpretation of their specific metabolic roles in persistence remains unresolved. Glucokinase, for example, catalyzes the specific phosphorylation of glucose into glucose phosphate, which can biochemically trap or retain glucose within the cell, fuel glycolysis, and/or facilitate the generation of NADPH. Fbp (fructose 1,6-bisphosphatase) can similarly serve both glycolysis and gluconeogenesis, while Lpd (lipoamide dehydrogenase) was shown to serve as a subunit of *M. tuberculosis*'s canonical pyruvate dehydrogenase complex, peroxynitrite reductase, and branched chain ketoacid dehydrogenase. Recent studies similarly demonstrated that HOAS/Kgd (2-hydroxy-3-oxoadipate synthase/ketoglutarate decarboxylase) was competent to support production of three products—2-hydroxy-3-oxoadipate, succinate semialdehyde, and succinate—but was found to mediate defense against glutamate toxicity and reactive nitrogen intermediates when present in *M. tuberculosis* cultured under standard in *in vitro* conditions (106).

Gene deletion studies have also identified specific roles for the core proteasome subunits (*prcA* and *prcB*), the stringent response regulator (*relA*), the methionine biosynthetic enzyme homoserine transacetylase (*metA*), and a mycolic acid cyclopropane synthetase (*pcaA*) in persistence in mice (107–111). Both *prcBA* and *relA* have been reported to facilitate adaptation to in vitro nutrient limitation in *M. tuberculosis* through roles in amino acid recycling and biosynthesis, respectively. Interestingly, however, expression of a hydrolase null allele of RelA, still competent to synthesize the stringent response alarmone (p)ppGpp, was found to be competent to complement the persistence defect of an isogenic *relA*-deficient strain in mice (112). Expression of a proteolytically null active site mutant was similarly shown to be sufficient to complement both the *in vitro* susceptibility to NO and *in vivo* persistence defects of *prcBA*-deficient *M. tuberculosis*, though complementation of other *in vitro* persistence defects associated with prolonged stationary phase incubation and nutrient starvation required the wild-type allele (107). The specific metabolic functions served by PrcBA and RelA, and ways in which they facilitate persistence, thus await further study.

In contrast, the persistence defects of *metA* and *pcaA*-deficient *M. tuberculosis* appear more straightforward. MetA catalyzes the first committed step in methionine biosynthesis. Deletion of *metA* results in rapid bactericidal death *in vitro* and in both the acute and chronic phases of mouse infection, the former of which can be chemically complemented with methionine supplementation alone (110). These results thus identify a likely essential role for methionine or methionine-derived metabolites in persistence. The function of *pcaA* is perhaps even more physiologically specific in that it encodes an enzyme required for the formation of the proximal cyclopropane ring of *M. tuberculosis* immunoreactive alpha-mycolic acids, loss of which was accompanied by alterations in cording morphology (a biomarker of virulence), lipid profile, and cytokine responses (111, 113, 114). These findings thus suggest that *pcaA* may facilitate persistence through effects on the composition and immunoreactivity of the cell surface lipids of *M. tuberculosis*.

Based on the foregoing considerations, it is interesting to reconsider historical evidence implicating fatty acid oxidation as an essential feature of persistence. The first line of evidence emerged from experimental studies by Segal and Bloch, who found that *M. tuberculosis* isolated *ex vivo* was primed to respire on fatty acids (115). This view was reinforced by the subsequent publication of its genome, which revealed over 250 enzymes involved in fatty acid metabolism, including 82 annotated as either fatty acid desaturases or acyl-CoA dehydrogenases (116). These numbers were interpreted to indicate extensive redundancy in the utilization of fatty acid substrates, though only 2 of *M. tuberculosis*'s over 100 β-oxidation genes have been determined to be essential *in vitro* (117). More specific, though circumstantial, evidence in support of a role for fatty acid metabolism in human infection emerged with the discovery of lipid droplets in *M. tuberculosis* recovered from the sputum of patients with active TB. These droplets were found to contain host-derived triacylglycerol (92) that could be mobilized when respiration was inhibited, presumably as a carbon and energy source (118). In addition, similar lipid inclusions could be modeled *in vitro* following incubation of *M. tuberculosis* in hypoxia (63). However, the strongest and perhaps most influential evidence in support of the essentiality of fatty acid utilization in persistence stemmed from the discovery of a selective survival defect of Δ*icl M. tuberculosis* during the chronic, but not acute, phase of infection in mice, whose interpretation was discussed above (97). Thus, while likely to be a feature of its metabolism during infection, direct evidence for the essentiality and nature (whether fueled by intra- or extracellular lipids) of fatty acid metabolism in persistence remains surprisingly scant.

Ambiguities notwithstanding, nucleic acid-based technologies have also enabled empiric genome-wide inventorying of metabolic genes required for persistence. The most comprehensive of these inventories was reported by Sassetti and Rubin, who used transposon-mutagenized libraries of *M. tuberculosis* to identify genes required for survival in resting and immune activated macrophages and in the spleens of mice infected by tail vein injection (91). These studies specifically enabled the identification of genes with competitive fitness defects in the acute and chronic phases of infection (Table 1).

Among the latter, work by Griffin and coworkers identified a gene cluster required for import of host cholesterol (44). This finding launched numerous follow-up genetic and biochemical studies showing that *M. tuberculosis* could both import and catabolize cholesterol and that this activity was essential for persistence in the

Table 1 Predicted essential genes for *in vivo* survival of *M. tuberculosis* at 8 weeks that are not significantly inhibited at 4 weeks[a]

Name	Rv#	Functional class
rv2808	2808	No prediction
cobC	2231c	Amino acid transport and metabolism
aftB	3805c	Capsule polysaccharide biosynthetic process
rv3472	3472	Conserved hypothetical protein
rv0199	0199	Conserved membrane protein
rv1974	1974	Conserved membrane protein
aceE	2241	Energy production and conversion— pyruvate dehydrogenase E1
rv0100	0100	Extracellular region
rv0098	0098	Fatty acid biosynthetic process
rv1021	1021	General functional prediction only
rv3649	3649	General functional prediction only
rv1939	1939	General functional prediction only
ctpD	1469	Inorganic ion transport and metabolism
mce1A	0169	Lipid transport and metabolism—mycolic acid transport
pks16	1013	Lipid transport and metabolism
rv3523	3523	Lipid transport and metabolism
rv3371	3371	Lipid transport and metabolism— triacylglycerol synthase
chp2	1184c	Plasma membrane—diacyltrehalose acyltransferase
ung	2976c	Replication, recombination, and repair
nrp	0101	Secondary metabolites biosynthesis, transport, metabolism
rv2857c	2857c	Secondary metabolites biosynthesis, transport, metabolism
pks12	2048c	Secondary metabolites biosynthesis, transport, metabolism
rv0687	0687	Secondary metabolites biosynthesis, transport, metabolism
rv1931c	1931c	Transcription
rv2912c	2912c	Transcription
proS	2845c	Translation

[a]Adapted from reference 91.

lungs of chronically infected animals and for growth within the interferon-gamma-activated macrophages (119–121). Cholesterol that is metabolized in *M. tuberculosis* (when used as a sole carbon source) is cleaved into pyruvate and propionyl-CoA and/or acetyl-CoA during aerobiosis. The resulting pyruvate can be oxidized into the TCA cycle. However, the propionyl-CoA that is generated must first be detoxified, primarily by the methylcitrate cycle (less so by the methylmalonyl pathway), into succinate and pyruvate before entering central carbon metabolism (120), while the carbon of the side chain of cholesterol can be assimilated into both phthiocerol dimycocerosates (PDIMs) and sulfolipid-1. The physiologic role and specific enzymes required for

cholesterol metabolism in persistence, however, remain unclear because it supports only weak *in vitro* growth as a carbon source, while a transposon mutant interrupted in Rv1106c (which is required for growth when cholesterol is provided as the sole carbon source) displayed no phenotype in either macrophage culture or guinea pig infection (122).

Looking beyond central carbon metabolism, gene deletion studies have identified essential roles for biosynthesis of the cofactors NAD and biotin in persistence. Silencing of either *nadE* or *bioA* resulted in clearance of *M. tuberculosis* from the lungs of mice when depleted during the chronic phase of infection (123, 124). NadE is a glutamine-dependent NAD(+) synthetase that catalyzes the last committed step in the NAD synthesis pathway. NAD(+) itself has long been implicated in survival in dormancy since Wayne and Lin found that glycine dehydrogenase and ICL activities were increased in their model of dormancy (125). Silencing of *bioA* resulted in a deficiency of biotinylated proteins in *M. tuberculosis*, leading the authors to posit that fatty acid biosynthesis would be impaired in the mutant (124). The fact that depletion resulted in a lethal phenotype in the chronic phase of infection in mice may thus serve as additional evidence in support of fatty acid metabolism as an essential feature of persistence. Fatty acid metabolism notwithstanding, these findings identify NAD+ and biotin as limiting cofactors, due to either increased turnover or demand, required for persistence during the chronic phase of infection in mice.

Interestingly, recent advances in proteomics and chemical biology have begun to deliver analogous systems level biochemical insights into persistence. Such studies have thus far focused on *in vitro* models of hypoxic *M. tuberculosis*. Comparing the quantitative proteomic composition of replicating *M. tuberculosis* against NRP-1, NRP-2, and re-aerated *M. tuberculosis*, Schubert and colleagues identified specific alterations in the levels of its respiratory enzymes (including its type I [Nuo] and type II [Ndh/NdhA], cytochrome *c* oxidase/reductase [Cta/Qcr], cytochrome *bd* oxidase [Cyd], and ATP synthase), consistent with prior biochemical, transcriptional and metabolomics studies (126). This study also identified additional linked changes in the levels of enzymes specifically involved in the acyl CoA, alanine/aspartate/glutamate, trehalose, cholesterol/lipid, and quinone biosyntheses, similarly consistent with genetic studies.

In a complementary biochemical approach, Ortega and colleagues used a more functional approach called activity-based protein profiling (127). This approach specifically enables proteome-wide profiling of the *in situ* activity (rather than abundance) of a given class of proteins within a cell or cell lysate based on their vulnerability to a covalently reactive, active site-specific probe. Using a serine hydrolase-specific probe, Ortega and colleagues identified decreases in the activity of three enzymes involved in the biosynthesis of *M. tuberculosis*'s cell envelope mycolic acids (the antigen 85 carboxyesterases, which generate trehalose mono- and dimycolates; Pks13, an enzyme involved in phthiocerol dymycocerosate; and TesA, a thioesterase) in hypoxic, compared to replicating, *M. tuberculosis*, and consistent with a prior lipidomic study using the same experimental model (127, 128).

Drug-Induced Persistence

In contrast to host-induced persistence, comparatively little attention has been paid to the metabolic features of drug-induced persistence. Screening a pool of signature-tagged *M. tuberculosis* transposon mutants, Dhar and McKinney identified *cydC*, a gene annotated to encode an ATP-binding cassette transporter required for assembly of the cytochrome *bd* oxidase, as a mediator of isoniazid-induced persistence or tolerance in mice (51). Disruption of *M. tuberculosis cydC* selectively accelerated bacterial clearance in isoniazid-treated mice without affecting growth or survival of untreated mice. This effect was specific for INH and could be genetically complemented *in vivo* with a wild-type allele. However, it could not be recapitulated *in vitro* using host-like conditions capable of inducing expression of *cydC*, providing further evidence for the limitations of *in vitro* systems alone. Nonetheless, it is interesting to note that, as mentioned above, *narG*, another alternative respiratory chain component, was also found to mediate isoniazid tolerance *in vitro* (60).

In a study examining the relationship between antibiotic tolerance and bacterial growth rate, Baek et al. identified *tgs1* in a transposon mutant screen for genes whose disruption resulted in a growth or survival advantage under hypoxia (129). *tgs1* is a well-characterized triglyceride synthase that constitutes the dominant Tgs activity under hypoxia. Moreover, targeted deletion of *tgs1* was shown to prevent triacylglyceride synthesis and redirect carbon to increase flux through the *M. tuberculosis* TCA cycle. This increase was subsequently shown to confer an increase in susceptibility of *M. tuberculosis* to a broad panel of antibiotics under conditions of *in vitro* hypoxia and in mice. It was thus proposed that redirection of metabolic flux away from the TCA cycle and toward the synthesis of triglycerides served as a mechanism of antibiotic-induced persistence

(or tolerance) in hypoxic *M. tuberculosis*. Shi et al. similarly proposed a model in which carbon and nitrogen are repurposed into triacylglycerol and glutamate for use during growth arrest and regrowth once favorable conditions were re-encountered (130).

Work by Nandakumar et al. more recently identified *M. tuberculosis* ICLs as a similarly broad metabolic mediator of antibiotic tolerance in replicating *M. tuberculosis* (101). This work specifically showed that (i) three mechanistically unrelated clinical antibiotics (isoniazid, rifampin, and streptomycin) all triggered an increase in expression of *M. tuberculosis* ICLs, in a carbon source-independent manner; (ii) absence of ICL activity led to a significant increase in susceptibility to all three antibiotics; and (iii) this heightened susceptibility could be functionally complemented with a chemical antioxidant. This study thus suggested that *M. tuberculosis* ICLs mediated antibiotic-induced persistence (or tolerance) by serving as a form of antioxidant defense in which increased flux through the glyoxylate shunt mitigates against the production of respiratory radicals arising from the generation of NADH in the oxidative arm of its TCA cycle.

Awaiting further studies, it is becoming apparent that, like its host-induced counterpart, antibiotic-induced persistence is an active cellular process, rather than a passive consequence of slowed or arrested growth, likely to be encoded by specific metabolic pathways.

MESSAGES

Accumulating evidence has left little doubt about the importance of persistence or metabolism in the biology and chemotherapy of TB. However, knowledge of the intersection of these two factors has only recently begun to emerge. The goal of this chapter is to reframe our understanding of each with respect to the other, their relationship to the fundamental biology of *M. tuberculosis*, and the potential union of these relationships to identify novel potential strategies against the pandemic.

One theme to emerge from this synthesis is the need for continued, but regulated, electron transport chain activity, a finding common to studies of persistence in other bacterial species. In *M. tuberculosis*, strains with deletion or inactivation of several individual components of the respiratory chain and glycolysis are attenuated by one log in the murine lung. Additionally, two of the most recent antitubercular drugs—BDQ and pretomanid—target the ATP synthase and respiratory chain and have activity during the chronic phase of infection. In terms of drug tolerance, this is consistent with investigations of persistence in *Escherichia coli* by several findings, including screens for factors involved in tolerance which turned up genes in central carbon metabolism and aerobic respiration (131). Other work found that metabolic stimulation of glycolysis kills drug-tolerant persisters by stimulating proton motive force both aerobically and anaerobically (132) and that disruption of stationary-phase respiration has a similar effect (133). The functional redundancy of the *M. tuberculosis* electron transport chain would complicate similar work, but the construction of conditional deletion strains offers an analytical approach to test these hypotheses in the future.

Respiration aside, however, knowledge of specific metabolic processes required for persistence remains scant and heavily dependent on the use of genomic orthologies derived from organisms and ecologies distinct from those of persistent *M. tuberculosis*. Further complicating this dependency is the modular nature of metabolic pathways and the physiologic functions they serve, which for most organisms have been limited to replication. Systems biologists have been able to define the objective function of *E. coli* in differing growth states (134). However, lacking a reliable, experimentally tractable model system, the use of such predictions is unlikely to yield insights that can be tested.

Limitations notwithstanding, it is interesting to note that the most represented, though understudied, class of annotated functions identified in screens for genes required for persistence in mice was that of transporters. Transporters are well known for a lack of strict substrate specificity. It is thus all the more surprising that loss of individual transporters of amino acids, lipids, carbohydrates, coenzymes, and inorganic ions resulted in measurable defects in persistence. Delineating the substrate specificities of these transporters thus represents a potentially fruitful, but understudied, source of drug targets in this important subpopulation.

Looking back, it has become clear that persistence may comprise a complex and heterogeneous set of physiologic states as potentially diverse as the conditions in which it can be found. So, just as any biochemical or thermodynamic event that disrupts the binding of an antibiotic to its target might manifest as drug tolerance, any event that limits the rate of binary fission has the potential to manifest as persistence. Knowledge of *M. tuberculosis*'s metabolic ledger in each of these states thus represents a key hurdle to overcoming the challenge of persistence.

Still, there is a notion that this heterogeneity may be unified by a common set of "persister essential" processes. The terminology that we use to classify complex traits such as "persistence" and "tolerance" gives the impression that inhibition of specific pathways might be controlling these broad phenotypes. However, it remains equally possible that there are as many avenues that facilitate entry into, dwell in, and exit from persistence as there are forms of persistence. Only further studies of core metabolic processes will allow us to resolve this ambiguity (135). However, until that time, the path forward will have to move at the pace that empirical research permits.

Acknowledgments. We apologize that many papers could not be discussed owing to the lack of space. The authors' research on this topic was supported by the NIH TB Research Unit Network (AI111143) and the Bill & Melinda Gates Foundation (OPP1024050, OPP1068025). The funders had no role in study design, data collection and interpretation, or the decision to submit the work for publication.

Citation. Hartman TE, Wang Z, Jansen RS, Gardete S, Rhee KY. 2017. Metabolic perspectives on persistence. Microbiol Spectrum 5(1):TBTB2-0026-2016.

References

1. **Gutierrez MC, Brisse S, Brosch R, Fabre M, Omaïs B, Marmiesse M, Supply P, Vincent V.** 2005. Ancient origin and gene mosaicism of the progenitor of *Mycobacterium tuberculosis*. *PLoS Pathog* 1:e5

2. **Russell DG, Barry CE III, Flynn JL.** 2010. Tuberculosis: what we don't know can, and does, hurt us. *Science* 328:852–856

3. **Nathan C.** 2012. Fresh approaches to anti-infective therapies. *Sci Transl Med* 4:140sr2

4. **Kester JC, Fortune SM.** 2014. Persisters and beyond: mechanisms of phenotypic drug resistance and drug tolerance in bacteria. *Crit Rev Biochem Mol Biol* 49: 91–101.

5. **Ehrt S, Rhee K.** 2013. *Mycobacterium tuberculosis* metabolism and host interaction: mysteries and paradoxes. *Curr Top Microbiol Immunol* 374:163–188.

6. **Gomez JE, McKinney JD.** 2004. *M. tuberculosis* persistence, latency, and drug tolerance. *Tuberculosis (Edinb)* 84:29–44.

7. **Kalscheuer R, Syson K, Veeraraghavan U, Weinrick B, Biermann KE, Liu Z, Sacchettini JC, Besra G, Bornemann S, Jacobs WR Jr.** 2010. Self-poisoning of *Mycobacterium tuberculosis* by targeting GlgE in an alpha-glucan pathway. *Nat Chem Biol* 6:376–384.

8. **Venugopal A, Bryk R, Shi S, Rhee K, Rath P, Schnappinger D, Ehrt S, Nathan C.** 2011. Virulence of *Mycobacterium tuberculosis* depends on lipoamide dehydrogenase, a member of three multienzyme complexes. *Cell Host Microbe* 9:21–31.

9. **Eoh H, Rhee KY.** 2014. Methylcitrate cycle defines the bactericidal essentiality of isocitrate lyase for survival of *Mycobacterium tuberculosis* on fatty acids. *Proc Natl Acad Sci USA* 111:4976–4981.

10. **Intlekofer AM, Dematteo RG, Venneti S, Finley LW, Lu C, Judkins AR, Rustenburg AS, Grinaway PB, Chodera JD, Cross JR, Thompson CB.** 2015. Hypoxia

induces production of L-2-hydroxyglutarate. *Cell Metab* 22:304–311

11. McCune RM Jr, McDermott W, Tompsett R. 1956. The fate of *Mycobacterium tuberculosis* in mouse tissues as determined by the microbial enumeration technique. II. The conversion of tuberculous infection to the latent state by the administration of pyrazinamide and a companion drug. *J Exp Med* **104**:763–802.

12. Ford CB, Shah RR, Maeda MK, Gagneux S, Murray MB, Cohen T, Johnston JC, Gardy J, Lipsitch M, Fortune SM. 2013. *Mycobacterium tuberculosis* mutation rate estimates from different lineages predict substantial differences in the emergence of drug-resistant tuberculosis. *Nat Genet* **45**:784–790

13. Gill WP, Harik NS, Whiddon MR, Liao RP, Mittler JE, Sherman DR. 2009. A replication clock for *Mycobacterium tuberculosis*. *Nat Med* **15**:211–214.

14. Stead WW, Eisenach KD, Cave MD, Beggs ML, Templeton GL, Thoen CO, Bates JH. 1995. When did *Mycobacterium tuberculosis* infection first occur in the New World? An important question with public health implications. *Am J Respir Crit Care Med* **151**:1267–1268.

15. Jasmer RM, Bozeman L, Schwartzman K, Cave MD, Saukkonen JJ, Metchock B, Khan A, Burman WJ, Tuberculosis Trials Consortium. 2004. Recurrent tuberculosis in the United States and Canada: relapse or reinfection? *Am J Respir Crit Care Med* **170**:1360–1366.

16. Hawken M, Nunn P, Godfrey-Faussett P, McAdam KPWJ, Morris J, Odhiambo J, Githui W, Gilks C, Hawken M, Gathua S, Nunn P, Hawken M, Brindle R, Batchelor B. 1993. Increased recurrence of tuberculosis in HIV-1-infected patients in Kenya. *Lancet* **342**:332–337.

17. Bryant JM, Harris SR, Parkhill J, Dawson R, Diacon AH, van Helden P, Pym A, Mahayiddin AA, Chuchottaworn C, Sanne IM, Louw C, Boeree MJ, Hoelscher M, McHugh TD, Bateson AL, Hunt RD, Mwaigwisya S, Wright L, Gillespie SH, Bentley SD. 2013. Whole-genome sequencing to establish relapse or re-infection with *Mycobacterium tuberculosis*: a retrospective observational study. *Lancet Respir Med* **1**:786–792.

18. Guerra-Assunção JA, Houben RM, Crampin AC, Mzembe T, Mallard K, Coll F, Khan P, Banda L, Chiwaya A, Pereira RP, McNerney R, Harris D, Parkhill J, Clark TG, Glynn JR. 2015. Recurrence due to relapse or reinfection with *Mycobacterium tuberculosis*: a whole-genome sequencing approach in a large, population-based cohort with a high HIV infection prevalence and active follow-up. *J Infect Dis* **211**:1154–1163.

19. Narayanan S, Swaminathan S, Supply P, Shanmugam S, Narendran G, Hari L, Ramachandran R, Locht C, Jawahar MS, Narayanan PR. 2010. Impact of HIV infection on the recurrence of tuberculosis in South India. *J Infect Dis* **201**:691–703.

20. Crampin AC, Mwaungulu JN, Mwaungulu FD, Mwafulirwa DT, Munthali K, Floyd S, Fine PE, Glynn JR. 2010. Recurrent TB: relapse or reinfection? The effect of HIV in a general population cohort in Malawi. *AIDS* **24**:417–426.

21. Vandiviere HM, Loring WE, Melvin I, Willis S. 1956. The treated pulmonary lesion and its tubercle bacillus.

II. The death and resurrection. *Am J Med Sci* **232**:30–37, passim

22. Zhang Y, Mitchison D. 2003. The curious characteristics of pyrazinamide: a review. *Int J Tuberc Lung Dis* **7**:6–21.

23. Mitchison D, Davies G. 2012. The chemotherapy of tuberculosis: past, present and future. *Int J Tuberc Lung Dis* **16**:724–732

24. Corper HJ, Cohn ML. 1951. The viability and virulence of old cultures of tubercle bacilli: studies on 30-year-old broth cultures maintained at 37 degrees C. *Tubercle* **32**:232–237.

25. Warner DF, Mizrahi V. 2006. Tuberculosis chemotherapy: the influence of bacillary stress and damage response pathways on drug efficacy. *Clin Microbiol Rev* **19**:558–570.

26. Keren I, Minami S, Rubin E, Lewis K. 2011. Characterization and transcriptome analysis of *Mycobacterium tuberculosis* persisters. *MBio* **2**:e00100–11

27. Pethe K, Sequeira PC, Agarwalla S, Rhee K, Kuhen K, Phong WY, Patel V, Beer D, Walker JR, Duraiswamy J, Jiricek J, Keller TH, Chatterjee A, Tan MP, Ujjini M, Rao SP, Camacho L, Bifani P, Mak PA, Ma I, Barnes SW, Chen Z, Plouffe D, Thayalan P, Ng SH, Au M, Lee BH, Tan BH, Ravindran S, Nanjundappa M, Lin X, Goh A, Lakshminarayana SB, Shoen C, Cynamon M, Kreiswirth B, Dartois V, Peters EC, Glynne R, Brenner S, Dick T. 2010. A chemical genetic screen in *Mycobacterium tuberculosis* identifies carbon-source-dependent growth inhibitors devoid of *in vivo* efficacy. *Nat Commun* **1**:57

28. Edson NL. 1951. The intermediary metabolism of the mycobacteria. *Bacteriol Rev* **15**:147–182.

29. McDonough KA, Kress Y, Bloom BR. 1993. Pathogenesis of tuberculosis: interaction of *Mycobacterium tuberculosis* with macrophages. *Infect Immun* **61**:2763–2773.

30. Rohde K, Yates RM, Purdy GE, Russell DG. 2007. *Mycobacterium tuberculosis* and the environment within the phagosome. *Immunol Rev* **219**:37–54.

31. Pieters J. 2008. *Mycobacterium tuberculosis* and the macrophage: maintaining a balance. *Cell Host Microbe* **3**:399–407

32. MacMicking JD, North RJ, LaCourse R, Mudgett JS, Shah SK, Nathan CF. 1997. Identification of nitric oxide synthase as a protective locus against tuberculosis. *Proc Natl Acad Sci USA* **94**:5243–5248.

33. MacMicking J, Xie QW, Nathan C. 1997. Nitric oxide and macrophage function. *Annu Rev Immunol* **15**:323–350

34. van der Wel N, Hava D, Houben D, Fluitsma D, van Zon M, Pierson J, Brenner M, Peters PJ. 2007. *M. tuberculosis* and *M. leprae* translocate from the phagolysosome to the cytosol in myeloid cells. *Cell* **129**:1287–1298.

35. Smith I. 2003. *Mycobacterium tuberculosis* pathogenesis and molecular determinants of virulence. *Clin Microbiol Rev* **16**:463–496.

36. Liu Y, Tan S, Huang L, Abramovitch RB, Rohde KH, Zimmerman MD, Chen C, Dartois V, VanderVen

BC, Russell DG. 2016. Immune activation of the host cell induces drug tolerance in *Mycobacterium tuberculosis* both *in vitro* and *in vivo*. *J Exp Med* 213:809–825.

37. Connolly LE, Edelstein PH, Ramakrishnan L. 2007. Why is long-term therapy required to cure tuberculosis? *PLoS Med* 4:e120

38. Wakamoto Y, Dhar N, Chait R, Schneider K, Signorino-Gelo F, Leibler S, McKinney JD. 2013. Dynamic persistence of antibiotic-stressed mycobacteria. *Science* 339: 91–95.

39. Maglica Ž, Özdemir E, McKinney JD. 2015. Single-cell tracking reveals antibiotic-induced changes in mycobacterial energy metabolism. *MBio* 6:e02236–14

40. Aldridge BB, Fernandez-Suarez M, Heller D, Ambravaneswaran V, Irimia D, Toner M, Fortune SM. 2012. Asymmetry and aging of mycobacterial cells lead to variable growth and antibiotic susceptibility. *Science* 335:100–104.

41. Barr DA, Kamdolozi M, Nishihara Y, Ndhlovu V, Khonga M, Davies GR, Sloan DJ. 2016. Serial image analysis of *Mycobacterium tuberculosis* colony growth reveals a persistent subpopulation in sputum during treatment of pulmonary TB. *Tuberculosis (Edinb)* 98: 110–115.

42. Murry JP, Rubin EJ. 2005. New genetic approaches shed light on TB virulence. *Trends Microbiol* 13:366–372.

43. Sassetti CM, Boyd DH, Rubin EJ. 2001. Comprehensive identification of conditionally essential genes in mycobacteria. *Proc Natl Acad Sci USA* 98:12712–12717.

44. Griffin JE, Gawronski JD, Dejesus MA, Ioerger TR, Akerley BJ, Sassetti CM. 2011. High-resolution phenotypic profiling defines genes essential for mycobacterial growth and cholesterol catabolism. *PLoS Pathog* 7: e1002251

45. Zhang YJ, Ioerger TR, Huttenhower C, Long JE, Sassetti CM, Sacchettini JC, Rubin EJ. 2012. Global assessment of genomic regions required for growth in *Mycobacterium tuberculosis*. *PLoS Pathog* 8:e1002946 [Erratum, doi:10.1371/annotation/4669e9e7-fd12-4a01-be2a-617b956ec0bb.]

46. Sassetti CM, Boyd DH, Rubin EJ. 2003. Genes required for mycobacterial growth defined by high density mutagenesis. *Mol Microbiol* 48:77–84.

47. Lamichhane G, Tyagi S, Bishai WR. 2005. Designer arrays for defined mutant analysis to detect genes essential for survival of *Mycobacterium tuberculosis* in mouse lungs. *Infect Immun* 73:2533–2540.

48. Fortune SM, Chase MR, Rubin EJ. 2006. Dividing oceans into pools: strategies for the global analysis of bacterial genes. *Microbes Infect* 8:1631–1636.

49. Kruh NA, Troudt J, Izzo A, Prenni J, Dobos KM. 2010. Portrait of a pathogen: the *Mycobacterium tuberculosis* proteome *in vivo*. *PLoS One* 5:e13938

50. Hisert KB, Kirksey MA, Gomez JE, Sousa AO, Cox JS, Jacobs WR Jr, Nathan CF, McKinney JD. 2004. Identification of *Mycobacterium tuberculosis* counterimmune (cim) mutants in immunodeficient mice by differential screening. *Infect Immun* 72:5315–5321.

51. Dhar N, McKinney JD. 2010. *Mycobacterium tuberculosis* persistence mutants identified by screening in isoniazid-treated mice. *Proc Natl Acad Sci USA* 107: 12275–12280

52. Shui W, Gilmore SA, Sheu L, Liu J, Keasling JD, Bertozzi CR. 2009. Quantitative proteomic profiling of host-pathogen interactions: the macrophage response to *Mycobacterium tuberculosis* lipids. *J Proteome Res* 8:282–289.

53. Bell C, Smith GT, Sweredoski MJ, Hess S. 2012. Characterization of the *Mycobacterium tuberculosis* proteome by liquid chromatography mass spectrometry-based proteomics techniques: a comprehensive resource for tuberculosis research. *J Proteome Res* 11:119–130.

54. Beste DJV, Espasa M, Bonde B, Kierzek AM, Stewart GR, McFadden J. 2009. The genetic requirements for fast and slow growth in mycobacteria. *PLoS One* 4:e5349

55. Beste DJV, Nöh K, Niedenführ S, Mendum TA, Hawkins ND, Ward JL, Beale MH, Wiechert W, McFadden J. 2013. 13C-flux spectral analysis of host-pathogen metabolism reveals a mixed diet for intracellular *Mycobacterium tuberculosis*. *Chem Biol* 20:1012–1021.

56. Darby CM, Ingólfsson HI, Jiang X, Shen C, Sun M, Zhao N, Burns K, Liu G, Ehrt S, Warren JD, Anderson OS, Brickner SJ, Nathan C. 2013. Whole cell screen for inhibitors of pH homeostasis in *Mycobacterium tuberculosis*. *PLoS One* 8:e68942 [Erratum, doi:10.1371/annotation/760b5b07-4922-42c4-b33a-162c1e9ae188.]

57. Gold B, Warrier T, Nathan C. 2015. A multi-stress model for high throughput screening against non-replicating *Mycobacterium tuberculosis*. *Methods Mol Biol* 1285:293–315

58. Gold B, Smith R, Nguyen Q, Roberts J, Ling Y, Lopez Quezada L, Somersan S, Warrier T, Little D, Pingle M, Zhang D, Ballinger E, Zimmerman M, Dartois V, Hanson P, Mitscher LA, Porubsky P, Rogers S, Schoenen FJ, Nathan C, Aubé J. 2016. Novel cephalosporins selectively active on nonreplicating *Mycobacterium tuberculosis*. *J Med Chem* 59:6027–6044.

59. Aly S, Wagner K, Keller C, Malm S, Malzan A, Brandau S, Bange FC, Ehlers S. 2006. Oxygen status of lung granulomas in *Mycobacterium tuberculosis*-infected mice. *J Pathol* 210:298–305.

60. Cunningham-Bussel A, Zhang T, Nathan CF. 2013. Nitrite produced by *Mycobacterium tuberculosis* in human macrophages in physiologic oxygen impacts bacterial ATP consumption and gene expression. *Proc Natl Acad Sci USA* 110:E4256–E4265.

61. Heng Y, Seah PG, Siew JY, Tay HC, Singhal A, Mathys V, Kiass M, Bifani P, Dartois V, Hervé M. 2011. *Mycobacterium tuberculosis* infection induces hypoxic lung lesions in the rat. *Tuberculosis (Edinb)* 91:339–341.

62. Via LE, Lin PL, Ray SM, Carrillo J, Allen SS, Eum SY, Taylor K, Klein E, Manjunatha U, Gonzales J, Lee EG, Park SK, Raleigh JA, Cho SN, McMurray DN, Flynn JL, Barry CE III. 2008. Tuberculous granulomas are hypoxic in guinea pigs, rabbits, and nonhuman primates. *Infect Immun* 76:2333–2340.

63. Wayne LG, Hayes LG. 1996. An *in vitro* model for sequential study of shiftdown of *Mycobacterium tubercu-*

losis through two stages of nonreplicating persistence. *Infect Immun* **64:**2062–2069.

64. Hartman T, Weinrick B, Vilchèze C, Berney M, Tufariello J, Cook GM, Jacobs WR Jr. 2014. Succinate dehydrogenase is the regulator of respiration in *Mycobacterium tuberculosis*. *PLoS Pathog* **10:**e1004510

65. Shi L, Sohaskey CD, Kana BD, Dawes S, North RJ, Mizrahi V, Gennaro ML. 2005. Changes in energy metabolism of *Mycobacterium tuberculosis* in mouse lung and under *in vitro* conditions affecting aerobic respiration. *Proc Natl Acad Sci USA* **102:**15629–15634.

66. Talaat AM, Lyons R, Howard ST, Johnston SA. 2004. The temporal expression profile of *Mycobacterium tuberculosis* infection in mice. *Proc Natl Acad Sci USA* **101:**4602–4607.

67. Timm J, Post FA, Bekker LG, Walther GB, Wainwright HC, Manganelli R, Chan WT, Tsenova L, Gold B, Smith I, Kaplan G, McKinney JD. 2003. Differential expression of iron-, carbon-, and oxygen-responsive mycobacterial genes in the lungs of chronically infected mice and tuberculosis patients. *Proc Natl Acad Sci USA* **100:**14321–14326

68. Wayne LG. 1977. Synchronized replication of *Mycobacterium tuberculosis*. *Infect Immun* **17:**528–530.

69. Wayne LG, Sohaskey CD. 2001. Nonreplicating persistence of mycobacterium tuberculosis. *Annu Rev Microbiol* **55:**139–163

70. McCormick CC, Li WP, Calero M. 2000. Oxygen tension limits nitric oxide synthesis by activated macrophages. *Biochem J* **350:**709–716.

71. Watanabe S, Zimmermann M, Goodwin MB, Sauer U, Barry CE III, Boshoff HI. 2011. Fumarate reductase activity maintains an energized membrane in anaerobic *Mycobacterium tuberculosis*. *PLoS Pathog* **7:**e1002287

72. Eoh H, Rhee KY. 2013. Multifunctional essentiality of succinate metabolism in adaptation to hypoxia in *Mycobacterium tuberculosis*. *Proc Natl Acad Sci USA* **110:**6554–6559

73. Diacon AH, Pym A, Grobusch M, Patientia R, Rustomjee R, Page-Shipp L, Pistorius C, Krause R, Bogoshi M, Churchyard G, Venter A, Allen J, Palomino JC, De Marez T, van Heeswijk RP, Lounis N, Meyvisch P, Verbeeck J, Parys W, de Beule K, Andries K, Mc Neeley DF. 2009. The diarylquinoline TMC207 for multidrug-resistant tuberculosis. *N Engl J Med* **360:**2397–2405.

74. Dawson R, Diacon AH, Everitt D, van Niekerk C, Donald PR, Burger DA, Schall R, Spigelman M, Conradie A, Eisenach K, Venter A, Ive P, Page-Shipp L, Variava E, Reither K, Ntinginya NE, Pym A, von Groote-Bidlingmaier F, Mendel CM. 2015. Efficiency and safety of the combination of moxifloxacin, pretomanid (PA-824), and pyrazinamide during the first 8 weeks of antituberculosis treatment: a phase 2b, open-label, partly randomised trial in patients with drug-susceptible or drug-resistant pulmonary tuberculosis. *Lancet* **385:**1738–1747.

75. Gler MT, Skripconoka V, Sanchez-Garavito E, Xiao H, Cabrera-Rivero JL, Vargas-Vasquez DE, Gao M, Awad M, Park SK, Shim TS, Suh GY, Danilovits M, Ogata H, Kurve A, Chang J, Suzuki K, Tupasi T, Koh WJ,

Seaworth B, Geiter LJ, Wells CD. 2012. Delamanid for multidrug-resistant pulmonary tuberculosis. *N Engl J Med* **366:**2151–2160.

76. Preiss L, Langer JD, Yildiz Ö, Eckhardt-Strelau L, Guillemont JE, Koul A, Meier T. 2015. Structure of the mycobacterial ATP synthase Fo rotor ring in complex with the anti-TB drug bedaquiline. *Sci Adv* **1:**e1500106

77. Andries K, Verhasselt P, Guillemont J, Göhlmann HW, Neefs JM, Winkler H, Van Gestel J, Timmerman P, Zhu M, Lee E, Williams P, de Chaffoy D, Huitric E, Hoffner S, Cambau E, Truffot-Pernot C, Lounis N, Jarlier V. 2005. A diarylquinoline drug active on the ATP synthase of *Mycobacterium tuberculosis*. *Science* **307:**223–227.

78. Koul A, Vranckx L, Dendouga N, Balemans W, Van den Wyngaert I, Vergauwen K, Göhlmann HW, Willebrords R, Poncelet A, Guillemont J, Bald D, Andries K. 2008. Diarylquinolines are bactericidal for dormant mycobacteria as a result of disturbed ATP homeostasis. *J Biol Chem* **283:**25273–25280.

79. Gengenbacher M, Rao SPS, Pethe K, Dick T. 2010. Nutrient-starved, non-replicating *Mycobacterium tuberculosis* requires respiration, ATP synthase and isocitrate lyase for maintenance of ATP homeostasis and viability. *Microbiology* **156:**81–87.

80. Rao SPS, Alonso S, Rand L, Dick T, Pethe K. 2008. The protonmotive force is required for maintaining ATP homeostasis and viability of hypoxic, nonreplicating *Mycobacterium tuberculosis*. *Proc Natl Acad Sci USA* **105:**11945–11950.

81. Diacon AH, Pym A, Grobusch MP, de los Rios JM, Gotuzzo E, Vasilyeva I, Leimane V, Andries K, Bakare N, De Marez T, Haxaire-Theeuwes M, Lounis N, Meyvisch P, De Paepe E, van Heeswijk RP, Dannemann B, TMC207-C208 Study Group. 2014. Multidrug-resistant tuberculosis and culture conversion with bedaquiline. *N Engl J Med* **371:**723–732.

82. Singh R, Manjunatha U, Boshoff HI, Ha YH, Niyomrattanakit P, Ledwidge R, Dowd CS, Lee IY, Kim P, Zhang L, Kang S, Keller TH, Jiricek J, Barry CE III. 2008. PA-824 kills nonreplicating *Mycobacterium tuberculosis* by intracellular NO release. *Science* **322:**1392–1395.

83. Manjunatha U, Boshoff HI, Barry CE. 2009. The mechanism of action of PA-824: novel insights from transcriptional profiling. *Commun Integr Biol* **2:**215–218.

84. Stover CK, Warrener P, VanDevanter DR, Sherman DR, Arain TM, Langhorne MH, Anderson SW, Towell JA, Yuan Y, McMurray DN, Kreiswirth BN, Barry CE, Baker WR. 2000. A small-molecule nitroimidazopyran drug candidate for the treatment of tuberculosis. *Nature* **405:**962–966.

85. Tyagi S, Nuermberger E, Yoshimatsu T, Williams K, Rosenthal I, Lounis N, Bishai W, Grosset J. 2005. Bactericidal activity of the nitroimidazopyran PA-824 in a murine model of tuberculosis. *Antimicrob Agents Chemother* **49:**2289–2293.

86. Dawson R, Diacon AH, Everitt D, van Niekerk C, Donald PR, Burger DA, Schall R, Spigelman M, Conradie A, Eisenach K, Venter A, Ive P, Page-Shipp L,

Variava E, Reither K, Ntinginya NE, Pym A, von Groote-Bidlingmaier F, Mendel CM. 2015. Efficiency and safety of the combination of moxifloxacin, pretomanid (PA-824), and pyrazinamide during the first 8 weeks of antituberculosis treatment: a phase 2b, open-label, partly randomised trial in patients with drug-susceptible or drug-resistant pulmonary tuberculosis. *Lancet* 385:1738–1747.

87. Diacon AH, Dawson R, von Groote-Bidlingmaier F, Symons G, Venter A, Donald PR, van Niekerk C, Everitt D, Winter H, Becker P, Mendel CM, Spigelman MK. 2012. 14-day bactericidal activity of PA-824, bedaquiline, pyrazinamide, and moxifloxacin combinations: a randomised trial. *Lancet* 380:986–993.

88. Betts JC, Lukey PT, Robb LC, McAdam RA, Duncan K. 2002. Evaluation of a nutrient starvation model of *Mycobacterium tuberculosis* persistence by gene and protein expression profiling. *Mol Microbiol* 43:717–731.

89. Rohde KH, Abramovitch RB, Russell DG. 2007. *Mycobacterium tuberculosis* invasion of macrophages: linking bacterial gene expression to environmental cues. *Cell Host Microbe* 2:352–364.

90. Fisher MA, Plikaytis BB, Shinnick TM. 2002. Microarray analysis of the *Mycobacterium tuberculosis* transcriptional response to the acidic conditions found in phagosomes. *J Bacteriol* 184:4025–4032.

91. Sassetti CM, Rubin EJ. 2003. Genetic requirements for mycobacterial survival during infection. *Proc Natl Acad Sci USA* 100:12989–12994.

92. Daniel J, Maamar H, Deb C, Sirakova TD, Kolattukudy PE. 2011. *Mycobacterium tuberculosis* uses host triacylglycerol to accumulate lipid droplets and acquires a dormancy-like phenotype in lipid-loaded macrophages. *PLoS Pathog* 7:e1002093

93. Garton NJ, Waddell SJ, Sherratt AL, Lee SM, Smith RJ, Senner C, Hinds J, Rajakumar K, Adegbola RA, Besra GS, Butcher PD, Barer MR. 2008. Cytological and transcript analyses reveal fat and lazy persister-like bacilli in tuberculous sputum. *PLoS Med* 5:e75

94. Rachman H, Strong M, Ulrichs T, Grode L, Schuchhardt J, Mollenkopf H, Kosmiadi GA, Eisenberg D, Kaufmann SH. 2006. Unique transcriptome signature of *Mycobacterium tuberculosis* in pulmonary tuberculosis. *Infect Immun* 74:1233–1242.

95. Ward SK, Abomoelak B, Marcus SA, Talaat AM. 2010. Transcriptional profiling of *Mycobacterium tuberculosis* during infection: lessons learned. *Front Microbiol* 1:121

96. Klotzsche M, Ehrt S, Schnappinger D. 2009. Improved tetracycline repressors for gene silencing in mycobacteria. *Nucleic Acids Res* 37:1778–1788.

97. McKinney JD, Höner zu Bentrup K, Muñoz-Elías EJ, Miczak A, Chen B, Chan WT, Swenson D, Sacchettini JC, Jacobs WR Jr, Russell DG. 2000. Persistence of *Mycobacterium tuberculosis* in macrophages and mice requires the glyoxylate shunt enzyme isocitrate lyase. *Nature* 406:735–738

98. Muñoz-Elías EJ, McKinney JD. 2005. *Mycobacterium tuberculosis* isocitrate lyases 1 and 2 are jointly required for *in vivo* growth and virulence. *Nat Med* 11:638–644.

99. Gould TA, van de Langemheen H, Muñoz-Elías EJ, McKinney JD, Sacchettini JC. 2006. Dual role of isocitrate lyase 1 in the glyoxylate and methylcitrate cycles in *Mycobacterium tuberculosis*. *Mol Microbiol* 61:940–947

100. Upton AM, Mushtaq A, Victor TC, Sampson SL, Sandy J, Smith DM, van Helden PV, Sim E. 2001. Arylamine N-acetyltransferase of *Mycobacterium tuberculosis* is a polymorphic enzyme and a site of isoniazid metabolism. *Mol Microbiol* 42:309–317.

101. Nandakumar M, Nathan C, Rhee KY. 2014. Isocitrate lyase mediates broad antibiotic tolerance in *Mycobacterium tuberculosis*. *Nat Commun* 5:4306

102. Marrero J, Rhee KY, Schnappinger D, Pethe K, Ehrt S. 2010. Gluconeogenic carbon flow of tricarboxylic acid cycle intermediates is critical for *Mycobacterium tuberculosis* to establish and maintain infection. *Proc Natl Acad Sci USA* 107:9819–9824.

103. Machová I, Snášel J, Zimmermann M, Laubitz D, Plocinski P, Oehlmann W, Singh M, Dostál J, Sauer U, Pichová I. 2014. *Mycobacterium tuberculosis* phosphoenolpyruvate carboxykinase is regulated by redox mechanisms and interaction with thioredoxin. *J Biol Chem* 289:13066–13078.

104. Marrero J, Trujillo C, Rhee KY, Ehrt S. 2013. Glucose phosphorylation is required for *Mycobacterium tuberculosis* persistence in mice. *PLoS Pathog* 9:e1003116

105. Ganapathy U, Marrero J, Calhoun S, Eoh H, de Carvalho LP, Rhee K, Ehrt S. 2015. Two enzymes with redundant fructose bisphosphatase activity sustain gluconeogenesis and virulence in *Mycobacterium tuberculosis*. *Nat Commun* 6:7912

106. Maksymiuk C, Balakrishnan A, Bryk R, Rhee KY, Nathan CF. 2015. E1 of α-ketoglutarate dehydrogenase defends *Mycobacterium tuberculosis* against glutamate anaplerosis and nitroxidative stress. *Proc Natl Acad Sci USA* 112:E5834–E5843. [Erratum, 112:E6257.]

107. Gandotra S, Lebron MB, Ehrt S. 2010. The *Mycobacterium tuberculosis* proteasome active site threonine is essential for persistence yet dispensable for replication and resistance to nitric oxide. *PLoS Pathog* 6:e1001040

108. Primm TP, Andersen SJ, Mizrahi V, Avarbock D, Rubin H, Barry CE III. 2000. The stringent response of *Mycobacterium tuberculosis* is required for long-term survival. *J Bacteriol* 182:4889–4898.

109. Dahl JL, Kraus CN, Boshoff HI, Doan B, Foley K, Avarbock D, Kaplan G, Mizrahi V, Rubin H, Barry CE III. 2003. The role of RelMtb-mediated adaptation to stationary phase in long-term persistence of *Mycobacterium tuberculosis* in mice. *Proc Natl Acad Sci USA* 100:10026–10031

110. Berney M, Berney-Meyer L, Wong KW, Chen B, Chen M, Kim J, Wang J, Harris D, Parkhill J, Chan J, Wang F, Jacobs WR Jr. 2015. Essential roles of methionine and S-adenosylmethionine in the autarkic lifestyle of *Mycobacterium tuberculosis*. *Proc Natl Acad Sci USA* 112:10008–10013

111. Glickman MS, Cox JS, Jacobs WR Jr. 2000. A novel mycolic acid cyclopropane synthetase is required for cording, persistence, and virulence of *Mycobacterium tuberculosis*. *Mol Cell* 5:717–727.

112. Flentie K, Garner AL, Stallings CL. 2016. *Mycobacterium tuberculosis* transcription machinery: ready to respond to host attacks. *J Bacteriol* 198:1360–1373.

113. Mak PA, Rao SP, Ping Tan M, Lin X, Chyba J, Tay J, Ng SH, Tan BH, Cherian J, Duraiswamy J, Bifani P, Lim V, Lee BH, Ling Ma N, Beer D, Thayalan P, Kuhen K, Chatterjee A, Supek F, Glynne R, Zheng J, Boshoff HI, Barry CE III, Dick T, Pethe K, Camacho LR. 2012. A high-throughput screen to identify inhibitors of ATP homeostasis in non-replicating *Mycobacterium tuberculosis*. *ACS Chem Biol* 7:1190–1197.

114. Rao V, Fujiwara N, Porcelli SA, Glickman MS. 2005. *Mycobacterium tuberculosis* controls host innate immune activation through cyclopropane modification of a glycolipid effector molecule. *J Exp Med* 201: 535–543.

115. Bloch H, Segal W. 1956. Biochemical differentiation of *Mycobacterium tuberculosis* grown *in vivo* and *in vitro*. *J Bacteriol* 72:132–141.

116. Cole ST, Brosch R, Parkhill J, Garnier T, Churcher C, Harris D, Gordon SV, Eiglmeier K, Gas S, Barry CE III, Tekaia F, Badcock K, Basham D, Brown D, Chillingworth T, Connor R, Davies R, Devlin K, Feltwell T, Gentles S, Hamlin N, Holroyd S, Hornsby T, Jagels K, Krogh A, McLean J, Moule S, Murphy L, Oliver K, Osborne J, Quail MA, Rajandream MA, Rogers J, Rutter S, Seeger K, Skelton J, Squares R, Squares S, Sulston JE, Taylor K, Whitehead S, Barrell BG. 1998. Deciphering the biology of *Mycobacterium tuberculosis* from the complete genome sequence. *Nature* 393:537–544.

117. Williams KJ, Boshoff HI, Krishnan N, Gonzales J, Schnappinger D, Robertson BD. 2011. The *Mycobacterium tuberculosis* β-oxidation genes echA5 and fadB3 are dispensable for growth *in vitro* and *in vivo*. *Tuberculosis (Edinb)* 91:549–555.

118. Daniel J, Deb C, Dubey VS, Sirakova TD, Abomoelak B, Morbidoni HR, Kolattukudy PE. 2004. Induction of a novel class of diacylglycerol acyltransferases and triacylglycerol accumulation in *Mycobacterium tuberculosis* as it goes into a dormancy-like state in culture. *J Bacteriol* 186:5017–5030.

119. Pandey AK, Sassetti CM. 2008. Mycobacterial persistence requires the utilization of host cholesterol. *Proc Natl Acad Sci USA* 105:4376–4380. [Erratum, 105:9130.]

120. Griffin JE, Pandey AK, Gilmore SA, Mizrahi V, McKinney JD, Bertozzi CR, Sassetti CM. 2012. Cholesterol catabolism by *Mycobacterium tuberculosis* requires transcriptional and metabolic adaptations. *Chem Biol* 19:218–227.

121. Nesbitt NM, Yang X, Fontán P, Kolesnikova I, Smith I, Sampson NS, Dubnau E. 2010. A thiolase of *Mycobacterium tuberculosis* is required for virulence and production of androstenedione and androstadienedione from cholesterol. *Infect Immun* 78:275–282.

122. Yang X, Gao J, Smith I, Dubnau E, Sampson NS. 2011. Cholesterol is not an essential source of nutrition for *Mycobacterium tuberculosis* during infection. *J Bacteriol* 193:1473–1476.

123. Kim J-H, O'Brien KM, Sharma R, Boshoff HI, Rehren G, Chakraborty S, Wallach JB, Monteleone M, Wilson DJ, Aldrich CC, Barry CE III, Rhee KY, Ehrt S, Schnappinger D. 2013. A genetic strategy to identify targets for the development of drugs that prevent bacterial persistence. *Proc Natl Acad Sci USA* 110:19095–19100.

124. Woong Park S, Klotzsche M, Wilson DJ, Boshoff HI, Eoh H, Manjunatha U, Blumenthal A, Rhee K, Barry CE III, Aldrich CC, Ehrt S, Schnappinger D. 2011. Evaluating the sensitivity of *Mycobacterium tuberculosis* to biotin deprivation using regulated gene expression. *PLoS Pathog* 7:e1002264

125. Wayne LG, Lin KY. 1982. Glyoxylate metabolism and adaptation of *Mycobacterium tuberculosis* to survival under anaerobic conditions. *Infect Immun* 37:1042–1049.

126. Schubert OT, Mouritsen J, Ludwig C, Röst HL, Rosenberger G, Arthur PK, Claassen M, Campbell DS, Sun Z, Farrah T, Gengenbacher M, Maiolica A, Kaufmann SH, Moritz RL, Aebersold R. 2013. The Mtb proteome library: a resource of assays to quantify the complete proteome of *Mycobacterium tuberculosis*. *Cell Host Microbe* 13:602–612.

127. Ortega C, Liao R, Anderson LN, Rustad T, Ollodart AR, Wright AT, Sherman DR, Grundner C. 2014. *Mycobacterium tuberculosis* Ser/Thr protein kinase B mediates an oxygen-dependent replication switch. *PLoS Biol* 12:e1001746

128. Galagan JE, Minch K, Peterson M, Lyubetskaya A, Azizi E, Sweet L, Gomes A, Rustad T, Dolganov G, Glotova I, Abeel T, Mahwinney C, Kennedy AD, Allard R, Brabant W, Krueger A, Jaini S, Honda B, Yu WH, Hickey MJ, Zucker J, Garay C, Weiner B, Sisk P, Stolte C, Winkler JK, Van de Peer Y, Iazzetti P, Camacho D, Dreyfuss J, Liu Y, Dorhoi A, Mollenkopf HJ, Drogaris P, Lamontagne J, Zhou Y, Piquenot J, Park ST, Raman S, Kaufmann SH, Mohney RP, Chelsky D, Moody DB, Sherman DR, Schoolnik GK. 2013. The *Mycobacterium tuberculosis* regulatory network and hypoxia. *Nature* 499:178–183.

129. Baek S-H, Li AH, Sassetti CM. 2011. Metabolic regulation of mycobacterial growth and antibiotic sensitivity. *PLoS Biol* 9:e1001065

130. Shi L, Sohaskey CD, Pheiffer C, Datta P, Parks M, McFadden J, North RJ, Gennaro ML. 2010. Carbon flux rerouting during *Mycobacterium tuberculosis* growth arrest. *Mol Microbiol* 78:1199–1215. [Erratum, 99:1179.]

131. Bertram R, Prax M. 2014. Metabolic aspects of bacterial persister cells. *Front Cell Infect Microbiol* 4:1–6.

132. Allison KR, Brynildsen MP, Collins JJ. 2011. Metabolite-enabled eradication of bacterial persisters by aminoglycosides. *Nature* 473:216–220.

133. Orman MA, Brynildsen MP. 2015. Inhibition of stationary phase respiration impairs persister formation in *E. coli*. *Nat Commun* 6:7983

134. Schuetz R, Kuepfer L, Sauer U. 2007. Systematic evaluation of objective functions for predicting intracellular fluxes in *Escherichia coli*. *Mol Syst Biol* 3:119

135. Dutta NK, Bandyopadhyay N, Veeramani B, Lamichhane G, Karakousis PC, Bader JS. 2014. Systems biology-based identification of *Mycobacterium tuberculosis* persistence genes in mouse lungs. *MBio* 5:e01066-13

Tuberculosis and the Tubercle Bacillus, 2nd ed.
Edited by William R. Jacobs, Jr., Helen McShane, Valerie Mizrahi, and Ian M. Orme
© 2018 American Society for Microbiology, Washington, DC
doi:10.1128/microbiolspec.TBTB2-0021-2016

Phenotypic Heterogeneity in *Mycobacterium tuberculosis*

32

Neeraj Dhar[1], John McKinney[1], and Giulia Manina[2]

INTRODUCTION

The terms "genotype" and "phenotype" were coined by the botanist and geneticist Wilhelm Johannsen at the beginning of the 20th century (1). Both words have a Greek etymology, meaning "generation of form" and "appearance of form," respectively. Hierarchically, the genotype predates the phenotype, considering that the genotype is defined as the genetic composition of a living entity, while the phenotype is defined as the perceivable characteristics of a living entity, which result from the interaction between the genetic composition and the environment. From unicellular to multicellular organisms, from bacteria to animals, the key for success, especially to evolve and adapt, lies in diversity. Diversity offers two main advantages: first, variants, exhibiting variety, could have a potential advantage against rapid adverse changes in environment, and, second, variants could potentially interact among themselves (mutualism) and perform more efficiently as a population than as individuals. Therefore, organisms have developed various means of generating and maintaining diversity. Changing the genetic content is a way of generating this diversity even though such changes are less frequent and can potentially be detrimental unless selected. Regardless, genetic diversity has been extensively documented even in monomorphic organisms such as *Mycobacterium tuberculosis*, and this often has a significant impact on the host-pathogen interaction and stimulation of host immune responses (2–5) as well as treatment outcomes (6). For example, some pathogens exhibit phase variation whereby diversity is generated by highly mutable loci (7). Genetic diversity in *M. tuberculosis* is being reviewed elsewhere (287) and will not be addressed here. In this review we focus exclusively on nongenetic modes of heterogeneity.

Microbes dividing asexually are quite clonal and this begets the misconception that individuals growing in the same environment will be identical to each other. However, this is not observed. Bacteria growing in the same environment, and encoding the same genetic information, exhibit clear phenotypic heterogeneity. This heterogeneity is not only readily apparent but also useful for long-term survival of the population and can be seen as a bet-hedging strategy against environmental stresses (8). This heterogeneity can be manifested as a simple two-state bistable population (9, 10) or a completely random heterogeneous population (11, 12). These phenotypic states could be generated by genetic mutations including adaptive mutagenesis (13–18); chromosomal changes or gene amplification (3, 19, 20) by programmed mechanisms such as bistability (9, 21); phase variation (7, 22); as a response to environmental perturbation (23–25) or randomly due to the noisy nature of gene expression (26, 27), each of these occurring on hugely different timescales (28). Furthermore, the magnitude and range of phenotypes observed could not be attained exclusively by genetic mutation, which usually occurs at a rate ranging from 10^{-8} to 10^{-10} per base pair per replication (18, 29, 30). Therefore, bacterial populations largely rely on diversity generated by nongenetic mechanisms. Phenotypic variation or "phenotypic heterogeneity," as we will refer to hereafter, is the simplest strategy to optimize individuals' fitness within fluctuating environments.

In the past few decades, huge advancements in single-cell technologies have not only allowed extensive documentation of phenotypic heterogeneity, but have also helped to resolve several previously unexplainable population-level behaviors (12, 31–35). This has led to increased appreciation of the role of cellular hetero-

[1]Global Health Institute, École Polytechnique Fédérale de Lausanne, CH-1015 Lausanne, Switzerland; [2]Microbial Individuality and Infection Group, Institut Pasteur, 75015 Paris, France.

geneity, as well as directed efforts toward development of new explorative strategies (36). In the following sections, we review the present understanding of phenotypic heterogeneity in *M. tuberculosis*, and highlight some of the novel tools and technologies being used to elucidate mycobacterial behavior at the single-cell level.

Peculiar Lifestyle of *M. tuberculosis*: A Persistent Pathogen

The interaction between the host and the microbe has been shaped and fine-tuned over the course of their coevolution, with the microbe expressing its arsenal of virulence factors, toxins, and immunomodulatory proteins and the host countering with a defense program, which includes immune cells, antibacterial reactive molecules, and inflammation. This interplay often results in four possible outcomes: (i) complete eradication of the microbe because of either the innate or adaptive immune mechanisms; (ii) proliferation of the pathogen leading to symptomatic infection and, in some cases, killing of the host; (iii) infection followed by a latent asymptomatic state that is characterized by suboptimal replication of the microbe with minimal host damage (a similar persistent state can also be generated following chemotherapy); and (iv) a commensal state wherein the microbe coexists with the host without causing any apparent damage (37). In reality, each of these outcomes may occur simultaneously in a host or during the course of infection, and tuberculosis (TB) is a case in point of such disease diversity.

As a facultative intracellular pathogen *M. tuberculosis* has developed a clever lifestyle to ensure its endurance within a fairly healthy host (38, 39). Human-to-human transmission occurs exclusively from hosts that for various health reasons do not represent any longer an appropriate niche for the bacilli. Tubercle bacilli disseminate from severely infected individuals through the airways. Upon inhalation by a new host, bacilli migrate to the lower respiratory tract accessing the alveoli. These initial steps are crucial inasmuch as the first contacts with innate immunity occur, influencing the likelihood of infection, which is inversely correlated to the number of systemic neutrophils, natural killer, and mucosal-associated invariant T cells. Different clinical isolates have exhibited differential activation of innate immunity (4, 39). Notably, bacterial membrane lipids can hinder the recognition by the innate immunity and, if the pathogen is not hampered at this stage, the colonization begins. Migratory dendritic cells then transport *M. tuberculosis* from the lung to the draining lymph nodes. Here naive T cells are activated to effector T cells, which return to the pulmonary site to activate permissive

macrophages that have accumulated in the interim. This promotes the progressive collection of macrophages and other immune cells into an organized structure, referred to as granuloma, which is one of the most characteristic features of clinical TB. *M. tuberculosis* is encapsulated in this structural lesion, wherein it resides primarily in the central acellular caseum. Depending on the balance between bacterial replication and host response, the caseum can either get calcified and fibrotic, restraining the pathogen, or necrotize and cavitate, leading to the pathogen's spread to different tissues and eventual transmission to other individuals (40). However, this process is neither simplistic nor homogeneous as has been demonstrated in several recent studies (41–45). Granulomas were found to be extremely heterogeneous in appearance and behavior within the same host, and characterized by widely varying outcomes, dependent on the local milieu of pro- and anti-inflammatory molecules (45). While host variation has a strong influence on the whole spectrum of TB heterogeneity, in this review we will mainly focus on the determinants of mycobacterial heterogeneity.

DRIVERS OF MYCOBACTERIAL PHENOTYPIC HETEROGENEITY

Stochastic Processes

The stochastic nature of biological phenomena makes it evident that no two bacteria can exhibit the same features and, as a result, the same phenotype. Minor differences in parameters such as cell size, partitioning of components, growth rates, gene expression, and stress responses can give rise to widely differing phenotypes (46) (Fig. 1). In most instances, these differences may not confer any advantage, but sometimes, for example, under stress conditions, such differences could be beneficial. Noise in gene expression has been shown to be a major contributor to heterogeneity. Most biological processes in bacteria such as transcription and translation involve very small numbers, which means that even small differences can lead to significant and detectable differences between genetically identical cells (27, 47, 48). Studies on stochasticity of gene expression have reinforced the importance of single-cell studies in microbiology (11, 49, 50). Elowitz et al. introduced the concepts of extrinsic and intrinsic noise. Extrinsic noise is due to fluctuations in the levels of components that affect gene expression, such as the number of RNA polymerases or the number of ribosomes per cell, whereas intrinsic noise is due to the stochastic nature of the biochemical process itself, for example,

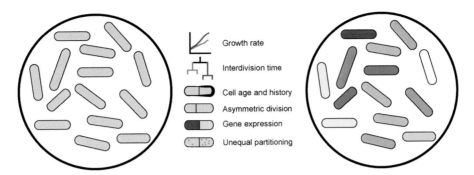

Figure 1 Causes and consequences of phenotypic heterogeneity. Bacterial isogenic populations arising from a single progenitor cell are usually expected to be homogeneous (left snapshot). However, single-cell analysis unveils significant cell-to-cell heterogeneity (right snapshot). Some of the causal factors leading to this heterogeneity are variations in growth rate, growth continuity, interdivision time, division symmetry, gene expression, protein distribution, and cell age generated either through deterministic or stochastic mechanisms.

the binding-unbinding of RNA polymerase to the promoter. Intrinsic fluctuations were found to exert their effects on much smaller timescales compared with extrinsic noise (51). Both transcription and protein production occur in stochastic bursts (49, 52–54), which are the predominant sources of noise. Protein noise tends to get smeared out because of the long half-life of proteins. However, often the noise can also get propagated to downstream pathways giving rise to cellular memory over the period of the bacterial cell cycle (48, 51). It has been experimentally demonstrated that higher transcription rates are associated with lower noise, whereas lower transcription rates accompanied with high translation give more variability (49). Negative feedback regulatory circuits tend to decrease noise, whereas a positive feedback circuit often increases variability (55). It has been suggested that bacteria use feedback regulation to generate multistable phenotypes in a population. Feedback-based multistability has been implicated to be a common mechanism adopted by bacteria to adapt to environmental fluctuations. Examples include induction of *lac* operon in *Escherichia coli*, mucoidy of *Pseudomonas*, competence development in *Bacillus subtilis*, sporulation and fruiting body formation in *Myxococcus xanthus*, and colicin expression in *E. coli* (56). Bistability was also found in mycobacterial stringent response through a positive feedback loop involving the *mprAB* operon. Furthermore, hysteresis was demonstrated in expression of *relA* as a function of the polyphosphate kinase (PPK1) levels (10, 57). However, a mathematical model built to analyze this stress-response network failed to reproduce bistability in biochemically relevant parameter range, despite incorporating multiple positive feedback loops. Only the inclusion of the posttranslational regulation of SigE

by anti-sigma factor RseA led to robust bistable systems (58).

A quantitative systemwide analysis of protein and mRNA levels in *E. coli* was performed with single-cell sensitivity using a fluorescent protein fusion library (59). Protein levels were found to span 5 orders of magnitude (10^{-1} to 10^4 molecules per cell), with more than 50% of the proteins being expressed at very low levels (<10 molecules per cell) reinforcing the importance of single-cell experiments in microbiology. For proteins expressed at low levels, protein noise was found to be inversely proportional to protein abundance and close to the intrinsic noise limit. However, at high expression levels, noise was found to be independent of protein abundance with extrinsic noise being the dominating factor. Interestingly, there was no correlation between mRNA and protein levels, which the authors attributed to the difference in half-lives. mRNAs have very short half-lives, usually a few minutes, and reflect the immediate history of transcription, whereas most proteins are stable with lifetimes usually longer than the interdivision time. Therefore, protein levels would be indicative of the long history of accumulated expression. In a study of analysis of global mRNA stability in *M. tuberculosis*, the average half-life of mRNAs was found to be 9.5 min, much longer than fast-growing species such as *E. coli* (~5.2 min) or even the nonpathogenic mycobacterium, *Mycobacterium smegmatis* (5.2 min). Interestingly, an inverse correlation was observed between abundance of transcript and half-life; thus, most housekeeping genes had shorter half-lives. On exposure to cold stress or to hypoxia there was global stabilization of all mRNA transcripts, resulting in average half-lives longer than 5 h (60). This could potentially pose a challenge for the bacterium to adapt to environments by repression of gene expression. While a similar analysis of protein stability has not yet been performed in *M. tuberculosis*, a targeted mass spectrometric method, "selected reaction monitoring," was used to quantify *M. tuberculosis* proteome. Protein abundance spanned over 4 orders of magnitude with a median concentration of 215 copies per cell. While proteins involved in the tricarboxylic acid cycle and lipid and amino acid metabolism were among the highly abundant proteins, there was not much variation in the fraction represented by ribosomal proteins in exponential phase versus dormancy (61). The observations that essential genes have lower levels of noise (62, 63) and that genes involved in housekeeping functions are predominantly controlled by negative autoregulation, which is a common noise-attenuating mechanism (56, 64), suggest that, to a large extent, noise is an evolvable trait and not just an artifact of biological processes (65, 66). Noise has important functional roles such as improving cellular regulation (32), enabling a range of probabilistic differentiation strategies, and facilitating evolutionary adaptation strategies (48). Ultimately, fast and sensitive single-cell assays are essential to discriminate mere stochastic noise from robust phenotypic switches. A clear understanding of stochastic gene expression on bacterial behavior at the individual and subpopulation level will be crucial to identify previously unexplored pathways critical for mycobacterial survival.

In a recent study, the stochastic pulsatile expression of an antioxidant enzyme KatG was observed to correlate with persistence against the antimycobacterial compound isoniazid (isonicotinylhydrazide; INH), which is activated into its potent form by KatG (12). The pulsatile nature of KatG expression could simply be due to low-frequency, high-amplitude stochastic bursting, but since it negatively correlates with survival in the presence of INH, it might cause selection of persister lineages characterized by infrequent pulsing, thus allowing a nonresponsive adaptation to drug survival. Similarly nonresponsive phenotypic resistance to antibiotics could also be generated by the error-prone biological processes that result in generation of quasispecies of the target molecule. For example, mistranslation was shown to increase phenotypic resistance to rifampicin in mycobacteria (67).

A recent study in *Salmonella* elegantly demonstrated the functional role of transcriptional heterogeneity in the pathogen influencing the immune activation of the host cell. Using a combination of flow cytometry and single-cell RNA-seq, the authors demonstrated how variation in expression of PhoPQ, a two-component system, affected the type I interferon (IFN) responses

in the host cell by modifying the lipopolysaccharide component (68). Thus, by analyzing pathogen heterogeneity at the single-cell level, this study convincingly highlights that the outcome of the host-pathogen interaction is affected not only by the variation in the immune activation or state of the host cell, but also by pathogen cell-to-cell heterogeneity. Similarly phenotypic specialization into distinct subpopulations based on spatial location and gene expression was shown in the case of mice infected with *Yersinia pseudotuberculosis* (69). Transcriptional noise also allows metabolic diversification, which could prove useful in environmentally challenging conditions and allows cells to survive substrate fluctuations (70, 71). In *B. subtilis* spores phenotypic diversity, in part, driven by variation in expression of a transcription factor, was found to affect the rate of spores to reinitiate growth (72).

Growth Phase

The process of mycobacterial infection, survival, and dissemination is neither synchronized nor uniform. Each interaction between the pathogen and the host cell potentially leads to diverse outcomes depending on the immune activation state of the host cell and the virulence and replication potential of the pathogen. This is likely reflected in the vast lesion diversity observed in any infected individual (40). Moreover, the coevolution of *M. tuberculosis* as a human pathogen has probably favored the development of genetic pathways, which have been fine-tuned to respond to each particular phase of the disease: responsive/anticipatory switching (73). Traditional "omics"-based approaches have been used to identify these pathways, which are differentially induced over the course of infection (74–79). Individual mycobacteria could express different antigens or enzymes depending on their growth and replicative state. For example, nutrient stress induces a unique set of starvation-responsive alleles and reprograms the metabolic state of the cell (80–83). To explore mycobacterial phenotypic heterogeneity, transcriptome studies have been used to identify suitable candidate genes and construct reporter strains to study the variation in expression at the single-cell level. Fluorescent protein-based reporters have been used extensively in the past mainly to quantify/visualize gene expression. However, in more recent studies, these constructs are being used to capture single-cell individuality with spatiotemporal resolution (24, 25, 35, 84, 85).

An acid- and phagosome-regulated locus (*aprABC*) was characterized and shown to be differentially induced depending on the pH of the medium. The authors then constructed a transcriptional reporter strain using the *aprA* promoter to drive green fluorescent protein (GFP) expression, which was used to infect resting and activated macrophages. Confocal imaging over the time course of infection revealed that, at the initial stages of infection, the bacteria expressed low levels of GFP and were homogeneous in their fluorescence. However, over the next 6 to 9 days, fluorescence induction was observed, which was also associated with a significant increase in heterogeneity of fluorescence suggestive of the bacteria experiencing the different phagosomal pH values (24). In a subsequent study, the authors demonstrated how acidic pH and carbon source cross talk to regulate *M. tuberculosis* growth and physiology and the central role of *phoPR* in modulating the growth rate by maintaining redox homeostasis (86). Similarly, with the aim of characterizing the environmental cue that *M. tuberculosis* encounters during infection, Tan et al. constructed a reporter strain based on genes that responded synergistically to both Cl⁻ and pH (25), which was also shown to be mediated through *phoP*. Since the transcriptional reporter, *rv2390c´*::GFP, was cloned into an episomal replicative plasmid, they included a second constitutively expressed fluorescent protein (mCherry) on the same construct to serve as an internal control for the GFP signal. They used this reporter strain to infect resting or activated macrophages, as well as immunocompetent and immune-deficient mice. GFP fluorescence was higher in activated macrophages than in resting macrophages. In the case of mice, the GFP fluorescence in wild-type immune competent mice was higher when compared with IFN-γ$^{-/-}$ mice, which fail to activate their macrophages and therefore acidify their phagosomes. The reporter strain was also induced to higher levels in inducible nitric oxide synthase-positive regions, highlighting the usefulness of such reporter strains to tease out the immune cues in the tissue microenvironments. Similar results were also obtained with a reporter based on the *dos* regulon, whose expression has been shown to be responsive to O₂ tension and nitric oxide. These reporters have been utilized to study *M. tuberculosis* adaptation in a vaccinated versus naive host immune environment (84). Rather surprisingly, lower induction of the pH and Cl⁻ responsive reporter was observed in the vaccinated mice in comparison with mock-treated mice, leading the authors to conclude that the preexisting immune response accelerated the development of a bacterial population that is more suited to survive in the host. Using vaccination studies in IFN-γ$^{-/-}$ mice, development of this adapted state was shown to depend on IFN-γ. To determine the replication status of *M. tuberculosis* in the host, they also constructed a reporter strain wherein the replisome component, single-stranded binding protein, was fused to GFP and expressed on a replicating plasmid. At 14 days postinfection, there was no difference in the fraction of actively replicating *M. tuberculosis* between mock-treated and vaccinated groups. However, at the 28-day time point, fewer *M. tuberculosis* in the vaccinated group were actively replicating, suggesting that vaccination leads to hastened onset of a nonreplicative state which may also promote drug tolerance (84, 87). In *Salmonella*, it was shown that bistable expression of a virulence gene conferred differences in growth rate and antibiotic susceptibility (88) and had an adaptive cooperative role for the maintenance of virulence in an animal model (89).

Phenotypic heterogeneity in a population can be generated through more simplistic ways, without invocation of specific pathways. Growth processes such as cell elongation, DNA replication, chromosome segregation, and cell division are discontinuous and unsynchronized. So at any given point of time in a population of cells, the individuals will be in different phases of growth and division in relation to each other and therefore heterogeneous. The chromosome replication and cell division cycles in mycobacteria were elegantly mapped recently at the single-cell level (90, 91). *M. smegmatis* was found to have a noncanonical cell cycle with the D period of the mother overlapping with the C period of the daughter cells in some cases. Cells with faster interdivision times were found to have no or a short B period. Single cells displayed marked cell-to-cell heterogeneity in their growth rates and interdivision times, accompanied with changes in the duration of the various cell cycle periods, leading to large variations in cell size, age, ploidy, and generation times in population distributions (90, 91). The observed inherent heterogeneity can therefore lead to diverse outcomes. For example, depending on their growth rate, individual bacteria could be in varying positions in the cell cycle and therefore exhibit differential susceptibility to DNA-damaging host antimicrobial effectors. Although the cell cycle has not yet been mapped in *M. tuberculosis*, characterizing the different cell cycle phases could potentially lead to a better understanding of the heterogeneity in this pathogen.

Growth Rate
Irrespective of its origin, growth rate variation reflects the global physiological state of microbial cells. Growth rate adjustments contingent on nutrient availability have been extensively documented in different microbial species. Broadly speaking, faster rates occur under

optimal conditions, whereas growth attenuation leading to growth arrest appears under restrictive conditions. The growth rate influences many cellular parameters, such as ribosomal content, concentration of RNA polymerases and transcription factors, overall macromolecular composition, mRNA lifetime, and cell size. The "growth-effect" is therefore not negligible and several processes, first and foremost gene expression, exhibit significant growth rate dependence (92). At steady state, the intracellular protein concentration is a net result of its production rate (rate of synthesis) minus the degradation rate and dilution. While during fast growth the dilution effect is dominant, at slower growth the contribution of dilution is negligible, and proteolytic complexes involved in degradation are dominant. As a result, at faster growth, the relative amount of any protein will decrease rapidly unless matched by high synthesis rates. On the contrary, at slower growth, some proteins can accumulate and, if they perturb growth, will induce growth arrest. In sum, growth rate fluctuations can dramatically impact cellular adaptation to stressful conditions, and possibly induce bi/multistable phenotypes, which are predicted to foster persistence-like behaviors (93). Heterogeneity in single-cell division time in yeast and bacteria was recently shown to result in increased population growth rates, suggesting that phenotypic heterogeneity can not only serve as a diversification strategy to generate fitter individuals, but could potentially also serve toward better population growth dynamics (94, 95). Growth rate heterogeneity is the most widely studied aspect in phenotypic heterogeneity of microbes because of the strong link between proliferation and virulence on one hand and the suggested association between growth arrest and drug tolerance on the other. *M. tuberculosis* encountering different microenvironments, intracellular versus extracellular, naive macrophage versus activated macrophage, closed cavity versus open cavity, high oxygen tension versus hypoxic lesions, nutrition-rich (fatty acid?) versus nutrition-poor environments, would be expected to exhibit very diverse growth rates. In addition, the replicative state of bacteria that persist in case of latent TB infections has been a longstanding question. Understanding this aspect and its underlying mechanisms has clear implications for disease management and treatment. Several population-level, indirect approaches have been used to address this question in the case of *M. tuberculosis* (30, 96–99) and have demonstrated the existence of diverse subpopulations (100–104). A recent study (35) attempted to capture this heterogeneity at the single-cell level using a GFP transcriptional reporter strain of *M. tuberculosis* rRNA

expression and use it as a single-cell correlate of growth and metabolic activity. Using real-time microscopy in conjunction with custom-made microfluidic devices (105), the authors were able to track individual cells over generations and measure their size and fluorescence over time. *M. tuberculosis* growing even *in vitro* in extremely optimal conditions was found to exhibit growth rate variation and heterogeneity in rRNA expression. This variation was further enhanced on exposure to diverse stress conditions, such as nutrient starvation, drug exposure, intracellular replication, or growth in mouse lungs (Fig. 2). Interestingly, active host immune response was found to exacerbate this heterogeneity and probably led to the formation of cryptic subpopulations of nongrowing but metabolically active bacteria (NGMA) that have been previously implicated in TB persistence and postchemotherapeutic relapses (Fig. 3). This approach now gives us a handle to directly observe and study this enigmatic population (106).

Another recent study (107) attempted to study mycobacterial replication dynamics at the single-cell level using the fluorescence dilution technique that was originally used to study phenotypic heterogeneity in *Salmonella* (108). This technique relies on expression of a fluorescent protein under the control of an inducible promoter. In a preinduced population, the level of protein in a cell decreases by half with each division. Using this approach to follow mycobacterial replication, the authors demonstrated actively growing and nongrowing *M. tuberculosis* subpopulations in murine macrophages. Their results suggested that macrophage uptake resulted in enrichment of slow-growing drug-tolerant persisters. However, other similar studies have suggested that replication rates of mycobacteria do not correlate with drug tolerance (12, 35, 98, 109).

Asymmetric Cell Division and Cell Aging

Cell division in rod-shaped bacteria produces two daughters that differ in their pole ages (110). Even in symmetrically dividing bacteria, such as *E. coli*, that give rise to two morphologically similar daughters, this division asymmetry often has a cost (111–114). In addition to polar aging, mycobacteria have an additional source of phenotypic variation. Mycobacteria divide asymmetrically and generate older pole siblings that are usually larger than their younger counterparts (90, 115–117). Even though alternate models have been proposed to explain how this asymmetry is generated (118), the functional consequences of division asymmetry toward increasing the phenotypic heterogeneity are obvious. This asymmetry can lead to differential partitioning of cellular components and resources or prefer-

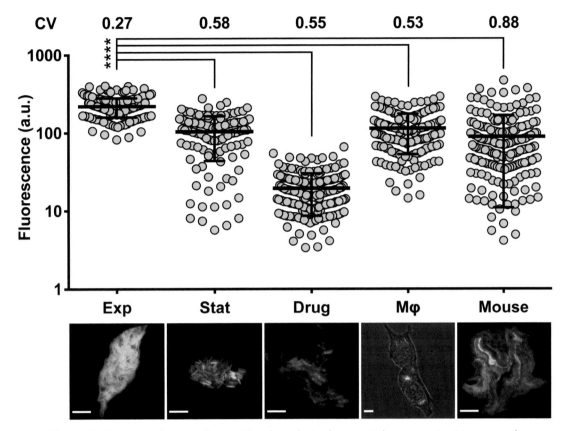

Figure 2 Stress conditions enhance *M. tuberculosis* phenotypic heterogeneity. Upper panel, single-cell rRNA-GFP fluorescence of *M. tuberculosis* isolated from different environments: Exp (exponential phase), Stat (stationary phase), Drug (treated with isoniazid), M (grown in macrophages), and Mouse (explanted from mouse lungs during the acute phase of infection). Each circle represents a single cell and the mean fluorescence ± SD is indicated (n = 200 per time point). Asterisks indicate significance difference of each data set in comparison with the control group, Exp ($P < 0.0001$), according to ANOVA followed by the Kruskal-Wallis test. The numbers shown on top are the coefficient of variation (CV) for each data set. Lower panel, representative snapshots from the corresponding conditions are shown. Green (rRNA-GFP) and red (constitutive dsRed) fluorescence channels are merged. Macrophages are also shown in phase contrast. Scale bars, 5 μm. Figure adapted from Manina et al. (35).

ential segregation of damaged components preferably to the older sibling as has been demonstrated in several other species (113, 119–121) (Fig. 1). In *M. tuberculosis*, the new pole siblings (younger) were observed to have higher rRNA-GFP concentration and had a slightly higher growth rate than their old-pole siblings (35), although at this point it is not clear to distinguish cause from effect. A recent study investigated the segregation of irreversibly oxidized proteins in mycobacteria at the single-cell level (122). Using fluorescently tagged ClpB protease chaperone as a proxy of these damaged proteins, it was shown that oxidized proteins get asymmetrically distributed between the progeny. This asymmetric distribution was associated with a fitness cost, because cells with higher oxidized protein content grew

more slowly and were less likely to recover after exposure to stresses such as antibiotics (122). Similar results were obtained when evaluating the role of DnaK in protein folding in mycobacteria (123). DnaK was found to be involved in the solubility of the large multimodular lipid synthases involved in cell wall biosynthesis. Using different fusion reporters to monitor protein folding, and by following the localization of DnaK fused to mCitrine, the authors were able to characterize different roles of DnaK in chaperone function, native protein folding, and aggregate processing where it relocalized with ClpB (123). Remarkably, AAA+ proteases are also involved in degradation of antitoxins belonging to type II toxin-antitoxin (TA) systems, which results in higher toxin concentration and growth inhibition. It is

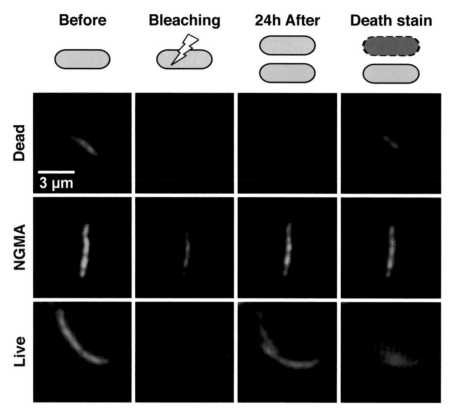

Figure 3 Identification of NGMA bacteria by single-cell techniques. A schematic of the fluorescence recovery after photobleaching (FRAP) method is shown on the top. *M. tuberculosis* expressing cytoplasmic rRNA-GFP were subjected to photobleaching using a laser, followed by staining with a dye that penetrates only cells with a compromised membrane. Metabolically active cells (green), bleached or metabolically inactive cells (gray), and dead cells (blue) are depicted. Representative snapshots of stationary-phase *M. tuberculosis* cells that were exposed to fresh 7H9 medium for 1 week. Top row, a nongrowing cell that does not recover fluorescence after photobleaching and stains positive for dead-cell stain (negative control). Middle row, a nongrowing cell that recovers fluorescence after photobleaching and stains negative for dead-cell stain and is therefore identified as nongrowing but metabolically active (NGMA). Bottom row, a growing cell that recovers fluorescence after photobleaching, stains negative for dead-cell stain, and continues to grow postbleaching.

therefore tempting to speculate that higher concentration of misfolded proteins inside older mycobacterial cells and coincident overexpression of AAA+ proteases might contribute to growth attenuation due to increased toxin levels. TA systems are emblematic of how heterogeneous behaviors can translate into multistable phenotypes, favoring diverse persistence mechanisms. In *E. coli* unequal partitioning of TA systems and its correlation with growth bistability and increased persister frequency was demonstrated both experimentally and theoretically (124–126). Furthermore, the secondary messenger (p)ppGpp alarmone, a major player of the stringent response to nutrient starvation, was shown to be stochastically expressed in single cells (127). This results in the activation of TA-encoded mRNA endonu-

cleases that halt translation, inhibit growth, and induce a persistent state (128).

Of note, 88 putative TA systems have been identified in *M. tuberculosis* chromosome by comparative genomics (129). The massive expansion of TA systems in *Mycobacterium* genus is more likely to be due to independent horizontal gene transfer, rather than to a unique ancestral event of acquisition. TA systems tend to be clustered in mycobacterial genome and mainly belong to conserved families (129). Typically, as in the case of the type II TA family, the balance between a stable toxin and an unstable antitoxin results in the TA system activity, which is then mediated through mRNA cleavage and inhibition of translation. A few novel TA systems have also been identified, such as the Rv0909-

Rv0910 module, which is the only one to be consistently represented throughout the *M. tuberculosis* complex and was found to inhibit growth instead of translation (129, 130). Transcriptional profiling of *M. tuberculosis* persister bacilli, which survived D-cycloserine exposure, revealed overexpression of 10 TA modules, some of which were also upregulated following nutrient starvation and hypoxia (131). In contrast to actively transcribed genes, leaderless transcripts were found to be predominant among genes coding for TA systems, and were expressed at low levels during exponential growth phase and at higher levels following starvation (132). Also, proteomic analysis of exponential versus starved bacilli suggested that the latter have increased expression of TA systems (133). In sum, bulk cell assays collectively imply that overexpression of TA systems may be coincident with adaption to various stress conditions. Given their potential implications to mycobacterial dormancy and persistence, TA systems have beckoned TB researchers and extensive investigation is still ongoing, although most attention has been hitherto placed on four main type II families.

The HigBA family exists either as a bipartite TA system or as a tripartite system, where an additional gene coding for a chaperone is present in the operon. HigB toxin is a ribosome-dependent RNase that targets tmRNA, causing growth arrest, and SecB chaperone helps to stabilize the HigA antitoxin by preventing its proteolytic degradation (134–136). Remarkably HigBA operon was upregulated *in vitro*, not only under heat shock, DNA damage, nutrient starvation, and hypoxia, but also in the persister subset of clinical isolates (137). *M. tuberculosis* genome also encodes nine MazEF systems. MazF3, MazF6, and MazF9 toxins were shown to sustain mycobacterial survival under oxidative stress and starvation and to promote drug persistence *in vitro*. Furthermore, the triple mutant strain displayed impaired virulence in guinea pig model of infection (138). It was shown that MazF7 toxin targets tRNA in a sequence- and structure-related fashion, affecting bacterial growth (139). *M. tuberculosis* also encodes three Rel TA modules, whose toxins, RelE, RelG, and RelK, were found to inhibit growth, and whose overexpression was induced under oxidative stress and nutrient limitation (140, 141). In particular, the RelBE system is responsible for mRNA degradation, which leads to changes in transcriptional and proteome profiles and cellular morphology (141).

VapBC operons represent the largest family of TA systems in mycobacteria. VapC toxins are RNases with a conserved N-terminal domain. Species belonging to *M. tuberculosis* complex have more than 40 VapBC loci organized in clusters, whereas other *Mycobacterium* species such as *M. avium*, *M. marinum*, and *M. smegmatis*, to cite a few, have only one module (129). VapBC systems were shown to affect growth by inhibiting translation (141–144), and VapC4 specifically cleaves three tRNA isoacceptors (145). Notably, the overexpression of VapC in *M. smegmatis* was found to downregulate carbon transport and metabolism. Accordingly, the VapBC null mutant displayed increased glycerol utilization, which corroborates the role of this TA system in regulating the metabolic flux in mycobacteria at the posttranscriptional level (146). It is noteworthy that transcriptional analysis of sputum from patients, who were treated with multidrug therapy for 6 months, displayed the presence of slowly growing bacilli, with marked upregulation of stress-associated sigma factors, transcription factors, and toxin-antitoxin genes, especially the VapBC family, and simultaneous downregulation of genes associated with growth, metabolism, and lipid synthesis (147).

Taken together, these studies imply a likely role of TA systems in *M. tuberculosis* response to different stress conditions, including host persistence and drug tolerance. Nevertheless, a number of critical questions remain unanswered. (i) Do the individual TA modules have any functional and stress-specific role or are they merely redundant? (ii) Which modules among the TA systems are the most relevant and what are their exact cellular targets? (iii) Does regulation of TA system activity belong to a programmed cell death process, which favors some individuals in the population? (iv) What is the actual contribution of TA systems to *M. tuberculosis* physiology, virulence, and drug tolerance? In sum, subtle fine-tuning of the regulation of TA systems may be part of the mycobacterial cellular decision-making process enabling adaptation to stressful conditions. Elucidating these issues will conceivably enable us to better understand *M. tuberculosis* pathogenesis and persistence mechanisms.

Host Microenvironment

Considering the intracellular lifestyle and its ability to persist in the latently infected individuals, the host environment is probably the largest contributor to mycobacterial phenotypic heterogeneity (Fig. 4). The clinical outcomes of the interaction between *M. tuberculosis* and the host are quite diverse and are influenced by numerous factors both on the host side and the pathogen's side. Most healthy individuals (90%) exposed to the bacilli are able to control the infection and remain asymptomatic. The remaining 10% of the individuals, because of various factors, develop clinical disease (148), which is manifested largely as pulmonary TB with sub-

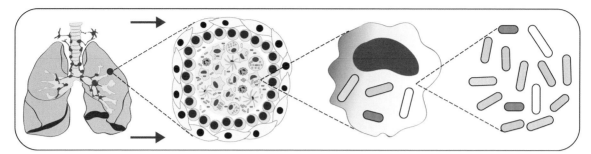

Figure 4 Host and pathogen heterogeneity contributes to TB diversity. Schematic of the increasingly heterogeneous environments *M. tuberculosis* resides in. Disease heterogeneity initiates in the major site of infection where host immunity gives rise to the typical granulomatous lesion (magnified from the lung parenchyma). This assembly of host cells consists of different types of macrophages, dendritic cells, neutrophils, lymphocytes, fibroblasts, and a necrotic caseous core. Bacilli can reside in discrete niches both intracellularly (magnified from the granuloma) and extracellularly, where they are subjected to a plethora of host immune effectors (red arrow) and antibiotics (blue arrow). Diverse environmental cues found within each microniche contribute to enhance the intrinsic phenotypic diversity of *M. tuberculosis* (right snapshot).

stantial cases of nonpulmonary involvement as well. Following the seeding of the pathogen into the lung and tissue remodeling, host cells aggregate to the site of infection to form a granuloma. From the early studies documenting the lesions from autopsies of TB patients (149), to the pioneering animal studies conducted by Arthur Dannenberg (150) and the more recent positron emission tomography (PET) and computed tomography (CT) analysis of lesions from animals and TB patients (42, 43, 151–155), it is clear that these lesions are heterogeneous and represent a continuum rather than discrete states, which is an outcome of the complex interaction at the pathological, immunological, and microbiological level (40).

Our understanding of the pathology of TB and granuloma development has been greatly aided by animal models, including zebrafish, rodents, rabbits, primates, as well as application of cutting-edge technologies (156–159). Despite this, even today it is not definitely clear whether the granuloma is beneficial to the bug or the host. Initially, it was believed that granuloma formation is a mechanism by which the host attempts to contain the infection and localize the inflammatory response. However, recent studies appear to suggest that mycobacteria play a more active role in manipulating the granuloma formation and, in fact, could be aiding the survival and dissemination of the pathogen (160). Granuloma development includes a sequence of maturation stages, during which different cell types are recruited at successive levels of nucleation. Inside the granuloma, macrophages can differentiate into epithelioid and foamy cells and, when infected, they can undergo either apoptosis or necrosis. Dendritic cells,

neutrophils, NK cells, and B and T cells are sequentially recruited, following activation of innate and adaptive immunity. Peripherally, epithelial cells rim the granuloma, and fibroblasts produce extracellular matrix, which harden the fibrotic structure. Immune cells drive the production of cytokines, proinflammatory and anti-inflammatory host-lipid mediators, and antimicrobial species, and changes in relative oxygen tension mediate the balance between bacterial proliferation, stasis, and lesion stability (40). Inside the granuloma, mycobacteria encounter reactive oxygen and nitrogen intermediates (ROI, RNI), hypoxia, and nutritive stress, and, combined with the host responses, create a highly variable and dynamic environment (161, 162). All these findings, besides affecting the global growth rate of the bacterium, influence the expression of diverse pathways (163) such as DosR regulon, antioxidant enzymes, DNA damage repair, metabolic rearrangements, redox modulators, efflux proteins, etc. The diverse lesion types and the heterogeneous response that *M. tuberculosis* encounters have been recently summarized very elegantly (40). Transcriptional profiling of human pulmonary TB granulomas has clearly demonstrated lesion-specific immune responses and dysregulation of host lipid metabolism (164, 165). The broad consensus is that the activation state of the macrophages, the local cytokine milieu, local concentration of antimicrobial effectors (ROI, RNI), and microenvironments of lipid-rich foamy cells all contribute toward making each granuloma unique and heterogeneous (165–169). Moreover, the lesions exhibit a wide spectrum and divergent trajectories within the same individual, suggesting that local immune responses rather than systemic immune responses are the determining factor in modulating lesion dynamics (40). These have been based on longitudinal FDG-PET/CT studies in mice, primates, and humans (42, 43, 154, 159, 170), which have demonstrated that most lesions are founded by a single bacterium and then follow diverse and often nonoverlapping trajectories. Therefore, at any point of time, an individual with active disease could have lesions with high bacterial burden as well as sterile lesions (42). The surprisingly similar heterogeneous nature of lesions was also observed in latently infected hosts although with lower bacterial burdens. The ability of lesions to control or sterilize the infection was correlated with its pathology; fibrocalcific lesions were associated with better bacterial control compared with regions of TB pneumonia. This heterogeneity in lesion progression and resolution was also observed in the case of chemotherapy of TB infection (43, 151, 171, 172), as well as in a model of TB reactivation (154).

Some of the components used by *M. tuberculosis* to manipulate the microenvironments have been identified in several studies (4, 39, 173, 174). At the host level, several players such as eicosanoids, leukotrienes, matrix metalloproteinase-9, tumor necrosis factor-α, and vascularization have been found to be influencing granuloma fate (160, 175, 176). The vascularization of the granuloma is especially important in contributing to lesional heterogeneity. Some of the earliest demonstrations of phenotypic heterogeneity in *M. tuberculosis* came from studies examining bacteria from lesions of TB patients (100). Bacilli from open cavities were observed to be culturable in the conventional 6- to 8-week period, whereas material from the closed cavities gave rise to normal-looking bacteria only on prolonged incubation for 12 to 18 weeks. Interestingly, the bacteria from the open cavities were more likely to be drug resistant than the ones isolated from closed cavities. This clearly demonstrates the heterogeneity in bacillary growth and behavior probably due to the differential host environment at the lesional level and at the level of vascularization. The open cavities are well circulated, and they are growth conducive with a strong propensity for development of drug resistance in the case of suboptimal drug dosing. On the other hand, in the closed lesions, the bacilli have been walled off without much access to oxygen and poor circulation. This probably causes the bacteria to enter into a state of slow growth or NGMA state. Since they are not actively replicating and are probably not being exposed to high concentrations of drug, they are less likely to acquire drug resistance. The lack of vascularization not only serves as an impediment for drug penetration but the

varying oxygen levels could serve to augment virulence of the pathogen and enhance drug tolerance as was shown in the case of *Salmonella* as well as mycobacteria (177, 178). Intervention of vascularization by anti-VEGF treatment appears to result in better bacterial control, although slightly different results were obtained in the zebrafish and rabbit models (178, 179). Distribution of the pathogen in distinct tissue regions has also been shown to promote diversification (180, 181).

Experimental support for the seminal observations by Vandiviere et al. was generated recently (44, 155) using matrix-assisted laser desorption ionization-mass spectrometry imaging, through which they were able to generate 2D spatial maps of drug distribution in the lesions from TB-infected patients. The capacity of anti-TB drugs to sterilize infections was correlated with its ability to penetrate lesions. INH and pyrazinamide were found to be homogeneously distributed across different tissues, from cavity walls to necrotic cores, and did not accumulate over time and repeated dosing. Moxifloxacin, on the other hand, was found to accumulate in cellular regions but was not able to penetrate into the acellular caseum, which could potentially be the reason for its failure to shorten TB treatment in clinical trials. RIF, on the other hand, was found to diffuse and accumulate in caseum and necrotic cores of cavities over multiple dosing, which could account for its sterilizing activity. Thus, spatial mapping of pharmacokinetics of TB drugs clearly demonstrates inter- and intralesional and cellular heterogeneity, differences that can clearly create heterogeneous subpopulations of bacteria eventually leading to development of drug-resistant mutants (182). Decreased drug permeability in a nutrition-starved *in vitro* nonreplicating *M. tuberculosis* model was also found to impart phenotypic resistance to compounds (183).

Intralesional heterogeneity was also demonstrated recently in a study using laser-capture microdissection, mass spectrometry, and confocal microscopy (45). Quantitative mass spectrometry of different granulomas from human TB patients helped in generating a spatial map of protein expression, which revealed the center of granulomas to have a proinflammatory environment and the surrounding tissue to have an anti-inflammatory signature. This spatial and anatomical heterogeneity led the authors to suggest that this organization allowed the localized restriction of antibacterial activity, and limited tissue destruction, as well (45). These two landmark studies therefore extend the heterogeneity observed between lesions in the same infected individual (42) to demonstrate anatomical and spatial heterogeneity within the same lesion.

In sum, investigating host-pathogen encounters in living cells at high spatiotemporal resolution will aid us to better understand the global dynamics of discrete infection foci and to design more reliable diagnostics and effective targeting strategies.

EXPLORATIVE TOOLS AND METHODOLOGIES

Over the past few decades, the field of microbiology has been enriched by studies investigating bacteria at the single-cell level and as constituents of complex and interactive communities (184–186). This has allowed microbiologists to reinterpret several themes in microbial physiology. With increasing awareness of the role of individuality in biological processes and the need to quantify and correlate with bacterial behavior, there have been huge advances made in tools and techniques enabling single-cell analysis. Here, we will attempt to highlight some of the most commonly used techniques and to present the advantages and disadvantages of each approach (Fig. 5).

Flow Cytometry and Omics

Flow cytometry represents one of the earliest and most widely used approaches to evaluate microbial populations at the single-cell level. The biggest advantage of this technique is the speed of analysis such that thousands of cells can be analyzed per sample, allowing the investigator to capture a quick snapshot at single-cell resolution enabling rare phenotypes to be detected and analyzed. With expanding repertoire of fluorescent proteins and dyes and advances in technology allowing multiparameter analysis, this technique is increasingly becoming more powerful (187). Although mainly used in immunological assays for profiling of the immune response during mycobacterial infection, several recent studies have developed and used fluorescent reporters to map mycobacterial phenotypic heterogeneity at the single-cell level. For example, flow-based assays have been used to report on nucleic acid content, intracellular pH (188), membrane potential (189), respiratory activity, redox state (85), antibacterial activity (190–192), metabolic activity (35), phage-based detection (193), and measurement of efflux. Another significant

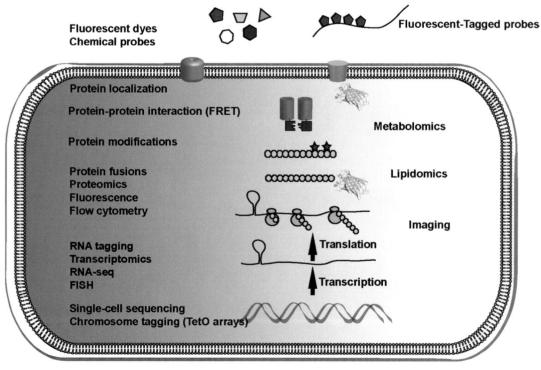

Figure 5 Cellular dynamic processes and single-cell techniques. The different biological processes that occur during cell growth and that often determine cell fate and some of the techniques that are used to track these processes at the single-cell level are depicted. Fluorescent approaches involve the use of fluorescent protein fusions or fluorescent-tagged molecules. Figure adapted from Spiller et al. (227).

advantage of flow cytometry is that culturing is not a prerequisite for analysis. Therefore, it can also be used for the elucidation of the NGMA bacteria or the viable but nonculturable bacteria often generated in drug-treated or stressed populations (106, 192, 194, 195) and was used to reveal the presence of nonreplicating subpopulations of bacteria using the fluorescence dilution technique (107, 108). Flow cytometry can also be combined with cell sorting wherein the cells or subpopulation of interest can be physically separated from the bulk population based on their unique characteristics. For example, using magnetic or flow sorting procedures, bone marrow-derived mesenchymal stem cell population was identified as a long-term protective niche for dormant *M. tuberculosis* (196, 197). The biggest disadvantage of flow cytometry is that it provides more of a snapshot of cells at that particular point of time, rather than a dynamic readout. It is not feasible to perform temporal studies on the same analyzed cell. An additional drawback is that, to be analyzed by flow, the cells have to be in a single-cell suspension; therefore, bacteria found in biofilms or structured communities have to be dispersed prior to analysis.

Application of omics-based approaches (genomics, transcriptomics, proteomics, lipidomics, metabolomics) to *M. tuberculosis* has led to significant understanding of this pathogen and the various adaptation strategies adopted during its intracellular lifestyle. However, for exploring bacterial phenotypic heterogeneity, these studies have to be applied at the single-cell level. The major technical challenges are the difficulty in isolating a single cell and the extremely low amount of experimental material. However, advances in single-cell isolation techniques and improvement in sensitivity of omic assays are making this feasible. While the majority of approaches use fluorescence-activated cell sorting (FACS) for cell separation (198, 199), micromanipulation using optical tweezers and microfluidics for cell isolation (200) or microdroplet-based separation (201) have recently been employed. For transcriptome studies, monitoring of a small number of transcripts at the single-cell level has been achieved by using various techniques such as RNA aptamers, split fluorescent proteins, molecular beacons, fluorescent *in situ* hybridization (FISH)-based approaches, or fluorescent proteins tagged to RNA-binding proteins (59, 202–208). Kang et al. used laser capture dissection microdissection to isolate a single bacterial cell and developed a novel procedure to amplify very low amounts of RNA to get enough material of cDNA to quantify by sequencing (209). They used this approach to quantify the transcriptional changes associated with exposure to an antibacterial agent at the single-cell level. With improvements in the technique and the sensitivity, it should be possible to use this technique more widely, to characterize individual cell expression patterns, and even to study the transcriptomics of NGMA mycobacteria (see reference 210 for potential applications). Proteomics involves not only measuring the protein concentration, but also the modifications, localization, and interactions. At bulk level, these are measured comparatively easily by using techniques such as gel electrophoresis, chromatography, or mass spectrometry (61, 211). However, as highlighted above, cells are very heterogeneous and often small variations in the level of protein can have a huge impact on cell fates (12, 32). Single-cell measurement of proteins can provide mechanistic insights into cellular behavior. Single-cell profiling of protein levels has been performed in *E. coli* with single-molecule sensitivity by using a YFP fusion library (59) and flow cytometry in combination with fluorescent antibodies, up to 20 different proteins in a single cell have been quantified (212, 213). Toward getting a complete proteomic profile, single-cell mass spectrometry is being developed wherein the single cell is isolated and lysed in an integrated microfluidic cell followed by capillary electrophoretic separation and electrospray mass spectrometry (214–216). The cellular metabolome, defined as the full complement of small-molecule metabolites (<2 kDa) present inside a cell, unlike proteins is more difficult to measure, because it fluctuates on very rapid timescales in response to the environment (217, 218). Technical advances in mass spectrometry and spectroscopy and the use of fluorescent biosensors now enable the detection of hundreds of metabolites in a single cell with sensitivity in the attomole range. Since sample handling is so critical, and to keep the metabolome of the analyzed cell unperturbed, the use of microfluidic device traps for cell trapping would be preferable (200, 218–220). These integrated microfluidic devices in combination with valves can enable cell capture, treatment, lysis, and subsequent analysis "on chip" within the reaction microchambers. Besides mass spectrometry and capillary electrophoresis, which are destructive techniques, other nondestructive approaches are being developed for single-cell metabolite analysis. These include Raman spectroscopy, secondary-ion mass spectrometry (SIMS and nanoscale SIMS [nanoSIMS]), and Fourier transform infrared spectroscopy (221, 222). NanoSIMS offers unprecedented resolution of metabolic potential of microorganisms such as N assimilation (71), for identification of phylogeny and quantification of substrate uptake when used in combination with FISH, localization of lipids, etc. (223). In a recent study, nanoSIMS was used to measure nitrogen fixation and photosynthesis in individual cyanobacteria to resolve the overlap of these two pathways at the single-cell level (224). Mass spectrometry has been used in several studies for determination of drug distribution in TB granulomas (44, 225). Therefore, based on the current state of technology, the analysis of the genome and transcriptome of mycobacteria at the single-cell level is clearly feasible using FACS or microdroplets in combination with microfluidic technologies (198–202). Advances made in the field of TB diagnostics for lysis of mycobacteria (226) can be applied in the context of microfluidics for better yield and recovery of nucleic acids and for on-chip amplification of the limited material. However, with regard to proteomics, lipidomics, and metabolomics, while the field has made tremendous advances in instrumentation sensitivity and sample preparation as a result of which variability in hundreds of proteins in mammalian cells has been captured at the single-cell level, it has been challenging to extend these studies at the complete proteome level to single bacteria. The main challenges include sample preparation and the low copy numbers of most molecules, which make it difficult to extend it to global-scale analysis. Targeted proteomics- or optics-based counting approaches (56) can potentially be applied for the analysis of mycobacterial heterogeneity at the single-cell level.

Time-Lapse Microscopy and Microfluidics

Several landmark advances in the past few decades in understanding microbial heterogeneity with single-cell resolution have come about through the use of time-lapse microscopy. While the application of flow cytometry, proteomics, and metabolomics to single cells is very informative, they provide more of a snapshot of cells at a given point of time. To fully understand the biological mechanism, usually it is not enough just to measure the distribution of the parameter within the population, but also to follow the temporal dynamics as to how these distributions change over time. Biological events occur in widely ranging timescales. Some events such as signal sensing/transduction occur within seconds, whereas transcriptional changes tend to occur in minutes and translational changes occur over several hours. Cell fates as a consequence of the response also need to be determined, which also can take place over hours or days (227). Time-lapse microscopy represents a unique approach that fulfills the criteria of single-cell as well as dynamic temporal kinetic resolution. However, the disadvantages of this approach are the requirement of fluorescent tagging, and that the throughput is

extremely low and only three to four parameters can be measured at the same time. This technique has greatly benefited from the advances in microscopy and the development of microscopy-compatible microfluidic devices. Fluorescent proteins have been optimized for expression in mycobacteria (85, 228) including photo-activatable variants (122). Fluorescent proteins have been used for labeling proteins by constructing translational fusions with the open reading frame of the gene of interest for studying protein localization, for evaluating transcriptional strength by constructing transcriptional fusions between the promoter of interest and the fluorescent reporter, protein diffusion, protein half-lives, for mRNA and protein counting, etc. (229). In the case of mycobacteria, some of the dynamic cellular processes that have been studied using fluorescent reporters include cell elongation (230); visualization of cell membrane (231) cell wall synthesis (232); cell division (90, 116, 117, 233–237); DNA replication (91, 238–241) for studying protein localization (122, 123, 242, 243); transcription (240), translation (240); and metabolic activity (35). Besides this, commercially available or customized chemical probes are being used for selective labeling of mycobacteria (115, 244–247). Using these novel fluorescent proteins/probes, different variations of fluorescence microscopy have been implemented such as Förster resonance energy transfer (FRET), fluorescence recovery after photobleaching (FRAP), fluorescence loss in photobleaching (FLIP), and fluorescence correlation spectroscopy (FCS) (35, 90, 248, 249). Single-cell FRET-based assay was used to demonstrate phagosomal rupture and cytosolic access by *M. tuberculosis*, which was dependent on expression of ESX-1 (249). FRET was also used to generate a genetically encoded ATP nanosensor and was used for long-term single-cell tracking of ATP levels in mycobacteria exposed to antibiotics by time-lapse microscopy (248). Fluorescence-based sensors have also been developed to provide single-cell readouts of mycobacterial redox potential (85) or intrabacterial pH (188). For example, using the redox-sensitive GFP, it was shown that the intracellular environment induces heterogeneity in the redox state of mycobacteria. In addition, exposure to antibiotics exerts an oxidative stress with a reduced-state subpopulation (less oxidized) contributing to drug tolerance (85). Time-lapse microscopy has also been used to study host-pathogen interaction at the single-cell level (35, 250). Quantitative time-lapse microscopy of mycobacteria has led to unique insights into bacterial behavior and responses. In a study looking at mycobacterial persistence against INH, time-lapse microscopy revealed that the persistent phase of stable number of cells was, in fact, a dynamic state of balanced division and death (12). Also, time-lapse analysis of mycobacterial growth and division suggested that growth occurred through the addition of new material at the poles and that different-sized daughters grew with different growth velocities (90, 115).

Imaging flow cytometry is another novel variation, which combines flow cytometry with imaging, wherein every particle of interest flowing through the cytometer is imaged. This technique, therefore, in addition to providing multiparameter fluorescence measurements, also achieves morphometric analysis such as cell size, localization studies, etc. (251).

While the study of single-cell behavior has accelerated by advances in imaging techniques, it would be fair to say that application of microfabrication and microfluidic technologies has been revolutionary for the field, from the manipulation and isolation of cells to multiparameter measurements. Microfluidics refers to the handling of fluids in micrometer-scale structures (10s to 100s micrometers). Under these conditions, the physical behavior of fluids is different than macroscale, and effects such as laminar flow, diffusion, fluidic resistance, surface tension, etc., become dominant (252). These systems allow precise control of the microenvironment and the ability to follow the response of microorganisms by using the different techniques mentioned earlier. These devices are fabricated by using various techniques such as soft lithography, laser ablation, injection molding, micromachining, etc. (252). But it is mainly the ease and the affordability of soft lithography that have made the application of microfluidics possible in so many areas of single-cell research (253, 254). Soft lithography is the set of techniques based on printing, molding, and embossing for creating microstructures using elastomeric polymers such as poly(dimethylsiloxane) (PDMS). PDMS has several useful properties: it is optically transparent, permeable to air, moderately stiff, intrinsically hydrophobic (but can be made hydrophilic by plasma treatment), adheres to other surfaces without or with minimal treatment, and is available commercially (253). Another useful feature of soft lithography is that, once the master is fabricated, several replicas can be made using PDMS. Several components also can be fabricated into the microfluidic device to improve the functionality of the device such as complex channel networks (to generate gradients, for example); pumps; sensors; valves to control flow; mixers to achieve online mixing (252, 253). These devices are often referred to as micro total analysis systems (μTAS) or lab-on-a-chip devices. In conjunction with time-lapse microscopy, microfluidic devices have

been used as chemostat devices for observing the growth and behavior of mycobacteria (35, 90, 115, 255–257); evaluate bactericidal activity of antimycobacterial compounds (12, 35, 248, 258–262), and, more recently, for TB diagnosis (263, 264). Microfluidics has also been used for separation of live and dead or antibiotic-treated mycobacteria by dielectrophoresis, a technique that enables the separation of polarizable particles suspended in a nonuniform electric field (265, 266) and for mimicking the space confinement of intracellular mycobacteria (267).

The main advantages of this approach are that they allow maintaining the cell under suitable conditions, in a homogeneous environment, and, because of the microscales, sample and reagent volume are minimized, which, apart from saving costs and reagents, also aids signal detection and avoids loss of signal by diffusion. This approach is also very amenable to massive parallelization of the setup. Complete integrated devices have been built that allow all the processes to be performed on the chip, from sample capture, to concentration, lysis, capturing the macromolecule of interest followed by analysis (268). As already highlighted in most of the methods above, microfluidics approaches have been combined with other traditional techniques, such as flow cytometry, mass spectrometry, optical microscopy, PCR, biochemical assays, etc.

These microfluidic devices, while undoubtedly very useful in allowing culture and documentation of phenotypic heterogeneity in mycobacterial populations, are still artificial models and do not recapitulate the intricate host microenvironments. It would be ideal to probe the bacterial heterogeneity inside the native environment in the host. This has been possible in some models such as the zebrafish. Zebrafish embryos and larvae can be infected with fluorescent mycobacterial strains and, given their transparency, size, and ease of manipulation, are very suitable models to investigate mycobacterial pathogenesis and antimicrobial tolerance by live imaging techniques (156).

In Vivo Investigation and Host-Mimicking Platforms

To untangle the physiology of different subpopulations under the intricate plethora of host stimuli, the ultimate and uppermost need is to probe the heterogeneity of bacterial behavior inside the host niche. This is undoubtedly the hardest challenge, and, over the past years, researchers have striven toward this objective by implementing different and often complementary approaches. Fluorescent reporter strains, as indicators of different intracellular functions, have been used to challenge wild-type as well as immunodeficient mice (35), or vaccinated and mock-treated mice (84), to analyze bacterial diversification in the lung over time.

Zebrafish has proved to be one of the most versatile and valuable tools. Zebrafish embryos and larvae can be infected either with fluorescent *M. marinum* or *Mycobacterium abscessus* and, given their transparency, size, and the abundance of reagents, are suitable models to investigate mycobacterial pathogenesis and antimicrobial tolerance by live imaging techniques (269, 270). Notably, the whole-animal zebrafish model has been used recently to visualize the phagocytosis of *M. marinum* by blood macrophages and the distribution dynamics of nanoparticle-delivered antibiotics by correlative light electron microscopy (271). Even though current technologies do not allow reaching this level of resolution in the mammalian host, huge advances have been made over the years in this context, contributing to changing our vision of infection dynamics. Our knowledge has benefited from the technologies that allow analysis of bacterial behavior within the complex tissue environment. In particular, PET/CT has enabled us to recapitulate the heterogeneous evolution of tubercular lesions and disease dynamics in live animals, including nonhuman and human primates (40, 42). Live imaging of the lung at the microscopic level still represents a major technical challenge, especially because of tissue impenetrability, autofluorescence, and constant motion, but the field is under constant development (272). Recently, the passive clearing technique for hydrogel-embedded tissues in conjunction with either spinning disk confocal or two-photon microscopy has enabled the imaging of healthy and infected tissue to a depth of 1 mm (273). Fluorescent bacilli have been visualized within the complex 3D granulomatous structures both in zebrafish and in mice. Thanks to this technique vascularization dynamics as well as neutrophils and tumor necrosis factor heterogeneity have been imaged at high resolution during infection. Whole-body *in vivo* imaging of fluorescent bacteria is used to test antimicrobial efficacy over time without euthanizing the animal (274). Nonetheless, the resolution limit of whole-animal imaging does not allow monitoring individual bacteria. Cirillo and colleagues proposed a compelling variant of *in vivo* imaging, so-called reporter enzyme fluorescence, which exploits the native expression of beta-lactamase by the tubercular bacilli. The mouse is perfused with a modified near-infrared fluorogenic substrate for beta-lactamase, and *M. tuberculosis* is directly tracked based on its ability to hydrolyze this molecule, monitoring the FRET reaction (275). Intravital imaging has been applied to improve the detection threshold of mycobacteria within the tissue geography. In particular, the use of a microendoscope endowed with an optical fiber in conjunction with whole-animal fluorescence imaging has enabled us to drive the resolution limit to a maximum of thousands of bacilli in the lung (276, 277).

A promising approach to study mycobacterial phenotypic heterogeneity within the organ's architecture, while circumventing the current technological limitations as well as the ethical constraints, dwells in biologically inspired engineering. Organs-on-a-chip are multicomponent microfluidic systems, where different cell types occupy separated but communicating sectors, aiming to globally reconstruct the physiology of the organ. Major progress has been made with respect to the lung-on-a-chip device, which already exists as a biomimicking system not only of the alveoli, but also of the small airways. By recapitulating the lung microenvironments and their physiology, this approach provides a concrete step toward the study of mycobacterial phenotypic heterogeneity within a noninvasive host-like environment where both disease pathogenesis and drug testing can be performed (278–280). By merging this technology with advanced live microscopy such as spinning disk confocal, 3D-structured illumination microscopy, two-photon, or light-sheet microscopy, and automated image analysis reconstruction tools will enable us to study the long-term infection dynamics of fluorescent bacteria in the host.

A further challenge is to study phenotypic heterogeneity of host-derived bacilli, without need to genetically modify the cells with fluorescent markers. NanoSIMS is conventionally used to measure the metabolites in environmental and nonculturable bacteria, by incorporating stable isotope-labeled substrates. Laser Raman spectroscopy is used later to quantify secondary ions at the single-cell level (71). This approach enables one to follow the metabolic dynamics of individual cells and can be coupled to downstream cell sorting and omics to further inspect the molecular signatures of the targeted cells subset. Even though nanoSIMS does not allow time-course analysis of the same cells, it is a promising technique to investigate the metabolic features of host-derived bacilli.

Scientific progress correlates with the innovation process. When innovation is rooted in science, there is an undeniable technical and scientific progress. The multidisciplinary trait that increasingly characterizes research nowadays will provide the fundamentals for original discoveries and paradigm shifts in the field of microbiology.

CONCLUDING REMARKS

Microbial populations are highly heterogeneous *per se*, both because of the inherent stochasticity of intracellular biochemical processes and variation in cellular components or processes. Nonetheless, intracellular fluxes are not the sole drivers of phenotypic heterogeneity, which is further leveraged by environmental clues (36), analogous to Conrad H. Waddington's epigenetic landscape (281), where eukaryotic cells are portrayed as marbles rolling down a hill toward the local altitude minima, influenced by the topology of the soil. Multistability is a common feature of many systems that have two or more relaxation states. From a physical perspective, multistable systems can be assumed within an energy landscape with different local minima. If an input signal provides sufficient activation energy to move the system from one minimum to another, the result will be a modification of the stability state. The parallelism between local minima and host microenvironments aids us in understanding how pathogens can undergo profound modifications pursuant to host-derived inputs (282). Collectively, infection sites, anatomic complexity, local tissue, cellular diversity, and xenobiotic compounds enhance the intrinsic pathogen's heterogeneity, obscuring our understanding of the infectious process. Diversity has strong implications both regarding single-lesion and overall disease progression, inasmuch as discrete infection foci essentially display different trajectories. In case of TB, the formation of granulomatous lesions creates microniche environments that allow the pathogen to persist either intracellularly or extracellularly surrounded by inflammatory cells at various states of immune activation. These structures constitute a barrier to antimicrobial defenses as well as to optimal drug penetration. While recent studies have underscored the heterogeneity and independent trajectories of individual lesions in an individual host, our understanding of phenotypic heterogeneity in *M. tuberculosis* is just in its infancy. By applying cutting-edge techniques to the study of host-pathogen interaction, we can begin to address the impact of phenotypic heterogeneity on the outcome of infection (185). Most of our current knowledge about phenotypic heterogeneity comes from experiments performed in laboratory settings. Some of the questions that need to be addressed are: What is the advantage of bacterial heterogeneity *in vivo*? Does phenotypic heterogeneity in the pathogen influence host responses? What are the main drivers of a pathogen's diversification in the host? And finally, can we design strategies to subvert this heterogeneity and ultimately dictate the infection outcome? Increased understanding of disease diversity will enable us to design original strategies to tackle persistent TB, either targeting the host (163, 283) or the pathogen (284). Three main approaches can be taken into consideration to tackle TB persistence: (i) selectively target subpopulations of persistent bacilli; (ii) resuscitate subpopulations of quiescent bacilli to make them more easily targetable; and (iii) prevent and/or modulate the formation of persisters by fine-tuning phenotypic heterogeneity. Addressing these issues in the natural environment of the host and evaluating its role in the disease process including drug persistence is going to be the next challenge. Beyond target identification at the subpopulation level and development of original targeting strategies against persistent TB, we should also revisit the data already at our disposal and the massive amount of information increasingly recorded with respect to phenotypic heterogeneity. By integrating interdisciplinary knowledge with computational studies, mathematical modeling and machine learning (285), we could envisage making a more fruitful use of our technology-based discoveries. Computational modeling has already been used in the TB field, for instance, to accelerate biomarker identification (286). Deep learning is used to uncover relationships between inputs and outputs, by translating complex numeric information into an output that is easily recognizable by our mind. This could virtually aid to generate more tangible understanding of the single-cell biology of TB, leading to more quantitative predictions, and aiding the move toward the concept of personalized medicine, which would represent a watershed with respect to current TB therapeutics.

Acknowledgments. The authors would like to apologize to those whose work could not be cited because of space limitations. This work was supported by the Swiss National Science Foundation (N.D., J.D.M.) and by the French Government's Investissement d'Avenir *program,* Laboratoire d'Excellence *Integrative Biology of Emerging Infectious Diseases (grant number ANR-10-LABX-62-IBEID) (G.M.).*

Citation. Dhar N, McKinney J, Manina G. 2016. Phenotypic heterogeneity in *Mycobacterium tuberculosis*. Microbiol Spectrum 4(6):TBTB2-0021-2016.

References

1. **Johannsen W.** 1911. The genotype conception of heredity. *Am Nat* **45:**129–159.
2. **Warner DF, Koch A, Mizrahi V.** 2015. Diversity and disease pathogenesis in *Mycobacterium tuberculosis. Trends Microbiol* **23:**14–21.
3. **Coscolla M, Gagneux S.** 2014. Consequences of genomic diversity in *Mycobacterium tuberculosis. Semin Immunol* **26:**431–444.
4. **Reed MB, Domenech P, Manca C, Su H, Barczak AK, Kreiswirth BN, Kaplan G, Barry CE III.** 2004. A glyco-

lipid of hypervirulent tuberculosis strains that inhibits the innate immune response. *Nature* **431**:84–87.

5. Barczak AK, Domenech P, Boshoff HIM, Reed MB, Manca C, Kaplan G, Barry CE III. 2005. *In vivo* phenotypic dominance in mouse mixed infections with *Mycobacterium tuberculosis* clinical isolates. *J Infect Dis* **192**: 600–606.

6. Liu Q, Via LE, Luo T, Liang L, Liu X, Wu S, Shen Q, Wei W, Ruan X, Yuan X, Zhang G, Barry CE III, Gao Q. 2015. Within patient microevolution of *Mycobacterium tuberculosis* correlates with heterogeneous responses to treatment. *Sci Rep* **5**:17507.

7. Bayliss CD. 2009. Determinants of phase variation rate and the fitness implications of differing rates for bacterial pathogens and commensals. *FEMS Microbiol Rev* **33**:504–520.

8. Beaumont HJ, Gallie J, Kost C, Ferguson GC, Rainey PB. 2009. Experimental evolution of bet hedging. *Nature* **462**:90–93.

9. Veening J-W, Smits WK, Kuipers OP. 2008. Bistability, epigenetics, and bet-hedging in bacteria. *Annu Rev Microbiol* **62**:193–210.

10. Sureka K, Ghosh B, Dasgupta A, Basu J, Kundu M, Bose I. 2008. Positive feedback and noise activate the stringent response regulator *rel* in mycobacteria. *PLoS ONE* **3**:e1771.

11. Elowitz MB, Levine AJ, Siggia ED, Swain PS. 2002. Stochastic gene expression in a single cell. *Science* **297**: 1183–1186.

12. Wakamoto Y, Dhar N, Chait R, Schneider K, Signorino-Gelo F, Leibler S, McKinney JD. 2013. Dynamic persistence of antibiotic-stressed mycobacteria. *Science* **339**: 91–95.

13. Lindsey HA, Gallie J, Taylor S, Kerr B. 2013. Evolutionary rescue from extinction is contingent on a lower rate of environmental change. *Nature* **494**:463–467.

14. Sánchez-Romero MA, Casadesús J. 2014. Contribution of phenotypic heterogeneity to adaptive antibiotic resistance. *Proc Natl Acad Sci USA* **111**:355–360.

15. Draghi JA, Parsons TL, Wagner GP, Plotkin JB. 2010. Mutational robustness can facilitate adaptation. *Nature* **463**:353–355.

16. Bjedov I, Tenaillon O, Gérard B, Souza V, Denamur E, Radman M, Taddei F, Matic I. 2003. Stress-induced mutagenesis in bacteria. *Science* **300**:1404–1409.

17. Rosenberg SM. 2001. Evolving responsively: adaptive mutation. *Nat Rev Genet* **2**:504–515.

18. McGrath M, Gey van Pittius NC, van Helden PD, Warren RM, Warner DF. 2014. Mutation rate and the emergence of drug resistance in *Mycobacterium tuberculosis*. *J Antimicrob Chemother* **69**:292–302.

19. Hendrickson H, Slechta ES, Bergthorsson U, Andersson DI, Roth JR. 2002. Amplification-mutagenesis: evidence that "directed" adaptive mutation and general hypermutability result from growth with a selected gene amplification. *Proc Natl Acad Sci USA* **99**:2164–2169.

20. Cui L, Neoh H-M, Iwamoto A, Hiramatsu K. 2012. Coordinated phenotype switching with large-scale chromosome flip-flop inversion observed in bacteria. *Proc Natl Acad Sci USA* **109**:E1647–E1656.

21. Dubnau D, Losick R. 2006. Bistability in bacteria. *Mol Microbiol* **61**:564–572.

22. van der Woude MW. 2011. Phase variation: how to create and coordinate population diversity. *Curr Opin Microbiol* **14**:205–211.

23. Vega NM, Allison KR, Khalil AS, Collins JJ. 2012. Signaling-mediated bacterial persister formation. *Nat Chem Biol* **8**:431–433.

24. Abramovitch RB, Rohde KH, Hsu F-F, Russell DG. 2011. *aprABC*: a *Mycobacterium tuberculosis* complex-specific locus that modulates pH-driven adaptation to the macrophage phagosome. *Mol Microbiol* **80**:678–694.

25. Tan S, Sukumar N, Abramovitch RB, Parish T, Russell DG. 2013. *Mycobacterium tuberculosis* responds to chloride and pH as synergistic cues to the immune status of its host cell. *PLoS Pathog* **9**:e1003282.

26. Kærn M, Elston TC, Blake WJ, Collins JJ. 2005. Stochasticity in gene expression: from theories to phenotypes. *Nat Rev Genet* **6**:451–464.

27. Raj A, van Oudenaarden A. 2008. Nature, nurture, or chance: stochastic gene expression and its consequences. *Cell* **135**:216–226.

28. Rando OJ, Verstrepen KJ. 2007. Timescales of genetic and epigenetic inheritance. *Cell* **128**:655–668.

29. Drake JW, Charlesworth B, Charlesworth D, Crow JF. 1998. Rates of spontaneous mutation. *Genetics* **148**: 1667–1686.

30. Ford CB, Lin PL, Chase MR, Shah RR, Iartchouk O, Galagan J, Mohaideen N, Ioerger TR, Sacchettini JC, Lipsitch M, Flynn JL, Fortune SM. 2011. Use of whole genome sequencing to estimate the mutation rate of *Mycobacterium tuberculosis* during latent infection. *Nat Genet* **43**:482–486.

31. Eldar A, Chary VK, Xenopoulos P, Fontes ME, Losón OC, Dworkin J, Piggot PJ, Elowitz MB. 2009. Partial penetrance facilitates developmental evolution in bacteria. *Nature* **460**:510–514.

32. Locke JC, Young JW, Fontes M, Hernández Jiménez MJ, Elowitz MB. 2011. Stochastic pulse regulation in bacterial stress response. *Science* **334**:366–369.

33. Norman TM, Lord ND, Paulsson J, Losick R. 2013. Memory and modularity in cell-fate decision making. *Nature* **503**:481–486.

34. Rotem E, Loinger A, Ronin I, Levin-Reisman I, Gabay C, Shoresh N, Biham O, Balaban NQ. 2010. Regulation of phenotypic variability by a threshold-based mechanism underlies bacterial persistence. *Proc Natl Acad Sci USA* **107**:12541–12546.

35. Manina G, Dhar N, McKinney JD. 2015. Stress and host immunity amplify Mycobacterium tuberculosis phenotypic heterogeneity and induce nongrowing metabolically active forms. *Cell Host Microbe* **17**:32–46.

36. Ackermann M. 2015. A functional perspective on phenotypic heterogeneity in microorganisms. *Nat Rev Microbiol* **13**:497–508.

37. Casadevall A, Pirofski LA. 2000. Host-pathogen interactions: basic concepts of microbial commensalism,

colonization, infection, and disease. *Infect Immun* 68: 6511–6518.

38. **Gomez JE, McKinney JD.** 2004. *M. tuberculosis* persistence, latency, and drug tolerance. *Tuberculosis (Edinb)* 84:29–44.

39. **Cambier CJ, Takaki KK, Larson RP, Hernandez RE, Tobin DM, Urdahl KB, Cosma CL, Ramakrishnan L.** 2014. Mycobacteria manipulate macrophage recruitment through coordinated use of membrane lipids. *Nature* 505:218–222.

40. **Lenaerts A, Barry CE III, Dartois V.** 2015. Heterogeneity in tuberculosis pathology, microenvironments and therapeutic responses. *Immunol Rev* 264:288–307.

41. **Gideon HP, Phuah J, Myers AJ, Bryson BD, Rodgers MA, Coleman MT, Maiello P, Rutledge T, Marino S, Fortune SM, Kirschner DE, Lin PL, Flynn JL.** 2015. Variability in tuberculosis granuloma T cell responses exists, but a balance of pro- and anti-inflammatory cytokines is associated with sterilization. *PLoS Pathog* 11:e1004603.

42. **Lin PL, Ford CB, Coleman MT, Myers AJ, Gawande R, Ioerger T, Sacchettini J, Fortune SM, Flynn JL.** 2014. Sterilization of granulomas is common in active and latent tuberculosis despite within-host variability in bacterial killing. *Nat Med* 20:75–79.

43. **Coleman MT, Chen RY, Lee M, Lin PL, Dodd LE, Maiello P, Via LE, Kim Y, Marriner G, Dartois V, Scanga C, Janssen C, Wang J, Klein E, Cho SN, Barry CE III, Flynn JL.** 2014. PET/CT imaging reveals a therapeutic response to oxazolidinones in macaques and humans with tuberculosis. *Sci Transl Med* 6:265ra167.

44. **Prideaux B, Via LE, Zimmerman MD, Eum S, Sarathy J, O'Brien P, Chen C, Kaya F, Weiner DM, Chen P-Y, Song T, Lee M, Shim TS, Cho JS, Kim W, Cho S-N, Olivier KN, Barry CE III, Dartois V.** 2015. The association between sterilizing activity and drug distribution into tuberculosis lesions. *Nat Med* 21:1223–1227.

45. **Marakalala MJ, Raju RM, Sharma K, Zhang YJ, Eugenin EA, Prideaux B, Daudelin IB, Chen PY, Booty MG, Kim JH, Eum SY, Via LE, Behar SM, Barry CE III, Mann M, Dartois V, Rubin EJ.** 2016. Inflammatory signaling in human tuberculosis granulomas is spatially organized. *Nat Med* 22:531–538.

46. **Schwabe A, Bruggeman FJ.** 2014. Contributions of cell growth and biochemical reactions to nongenetic variability of cells. *Biophys J* 107:301–313.

47. **Avery SV.** 2006. Microbial cell individuality and the underlying sources of heterogeneity. *Nat Rev Microbiol* 4:577–587.

48. **Eldar A, Elowitz MB.** 2010. Functional roles for noise in genetic circuits. *Nature* 467:167–173.

49. **Ozbudak EM, Thattai M, Kurtser I, Grossman AD, van Oudenaarden A.** 2002. Regulation of noise in the expression of a single gene. *Nat Genet* 31:69–73.

50. **Choi PJ, Cai L, Frieda K, Xie XS.** 2008. A stochastic single-molecule event triggers phenotype switching of a bacterial cell. *Science* 322:442–446.

51. **Rosenfeld N, Young JW, Alon U, Swain PS, Elowitz MB.** 2005. Gene regulation at the single-cell level. *Science* 307:1962–1965.

52. **Golding I, Paulsson J, Zawilski SM, Cox EC.** 2005. Real-time kinetics of gene activity in individual bacteria. *Cell* 123:1025–1036.

53. **Yu J, Xiao J, Ren X, Lao K, Xie XS.** 2006. Probing gene expression in live cells, one protein molecule at a time. *Science* 311:1600–1603.

54. **Cai L, Friedman N, Xie XS.** 2006. Stochastic protein expression in individual cells at the single molecule level. *Nature* 440:358–362.

55. **Alon U.** 2007. Network motifs: theory and experimental approaches. *Nat Rev Genet* 8:450–461.

56. **Smits WK, Kuipers OP, Veening J-W.** 2006. Phenotypic variation in bacteria: the role of feedback regulation. *Nat Rev Microbiol* 4:259–271.

57. **Ghosh S, Sureka K, Ghosh B, Bose I, Basu J, Kundu M.** 2011. Phenotypic heterogeneity in mycobacterial stringent response. *BMC Syst Biol* 5:18.

58. **Tiwari A, Balázsi G, Gennaro ML, Igoshin OA.** 2010. The interplay of multiple feedback loops with post-translational kinetics results in bistability of mycobacterial stress response. *Phys Biol* 7:036005.

59. **Taniguchi Y, Choi PJ, Li GW, Chen H, Babu M, Hearn J, Emili A, Xie XS.** 2010. Quantifying *E. coli* proteome and transcriptome with single-molecule sensitivity in single cells. *Science* 329:533–538.

60. **Rustad TR, Minch KJ, Brabant W, Winkler JK, Reiss DJ, Baliga NS, Sherman DR.** 2013. Global analysis of mRNA stability in *Mycobacterium tuberculosis*. *Nucleic Acids Res* 41:509–517.

61. **Schubert OT, Mouritsen J, Ludwig C, Röst HL, Rosenberger G, Arthur PK, Claassen M, Campbell DS, Sun Z, Farrah T, Gengenbacher M, Maiolica A, Kaufmann SHE, Moritz RL, Aebersold R.** 2013. The Mtb proteome library: a resource of assays to quantify the complete proteome of *Mycobacterium tuberculosis*. *Cell Host Microbe* 13:602–612.

62. **Silander OK, Nikolic N, Zaslaver A, Bren A, Kikoin I, Alon U, Ackermann M.** 2012. A genome-wide analysis of promoter-mediated phenotypic noise in *Escherichia coli*. *PLoS Genet* 8:e1002443

63. **Singh GP.** 2013. Coupling between noise and plasticity in *E. coli*. *G3 (Bethesda)* 3:2115–2120.

64. **Thieffry D, Huerta AM, Pérez-Rueda E, Collado-Vides J.** 1998. From specific gene regulation to genomic networks: a global analysis of transcriptional regulation in *Escherichia coli*. *BioEssays* 20:433–440.

65. **Fraser HB, Hirsh AE, Giaever G, Kumm J, Eisen MB.** 2004. Noise minimization in eukaryotic gene expression. *PLoS Biol* 2:e137.

66. **Wang Z, Zhang J.** 2011. Impact of gene expression noise on organismal fitness and the efficacy of natural selection. *Proc Natl Acad Sci USA* 108:E67–E76.

67. **Javid B, Sorrentino F, Toosky M, Zheng W, Pinkham JT, Jain N, Pan M, Deighan P, Rubin EJ.** 2014. Mycobacterial mistranslation is necessary and sufficient for rifampicin phenotypic resistance. *Proc Natl Acad Sci USA* 111:1132–1137.

68. **Avraham R, Haseley N, Brown D, Penaranda C, Jijon HB, Trombetta JJ, Satija R, Shalek AK, Xavier RJ,**

Regev A, Hung DT. 2015. Pathogen cell-to-cell vari-ability drives heterogeneity in host immune responses. *Cell* 162:1309–1321.

69. Davis KM, Mohammadi S, Isberg RR. 2015. Commu-nity behavior and spatial regulation within a bacterial microcolony in deep tissue sites serves to protect against host attack. *Cell Host Microbe* 17:21–31.

70. Guantes R, Benedetti I, Silva-Rocha R, de Lorenzo V. 2016. Transcription factor levels enable metabolic di-versification of single cells of environmental bacteria. *ISME J* 10:1122–1133.

71. Schreiber F, Littmann S, Lavik G, Escrig S, Meibom A, Kuypers MM, Ackermann M. 2016. Phenotypic hetero-geneity driven by nutrient limitation promotes growth in fluctuating environments. *Nat Microbiol* 1:16055.

72. Sturm A, Dworkin J. 2015. Phenotypic diversity as a mechanism to exit cellular dormancy. *Curr Biol* 25: 2272–2277.

73. Mitchell A, Romano GH, Groisman B, Yona A, Dekel E, Kupiec M, Dahan O, Pilpel Y. 2009. Adaptive prediction of environmental changes by microorgan-isms. *Nature* 460:220–224.

74. Shi L, Jung Y-J, Tyagi S, Gennaro ML, North RJ. 2003. Expression of Th1-mediated immunity in mouse lungs induces a *Mycobacterium tuberculosis* transcription pattern characteristic of nonreplicating persistence. *Proc Natl Acad Sci USA* 100:241–246.

75. Talaat AM, Lyons R, Howard ST, Johnston SA. 2004. The temporal expression profile of Mycobacte-rium tuberculosis infection in mice. *Proc Natl Acad Sci USA* 101:4602–4607.

76. Rachman H, Strong M, Ulrichs T, Grode L, Schuchhardt J, Mollenkopf H, Kosmiadi GA, Eisenberg D, Kaufmann SHE. 2006. Unique transcriptome signature of *Myco-bacterium tuberculosis* in pulmonary tuberculosis. *In-fect Immun* 74:1233–1242.

77. Rogerson BJ, Jung YJ, LaCourse R, Ryan L, Enright N, North RJ. 2006. Expression levels of *Mycobacterium tuberculosis* antigen-encoding genes versus production levels of antigen-specific T cells during stationary level lung infection in mice. *Immunology* 118:195–201.

78. Rohde KH, Abramovitch RB, Russell DG. 2007. *Myco-bacterium tuberculosis* invasion of macrophages: linking bacterial gene expression to environmental cues. *Cell Host Microbe* 2:352–364.

79. Flentie K, Garner AL, Stallings CL. 2016. *Mycobac-terium tuberculosis* transcription machinery: ready to respond to host attacks. *J Bacteriol* 198:1360–1373.

80. Shi L, Sohaskey CD, Kana BD, Dawes S, North RJ, Mizrahi V, Gennaro ML. 2005. Changes in energy me-tabolism of *Mycobacterium tuberculosis* in mouse lung and under in vitro conditions affecting aerobic respira-tion. *Proc Natl Acad Sci USA* 102:15629–15634.

81. Shi L, Sohaskey CD, Pfeiffer C, Datta P, Parks M, McFadden J, North RJ, Gennaro ML. 2010. Carbon flux rerouting during *Mycobacterium tuberculosis* growth arrest. *Mol Microbiol* 78:1199–1215.

82. Balázsi G, Heath AP, Shi L, Gennaro ML. 2008. The temporal response of the *Mycobacterium tuberculo-sis* gene regulatory network during growth arrest. *Mol Syst Biol* 4:225.

83. Baek S-H, Li AH, Sassetti CM. 2011. Metabolic regula-tion of mycobacterial growth and antibiotic sensitivity. *PLoS Biol* 9:e1001065.

84. Sukumar N, Tan S, Aldridge BB, Russell DG. 2014. Exploitation of *Mycobacterium tuberculosis* reporter strains to probe the impact of vaccination at sites of in-fection. *PLoS Pathog* 10:e1004394.

85. Bhaskar A, Chawla M, Mehta M, Parikh P, Chandra P, Bhave D, Kumar D, Carroll KS, Singh A. 2014. Reengineering redox sensitive GFP to measure myco-thiol redox potential of Mycobacterium tuberculosis during infection. *PLoS Pathog* 10:e1003902.

86. Baker JJ, Johnson BK, Abramovitch RB. 2014. Slow growth of *Mycobacterium tuberculosis* at acidic pH is regulated by *phoPR* and host-associated carbon sources. *Mol Microbiol* 94:56–69.

87. Liu Y, Tan S, Huang L, Abramovitch RB, Rohde KH, Zimmerman MD, Chen C, Dartois V, VanderVen BC, Russell DG. 2016. Immune activation of the host cell induces drug tolerance in *Mycobacterium tu-berculosis* both *in vitro* and *in vivo*. *J Exp Med* 213: 809–825.

88. Arnoldini M, Vizcarra IA, Peña-Miller R, Stocker N, Diard M, Vogel V, Beardmore RE, Hardt WD, Ackermann M. 2014. Bistable expression of viru-lence genes in salmonella leads to the formation of an antibiotic-tolerant subpopulation. *PLoS Biol* 12: e1001928.

89. Diard M, Garcia V, Maier L, Remus-Emsermann MN, Regoes RR, Ackermann M, Hardt WD. 2013. Stabiliza-tion of cooperative virulence by the expression of an avirulent phenotype. *Nature* 494:353–356.

90. Santi I, Dhar N, Bousbaine D, Wakamoto Y, McKinney JD. 2013. Single-cell dynamics of the chromosome rep-lication and cell division cycles in mycobacteria. *Nat Commun* 4:2470.

91. Santi I, McKinney JD. 2015. Chromosome organization and replisome dynamics in Mycobacterium smegmatis. *MBio* 6:e01999-14.

92. Klumpp S, Zhang Z, Hwa T. 2009. Growth rate-dependent global effects on gene expression in bac-teria. *Cell* 139:1366–1375.

93. Ray JCJ, Tabor JJ, Igoshin OA. 2011. Non-transcriptional regulatory processes shape transcriptional network dy-namics. *Nat Rev Microbiol* 9:817–828.

94. Cerulus B, New AM, Pougach K, Verstrepen KJ. 2016. Noise and epigenetic inheritance of single-cell division times influence population fitness. *Curr Biol* 26:1138–1147.

95. Hashimoto M, Nozoe T, Nakaoka H, Okura R, Akiyoshi S, Kaneko K, Kussell E, Wakamoto Y. 2016. Noise-driven growth rate gain in clonal cellular popula-tions. *Proc Natl Acad Sci USA* 113:3251–3256.

96. Muñoz-Elías EJ, Timm J, Botha T, Chan WT, Gomez JE, McKinney JD. 2005. Replication dynamics of *Myco-bacterium tuberculosis* in chronically infected mice. *In-fect Immun* 73:546–551.

97. Gill WP, Harik NS, Whiddon MR, Liao RP, Mittler JE, Sherman DR. 2009. A replication clock for *Mycobacterium tuberculosis*. *Nat Med* 15:211–214.

98. Raffetseder J, Pienaar E, Blomgran R, Eklund D, Patcha Brodin V, Andersson H, Welin A, Lerm M. 2014. Replication rates of *Mycobacterium tuberculosis* in human macrophages do not correlate with mycobacterial antibiotic susceptibility. *PLoS One* 9:e112426.

99. Ufimtseva E. 2015. *Mycobacterium*-host cell relationships in granulomatous lesions in a mouse model of latent tuberculous infection. *BioMed Res Int* 2015: 948131.

100. Vandiviere HM, Loring WE, Melvin I, Willis S. 1956. The treated pulmonary lesion and its tubercle bacillus. II. The death and resurrection. *Am J Med Sci* 232: 30–37; passim

101. Dhillon J, Fourie PB, Mitchison DA. 2014. Persister populations of *Mycobacterium tuberculosis* in sputum that grow in liquid but not on solid culture media. *J Antimicrob Chemother* 69:437–440.

102. Mukamolova GV, Turapov O, Malkin J, Woltmann G, Barer MR. 2010. Resuscitation-promoting factors reveal an occult population of tubercle Bacilli in Sputum. *Am J Respir Crit Care Med* 181:174–180.

103. Nikitushkin VD, Demina GR, Shleeva MO, Kaprelyants AS. 2013. Peptidoglycan fragments stimulate resuscitation of "non-culturable" mycobacteria. *Antonie van Leeuwenhoek* 103:37–46.

104. Garton NJ, Waddell SJ, Sherratt AL, Lee SM, Smith RJ, Senner C, Hinds J, Rajakumar K, Adegbola RA, Besra GS, Butcher PD, Barer MR. 2008. Cytological and transcript analyses reveal fat and lazy persister-like bacilli in tuberculous sputum. *PLoS Med* 5:0364–0645.

105. Dhar N, Manina G. 2015. Single-cell analysis of mycobacteria using microfluidics and time-lapse microscopy. *Methods Mol Biol* 1285:241–256.

106. Manina G, McKinney JD. 2013. A single-cell perspective on non-growing but metabolically active (NGMA) bacteria. *Curr Top Microbiol Immunol* 374: 135–161.

107. Mouton JM, Helaine S, Holden DW, Sampson SL. 2016. Elucidating population-wide mycobacterial replication dynamics at the single-cell level. *Microbiology* 162:966–978.

108. Helaine S, Cheverton AM, Watson KG, Faure LM, Matthews SA, Holden DW. 2014. Internalization of *Salmonella* by macrophages induces formation of non-replicating persisters. *Science* 343:204–208.

109. Adams KN, Takaki K, Connolly LE, Wiedenhoft H, Winglee K, Humbert O, Edelstein PH, Cosma CL, Ramakrishnan L. 2011. Drug tolerance in replicating mycobacteria mediated by a macrophage-induced efflux mechanism. *Cell* 145:39–53.

110. Nyström T. 2007. A bacterial kind of aging. *PLoS Genet* 3:e224.

111. Stewart EJ, Madden R, Paul G, Taddei F. 2005. Aging and death in an organism that reproduces by morphologically symmetric division. *PLoS Biol* 3:e45.

112. Wang P, Robert L, Pelletier J, Dang WL, Taddei F, Wright A, Jun S. 2010. Robust growth of *Escherichia coli*. *Curr Biol* 20:1099–1103.

113. Lindner AB, Madden R, Demarez A, Stewart EJ, Taddei F. 2008. Asymmetric segregation of protein aggregates is associated with cellular aging and rejuvenation. *Proc Natl Acad Sci USA* 105:3076–3081.

114. Clark MW, Yie AM, Eder EK, Dennis RG, Basting PJ, Martinez KA II, Jones BD, Slonczewski JL. 2015. Periplasmic acid stress increases cell division asymmetry (polar aging) of *Escherichia coli*. *PLoS One* 10:e0144650.

115. Aldridge BB, Fernandez-Suarez M, Heller D, Ambravaneswaran V, Irimia D, Toner M, Fortune SM. 2012. Asymmetry and aging of mycobacterial cells lead to variable growth and antibiotic susceptibility. *Science* 335:100–104.

116. Joyce G, Williams KJ, Robb M, Noens E, Tizzano B, Shahrezaei V, Robertson BD. 2012. Cell division site placement and asymmetric growth in mycobacteria. *PLoS One* 7:e44582.

117. Singh B, Nitharwal RG, Ramesh M, Pettersson BMF, Kirsebom LA, Dasgupta S. 2013. Asymmetric growth and division in Mycobacterium spp.: compensatory mechanisms for non-medial septa. *Mol Microbiol* 88: 64–76.

118. Kieser KJ, Rubin EJ. 2014. How sisters grow apart: mycobacterial growth and division. *Nat Rev Microbiol* 12:550–562.

119. Aguilaniu H, Gustafsson L, Rigoulet M, Nyström T. 2003. Asymmetric inheritance of oxidatively damaged proteins during cytokinesis. *Science* 299:1751–1753.

120. Winkler J, Seybert A, König L, Pruggnaller S, Haselmann U, Sourjik V, Weiss M, Frangakis AS, Mogk A, Bukau B. 2010. Quantitative and spatio-temporal features of protein aggregation in *Escherichia coli* and consequences on protein quality control and cellular ageing. *EMBO J* 29:910–923.

121. Bufalino MR, DeVeale B, van der Kooy D. 2013. The asymmetric segregation of damaged proteins is stem cell-type dependent. *J Cell Biol* 201:523–530.

122. Vaubourgeix J, Lin G, Dhar N, Chenouard N, Jiang X, Botella H, Lupoli T, Mariani O, Yang G, Ouerfelli O, Unser M, Schnappinger D, McKinney J, Nathan C. 2015. Stressed mycobacteria use the chaperone ClpB to sequester irreversibly oxidized proteins asymmetrically within and between cells. *Cell Host Microbe* 17:178–190.

123. Fay A, Glickman MS. 2014. An essential nonredundant role for mycobacterial DnaK in native protein folding. *PLoS Genet* 10:e1004516.

124. Feng J, Kessler DA, Ben-Jacob E, Levine H. 2014. Growth feedback as a basis for persister bistability. *Proc Natl Acad Sci USA* 111:544–549.

125. Fasani RA, Savageau MA. 2013. Molecular mechanisms of multiple toxin-antitoxin systems are coordinated to govern the persister phenotype. *Proc Natl Acad Sci USA* 110:E2528–E2537.

126. Rotem E, Loinger A, Ronin I, Levin-Reisman I, Gabay C, Shoresh N, Biham O, Balaban NQ. 2010.

Regulation of phenotypic variability by a threshold-based mechanism underlies bacterial persistence. *Proc Natl Acad Sci USA* **107:**12541–12546.

127. Maisonneuve E, Castro-Camargo M, Gerdes K. 2013. (p)ppGpp controls bacterial persistence by stochastic induction of toxin-antitoxin activity. *Cell* **154:**1140–1150.

128. Germain E, Roghanian M, Gerdes K, Maisonneuve E. 2015. Stochastic induction of persister cells by HipA through (p)ppGpp-mediated activation of mRNA endonucleases. *Proc Natl Acad Sci USA* **112:**5171–5176.

129. Ramage HR, Connolly LE, Cox JS. 2009. Comprehensive functional analysis of *Mycobacterium tuberculosis* toxin-antitoxin systems: implications for pathogenesis, stress responses, and evolution. *PLoS Genet* **5:**e1000767.

130. Sala A, Bordes P, Genevaux P. 2014. Multiple toxin-antitoxin systems in *Mycobacterium tuberculosis*. *Toxins (Basel)* **6:**1002–1020.

131. Keren I, Minami S, Rubin E, Lewis K. 2011. Characterization and transcriptome analysis of Mycobacterium tuberculosis persisters. *MBio* **2:**e00100-11.

132. Cortes T, Schubert OT, Rose G, Arnvig KB, Comas I, Aebersold R, Young DB. 2013. Genome-wide mapping of transcriptional start sites defines an extensive leaderless transcriptome in *Mycobacterium tuberculosis*. *Cell Reports* **5:**1121–1131 (Erratum **6:**415).

133. Albrethsen J, Agner J, Piersma SR, Højrup P, Pham TV, Weldingh K, Jimenez CR, Andersen P, Rosenkrands I. 2013. Proteomic profiling of *Mycobacterium tuberculosis* identifies nutrient-starvation-responsive toxin-antitoxin systems. *Mol Cell Proteomics* **12:**1180–1191.

134. Fivian-Hughes AS, Davis EO. 2010. Analyzing the regulatory role of the HigA antitoxin within *Mycobacterium tuberculosis*. *J Bacteriol* **192:**4348–4356.

135. Bordes P, Cirinesi AM, Ummels R, Sala A, Sakr S, Bitter W, Genevaux P. 2011. SecB-like chaperone controls a toxin-antitoxin stress-responsive system in *Mycobacterium tuberculosis*. *Proc Natl Acad Sci USA* **108:**8438–8443.

136. Schuessler DL, Cortes T, Fivian-Hughes AS, Lougheed KEA, Harvey E, Buxton RS, Davis EO, Young DB. 2013. Induced ectopic expression of HigB toxin in *Mycobacterium tuberculosis* results in growth inhibition, reduced abundance of a subset of mRNAs and cleavage of tmRNA. *Mol Microbiol* **90:**195–207.

137. Torrey HL, Keren I, Via LE, Lee JS, Lewis K. 2016. High persister mutants in *Mycobacterium tuberculosis*. *PLoS One* **11:**e0155127.

138. Tiwari P, Arora G, Singh M, Kidwai S, Narayan OP, Singh R. 2015. MazF ribonucleases promote *Mycobacterium tuberculosis* drug tolerance and virulence in guinea pigs. *Nat Commun* **6:**6059.

139. Schifano JM, Cruz JW, Vvedenskaya IO, Edifor R, Ouyang M, Husson RN, Nickels BE, Woychik NA. 2016. tRNA is a new target for cleavage by a MazF toxin. *Nucleic Acids Res* **44:**1256–1270.

140. Korch SB, Contreras H, Clark-Curtiss JE. 2009. Three *Mycobacterium tuberculosis* Rel toxin-antitoxin modules inhibit mycobacterial growth and are expressed

in infected human macrophages. *J Bacteriol* **191:**1618–1630.

141. Korch SB, Malhotra V, Contreras H, Clark-Curtiss JE. 2015. The *Mycobacterium tuberculosis relBE* toxin:antitoxin genes are stress-responsive modules that regulate growth through translation inhibition. *J Microbiol* **53:**783–795.

142. Robson J, McKenzie JL, Cursons R, Cook GM, Arcus VL. 2009. The *vapBC* operon from *Mycobacterium smegmatis* is an autoregulated toxin-antitoxin module that controls growth via inhibition of translation. *J Mol Biol* **390:**353–367.

143. Ahidjo BA, Kuhnert D, McKenzie JL, Machowski EE, Gordhan BG, Arcus V, Abrahams GL, Mizrahi V. 2011. VapC toxins from *Mycobacterium tuberculosis* are ribonucleases that differentially inhibit growth and are neutralized by cognate VapB antitoxins. *PLoS One* **6:**e21738.

144. Andrews ES, Arcus VL. 2015. The mycobacterial PhoH2 proteins are type II toxin antitoxins coupled to RNA helicase domains. *Tuberculosis (Edinb)* **95:**385–394.

145. Cruz JW, Sharp JD, Hoffer ED, Maehigashi T, Vvedenskaya IO, Konkimalla A, Husson RN, Nickels BE, Dunham CM, Woychik NA. 2015. Growth-regulating *Mycobacterium tuberculosis* VapC-mt4 toxin is an isoacceptor-specific tRNase. *Nat Commun* **6:**7480.

146. McKenzie JL, Robson J, Berney M, Smith TC, Ruthe A, Gardner PP, Arcus VL, Cook GM. 2012. A VapBC toxin-antitoxin module is a posttranscriptional regulator of metabolic flux in mycobacteria. *J Bacteriol* **194:**2189–2204.

147. Walter ND, Dolganov GM, Garcia BJ, Worodria W, Andama A, Musisi E, Ayakaka I, Van TT, Voskuil MI, de Jong BC, Davidson RM, Fingerlin TE, Kechris K, Palmer C, Nahid P, Daley CL, Geraci M, Huang L, Cattamanchi A, Strong M, Schoolnik GK, Davis JL. 2015. Transcriptional adaptation of drug-tolerant *Mycobacterium tuberculosis* during treatment of human tuberculosis. *J Infect Dis* **212:**990–998.

148. Comstock GW. 1982. Epidemiology of tuberculosis. *Am Rev Respir Dis* **125:**8–15.

149. Canetti G. 1968. Biology of the mycobacterioses. Pathogenesis of tuberculosis in man. *Ann N Y Acad Sci* **154**(1 Biology of My):13–18.

150. Dannenberg AM Jr. 2006. *Pathogenesis of Human Pulmonary Tuberculosis*. ASM Press, Washington, DC.

151. Via LE, Schimel D, Weiner DM, Dartois V, Dayao E, Cai Y, Yoon Y-S, Dreher MR, Kastenmayer RJ, Laymon CM, Carny JE, Flynn JL, Herscovitch P, Barry CE III. 2012. Infection dynamics and response to chemotherapy in a rabbit model of tuberculosis using [^{18}F]2-fluoro-deoxy-D-glucose positron emission tomography and computed tomography. *Antimicrob Agents Chemother* **56:**4391–4402.

152. Via LE, Weiner DM, Schimel D, Lin PL, Dayao E, Tankersley SL, Cai Y, Coleman MT, Tomko J, Paripati P, Orandle M, Kastenmayer RJ, Tartakovsky M, Rosenthal A, Portevin D, Eum SY, Lahouar S, Gagneux S, Young DB, Flynn JL, Barry CE III. 2013. Differential virulence and disease progression following *Mycobacte-*

rium tuberculosis complex infection of the common marmoset (*Callithrix jacchus*). *Infect Immun* 81:2909–2919.

153. Bagci U, Foster B, Miller-Jaster K, Luna B, Dey B, Bishai WR, Jonsson CB, Jain S, Mollura DJ. 2013. A computational pipeline for quantification of pulmonary infections in small animal models using serial PET-CT imaging. *EJNMMI Res* 3:55.

154. Murawski AM, Gurbani S, Harper JS, Klunk M, Younes L, Jain SK, Jedynak BM. 2014. Imaging the evolution of reactivation pulmonary tuberculosis in mice using 18F-FDG PET. *J Nucl Med* 55:1726–1729.

155. Dartois V. 2014. The path of anti-tuberculosis drugs: from blood to lesions to mycobacterial cells. *Nat Rev Microbiol* 12:159–167.

156. Ramakrishnan L. 2013. The zebrafish guide to tuberculosis immunity and treatment. *Cold Spring Harb Symp Quant Biol* 78:179–192.

157. Kramnik I, Dietrich WF, Demant P, Bloom BR. 2000. Genetic control of resistance to experimental infection with virulent *Mycobacterium tuberculosis*. *Proc Natl Acad Sci USA* 97:8560–8565.

158. Manabe YC, Kesavan AK, Lopez-Molina J, Hatem CL, Brooks M, Fujiwara R, Hochstein K, Pitt MLM, Tufariello J, Chan J, McMurray DN, Bishai WR, Dannenberg AM Jr, Mendez S. 2008. The aerosol rabbit model of TB latency, reactivation and immune reconstitution inflammatory syndrome. *Tuberculosis (Edinb)* 88:187–196.

159. Lin PL, Rodgers M, Smith L, Bigbee M, Myers A, Bigbee C, Chiosea I, Capuano SV, Fuhrman C, Klein E, Flynn JL. 2009. Quantitative comparison of active and latent tuberculosis in the cynomolgus macaque model. *Infect Immun* 77:4631–4642.

160. Pagán AJ, Ramakrishnan L. 2014. Immunity and immunopathology in the tuberculous granuloma. *Cold Spring Harb Perspect Med* 5:a018499.

161. Seimon TA, Kim M-J, Blumenthal A, Koo J, Ehrt S, Wainwright H, Bekker L-G, Kaplan G, Nathan C, Tabas I, Russell DG. 2010. Induction of ER stress in macrophages of tuberculosis granulomas. *PLoS One* 5:e12772.

162. Sallusto F. 2016. Heterogeneity of Human CD4(+) T Cells Against Microbes. *Annu Rev Immunol* 34:317–334.

163. Nathan C. 2012. Fresh approaches to anti-infective therapies. *Sci Trans Med* 4:140sr2–140sr2.

164. Subbian S, Tsenova L, Kim M-J, Wainwright HC, Visser A, Bandyopadhyay N, Bader JS, Karakousis PC, Murrmann GB, Bekker L-G, Russell DG, Kaplan G. 2015. Lesion-specific immune response in granulomas of patients with pulmonary tuberculosis: a pilot study. *PLoS One* 10:e0132249.

165. Kim M-J, Wainwright HC, Locketz M, Bekker L-G, Walther GB, Dittrich C, Visser A, Wang W, Hsu F-F, Wiehart U, Tsenova L, Kaplan G, Russell DG. 2010. Caseation of human tuberculosis granulomas correlates with elevated host lipid metabolism. *EMBO Mol Med* 2:258–274.

166. Peyron P, Vaubourgeix J, Poquet Y, Levillain F, Botanch C, Bardou F, Daffé M, Emile J-F, Marchou B,

Cardona P-J, de Chastellier C, Altare F. 2008. Foamy macrophages from tuberculous patients' granulomas constitute a nutrient-rich reservoir for *M. tuberculosis* persistence. *PLoS Pathog* 4:e1000204.

167. Mattila JT, Ojo OO, Kepka-Lenhart D, Marino S, Kim JH, Eum SY, Via LE, Barry CE III, Klein E, Kirschner DE, Morris SM Jr, Lin PL, Flynn JL. 2013. Microenvironments in tuberculous granulomas are delineated by distinct populations of macrophage subsets and expression of nitric oxide synthase and arginase isoforms. *J Immunol* 191:773–784.

168. Irwin SM, Driver E, Lyon E, Schrupp C, Ryan G, Gonzalez-Juarrero M, Basaraba RJ, Nuermberger EL, Lenaerts AJ. 2015. Presence of multiple lesion types with vastly different microenvironments in C3HeB/FeJ mice following aerosol infection with *Mycobacterium tuberculosis*. *Dis Model Mech* 8:591–602.

169. Martin CJ, Carey AF, Fortune SM. 2016. A bug's life in the granuloma. *Semin Immunopathol* 38:213–220.

170. Lin PL, Dartois V, Johnston PJ, Janssen C, Via L, Goodwin MB, Klein E, Barry CE III, Flynn JL. 2012. Metronidazole prevents reactivation of latent *Mycobacterium tuberculosis* infection in macaques. *Proc Natl Acad Sci USA* 109:14188–14193.

171. Chen RY, Dodd LE, Lee M, Paripati P, Hammoud DA, Mountz JM, Jeon D, Zia N, Zahiri H, Coleman MT, Carroll MW, Lee JD, Jeong YJ, Herscovitch P, Lahouar S, Tartakovsky M, Rosenthal A, Somaiyya S, Lee S, Goldfeder LC, Cai Y, Via LE, Park S-K, Cho S-N, Barry CE III. 2014. PET/CT imaging correlates with treatment outcome in patients with multidrug-resistant tuberculosis. *Sci Trans Med* 6:265ra166.

172. Via LE, England K, Weiner DM, Schimel D, Zimmerman MD, Dayao E, Chen RY, Dodd LE, Richardson M, Robbins KK, Cai Y, Hammoud D, Herscovitch P, Dartois V, Flynn JL, Barry CE III. 2015. A sterilizing tuberculosis treatment regimen is associated with faster clearance of bacteria in cavitary lesions in marmosets. *Antimicrob Agents Chemother* 59:4181–4189.

173. Cambier CJ, Falkow S, Ramakrishnan L. 2014. Host evasion and exploitation schemes of *Mycobacterium tuberculosis*. *Cell* 159:1497–1509.

174. Al Shammari B, Shiomi T, Tezera L, Bielecka MK, Workman V, Sathyamoorthy T, Mauri F, Jayasinghe SN, Robertson BD, D'Armiento J, Friedland JS, Elkington PT. 2015. The extracellular matrix regulates granuloma necrosis in Tuberculosis. *J Infect Dis* 212:463–473.

175. Tobin DM, Roca FJ, Oh SF, McFarland R, Vickery TW, Ray JP, Ko DC, Zou Y, Bang ND, Chau TTH, Vary JC, Hawn TR, Dunstan SJ, Farrar JJ, Thwaites GE, King M-C, Serhan CN, Ramakrishnan L. 2012. Host genotype-specific therapies can optimize the inflammatory response to mycobacterial infections. *Cell* 148:434–446.

176. Mayer-Barber KD, Andrade BB, Oland SD, Amaral EP, Barber DL, Gonzales J, Derrick SC, Shi R, Kumar NP, Wei W, Yuan X, Zhang G, Cai Y, Babu S, Catalfamo M, Salazar AM, Via LE, Barry CE III, Sher A. 2014. Host-directed therapy of tuberculosis based

on interleukin-1 and type I interferon crosstalk. *Nature* **511**:99–103.

177. Jennewein J, Matuszak J, Walter S, Felmy B, Gendera K, Schatz V, Nowottny M, Liebsch G, Hensel M, Hardt W-D, Gerlach RG, Jantsch J. 2015. Low-oxygen tensions found in Salmonella-infected gut tissue boost Salmonella replication in macrophages by impairing antimicrobial activity and augmenting Salmonella virulence. *Cell Microbiol* **17**:1833–1847.

178. Oehlers SH, Cronan MR, Scott NR, Thomas MI, Okuda KS, Walton EM, Beerman RW, Crosier PS, Tobin DM. 2015. Interception of host angiogenic signalling limits mycobacterial growth. *Nature* **517**: 612–615.

179. Datta M, Via LE, Kamoun WS, Liu C, Chen W, Seano G, Weiner DM, Schimel D, England K, Martin JD, Gao X, Xu L, Barry CE III, Jain RK. 2015. Anti-vascular endothelial growth factor treatment normalizes tuberculosis granuloma vasculature and improves small molecule delivery. *Proc Natl Acad Sci USA* **112**:1827–1832.

180. Jorth P, Staudinger BJ, Wu X, Hisert KB, Hayden H, Garudathri J, Harding CL, Radey MC, Rezayat A, Bautista G, Berrington WR, Goddard AF, Zheng C, Angermeyer A, Brittnacher MJ, Kitzman J, Shendure J, Fligner CL, Mittler J, Aitken ML, Manoil C, Bruce JE, Yahr TL, Singh PK. 2015. Regional isolation drives bacterial diversification within Cystic Fibrosis lungs. *Cell Host Microbe* **18**: 307–319.

181. Markussen T, Marvig RL, Gómez-Lozano M, Aanæs K, Burleigh AE, Høiby N, Johansen HK, Molin S, Jelsbak L. 2014. Environmental heterogeneity drives within-host diversification and evolution of *Pseudomonas aeruginosa*. *MBio* **5**:e01592-14.

182. Moreno-Gamez S, Hill AL, Rosenbloom DIS, Petrov DA, Nowak MA, Pennings PS. 2015. Imperfect drug penetration leads to spatial monotherapy and rapid evolution of multidrug resistance. *Proc Natl Acad Sci USA* **112**:E2874–E2883.

183. Keren I, Minami S, Rubin E, Lewis K. 2011. Characterization and transcriptome analysis of *Mycobacterium tuberculosis* persisters. *mBio* **2**:e00100-11.

184. Dhar N, McKinney JD. 2007. Microbial phenotypic heterogeneity and antibiotic tolerance. *Curr Opin Microbiol* **10**:30–38.

185. Bumann D. 2015. Heterogeneous host-pathogen encounters: act locally, think globally. *Cell Host Microbe* **17**:13–19.

186. Kreibich S, Hardt W-D. 2015. Experimental approaches to phenotypic diversity in infection. *Curr Opin Microbiol* **27**:25–36.

187. Müller S, Nebe-von-Caron G. 2010. Functional single-cell analyses: flow cytometry and cell sorting of microbial populations and communities. *FEMS Microbiol Rev* **34**:554–587.

188. Vandal OH, Pierini LM, Schnappinger D, Nathan CF, Ehrt S. 2008. A membrane protein preserves intrabacterial pH in intraphagosomal *Mycobacterium tuberculosis*. *Nat Med* **14**:849–854.

189. Rao SPS, Alonso S, Rand L, Dick T, Pethe K. 2008. The protonmotive force is required for maintaining ATP homeostasis and viability of hypoxic, nonreplicating *Mycobacterium tuberculosis*. *Proc Natl Acad Sci USA* **105**:11945–11950.

190. DeCoster DJ, Vena RM, Callister SM, Schell RF. 2005. Susceptibility testing of *Mycobacterium tuberculosis*: comparison of the BACTEC TB-460 method and flow cytometric assay with the proportion method. *Clin Microbiol Infect* **11**:372–378.

191. Pina-Vaz C, Costa-de-Oliveira S, Rodrigues AG. 2005. Safe susceptibility testing of *Mycobacterium tuberculosis* by flow cytometry with the fluorescent nucleic acid stain SYTO 16. *J Med Microbiol* **54**:77–81.

192. Hendon-Dunn CL, Doris KS, Thomas SR, Allnutt JC, Marriott AAN, Hatch KA, Watson RJ, Bottley G, Marsh PD, Taylor SC, Bacon J. 2016. A flow cytometry method for rapidly assessing *M. tuberculosis* responses to antibiotics with different modes of action. *Antimicrob Agents Chemother* **60**:3869–3883.

193. Jain P, Hartman TE, Eisenberg N, O'Donnell MR, Kriakov J, Govender K, Makume M, Thaler DS, Hatfull GF, Sturm AW, Larsen MH, Moodley P, Jacobs WR Jr. 2012. (2)GFP10, a high-intensity fluorophage, enables detection and rapid drug susceptibility testing of *Mycobacterium tuberculosis* directly from sputum samples. *J Clin Microbiol* **50**:1362–1369.

194. Oliver JD. 2005. The viable but nonculturable state in bacteria. *J Microbiol* **43**:93–100.

195. Soejima T, Iida K, Qin T, Taniai H, Yoshida S. 2009. Discrimination of live, anti-tuberculosis agent-injured, and dead *Mycobacterium tuberculosis* using flow cytometry. *FEMS Microbiol Lett* **294**:74–81.

196. Das B, Kashino SS, Pulu I, Kalita D, Swami V, Yeger H, Felsher DW, Campos-Neto A. 2013. CD271(+) bone marrow mesenchymal stem cells may provide a niche for dormant *Mycobacterium tuberculosis*. *Sci Transl Med* **5**:170ra13.

197. Beamer G, Major S, Das B, Campos-Neto A. 2014. Bone marrow mesenchymal stem cells provide an antibiotic-protective niche for persistent viable *Mycobacterium tuberculosis* that survive antibiotic treatment. *Am J Pathol* **184**:3170–3175.

198. Swan BK, Martinez-Garcia M, Preston CM, Sczyrba A, Woyke T, Lamy D, Reinthaler T, Poulton NJ, Masland EDP, Gomez ML, Sieracki ME, DeLong EF, Herndl GJ, Stepanauskas R. 2011. Potential for chemolithoautotrophy among ubiquitous bacteria lineages in the dark ocean. *Science* **333**:1296–1300.

199. Wilson MC, Mori T, Rückert C, Uria AR, Helf MJ, Takada K, Gernert C, Steffens UAE, Heycke N, Schmitt S, Rinke C, Helfrich EJN, Brachmann AO, Gurgui C, Wakimoto T, Kracht M, Crüsemann M, Hentschel U, Abe I, Matsunaga S, Kalinowski J, Takeyama H, Piel J. 2014. An environmental bacterial taxon with a large and distinct metabolic repertoire. *Nature* **506**:58–62.

200. Leung K, Zahn H, Leaver T, Konwar KM, Hanson NW, Pagé AP, Lo C-C, Chain PS, Hallam SJ, Hansen CL. 2012. A programmable droplet-based microfluidic device applied to multiparameter analysis of single microbes and microbial communities. *Proc Natl Acad Sci USA* **109**: 7665–7670.

201. Dichosa AEK, Daughton AR, Reitenga KG, Fitzsimons MS, Han CS. 2014. Capturing and cultivating single bacterial cells in gel microdroplets to obtain near-complete genomes. *Nat Protoc* 9:608–621.

202. Levsky JM, Shenoy SM, Pezo RC, Singer RH. 2002. Single-cell gene expression profiling. *Science* 297:836–840.

203. Golding I, Paulsson J, Zawilski SM, Cox EC. 2005. Real-time kinetics of gene activity in individual bacteria. *Cell* 123:1025–1036.

204. Maamar H, Raj A, Dubnau D. 2007. Noise in gene expression determines cell fate in *Bacillus subtilis*. *Science* 317:526–529.

205. Raj A, Peskin CS, Tranchina D, Vargas DY, Tyagi S. 2006. Stochastic mRNA synthesis in mammalian cells. *PLoS Biol* 4:e309–e313.

206. Tyagi S. 2009. Imaging intracellular RNA distribution and dynamics in living cells. *Nat Methods* 6:331–338.

207. Paige JS, Wu KY, Jaffrey SR. 2011. RNA mimics of green fluorescent protein. *Science* 333:642–646.

208. Wu B, Piatkevich KD, Lionnet T, Singer RH, Verkhusha VV. 2011. Modern fluorescent proteins and imaging technologies to study gene expression, nuclear localization, and dynamics. *Curr Opin Cell Biol* 23:310–317.

209. Kang Y, Norris MH, Zarzycki-Siek J, Nierman WC, Donachie SP, Hoang TT. 2011. Transcript amplification from single bacterium for transcriptome analysis. *Genome Res* 21:925–935.

210. Westermann AJ, Gorski SA, Vogel J. 2012. Dual RNA-seq of pathogen and host. *Nat Rev Microbiol* 10:618–630.

211. Schubert OT, Ludwig C, Kogadeeva M, Zimmermann M, Rosenberger G, Gengenbacher M, Gillet LC, Collins BC, Röst HL, Kaufmann SHE, Sauer U, Aebersold R. 2015. Absolute proteome composition and dynamics during dormancy and resuscitation of *Mycobacterium tuberculosis*. *Cell Host Microbe* 18:96–108.

212. Chattopadhyay PK, Gierahn TM, Roederer M, Love JC. 2014. Single-cell technologies for monitoring immune systems. *Nat Immunol* 15:128–135.

213. Jahn M, Seifert J, von Bergen M, Schmid A, Bühler B, Müller S. 2013. Subpopulation-proteomics in prokaryotic populations. *Curr Opin Biotechnol* 24:79–87.

214. Mellors JS, Jorabchi K, Smith LM, Ramsey JM. 2010. Integrated microfluidic device for automated single cell analysis using electrophoretic separation and electrospray ionization mass spectrometry. *Anal Chem* 82:967–973.

215. Urban PL, Jefimovs K, Amantonico A, Fagerer SR, Schmid T, Mädler S, Puigmarti-Luis J, Goedecke N, Zenobi R. 2010. High-density micro-arrays for mass spectrometry. *Lab Chip* 10:3206–3209.

216. Wu M, Singh AK. 2012. Single-cell protein analysis. *Curr Opin Biotechnol* 23:83–88.

217. Zimmermann M, Kuehne A, Boshoff HI, Barry CE III, Zamboni N, Sauer U. 2015. Dynamic exometabolome analysis reveals active metabolic pathways in non-replicating mycobacteria. *Environ Microbiol* 17:4802–4815.

218. Zenobi R. 2013. Single-cell metabolomics: analytical and biological perspectives. *Science* 342:1243259.

219. Di Carlo D, Wu LY, Lee LP. 2006. Dynamic single cell culture array. *Lab Chip* 6:1445–1449.

220. Schmitz CHJ, Rowat AC, Köster S, Weitz DA. 2009. Dropspots: a picoliter array in a microfluidic device. *Lab Chip* 9:44–49.

221. Rubakhin SS, Lanni EJ, Sweedler JV. 2013. Progress toward single cell metabolomics. *Curr Opin Biotechnol* 24:95–104.

222. Lanni EJ, Rubakhin SS, Sweedler JV. 2012. Mass spectrometry imaging and profiling of single cells. *J Proteomics* 75:5036–5051.

223. Musat N, Foster R, Vagner T, Adam B, Kuypers MMM. 2012. Detecting metabolic activities in single cells, with emphasis on nanoSIMS. *FEMS Microbiol Rev* 36:486–511.

224. Mohr W, Vagner T, Kuypers MMM, Ackermann M, Laroche J. 2013. Resolution of conflicting signals at the single-cell level in the regulation of cyanobacterial photosynthesis and nitrogen fixation. *PLoS One* 8: e66060–e66067.

225. Prideaux B, Dartois V, Staab D, Weiner DM, Goh A, Via LE, Barry CE III, Stoeckli M. 2011. High-sensitivity MALDI-MRM-MS imaging of moxifloxacin distribution in tuberculosis-infected rabbit lungs and granulomatous lesions. *Anal Chem* 83:2112–2118.

226. Boehme CC, Nabeta P, Hillemann D, Nicol MP, Shenai S, Krapp F, Allen J, Tahirli R, Blakemore R, Rustomjee R, Milovic A, Jones M, O'Brien SM, Persing DH, Ruesch-Gerdes S, Gotuzzo E, Rodrigues C, Alland D, Perkins MD. 2010. Rapid molecular detection of tuberculosis and rifampin resistance. *N Engl J Med* 363: 1005–1015.

227. Spiller DG, Wood CD, Rand DA, White MRH. 2010. Measurement of single-cell dynamics. *Nature* 465:736–745.

228. Carroll P, Schreuder LJ, Muwanguzi-Karugaba J, Wiles S, Robertson BD, Ripoll J, Ward TH, Bancroft GJ, Schaible UE, Parish T. 2010. Sensitive detection of gene expression in mycobacteria under replicating and non-replicating conditions using optimized far-red reporters. *PLoS One* 5:e9823.

229. Chudakov DM, Matz MV, Lukyanov S, Lukyanov KA. 2010. Fluorescent proteins and their applications in imaging living cells and tissues. *Physiol Rev* 90:1103–1163.

230. Meniche X, Otten R, Siegrist MS, Baer CE, Murphy KC, Bertozzi CR, Sassetti CM. 2014. Subpolar addition of new cell wall is directed by DivIVA in mycobacteria. *Proc Natl Acad Sci USA* 111:E3243–E3251.

231. Hayashi JM, Luo C-Y, Mayfield JA, Hsu T, Fukuda T, Walfield AL, Giffen SR, Leszyk JD, Baer CE, Bennion OT, Madduri A, Shaffer SA, Aldridge BB, Sassetti CM, Sandler SJ, Kinoshita T, Moody DB, Morita YS. 2016. Spatially distinct and metabolically active membrane domain in mycobacteria. *Proc Natl Acad Sci USA* 113: 5400–5405.

232. Gee CLC, Papavinasasundaram KGK, Blair SRS, Baer CEC, Falick AMA, King DSD, Griffin JEJ, Venghatakrishnan H, Zukauskas A, Wei J-RJ, Dhiman RKR, Crick DCD, Rubin EJE, Sassetti CMC, Alber T.

2012. A phosphorylated pseudokinase complex controls cell wall synthesis in mycobacteria. *Sci Signal* 5:ra7.

233. Hett EC, Chao MC, Steyn AJ, Fortune SM, Deng LL, Rubin EJ. 2007. A partner for the resuscitation-promoting factors of *Mycobacterium tuberculosis*. *Mol Microbiol* 66:658–668.

234. Plocinska R, Purushotham G, Sarva K, Vadrevu IS, Pandeeti EVP, Arora N, Plocinski P, Madiraju MV, Rajagopalan M. 2012. Septal localization of the *Mycobacterium tuberculosis* MtrB sensor kinase promotes MtrA regulon expression. *J Biol Chem* 287:23887–23899.

235. Plocinski P, Ziolkiewicz M, Kiran M, Vadrevu SI, Nguyen HB, Hugonnet J, Veckerle C, Arthur M, Dziadek J, Cross TA, Madiraju M, Rajagopalan M. 2011. Characterization of CrgA, a new partner of the *Mycobacterium tuberculosis* peptidoglycan polymerization complexes. *J Bacteriol* 193:3246–3256.

236. Chauhan A, Lofton H, Maloney E, Moore J, Fol M, Madiraju MVVSM, Rajagopalan M. 2006. Interference of *Mycobacterium tuberculosis* cell division by Rv2719c, a cell wall hydrolase. *Mol Microbiol* 62:132–147.

237. Rajagopalan M, Maloney E, Dziadek J, Poplawska M, Lofton H, Chauhan A, Madiraju MVVS. 2005. Genetic evidence that mycobacterial FtsZ and FtsW proteins interact, and colocalize to the division site in *Mycobacterium smegmatis*. *FEMS Microbiol Lett* 250:9–17.

238. Maloney E, Madiraju SC, Rajagopalan M, Madiraju M. 2011. Localization of acidic phospholipid cardiolipin and DnaA in mycobacteria. *Tuberculosis (Edinb)* 91 (Suppl 1):S150–S155.

239. Ginda K, Bezulska M, Ziółkiewicz M, Dziadek J, Zakrzewska-Czerwińska J, Jakimowicz D. 2013. ParA of *Mycobacterium smegmatis* co-ordinates chromosome segregation with the cell cycle and interacts with the polar growth determinant DivIVA. *Mol Microbiol* 87:998–1012.

240. Harris KK, Fay A, Yan H-G, Kunwar P, Socci ND, Pottabathini N, Juventhala RR, Djaballah H, Glickman MS. 2014. Novel imidazoline antimicrobial scaffold that inhibits DNA replication with activity against mycobacteria and drug resistant Gram-positive cocci. *ACS Chem Biol* 9:2572–2583.

241. Trojanowski D, Ginda K, Pióro M, Hołówka J, Skut P, Jakimowicz D, Zakrzewska-Czerwińska J. 2015. Choreography of the *Mycobacterium* replication machinery during the cell cycle. *MBio* 6:e02125-14.

242. Baer CE, Iavarone AT, Alber T, Sassetti CM. 2014. Biochemical and spatial coincidence in the provisional Ser/Thr protein kinase interaction network of *Mycobacterium tuberculosis*. *J Biol Chem* 289:20422–20433.

243. Carel C, Nukdee K, Cantaloube S, Bonne M, Diagne CT, Laval F, Daffé M, Zerbib D. 2014. *Mycobacterium tuberculosis* proteins involved in mycolic acid synthesis and transport localize dynamically to the old growing pole and septum. *PLoS One* 9:e97148.

244. Backus KM, Boshoff HI, Barry CS, Boutureira O, Patel MK, D'Hooge F, Lee SS, Via LE, Tahlan K, Barry CE III, Davis BG. 2011. Uptake of unnatural trehalose analogs as a reporter for *Mycobacterium tuberculosis*. *Nat Chem Biol* 7:228–235.

245. Neres J, Pojer F, Molteni E, Chiarelli LR, Dhar N, Boy-Röttger S, Buroni S, Fullam E, Degiacomi G, Lucarelli AP, Read RJ, Zanoni G, Edmondson DE, De Rossi E, Pasca MR, McKinney JD, Dyson PJ, Riccardi G, Mattevi A, Cole ST, Binda C. 2012. Structural basis for benzothiazinone-mediated killing of *Mycobacterium tuberculosis*. *Sci Transl Med* 4:150ra121.

246. Siegrist MS, Swarts BM, Fox DM, Lim SA, Bertozzi CR. 2015. Illumination of growth, division and secretion by metabolic labeling of the bacterial cell surface. *FEMS Microbiol Rev* 39:184–202.

247. Xue L, Karpenko IA, Hiblot J, Johnsson K. 2015. Imaging and manipulating proteins in live cells through covalent labeling. *Nat Chem Biol* 11:917–923.

248. Maglica Ž, Özdemir E, McKinney JD. 2015. Single-cell tracking reveals antibiotic-induced changes in mycobacterial energy metabolism. *MBio* 6:e02236-14.

249. Simeone R, Bobard A, Lippmann J, Bitter W, Majlessi L, Brosch R, Enninga J. 2012. Phagosomal rupture by *Mycobacterium tuberculosis* results in toxicity and host cell death. *PLoS Pathog* 8:e1002507.

250. Barisch C, López-Jiménez AT, Soldati T. 2015. Live imaging of *Mycobacterium marinum* infection in *Dictyostelium discoideum*. *Methods Mol Biol* 1285:369–385.

251. Johansson J, Karlsson A, Bylund J, Welin A. 2015. Phagocyte interactions with *Mycobacterium tuberculosis*–Simultaneous analysis of phagocytosis, phagosome maturation and intracellular replication by imaging flow cytometry. *J Immunol Methods* 427:73–84.

252. Beebe DJ, Mensing GA, Walker GM. 2002. Physics and applications of microfluidics in biology. *Annu Rev Biomed Eng* 4:261–286.

253. Whitesides GM, Ostuni E, Takayama S, Jiang X, Ingber DE. 2001. Soft lithography in biology and biochemistry. *Annu Rev Biomed Eng* 3:335–373.

254. Weibel DB, Diluzio WR, Whitesides GM. 2007. Microfabrication meets microbiology. *Nat Rev Microbiol* 5:209–218.

255. Sala C, Dhar N, Hartkoorn RC, Zhang M, Ha YH, Schneider P, Cole ST. 2010. Simple model for testing drugs against nonreplicating *Mycobacterium tuberculosis*. *Antimicrob Agents Chemother* 54:4150–4158.

256. Kolly GS, Boldrin F, Sala C, Dhar N, Hartkoorn RC, Ventura M, Serafini A, McKinney JD, Manganelli R, Cole ST. 2014. Assessing the essentiality of the decaprenyl-phospho-d-arabinofuranose pathway in *Mycobacterium tuberculosis* using conditional mutants. *Mol Microbiol* 92:194–211.

257. Golchin SA, Stratford J, Curry RJ, McFadden J. 2012. A microfluidic system for long-term time-lapse microscopy studies of mycobacteria. *Tuberculosis (Edinb)* 92:489–496.

258. Makarov V, Manina G, Mikusova K, Möllmann U, Ryabova O, Saint-Joanis B, Dhar N, Pasca MR, Buroni S, Lucarelli AP, Milano A, De Rossi E, Belanova M, Bobovska A, Dianiskova P, Kordulakova J, Sala C, Fullam E, Schneider P, McKinney JD, Brodin P, Christophe T, Waddell S, Butcher P, Albrethsen J, Rosenkrands I, Brosch R, Nandi V, Bharath S, Gaonkar S, Shandil RK, Balasubramanian V, Balganesh T,

Tyagi S, Grosset J, Riccardi G, Cole ST. 2009. Benzothiazinones kill *Mycobacterium tuberculosis* by blocking arabinan synthesis. *Science* 324:801–804.

259. Koul A, Vranckx L, Dhar N, Göhlmann HWH, Özdemir E, Neefs J-M, Schulz M, Lu P, Mørtz E, McKinney JD, Andries K, Bald D. 2014. Delayed bactericidal response of *Mycobacterium tuberculosis* to bedaquiline involves remodelling of bacterial metabolism. *Nat Commun* 5:3369.

260. Dhar N, Dubée V, Ballell L, Cuinet G, Hugonnet J-E, Signorino-Gelo F, Barros D, Arthur M, McKinney JD. 2015. Rapid cytolysis of *Mycobacterium tuberculosis* by faropenem, an orally bioavailable β-lactam antibiotic. *Antimicrob Agents Chemother* 59:1308–1319.

261. Neres J, Hartkoorn RC, Chiarelli LR, Gadupudi R, Pasca MR, Mori G, Venturelli A, Savina S, Makarov V, Kolly GS, Molteni E, Binda C, Dhar N, Ferrari S, Brodin P, Delorme V, Landry V, de Jesus Lopes Ribeiro AL, Farina D, Saxena P, Pojer F, Carta A, Luciani R, Porta A, Zanoni G, De Rossi E, Costi MP, Riccardi G, Cole ST. 2015. 2-Carboxyquinoxalines kill *Mycobacterium tuberculosis* through noncovalent inhibition of DprE1. *ACS Chem Biol* 10:705–714.

262. Batt SM, Cacho Izquierdo M, Castro Pichel J, Stubbs CJ, Vela-Glez Del Peral L, Pérez-Herrán E, Dhar N, Mouzon B, Rees M, Hutchinson JP, Young RJ, McKinney JD, Barros-Aguirre D, Ballell L, Besra GS, Argyrou A. 2015. Whole cell target engagement identifies novel inhibitors of *Mycobacterium tuberculosis* decaprenylphosphoryl-β-D-ribose oxidase. *ACS Infect Dis* 1:615–626.

263. Jing W, Jiang X, Zhao W, Liu S, Cheng X, Sui G. 2014. Microfluidic platform for direct capture and analysis of airborne *Mycobacterium tuberculosis*. *Anal Chem* 86:5815–5821.

264. Lyu F, Xu M, Cheng Y, Xie J, Rao J, Tang SKY. 2015. Quantitative detection of cells expressing BlaC using droplet-based microfluidics for use in the diagnosis of tuberculosis. *Biomicrofluidics* 9:044120.

265. Zhu K, Kaprelyants AS, Salina EG, Markx GH. 2010. Separation by dielectrophoresis of dormant and nondormant bacterial cells of *Mycobacterium smegmatis*. *Biomicrofluidics* 4:022809.

266. Elitas M, Martinez-Duarte R, Dhar N, McKinney JD, Renaud P. 2014. Dielectrophoresis-based purification of antibiotic-treated bacterial subpopulations. *Lab Chip* 14:1850–1857.

267. Luthuli BB, Purdy GE, Balagaddé FK. 2015. Confinement-induced drug-tolerance in mycobacteria mediated by an efflux mechanism. *PLoS One* 10:e0136231.

268. Maerkl SJ. 2009. Integration column: microfluidic high-throughput screening. *Integr Biol Camb* 1:19–29.

269. Takaki K, Cosma CL, Troll MA, Ramakrishnan L. 2012. An in vivo platform for rapid high-throughput antitubercular drug discovery. *Cell Reports* 2:175–184.

270. Bernut A, Dupont C, Sahuquet A, Herrmann JL, Lutfalla G, Kremer L. 2015. Deciphering and imaging pathogenesis and cording of *Mycobacterium abscessus* in Zebrafish embryos. *J Vis Exp* (103):e53130.

271. Fenaroli F, Westmoreland D, Benjaminsen J, Kolstad T, Skjeldal FM, Meijer AH, van der Vaart M, Ulanova L, Roos N, Nyström B, Hildahl J, Griffiths G. 2014. Nanoparticles as drug delivery system against tuberculosis in zebrafish embryos: direct visualization and treatment. *ACS Nano* 8:7014–7026.

272. Looney MR, Bhattacharya J. 2014. Live imaging of the lung. *Annu Rev Physiol* 76:431–445.

273. Cronan MR, Rosenberg AF, Oehlers SH, Saelens JW, Sisk DM, Jurcic Smith KL, Lee S, Tobin DM. 2015. CLARITY and PACT-based imaging of adult zebrafish and mouse for whole-animal analysis of infections. *Dis Model Mech* 8:1643–1650.

274. Kong Y, Yang D, Cirillo SLG, Li S, Akin A, Francis KP, Maloney T, Cirillo JD. 2016. Application of fluorescent protein expressing strains to evaluation of antituberculosis therapeutic efficacy in vitro and in vivo. *PLoS One* 11:e0149972.

275. Kong Y, Yao H, Ren H, Subbian S, Cirillo SLG, Sacchettini JC, Rao J, Cirillo JD. 2010. Imaging tuberculosis with endogenous beta-lactamase reporter enzyme fluorescence in live mice. *Proc Natl Acad Sci USA* 107:12239–12244.

276. Egen JG, Rothfuchs AG, Feng CG, Horwitz MA, Sher A, Germain RN. 2011. Intravital imaging reveals limited antigen presentation and T cell effector function in mycobacterial granulomas. *Immunity* 34:807–819.

277. Nooshabadi F, Yang H-J, Bixler JN, Kong Y, Cirillo JD, Maitland KC. 2016. Intravital fluorescence excitation in whole-animal optical imaging. *PLoS One* 11:e0149932.

278. Bhatia SN, Ingber DE. 2014. Microfluidic organs-on-chips. *Nat Biotechnol* 32:760–772.

279. Esch EW, Bahinski A, Huh D. 2015. Organs-on-chips at the frontiers of drug discovery. *Nat Rev Drug Discov* 14:248–260.

280. Benam KH, Villenave R, Lucchesi C, Varone A, Hubeau C, Lee HH, Alves SE, Salmon M, Ferrante TC, Weaver JC, Bahinski A, Hamilton GA, Ingber DE. 2016. Small airway-on-a-chip enables analysis of human lung inflammation and drug responses *in vitro*. *Nat Methods* 13:151–157.

281. Waddington CH. 1957. *The Strategy of Genes*. George Allen & Unwin, London.

282. Lorenzi T, Chisholm RH, Desvillettes L, Hughes BD. 2015. Dissecting the dynamics of epigenetic changes in phenotype-structured populations exposed to fluctuating environments. *J Theor Biol* 386:166–176.

283. Hawn TR, Shah JA, Kalman D. 2015. New tricks for old dogs: countering antibiotic resistance in tuberculosis with host-directed therapeutics. *Immunol Rev* 264:344–362.

284. Dar RD, Hosmane NN, Arkin MR, Siliciano RF, Weinberger LS. 2014. Screening for noise in gene expression identifies drug synergies. *Science* 344:1392–1396.

285. LeCun Y, Bengio Y, Hinton G. 2015. Deep learning. *Nature* 521:436–444.

286. Marino S, Gideon HP, Gong C, Mankad S, McCrone JT, Lin PL, Linderman JJ, Flynn JL, Kirschner DE. 2016. Computational and Empirical Studies Predict *Mycobacterium tuberculosis*-Specific T Cells as a Biomarker for Infection Outcome. *PLOS Comput Biol* 12:e1004804.

287. Jacobs WR Jr, McShane H, Mizrahi V, Orme IM (ed). *Tuberculosis and the Tubercle Bacillus*, 2nd ed. ASM Press, Washington, DC, in press.

Tuberculosis and the Tubercle Bacillus, 2nd ed.
Edited by William R. Jacobs, Jr., Helen McShane, Valerie Mizrahi, and Ian M. Orme
© 2018 American Society for Microbiology, Washington, DC
doi:10.1128/microbiolspec.TBTB2-0030-2016

Mycobacterium tuberculosis in the Face of Host-Imposed Nutrient Limitation

33

Michael Berney and Linda Berney-Meyer

INTRODUCTION

Interactions of bacteria with the human host are, in the vast majority of cases, beneficial for both partners (1). In fact, humans are dependent on their microbial associates for nutrition, defense, and development (1). However, a minority of bacteria use the human organism as a vessel to proliferate and spread and, as a consequence, leave behind collateral damage of varying degrees. These so-called pathogens have typically evolved to inhabit niches in the human body with little competition from their commensal counterparts (2). Many of these human pathogens are intracellular bacteria, meaning that their preferred niche of proliferation and persistence is within human cells. Intracellular pathogens invade phagocytic or nonphagocytic host cells, where they replicate in specialized phagosomal compartments or in the cytosol. After having made their way into their preferred niche, they try to benefit from host nutrients and other metabolites to satisfy their bioenergetic and biosynthetic requirements (3). The dynamic metabolic interplay between pathogen and host is essential for virulence, disease progression, and infection control.

Emerging evidence suggests that the host immune system actively depletes nutrients from the cytosol or phagosome of phagocytic cells to starve the invading microbes (3–7). Such processes could be collectively described as "nutritional immunity." The first scientifically described mechanism that falls under this term was host-mediated restriction of Fe by NRAMP and transferrin (6, 8). However, more recently it became clear that the host also restricts access to other transition metals, including Mn, Zn, and Cu (9), as well as carbon

(10, 11) and amino acids (7, 10, 12). For example, the mammalian enzyme indoleamine 2,3-dioxygenase (IDO) actively degrades tryptophan and is activated during pathogen infection to starve the intruders of this essential amino acid (13–15). In response to host nutrient deprivation, many human pathogens, e.g., *Legionella pneumophila* (16), *Francisella tularensis* (17), and *Listeria monocytogenes* (18), have acquired elaborate mechanisms to circumvent nutritional immunity and access essential metabolites. Such nutritional virulence mechanisms (19) allowed these pathogens to evolve into natural auxotrophs for up to 10 amino acids (16, 17), a characteristic that results in partial dependency on the host. However, it remains largely unknown what *M. tuberculosis* can and cannot scavenge from the host.

The mechanisms governing *M. tuberculosis* entry into the host, replication, and dissemination are still poorly understood. Nevertheless, based on studies with *M. tuberculosis* in macrophages and animal models, as well as *Mycobacterium marinum* in the zebra fish model, a (probably simplified) picture emerges wherein the main niche of replication of *M. tuberculosis* is the phagosome of human alveolar macrophages (20). It was suggested that during the 70,000 years of coevolution of *M. tuberculosis* with its human host (21), the pathogen has developed tactics to make a stealthy entry past the commensal barrier of the upper lungs to the lower alveolar spaces, which harbor few, if any, commensals (2, 22). In the lower alveolar space, it is thought that *M. tuberculosis* uses a masking lipid, phthiocerol dimycocerosate, to avoid the microbicidal macrophages and a recruiting lipid, phenolic glyco-

Albert Einstein College of Medicine, Department of Microbiology and Immunology, New York, NY 10461.

lipid, to infect the permissive ones (2, 22). Once in their preferred niche, they replicate and, mediated by mechanisms such as the type VII secretion system ESX1, induce coordinated macrophage death and phagocytosis by new macrophages, leading to granuloma formation (23–26). This process seems to enable a tremendous expansion in bacterial numbers. To achieve this, *M. tuberculosis* must access essential elements such as carbon, nitrogen, phosphorus, and trace elements.

There are possibly three stages of *M. tuberculosis* infection that provide completely different diets to the pathogen: first, active proliferation in the macrophages; second, persistence in the granuloma; and third, possibly extracellular growth in caseating lesions. Determining nutrient availability and nutrient uptake by the pathogen during these stages is extremely challenging. The first stage can be studied to a certain extent *in vitro* (e.g., with a macrophage infection model and metabolomics); however, the difficulties in distinguishing between cytosolic and phagosomal metabolites in pathogen-infected host cells are not yet resolved. The second and third stages can only be satisfyingly studied *in vivo*. Therefore, we have to rely on indirect evidence that can be garnered from *in vivo* experiments with auxotrophic strains. In this article, we will review *M. tuberculosis* nutritional requirements and vulnerabilities with a focus on amino acids and coenzymes. We aim to summarize and discuss the current data acquired from *in vitro* studies in macrophages and *in vivo* studies in animal models, with a focus on nutrient use by the pathogen and strategies of the host to limit the pathogen's growth. Knowledge about *M. tuberculosis*'s *in vivo* diet will help to unravel the microenvironment at different stages of infection, elucidate metabolic signaling and nutritional checkpoints in disease progression, identify mechanisms of nutritional immunity, and most importantly, identify metabolic vulnerabilities and much needed new chemotherapeutic strategies.

M. TUBERCULOSIS'S IN VIVO GROWTH REQUIREMENTS

Lessons from Metabolomics

M. tuberculosis in macrophages

Defining the nutritional environment of intracellular pathogens is technically extremely challenging in terms of the infection models and the available analytical methods. At present, the analysis of metabolic host-pathogen interactions is most easily studied using infected host cells because they represent fairly well-defined metabolic entities (3, 27, 28). The main approach is to infect

human cells (e.g., monocytes or macrophages) with a virulent strain of the pathogen and measure the changes in metabolites over time. With the development of high-sensitivity small-molecule mass spectrometry, it is possible to accurately measure bacterial and host cell metabolite abundance. The advantages of this approach are high sensitivity and the simultaneous measurement of hundreds of metabolites.

Several studies have been conducted to look at metabolic changes in macrophages upon *M. tuberculosis* infection. One study used gas chromatography mass spectrometry to measure changes in metabolites in THP-1 macrophages infected with the virulent strains *M. tuberculosis* H37Rv and B36 or the avirulent strains *Mycobacterium bovis* BCG and *M. tuberculosis* H37Ra (29). This analysis indicated that in cells infected with virulent *M. tuberculosis*, the abundance of glycine, aspartate, proline, isoleucine, alanine, ornithine, threonine, cysteine, and lysine decreased, whereas glutamate, serine, and valine increased (29). However, it is unknown if these results are indicative of the nutritional environment that *M. tuberculosis* experiences in the phagosome. In nearly all studies conducted so far, metabolites were extracted from homogenized cells, an approach that does not take into account the metabolic differences of the microenvironments (e.g., cytosol versus pathogen-containing vacuole) in macrophages.

To this end, Beste and coworkers (30) performed an elegant experiment using ^{13}C-flux analysis to determine which metabolites can be taken up by *M. tuberculosis* when residing in THP-1 macrophages. This study indicated that *M. tuberculosis* is able to take up alanine, glutamate/glutamine, and asparagine/aspartate from the THP-1 cells. Consistent with this finding, Gouzy and coworkers identified specific transporters for asparagine and aspartate in *M. tuberculosis* (31, 32). *In vivo* data showed that *M. tuberculosis* does not rely on these transporters for replication in mouse organs, which is supported by the fact that *M. tuberculosis* harbors the biosynthetic machinery to produce both amino acids and that natural auxotrophs of these amino acids are absent in clinical isolates. Still, the same group demonstrated that asparagine plays a role in the pH homeostasis of *M. tuberculosis* in the phagosome via the release of ammonia by the activity of asparaginase AnsA. The *ansA* deletion strains also displayed a 1-log decrease in organ burden compared to the wild-type (WT) strain in infected mice, indicating that this process might be important *in vivo*. Taken together and based on the current literature, we know that several amino acids can be taken up by the pathogen from the host, but none of them is essential for replication and survival in the host. This suggests that *M. tuberculosis* uses nitrogen cocatabolism for nitrogen assimilation, much like its strategy of carbon cocatabolism (33, 34).

Another limitation of the cell-line-based approach is that most of the host cells used in these assays are from cancer cell lines, which have an entirely different metabolic signature than WT cells, and therefore the metabolic environment experienced by the pathogen is different and potentially changes the microbes' own metabolic response (3, 28, 35). This problem could be prevented, for example, by using macrophages derived from peripheral blood mononuclear cells; however, the difficulty of distinguishing between cytosolic and phagosomal metabolites still remains. In more recent years, imaging mass spectrometry, such as dynamic secondary ion mass spectrometry (SIMS microscopy) and matrix-assisted laser desorption ionization imaging mass spectrometry (see reference 36 for a comprehensive review), has been used on *M. tuberculosis*-infected macrophages (32) and organ tissues (37, 38). Gouzy and coworkers were able to show, using NanoSIMS, that *M. tuberculosis* can scavenge labeled aspartate and asparagine from THP-1 cells (31, 32). In the current state, these methods are costly and mostly used to detect specific metabolites because the deconvolution of metabolite signals in the complex matrices is challenging (39). In some circumstances, isotopic labeling can overcome isobaric interference, but even these approaches will need validation on a sample-by-sample basis (39). Nevertheless, further advancements in imaging mass-spectrometry technology might soon allow the label-free detection of *in situ* metabolic profiles of pathogens within host cell vacuoles and within tissue samples.

M. tuberculosis in host tissue

Metabolic changes in host tissues in response to *M. tuberculosis* infection have been measured in mice and guinea pigs. A ^{1}H nuclear magnetic resonance-based metabolomics profiling approach in infected mouse organs showed a significant increase in tissue concentration of several amino acids (alanine, aspartate, glutamate, leucine, lysine, isoleucine, phenylalanine, tyrosine, and glutamine) (40). However, it is unclear if these differences in metabolite concentration stem from the infected or uninfected areas in these organs, and hence they may not be indicative of the nutritional environment *M. tuberculosis* finds itself in. Somashekar and coworkers (41) showed by high-resolution magic angle spinning nuclear magnetic resonance spectroscopy that lung granulomas from *M. tuberculosis*-infected

guinea pigs have elevated abundance of lactate, alanine, acetate, glutamate, glutathionine, aspartate, creatine, phosphocholine, glycerophosphocholine, betaine, trimethylamine N-oxide, myo-inositol, scyllo-inositol, and dihydroxyacetone.

In summary, metabolomics approaches so far have given us some indication of the metabolic changes in host tissues in response to *M. tuberculosis* infection. However, the immediate metabolic environment of a tubercle bacillus, when it is growing within a pathogen-containing vacuole in alveolar macrophages, is still elusive, and more sophisticated methods and alternative approaches are needed to measure metabolic exchanges between the pathogen-containing vacuole, the cytosol, and bacteria.

Lessons from Auxotrophic Strains

Amino acid auxotrophies

Auxotrophy is the inability of an organism to synthesize a particular organic compound required for its growth. Early on, with the advent of molecular genetics, the use of bacterial strains with auxotrophies led to breakthrough findings about the exchange of genetic material in bacteria (42–45). Using *Escherichia coli* auxotrophic strains, Tatum and Lederberg, as well as B.D. Davis, discovered the process of conjugation (43, 46), an achievement for which Tatum and Lederberg later received the Nobel Prize in Physiology or Medicine.

Typically, auxotrophic strains are relatively easy to construct because mutants can be chemically complemented by the biosynthetic end product as long as the bacterium can transport sufficient amounts of the metabolite. Bacterial auxotrophs were also among the first mutants to be constructed when genetic tools were pioneered for mycobacteria (47, 48). Most of the auxotrophic strains constructed were attenuated in mouse models (7, 49–57), which led to the idea of using such strains as live vaccine candidates, especially because the efficacy of *M. bovis* BCG, the only vaccine available against tuberculosis (TB), is limited and in many cases not protective. Unfortunately, most of these live attenuated *M. tuberculosis* strains provided only little to no improvement in protection compared to BCG. Still, some of these auxotrophic strains have proven extremely valuable as avirulent strains of *M. tuberculosis* that can be used and manipulated under less restrictive biosafety level II conditions (58). Interestingly, despite the wealth of auxotrophic mutants, they have rarely been considered as metabolic probes *in vivo*. Arguably, an auxotrophic strain is the perfect biosensor to inform about the availability of nutrients *in vivo*. Here, we will review the literature on auxotrophic strains in the context of *in vivo* nutrition.

Aspartate and asparagines

To date, no aspartate or asparagine auxotrophs of *M. tuberculosis* have been isolated, although considerable advances have been made in understanding the role of these metabolites in *M. tuberculosis* pathogenesis. Gouzy and coworkers have inactivated the only aspartate transporter in *M. tuberculosis*, AnsP1, and shown that the mutant (Δ*ansP1*) could not grow on aspartate as the sole nitrogen source (32). Furthermore, using NanoSIMS, these authors demonstrated that *M. tuberculosis* can scavenge labeled aspartate from THP-1 cells, and a mouse infection experiment showed growth of Δ*ansP1* in lungs and spleens, albeit to a lower organ burden (1-log decrease) compared to the parental strain (32). The fact that the Δ*ansP1* mutant could still replicate *in vivo* argues that aspartate is mainly produced biosynthetically by the bacterium and not taken up from the host. Moreover, the studies by Gouzy et al. suggest that the role of host-derived aspartate and asparagine in TB pathogenesis has to do with pH homeostasis rather than nutrition per se (31, 32). The asparagine transporter mutant Δ*ansP2* was still virulent in mice, but inactivation of asparaginase (encoded by *ansA*) of *M. tuberculosis*, the enzyme that converts asparagine to aspartate and ammonium, led to a strong *in vivo* phenotype and strong susceptibility to low pH (31). It remains to be seen if host-derived aspartate and asparagine also have a nutritional role in TB pathogenesis. Constructing auxotrophic mutants and testing them *in vivo* could help to delineate their role in extracellular pH control and nutrition.

Arginine

Gordhan and coworkers constructed an *argF* mutant strain, Δ*argF*, by homologous recombination (55). ArgF encodes an ornithine carbamoyltransferase that converts ornithine to citrulline. Interestingly, *M. tuberculosis* Δ*argF* could not be rescued by citrulline but was chemically complemented by the downstream metabolites argininosuccinate and arginine, indicating that the mutation had polar effects on *argG* (55). One interesting feature of this mutant is its rapid death and culture sterilization *in vitro* (55). *In vivo* experiments in immunocompetent DBA/2 mice or immunocompromised SCID mice showed strong virulence attenuation; however, the SCID mice still succumbed to Δ*argF* infection, indicating that the mutant could potentially scavenge arginine from the host (55). However, evidence of complementation is absent, and colonies isolated from diseased SCID mice were not analyzed for potential suppressor mutants (55).

Macrophages have dedicated arginine transporters (e.g., SLC7A2) (59) to fuel nitric oxide (NO) production by NO synthase (iNOS) (58). Pathogen entry triggers NO production and therefore arginine depletion (59). Second, arginine concentration is controlled by arginases (Arg1 and Arg2) (58), and it is thought that arginases control arginine homeostasis to regulate NO levels (60, 61). When Arg1 knockout mice were infected with *M. tuberculosis*, the bacterial replication stopped earlier (1 log difference) than in WT mice (62). This was ascribed to an increase in NO production in the absence of arginine-degrading arginase 1 (62). To our knowledge, it is unknown if arginine depletion is an antibacterial mechanism or if it is just a side effect of antibacterial NO production and homeostasis. Hence, it would be interesting to test if an *M. tuberculosis* arginine auxotroph can grow in an iNOS/Arg1 double-knockout mouse that theoretically loses its ability to lower arginine concentrations.

Cysteine

Senaratne and coworkers constructed a cysteine auxotrophic strain by deleting *cysH* from *M. tuberculosis* (63). CysH encodes a phosphoadenosine phosphosulfate (PAPS) reductase that converts PAPS to sulfite and is involved in sulfur assimilation. The *cysH* deletion mutant (Δ*cysH*) was attenuated in immunocompetent mice but not in immunocompromised animals, suggesting that chemical complementation of this auxotroph is dependent on the adaptive immune system. Both methionine and cysteine complemented the mutant *in vitro*, but the nature of the *in vivo* complementation is still unknown. Given the early position of CysH in the sulfur assimilation pathway, it is possible that this mutant is able to scavenge sulfide, taurine, or cysteine from the host. Methionine was long believed to be an amino acid that could be scavenged from mouse tissue, but recently we showed that this is not the case (57). Taken together, the current literature suggests that *M. tuberculosis* Δ*cysH* can scavenge a yet unknown sulfur-containing compound from the host other than sulfate.

Methionine

Methionine auxotrophy was among the first auxotrophies described in mycobacterial research. Two transposon mutants of *M. bovis* BCG that could grow in the presence of methionine, but not with sulfide or cysteine, were isolated and shown to survive in mice just as well as the WT strain (47, 64). This led the authors to hypothesize that methionine can be scavenged from the host. The studies showed that the transposon insertions were in genes encoding for the proteins SubI and CysA, both subunits of the sulfate uptake permease (31).

Contrary opinions exist about the ability of mycobacteria to scavenge cysteine from the medium. Whereas it has been corroborated that a *cysA* mutant of BCG could not be complemented by cysteine, a *cysH* mutant of *M. tuberculosis* could be complemented. It is possible that there are species-specific differences in cysteine biosynthesis or that differences in experimental setups led to this discrepancy. However, what both mutants had in common was their ability to grow normally in the presence of methionine. Methionine biosynthesis is linked to sulfur metabolism by transsulfurylation, which is catalyzed by the two enzymes cystathione γ-synthase (*metB*) and cystathione β-lyase (*metC*). This branch uses cysteine and O-acetyl-homoserine to yield cystathione and then homocysteine in a two-step reaction. Deletion of *metB* in *M. tuberculosis* did not lead to auxotrophy (50), which suggests an alternative pathway. *M. tuberculosis* and other actinobacteria (65) also encode a cysteine-independent enzyme, O-acetylhomoserine sulfhydrylase encoded by *metY* (Rv3340), that catalyzes a sulfhydrylation reaction converting O-acetyl-homoserine and sulfide to homocysteine. Given the distance of CysA and CysH enzymes from the methionine biosynthesis pathway, it is unlikely that these strains are only methionine auxotrophs, and hence other metabolites can potentially lead to *in vivo* complementation of these mutants. We have recently shown that *M. tuberculosis* Δ*metA*, a strain deficient in catalyzing the first reaction of methionine biosynthesis, could be chemically complemented by all intermediates of methionine biosynthesis (O-acetylhomoserine, homocysteine, methionine, or S-adenosylmethionine) *in vitro*, but no viable bacilli could be retrieved from immunocompetent and immunocompromised mice 3 weeks after infection or later (57). Hence, our study clearly showed that *M. tuberculosis* is unable to scavenge methionine or any of the pathway intermediates from mouse organs or human macrophages. Another interesting characteristic of the *metA* mutant was rapid killing and culture sterilization, which makes this pathway very attractive for drug discovery.

Histidine

A histidine auxotroph of *M. tuberculosis* was constructed by deleting *hisDC*, the first two genes of the *his* operon (66). This strain was attenuated in macrophages and rapidly killed when starved for histidine (66). However, the strain could survive prolonged periods in total starvation (water without any supplements) (66). The author concluded that histidine is not available to *M. tuberculosis* in THP-1 macrophages and that complete starvation of the histidine auxotroph might not reflect the *in vivo* situation because CFUs were clearly dropping in macrophages but not in water (66). Furthermore, it needs to be mentioned here that the *hisDC* mutant was not complemented, and hence the genotype-phenotype link is not yet confirmed.

Proline

A proline auxotroph in *M. tuberculosis* was created by deleting *proC* by homologous recombination and replacing the gene with a hygromycin cassette (66). This mutation was bactericidal in unsupplemented medium, and the mutant was attenuated in mice (66). Interestingly, CFU data showed that the mutant could still replicate in mouse organs, albeit at a very slow rate (66), which implies that proline can be scavenged *in vivo*. However, the mutation was not complemented, and colonies isolated from mice were not checked for suppressor mutations (66). It is conceivable that the *pruB*-encoded proline dehydrogenase (67, 68) is potentially capable of reversing the reaction and producing proline in the absence of ProC. Future experiments will need to confirm *proC* and proline biosynthesis as viable drug targets.

Lysine

Construction of a lysine auxotrophic strain of *M. tuberculosis* was surprisingly difficult. Pavelka and Jacobs created *lysA* deletion mutants of *Mycobacterium smegmatis* and *M. bovis* BCG by allelic exchange using lysine-supplemented plates for rescue (69). However, no *lysA* mutants of *M. tuberculosis* could be isolated by this strategy until the lysine concentration in the medium was increased to 1 mg/ml and Tween 80 was added to the medium (69). The *lysA* mutants grew considerably slower than WT on solid media and in liquid media and always required Tween 80 for growth (69). Such dependence on detergent and a high concentration of supplement points to inefficient lysine uptake in this mutant. Whereas *M. smegmatis* efficiently transports lysine across the cell wall, *M. bovis* BCG and *M. tuberculosis* seem to lack a dedicated high-affinity lysine permease (M. Berney and G. M. Cook, unpublished results). Moreover, Pavelka and Jacob's results point to a difference in lysine uptake activity between *M. bovis* BCG and *M. tuberculosis*. The *M. tuberculosis lysA* auxotroph was strongly attenuated *in vivo* as it was rapidly cleared from mouse lungs after high-dose intravenous infections. Even when the same mice were injected with this strain three consecutive times, the lung burden dropped by 2 to 3 logs within 20 days, which strongly argues that lysine cannot be scavenged from the mouse organs. The attenuation described above made the *M. tuberculosis lysA* mutant attractive as a live attenuated vaccine candidate (53). The strain was made safer by adding a second auxotrophy (pantothenate) by knocking out *panCD* (70). This double mutant was then shown to be safe in guinea pigs as well as in non-human primates (71) and has since been approved for biosafety level II work by dozens of institutional biosafety committees from research organizations and universities (71).

Threonine

Covarrubias et al. (72) constructed a threonine auxotroph of *M. tuberculosis* by deleting *thrC*, the last enzyme in threonine biosynthesis. This mutant could not grow in the absence of threonine and grew slowly even in the presence of threonine. A systematic investigation of this mutant *in vitro* and *in vivo* has yet to be conducted to determine if threonine can be scavenged from the host or if threonine auxotrophy is lethal.

Leucine

Leucine auxotrophy in *M. tuberculosis* is one of the best-described amino acid auxotrophies in mycobacteriology (49). This stems from early studies showing that deletion of *leuD* yielded *M. tuberculosis* that was unable to establish an infection when delivered by aerosol to immunocompetent or immunocompromised mice and that the mutant was cleared quickly from mouse organs when given intravenously (49). Subsequently, a *leuD* strain was proposed as a live attenuated vaccine strain and was continuously improved to make it safer by knocking out two subunits in the leucine biosynthesis pathway (ΔleuC and ΔleuD) and by adding a second auxotrophy for pantothenate (ΔpanCD) (58, 73). Many labs now use this double auxotroph in biosafety level II laboratory conditions.

Isoleucine and valine

The biosynthetic pathways for the branched-chain amino acids isoleucine, valine, and leucine share several enzymes. Deletion of *ilvB1*, encoding the acetohydroxyacid synthase, the key enzyme in branched-chain amino acid biosynthesis, leads to multiple auxotrophies for isoleucine, valine, and leucine (74). Although several potential homologs are encoded in the *M. tuberculosis* genome (IlvB1, IlvB2, IlvG, IlvX), deletion of *ilvB1* led to complete loss of viability and killing in

the absence of the three amino acids *in vitro* (74). Intravenous injection of this mutant into BALB/c mice showed that *M. tuberculosis* Δ*ilvB1* is unable to proliferate in lungs or spleen. However, the strain was not cleared from the organs as has been observed for other auxotrophic *M. tuberculosis* strains (56). The authors concluded that there is potentially a homologous enzyme that is only activated *in vivo* and that can partially complement the loss of IlvB1 during mouse infection.

Tryptophan

The picture emerges that *M. tuberculosis* lacks the ability to take up most essential amino acids from the host. This is supported by the fact that no natural amino acid auxotrophs have been identified to date and that *M. tuberculosis* harbors the biosynthetic machinery for all 20 amino acids. The question remains of which immune mechanisms are responsible for amino acid deprivation in the infected host cells. Does the deprivation simply result from the fact that *M. tuberculosis* resides in a host-derived, nutrient-depleted vacuole, or are there other active amino acid depletion mechanisms at work? A recent publication on tryptophan auxotrophy helped to shed some light on this question (7). The first tryptophan auxotroph was isolated in 1999 by Parish et al. by deleting *trpD* from the *M. tuberculosis* H37Rv genome (48); the deletion was subsequently shown to be bactericidal *in vitro* in the absence of tryptophan supplementation, and the resulting mutant was deficient in growth in SCID mice and THP-1 macrophages (50, 66). Much later, by screening with "TraSH," a method for mapping transposon insertion sites, several tryptophan biosynthetic genes associated with the bacterium's ability to survive in MHC-II class knockout mice were identified (7). These mice are deficient in producing CD4 T cells, and it is well documented that CD4 T cells produce interferon (IFN), which in turn potently stimulates expression of IDO. IDO degrades tryptophan to kynurenine, thereby depleting tryptophan from macrophages and inhibiting the replication of various intracellular pathogens such as *Toxoplasma gondii* and *Chlamydia pneumoniae* (13–15).

The study by Zhang et al. was the first to suggest that tryptophan can be scavenged by *M. tuberculosis* from the host, albeit only when the host IDO degradative pathway is inhibited (7). Apart from arginine depletion by NOS and arginase (60) (see above), this is the only well-characterized immune mechanism that depletes an amino acid. It is interesting to note the difference in phenotype of a *trpD* mutant in the SCID mouse (no growth of Δ*trpD*) compared to results in the MHC-II knockout mouse (growth of Δ*trpD* and Δ*trpE*). Both types of mice should be deficient in producing CD4 T cells and therefore IFN-γ. This discrepancy might argue that upon *M. tuberculosis* infection, SCID mice, which are deficient in mounting an adaptive immune response, still produce IDO. Indeed, it has been shown that IFN-γ is produced in SCID mice, possibly by natural killer cells (75–77). However, it is unclear if and why this mechanism would be absent in MHC-II knockout mice.

Glutamine

Glutamine synthetase (GS) is an integral part of central nitrogen metabolism in bacteria because it assimilates inorganic ammonium by condensation with glutamate to produce glutamine in an ATP-dependent manner. In *M. tuberculosis*, GS is encoded by *glnA1* (78, 79). Three other isoforms of GS are encoded in the *M. tuberculosis* genome (*glnA2*, *glnA3*, and *glnA4*), and all were shown to catalyze glutamine synthase activity *in vitro*, but only GlnA1 is abundantly expressed (78) and essential for bacterial homeostasis.

In addition to its role in bacterial nitrogen metabolism, *M. tuberculosis* GS plays an essential role in cell wall biosynthesis via the production of a poly-L-glutamate-glutamine, a cell wall component exclusively found in pathogenic mycobacteria (80). Interestingly, GS is found in high abundance extracellularly, possibly due to its high expression level and protein stability in the extracellular space (81). Deletion of *glnA1* in *M. tuberculosis* yielded a mutant with no detectable GS protein or GS activity and that was auxotrophic for L-glutamine (79). This glutamine auxotroph was rapidly killed *in vitro* in unsupplemented medium, attenuated for intracellular growth in human THP-1 macrophages, and no bacteria could be recovered from guinea pigs 10 weeks after infection. This argues that glutamine is not available for *M. tuberculosis* in guinea pig lungs. However, Beste and coworkers presented data showing glutamine to be taken up into WT *M. tuberculosis* cells from within macrophages (30). These discrepancies illustrate the knowledge gaps we still face in our understanding of *M. tuberculosis*-host metabolic cross-talk, and it remains to be tested if glutamine can be scavenged during latent infection or in immunocompromised animals. Nevertheless, *M. tuberculosis* GS is being actively pursued as a drug target, and several compounds have shown inhibition and *in vivo* efficacy. It is thought that the extracellular location of the bulk of the enzyme might obviate problems associated with the uptake of compounds across the notoriously impermeable mycobacterial cell wall (82).

Glutamate

Glutamic acid is a central player in nitrogen metabolism in *M. tuberculosis* (83). Emerging evidence in bacteriology suggests that glutamate, glutamine, and alpha-ketoglutarate are the three main metabolites of a metabolic feedback loop that integrates information from carbon and nitrogen metabolism and aids in the control of the carbon-nitrogen ratio in the cell (84). The standard medium for growing *M. tuberculosis*, 7H9, contains ample amounts of glutamate (3.4 mM), indicating a growth-enhancing role of this amino acid for this pathogen. It has been shown that *in vitro*, glutamate is a preferred nitrogen source, because *M. tuberculosis* grows faster on it than with ammonium (85, 86).

Creating a true glutamate auxotroph might be challenging because this amino acid is the substrate or product of many cellular reactions. Glutamine oxoglutarate aminotransferase (GOGAT) is a major glutamate-producing enzyme and is important in the nitrogen-sensing cycle that is regulated by GarA and PknG (87–89). Deletion of *gltBD*, the genes encoding the small and large subunit of GOGAT in *M. bovis* BCG, severely impaired growth of the mutant in ammonium-containing medium but did not completely abrogate it, indicating that other glutamate-producing processes can partially complement the loss of GOGAT function (90). Addition of glutamate, aspartate, and asparagine rescued the mutant to some degree, but only a combination of ammonium and high levels of glutamate brought growth of Δ*gltBD* back to WT levels (90). Both aspartate and asparagine can be converted to glutamate by the bacterium.

The Δ*gltBD* strain was able to grow in bone marrow-derived macrophages, indicating that its partial glutamate auxotrophy is complemented during infection (89). On the contrary, a BCG mutant lacking the major glutamate catabolic enzyme glutamate dehydrogenase (Gdh) was severely attenuated for survival in RAW 264.7 macrophages and growth in bone marrow-derived macrophages (89). *M. bovis* BCG Δ*gdh* was also unable to grow with cholesterol as the sole carbon source (89), indicating that glutamate anaplerosis (glutamate feeds into the TCA cycle via alpha-ketoglutarate) is important during growth on lipids and fatty acids. In fact, an *M. tuberculosis* strain (Δ*pykA*) deficient for growth on fermentable carbon sources was recently shown to be unable to grow on fatty acids unless the medium was supplemented with glutamate (34). However, the *pykA* mutant was not attenuated in a mouse model, suggesting that metabolites such as glutamate or acetate can be scavenged from the host (34). An isotopologue labeling experiment in human THP-1 macrophages suggests *M. tuberculosis*'s ability to scavenge glutamate (30), but proof of glutamate utilization during animal infection is still missing. Constructing Δ*gltBD* and Δ*gdh* in *M. tuberculosis* and testing them in a mouse model could potentially shed some light on *M. tuberculosis*'s ability to scavenge glutamate from the host; however, ultimately, a true glutamate auxotroph has to be constructed to definitively answer this question, an endeavor that may entail the combination of multiple mutations in one strain.

Amino acids for which no auxotrophs have been constructed yet

Out of the 20 amino acids, auxotrophs for alanine, asparagine, aspartate, glycine, phenylalanine, serine, and tyrosine have, to our knowledge, not yet been isolated. Some of these metabolites (e.g., aspartate) are products of many enzymatic reactions, and therefore construction of auxotrophic strains can be challenging. Still, some of the biosynthetic pathways that produce these amino acids are worth looking at as potential drug targets even if multiple enzymes might have to be inhibited to achieve synthetic lethality.

Cofactor auxotrophies

Nicotinamide

M. tuberculosis produces nicotinamide adenine dinucleotide (NAD) by *de novo* biosynthesis but also encodes a functional salvage pathway (54, 91). This pathway allows the bacterium to use exogenous nicotinamide to complement NAD auxotrophy (54, 91). Two studies have investigated NAD auxotrophy in *M. tuberculosis* pathogenesis (54, 91), and both concluded that nicotinamide can be scavenged from the host, thereby allowing strains that are deficient in *de novo* biosynthesis of NAD to grow normally in mice and remain virulent. However, if the last two enzymes in NAD biosynthesis (NadD or NadE) are targeted, *M. tuberculosis* cannot be chemically rescued anymore, because these enzymes are also needed to produce NAD regardless of whether the precursors are made *de novo* or are salvaged (54, 91). *nadE* and *nadD* deletions are bactericidal, and conditional knockdowns cannot grow or survive during any stage of infection (92, 93). This makes NadD and NadE potential drug targets (93), yet the existence of human homologs could potentially complicate the finding of suitable inhibitors. To date, nicotinamide remains one of the few metabolites that have been convincingly shown to be scavenged from the host.

Pantothenate (vitamin B₅)

Pantothenic acid is synthesized in bacteria, plants, and fungi, whereas it is a nutritional requirement in higher animals. This vitamin is a precursor of the essential cofactor coenzyme A (CoA). Sambandamurthy et al. (56) constructed a pantothenate auxotrophic strain of *M. tuberculosis* by deleting *panC* and *panD*, reasoning that such a mutant should be severely impaired in global lipid biosynthesis. This mutant was attenuated in immunocompetent mice, showing a very slow reduction of CFUs in lungs (1 log/250 days) after high-dose intravenous infection. In SCID mice, which lack an adaptive immune response, the *panCD* mutant was able to replicate, albeit at a very slow rate. This is a very interesting observation and indicates that, in the absence of adaptive immunity, *M. tuberculosis* can potentially scavenge pantethine from the host. However, the possibility of a suppressor mutation was not ruled out.

Interestingly, recent work from our laboratory has shown that pantothenate auxotrophy is bacteriostatic for prolonged periods in unsupplemented standard medium, indicating that the consumption of this vitamin is very slow and/or that it can be efficiently recycled (57; M. Berney, unpublished results). Indeed, a *panK* conditional knockdown strain did not show significant attenuation in a mouse infection model even in the absence of inducer, which means that inactivation of pantothenate biosynthesis is not immediately bactericidal and that PanK is not a good drug target (94). Whether the CoA biosynthetic pathway harbors any viable drug targets remains to be assessed. Nevertheless, the *panCD* mutant showed great potential as a vaccine strain because it gave better protection in mice and was safer than BCG (56). Subsequently, a *panCD* deletion was used to create several *M. tuberculosis* strains (Δ*panCD* Δ*lysA*, Δ*panCD* Δ*leuD*, Δ*panCD* Δ*RD1*) that were tested in guinea pigs and non-human primates for their vaccine potential (56, 70, 71, 73, 95). In all these experiments, the auxotrophic strains were safer than BCG and showed protection similar to the current BCG vaccine. From a nutritional point of view, it could be interesting to pursue the slow growth phenotype of Δ*panCD* in SCID mice because it indicates the existence of an immune mechanism that restricts *M. tuberculosis* from accessing dietary pantethine from the host.

Pyridoxamine (vitamin B₆)

M. tuberculosis synthesizes pyridoxal 5-phosphate (PLP), the bioactive form of vitamin B₆, by a bifunctional enzyme complex called PLP synthase, a class I glutamine amidotransferase composed of the synthase domain Pdx1 and the glutaminase domain Pdx2. In mycobacteria, PLP is predicted to be the cofactor of 58 proteins, many of which are predicted to be essential. Pyridoxamine is a vitamer of vitamin B_6 and a supplement in the standard medium of *M. tuberculosis*. Dick and coworkers constructed a *pdx1* knockout strain in *M. tuberculosis* that is a vitamin B_6 auxotroph (52). Chemical complementation was reached at the relatively low concentration of 5 μM pyridoxine (52). Vitamin B_6 auxotrophy was bactericidal in unsupplemented medium under a variety of conditions (exponential growth, stationary phase, hypoxia), albeit at a slow rate compared to other auxotrophs (52). *M. tuberculosis* Δ*pdx1* was unable to establish an infection in immunocompetent mice after aerosol infection, and the mutant was cleared from the lungs after 30 days (52). To our knowledge, the same mutant was not tested in immunocompromised mice; hence, it is unknown if vitamin B_6 is actively withheld from the pathogen by the immune system.

Pdx1 looks like a promising drug target, but an assessment of its essentiality during latent infection (such as by conditional knockdown) and in immunocompromised mice has yet to be conducted. To this end, it is interesting to note that *pdx1* was recently deleted in the vaccine strain *M. bovis* BCG Δ*ureC::hly* to increase safety (96). In mice that received vitamin B_6 supplements, BCG Δ*ureC::hly* Δ*pdx1* exhibited prolonged survival in the draining lymph nodes, but not in spleens (96), which argues that pyridoxine can be scavenged from the host if it is available in high enough concentrations. The authors further concluded that the improved survival of the auxotrophic BCG Δ*ureC::hly* Δ*pdx1* strain, due to administration of vitamin B_6, supported the generation of memory T cells, which persisted after clearance of the vaccine strain (96).

Biotin (vitamin B_7)

Biotin is an essential cofactor for enzymes in metabolic pathways such as fatty acid biosynthesis, anaplerosis, and amino acid metabolism (97). Biotin auxotrophy was the first auxotrophy in *M. tuberculosis* that was shown to be bactericidal during latent infection in mice (51). This was an important milestone because it showed that, even in this putatively more quiescent stage of pathogenesis, auxotrophy could lead to death. Woong Park and coworkers constructed a BioA conditional knockdown strain with a tetracycline-responsive genetic switch to turn on or off the *bioA*-encoded 7,8-diaminopelargonic acid synthase (BioA) (51). This strain allowed BioA expression to be controlled during different stages of infection and demonstrated that *M. tuberculosis* is not able to scavenge biotin from the mouse at any stage of infection (51). Such information is particularly useful for drug target discovery, because new anti-TB drugs should kill both actively growing bacteria and nongrowing, persistent bacteria. This same group and others have already developed some promising lead compounds that inhibit BioA and that are efficacious against *M. tuberculosis* whole cells (98). Using conditional knockdowns, these investigators have developed a new drug screen called the "target-based whole cell screen." The advantage of using a conditional knockdown is that the bacterium can be sensitized to a drug by partially depleting the target enzyme, thereby detecting potential lead scaffolds that might be ignored in traditional, whole-cell drug screens due to their high MICs (98–100).

Folate (vitamin B_9)

Folates are essential cofactors in many one-carbon transfer reactions and are required for the production of purines, pyrimidines, and certain amino acids. The essentiality of reduced folates in cellular metabolism made folate biosynthesis a clinically important target of drugs to treat cancer as well as bacterial (including *M. tuberculosis*), fungal, and parasitic infections. Inhibitors of folate biosynthesis have been studied as TB chemotherapeutics since the discovery in the 1940s that para-aminosalicylic acid (PAS) has antitubercular activity (101–104). Although it was initially believed that the main mechanism of action of PAS is via inhibition of dihydropteroate synthase (DHPS), it was shown recently that PAS acts as a prodrug by poisoning folate-dependent pathways (103). Among the enzymes involved in folate biosynthesis, dihydrofolate reductase has been the target of numerous drug screens (101, 105, 106). Some of these drugs, such as sulfamethoxazole or dapsone, have some efficacy *in vivo*, which argues that folate or its precursors cannot be scavenged from the host in sufficient amounts to relieve the metabolic block. However, in the case of PAS, the exact mode of action is still unknown, and it is suggested that multiple targets are affected by this drug. A genetic approach with auxotrophic strains or conditional knockdowns could shed some light on the availability of folate intermediates in host tissues.

Cobalamin (vitamin B_{12})

To date, it is still unclear if *M. tuberculosis* relies on vitamin B_{12} uptake during pathogenesis. *M. tuberculosis* encodes genes for *de novo* vitamin B_{12} biosynthesis (107), but it has been suggested that the production of this cofactor is hampered or even abrogated due to the absence and mutation of certain genes (108, 109). Based on bioinformatics analyses, it is possible that *M. tuberculosis* produces B_{12}, but a growth condition has yet to be identified where endogenous B_{12} production is induced, and Gopinath and coworkers argue that this induction might only happen *in vivo* (108). Three unrelated B_{12}-dependent enzymes and one B_{12} transporter have been identified in *M. tuberculosis* (108, 109). Investigations into their functions helped in understanding several aspects of B_{12} metabolism in this pathogen.

Growth of *M. tuberculosis* on odd-chain fatty acids or cholesterol as single carbon sources was shown to depend on the detoxification of propionate catabolite accumulation (110–112). This is an important finding because *M. tuberculosis* is believed to rely primarily on a lipid-rich diet *in vivo*, which requires β-oxidation that produces propionyl-CoA as well as acetyl-CoA. Accumulation of toxic propionyl-CoA can be prevented by a functioning methylmalonyl-CoA pathway or methylcitrate cycle (111). The methylmalonyl-CoA pathway is B_{12} dependent, due to methylmalonyl-CoA mutase (MCM) (111), whereas the methylcitrate cycle is B12 independent. Although MCM is not essential for virulence, it is intriguing that *M. tuberculosis* keeps a B_{12}-dependent and a B_{12}-independent mechanism to detoxify propionyl-CoA. This redundancy is also observed in the last step of methionine biosynthesis, where MetH encodes a vitamin B_{12}-dependent methionine synthase and MetE encodes a B_{12}-independent enzyme (113).

Being able to quickly respond to changes in B_{12} availability might highlight the importance of methionine biosynthesis and detoxification of propionyl-CoA for the bacterium. We have shown that inactivation of methionine biosynthesis is extremely lethal to *M. tuberculosis* (57). Controlling methionine and S-adenosylmethionine biosynthesis with such a metabolic switch could argue that B_{12} is a metabolic checkpoint during infection. However, some clinical isolates, for example, *M. tuberculosis* CDC1551, carry an inactive (through truncation or other mutation) version of MetH (113). This strain is susceptible to B_{12} (113), because it inhibits transcription of MetE and, with it, the biosynthesis of the essential amino acid methionine and the cofactor S-adenosylmethionine (57). Since this strain is still virulent, B_{12} obviously does not play a role in its pathogenesis. Still, *M. tuberculosis* encodes a dedicated B_{12} transporter (114), which enables the pathogen to take advantage of B_{12} availability when it might occur.

Other auxotrophies: purine

Two purine auxotrophic strains were constructed and characterized in *M. tuberculosis* and *M. bovis* BCG with the goal to create new live vaccines (115). Deletion of the gene *purC* rendered both strains unable to grow in the absence of hypoxanthine (115). In macrophages, both the *M. tuberculosis* and BCG auxotrophs could not proliferate, but there was a difference in survival (115). Whereas the *M. tuberculosis* Δ*purC* strain persisted, the Δ*purC* mutant of BCG was killed gradually (115). After intravenous injection into BALB/c mice, the *M. tuberculosis* Δ*purC* mutant persisted in lungs, spleens, and livers for about 20 days, after which the CFU burden in all organs started to drop and became undetectable after 60 days (115). The temporary persistence of the *M. tuberculosis purC* mutant in BALB/c mice is most likely due to residual hypoxanthine/purine after growth in supplemented medium before injection. Temporary persistence of an *M. tuberculosis* auxotroph *in vivo* might be a useful trait for a live vaccine because it is thought that persistence of vaccine strains through limited replication *in vivo* generates better protective immunity against *M. tuberculosis* (116). The *purC* mutant was also tested in a guinea pig model to evaluate its protective efficacy against *M. tuberculosis* infection. Protection after subcutaneous vaccination with 10^7 CFU/ml *M. tuberculosis* Δ*purC* was similar to BCG in the lungs, but the *M. tuberculosis* mutant was less protective than BCG in the spleen. Taken together, these data lead to the conclusion that *M. tuberculosis* cannot scavenge purine or hypoxanthine from the host in amounts sufficient for normal growth.

CONCLUSIONS AND FUTURE PERSPECTIVES

Based on the current literature, *M. tuberculosis* has the capacity to take up most amino acids and cofactors *in vitro*. However, this ability to scavenge essential building blocks does not translate to the *in vivo* situation in the presence of intact innate and adaptive immunity. For example, *M. tuberculosis* is predicted to have up to five putative arginine transporters (117), yet an arginine auxotroph is unable to survive in a mouse infection model (55). Moreover, to our knowledge, only one example is known to date where absence of adaptive immunity aids the proliferation of an *M. tuberculosis* auxotroph (tryptophan) (7). This does not necessarily mean that *M. tuberculosis* lacks the ability to take up amino acids from the host, but it argues that not enough metabolites can be scavenged to chemically complement the auxotrophies. It is conceivable that *M. tuberculosis* feeds on a complex host diet whenever it is available but that this happens at concentrations that are orders of magnitude smaller than what is needed to offset an auxotrophy. Nutritional immunity is likely responsible for this phenomenon. In other intracellular pathogens that are naturally amino acid dependent, such as *L. pneumophila* (16), *F. tularensis* (17), and *L. monocytogenes* (18), auxotrophy always comes with a sophisticated virulence mechanism allowing the pathogen to circumvent nutritional immunity by manipulating the host to provide large amounts of the needed growth factor. The human pathogens evolved to access host nutrients by stimulating host protein degradation, manipulation of autophagy, or degradation of complex metabolites such as glutathionine. Such mechanisms have been described as nutritional virulence (19) and are direct reactions to nutritional immunity. These adaptations might also have evolutionary consequences because the loss of genes required for synthesis of an amino acid results in partial dependency on the host, and the bacteria will coevolve with the host (118).

Mycobacterium leprae, a close relative of *M. tuberculosis*, is an extreme example of genome reduction (119). Its metabolism is so much adapted to the host that it cannot be cultured axenically. Indeed, genetic links between new metabolic capacities and virulence factors illustrate that metabolic pathways are acquired as part of a pathogen's evolution toward colonizing new niches with new food sources (120). Such mechanisms are, to date, unknown in *M. tuberculosis*, and it will be interesting to see if any of the five type VII secretion systems present in the *M. tuberculosis* genome (ESX-1 to ESX-5) (121) are involved in nutrient acquisition. To this end, the ESX-3 gene products were proposed to be involved in iron acquisition (122), and ESX-1 is involved in phagosomal escape, potentially giving access to cytosolic nutrients. The phagosomal milieu is generally inherently nonpermissive for bacterial growth in comparison to the cytosol (123). For example, *L. monocytogenes*, which is naturally auxotrophic for several amino acids and vitamins (124), replicates within the cytoplasm, but hemolysin-negative mutants, which are unable to escape from the phagosome, do not grow (125). However, although the cytosol is believed to be amino acid replete, it is questionable if the nutrient abundance is enough to allow considerable replication of pathogens. According to Abu Kwaik and Bumann (126), extensive proliferation based on host-derived amino acids and energy sources is only possible if nutrients are replenished through active transport into the phagocytes.

The amino acid and cofactor independence of *M. tuberculosis* allows this bacterium to dwell on a minimal diet of carbon, nitrogen, and trace elements in the host. Intracellular pathogens compete with the host cell for the same nutrient pools, and hence, a strategy of using a minimal amount of host metabolites means not leaving a trail, thereby potentially gaining more time for proliferation as an unrecognized intruder. This feature might also be connected to *M. tuberculosis*'s ultra-slow growth rate. Slow growth allows *M. tuberculosis* to preferentially use lipids as carbon and energy sources while making the whole set of essential amino acids by itself. It is intriguing to note that most intracellular pathogens that are natural auxotrophs grow considerably faster in the host. For example, *F. tularensis* divides every 3 hours in human alveolar macrophages (129), *L. pneumophila* every 2 hours (130), and *L. monocytogenes* doubles in less than an hour (131); in contrast, the maximum specific growth rate of *M. tuberculosis* in the same type of macrophage is 24 hours. Faster growth means higher energetic needs, and amino acid and cofactor biosyntheses are energetically expensive processes, so uptake of the finished building blocks can be a huge energetic advantage. This is reflected in the slower growth rate of bacteria when growing on minimal medium compared to a rich medium that contains many building blocks. For example, the doubling time of *E. coli* triples from 20 minutes in Luria broth to 1 hour on minimal medium (127). Fast proliferation, though, also means the need for fast replenishment of those nutrients, which many intracellular pathogens achieve by manipulating the host to provide more of the precious food. In contrast, it seems as if the intracellular lifestyle of *M. tuberculosis* is more focused on remaining as metabolically quiet as possible, thereby subverting many potential assaults by the immune system. Collectively, the literature reviewed here suggests that nutritional independence from the host is an important virulence mechanism of *M. tuberculosis* that holds great promise for new drug target discovery.

Several new studies show that amino acid and cofactor auxotrophy in *M. tuberculosis* can be bactericidal and lead to rapid killing *in vitro* and *in vivo* (7, 57, 92), which leads to the conclusion that unbalanced growth/metabolism is a bactericidal event that should be considered for drug target discovery. Intriguingly, Parish (66) showed that killing of *M. tuberculosis* auxotrophs was very slow in a general starvation medium such as phosphate-buffered saline but more rapid in unsupplemented medium (medium that only lacks a particular nutrient). This phenomenon is called "unbalanced growth" and was first discussed in a paper by Cohen and Barner published in 1954 on thymine-less death in *E. coli* (128). The authors state, "The induction of unbalanced growth in this case [i.e., thymine auxotroph in thymine-depleted medium] leads to death; the inhibition of all growth, as a result of the omission of many metabolites, permits survival." In fact, most, if not all, antibiotics on the market kill replicating cells much more efficiently than nonreplicating cells.

These considerations also lead to the question of whether complete starvation (e.g., using water or phosphate-buffered saline) is a good model of the *in vivo* environment of *M. tuberculosis*. Mouse experiments with several amino acid auxotrophs show clearance of *M. tuberculosis* from lungs, spleens, and liver whether infected by aerosol or intravenously (49, 53). Hence, the current data clearly argue that the *in vivo* nutritional environment is more akin to unsupplemented medium (possibly due to the constant availability of a carbon source) and is not perceived by the pathogen as complete starvation. However, this still has to be systematically investigated because the lethality of inactivating amino acid biosynthesis has not been shown during the latent phase of infection. The natural route of *M. tuberculosis* infection is via aerosol into the lungs, and most auxotrophs examined so far were unable to proliferate in the lung and therefore could not establish a latent infection. With the latest genetic tools for mycobacteria, conditional knockdowns, we can now examine auxotrophies during different stages of infection, e.g., active and latent, as has been nicely shown for three auxotrophs so far: a biotin auxotroph, a nicotinamide auxotroph, and a methionine auxotroph (M. Berney, unpublished data). Using this technology in a systematic fashion will allow us to learn about new mechanisms of nutritional immunity in TB pathogenesis.

The ultimate goal of this research must be to defeat the TB disease. *M. tuberculosis*'s strong dependence on its own amino acid and coenzyme biosynthesis machinery allows it to be independent from the host, stay metabolically flexible, and keep a low profile during infection. At the same time, the absence of virulence mechanisms to acquire large amounts of host amino acids and cofactors makes the biosynthetic machinery an attractive vulnerability for drug targeting. Inhibition of biosynthetic pathways holds great promise for discovering new drug targets because it seems that *M. tuberculosis* finds itself in an amino acid- and cofactor-deprived environment in the host. However, not all biosynthetic pathways are suitable for targeting. For example, some amino acids, such as alanine and gluta-

mate, can be produced by multiple enzymes, which makes the search for suitable inhibitors more difficult. Much work is ahead of us to identify the right pathways and the right enzymes that lead to rapid killing and that, most importantly, are going to be amenable to drug targeting.

Citation. Berney M, Berney-Meyer L. 2017. *Mycobacterium tuberculosis* in the face of host-imposed nutrient limitation. Microbiol Spectrum 5(3):TBTB2-0030-2016.

References

1. Chaston J, Goodrich-Blair H. 2010. Common trends in mutualism revealed by model associations between invertebrates and bacteria. *FEMS Microbiol Rev* 34:41–58.
2. Cambier CJ, Falkow S, Ramakrishnan L. 2014. Host evasion and exploitation schemes of *Mycobacterium tuberculosis*. *Cell* 159:1497–1509.
3. Eisenreich W, Heesemann J, Rudel T, Goebel W. 2013. Metabolic host responses to infection by intracellular bacterial pathogens. *Front Cell Infect Microbiol* 3:24.
4. Zhang YJ, Rubin EJ. 2013. Feast or famine: the host-pathogen battle over amino acids. *Cell Microbiol* 15:1079–1087.
5. Appelberg R. 2006. Macrophage nutriprive antimicrobial mechanisms. *J Leukoc Biol* 79:1117–1128.
6. Hood MI, Skaar EP. 2012. Nutritional immunity: transition metals at the pathogen-host interface. *Nat Rev Microbiol* 10:525–537.
7. Zhang YJ, Reddy MC, Ioerger TR, Rothchild AC, Dartois V, Schuster BM, Trauner A, Wallis D, Galaviz S, Huttenhower C, Sacchettini JC, Behar SM, Rubin EJ. 2013. Tryptophan biosynthesis protects mycobacteria from CD4 T-cell-mediated killing. *Cell* 155:1296–1308.
8. Barber MF, Elde NC. 2014. Escape from bacterial iron piracy through rapid evolution of transferrin. *Science* 346:1362–1366.
9. Kehl-Fie TE, Skaar EP. 2010. Nutritional immunity beyond iron: a role for manganese and zinc. *Curr Opin Chem Biol* 14:218–224.
10. MacMicking JD. 2014. Cell-autonomous effector mechanisms against mycobacterium tuberculosis. *Cold Spring Harb Perspect Med* 4:a018507.
11. Michelucci A, Cordes T, Ghelfi J, Pailot A, Reiling N, Goldmann O, Binz T, Wegner A, Tallam A, Rausell A, Buttini M, Linster CL, Medina E, Balling R, Hiller K. 2013. Immune-responsive gene 1 protein links metabolism to immunity by catalyzing itaconic acid production. *Proc Natl Acad Sci USA* 110:7820–7825.
12. Tattoli I, Sorbara MT, Vuckovic D, Ling A, Soares F, Carneiro LA, Yang C, Emili A, Philpott DJ, Girardin SE. 2012. Amino acid starvation induced by invasive bacterial pathogens triggers an innate host defense program. *Cell Host Microbe* 11:563–575.
13. Silva NM, Rodrigues CV, Santoro MM, Reis LF, Alvarez-Leite JI, Gazzinelli RT. 2002. Expression of

indoleamine 2,3-dioxygenase, tryptophan degradation, and kynurenine formation during *in vivo* infection with *Toxoplasma gondii*: induction by endogenous gamma interferon and requirement of interferon regulatory factor 1. *Infect Immun* **70:**859–868.

14. **Fujigaki S, Saito K, Takemura M, Maekawa N, Yamada Y, Wada H, Seishima M.** 2002. L-tryptophan-L-kynurenine pathway metabolism accelerated by *Toxoplasma gondii* infection is abolished in gamma interferon-gene-deficient mice: cross-regulation between inducible nitric oxide synthase and indoleamine-2,3-dioxygenase. *Infect Immun* **70:**779–786.

15. **Rottenberg ME, Gigliotti Rothfuchs A, Gigliotti D, Ceausu M, Une C, Levitsky V, Wigzell H.** 2000. Regulation and role of IFN-gamma in the innate resistance to infection with *Chlamydia pneumoniae*. *J Immunol* **164:**4812–4818.

16. **Price CT, Richards AM, Von Dwingelo JE, Samara HA, Abu Kwaik Y.** 2014. Amoeba host-*Legionella* synchronization of amino acid auxotrophy and its role in bacterial adaptation and pathogenic evolution. *Environ Microbiol* **16:**330–338.

17. **Meibom KL, Charbit A.** 2010. *Francisella tularensis* metabolism and its relation to virulence. *Front Microbiol* **1:**140.

18. **Schneebeli R, Egli T.** 2013. A defined, glucose-limited mineral medium for the cultivation of *Listeria* spp. *Appl Environ Microbiol* **79:**2503–2511.

19. **Abu Kwaik Y, Bumann D.** 2013. Microbial quest for food *in vivo*: 'nutritional virulence' as an emerging paradigm. *Cell Microbiol* **15:**882–890.

20. **Flynn JL, Chan J, Lin PL.** 2011. Macrophages and control of granulomatous inflammation in tuberculosis. *Mucosal Immunol* **4:**271–278.

21. **Comas I, Coscolla M, Luo T, Borrell S, Holt KE, Kato-Maeda M, Parkhill J, Malla B, Berg S, Thwaites G, Yeboah-Manu D, Bothamley G, Mei J, Wei L, Bentley S, Harris SR, Niemann S, Diel R, Aseffa A, Gao Q, Young D, Gagneux S.** 2013. Out-of-Africa migration and Neolithic coexpansion of *Mycobacterium tuberculosis* with modern humans. *Nat Genet* **45:**1176–1182.

22. **Cambier CJ, Takaki KK, Larson RP, Hernandez RE, Tobin DM, Urdahl KB, Cosma CL, Ramakrishnan L.** 2014. Mycobacteria manipulate macrophage recruitment through coordinated use of membrane lipids. *Nature* **505:**218–222.

23. **van der Wel N, Hava D, Houben D, Fluitsma D, van Zon M, Pierson J, Brenner M, Peters PJ.** 2007. *M. tuberculosis* and *M. leprae* translocate from the phagolysosome to the cytosol in myeloid cells. *Cell* **129:**1287–1298.

24. **Davis JM, Ramakrishnan L.** 2009. The role of the granuloma in expansion and dissemination of early tuberculous infection. *Cell* **136:**37–49.

25. **Clay H, Davis JM, Beery D, Huttenlocher A, Lyons SE, Ramakrishnan L.** 2007. Dichotomous role of the macrophage in early *Mycobacterium marinum* infection of the zebrafish. *Cell Host Microbe* **2:**29–39.

26. **Fortune SM, Rubin EJ.** 2007. The complex relationship between mycobacteria and macrophages: it's not all bliss. *Cell Host Microbe* **2:**5–6.

27. **Eisenreich W, Dandekar T, Heesemann J, Goebel W.** 2010. Carbon metabolism of intracellular bacterial pathogens and possible links to virulence. *Nat Rev Microbiol* **8:**401–412.

28. **Fuchs TM, Eisenreich W, Heesemann J, Goebel W.** 2012. Metabolic adaptation of human pathogenic and related nonpathogenic bacteria to extra- and intracellular habitats. *FEMS Microbiol Rev* **36:**433–462.

29. **Cheng J, Che N, Li H, Ma K, Wu S, Fang J, Rong Gao JL, Yan X, Fangting CL, Dong F.** 2013. Gas chromatography time-of-flight mass-spectrometry-based metabolomic analysis of human macrophages infected by *M. tuberculosis*. *Anal Lett* **46:**1922–1936.

30. **Beste DJ, Nöh K, Niedenführ S, Mendum TA, Hawkins ND, Ward JL, Beale MH, Wiechert W, McFadden J.** 2013. 13C-flux spectral analysis of host-pathogen metabolism reveals a mixed diet for intracellular *Mycobacterium tuberculosis*. *Chem Biol* **20:**1012–1021.

31. **Gouzy A, Larrouy-Maumus G, Bottai D, Levillain F, Dumas A, Wallach JB, Caire-Brandli I, de Chastellier C, Wu TD, Poincloux R, Brosch R, Guerquin-Kern JL, Schnappinger D, Sório de Carvalho LP, Poquet Y, Neyrolles O.** 2014. *Mycobacterium tuberculosis* exploits asparagine to assimilate nitrogen and resist acid stress during infection. *PLoS Pathog* **10:**e1003928.

32. **Gouzy A, Larrouy-Maumus G, Wu TD, Peixoto A, Levillain F, Lugo-Villarino G, Guerquin-Kern JL, de Carvalho LP, Poquet Y, Neyrolles O.** 2013. *Mycobacterium tuberculosis* nitrogen assimilation and host colonization require aspartate. *Nat Chem Biol* **9:**674–676.

33. **de Carvalho LP, Fischer SM, Marrero J, Nathan C, Ehrt S, Rhee KY.** 2010. Metabolomics of *Mycobacterium tuberculosis* reveals compartmentalized co-catabolism of carbon substrates. *Chem Biol* **17:**1122–1131.

34. **Noy T, Vergnolle O, Hartman TE, Rhee KY, Jacobs WR Jr, Berney M, Blanchard JS.** 2016. Central role of pyruvate kinase in carbon co-catabolism of *Mycobacterium tuberculosis*. *J Biol Chem* **291:**7060–7069.

35. **Mehrotra P, Jamwal SV, Saquib N, Sinha N, Siddiqui Z, Manivel V, Chatterjee S, Rao KV.** 2014. Pathogenicity of *Mycobacterium tuberculosis* is expressed by regulating metabolic thresholds of the host macrophage. *PLoS Pathog* **10:**e1004265.

36. **Watrous JD, Dorrestein PC.** 2011. Imaging mass spectrometry in microbiology. *Nat Rev Microbiol* **9:**683–694.

37. **Marakalala MJ, Raju RM, Sharma K, Zhang YJ, Eugenin EA, Prideaux B, Daudelin IB, Chen PY, Booty MG, Kim JH, Eum SY, Via LE, Behar SM, Barry CE III, Mann M, Dartois V, Rubin EJ.** 2016. Inflammatory signaling in human tuberculosis granulomas is spatially organized. *Nat Med* **22:**531–538.

38. **Prideaux B, Via LE, Zimmerman MD, Eum S, Sarathy J, O'Brien P, Chen C, Kaya F, Weiner DM, Chen PY, Song T, Lee M, Shim TS, Cho JS, Kim W, Cho SN, Olivier KN, Barry CE III, Dartois V.** 2015. The association between sterilizing activity and drug distribution into tuberculosis lesions. *Nat Med* **21:**1223–1227.

39. **Fletcher JS, Kotze HL, Armitage EG, Lockyer NP, Vickerman JC.** 2013. Evaluating the challenges associated with time-of-flight secondary ion mass spectrometry for

metabolomics using pure and mixed metabolites. *Metabolomics* 9:533–544.

40. Shin JH, Yang JY, Jeon BY, Yoon YJ, Cho SN, Kang YH, Ryu DH, Hwang GS. 2011. (1)H NMR-based metabolomic profiling in mice infected with *Mycobacterium tuberculosis*. *J Proteome Res* 10:2238–2247.

41. Somashekar BS, Amin AG, Rithner CD, Troudt J, Basaraba R, Izzo A, Crick DC, Chatterjee D. 2011. Metabolic profiling of lung granuloma in *Mycobacterium tuberculosis* infected guinea pigs: *ex vivo* 1H magic angle spinning NMR studies. *J Proteome Res* 10: 4186–4195.

42. Lederberg J, Tatum EL. 1953. Sex in bacteria; genetic studies, 1945–1952. *Science* 118:169–175.

43. Lederberg J, Tatum EL. 1946. Gene recombination in *Escherichia coli*. *Nature* 158:558.

44. Lederberg J, Tatum EL. 1946. Detection of biochemical mutants of microorganisms. *J Biol Chem* 165:381.

45. Tatum EL, Lederberg J. 1947. Gene recombination in the bacterium *Escherichia coli*. *J Bacteriol* 53:673–684.

46. Davis BD. 1950. Nonfiltrability of the agents of genetic recombination in *Escherichia coli*. *J Bacteriol* 60:507–508.

47. McAdam RA, Weisbrod TR, Martin J, Scuderi JD, Brown AM, Cirillo JD, Bloom BR, Jacobs WR Jr. 1995. *In vivo* growth characteristics of leucine and methionine auxotrophic mutants of *Mycobacterium bovis* BCG generated by transposon mutagenesis. *Infect Immun* 63: 1004–1012.

48. Parish T, Gordhan BG, McAdam RA, Duncan K, Mizrahi V, Stoker NG. 1999. Production of mutants in amino acid biosynthesis genes of *Mycobacterium tuberculosis* by homologous recombination. *Microbiology* 145:3497–3303.

49. Hondalus MK, Bardarov S, Russell R, Chan J, Jacobs WR Jr, Bloom BR. 2000. Attenuation of and protection induced by a leucine auxotroph of *Mycobacterium tuberculosis*. *Infect Immun* 68:2888–2898.

50. Smith DA, Parish T, Stoker NG, Bancroft GJ. 2001. Characterization of auxotrophic mutants of *Mycobacterium tuberculosis* and their potential as vaccine candidates. *Infect Immun* 69:1142–1150.

51. Woong Park S, Klotzsche M, Wilson DJ, Boshoff HI, Eoh H, Manjunatha U, Blumenthal A, Rhee K, Barry CE III, Aldrich CC, Ehrt S, Schnappinger D. 2011. Evaluating the sensitivity of *Mycobacterium tuberculosis* to biotin deprivation using regulated gene expression. *PLoS Pathog* 7:e1002264.

52. Dick T, Manjunatha U, Kappes B, Gengenbacher M. 2010. Vitamin B6 biosynthesis is essential for survival and virulence of *Mycobacterium tuberculosis*. *Mol Microbiol* 78:980–988.

53. Pavelka MS Jr, Chen B, Kelley CL, Collins FM, Jacobs WR Jr. 2003. Vaccine efficacy of a lysine auxotroph of *Mycobacterium tuberculosis*. *Infect Immun* 71:4190–4192.

54. Vilchèze C, Weinrick B, Wong KW, Chen B, Jacobs WR Jr. 2010. NAD+ auxotrophy is bacteriocidal for the tubercle bacilli. *Mol Microbiol* 76:365–377.

55. Gordhan BG, Smith DA, Alderton H, McAdam RA, Bancroft GJ, Mizrahi V. 2002. Construction and phenotypic characterization of an auxotrophic mutant of *Mycobacterium tuberculosis* defective in L-arginine biosynthesis. *Infect Immun* 70:3080–3084.

56. Sambandamurthy VK, Wang X, Chen B, Russell RG, Derrick S, Collins FM, Morris SL, Jacobs WR Jr. 2002. A pantothenate auxotroph of *Mycobacterium tuberculosis* is highly attenuated and protects mice against tuberculosis. *Nat Med* 8:1171–1174.

57. Berney M, Berney-Meyer L, Wong KW, Chen B, Chen M, Kim J, Wang J, Harris D, Parkhill J, Chan J, Wang F, Jacobs WR Jr. 2015. Essential roles of methionine and S-adenosylmethionine in the autarkic lifestyle of *Mycobacterium tuberculosis*. *Proc Natl Acad Sci USA* 112: 10008–10013.

58. Jain P, Hsu T, Arai M, Biermann K, Thaler DS, Nguyen A, González PA, Tufariello JM, Kriakov J, Chen B, Larsen MH, Jacobs WR Jr. 2014. Specialized transduction designed for precise high-throughput unmarked deletions in *Mycobacterium tuberculosis*. *MBio* 5: e01245-14

59. Thompson RW, Pesce JT, Ramalingam T, Wilson MS, White S, Cheever AW, Ricklefs SM, Porcella SF, Li L, Ellies LG, Wynn TA. 2008. Cationic amino acid transporter-2 regulates immunity by modulating arginase activity. *PLoS Pathog* 4:e1000023.

60. Murray PJ. 2016. Amino acid auxotrophy as a system of immunological control nodes. *Nat Immunol* 17: 132–139.

61. Qualls JE, Murray PJ. 2016. Immunometabolism within the tuberculosis granuloma: amino acids, hypoxia, and cellular respiration. *Semin Immunopathol* 38:139–152.

62. El Kasmi KC, Qualls JE, Pesce JT, Smith AM, Thompson RW, Henao-Tamayo M, Basaraba RJ, König T, Schleicher U, Koo MS, Kaplan G, Fitzgerald KA, Tuomanen EI, Orme IM, Kanneganti TD, Bogdan C, Wynn TA, Murray PJ. 2008. Toll-like receptor-induced arginase 1 in macrophages thwarts effective immunity against intracellular pathogens. *Nat Immunol* 9:1399–1406.

63. Senaratne RH, De Silva AD, Williams SJ, Mougous JD, Reader JR, Zhang T, Chan S, Sidders B, Lee DH, Chan J, Bertozzi CR, Riley LW. 2006. 5′-Adenosinephosphosulphate reductase (CysH) protects *Mycobacterium tuberculosis* against free radicals during chronic infection phase in mice. *Mol Microbiol* 59: 1744–1753.

64. Wooff E, Michell SL, Gordon SV, Chambers MA, Bardarov S, Jacobs WR Jr, Hewinson RG, Wheeler PR. 2002. Functional genomics reveals the sole sulphate transporter of the *Mycobacterium tuberculosis* complex and its relevance to the acquisition of sulphur *in vivo*. *Mol Microbiol* 43:653–663.

65. Hwang BJ, Yeom HJ, Kim Y, Lee HS. 2002. *Corynebacterium glutamicum* utilizes both transsulfuration and direct sulfhydrylation pathways for methionine biosynthesis. *J Bacteriol* 184:1277–1286.

66. Parish T. 2003. Starvation survival response of *Mycobacterium tuberculosis*. *J Bacteriol* 185:6702–6706.

67. Berney M, Weimar MR, Heikal A, Cook GM. 2012. Regulation of proline metabolism in mycobacteria and its role in carbon metabolism under hypoxia. *Mol Microbiol* **84:**664–681.

68. Lagautriere T, Bashiri G, Paterson NG, Berney M, Cook GM, Baker EN. 2014. Characterization of the proline-utilization pathway in *Mycobacterium tuberculosis* through structural and functional studies. *Acta Crystallogr D Biol Crystallogr* **70:**968–980.

69. Pavelka MS Jr, Jacobs WR Jr. 1999. Comparison of the construction of unmarked deletion mutations in *Mycobacterium smegmatis*, *Mycobacterium bovis* bacillus Calmette-Guérin, and *Mycobacterium tuberculosis* H37Rv by allelic exchange. *J Bacteriol* **181:**4780–4789.

70. Sambandamurthy VK, Derrick SC, Jalapathy KV, Chen B, Russell RG, Morris SL, Jacobs WR Jr. 2005. Long-term protection against tuberculosis following vaccination with a severely attenuated double lysine and pantothenate auxotroph of *Mycobacterium tuberculosis*. *Infect Immun* **73:**1196–1203.

71. Larsen MH, Biermann K, Chen B, Hsu T, Sambandamurthy VK, Lackner AA, Aye PP, Didier P, Huang D, Shao L, Wei H, Letvin NL, Frothingham R, Haynes BF, Chen ZW, Jacobs WR Jr. 2009. Efficacy and safety of live attenuated persistent and rapidly cleared *Mycobacterium tuberculosis* vaccine candidates in non-human primates. *Vaccine* **27:**4709–4717.

72. Covarrubias AS, Högbom M, Bergfors T, Carroll P, Mannerstedt K, Oscarson S, Parish T, Jones TA, Mowbray SL. 2008. Structural, biochemical, and *in vivo* investigations of the threonine synthase from *Mycobacterium tuberculosis*. *J Mol Biol* **381:**622–633.

73. Sampson SL, Dascher CC, Sambandamurthy VK, Russell RG, Jacobs WR Jr, Bloom BR, Hondalus MK. 2004. Protection elicited by a double leucine and pantothenate auxotroph of *Mycobacterium tuberculosis* in guinea pigs. *Infect Immun* **72:**3031–3037.

74. Awasthy D, Gaonkar S, Shandil RK, Yadav R, Bharath S, Marcel N, Subbulakshmi V, Sharma U. 2009. Inactivation of the ilvB1 gene in *Mycobacterium tuberculosis* leads to branched-chain amino acid auxotrophy and attenuation of virulence in mice. *Microbiology* **155:**2978–2987.

75. Wherry JC, Schreiber RD, Unanue ER. 1991. Regulation of gamma interferon production by natural killer cells in scid mice: roles of tumor necrosis factor and bacterial stimuli. *Infect Immun* **59:**1709–1715.

76. Hayward AR, Chmura K, Cosyns M. 2000. Interferon-gamma is required for innate immunity to *Cryptosporidium parvum* in mice. *J Infect Dis* **182:**1001–1004.

77. Bell LV, Else KJ. 2011. Regulation of colonic epithelial cell turnover by IDO contributes to the innate susceptibility of SCID mice to *Trichuris muris* infection. *Parasite Immunol* **33:**244–249.

78. Harth G, Maslesa-Galić S, Tullius MV, Horwitz MA. 2005. All four *Mycobacterium tuberculosis* glnA genes encode glutamine synthetase activities but only GlnA1 is abundantly expressed and essential for bacterial homeostasis. *Mol Microbiol* **58:**1157–1172.

79. Tullius MV, Harth G, Horwitz MA. 2003. Glutamine synthetase GlnA1 is essential for growth of *Mycobacterium tuberculosis* in human THP-1 macrophages and guinea pigs. *Infect Immun* **71:**3927–3936.

80. Harth G, Horwitz MA. 2003. Inhibition of *Mycobacterium tuberculosis* glutamine synthetase as a novel antibiotic strategy against tuberculosis: demonstration of efficacy *in vivo*. *Infect Immun* **71:**456–464.

81. Tullius MV, Harth G, Horwitz MA. 2001. High extracellular levels of *Mycobacterium tuberculosis* glutamine synthetase and superoxide dismutase in actively growing cultures are due to high expression and extracellular stability rather than to a protein-specific export mechanism. *Infect Immun* **69:**6348–6363.

82. Mowbray SL, Kathiravan MK, Pandey AA, Odell LR. 2014. Inhibition of glutamine synthetase: a potential drug target in *Mycobacterium tuberculosis*. *Molecules* **19:**13161–13176.

83. Gouzy A, Poquet Y, Neyrolles O. 2014. Nitrogen metabolism in *Mycobacterium tuberculosis* physiology and virulence. *Nat Rev Microbiol* **12:**729–737.

84. Doucette CD, Schwab DJ, Wingreen NS, Rabinowitz JD. 2011. α-Ketoglutarate coordinates carbon and nitrogen utilization via enzyme I inhibition. *Nat Chem Biol* **7:**894–901.

85. Lyon RH, Hall WH, Costas-Martinez C. 1970. Utilization of amino acids during growth of *Mycobacterium tuberculosis* in rotary cultures. *Infect Immun* **1:**513–520.

86. Song H, Niederweis M. 2012. Uptake of sulfate but not phosphate by *Mycobacterium tuberculosis* is slower than that for *Mycobacterium smegmatis*. *J Bacteriol* **194:**956–964.

87. Cowley S, Ko M, Pick N, Chow R, Downing KJ, Gordhan BG, Betts JC, Mizrahi V, Smith DA, Stokes RW, Av-Gay Y. 2004. The *Mycobacterium tuberculosis* protein serine/threonine kinase PknG is linked to cellular glutamate/glutamine levels and is important for growth *in vivo*. *Mol Microbiol* **52:**1691–1702.

88. Ventura M, Rieck B, Boldrin F, Degiacomi G, Bellinzoni M, Barilone N, Alzaidi F, Alzari PM, Manganelli R, O'Hare HM. 2013. GarA is an essential regulator of metabolism in *Mycobacterium tuberculosis*. *Mol Microbiol* **90:**336–366.

89. Gallant JL, Viljoen AJ, van Helden PD, Wiid IJ. 2016. Glutamate dehydrogenase is required by *Mycobacterium bovis* BCG for resistance to cellular stress. *PLoS One* **11:**e0147706.

90. Viljoen AJ, Kirsten CJ, Baker B, van Helden PD, Wiid IJ. 2013. The role of glutamine oxoglutarate aminotransferase and glutamate dehydrogenase in nitrogen metabolism in *Mycobacterium bovis* BCG. *PLoS One* **8:**e84452.

91. Boshoff HI, Xu X, Tahlan K, Dowd CS, Pethe K, Camacho LR, Park TH, Yun CS, Schnappinger D, Ehrt S, Williams KJ, Barry CE III. 2008. Biosynthesis and recycling of nicotinamide cofactors in *Mycobacterium tuberculosis*. An essential role for NAD in nonreplicating bacilli. *J Biol Chem* **283:**19329–19341.

92. Kim JH, O'Brien KM, Sharma R, Boshoff HI, Rehren G, Chakraborty S, Wallach JB, Monteleone M, Wilson

DJ, Aldrich CC, Barry CE III, Rhee KY, Ehrt S, Schnappinger D. 2013. A genetic strategy to identify targets for the development of drugs that prevent bacterial persistence. *Proc Natl Acad Sci USA* 110:19095–19100.

93. Rodionova IA, Schuster BM, Guinn KM, Sorci L, Scott DA, Li X, Kheterpal I, Shoen C, Cynamon M, Locher C, Rubin EJ, Osterman AL. 2014. Metabolic and bactericidal effects of targeted suppression of NadD and NadE enzymes in mycobacteria. *MBio* 5:e00747-13.

94. Reddy BK, Landge S, Ravishankar S, Patil V, Shinde V, Tantry S, Kale M, Raichurkar A, Menasinakai S, Mudugal NV, Ambady A, Ghosh A, Tunduguru R, Kaur P, Singh R, Kumar N, Bharath S, Sundaram A, Bhat J, Sambandamurthy VK, Björkelid C, Jones TA, Das K, Bandodkar B, Malolanarasimhan K, Mukherjee K, Ramachandran V. 2014. Assessment of *Mycobacterium tuberculosis* pantothenate kinase vulnerability through target knockdown and mechanistically diverse inhibitors. *Antimicrob Agents Chemother* 58:3312–3326.

95. Sambandamurthy VK, Jacobs WR Jr. 2005. Live attenuated mutants of *Mycobacterium tuberculosis* as candidate vaccines against tuberculosis. *Microbes Infect* 7:955–961.

96. Gengenbacher M, Vogelzang A, Schuerer S, Lazar D, Kaiser P, Kaufmann SH. 2014. Dietary pyridoxine controls efficacy of vitamin B6-auxotrophic tuberculosis vaccine bacillus Calmette-Guérin ΔureC:hly Δpdx1 in mice. *MBio* 5:e01262-14.

97. Salaemae W, Booker GW, Polyak SW. 2016. The role of biotin in bacterial physiology and virulence: a novel antibiotic target for *Mycobacterium tuberculosis*. *Microbiol Spectr* 4:VMBF-0008-2015.

98. Park SW, Casalena DE, Wilson DJ, Dai R, Nag PP, Liu F, Boyce JP, Bittker JA, Schreiber SL, Finzel BC, Schnappinger D, Aldrich CC. 2015. Target-based identification of whole-cell active inhibitors of biotin biosynthesis in *Mycobacterium tuberculosis*. *Chem Biol* 22:76–86.

99. Kana BD, Karakousis PC, Parish T, Dick T. 2014. Future target-based drug discovery for tuberculosis? *Tuberculosis (Edinb)* 94:551–556.

100. Gengenbacher M, Dick T. 2015. Antibacterial drug discovery: doing it right. *Chem Biol* 22:5–6.

101. Nixon MR, Saionz KW, Koo MS, Szymonifka MJ, Jung H, Roberts JP, Nandakumar M, Kumar A, Liao R, Rustad T, Sacchettini JC, Rhee KY, Freundlich JS, Sherman DR. 2014. Folate pathway disruption leads to critical disruption of methionine derivatives in *Mycobacterium tuberculosis*. *Chem Biol* 21:819–830.

102. Minato Y, Thiede JM, Kordus SL, McKlveen EJ, Turman BJ, Baughn AD. 2015. *Mycobacterium tuberculosis* folate metabolism and the mechanistic basis for para-aminosalicylic acid susceptibility and resistance. *Antimicrob Agents Chemother* 59:5097–5106.

103. Chakraborty S, Gruber T, Barry CE III, Boshoff HI, Rhee KY. 2013. Para-aminosalicylic acid acts as an alternative substrate of folate metabolism in *Mycobacterium tuberculosis*. *Science* 339:88–91.

104. Lehmann J. 1946. Para-aminosalicylic acid in the treatment of tuberculosis. *Lancet* 247:15–16.

105. Kumar A, Zhang M, Zhu L, Liao RP, Mutai C, Hafsat S, Sherman DR, Wang MW. 2012. High-throughput screening and sensitized bacteria identify an *M. tuberculosis* dihydrofolate reductase inhibitor with whole cell activity. *PLoS One* 7:e39961.

106. Kumar A, Guardia A, Colmenarejo G, Pérez E, Gonzalez RR, Torres P, Calvo D, Gómez RM, Ortega F, Jiménez E, Gabarro RC, Rullás J, Ballell L, Sherman DR. 2015. A focused screen identifies antifolates with activity on *Mycobacterium tuberculosis*. *ACS Infect Dis* 1:604–614.

107. Cole ST, Brosch R, Parkhill J, Garnier T, Churcher C, Harris D, Gordon SV, Eiglmeier K, Gas S, Barry CE III, Tekaia F, Badcock K, Basham D, Brown D, Chillingworth T, Connor R, Davies R, Devlin K, Feltwell T, Gentles S, Hamlin N, Holroyd S, Hornsby T, Jagels K, Krogh A, McLean J, Moule S, Murphy L, Oliver K, Osborne J, Quail MA, Rajandream MA, Rogers J, Rutter S, Seeger K, Skelton J, Squares R, Squares S, Sulston JE, Taylor K, Whitehead S, Barrell BG. 1998. Deciphering the biology of *Mycobacterium tuberculosis* from the complete genome sequence. *Nature* 393:537–544.

108. Gopinath K, Moosa A, Mizrahi V, Warner DF. 2013. Vitamin B(12) metabolism in *Mycobacterium tuberculosis*. *Future Microbiol* 8:1405–1418.

109. Young DB, Comas I, de Carvalho LP. 2015. Phylogenetic analysis of vitamin B12-related metabolism in *Mycobacterium tuberculosis*. *Front Mol Biosci* 2:6.

110. Griffin JE, Pandey AK, Gilmore SA, Mizrahi V, McKinney JD, Bertozzi CR, Sassetti CM. 2012. Cholesterol catabolism by *Mycobacterium tuberculosis* requires transcriptional and metabolic adaptations. *Chem Biol* 19:218–227.

111. Savvi S, Warner DF, Kana BD, McKinney JD, Mizrahi V, Dawes SS. 2008. Functional characterization of a vitamin B12-dependent methylmalonyl pathway in *Mycobacterium tuberculosis*: implications for propionate metabolism during growth on fatty acids. *J Bacteriol* 190:3886–3895.

112. Lee W, VanderVen BC, Fahey RJ, Russell DG. 2013. Intracellular *Mycobacterium tuberculosis* exploits host-derived fatty acids to limit metabolic stress. *J Biol Chem* 288:6788–6800.

113. Warner DF, Savvi S, Mizrahi V, Dawes SS. 2007. A riboswitch regulates expression of the coenzyme B12-independent methionine synthase in *Mycobacterium tuberculosis*: implications for differential methionine synthase function in strains H37Rv and CDC1551. *J Bacteriol* 189:3655–3659.

114. Gopinath K, Venclovas C, Ioerger TR, Sacchettini JC, McKinney JD, Mizrahi V, Warner DF. 2013. A vitamin B_{12} transporter in *Mycobacterium tuberculosis*. *Open Biol* 3:120175.

115. Jackson M, Phalen SW, Lagranderie M, Ensergueix D, Chavarot P, Marchal G, McMurray DN, Gicquel B, Guilhot C. 1999. Persistence and protective efficacy of a *Mycobacterium tuberculosis* auxotroph vaccine. *Infect Immun* 67:2867–2873.

116. Senaratne RH, Mougous JD, Reader JR, Williams SJ, Zhang T, Bertozzi CR, Riley LW. 2007. Vaccine

efficacy of an attenuated but persistent *Mycobacterium tuberculosis* cysH mutant. *J Med Microbiol* **56**:454–458.

117. **Niederweis M.** 2008. Nutrient acquisition by mycobacteria. *Microbiology* **154**:679–692.

118. **Yu XJ, Walker DH, Liu Y, Zhang L.** 2009. Amino acid biosynthesis deficiency in bacteria associated with human and animal hosts. *Infect Genet Evol* **9**:514–517.

119. **Gómez-Valero L, Rocha EP, Latorre A, Silva FJ.** 2007. Reconstructing the ancestor of *Mycobacterium leprae*: the dynamics of gene loss and genome reduction. *Genome Res* **17**:1178–1185.

120. **Rohmer L, Hocquet D, Miller SI.** 2011. Are pathogenic bacteria just looking for food? Metabolism and microbial pathogenesis. *Trends Microbiol* **19**:341–348.

121. **Houben EN, Korotkov KV, Bitter W.** 2014. Take five: type VII secretion systems of mycobacteria. *Biochim Biophys Acta* **1843**:1707–1716.

122. **Tufariello JM, Chapman JR, Kerantzas CA, Wong KW, Vilchèze C, Jones CM, Cole LE, Tinaztepe E, Thompson V, Fenyö D, Niederweis M, Ueberheide B, Philips JA, Jacobs WR Jr.** 2016. Separable roles for *Mycobacterium tuberculosis* ESX-3 effectors in iron acquisition and virulence. *Proc Natl Acad Sci USA* **113**:E348–E337.

123. **Marquis H, Bouwer HG, Hinrichs DJ, Portnoy DA.** 1993. Intracytoplasmic growth and virulence of *Listeria monocytogenes* auxotrophic mutants. *Infect Immun* **61**:3756–3760.

124. **Premaratne RJ, Lin WJ, Johnson EA.** 1991. Development of an improved chemically defined minimal medium for *Listeria monocytogenes*. *Appl Environ Microbiol* **57**:3046–3048.

125. **Portnoy DA, Jacks PS, Hinrichs DJ.** 1988. Role of hemolysin for the intracellular growth of *Listeria monocytogenes*. *J Exp Med* **167**:1459–1471.

126. **Abu Kwaik Y, Bumann D.** 2015. Host delivery of favorite meals for intracellular pathogens. *PLoS Pathog* **11**:e1004866.

127. **Ihssen J, Egli T.** 2005. Global physiological analysis of carbon- and energy-limited growing *Escherichia coli* confirms a high degree of catabolic flexibility and preparedness for mixed substrate utilization. *Environ Microbiol* **7**:1568–1581.

128. **Cohen SS, Barner HD.** 1954. Studies on unbalanced growth in *Escherichia coli*. *Proc Natl Acad Sci USA* **40**:885–893.

129. **Hall JD, Craven RR, Fuller JR, Pickles RJ, Kawula TH.** 2007. *Francisella tularensis* replicates within alveolar type II epithelial cells in vitro and in vivo following inhalation. *Infect Immun* **75**:1034–1039.

130. **Horwitz MA.** 1983. The Legionnaires' disease bacterium (*Legionella pneumophila*) inhibits phagosome-lysosome fusion in human monocytes. *J Exp Med* **158**:2108–2126.

131. **Marquis H, Bouwer HG, Hinrichs DJ, Portnoy DA.** 1993. Intracytoplasmic growth and virulence of *Listeria monocytogenes* auxotrophic mutants. *Infect Immun* **61**:3756–3760.

Index

A

Acid-fast (AF) mycobacteria, 519, 528–529
  AF-negative *M. tuberculosis* and cell wall alterations, 527–528
  brief history of AF staining, 520–522
  chemical structures of mycolic acids, 520
  clinical diagnosis of TB, 522–523
  importance of mycolic acids, 523–524
  Koch paradox, 523
  lipid accumulation, 526–527
  loss of AF property, 526–527, 528
  mycobacterial cell envelope, 523–526
  non-mycolic acid-containing components, 524–526
  process for loss of acid-fastness, 525
Acquired immunity, 35, 43
  CD4 T cells in HIV-TB coinfection, 248–251
  HIV-TB coinfection, 248–252
  TB-immune reconstitution inflammatory syndrome (TB-IRIS), 255–256
Adjunctive therapeutic vaccination, TB disease, 196–197
Alveolar epithelial cells (AECs), 3, 4
Alveolar macrophage (AM), 3, 4–5; *see also* Macrophages
M. tuberculosis infection, 215–216
Alzheimer's disease, 630
Amikacin, drug resistance, 503, 505
Amino acids, auxotrophs, 701–706
Amyloid diseases, 630
Anhui Zhifei Longcom Biologic Pharmacy Co. Ltd., 202

Animal models, 131, 139; *see also* Experimental infection models; Guinea pigs; Mouse models
  assessment of new drugs, 136–137
  assessment of vaccines, 135
  cattle, 134
  common experimental designs, 280
  efficacy testing, 277–284
  ethical and husbandry issues, 138–139
  guinea pigs, 132
  host response and pathogenesis, 134–135
  limitations of, 137–139
  mechanism of protection, 136
  mice, 132, 278–280
  mini pigs, 134
  non-human primates (NHP), 132–133
  pathology of tuberculosis, 117–121
  practical applications of, 134–137
  primary host response to *M. tuberculosis* infection, 122–123
  process and capacity, 135–136
  rabbits, 133
  rats, 133–134
  Treg cell responses in experimental, 80–87
  Treg cells in guinea pig model of TB, 85–86
  Treg cells in mouse models of TB, 80–85
  Treg cells in non-human primate models of TB, 86–87
  tuberculosis disease progression in, 122
  vaccine testing protocols, 136, 137
  zebrafish, 133, 685, 686
Anopheles, 17
Antibiotics, golden era of, 317

Antibiotics treatment, extracellular *M. tuberculosis* in, 535
Antibiotic tolerance, 596
Antibodies
  BCG vaccination and, 220
  M. tuberculosis infection, 219–220, 221
  role in anti-*M. tuberculosis* infection, 219
  tuberculosis, 225–226
Antigen-presenting cells (APCs)
  development of memory T cells, 98
  function of, 74, 75
Antiretroviral therapy (ART), 389
  HIV, 239
  HIV-TB coinfection, 250
  HIV-TB immune constitution inflammatory syndrome (IRIS), 252–253, 255–256
  influence on T cell responses in coinfection, 251
Apoptosis, 563
Archaebacteria, 455
Archivel Farma SL, 202
Arginine auxotrophs, 702
Aristotle, 413
Asparagine auxotrophs, 702
Aspartate auxotrophs, 702
Association of Internal Medicine, 520
AstraZeneca, 282
ATP synthesis, 308–309
Auramine O, staining of *M. tuberculosis*, 522–523, 526–527
Austin, Robert, 597
Autophagy, 8, 10

Auxotrophies, 701; *see also* Nutrient use of
    pathogens
  amino acid, 701–706
  arginine, 702
  asparagines, 702
  aspartate, 702
  biotin (vitamin B$_7$), 707
  cobalamin (vitamin B$_{12}$), 707–708
  cofactor, 706–708
  cysteine, 702
  folate (vitamin B$_9$), 707
  glutamate, 705–706
  glutamine, 705
  histidine, 703
  isoleucine, 704
  leucine, 704
  lysine, 703–704
  methionine, 702–703
  nicotinamide, 706
  pantothenate (vitamin B$_5$), 706
  proline, 703
  purine, 708
  pyridoxamine (vitamin B$_6$), 706–707
  threonine, 704
  tryptophan, 704–705
  valine, 704

B

Bacillus Calmette-Guérin (BCG), original
    vaccine, 95, 117
Bacillus subtilis, 582, 673
Bacterial cell biology, tuberculosis
    research, 185
Bacterial clearance, 16–17
Bacterial replisome, components of,
    584–586
B cells
  M. tuberculosis infection, 217, 219–220
  tuberculosis (TB), 225–226
Bedaquiline
  animal model, 278
  drug candidate, 271, 273
  mice, 279
  proof-of-concept molecule, 333
  TB drug, 298–300, 302, 306–307, 309
Biofilms, *see* Mycobacterial biofilms
Biology
  animal- and human-associated MTBC
      lineages, 481–482
  genetic diversity of TB bacilli, 477–484
  M. canettii and MTBC, 482
  M. tuberculosis strains, 482–484
  variations from genomics, 480–481
Biomarkers
  classes of TB, 371
  human tuberculosis (TB), 226–227
  transcriptomic profiling, 226–227
  treatment response, 227
Biomedical Primate Research Center
    (Netherlands), 165, 167
Biosynthesis, menaquinone, 302–303, 304
Biotin (vitamin B$_7$), 707
British Medical Research Council, 654
Bronchoalveolar lavage (BAL), 215, 242

C

Callithrix jacchus (common marmoset),
    172, 284
Canadian Tuberculosis Standards, 379

Candida albicans, 321
Canetti, Georges, 496
Capreomycin, drug resistance, 503, 505
Carbon starvation, screening, 341, 342
Carbonyl cyanide *m*-chlorophenyl hydrazine
    (CCCP), 298
Cattle
  animal model, 134
  experimental infection of, 177–178
  as model of TB in humans, 178
  new TB vaccines tested in, 181
  potential correlates of protection, 183
Caulobacter crescentus, 594
Cavity formation, pathology of tuberculosis,
    119, 120
CD4 T and T helper 1 (Th1) cells, memory
    immunity, 95–96, 102–104
CD4 T and T helper 17 (Th17) cells,
    memory immunity, 104–105
CD8 memory T cells, 105–106
Cellular immunity, 143
Centers for Disease Control and Prevention
    (CDC), 379
Chagas' disease, 454
Chemokines
  CCR (CC receptors) and ligands, 49–52
  CCR1, 49–50
  CCR2, 50
  CCR4, 50
  CCR5, 50–51
  CCR6, 51
  CCR7, 51–52
  CXCR1, 52
  CXCR2, 52
  CXCR3, 52–53
  CXCR5, 53
  CXC receptors and ligands, 52–53
  HIV-TB coinfection, 241
  M. tuberculosis infection, 49–53
  positive and negative roles in TB, 36
  role in adaptive response to
      M. tuberculosis infection, 38
  role in innate response to *M. tuberculosis*
      infection, 37
Chemotherapy
  latent TB infection (LTBI), 284–286
  M. tuberculosis persistence, 653–658, 662
Chicago Center for Biomedical
    Research, 171
Chlamydia trachomatis, 609
Chlorpromazine, 299
Cholesterol, *M. tuberculosis* in macrophages,
    645, 646
Ciprofloxacin, drug resistance, 505
Clinical testing, *see* Vaccine candidates
Clofazimine
  animal models, 278–279
  drug candidate, 272, 300
  mice, 281
Clostridium difficile, 611
Cobalamin (vitamin B$_{12}$), 707–708
Cofactors, auxotrophies, 706–708
Collaborative Drug Discovery, 329
Commercial liquid culture, 364
Comparative genomic analysis, 185
Comparative transcriptome analysis, 185
Computed tomography (CT), 171
Congenic mice, 145
Consumption, 453

Cox models, cumulative risk curves, 405
Crohn's disease, 428
Cyclophosphamide, 97
D-Cycloserine, drug resistance, 505
Cynomolgus macaques
  comparing TB in humans to, 164
  Golden Age of research, 163, 166
  Macaca fascicularis, 163, 172
  TB studies, 166–167, 168
  21st century TB research, 166
Cysteine auxotrophs, 702
Cytokines
  enhancing HIV-1 replication, 246, 247
  HIV-1 replication, 246, 247
  IL-6 (interleukin-6), 40–41
  IL-10, 48–49
  IL-12 family, 42–45
  IL-18, 42
  IL-1R/IL18R/MyD88, 41
  IL-22, 46
  IL-23, 44
  IL-23-dependent, 45–46
  IL-27, 44–45
  IL-35, 45
  interferons, 37–40
  M. tuberculosis infection, 34–49
  positive and negative roles in TB, 35
  proflammatory IL-1, 41–42
  regulatory, 47–49
  role in adaptive response to
      M. tuberculosis infection, 38
  role in innate response to *M. tuberculosis*
      infection, 37
  transforming growth factor β (TGFβ), 48
  tumor necrosis factor alpha (TNFα),
      34–37
  type II interferon (INFγ), 38–39
  type I INF, 39–40
Cytomegalovirus (CMV) infection, 249,
    251, 255

D

Damage-associated molecular pattern
    molecules (DAMPs), 11
Dannenberg, Arthur, 680
Dartmouth University, 202
Deer, experimental infection of, 177, 179
Dehydrogenases
  NADH:menaquinone oxidoreductases,
      299–300
  oxidative phosphorylation, 301–302
  succinate:quinone oxidoreductase,
      300–301
Delamanid, drug candidate, 271, 273
Dendritic cells (DCs)
  development of memory T cells, 98
  HIV-TB coinfection, 241, 244
  lung, 5
  M. tuberculosis infection, 11–12
Diabetes mellitus, 222–223, 630
Diagnostics for TB
  acid-fast (AF) staining in clinical
      diagnosis, 522–523
  classes of TB biomarkers, 371
  commercial liquid culture, 364
  current, for active TB, 363–366
  current, for drug-resistant TB, 366–369
  line probe assays for detecting resistance,
      367–368

loop-mediated amplification test, 365–366
maximizing impact of new diagnostics, 361, 373–374
pipeline of future, 369–371
rapid speciation strip tests, 364
smear microscopy, 363–364
tests impacting patient outcomes, 373
translational challenges, 371, 372
unmet needs and gaps, 369
urine lipoarabinomannan rapid test, 366
Xpert MTB/RIF, 365, 368
Diagnostics of TB, *see also* GeneXpert MTB/RIF technology
background, 390–391
GeneXpert technology, 391
impact of GeneXpert MTB/RIF, 399–401
Disease burden, impact of GeneXpert MTB/RIF, 400
DIVA (differentiating infected from vaccinated animals) tests, domestic livestock, 184–186
Diversity outbred mice, 146
DNA replication
bacterial, 582–583, 586
B-family DNA polymerase, 591
components of bacterial replisome, 584–586
components of mycobacterial replisome/repair, 587
coordinating, and cell division, 594–595
DnaE1 PHP domain proofreading activity in maintaining fidelity, 588–590
DnaE1 versus DnaE2, 590–591
DNA polymerases at replication fork, 591–592
mycobacterial C-family DNA polymerases, 586, 588–591
mycobacterial persistence and, 596–599
mycobacterial replication rate, 592–594
persistence and resistance, 597–599
PHP (polymerase and histidinol phosphatase) domain, 586, 588
replication rate, 592
structure of C-family polymerases, 589
subcomplex division of bacterial replisome, 588
targeting replisome for new TB drug development, 595–596
DNA synthesis, 334–335
Domestic livestock, 177, 186
antigen mining, 184–186
bacterial cell biology, 185
cattle, 177–178
comparative genomic analysis, 185
comparative transcriptome analysis, 185
deer, 177, 179
development and evaluation of TB vaccines, 179–182
DIVA (differentiating infected from vaccinated animals) tests, 184–186
DIVA skin test development, 185–186
experimental infection models, 177–179
goats, 178–179
immune correlates of protection and disease, 182–184
tuberculosis (TB) in, 177
Dormancy
definition, 654
secretion, 610, 611, 619

Drosophila melanogaster, 17
Drug development
clinical trials, 272–273
macaque models for evaluation, 170–171
targeting replisome for new, 595–596
Drug-resistant *M. tuberculosis* strains
evolution of, 502–508
evolution of MDR-TB, 503, 506
evolution of resistance to second-line drugs, 506–507
impact of GeneXpert MTB/RIF, 401, 402–404
microevolution during TB infection, 507–508
resistance to first-line drugs, 504
resistance to second-line drugs, 505
suggested model for genetic diversity of subpopulations, 507
Drug susceptibility testing (DST), 363
commercial liquid culture-based DST, 366–367
genotypic tests for, 367
line probe assays for resistance detection, 367–368
noncommercial methods, 367
phenotypic tests for, 366
pipeline of diagnostics, 370
Drug targets, menaquinone biosynthesis, 302–303, 304
Drug tolerance, definition, 654
Drug-tolerant cells
class I persisters, 321–322
class II persisters, 322–325, 329–346
population of nonreplicating, 322–325, 329–346
Dual-active molecules, 331–332
canonical and noncanonical targets of, 334

E

Ebola virus, 454
Efficacy, *see* Preclinical efficacy testing
Ehrlich, P., 520
Electron flow, *M. tuberculosis*, 296
Enterococcus faecalis, 610
Erdman strain, *M. tuberculosis*, 166, 167, 168, 170, 171–172
Escherichia coli, 12, 309, 321, 464, 467, 535, 536, 557, 583, 590, 599, 610, 638, 662, 673, 676, 701
ESX-1 (ESAT-6 secretion system-1), 627, 631–632
damage of *M. tuberculosis*-containing phagosome, 628–630
innate immune mechanisms, 631
interventions by target, 631
phagosome disruption by, 628
regulations of, 630–631
role in TB pathogenesis, 630
Ethambutol
drug resistance, 502, 503, 504
tolerance of infected cells, 640
Ethical issues, animal models, 138–139
Ethionamide, drug resistance, 505
Eubacteria, 455
Evolution of MTBC
animal-related *M. tuberculosis* complex (MTBC) strains, 461

biogeographical structure of *M. tuberculosis* Beijing lineage, 463
correspondence table of strains by typing methods, 457
diagram of proposed evolutionary pathway, 456
fingerprint era, 454–455
genome-based phylogeny of MTBC, 459
global phylogeny of MTBC isolates, 465
global picture, 458–461
history and early (mis)conceptions, 453–454
limitations, 466–467
multilocus era, 455–458
pattern for evolving populations, 466
pregenomic era, 454–458
relativity of clock, 464–467
spoligotyping, 455, 457, 461
substitution rate estimates, 464–466
taxonomic nomenclature, 464
whole-genome phylogeny of strains of MTBC, 460
zooming into lineages, 461–464
Evolution of *Mycobacterium tuberculosis*
drug-resistant strains, 502–508
global spread of *M. tuberculosis* L2 Beijing and L4 strains, 499–500
L2 Beijing sublineage, 500–501
L4 sublineage, 501–502
lessons from *M. canettii*, 496–498
molecular key events in evolution, 497
neighbor-joining phylogeny scheme, 499
professional pathogenicity, 498–502
Expanded Program on Immunization (EPI), World Health Organization, 193
Experimental infection models
cattle, 177–178
deer, 179
goats, 178–179
Experimental medicine
controlled human challenge models, 205
examples of, 205
potential outcomes on studies, 204–205
preclinical studies in, 205–206
product development and, 204
role in TB vaccine development, 203–206
scientific community, 206
Extensively drug-resistant (XDR) strains, 533

F

Fatty acids, *M. tuberculosis* in macrophages, 644–645
Fauci, Anthony, 117
Flow cytometry, 682–684, 685
Fluorescence-activated cell sorting (FACS), 683
Fluorescence recovery after photobleaching (FRAP), 678, 684
Foam cell formation, human post-primary TB, 125
Folate (vitamin B$_9$), 707
Foxp3 (transcription factor forkhead box P3)
coexpression with CD25, 74, 75–76, 78–79
function of, 73
host defense against *M. tuberculosis*, 82
Francisella tularensis, 609, 699, 709

G

Gabbett, H. S., 520–521
Genetic deficiency, mycobacterial disease, 38
Genetic diversity
  biological impact of, 480
  intrapatient, 479–480
  M. tuberculosis complex (MTBC),
    477–484
Genetics and genomics
  advance vaccine development, 430
  candidate gene studies, 417–418,
    420–426
  clinical translation of host genomic
    insights, 429–430
  DNA sequence variation, 414, 418
  epidemiology of TB, 429
  epigenetic variation, 414, 429
  future prospects, 427–430
  genetic studies of mice, 145–146
  genome-wide association studies (GWAS),
    418–419, 427
  heritability of TB susceptibility, 413–416
  host "omics" in TB, 414
  host-pathogen coevolution, 428
  identification of genetic variants with TB,
    416–427
  karyogram of host-genetic correlates, 427
  linkage studies, 416–417
  Mendelian susceptibility to mycobacterial
    disease (MSMD), 413, 415, 416
  M. tuberculosis infection in macrophages,
    643–644
  phenotype definitions, 429
  population-specific associations, 428
  predictive tools, 429–430
  role of Mendelian randomization
    studies, 430
  sequence-based approaches to identifying
    loci, 428
  therapeutic tools, 430
  transcriptomic assays, 430
  transcriptomic studies of TB, 414,
    419, 427
  twin studies, 413, 415
GeneXpert MTB/RIF technology
  background, 391
  challenges and opportunities during
    national implementation, 394–396
  cumulative risk curves, 405
  expansion in other countries, 399
  failures in, 399
  financial modeling, 398
  future for, 401, 405
  historical context of national
    implementation, 391–396
  impact on diagnostics, 399–401
  impact on national programs, 396–398
  innovations in South Africa, 397
  nucleic acid amplification testing (NAAT)
    strategies, 390, 391, 392
  procurement strategies, 398
  South African national implementation of,
    393–394
  treatment outcomes, 401, 402–404
  Xpert Omni, 392, 401, 405
  Xpert ULTRA, 392, 395, 397, 401
GeneXpert Omni, 365
Genome-wide association studies (GWAS)
  host-genetic evidence, 417

  revisiting heritability in post-GWAS
    era, 416
  TB susceptibility, 413, 418–419, 427
Genomics, *see* Genetics and genomics
Genotype, 671
GlaxoSmithKline, 199
Global TB epidemic, 389–390
Glutamate auxotroph, 705–706
Glutamine synthetase (GS), 705
Goats, experimental infection of, 177,
    178–179
Gordonia otitidis, 498
Granulocyte-macrophage colony-stimulating
    factor (GM-CSF), 144
Granulocytes, *M. tuberculosis* infection,
    14–16
Granulomas
  development, 680–681, 684, 687
  guinea pig model, 152
  in vitro models, 549–550
  lung of human with primary tuberculosis,
    118, 120–121
  morphological features of, 533
  M. tuberculosis infection, 217, 636
  progressive caseating, 126
  restricting *M. tuberculosis* movement,
    35–36
  term, 16
Granulomatous inflammation, 123
Guinea pigs, 150–155; *see also* Animal
    models
  animal model, 132
  anti-TB treatment, 86
  BCG vaccination, 86
  devices for aerosol exposure, 147
  gating host cells from lung, 153
  granulomas in lungs, 118, 124, 126
  human-to-guinea pig transmission, 153
  immunopathology of, 152
  magnetic resonance imaging of infected
    lungs, 155
  preclinical efficacy models, 282
  response to infection, 123, 124, 154
  TB disease progression, 122
  Treg cells in, 80, 85–86
  vaccines, 153–154

H

H37Rv strain of *Mycobacterium
  tuberculosis*, 166, 167, 168, 170,
    172, 215
Harvard School of Public Health, 467
Helicobacter pylori, 462, 464, 594
Heritability, *see* Genetics and genomics
Heterogeneity, *see* Phenotypic heterogeneity
Histidine auxotroph, 703
HIV-1 (human immunodeficiency virus
    type 1)
  functional impairment of CD4 T cells,
    250–251
  heterogeneity at site of *M. tuberculosis*
    disease, 247
  immunity to TB, 50
  infected people, 239
  interferons and, 39
  mediating immunosuppression, 239–241
  M. tuberculosis infection risk, 172, 475
  replication at site of *M. tuberculosis*
    disease, 245–247

  tuberculosis epidemic and, 389
  tuberculosis resurgence, 222
HIV-TB-associated immune reconstitution
    inflammatory syndrome (IRIS)
  acquired immunity and TB-IRIS, 255–256
  hypercytokinemia in TB-IRIS, 253, 255
  innate immunity and TB-IRIS, 252–253
  model of innate receptor signaling in
    TB-IRIS, 254
HIV-TB coinfection
  acquired immunity, 248–252
  CD4 T cells in, 248–251
  cytotoxic lymphocytes in, 251–252
  dendritic cells in, 244
  dissemination and mycobacteremia in, 248
  immune activation in, 247–248
  immune reconstitution inflammatory
    syndrome (IRIS), 252–256
  macrophages in, 241–243
  natural killer (NK) cells in, 244–245
  neutrophils in, 243–244
  spectrum of disease in, 240
Hollow fiber systems
  diagram, 276
  tuberculosis (TB) model, 275–277
Homeostatic regulation, 73
Homo sapiens
  M. tuberculosis, 653
  tuberculosis in, 453–454, 458, 460–462,
    467
Host genetic studies, tuberculosis, 429
Host-mimicking platforms, 685–686
Host-pathogen coevolution, 428
Host response, application of animal models,
    134–135
Human immunology of tuberculosis
  acquisition of *M. tuberculosis* infection,
    213, 215–221
  adaptive responses and spectrum of
    infection, 217–220
  alveolar macrophages, 215–216
  antibody responses, 219–220, 221
  B cells, 217, 219–220
  biomarkers in human TB, 226–227
  granuloma, 2178
  immunity to *M. tuberculosis*, 213
  innate T cells, 216–217
  neutrophils, 216
  progression from infection to TB disease,
    222–226
  spectrum of pulmonary TB lesions, 218
  stages of response to infection, 214
  T cells, 217–218
Human models
  challenge models, 205
  in vitro, 545–546
Human tuberculosis (TB)
  balance of Treg activity, 77
  cavity formation in lungs, 119, 120
  CD39+ Treg cell subsets in, 77–78
  granuloma in lung, 118, 120–121
  in vitro expansion of mycobacteria-
    specific Treg cells, 76–77
  novel TB vaccine candidate MVA85A,
    77–78
  post-primary lung reinfection, 124–125
  TB disease progression, 122
  Treg at site of infection, 79–80
  Treg cell responses in, 74–80

Treg cells and anti-TB treatment, 78–79
Treg cells and clinical *M. tuberculosis* strains, 78
Treg-mediated manipulation of immune cell activation, 75–79
Treg responses in cell and fluid samples, 79–80
Treg responses in tissue, 79
Husbandry issues, animal models, 138–139
Hypercytokinemia, TB-immune reconstitution inflammatory syndrome (TB-IRIS), 253, 255
Hypoxia, 341
  redox homeostasis during, 307–308
  relationship to metronidazole activity, 318
  screening, 341, 342

I

Imidazopyridine amide, TB drug, 300, 305
Immune response, *see* Memory immune response
Immunity, *see also* Regulation of TB immunity
  cytokines and chemokines in, 33–34
  HIV infection and TB, 50
  interleukin-6 (IL-6), 40–41
  working model of, 42, 45
Immunodeficient mice, 145
Immunopathology, guinea pig model, 152
Immunosuppression, HIV-1 mediating, 239–241
Immunotherapy, vaccine development, 197
Inactivated whole-cell and fragmented TB vaccines, 202
Infectious Diseases Research Institute, 199
Inflammation, TB progression, 224–225
Infliximab, 36
Innate immunity, 16–17, 35, 106–107
  HIV-TB coinfection, 241–245
  mouse model, 145
  TB-immune reconstitution inflammatory syndrome (TB-IRIS), 252–253, 254
Institut Pasteur, 496
Interferon gamma (IFN-γ) response assay (IGRA), 16, 193, 214, 220, 221, 225
  latent TB infection, 381–385
  reducing test variability with, 385
Interferons (IFN-γ)
  M. tuberculosis infection, 37–40
  protection against TB, 102–104
  roles in TB, 35
  type I, 39–40
  type II IFN-γ, 38–39
Interleukin-12 (IL-12) cytokine family, 42–45
  IL-12, 43–44
  IL-23, 44
  IL-27, 44–45
  IL-35, 45
Interleukin 17 (IL-17), memory immunity, 104–105
Interleukin-1 cytokine family, 41–42
  IL-1, 41–42
  IL-18, 42
  IL-1R/IL18R/MyD88, 41
Interleukin-23 (IL-23) dependent cytokines, 45–46
  IL-17, 45–46, 104–105
  IL-22, 46

Interleukin-6 (IL-6)
  cytokine, 40–41
  roles in tuberculosis (TB), 35
International Tuberculosis Host Genetics Consortium (ITHGC), 413, 416, 428
Intracellular receptors, *M. tuberculosis* infection, 10
In vitro models
  granuloma models, 549–550
  human, 545–546
  investigating MTB infection, 548–550
  mouse, 542–544
  non-human primate (NHP), 544–545
  zebrafish, 550
IPEX syndrome (immune dysregulation, polyendocrinopathy, enteropathy, X-linked syndrome), 73, 74
Isocitrate lyase (Icl), *M. tuberculosis* in macrophages, 644, 645–647
Isoleucine auxotroph, 704
Isoniazid, 86
  animal models for testing, 278–280
  drug candidate, 272, 274
  drug resistance, 503, 504, 505, 506
  guinea pigs, 282
  latent TB infection, 285–286
  line probe assays for detecting resistance, 367–368
  non-human primates, 283–284
  phenotypic heterogeneity of *M. tuberculosis* with, 674, 677
  staining of *M. tuberculosis*, 519, 523
  tolerance of infected cells, 639–641
Isoniazid preventive therapy (IPT), HIV, 239

J

Jeffreys, Sir Alec, 455
Johannsen, Wilhelm, 671

K

Kanamycin, drug resistance, 503, 505
Kaplan-Meier analysis, vaccine, 138
Kinyoun, J., 521–522
Koch, Robert, 224, 390, 520
Koch paradox, 519, 523
Koch phenomena, 126

L

Laënnec, Rene, 121
Lamers, Meindert H., 581–599
Lansoprazole, TB drug, 300, 305
Latency, definition, 654
Latent TB infection (LTBI), 217, 226, 227, 239, 379, 385–386
  human model, 593–594
  IGRAs, 381–385
  immunological principles underlying IGRA, 382
  modeling chemotherapy of, 284–286
  mouse model and clinical guidelines, 285
  new skin tests, 385
  purified protein derivative (PPD)-based TST, 381
  testing methods for, 380
Legionella pneumophila, 699, 709
Leishmania, 146
Lentivirus genus, 239
Leucine auxotroph, 704
Levofloxacin, drug candidate, 272–273

Line probe assays (LPAs)
  detecting resistance to anti-TB drugs, 367–368
  detecting resistance to second-line anti-TB drugs, 368–369
Linezolid
  drug candidate, 272
  mice, 279
  non-human primates, 283
Lipidomics, 683–684
Lipid synthesis, 332–334
Lipid utilization, *M. tuberculosis* in macrophages, 644, 647
Lipoarabinomannan (LAM)
  improving detection, 369
  rapid urine test, 366
Liquid culture, TB diagnostics, 364
Listeria monocytogenes, 102, 203, 609, 611, 699, 709
Little, Clarence, 143
Loop-mediated amplification test, 365–366
Low oxygen recovery assay (LORA), 323
Lung, 3–6
  cellular components, 4–5
  M. tuberculosis interaction with, 6–16
  mucus and surfactant, 5
  pathology of C3HeB/FeJ mice, 281
  post-primary reinfection, 124–125
  post-primary TB in human, 125–127
  schematic of, 4
  soluble components in surfactant hypophase, 5–6
  spectrum of human pulmonary TB lesions, 218
Lung macrophages, 4–5
  cell death, 11
  release of exosomes, 10–11
Lymphotactin (XCL1), 144
Lysine auxotroph, 703–704

M

Macaca fascicularis (cynomolgus macaque), 163, 172
Macaca mulatta (rhesus macaque), 163, 173
Macaque models
  Golden Age of TB research, 163, 165
  historical use of, 163–165
  M. tuberculosis/simian immunodeficiency virus coinfection, 171–172
  TB drug evaluation, 170–171
  TB pathogenesis study, 171
  TB vaccine evaluation, 167, 170
  Treg cells in macaques, 86–87
  validation of, 163
Macrophages, *see also Mycobacterium tuberculosis* in macrophage; *Mycobacterium tuberculosis*-macrophage biology
  basic principles of macrophage biology, 546–548
  cell death, 11
  exosome release from, 10–11
  HIV-TB coinfection, 241–243
  human *in vitro* models, 545–546
  lung, 4–5
  mouse *in vitro* models, 542–544
  M. tuberculosis and, 541–542
  M. tuberculosis growth in, 700–701

Macrophages *(Continued)*
mycobacterial growth and HIV-1 viral
replication, 243
non-human primate *in vitro* models,
544–545
Magnetic resonance imaging (MRI), infected
guinea pig lungs, 155
Major histocompatibility complex (MHC),
38, 39, 49, 74, 97
Malnutrition, 223–224
Marmosets *(Callithrix jacchus)*, 172, 284
McMaster (Ad5Ag85A), 201
Memory immune response
against tuberculosis (TB), 96–97
alternative mediators of memory
immunity, 105–107
CD4T and Th17 cells, 104–105
CD4T and T helper (Th) 1 cells, 95–96,
102–104
CD8 T cells, 105–106
development after TB infection or
vaccination, 98
γδ T cells, 106
generation of memory T cells, 97–99
innate memory, 106–107
memory T cell heterogeneity, 99–102
models of T cell fate, 98–99
natural killer (NK) cell memory, 107
novel TB vaccines, 107–108
resident memory T cells, 101–102
stem cell-like memory T cells, 102
T cell memory and TB vaccination,
107–108
T cell memory phenotypes, 100
trained immunity in monocytes, 107
Memory T cells, 95
CD8, 105–106
development after infection or
vaccination, 98
enzyme-linked immunospot (ELISPOT)
method, 182
generation of, 97–99
heterogeneity, 99–102
models of fate, 98–99
phenotypes, 100
proposed models of differentiation, 99
resident, 101–102
stem cell-like, 102
TB vaccination and, 107–108
vaccine efficacy, 182
Menaquinone biosynthesis, 302–303, 304
Mendelian susceptibility to mycobacterial
disease (MSMD), 413, 415, 416, 417
Merck Research Laboratories, 596
Metabolomics, 683–684, 700–701
Methionine auxotrophs, 702–703
Methyl citrate cycle, *M. tuberculosis* in
macrophages, 644, 645–647
Metronidazole, 278
hypoxia and activity of, 318
mice, 279, 286
non-human primates, 283
proof-of-concept molecule, 333
rabbits, 283
Microbiology, explorative tools and
methodologies, 682–686
Micrococcus luteus, 611
Microfluidics, 684–685
MicroRNAs (miRNAs), 10

Microscopy, time-lapse, 684–685
Millennium Development Goals, 389
Minimal unit of infection, 635, 648
Mini pigs, animal model, 134
Modified Henderson apparatus, 167, 173
Monocytes
trained immunity in, 107
tuberculosis, 224–225
Moorella, 458
Morbidity, impact of GeneXpert MTB/
RIF, 400
Mortality, impact of GeneXpert MTB/RIF,
400–401
Mouse models, 143–150, 278–280; *see also*
Animal models
animal model, 132, 137
anti-TB treatment, 85
C3HeB/FeJ mice, 280–281
clinical *M. tuberculosis* strains, 83
common experimental designs, 280
Cornell model, 284–286
devices for aerosol exposure, 147
experimental infection of, 279–280
gene-disrupted mice, 144–145
genetic studies in mice, 145–146
immunodeficient, transgenic and congenic
mice, 145
innate immunity, 145
in vitro, 542–544
latent TB infection (LTBI), 285
low-dose aerosol exposure to
M. tuberculosis, 148
lung inflammatory response, 149
mouse response to infection, 146–150
obstructive alveolar pneumonia, 126
persistence in *M. tuberculosis* infection,
654–655, 657–659
preclinical efficacy models, 278–281
proposed regulation T cell suppression,
84
TB disease progression, 122
Treg cells and TB vaccination, 83–84
Treg cells in, 80–85
Treg cells in chronic TB infection, 82–83
Treg cells in early TB infection, 81–82
Moxifloxacin
animal model, 279
drug candidate, 272, 331
drug resistance, 505
guinea pigs, 282
proof-of-concept molecule, 333
Mucosal associated invariant T (MAIT)
cells, 5
M. tuberculosis infection, 216–217, 549
Multidrug-resistant (MDR) strains, 533
Mutagenesis, *M. tuberculosis*, 595
MVA85A (modified vaccinia Ankara virus
expressing antigen 85A)
TB vaccine candidate, 77–78, 96, 104,
108, 182, 200–201
testing protocols, 136
trial in South Africa, 137–138, 153–154
Mycobacteria
C-family DNA polymerases, 586, 588–591
DNA synthesis, 334–335, 336
evaluating bactericidal action against
nonreplicating, 329
fluoroquinolones, 339
folate synthesis, 338

high-throughput screens targeting
phenotypically tolerant, 322–323,
325
4-hydroxyquinolines, 338, 339
8-hydroxyquinolines, 338, 339
lipid synthesis, 332–334, 336
membrane depolarizers, 343–346
metabolism and respiration, 309–310
oxidative phosphorylation, 295
peptidoglycan synthesis, 335, 337, 338
persistence and resistance, 597–599
population heterogeneity as function of
applied stress, 598
protein synthesis, 335, 337
proteolysis/proteostasis pathway, 339–341
quinolines, 338–339
replication machinery, 583, 586
respiration, 309–310
RNA synthesis, 335, 336
screening, 341–343
strategies for evaluating
nonreplicating, 323
targeting oxygen reduction in, 303,
305–308
Mycobacterial biofilms, 533, 535, 536
extracellular *M. tuberculosis* in necrotizing
lesions, 535–536
formation, 535, 536, 537
Mycobacterial replisome, working model
of, 582
Mycobacteria orygis, 460
Mycobacteria other than tuberculosis
(MOTT), 495
Mycobacteriology, 460, 467
Mycobacterium africanum, 453, 455–
460, 477
Mycobacterium avium, 13, 52, 679
Mycobacterium bovis, 476, 477
bovine tuberculosis (TB), 177
Ravenel strain, 133
Mycobacterium bovis bacille Calmette-
Guérin (BCG), 6, 12, 13, 15, 703
BCG vaccine-induced protection, 43, 46
C3HeB/FeJ mice, 281
cattle model, 134
expansions of Treg cells, 76
responses of innate immune cells to, 12
vaccine, 95, 117, 179–180, 627
Mycobacterium canettii, 456, 458, 460, 476,
477, 479, 481–483, 485
drug resistance, 502
lessons to learn from, 496–498
Mycobacterium caprae, 460, 461, 476, 477,
479, 496
Mycobacterium flavescens, 382
Mycobacterium haemophilum, 495
Mycobacterium kansasii, 382, 495
Mycobacterium leprae, 382, 428, 495, 709
replisome components, 584–586, 587
Mycobacterium lepromatosis, 495
Mycobacterium marinum, 14, 382, 495,
679
mycolic acids, 523
virulence, 610
zebrafish model, 36, 133, 699
Mycobacterium microti, 382, 453–454, 460,
461, 476, 477, 479–481, 485,
496, 498
Mycobacterium mungi, 461, 496

Mycobacterium orygis, 460, 476, 479, 496, 498
Mycobacterium phlei, 6, 295
Mycobacterium pinnipedii, 460, 461, 476, 477, 479
Mycobacterium prototuberculosis, 458
Mycobacterium smegmatis, 10, 308–309, 535, 536, 609, 673, 675, 679, 703
    replisome components, 584–586, 587
Mycobacterium suricattae, 496
Mycobacterium szulgai, 382
Mycobacterium tuberculosis, 3;
    see also HIV-TB coinfection
    ATP synthesis by F_1F_0 ATP synthase, 308–309
    chemokines and cytokines in adaptive response to, 38
    chemokines and cytokines in innate response to, 37
    chemokines in, infection, 49–53
    cytokines in, infection, 34–49
    emerging strains inducing regulatory T cells in lungs, 150
    Erdman strain, 166, 167, 168, 170, 171–172
    fate upon macrophage infection, 9
    H37Rv strain, 166, 167, 168, 170, 172
    HIV-1 heterogeneity at site of disease, 247
    HIV-1 replication at site of disease, 245–247
    hypothesized states of response to infection, 214
    immune system, 95
    interactions with macrophages, 6–8, 10–11
    interaction with granulocytes, 14–16
    interaction with lung, 6–16
    latent TB infection (LTBI), 217, 226, 227
    macrophage receptors, 7
    mouse response to infection, 146–150
    mutagenesis in, 595
    oxidative phosphorylation in, 295
    pathology of, 117–121, 125–127, 672
    physiology for nonreplicating persistence, 567–571
    prevention of infection, 193–195
    primary host response to infection, 122–123
    protein phosphorylation in, 557, 559–560
    pulmonary innate immune cells during infection, 4
    replisome components, 584–586, 587
    respiration overview in, 295
    responses of innate immune cells to, 12
    schematic of electron transfer components, 296
    spectrum of infection, 379–380
    targeting primary dehydrogenases in, 299–302
    targeting proton motive force (PMF) in, 295–299
    vaccination, 95–96
Mycobacterium tuberculosis complex (MTBC), *see also* Evolution of MTBC
    biological differences among *M. tuberculosis* strains, 482–484
    biological differences between animal and human MTBC lineages, 481–482

biological differences between *M. canettii* and, 482
biological impact of genetic diversity, 480
evidence for potential of biological variation, 480–481
geographical distribution of Beijing isolates, 483
global emergence of multidrug-resistant TB strains, 475–477
global genetic diversity, 477–484
global phylogenetic structure of MTBC strains, 476
global phylogeny of MTBC isolates, 465
intrapatient diversity, 479–480
phylogenetic reconstruction of MTBC Beijing lineage population, 478
Mycobacterium tuberculosis infection, *see also* Protein phosphorylation
    apoptosis, 563
    cell wall remodeling, 569–570
    defense against host-generated reactive oxygen and nitrogen species, 563–564
    growth arrest, 567–569
    Ser/Thr protein kinases (STPKs) coordinating physiology of, 567–571
    slowing central metabolism, 570–571
    STPK cell signaling network, 568
    subversion of innate immune response, 560–564
Mycobacterium tuberculosis in macrophage
    bottleneck response, 637
    chemical genetics of infection, 643–644
    cholesterol, 645, 646
    construction of reporter strains, 638–639, 640
    drug sensitivity of, 641
    environmental cues and responses, 638
    fatty acids, 644–645
    flow cytometry gating strategy, 642
    flow sorting strategy, 641
    guilt-by-association analysis, 637
    life and death dynamics, 637
    lipid acquisition from host cell, 647
    lipid utilization by, 644
    manipulating host cell for nutritional purposes, 647–648
    minimal unit of infection, 635, 648
    phagocytosis, 636
    replication clock plasmid, 637
    response of *M. tuberculosis* to intracellular environment, 636–638
    role of isocitrate lyase (Icl) and methyl citrate cycle (MCC), 645–647
    single-cell suspension, 639–642
Mycobacterium tuberculosis-macrophage biology
    downstream proinflammatory signaling, 547–548
    innate immune sensing, 547–548
    modulation of cell death pathways, 547
    phagosome maturation arrest, 546
    principles of, 546–548
    survival in the face of host antimycobacterial molecules, 546–547
Mycobacterium tuberculosis sensu stricto, 454, 476, 477
Mycobacterium ulcerans, 495
Mycobacterium vaccae, 197

Mycolic acids
    chemical structures of, 520
    importance of, 523–524
    loss of acid-fastness, 519, 529
Myxococcus xanthus, 673

N

NADH:menaquinone oxidoreductases, 299–300
National Institute for Health and Care Excellence (UK), 379
National Institute of Allergy and Infectious Diseases, 117
National Primate Research Centers (NPRCs), 164, 165, 166, 170, 171, 172
National TB Costing Model, 395, 398
Natural killer (NK) cells
    HIV-TB coinfection, 244–245
    memory, 107
    M. tuberculosis infection, 12–14
Natural resistance-associated macrophage protein (*Nramp*), 146
Neanderthals, 467
Necrosis-associated extracellular clusters (NECs), 151, 153
Necrotizing lesions
    biofilms as perspective of extracellular *M. tuberculosis* in, 535–536
    characteristic of active pulmonary TB, 533–534
    extracellular *M. tuberculosis* in, 534–535
Neelsen, F., 520
Neisseria meningitidis, 197
Neutrophils
    HIV-TB coinfection, 243–244
    lung, 5
    M. tuberculosis infection, 12, 39, 216, 548
    response to *M. tuberculosis*, 125
Niclosamide, 343–344, 346
Nicotinamide, 706
Nigericin, 297, 298
Nile red stain, 526–527
Nitro-containing compounds, dual- and nonreplicating active, 343, 344
3-Nitropropionate, 300, 301
Nocardia farcinica, 13
Nongrowing but metabolically active bacteria (NGMA), 676
    identification of, 678, 681, 683
Non-human primate models, *see also* Animal models
    animal model, 132–133
    comparison of rhesus and cynomolgus macaque models, 165–167
    cynomolgus macaques, 166–167, 169
    future research strategies, 172
    historical use of macaque models, 163–165
    in vitro, 544–545
    macaque models for study of TB pathogenesis, 171
    macaque models for TB drug evaluation, 170–171
    macaque models for TB vaccine evaluation, 167, 170
    M. tuberculosis/simian immunodeficiency virus coinfection, macaque models, 171–172

Non-human primate models *(Continued)*
    preclinical efficacy models, 283–284
    rhesus macaques, 165, 166, 168
    Treg cells in, 80, 86–87
    validation of macaques in TB
        research, 163
Nonreplicating (NR) models, selecting and
        designing, 323, 324
Nonreplicating persistence (NRP)
    M. tuberculosis physiology for, 567–571
    sensing when to exit NRP, 571–572
Nonreplication, diversity in, 319–321
Nontuberculous mycobacteria (NTM), 495
Nucleic acid amplification testing (NAAT),
        390, 391, 392; *see also* GeneXpert
        MTB/RIF technology
Nutrient use of pathogens, *see also*
        Auxotrophies
    amino acid auxotrophies, 701–706
    cofactor auxotrophies, 706–708
    future perspectives, 708–710
    lessons from auxotrophic strains, 701–708
    lessons from metabolomics, 700–701
    M. tuberculosis in host tissue, 701
    M. tuberculosis in macrophages, 700–701

O
Ofloxacin, drug resistance, 505
Oxford University, 200
Oxidative phosphorylation
    growth reactivation, 301–302
    M. tuberculosis, 295

P
Pääbo, Svante, 467
Paleomicrobiology, 467
PAMP (pathogen-associated molecular
        pattern), *M. tuberculosis*-derived, 246
Pantothenate (vitamin B$_5$), 706
Paradigm, 121
Parkinson diseases, 630
Pathogenesis
    application of animal models, 134–135
    macaque models for studying TB, 171
    persistence, 672
Pathogens, *see* Nutrient use of pathogens
Pathology of tuberculosis, 117–121,
        125–127
    alveolar pneumonia, 126
    cavity formation, 119, 120
    disease progression in animal models, 122
    granuloma within the lung, 118
    hypersensitivity of pathogenesis of post-
        primary TB, 123–125
    intrapulmonary spread of mixed
        inflammatory cells, 121
    lipid pneumonia, 121, 125
    obstructive lobular pneumonia, 121, 123
    post-primary lung reinfection, 124–125
    primary host response to *M. tuberculosis*
        infection, 122–123
Pattern recognition, 145
Penicillin, 317–318
Peripheral blood mononuclear cells
        (PBMCs), 4
Peroxisome proliferator-associated receptor
        gamma (PPARγ), 4, 10
Persistence
    definition, 654

drug-induced, 662
gene deletion studies, 659–661
host-induced, 657–662
measurements, 656–662
messages, 662–663
methods, 656
models, 654–656
pathogenicity of *M. tuberculosis*, 653, 672
physiology of *M. tuberculosis*, 653
predicted genes for *in vivo* survival of
        M. tuberculosis, 661
terms, 653–654
Persisters, 317
    class I, 321–322
    class II, 322–325, 329–346
    diversity in nonreplicating cells, 319–321
    killing class II persisters, 329, 331–341
Phagocytosis, 636
Phagosome maturation, 8, 9
Phenotype, 671
Phenotype definitions, 429
Phenotypically tolerant *M. tuberculosis*,
        317–319
    class I persisters, 321–322
    class II persisters, 322–325, 329–346
    compound transformation during
        screening and secondary assays,
        325, 329
    conditions for replication rates of, 326
    designing high-throughput screens to
        target, 322–325
    diversity in nonreplication, 319–321
    evaluating bactericidal action against
        nonreplicating mycobacteria, 329
    fluoroquinolones, 339
    future studies, 347–348
    high-throughput screening (HTS),
        341–343
    key observations, 319
    key recommendations, 348
    killing class II persisters, 329, 331–341
    membrane depolarizers, 343–346
    modeling hypoxia and metronidazole
        activity relationship, 318
    molecules targeting nonreplicating
        mycobacteria, 346, 347
    nitro-containing compounds, 343
    postscreening assays, 327, 328
    proof-of-concept molecules, 331–332
    proteolysis/proeostasis pathway, 339–341
    quinolines and derivatives, 338–339
    screening assays, 325, 329, 330
    selecting and designing nonreplicating
        models, 324
    strategies for evaluating viability of
        nonreplicating, 323
Phenotypic drug resistance, 317
Phenotypic heterogeneity, 671–672
    asymmetric cell division and cell aging,
        676–679
    causes and consequences of, 673
    flow cytometry and omics, 682–684
    fluorescence recovery after photobleaching
        (FRAP), 678, 684
    growth phase, 674–675
    growth rate, 675–676
    host microenvironment, 679–682
    host-mimicking platforms, 685–686
    in vivo investigation, 685–686

stochastic processes, 672–674
stress conditions enhancing, 677
time-lapse microscopy and microfluidics,
        684–685
tools and methodology, 682–686
Phenotypic tolerance, 317
Phosphorylation, *see* Protein
        phosphorylation
Pneumonia, tuberculosis as obstructive
        lobular, 121, 123
Positron emission tomography/computed
        tomography (PET/CT), 171, 213,
        283, 680–681, 686
Post-primary tuberculosis, 124–125
Preclinical efficacy testing, 271, 274
    animal infection models of active TB,
        277–284
    drug candidates, 272–273
    dynamic drug concentration models,
        275–277
    goals of, 274–275
    guinea pigs, 282
    hollow fiber system model of TB, 275–277
    in vitro models, 275–277
    mice, 278–281
    modeling chemotherapy of latent TB
        infection (LTBI), 284–286
    non-human primates, 283–284
    rabbits, 283
    rats, 281–282
    static drug concentration models, 275
Preclinical studies, role in experimental
        medicine studies, 205–206
Pretomanid
    drug candidate, 273
    guinea pigs, 282
    mice, 279
Prime, vaccine development, 197
Prime-boost, vaccine development, 197
Programmed cell death protein-1 (PD-1),
        101–102
Proline auxotroph, 703
Proof-of-concept molecules
    dual actives with *in vivo* efficacy, 331–332
    nonreplicating actives with *in vivo*
        efficacy, 332
    nonreplicating activity, 333
    selective nonreplicating activity, 331
Protein-adjuvant TB vaccines, 198–200
Protein kinase activity, 557
Protein phosphorylation, *see also*
        Mycobacterium tuberculosis infection
    apoptosis, 563
    biochemically verified substrates of
        M. tuberculosis serine/threonine
        protein kinases (STPKs), 558–559
    effect on *M. tuberculosis* STPKs, 566
    growth and persistence phenotypes of
        M. tuberculosis STPKs, 562
    hierarchy of *M. tuberculosis* STPK
        activation, 561
    inhibition of phagosome-lysosome fusion,
        561, 563
    M. tuberculosis, 557, 559–560
    STPKs coordinating *M. tuberculosis*
        physiology, 567–571
    STPKs regulating *M. tuberculosis*
        morphology, 564–565, 567
Proteomics, 679, 683–684

Proton motive force (PMF), 297
mechanisms, 297
targeting, in *M. tuberculosis*, 295–299
traditional inhibitors of PMF
generation, 298
Pseudomonas, 673
Pseudomonas aeruginosa, 13, 321, 467, 536, 591, 594
Pseudomonas putida, 591
Pseudonocardia dioxanivorans, 498
PubChem, 329
Purine auxotroph, 708
Pyrazinamide, 528, 681
drug resistance, 502, 504
proof-of-concept molecule, 333
tolerance of infected cells, 640
Pyridoxamine (vitamin B$_6$), 706–707
Pyrizinamide, 86

Q

QuantiFERON-TB (QFT) Gold In-Tube
assay, 382, 384, 385
QuantiFERON-TB Gold-Plus (QFT-Plus), 383
QuantiFERON technology, 382–384, 385
Quinolinyl pyrimidines (QPs), TB drug, 300, 305

R

Rabbits
animal model, 133
granulomas in lungs, 126
preclinical efficacy models, 283
response to infection, 123, 124
TB disease progression, 122
Rapid speciation strip tests, 364
Rats
animal model, 133–134
preclinical efficacy models, 281–282
Recombinant mycobacterial vaccines, 202–203
Regulation of TB immunity, *see also* Animal
models; Human tuberculosis (TB)
antigen-presenting cells (APCs), 74, 75
human regulatory T (Treg) cells and anti-TB treatment, 78–79
human Treg cells and clinical
M. tuberculosis strains, 78
in vitro expansion of mycobacteria-specific Treg cells, 76–77
mechanisms of Treg suppression, 74
naturally occurring and induced Treg cells, 73–74
Treg activity balance, 77
Treg cell, 73–74
Treg cell responses in experimental animal
models of TB, 80–87
Treg cell responses in human TB, 74–80
Treg-mediated manipulation of immune
cell activation, 75–79
Treg responses at *M. tuberculosis* infection
site, 79–80
Treg suppression of APCs, 75
Regulatory cytokines
IL-4, IL-5, and IL-13, 47–48
interleukin IL-10, 48–49
transforming growth factor β (TGFβ), 48
Replication rate, 592; *see also* DNA
replication

mycobacterial, 592–594
Research Institute of Influenza
(St. Petersburg, Russia), 202
Respiration, *M. tuberculosis*, 295
Restriction fragment length polymorphism
(RFLP) method, 454–455, 583
Retroviridae family, 239
Rhesus macaques, 163; *see also* Macaque
models
comparing TB in humans to, 164
"Golden Age" of TB research using, 165, 166
Macaca mulatta, 163, 173
TB studies, 166, 167, 168
21st century TB research, 166
Rhizobium leguminosarum, 613
Rifampin, 86, 527–528
animal models, 279–280
drug candidate, 272, 274, 278, 331
drug resistance, 503, 504, 674
guinea pigs, 282
latent TB infection, 285–286
line probe assays for detecting resistance, 367–368
non-human primates, 283
proof-of-concept molecule, 333
tolerance of infected cells, 639–641
Xpert MTB/RIF for resistance to, 368
Rifapentine
drug candidate, 272
guinea pigs, 282
latent TB infection (LTBI), 285–286

S

Salmonella, 146, 321, 674, 676
Salmonella enterica serovar Typhi, 462
Salmonella typhimurium, 557
Sanofi Pasteur, 199
Scavenger receptors (SRs), 8
SciFinder, 329
Screening
acidic pH, 341, 342
biofilms, 341, 343
hypoxia, 341, 342
multiple physiological stresses, 341, 342
Screening assays
compound transformation during, 330
designing high-throughput screens for
phenotypically tolerant mycobacteria, 322–323, 325
post-, 327, 328
potential compound transformation
during, 325, 329
Secretion (SecA1) pathway
cell wall synthesis and remodeling
factors, 609
conserved, 607–608
conserved SecA1 exportome, 608–611
entering dormancy, 610
exported virulence factors, 610
lipoproteins, 609–610
models of SecA1 export, 608
reactivation/resuscitation from
dormancy, 611
Secretion (SecA2) pathway
dormancy, 619
features of SecA2-dependent
substrates, 613
identification, 611–612

immunomodulation and, 618–619
inhibition of apoptosis, 618
KatB (catalase-peroxidase), 616
Mce transporters, 614–615
mechanism, 612–613
models of SecA2 export, 608
multiple components of Mce
transporters, 615
phagosome maturation arrest, 617
PknG (eukaryotic-like serine-threonine
kinase), 616
protein export pathway, 611–613
reactive radicals and, 619
SBPs (solute binding proteins), 613–614
secA2 mutant as vaccine candidate, 619–620
SecA2 and DosR regulon, 616–617
SecA2 exportome, 613–616
SodA (Fe-superoxide dismutase), 615–616
virulence and, 617–619
Secretion system, *see also* ESX-1 (ESAT-6
secretion system-1)
ESAT-6 (ESX-1), 627, 631–632
Shuman, Stewart, 591
Simian immunodeficiency virus (SIV),
M. tuberculosis and, coinfection
macaque models, 171–172
Smear microscopy, diagnostics for active TB, 363–364
Solute carrier, 146
South Africa
challenges and opportunities of
implementation, 394, 396
GeneXpert implementation, 397
GeneXpert placement, 394
national implementation of Xpert NTB/
RIF assay, 393–394
tuberculosis in, 391, 393
South African Tuberculosis Vaccine Initiative
(SATVI), 104, 105
Spectroscopy, 683–684, 701
Spoligotyping, 455, 457, 461
Staphylococcus aureus, 609, 611
Statens Serum Institut, Denmark, 198
Stead, W. W., 654
Stem cell-like memory T cells, 102
Streptococcus gordonii, 611
Streptococcus parasanguinis, 611
Streptococcus pneumoniae, 197, 536
Streptomyces coelicolor, 591
Streptomycin, drug resistance, 502, 505
Succinate:quinone oxidoreductase, 300–301
Swedish Institute of Infectious Disease
Control, 167
Systems biology, tuberculosis, 429

T

TB-associated immune reconstitution
inflammatory syndrome (TB-IRIS), 76
T cells, *see also* Memory T cells
cytotoxic, in TB-immune reconstitution
inflammatory syndrome (TB-IRIS), 255–256
M. tuberculosis infection, 217–219, 548–549
responses to tuberculosis (TB), 225
Technical Expert Group, 365
Thioalkalivibrio, 458
Thiorhodovibrio, 458

Thioridazine, 297, 299
Threonine auxotroph, 704
Time-lapse microscopy, 684–685
Tissue remodeling, tuberculosis (TB), 225
Toll-like receptor 9 (TLR9), 4
Toll-like receptors (TLRs), 7–8, 39, 145
Trained immunity, 13, 17, 107
Transcriptional profiling, *M. tuberculosis* in macrophages, 636–638
Transcriptome studies, 674, 683–684
Transcriptomic profiling, biomarkers, 226–227
Transforming growth factor β (TGFβ), 48
Transgenic mice, 145
TraSH screening method, 704
Treatment outcomes, impact of GeneXpert MTB/RIF, 401, 402–404
Trifluoperazine, 299, 300
Trudeau, E. L., 131
Tryptophan auxotroph, 704–705
Tuberculin skin testing (TST), 213, 214, 215, 220, 221, 225
    administering and reading TST, 381
    latent TB infection, 380
    purified protein derivative (PPD)-based TST, 381
Tuberculosis (TB), *see also* Animal models; HIV-TB coinfection; Human tuberculosis (TB); Vaccine candidates
    adjunctive therapeutic vaccination, 196–197
    anti-TB vaccine design, 39
    biomarkers in human, 226–227
    diabetes mellitus, 222–223
    diversity, 680
    global epidemic, 389–390
    HIV-1 heterogeneity at site of disease, 247
    HIV-1 replication at site of disease, 245–247
    HIV and, 172, 222
    lung, 3–6
    malnutrition, 223–224
    necrotizing lesions in active pulmonary, 533–534
    positive and negative roles of chemokines in, 36
    positive and negative roles of cytokines in, 35
    post-primary, 119–121, 123–127
    preventing recurrent TB, 196–197
    prevention of disease, 195–196
    progression from infection to disease, 222–226
    proposed framework for spectrum of infection, 380
    protective memory against, 96–97
    risk factors for, 222
    systems biology of, 429
    targeting replisome for new drug development, 595–596
    Treg cell responses in human, 74–80
    vaccine, 40, 43, 45, 46, 49
    vaccine development strategies, 197–198
    vitamin D deficiency, 223
Tuberculosis (TB) vaccination
    animal models, 80
    guinea pig model, 86
    mouse models, 83–84
Tumor necrosis factor alpha (TNFα), 34–37

roles in TB, 35
Type I interferons (IFN-γ), tuberculosis, 224

U

University of Pittsburgh, 166–167, 171
University of Zaragoza and Biofabri, 202
Urine lipoarabinomannan rapid test, 366
U.S. Department of Agriculture, 139
U.S. Food and Drug Administration (FDA), 382

V

Vaccae, vaccine candidate, 197, 198, 202
Vaccination
    adjunctive therapeutic vaccination, 196–197
    BCG and disease protection, 194
    clinical trials of TB candidates, 197–203
    M. tuberculosis, 95–96
    prevention of *M. tuberculosis* infection, 193–195
    prevention of recurrent TB disease, 196–197
    prevention of TB disease, 195–196
Vaccine candidates, 198
    Ad5Ag85A, 201
    Crucell Ad35, 201
    DAR-901, 202
    development strategies, 197–198
    experimental medicine role in development, 203–206
    global clinical pipeline of, 198
    H1:IC31 and H1:CAF01, 198
    H4:IC31, 199
    H56:IC31, 198–199
    ID93+GLA-SE, 199
    inactivated whole-cell and fragmented TB vaccines, 202
    M72/AS01E, 199–200
    MTBVAC, 202–203
    MVA85A, 200–201
    Protein-adjuvant TB vaccines, 198–200
    recombinant mycobacterial vaccines, 202–203
    RUTI, 202
    secA2 mutant as, 619–620
    TB/Flu-04L, 202
    Vaccae, 202
    VAP 1002, 203
    viral-vectored vaccines, 200–202
    VPM 1002, 203
Vaccines, *see also* Vaccine candidates
    Ad85A (human adenovirus 5 expressing Ag85A), 181–182
    animal models and testing protocols, 136, 137
    animal models for assessment of, 135
    antibody-inducing, 220
    BCG protection, 40, 43, 45, 46, 49, 220
    BCG vaccination in animals, 100
    BCG vaccination in guinea pigs, 86
    BCG vaccination in humans, 76, 100
    BCG vaccination in mice, 83–84
    biomarkers correlating disease severity, 184
    biomarkers predicting efficacy, 182
    guinea pig model, 153–154
    macaque models of evaluating TB vaccine, 167, 170

mechanism of protection, 136
    memory immunity by novel TB, 107–108
    Mycobacterium bovis bacillus Calmette-Guérin (BCG), 95, 117, 179–180
    new-generation TB, 180–182
    novel TB candidate MVA85A, 77–78, 96, 104, 108, 200–201
    predictivity of animal models, 137–138
    proof of concept for, 194, 196, 203–206
    role of experimental medicine in vaccine development, 203–206
    schedules of BCG and virally vectored, 183–184
    types of new, tested in cattle, 181
Vakzine Projekt Management GmbH, 203
Valine auxotroph, 704
Valinomycin, 297, 298
Vertex Pharmaceuticals, 643
Vibrio cholerae, 465
Viral-vectored vaccines, 200–202
Vitamin B$_5$ (pantothenate), 706
Vitamin B$_6$ (pyridoxamine), 706–707
Vitamin B$_7$ (biotin), 707
Vitamin B$_9$ (folate), 707
Vitamin B$_{12}$ (cobalamin), 707–708
Vitamin D deficiency, 223

W

Wallgren, Arvid, 215
Wayne model, hypoxia, 318, 323, 325
Whole-genome sequencing (WGS)
    emergence of, 495
    M. tuberculosis L2 Beijing sublineage, 500
    resistant strains, 502, 506–507
World Health Organization (WHO), 193, 226, 239
    global TB epidemic, 389–390
    line probe assay recommendations, 368–369
    TB disease control, 379, 533
    TB screening, 363, 364

X

XLAAD (X-linked autoimmunity allergic dysregulation syndrome), 73
Xpert MTB/RIF, *see also* GeneXpert MTB/RIF technology
    background of, 391
    diagnostics for TB, 365, 368
    maximizing impact of new diagnostics, 371, 373–374
    timeline of availability, 374

Y

Yersinia pseudotuberculosis, 674

Z

Zebrafish
    animal models, 133, 685, 686
    granuloma formation, 135
    in vitro model, 550
    M. marinum, 36, 133, 699
Ziehl, F., 520
ZN (Ziehl-Neelsen) stain, 519; *see also* AF (acid-fast) mycobacteria
    clinical diagnosis of TB, 522–523
    history of acid-fast (AF) staining, 520–522
    M. tuberculosis, 521, 528